PATHOLOGY AND IMMUNOLOGY
OF TRANSPLANTATION AND REJECTION

# Pathology and Immunology of Transplantation and Rejection

EDITED BY

SATHIA THIRU FRCP, FRCPath
*Department of Pathology*
*University of Cambridge*
*School of Clinical Medicine*
*Addenbrooke's Hospital*
*Cambridge*

AND

HERMAN WALDMANN MRCP, FRCPath, FRS
*Dunn School of Pathology*
*University of Oxford*
*South Parks Road*
*Oxford*

**Blackwell Science**

© 2001
Blackwell Science Ltd
Editorial Offices:
Osney Mead, Oxford OX2 0EL
25 John Street, London WC1N 2BS
23 Ainslie Place, Edinburgh EH3 6AJ
350 Main Street, Malden
  MA 02148 5018, USA
54 University Street, Carlton
  Victoria 3053, Australia
10, rue Casimir Delavigne
  75006 Paris, France

Other Editorial Offices:
Blackwell Wissenschafts-Verlag GmbH
Kurfürstendamm 57
10707 Berlin, Germany

Blackwell Science KK
MG Kodenmacho Building
7–10 Kodenmacho Nihombashi
Chuo-ku, Tokyo 104, Japan

First published 2001

Set by Best-set Typesetter Ltd, Hong Kong
Printed and bound in Great Britain
by MPG Books Ltd, Bodmin, Cornwall

A catalogue record for this title
is available from the British Library

ISBN 0-632-03676-1

Library of Congress
Cataloging-in-publication Data

Pathology and immunology of
transplantation and rejection / edited by
Sathia Thiru and Herman Waldmann.
      p. ;    cm.
    Includes bibliographical references.
    ISBN 0-632-03676-1
    1. Transplantation immunology.
  2. Transplantation of organs, tissues,
  etc. —Complications.   3. Graft versus
  host disease.  I. Thiru, Sathia.
  II. Waldmann, Herman.
    [DNLM:    1. Transplantation
  Immunology.   2. Histocompatibility
  Testing—methods.
  3. Immunosuppression—methods.
  4. Transplantation—pathology.
  WO 680 I331 2000]
  QR188.8. I476 2000
  617.9′5—dc21              99-053903

DISTRIBUTORS
Marston Book Services Ltd
PO Box 269
Abingdon, Oxon OX14 4YN
(*Orders*: Tel:  01235 465500
            Fax: 01235 465555)

USA
Blackwell Science, Inc.
Commerce Place
350 Main Street
Malden, MA 02148 5018
(*Orders*: Tel:  800 759 6102
            781 388 8250
            Fax: 781 388 8255)

Canada
Login Brothers Book Company
324 Saulteaux Crescent
Winnipeg, Manitoba R3J 3T2
(*Orders*: Tel:  204 837 2987)

Australia
Blackwell Science Pty Ltd
54 University Street
Carlton, Victoria 3053
(*Orders*: Tel:  3 9347 0300
            Fax: 3 9347 5001)

For further information on
Blackwell Science, visit our website:
www.blackwell-science.com

# Contents

# List of contributors

JEAN-FRANÇOIS BACH MD, DSc, *Head of Immunology Department, Inserm U25, Hospital Necker, 161 Rue de Sèvres, 75743 Paris Cedex 15, France*

BENJAMIN A. BRADLEY MBChB, MSc, PhD, MA (Contab), FRCPath, FRCP, *Head of Division of Transplantation Sciences, Southmead Health Services, Westbury-on-Trym, Bristol BS10 5NB, UK*

JOHN R. BRADLEY BMedSci, BM, BS, DM, FRCP, *Department of Medicine, University of Cambridge School of Clinical Medicine, Addenbrooke's Hospital, Hills Road, Cambridge CB2 2QQ, UK*

I. GABRIELLE M. BRONS PhD, *Department of Surgery, University of Cambridge Clinical School, Level 9, Addenbrooke's Hospital, Hills Road, Cambridge CB2 2QQ, UK*

MIKE BUNCE PhD, *Oxford Transplantation Centre, Churchill Hospital, Oxford OX3 7LJ, UK*

WILLIAM J. BURLINGHAM PhD, *Clinical Sciences Centre, University of Wisconsin, 600 Highland Avenue, Madison, WI 52792, USA*

NATHANIEL CARY MA, MD, MB, BS, FRCPath, DMJPath, *Consultant Forensic Pathologist, Department of Forensic Medicine, Guy's, King's and St Thomas' School of Medicine, Guy's Hospital, London SE1 9RT, UK*

STEVEN J. CHADBAN BMed, PhD, FRACP, *Department of Medicine, University of Cambridge School of Clinical Medicine, Addenbrooke's Hospital, Hills Road, Cambridge CB2 2QQ, UK*

LUCIENNE CHATENOUD MD, DSc, *Inserm U25, Hospital Necker, 161 Rue de Sèvres, 75743 Paris Cedex 15, France*

STEPHEN COBBOLD MA, PhD, *Dunn School of Pathology, South Parks Road, Oxford OX1 3RE, UK*

MARGARET J. DALLMAN DPhil, *Department of Biology, Imperial College of Science, Technology and Medicine, Prince Consort Road, London SW7 2BB, UK*

JEREMY P. DIAMOND FRCS, FCOphth, *Lecturer in Ophthalmology, School of Medical Sciences, University of Bristol, Lower Maudlin Street, Bristol BS1 2LX, UK*

J. PETER DONNELLY PhD, *Department of Haematology, University Hospital, Nijmegen, PO Box 8171, 6500 HB, Nijmegen, the Netherlands*

ANTHONY DORLING PhD, MRCP, *Imperial College School of Medicine, Hammersmith Hospital, Du Cane Road, London W12 0NN, UK*

DAVID L. EASTY MD, FRCS, FRCOphth, *Emeritus Professor of Ophthalmology, Department of Ophthalmology, School of Medical Sciences, University of Bristol, University Walk, Bristol BS8 1TD, UK*

MARK FARRINGTON MB, BChir, FRCPath, *Clinical Microbiology and Public Health Laboratory, Addenbrooke's Hospital, Hills Road, Cambridge CB2 2QW, UK*

JULIET E. FOWERAKER PhD, MRCPath, *Consultant Microbiologist, Department of Microbiology, Papworth Hospital, Papworth Everard, Cambridge CB3 8RE, UK*

SHERYL L. FULLER-ESPIE BS, PhD, DIC, *Department of Biology, Cabrini College, 610 King of Prussia Road, Radnor, PA 19087, USA*

JIM GRAY FIMLS, PhD, MRCPath, *Public Health Laboratory, Addenbrooke's Hospital, Hills Road, Cambridge CB2 2QQ, UK*

GEOFFREY HALE BA, PhD, *Dunn School of Pathology, South Parks Road, Oxford OX1 3RE, UK*

ROBERT I. LECHLER PhD, FRCP, *Professor of Molecular Immunology and Honorary Consultant in Medicine, University of London, Imperial College School of Medicine, Hammersmith Hospital, Du Cane Road, London W12 0NN, UK*

SAMUEL W. B. NEWSOM MD, MA, MB, BChir, FRCPath, *former Consultant Microbiologist, Department of Microbiology, Papworth Hospital, Papworth Everard, Cambridge CB2 8RE, UK*

SUSAN M. NICHOLLS PhD, *Research Fellow, Department of Ophthalmology, School of Medical Sciences, University of Bristol, University Walk, Bristol BS8 1TD, UK*

ELIZABETH SIMPSON MA, VETMB, FMedSci, *Head, Transplantation Biology Group, MRC Clinical Sciences Centre, Imperial College School of Medicine, Hammersmith Hospital, Du Cane Road, London W12 0NN, UK*

KENNETH G. C. SMITH BMedSci, MB, BS, PhD, FRACP, FRCPA, *Cambridge Institute for Medical Research, University of Cambridge School of Clinical Medicine, Addenbrooke's Hospital, Hills Road, Cambridge CB2 2QQ, UK*

MARGARET A. STANLEY PhD, *Lecturer in Pathology, Department of Pathology, Tennis Court Road, Cambridge CB2 1QP, UK*

SUSAN STEWART MA, MB, BChir, FRCPath, *Consultant Histopathologist, Department of Histopathology, Papworth Hospital, Papworth Everard, Cambridge CB3 8RE, UK*

SATHIA THIRU FRCP, FRCPath, *Lecturer and Honorary Consultant Pathologist, Department of Pathology, University of Cambridge School of Clinical Medicine, Addenbrooke's Hospital, Hills Road, Cambridge CB2 2QQ, UK*

HERMAN WALDMANN MRCP, FRCPath, FRS, *Dunn School of Pathology, University of Oxford, South Parks Road, Oxford OX1 3RE, UK*

KEN I. WELSH *Oxford Transplantation Centre, Churchill Hospital, Oxford OX3 7LJ, UK*

DEREK WIGHT FRCPath, *Consultant Histopathologist, Department of Histopathology, Addenbrooke's Hospital, Hills Road, Cambridge CB2 2QQ, UK*

TIM WREGHITT MA, PhD, FRCPath, *Honorary Consultant Microbiologist, Public Health Laboratory, Level 6, Addenbrooke's Hospital, Hills Road, Cambridge CB2 2QQ, UK*

# Foreword

Therapeutic transplantation of solid organs has been regarded as primarily the province of surgeons, at least by the surgeons themselves, but the whole modern edifice of transplantation could not have evolved without the participation of pathologists. From the beginning of transplantation in the 1950s it become clear that there were two problems to be overcome.

The first was surgical—the goal being to remove an organ as healthy as possible from the donor and transfer it to the recipient without significant damage and to provide the graft with a satisfactory habitat and a good blood supply. For the most part the surgery of transplantation has reached a successful solution. There are, of course, still difficulties, particularly associated with the shortage of organs and the increasing waiting list. Recently there has been a tendency to use organs that are not perfect, for example, from elderly donors or livers with fatty infiltration. These defects are recognized and can be addressed.

The second problem, the immunology and pathology of transplantation, however, is still far from being fully understood. Not surprisingly, rejection, particularly chronic rejection, cannot be prevented in all cases. Before the advent of cyclosporin, when azathioprine and steroids were the main form of immunosuppression, only 50% of grafts had functional survival at 1 year. Now, with modern immunosuppression, which followed the watershed advantages of cyclosporin, we expect between 80% and 90% of grafts to be func-

tional at 1 year, although by 10 years this will figure will have dropped to between 50% and 60%.

Dr Thiru and Professor Waldmann have produced a magnum opus explaining what is known of the immunology of transplantation, describing the pathology and covering the whole field from bone marrow transplantation to heart grafting, including viral and bacterial infections and the prospect for transplanting organs from animal to man.

With so many authors involved, it is a tribute to their editing and persuasive skills that they have managed to produce a publication that is up to date and will be an important source of reference to all those interested in tissue and organ transplantation. Chapters are authoritative and comprehensive and each has an extensive list of references. It is only by understanding what we know of the immunology and pathology of transplantation and, therefore, acknowledging and realizing the large defects in our knowledge that we can hope to make advances in the results of organ transplantation. The eventual goal is to induce immunological tolerance, so that our patients are not burdened by the continuous requirements of daily medicines, each of which has important and deleterious side effects, and makes them perpetually vulnerable to infections and malignancies. I am sure this book will achieve the success that it deserves.

Sir Roy Calne

# Preface

Organ transplantation is the treatment of choice in a variety of disabling and life-threatening disease processes. Kidney, liver, heart, lung, cornea and bone marrow transplantation are well established in a number of specialist centres, although pancreas and skin transplantation are less widely established.

Survival rates, particularly short-term survival, have improved considerably over the past two decades and this success has been due to increased insight into the immunological and pathogenetic mechanisms involved in acute rejection, in the development of effective immunosuppressive agents with the better use of combination therapy, improved methods of organ preservation and tissue matching, and better monitoring and management of the complications that can arise in immunosuppressed patients. Success of short-term survival highlights the fact that chronic rejection remains a major problem in long-term allograft survival. Until recently, there has not been much interest in research into the pathogenetic mechanisms involved, and, until these are better understood, prevention of chronic rejection remains a hurdle. Advances in allotransplantation have resulted in an increased demand for organ grafts. The severe shortage of human organs available for transplantation has led to an active interest in xenotransplantation. Although transplantation of animal tissues into humans has been attempted at various times in the 20th century, systematic and organized research into xenotransplantation is a new field. Techniques that allow genetic or biochemical manipulation of animal tissues to render xenografts less susceptible to rejection and insights into the mechanisms of hyperacute and acute humoral rejection have made xenotransplantation of vascularized organs increasingly feasible.

This book has made an attempt to cover all of these aspects of transplantation as clearly as possible. Given that the subject is vast and still evolving, the work is not by any means a complete thesis on the subject. A very great debt of gratitude is owed to all the authors, some more prominent than others, who have produced up to date and comprehensive contributions of their specialist subject. Apologies are due to authors who have had to revise and update their chapters because of delays in finalizing the entire volume. This book will be of interest to immunologists, surgeons, physicians and pathologists involved in experimental and clinical transplantation, as well as to those contemplating a future career in the field of transplantation.

Sathia Thiru
Cambridge

# Chapter 1/Immunobiology of graft rejection

MARGARET J. DALLMAN

## Introduction

Transplantation of an organ from one individual to another induces many changes both in the host and in the graft. Some of these changes are a simple consequence of the trauma associated with surgery, while others involve specific recognition of antigenic differences between donor and recipient. The net result of these changes is normally a destructive immune response which, if unabated, will result in immune rejection and loss of the transplant. The problems associated with transplantation of material between genetically different individuals have been underscored by many workers since originally being highlighted by workers such as Little and Tyzer (1916). The immunological nature of tissue rejection was clearly demonstrated over 50 years ago by Gibson and Medawar (1943) and Medawar (1944, 1945) in work in which skin grafts were performed between genetically disparate humans or rabbits. These authors showed that the rejection process displayed marked specificity and memory for donor tissue and was accompanied by infiltration with leucocytes. Since this

time, our understanding of the immune system has developed considerably and we are now able to describe more fully the molecular and cellular events which result in graft rejection. The aim of this chapter is to review our current understanding of immunity to skin and organ grafts, highlighting recent technical and intellectual advances that have advanced knowledge in this area.

Perhaps the most interesting technical advance which has allowed new experimental approaches in the field of transplantation is the development of mice bearing defined mutations in genes of the immune system. Such 'knockout' mice in theory allow the investigator to define the activity of a protein by investigating the functioning of the immune system in its absence, a classical approach which has been very valuable in many organisms. While some interesting and important data have accumulated from experiments with knockout mice, their use in understanding immunity has been complicated by adaptability and redundancy, hallmark features of the immune system. As we will see, results from transplantation experiments using knockout mice have not always been easy

1

to interpret and certainly can be confounded by the elasticity of the immune system and its ability to circumvent any deficiency using mechanisms that might not normally be employed.

This chapter assumes a basic level of understanding of the cells and molecules involved in immune responses, but the reader is referred to other books and reviews for general descriptions of the immune system (Halloran *et al.* 1993; Janeway & Travers 1996).

## The trauma of transplantation

The response to a transplant occurs in a series of relatively well-defined stages, as shown in Fig. 1.1, the first of which involves the rather severe physical assault that the graft undergoes during harvest from the donor and transplantation into the recipient. As a result of this, a variety of genes become activated and inflammatory cells infiltrate the graft. The induction of several soluble proteins or cytokines, or transcripts of cytokines, such as IL-6 and IL-1, can be demonstrated at early time points following transplantation even in situations in which there is no antigenic difference between donor and recipient (syngeneic grafts) and in which an immune response is therefore not generated (Dallman *et al.* 1991a; Tono *et al.* 1992). Probably as a result of this, in combination with an up-regulated expression of adhesion proteins on the vascular endothelium of the graft, an early infiltrate of inflammatory cells, including macrophages, develops (McLean *et al.* 1997). These early events alone do not result in graft rejection and are observed in syngeneic grafts. Their influence on early graft function and later importance in rejection should an immune response ensue are, however, unclear.

## Presentation of antigen to recipient T cells

### Antigens involved in graft rejection

Histocompatibility antigens determine the outcome of tissue grafts between different members of the same species (allografts). In all vertebrate species histocompatibility antigens can be divided into a single major

histocompatibility complex or system (MHC) and numerous minor systems. Incompatibility for such antigens between a donor and a recipient of a graft leads to an immune response against the graft. Most vigorous rejection is observed where MHC incompatibilities between donor and recipient occur and, in a non-sensitized recipient, rejection in the presence of compatibility for the MHC may not occur or may be delayed. However, as demonstrated in mice, multiple minor histocompatibility differences may result in skin or cardiac allograft rejection with as rapid kinetics as that seen for transplantation across the MHC (Peugh *et al.* 1986). Further, in humans, bone marrow transplants between HLA-identical siblings can be rejected where a disparity in even a few minor antigens is present (Goulmy 1985).

There is considerable similarity between the MHC in different species with respect to both immunogenetics and biochemistry. The genes within the MHC are divided into class I, II and III types (Klein *et al.* 1981; Campbell & Trowsdale 1993). The class I cell surface glycoproteins are comprised of two chains: the heavy chain (MW 45 kDa), which is polymorphic and encoded within the MHC; and a non-variable light chain, $\beta_2$ microglobulin (MW 12 kDa) which is not encoded within the MHC. Such MHC class I proteins are expressed on virtually all nucleated cells and are, in general, responsible for activating T cells bearing the CD8 surface protein (CD8+ cells, see below). The class II genes also encode glycoproteins which in the main are present on the cell surface; these are composed of two chains of similar molecular weight (alpha chain MW 35 kDa, beta chain MW 28 kDa) and stimulate T cells bearing the CD4 surface protein (CD4+ cells). The tissue distribution of class II expression is far more restricted than that of class I, being expressed constitutively only by B lymphocytes, dendritic cells and some endothelial cells. However, during the course of an immune response most other cell types, with a few exceptions, may be induced to express MHC class II molecules (Lampert *et al.* 1981; Mason *et al.* 1981; Dallman *et al.* 1982; Fellous *et al.* 1982; de Waal *et al.* 1983; Wong *et al.* 1984; Fuggle *et al.* 1986). During the synthesis and transport of MHC class I and II proteins to the cell surface they become associated with small

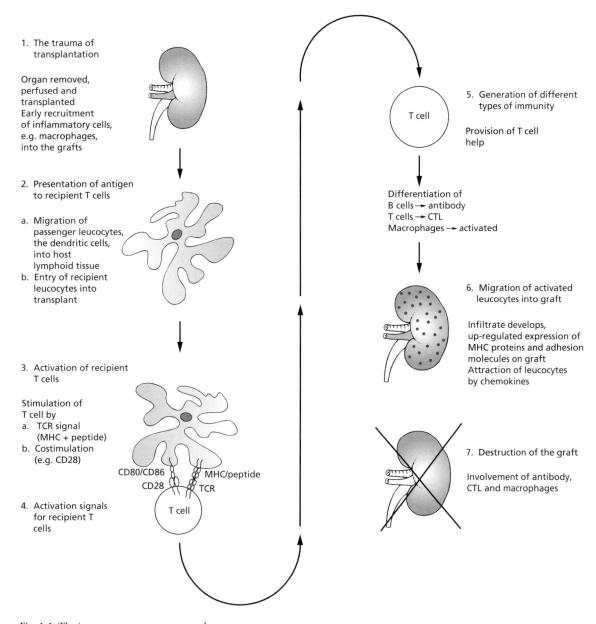

1. The trauma of transplantation

   Organ removed, perfused and transplanted Early recruitment of inflammatory cells, e.g. macrophages, into the grafts

2. Presentation of antigen to recipient T cells

   a. Migration of passenger leucocytes, the dendritic cells, into host lymphoid tissue
   b. Entry of recipient leucocytes into transplant

3. Activation of recipient T cells

   Stimulation of T cell by
   a. TCR signal (MHC + peptide)
   b. Costimulation (e.g. CD28)

   CD80/CD86    MHC/peptide
   CD28    TCR
   T cell

4. Activation signals for recipient T cells

T cell

5. Generation of different types of immunity

   Provision of T cell help

   Differentiation of
   B cells → antibody
   T cells → CTL
   Macrophages → activated

6. Migration of activated leucocytes into graft

   Infiltrate develops, up-regulated expression of MHC proteins and adhesion molecules on graft Attraction of leucocytes by chemokines

7. Destruction of the graft

   Involvement of antibody, CTL and macrophages

**Fig. 1.1** The immune response to a transplant.

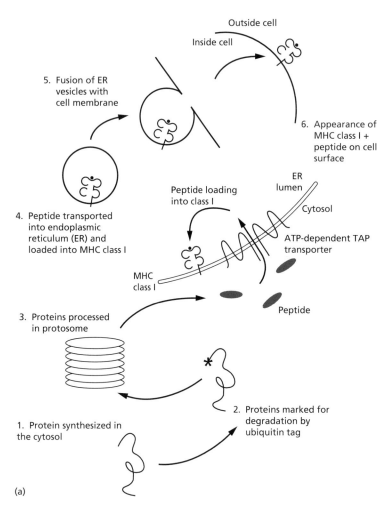

5. Fusion of ER
   vesicles with
   cell membrane

Outside cell

Inside cell

6. Appearance of
   MHC class I +
   peptide on cell
   surface

4. Peptide transported
   into endoplasmic
   reticulum (ER) and
   loaded into MHC class I

Peptide loading
into class I

ER
lumen

Cytosol

ATP-dependent TAP
transporter

MHC
class I

Peptide

3. Proteins processed
   in protosome

1. Protein synthesized in
   the cytosol

2. Proteins marked for
   degradation by
   ubiquitin tag

(a)

**Fig. 1.2** Antigen processing and presentation: (a) the class I pathway.

peptides, derived from (primarily) intracellularly and extracellularly derived proteins, respectively (Fig. 1.2). It is the combination of MHC and peptide that is recognized by the antigen receptor (TCR) on the T cell. One type of class II protein, HLA-DM, does not appear on the cell surface, but has a role in loading peptide into other class II proteins before they emigrate to the cell surface (Roche 1995).

Our understanding of such antigen processing and presentation pathways has increased enormously in recent years (Grey & Chestnut 1985; Monaco 1992, 1993, 1995; Germain & Margulies 1993; Cresswell

1994; Belich & Trowsdale 1995) and this, together with the structural resolution of MHC and TCR proteins (Fig. 1.3) (Bjorkman *et al.* 1987; Garcia *et al.* 1996; Bjorkman 1997), represents two of the most important advances in immunology in the last decade.

Mice with disrupted expression of either $\beta_2$ microglobulin (in which surface expression of the whole class I protein is inhibited, class I –/– mice) or class II genes (class II –/– mice) have been generated and used as either donor or recipient in transplantation studies. The literature regarding such experiments is quite complex; in many situations a lack of class I or II

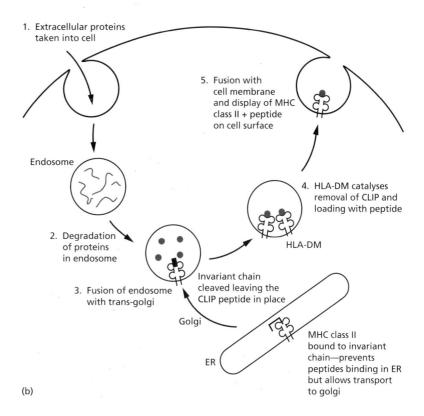

1. Extracellular proteins taken into cell

5. Fusion with cell membrane and display of MHC class II + peptide on cell surface

Endosome

4. HLA-DM catalyses removal of CLIP and loading with peptide

2. Degradation of proteins in endosome

HLA-DM

3. Fusion of endosome with trans-golgi

Invariant chain cleaved leaving the CLIP peptide in place

Golgi

ER

MHC class II bound to invariant chain—prevents peptides binding in ER but allows transport to golgi

**Fig. 1.2** *Continued.* (b) The class II pathway.          (b)

antigens alone on donor tissue has little effect on graft survival (Auchincloss *et al.* 1993; Dierich *et al.* 1993; Li & Faustman 1993; Henretta *et al.* 1995; Mannon *et al.* 1995). However, in other experiments graft survival may be prolonged or permanent when donor tissue lacks either class I (Markmann *et al.* 1992; Henretta *et al.* 1995) or class II (Campos *et al.* 1995; Henretta *et al.* 1995) or both class I and II antigens (Osorio *et al.* 1993; Campos *et al.* 1995; Mannon *et al.* 1995). It is clear from these experiments that different results are obtained when different types of grafts are used, probably reflecting a greater or lesser involvement of either CD4+ or CD8+ cells (Campos *et al.* 1995; Henretta *et al.* 1995). However, the interpretation of some of these apparently straightforward experiments is complicated by the suggestion that grafts from class I –/– mice may be reconstituted in their expression of class I by serum $\beta_2$ microglobulin in the recipient or

may express residual cell surface class I protein in the absence of $\beta_2$ microglobulin (Li & Faustman 1993; Lee *et al.* 1997).

The class III genes that have been characterized encode proteins with a variety of different functions and, while they themselves do not stimulate T cells in the same way as class I and II proteins, many have important activities in generating and influencing immunity. For example, proteins involved in processing antigen and loading peptide into class I antigens and the cytokines TNFα and TNFβ are encoded in the class III region (Campbell & Trowsdale 1993).

One of the most notable aspects of the MHC, and the one that creates serious problems for the transplant clinician, is the very high degree of polymorphism in the class I and II genes. The intimate involvement of the MHC in the cellular interactions of the immune response suggests that extensive polymorphism has

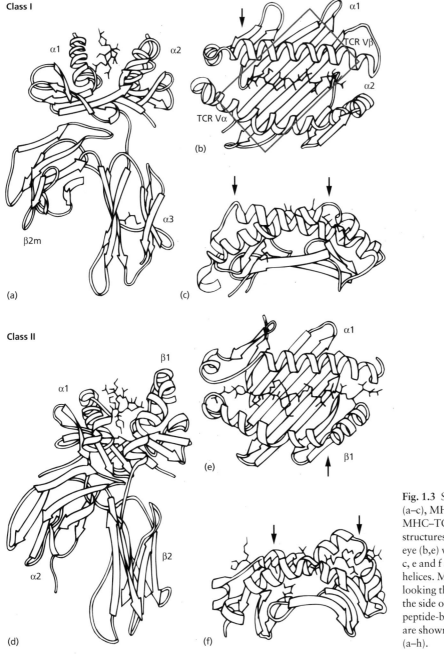

**Class I**

α1    α2

α3

β2m

(a)

α1

TCR Vβ

TCR Vα

α2

(b)

(c)

**Class II**

β1

α1

α2

β2

(d)

α1

β1

(e)

(f)

**Fig. 1.3** Structures of MHC class I (a–c), MHC class II (d–f) and MHC–TCR interactions (g,h). MHC structures are side (a,c,d,f) or bird's eye (b,e) view. The black arrows in b, c, e and f are high points on the MHC helices. MHC–TCR interactions are looking through the groove (g) or at the side of the α helix forming the peptide-binding groove (h). Peptides are shown as sticks with side chains (a–h).

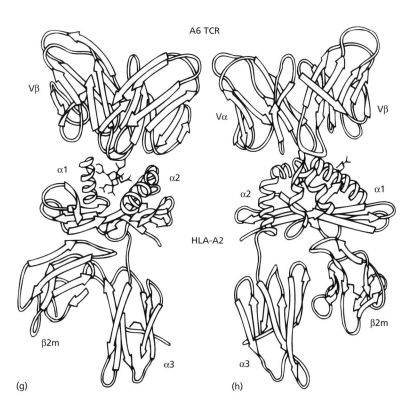

**Fig. 1.3** *Continued.*    (g)    (h)

evolved as a product of immune defence mechanisms against infection (Klein *et al.* 1981). Indeed, certain species have very limited polymorphism at either class I or II loci and can be devastated by infections which closely related species with a polymorphic MHC have little problem in clearing (O'Brien *et al.* 1985). The practical result of this polymorphism for the transplant clinician is that, in organ transplantation between unrelated individuals, truly MHC-identical donors and recipients are extremely uncommon and, even where they are found, minor histocompatibility antigens are different. Indeed, it is only possible clinically to graft tissue which is both MHC- and minor histocompatibility antigen-identical when it is carried out between monozygotic twins. Immunosuppression is therefore routinely needed in clinical transplantation and even so rejection, either as an acute reaction or as a more chronic process, occurs in many patients.

## Minor histocompatibility antigens

The nature of minor histocompatibility antigens was for many years elusive. While T cells clearly could recognize and respond to cells from MHC-identical individuals it was almost impossible to raise antibodies against the antigens involved, making biochemical characterization very difficult. The knowledge that T cells recognize small peptides from antigens, together with the powerful techniques of molecular biology, has allowed several groups recently to characterize certain minor histocompatibility antigens (Scott *et al.* 1995; Wang *et al.* 1995). It has become clear that minor histocompatibility antigens comprise peptides from self proteins that have a low level of polymorphism within a species, presented in the MHC groove. This explains why it has been difficult to raise antibodies, which normally recognize conformational determinants on proteins, to minor antigens. The most well-characterized minor histocompatibility antigens are the male-specific H-Y antigens, which are derived from a group of proteins encoded on the Y chromosome and which can induce graft rejection in female mice of male skin originating from otherwise genetically identical individuals (Scott *et al.* 1995, 1997; Wang *et al.* 1995; Greenfield *et al.* 1996).

## Migration of passenger leucocytes into recipient lymphoid organs

Isolated MHC proteins or minor histocompatibility antigens can have a remarkably low level of immunogenicity but found as integrated cell surface proteins may be highly immunogenic. The level of immunogenicity varies, however, with the cell type on which they are found. Several years ago, cells with the characteristics of bone marrow-derived leucocytes were demonstrated in most non-lymphoid tissues (Hart & Fabre 1981). These so-called passenger leucocytes migrate rapidly out of a tissue following transplantation to the recipient lymphoid organs, where they are able to interact with and stimulate the host immune response (Larsen *et al.* 1990a,b). Passenger leucocytes have the characteristics of immature dendritic cells (Reis e Sousa *et al.* 1993), which upon migration rapidly mature into antigen-presenting cells with the ability to stimulate T cells (Steinman & Witmer 1978; Steinman *et al.* 1983; Steinman 1991). Mature dendritic cells express a high level of both MHC class I and II antigens and as such are able to stimulate both CD4+ and CD8+ cells. As described below, such cells also have a number of additional features which make them uniquely potent in stimulating naïve, previously unactivated, T cells. These features earn the dendritic cell the title of 'professional' antigen-presenting cell. Such cells certainly can provide an important stimulus for graft rejection as their removal from the graft prior to transplantation can prolong the survival of that graft (Billingham 1971; Lafferty *et al.* 1976; Lechler & Batchelor 1982). However, this is not always the case, suggesting that there is a second route to sensitization of the recipient. Indeed, it has become clear that foreign graft-derived antigens can be presented to the recipient immune system by dendritic cells in more than one

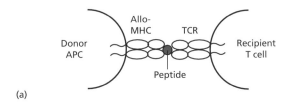

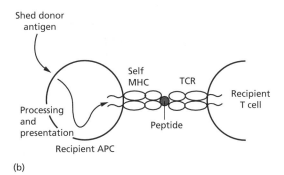

**Fig. 1.4** Pathways of (a) direct and (b) indirect antigen presentation.

way, termed direct and indirect antigen presentation (Fig. 1.4).

## Direct antigen presentation

Following migration of graft-derived dendritic cells into the recipient lymphoid tissue, they may directly stimulate T cells of the host. This may initially seem counter-intuitive because we know that the T cell repertoire is skewed towards recognition of peptide in the context of self MHC proteins. However, it is clear experimentally that allogeneic MHC (allo-MHC) provides a uniquely strong stimulus to the immune system and indeed a very high frequency, up to 1–10%, of T cells respond to any allo-MHC. The allo-MHC will, like all MHC proteins, contain peptides derived from the donor tissue. Such 'self' peptides originate mainly from normal non-polymorphic proteins (Rotzschke *et al.* 1991) or MHC itself (Golding & Singer 1984; Parham *et al.* 1987) and in the context of self MHC would not induce an immune response. However, when the MHC is allogeneic (i.e. when a graft is placed in an MHC-disparate recipient) the sum of the MHC +

peptide may now be recognized as not-self and stimulate a T cell(s). The real job of such T cells is obviously not to respond to alloantigen, but to deal with invading organisms. Their ability to respond to alloantigen is therefore simply caused by a rather inconvenient cross-reactivity of their receptor for self MHC + foreign peptide with allo-MHC + self peptide. For many T cells which have perfectly respectable reactivity for a foreign peptide + self MHC, it is possible to demonstrate cross-reactivity on one or more alloantigens. In addition to this, different ranges of peptides may be displayed by the foreign and self MHC proteins as a result of the different peptide-binding capacities of each MHC groove. Those peptides not normally displayed in self MHC will not have had an opportunity to induce tolerance in the recipient and thus may induce an immune response when presented on allo-MHC proteins. That populations of alloreactive cytotoxic T lymphocytes (CTL) induced by direct antigen presentation are able to recognize a wide spectrum of different peptide–MHC aggregates and even empty MHC molecules as has been elegantly demonstrated by Rotzschke *et al.* (1991). In these studies, peptides were acid-eluted from the MHC and characterized for their ability to trigger killing by alloantigen-primed mouse CTL and for their distribution in cells of both mouse and other species.

The most likely explanation for the unusually high number of T cells that react to any given allo-MHC is that a very large number of different self peptides will be derived from the graft and the combination of these with the allo-MHC will stimulate a very large number of different T cell clones in the recipient (Dorling & Lechler 1996).

## Indirect antigen presentation

Several pieces of evidence suggest that allo-MHC antigens can be treated in precisely the same way as any other foreign antigen and be presented in association with self MHC (Butcher & Howard 1982; Rock *et al.* 1983; Golding & Singer 1984; Sherwood *et al.* 1986; Fangmann *et al.* 1992; Liu *et al.* 1992). From our understanding of processing and presentation it seems likely that most allo-MHC peptides will be presented in the context of class II MHC antigens, because it is this pathway that deals with proteins exogenous to the cell.

There is, however, some crossover between class II and I pathways such that allo-MHC peptides may also be presented in the context of self class I antigens (Pfeiffer *et al.* 1995; Malaviya *et al.* 1996). That indirect presentation may have practical significance in transplantation is suggested by experiments of Fabre and colleagues (Fangmann *et al.* 1992) which show that peptides derived from rat class I antigens are able to immunize animals via the indirect pathway. Such immunized animals display accelerated rejection of a subsequent skin graft carrying the class I antigens from which the peptides were derived. Further information comes from experiments in which skin grafts from class II –/– mice are transplanted on to normal mice. Antigen-presenting cells from these grafts cannot stimulate CD4+ cells directly because of the absence of class II antigen, yet graft rejection still occurs and is CD4+ cell-dependent. In this case the CD4+ cells are presumed to have been stimulated by indirect presentation of donor alloantigens on self MHC (Auchincloss *et al.* 1993; Lee *et al.* 1994, 1997). The actual importance of this pathway in primary graft rejection by normal animals remains somewhat unclear, although it has been suggested that indirect antigen presentation provides the continued antigenic stimulus required for chronic graft rejection (Cramer *et al.* 1989) and may also play a dominant part in acute rejection (Auchincloss & Sultan 1996).

## Entry of naïve recipient leucocytes into graft tissue

While dendritic cells are able to migrate out of a graft into the local lymphoid tissue to stimulate an immune response, it is also apparent that naïve recipient-derived leucocytes may migrate into the graft. This is particularly obvious following small-bowel transplantation when recipient-derived leucocytes, including T lymphocytes, migrate into the mesenteric lymph nodes and Peyer's patches of the graft and generate a response within 24 h of grafting (Ingham-Clark *et al.* 1990; Kim *et al.* 1991; Toogood *et al.* 1997). It is certainly possible that such cells may readily become activated via direct antigen presentation as the gut-associated lymphoid tissue will be rich in mature dendritic cells. The extent to which naïve T cells enter other types of transplant and then become activated *in situ* is rather unclear because while all tissues contain dendritic cells these are in general immature and lack the full stimulatory capacity of migrant dendritic cells.

The work of Pober and colleagues, and more recently other groups, has suggested that the vascular endothelium may provide another source of stimulation to the host immune system (Hughes *et al.* 1990; Pober & Cotran 1991). Using cell culture systems these workers have demonstrated that vascular endothelial cells, devoid of dendritic cells, are able to cause marked proliferation of allogeneic lymphocytes and induce the differentiation of cytotoxic effector cells. Interestingly, in humans, endothelial cells constitutively express MHC class II antigens whereas in rodents they do not, suggesting that such cells may play a more important part in induction of the immune response in humans than in rodents. The ability of endothelial cells to stimulate truly naïve T cells remains somewhat controversial, however, particularly because they appear to lack some cell surface proteins which may be critical in T cell activation (Page *et al.* 1994a,b).

## Activation signals for recipient T cells

Following the discovery that lymphocytes could be subdivided into two major populations, the T and B

cells, it became clear that T cells were required for graft rejection in animals that had not previously been exposed to the donor antigens. Animals deprived of T cells through genetic mutation or through experimental manipulation are unable to reject grafts (Rolstad & Ford 1974; Rygaard 1974; Hall *et al.* 1978).

### TCR signals

Without an interaction of the TCR with its cognate antigen, T cells remain quiescent and can recirculate through the lymphoid tissues waiting for their antigen to come along for many years (Gowans 1959; Butcher & Picker 1996). Most T cells bear a TCR comprised of two similar chains, the α and β chains (Hedrick *et al.* 1984), which are complexed with several more proteins, the γ, δ, ε and ζ chains of the CD3 complex (Weiss *et al.* 1986). The TCR confers specificity of antigen–MHC binding (Fig. 1.5) while the ζ chains of the CD3 complex transduce signals of activation to the T cell. A number of intracellular signalling pathways are activated, resulting in *de novo* expression of a range of genes, including those encoding cytokines and new cell surface proteins. The signalling pathways are increasingly well characterized (Cantrell 1996) and indeed are the target of some immunosuppressive drugs (Morris 1991, 1993).

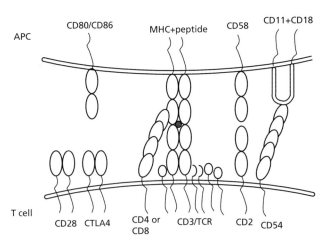

Fig. 1.5 Cell surface interactions between antigen-presenting cells (APC) and T cells.

## Second or costimulatory signals

The fate of a CD4+ T cell once in receipt of a TCR signal appears to depend critically on whether or not it secures other so-called costimulatory or second signals. Without these second signals a T cell may very well become anergic or unresponsive (Jenkins & Schwartz 1987; Jenkins *et al.* 1987; Schwartz 1990, 1997), a state which may also result in an ability to prevent the activation of its neighbouring T cells (Lombardi *et al.* 1994). The fact that deprivation of second signals results in an unresponsive and even regulatory fate for T cells has attracted enormous interest as harnessing and application of such an approach could be of major importance in preventing graft rejection. There are many cell surface proteins on a T cell that potentially contribute to its activation in this way (see Fig. 1.5). The CD4 and CD8 proteins act by binding to class II and I, respectively, on the antigen-presenting cell. Both CD4 and CD8 are linked to intracellular proteins which are involved in transducing further signals to the T cell. A series of additional proteins on the T cell surface, such as CD54, CD2, CD11a/CD18 and CD5, act to increase the affinity of interaction between the T cell and its antigen-presenting cell and may also transduce further signals to the T cell.

Recent interest in the area of costimulation has centred on the role of the CD28 pathway (June *et al.* 1987; Harding *et al.* 1992; Lenschow *et al.* 1996b; Chambers & Allison 1997). CD28 is a homodimeric glycoprotein which is present on the surface of T cells and which interacts with two counter-receptors, CD80 and CD86, which may be expressed on the surface of APCs. CD80 and CD86 are very similar in overall structure although they have different patterns of expression and bind with distinct affinities to CD28 (Larsen *et al.* 1994; Lenschow *et al.* 1994; Linsley *et al.* 1994; Morton *et al.* 1996). CD86, expressed constitutively at a low level by professional APCs (e.g. dendritic cells) and up-regulated rapidly following interaction with the T cell, has a rather low affinity for CD28 whereas CD80 is expressed with slower kinetics, only following interaction of an APC with the T cell, and has an ~ 10-fold greater binding affinity for CD28 than does CD86 (van der Merwe *et al.* 1997). The result of

ligation of CD28 by either CD86 or CD80 appears to be increased cytokine synthesis and proliferation following signalling through as yet incompletely defined intracellular pathways (Lindsten *et al.* 1989; Thompson *et al.* 1989; Rudd *et al.* 1994; Rudd 1996). The reason for the apparent redundancy in expression of the costimulatory proteins CD80 and CD86 is as yet unknown, but it is likely, and indeed there is some evidence (see below), that they may have subtly different roles in the development of immunity. To complicate the situation further an additional protein, CTLA4, is expressed by T cells following activation which, while structurally related to CD28, appears to be critically involved in regulating the T cell such that it does not respond indefinitely to antigen (Tivol *et al.* 1995; Karandiker *et al.* 1996). CTLA4 also binds to both CD80 and CD86, not only showing a higher affinity for CD80 than CD86 but also a higher affinity for both than does CD28. Clearly the integration of signals resulting from all of these interactions is complex and as yet poorly understood (Chambers & Allison 1997).

The requirement of CD28 signals for CD4+ T cells in secondary immune responses or for CD8+ T cells is less clear. The prevailing view for CD4+ cells is that if they have not recently been stimulated by antigen (i.e. they have developed into memory cells) they will require costimulation for reactivation. Experimentally it can be shown that in certain situations virus-reactive CD8+ cells require neither costimulation through CD28 nor CD28-dependent help (Kudig *et al.* 1996; Zimmerman *et al.* 1997). However, to achieve this they may require massive TCR stimulation provided, for instance, by a replicating virus, a situation which may infrequently occur during other immune responses. Even for CD4+ cells overwhelming stimulation through the TCR may obviate the requirement for CD28-mediated costimulation. Indeed, mice with a disrupted CD28 gene do make impaired immune responses yet can reject skin grafts, albeit in a delayed fashion (Kawai *et al.* 1996). Nevertheless, blocking this pathway in normal animals may have dramatic effects on the generation of immune responses and indeed may result in prolonged graft survival or even tolerance of grafts (Lenschow *et al.* 1992; Turka *et al.* 1992; Pearson *et al.* 1994). The potential for blocking this route of immunity in the treatment of transplant patients is as yet unexplored but remains exciting.

Upon activation T cells express another cell surface protein, gp39 (CD40 ligand). Interaction of this protein with its counter-receptor, CD40, appears to be critical for the activation of B cells, dendritic cells and monocytes. In an interesting recent report Larsen *et al.* (1996a) showed that blocking this interaction could prolong graft survival in a mouse cardiac transplant model. Even more impressive, however, are more recent data from this group showing that combined block of CD28 and gp39 interactions can induce permanent survival of an allogeneic skin graft in mice with no long-term deterioration of graft integrity (Larsen *et al.* 1996b). Curiously, tolerance to the graft antigens could not be demonstrated in these mice despite the excellent survival of the transplant itself.

In addition to this large number of cell–cell based interactions, T cells also receive important signals through the binding of soluble proteins, the cytokines, to specific cell surface cytokine receptors. Cytokines such as IL-1 and IL-12, derived primarily from macrophages, seem to sensitize T cells through up-regulating the expression of receptors for other cytokines, to the proliferative and differentiative effects of the (primarily) T cell derived cytokines such as IL-2 and IL-4. A whole cascade of cytokines are produced that amplify both immune and inflammatory processes following transplantation (reviewed extensively by Dallman & Clark 1992; Nickerson *et al.* 1994; Dallman 1995; Strom *et al.* 1996; see below).

## Generation of different types of immunity

### CD4+ and CD8+ cells

A fundamental aspect of immunity is the initiation of the response by helper T cells. In general, such cells bear the CD4 surface protein but in certain situations CD8+ cells are able to meet all the requirements of a helper T cell. Once activated these helper T cells are able to recruit and activate other cells, inducing their differentiation into effector cells.

That CD4+ cells are normally required to initiate

graft rejection has been shown by many workers using a variety of experimental approaches (Loveland *et al.* 1981; Dallman *et al.* 1982; Gurley *et al.* 1983; Hall *et al.* 1983; Lowry *et al.* 1983), although, depending on the mismatch between donor and recipient, CD8+ cells may be additionally required or may act independently of CD4+ cells (Tilney *et al.* 1984; Rosenberg *et al.* 1986, 1987; Sprent *et al.* 1986; Rosenberg 1993).

The most recent work that addresses the roles of CD4+ and CD8+ cells in transplantation responses involves the use of mice deprived of these populations through genetic manipulation. Mice lacking class I or II antigens are severely depleted of CD8+ or CD4+ cells, respectively, as are those mice in which either the CD4 or CD8 gene has been disrupted (Dierich *et al.* 1993; Lamouse-Smith *et al.* 1993; Schilham *et al.* 1993; Apasov & Sitkovsky 1994; Mannon *et al.* 1995; Dalloul *et al.* 1996a,b; Kreiger *et al.* 1996). The effects on graft rejection of a lack of CD4+ or CD8+ cells produced in this manner are not always predictable and depend often on the nature of the antigenic mismatch between donor and recipient. Further, despite an apparent depletion of CD8+ cells in class I –/– mice, CD8+ cytotoxic T lymphocytes (CTLs) can be generated in large numbers following transplantation and may be involved in the rejection process (Schilham *et al.* 1993; Apasov & Sitkovsky 1994; Lee *et al.* 1994) and CD4– and CD8– T cells may develop and function normally in CD4 –/– CD8 –/– mice (Schilham *et al.* 1993).

It is probably fair to say that results from the use of knockout mice have not altered our ideas about the roles of these two T cell subsets in initiating graft rejection; in other words CD4+ cells seem normally to play a central part in directing graft rejection. However, there are clearly experimental situations, usually when there is a dominant or sole MHC class I mismatch, in which CD8+ cells are also required for rejection to proceed with normal kinetics or can act independently of the CD4+ cell.

### T1- and T2-driven immunity

A critical role of the helper cell is to produce cytokines which direct the proliferation and differentiation of effector cells. Following stimulation of the immune system, a response develops in which either humoral or cell-mediated immunity tends to dominate (Parish 1972; Katsura 1977) and it has become clear that cytokines have an important role in determining which type of immunity emerges (Mosmann *et al.* 1986; Mosmann & Coffman 1989; Del Prete *et al.* 1991; McKnight *et al.* 1991; Mosmann & Moore 1991) (Fig. 1.6). Following continued stimulation of T cells, they will differentiate to produce varying patterns of cytokines. It should be made clear not only that early on during an immune response many T cells will make a wide range of cytokines and it is only later that any obvious divergence of such populations can be observed, but also that it is the view of some workers that we have through this paradigm over-simplified our view of the immune response (Kelso 1995).

IFN-γ is the hallmark cytokine of T1 cells and a predominance of this population results in the appearance of cell-mediated immunity involving the generation of both specific CTL and activated macrophages. T2 cells, on the other hand, make cytokines such as IL-4, IL-5 and IL-6 which are critical for the induction of humoral immunity, and in particular selected immunoglobulin isotypes, and eosinophilia. Recently it has become apparent that both CD4+ and CD8+ cells can produce these distinct patterns of cytokines.

Exactly how a T1 or T2 dominated response is determined is somewhat uncertain, but factors such as the local cytokine milieu (Gajewski & Fitch 1988; Gajewski *et al.* 1989; Swain *et al.* 1990, 1991; Hsieh *et al.* 1992, 1993), involvement of APCs other than dendritic cells (Macatonia *et al.* 1993a,b) and the type of CD28 signal delivered (i.e. either through CD80 or CD86) (Freeman *et al.* 1995; Kuchroo *et al.* 1995; Lenschow *et al.* 1996a; Ranger *et al.* 1996) may all be important.

Within the transplantation community particular interest has focused on the possibility that, while a T1-driven response may inevitably be damaging and result in graft rejection, a T2-driven response may not be and indeed may be associated with the induction of tolerance to a graft (reviewed by Dallman 1993, 1995; Nickerson *et al.* 1994; Strom *et al.* 1996). A number of groups have found that tolerance or reduced donor-directed reactivity is associated with a decrease in expression of the T1 associated cytokines IL-2 and IFN-γ (Mohler & Streilein 1989; Burdick & Clow 1990; Dallman *et al.* 1991b; Bugeon *et al.* 1992; Takeuchi *et al.* 1992; Alard *et al.* 1993). It has been tempting to speculate that this is accompanied by, or even caused by, the expansion of regulatory T2 cells. Indeed, there is some evidence that the expression of cytokines such as IL-4, IL-5 and IL-10 is preserved during the development of tolerance (Gorczynski

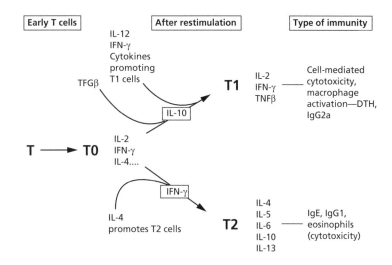

**Fig. 1.6** T1 and T2 cell differentiation. IL-10 blocks T1 differentiation and IFN-γ blocks differentiation.

1992; Takeuchi *et al.* 1992; Dallman *et al.* 1993), although it must be said that cells other than T2 cells can produce such cytokines, meaning that their detection does not automatically infer the presence or action of the T2 population. As we will see in the following sections, an immune response to a transplant is complex; both humoral and cellular mechanisms can effect graft destruction. It is likely that any type of immunity, T1- or T2-driven, would result in graft rejection. Indeed, in models of complete tolerance, rather than prolonged graft survival almost a complete shutdown of T cell cytokine production is observed (Pearson *et al.* 1994; Josien *et al.* 1995).

Several groups have looked at the role of key T cell derived cytokines by performing experiments in which their over-expression or absence is tested. Using IL-4 knockout mice, two groups have now shown that tolerance can be induced using reagents that block CD28 signalling in the absence of IL-4 (Nickerson *et al.* 1996; Lakkis *et al.* 1997). Perhaps the most important finding in these studies was that Nickerson *et al.* (1996) showed that tolerance was in fact less easily induced in heterozygous IL-4 +/− mice than in homozygous IL-4 −/− mice. The implication of this is that the presence of IL-4 itself can be damaging to the graft. In other experiments it was shown, again using knockout mice, that neither IL-2 nor IFN-γ is required for rejection (Steiger *et al.* 1995; Konieczny *et al.* 1996; Saleem *et al.* 1996; Strom *et al.* 1996). Interpretation of such experiments is again complicated by the fact that cytokines can often substitute for one another and it is therefore unclear whether or not the phenotype of these mice accurately reflects the importance of these cytokines in normal mice. For instance, IL-15 can substitute many of the actions of IL-2 and IL-13 for IL-4. Indeed, in the experiments described above IL-15 transcripts were found in grafts put into the IL-2 knockout mice and IL-13 transcripts in those transplanted into IL-4 knockout mice. The results of these experiments do not therefore address the relative involvement of T1 and T2 cells in rejection and tolerance.

An alternative approach to this issue has been used by several groups in experiments in which cytokines have been injected or over-expressed in animal transplant models in an attempt to deviate the immune system towards a T1 or T2 response. Injection of IL-2 or IFN-γ can prevent the induction of tolerance (Dallman *et al.* 1991b; Bugeon *et al.* 1992). However, injection or over-expression of IL-4 cannot induce tolerance and while this treatment may marginally prolong graft survival (M. Dallman *et al.*, unpublished data) it may actually inhibit tolerance induction (Nickerson *et al.* 1996).

The most plausible conclusion from all of these studies is that immunity driven by either T1 or T2 cells is damaging although that driven by T2 cells may be less damaging than that driven by T1 cells.

## Migration of activated leucocytes into the graft

In order to enter any site of inflammation or immune response, leucocytes must migrate across the vascular endothelium. This migration process is controlled by the elaboration of cell attractants or chemokines and by cell–cell interactions between the leucocyte and the endothelium.

### Cell–cell interactions

The adhesion of leucocytes to the endothelium is a complex multistep process that involves a series of interactions between the surface of the leucocyte and the endothelial cell or its extracellular matrix (reviewed by Butcher & Picker 1996; Kirby 1996). The proteins involved fall into three groups: the selectins, members of the integrin family and immunoglobulin (Ig) super-families. Initial interaction and rolling of leucocytes along the endothelium allows the leucocyte to sample the endothelial environment while maintaining its ability to detach and travel somewhere else. This step is largely controlled by the selectins although α4 integrins, for instance, may also have a role at this stage. Under the correct conditions this interaction will lead to signalling to the leucocyte, thereby slowing down and arresting the rolling process and allowing extravasation. These latter stages are regulated mainly by the integrins and adhesion proteins of the Ig superfamily.

The expression of many adhesion proteins involved

in these interactions is up-regulated by proinflammatory cytokines. Indeed, ischaemic damage alone results in increased expression of several cytokines and of these, IL-1, for instance, up-regulates the expression of members of the selectin family (Pober *et al.* 1986; Collins *et al.* 1995). Other adhesion proteins, such as ICAM-1 and VCAM-1 of the Ig superfamily and endothelial-specific selectin (E-selectin) are known to be up-regulated by the type of cytokines induced following the trauma of transplantation. Even before an immune response has been generated the graft therefore becomes attractive to circulating leucocytes, although naïve lymphocytes at least tend not to home into non-lymphoid sites. Antigen-activated lymphocytes, however, have an altered recirculation pattern and are now perfectly happy to migrate into extralymphoid sites (Butcher 1986; Picker & Butcher 1992; Mackay 1993). Indeed they may show tissue-selective homing and show preference for sites in which they are most likely to re-encounter their specific antigen.

One practical aspect of this process in terms of transplantation is that it may be possible to block the proteins involved in leucocyte extravasation, thereby slowing or preventing the rejection process. Indeed, interruption of these adhesion pathways either by antibodies or by inhibiting their expression has been attempted in both experimental and clinical transplantation (Heagy *et al.* 1984; Cosimi *et al.* 1990; Haug *et al.* 1993; Hourmant *et al.* 1996). In general, cocktails of antibodies have a greater beneficial effect than do single antibodies (Yang *et al.* 1995; Iwata *et al.* 1996), although the results are variable and in one case a combination of antibodies to ICAM-1 and LFA-1 has been shown to result in accelerated rejection of rat cardiac allografts (Morikawa *et al.* 1994).

## Chemokines

A large number of chemokines have been identified and include RANTES, IL-8 and MCP-1 (Oppenheim *et al.* 1991, 1996); these chemokines are involved in the attraction of T cells and eosinophils, neutrophils and basophils, and monocytes, respectively. Initial excitement surrounding the involvement of chemokines in

extravasation of leucocytes has been tempered somewhat by the finding that chemokine receptors are expressed at low levels by resting leucocytes (Bacon & Schall 1996). However, in certain situations they appear to play an important role in the development of graft infiltrates (Grandaliano *et al.* 1997).

## Destruction of the graft

The immune system generates a wide variety of effector mechanisms depending on the challenge it meets. In certain infections a single mechanism appears to be essential in the clearance of the organism and the absence of that mechanism renders the host susceptible to disease. For example, in the clearance of lymphocytic choriomeningitis virus (LCMV) infections in mice, cytotoxic cells are absolutely required and disabling this arm of immunity by disrupting the perforin gene leads to death in infected animals (Kagi *et al.* 1995). Unfortunately, most of the known effector mechanisms of the immune system seem to be capable of damaging a graft such that the absence of any single effector mechanism has little beneficial effect on graft survival. This is most likely to be the reason that it is so difficult to prevent graft rejection without disabling the central components of the immune system. Described below are the various effector systems that can damage tissue. Their role in hyperacute, acute and chronic rejection are discussed.

### Antibody

Antibody may cause tissue damage not only through the fixation of complement, but also through the activity of K cells in antibody-dependent cellular cytotoxicity (ADCC). In the latter case, the antibody acts as a bridge between the target tissue and the effector cell, activating the lytic machinery of the K cell and thus resulting in tissue damage (Perlmann & Holm 1969). Many different leucocytes appear to be able to express K cell activity but, although ADCC activity may be recovered from grafts (Tilney *et al.* 1975), their role *in vivo* in graft rejection is not firmly established.

Patients previously exposed to MHC antigens through transplant, blood transfusions or pregnancy often develop antibodies reactive with those MHC antigens. Such preformed antibodies can undoubtedly cause hyperacute rejection where the organ fails immediately following revascularization (Kissmeyer-Nielsen *et al.* 1966; Williams *et al.* 1968; Patel & Terasaki 1969; Morris & Ting 1982). Rejection is accompanied by deposition of antibody and complement and accumulation of polymorphonuclear leucocytes within the graft (Williams *et al.* 1968). Hyperacute rejection is now pre-empted through the use of pretransplant screening by a cross-match test for antibodies directed towards donor antigens. However, the conventional cross-match test detects not only harmful MHC directed cytotoxic antibodies, but also harmless autoantibodies (Ting & Morris 1977, 1981). In most cases it is now possible to distinguish auto- from alloreactive antibodies and thus it is has become possible to transplant an increasing number of patients across an apparent positive cross-match, but in whom the reactivity is caused by autoantibodies.

Liver transplantation appears to be an exception to the rules regarding transplantation across a positive cross-match. In fact liver transplants are carried out with little regard to the immune system and are performed successfully not only across positive cross-matches but also with little or no attempt at MHC matching between donor and recipient. The reasons for the refractoriness to immune rejection displayed by liver grafts is not fully understood and may be partly a result of the size and enormous capacity for regeneration displayed by the liver. However, the immune response to liver transplants also differs from that to other grafts with spontaneous tolerance developing in several rat and mouse strain combinations. An understanding of this phenomenon may help us design new strategies of tolerance induction (Kamada *et al.* 1981; Kamada & Wight 1984; Farges *et al.* 1994, 1995).

Many of the changes associated with acute rejection, such as arteriolar thrombosis, interstitial haemorrhage and fibrinoid necrosis of the arteriolar walls, may result from the deposition of antibody and fixation of complement (Dunnill 1984). However, the appearance of donor-specific antibody does not necessarily accompany graft rejection and its presence may be compatible with unimpaired graft function (Ting & Morris 1978;

Baldwin *et al.* 1991). On the other hand, in at least one experimental model in which donor and recipient rats differ only at MHC class I loci, acute rejection of kidney grafts associates with and can be initiated by donor-specific antibody (Gracie *et al.* 1990).

Donor-specific antibodies may also be found in the circulation and immunoglobulin deposits may be seen in vessel walls during chronic rejection, but it is not clear whether or how the presence of such antibodies may be causally related to graft dysfunction (Yilmaz *et al.* 1992).

An area of increasing interest is that of xenotransplantation in which the use of animal donors is being considered for human transplantation. There are certainly many problems associated with this approach, not the least of which is the presence, in human circulation, of antibodies that react with the cells of many animal species including the pig, which is currently the donor animal of choice in xenotransplantation. These antibodies show a predominant reactivity to particular sugars on cell surface proteins; these are caused by the activity of the $\alpha$-1,3-galactosyltransferase gene present in pigs, and indeed many other species, but not in humans (Galili *et al.* 1984, 1985; Cooper *et al.* 1993; Sandrin *et al.* 1993; Parker *et al.* 1994). Such 'natural antibodies' result in hyperacute rejection of pig tissue by the human (Platt & Bach 1991; Platt *et al.* 1991).

## Cellular mechanisms

The involvement of cell-mediated mechanisms is usually invoked in acute or chronic graft rejection but, although hyperacute rejection has almost always been attributed to antibody, in certain situations a very rapid rejection may occur even when the role of antibody has been excluded. In these situations a cellular mechanism of rejection has been implicated (Kirkman *et al.* 1979).

### NATURAL KILLER CELLS

Unlike cytotoxic T cells, described below, the natural killer (NK) cell apparently does not need to interact with antigen in order to become lytic to target cells, although it is clear that its activity can be increased by certain cytokines. NK cells may be recovered from the blood or spleen and are able to lyse NK-sensitive targets which tend to be of tumour origin (Herberman *et al.* 1979). While clearly a potent source of cytotoxic activity, a role for the NK cell in organ graft rejection remains to be established. Indeed, several laboratories using different experimental models have found that grafts survive indefinitely in the presence of demonstrable NK effector activity (Mason & Morris 1984; Bradley *et al.* 1985; Armstrong *et al.* 1987). On the other hand, NK cells have quite clearly been shown to be involved in the rejection of bone marrow transplants (Murphy *et al.* 1987a,b). The method of target cell recognition employed by the NK cell is increasingly understood (Colonna *et al.* 1993; Leibson 1995; Long & Wagtmann 1997). For the NK cell, interaction with MHC on a target cell may actually result in the delivery of a negative signal to the NK cell, preventing the activation of its lytic machinery. The absence of self class I MHC antigens triggers the NK cell to attack its target, a finding which is consistent with the observation that NK cells are capable of rejecting bone marrow cells which express little or no class I antigen (Bix *et al.* 1991).

SPECIFIC CYTOTOXIC T CELLS

In cell culture systems, MHC mismatched lymphocytes proliferate and produce cytokines in response to one another in the so-called mixed lymphocyte reaction (MLR). The resulting cytokine production allows the differentiation of cytotoxic T lymphocytes (CTLs) that lyse target cells bearing the mismatched MHC antigens (Hayry & Defendi 1970; Hodes & Svedmyr 1970). The fact that a very powerful yet totally antigen-specific response is generated in such MLRs has made the CTL the prime suspect as the central effector mechanism in graft destruction.

There is considerable evidence to suggest that CTLs may be involved in graft rejection. First, CTLs may be recovered from allografts that are undergoing rejection but they are present only at low levels in grafts of animals that have been treated with cyclosporin to prevent rejection (Mason & Morris 1984; Bradley *et*

*al.* 1985). Secondly, cloned populations of CTLs are capable of causing the type of tissue damage associated with rejection (Engers *et al.* 1982; Tyler *et al.* 1984). Thirdly, most class I MHC antigen directed CTL expresses the CD8 protein and graft rejection may often be delayed in the absence of CD8+ cells (Lowry *et al.* 1983; Cobbold *et al.* 1984; Tilney *et al.* 1984; Madsen *et al.* 1987, 1988).

Conversely, graft destruction may occur in the absence of demonstrable CTL activity and the presence of such cells within a graft may not always lead to graft destruction. The male-specific minor histocompatibility antigen, H-Y, was first detected by the rejection of male skin grafts by female mice of the same strain. Using a variety of mouse strains it has been found that although female mice often reject male skin they do not always mount a detectable cytotoxic T cell response. Furthermore, in some strains of mice the females are able to generate H-Y specific cytotoxic cells but do not reject male-derived skin grafts (Hurme *et al.* 1978a,b).

Other experiments have demonstrated the presence of cytotoxic effector cells within a graft that is not rejected (Armstrong *et al.* 1987; Dallman *et al.* 1987). Rats given a donor-specific preoperative blood transfusion may retain a subsequent renal allograft indefinitely, yet cells extracted from such grafts show high and persistent donor-specific CTL activity. The simple conclusion from these studies is that CTLs cannot always reject grafts. The possibility that the action of these CTLs may be blocked in the graft itself, only being released on removal from the graft, or that the activity of CTLs in cell culture does not accurately reflect their potential in the animal must be considered. These results do, however, remain intriguing and provide direct evidence of the presence of cytotoxic effector cells within an organ graft that is not ultimately rejected.

Cytotoxic T cells are able to kill their targets through the elaboration of perforins and granzymes, through activation of the Fas death pathway in the target cell or through secretion of the cytokine TNFα. Their involvement in graft rejection has been further questioned by the finding that mice deficient in perforin (perforin knockouts) are able to reject tumour (Walsh *et al.* 1996), skin (Selvaggi *et al.* 1996) and organ (Schulz *et al.* 1995) grafts, even when the grafts are resistant to Fas and TNFα-mediated killing (Walsh *et al.* 1996). In the experiments of Schulz *et al.* (1995), however, grafts mismatched only at the class I MHC are rejected more slowly in perforin knockout mice indicating that, for class I different grafts at least, cytotoxic cells have an important role in rejection.

Even if CTLs themselves do not mediate the tissue damage that ultimately results in graft loss, they may still be important in the immune response to the graft. Through the elaboration of high levels of IFN-γ they are able to recruit and activate cells involved in delayed-type hypersensitivity (DTH) reactions, thus initiating acute or chronic rejection.

### MACROPHAGES AND DELAYED-TYPE HYPERSENSITIVITY REACTIONS

T cells initiate a DTH reaction (Loveland & McKenzie 1982), which involves an essentially non-specific effector phase (as described by Koch in 1891 in the tuberculin skin reaction; see Florey & Jennings 1970), characterized by an infiltrate of lymphocytes and cells of the monocyte–macrophage lineage. Damage happens during a DTH reaction through the elaboration of various noxious substances including reactive nitrogen and oxygen intermediates and TNFα by the macrophage. As macrophages do not themselves carry antigen receptors the specificity of rejection, if mediated by macrophages, must rely on activity of the T cell. This means that the effector step in graft destruction would not itself be antigen-specific, a suggestion difficult to reconcile with data indicating that graft damage may on occasion be incredibly specific (Mintz & Silvers 1967, 1970; Rosenberg & Singer 1992). In other situations, however, tissue destruction can be rather non-specific, involving destruction of bystander cells, suggesting again that the circumstance of the graft may determine the effector mechanism involved in its destruction.

Support for the role of DTH reactions in graft rejection comes from the studies on rejection of H-Y disparate grafts. Although cytotoxic cell responses do not always correlate with graft rejection, the generation of

DTH reactions to H-Y antigens follows closely the ability of female mice to reject male skin (Liew & Simpson 1980). In addition, irradiated rats reconstituted with CD4 cells can reject heart grafts without developing a detectable specific cytotoxic cell response within the transplant (Lowry *et al.* 1983).

The high level of inflammatory mediators and the type of changes within grafts undergoing chronic rejection suggest a role for activated macrophages in this process (Hayry *et al.* 1993; Paul & Benediktsson 1993; Chen *et al.* 1996; Paul *et al.* 1996). Cytokines such as IL-1, TNFα, TGFβ and PDGF lead to smooth muscle proliferation; TGFβ and PDGF result in an increased synthesis of extracellular matrix proteins. These cytokines are products of activated macrophages and may result in the atherosclerotic and fibrotic changes associated with chronic graft failure.

In summary, there is evidence in favour of and against the involvement of the specific CTL and DTH effector mechanisms in graft rejection. It has been suggested by several workers (Snider & Steinmuller 1987; Rosenberg & Singer 1992) that a specifically activated effector T cell population, through the elaboration of cytokines such as IFN-γ, may recruit cells to mediate tissue destruction through non-specific or DTH mechanisms. It seems likely that neither CTL nor DTH mechanisms are unique in their ability to cause acute graft rejection, that frequently both are involved but also that in the absence of one mechanism the other may develop and cause graft rejection.

### CYTOKINES

Undoubtedly the primary role of cytokines in the immune response to a graft is to initiate proliferation, differentiation and homing of leucocytes in the generation of immunity. However, certain cytokines may also damage tissue directly. As described above, TNFα, produced by CTL cells and macrophages, may damage a graft. Blocking the effects of TNF, using neutralizing antibodies, can prolong organ graft survival (Imagawa *et al.* 1990, 1991; Bolling *et al.* 1992). The rather minimal effects of these antibodies, however, suggest that the TNFs may not contribute centrally to graft rejection. Islets appear to be particularly susceptible to damage mediated by proinflammatory cytokines such that these may be a more important component in the rejection of islet transplants (Mandrup-Poulsen *et al.* 1986, 1989; Rabinovitch *et al.* 1988; Wolf *et al.* 1989).

## Target cells of destructive immunity

Damage to the vascular endothelium, which may express both class I and II MHC antigens, is likely to result in rapid cell necrosis and graft loss (Kauntz *et al.* 1963). Indeed, the predominantly vascular changes that occur during rejection of an organ graft suggest that this is the case (Porter *et al.* 1964; Laden & Sinclair 1971; Dvorak *et al.* 1979). It is possible that parenchymal cells may also be targets for tissue destruction, but this is more likely to be secondary to the initial attack on endothelium. The increase in expression of both class I and II MHC antigens following transplantation could increase susceptibility of both endothelium and parenchymal cells to destruction. The marked arterial changes seen as a manifestation of both acute and chronic rejection would also suggest the importance of the endothelium as the main target of the response, and indeed in the case of chronic rejection the fibrotic changes seen histologically could well be caused mainly by ischaemia resulting from gradual vascular obliteration.

## Conclusions

The immune response to a transplant is complex. Virtually any cell involved in immunity has been implicated in graft rejection, its importance in the process depending on factors such as the donor recipient incompatibility, the type of graft or the type of immunosuppression. It is therefore very difficult to provide immunosuppression adequate to prevent graft rejection without disabling, at a central point, the immune system. The unfortunate consequence of this is that patients become susceptible to infection and are at increased risk of cancer. The only true solution to this problem is the development of strategies to induce donor-specific tolerance in the recipient. While this is straightforward in rodents it remains an elusive goal in humans.

## References

Alard, P., Lantz, O., Perrot, J.Y. *et al.* (1993) A possible role for specific 'anergy' in immunologic hyporeactivity to donor stimulation in human kidney allograft recipients. *Transplantation* 55, 277–283.

Apasov, S.G. & Sitkovsky, M.V. (1994) Development and antigen specificity of CD8+ cytotoxic T lymphocytes in beta 2-microglobulin-negative, MHC class 1-deficient mice in response to immunization with tumor cells. *Journal of Immunology* 152, 2087–2097.

Armstrong, H.E., Bolton, E.M., McMillan, I., Spencer, S.C. & Bradley, J.A. (1987) Prolonged survival of actively enhanced rat renal allografts despite accelerated cellular infiltration and rapid induction of both class I and class II MHC antigens. *Journal of Experimental Medicine* 165, 891–907.

Auchincloss, H. & Sultan, H. (1996) Antigen processing and presentation in transplantation. *Current Opinion in Immunology* 8, 681–687.

Auchincloss, H., Lee, R., Shea, S. *et al.* (1993) The role of 'indirect' recognition in intiating rejection of skin grafts from major histocompatibility complex class II-deficient mice. *Proceedings of the National Academy of Science (USA)* 90, 3373–3377.

Bacon, K.B. & Schall, T.J. (1996) Chemokines as mediators of allergic inflammation. *International Archives of Allergy Immunology* 109, 97–109.

Baldwin, W.M.I., Pruitt, S.K. & Sanfilippo, F. (1991) Alloantibodies: Basic and clinical concepts. *Transplantation Reviews* 5, 100–109.

Belich, M.P. & Trowsdale, J. (1995) Proteosome and class I antigen processing and presentation. *Molecular Biology Reports* 21, 53–56.

Billingham, R.E. (1971) The passenger cell concept in transplantation. *Cellular Immunology* 1, 1–12.

Bix, M., Liao, N.S., Zijlstra, M. *et al.* (1991) Rejection of class I MHC-deficient haemopoietic cells by irradiated MHC-matched mice. *Nature* 349, 329–331.

Bjorkman, P.J. (1997) MHC restriction in three dimensions: a view of the T cell receptor/ligand interactions. *Cell* 89, 167–170.

Bjorkman, P.J., Saper, M.A., Samraoni, B. *et al.* (1987) Structure of the human class I histocompatibility antigen, HLA-A2. *Nature* 329, 506–512.

Bolling, S., Kunkel, S.L. & Lin, H. (1992) Prolongation of cardiac allograft survival in rats by anti-TNF and cyclosporin combination therapy. *Transplantation* 53, 283–286.

Bradley, J.A., Mason, D.W. & Morris, P.J. (1985) Evidence that rat renal allografts are rejected by cytotoxic T cells and not by non-specific effectors. *Transplantation* **39**, 169–175.

Bugeon, L., Cuturi, M.-C., Hallet, M.-M. *et al.* (1992) Peripheral tolerance of an allograft in adult rats—characterization by low interleukin-2 and interferon-γ mRNA levels and by strong accumulation of major histocompatibility complex transcripts in the graft. *Transplantation* **54**, 219–225.

Burdick, J.F. & Clow, L.W. (1990) Rejection of primarily vascularized heart grafts. III Depression of the interleukin 2 mechanism early after grafting. *Transplantation* **50**, 476–481.

Butcher, E.C. (1986) The regulation of lymphocyte traffic. *Current Topics in Microbiological Immunology* **128**, 85–122.

Butcher, E.C. & Picker, L.J. (1996) Lymphocyte homing and homeostasis. *Science* **272**, 60–66.

Butcher, G.W. & Howard, J.C. (1982) Genetic control of transplant rejection. *Transplantation* **34**, 161–166.

Campbell, R.D. & Trowsdale, J. (1993) Map of the human major histocompatibility complex. *Immunology Today* **14**, 349–352.

Campos, L., Naji, A., Deli, B.C. *et al.* (1995) Survival of MHC-deficient mouse heterotopic cardiac allografts. *Transplantation* **59**, 187–191.

Cantrell, D. (1996) T cell antigen receptor signal transduction pathways. *Annual Review of Immunology* **14**, 259–274.

Chambers, C.A. & Allison, J.P. (1997) Co-stimulation in T cell responses. *Current Opinion in Immunology* **9**, 396–404.

Chen, J., Myllarniemi, M., Akyurek, L.M. *et al.* (1996) Identification of differentially expressed genes in rat aortic allograft vasculopathy. *American Journal of Pathology* **149**, 597–611.

Cobbold, S.P., Jayasuriya, A., Nash, A., Prospero, T.D. & Waldmann, H. (1984) Therapy with monoclonal antibodies by elimination of T cell subsets *in vivo*. *Nature* **312**, 548–551.

Collins, T., Read, M.A., Neish, A.S. *et al.* (1995) Transcriptional regulation of endothelial cell adhesion molecules: NF-kappa B and cytokine-inducible enhancers. *FASEB Journal* **9**, 899–909.

Colonna, M., Brooks, E.G., Falco, M., Ferrara, G.B. & Strominger, J.L. (1993) Generation of allospecific natural killer cells by stimulation across a polymorphism of HLA-C. *Science* **260**, 1121–1124.

Cooper, D.K.C., Good, A.H., Koren, E. *et al.* (1993) Identification of a-galactosyl and other carbohydrate epitopes that are bound by human anti-pig antibodies: relevance to discordant xenografting in man. *Transplant Immunology* **1**, 198–205.

Cosimi, A.B., Conti, D., Delmonico, F. & Lea. (1990) In vivo effects of monoclonal antibody to ICAM-1 (CD54) in nonhuman primates with renal allografts. *Journal of Immunology* **144**, 4604–4612.

Cramer, D.V., Qian, S., Harnaha, J. *et al.* (1989) Cardiac transplantation in the rat I. The effect of histocompatibility differences on graft arteriosclerosis. *Transplantation* **47**, 414–419.

Cresswell, P. (1994) Assembly, transport and function of MHC class II molecules. *Annual Review of Immunology* **12**, 259–293.

Dallman, M.J. (1993) Cytokines as mediators of organ graft rejection and tolerance. *Current Opinion in Immunology* **5**, 788–793.

Dallman, M.J. (1995) Cytokines and transplantation: Th1/Th2 regulation of the immune response to solid organ transplants in the adult. *Current Opinion in Immunology* **7**, 632–638.

Dallman, M.J. & Clark, G.J. (1992) Cytokine and their receptors in transplantation. *Current Opinion in Immunology* **3**, 729–734.

Dallman, M.J., Mason, D.W. & Webb, M. (1982) Induction of Ia antigens on murine epidermal cells during the rejection of skin allografts. *European Journal of Immunology* **12**, 511–518.

Dallman, M.J., Wood, K.J. & Morris, P.J. (1987) Specific cytotoxic T cells are found in the non-rejected kidneys of blood transfused rats. *Journal of Experimental Medicine* **165**, 566–571.

Dallman, M.J., Larsen, C.P. & Morris, C.P. (1991a) Cytokine gene transcription in vascularised organ grafts–analysis using semiquantitative polymerase chain reaction. *Journal of Experimental Medicine* **174**, 493–496.

Dallman, M.J., Shiho, O., Page, T.H., Wood, K.J. & Morris, P.J. (1991b) Peripheral tolerance to alloantigen results from altered regulation of the interleukin 2 pathway. *Journal of Experimental Medicine* **173**, 79–87.

Dallman, M.J., Wood, K.J., Hamano, K. *et al.* (1993) Cytokines and peripheral tolerance to alloantigen. *Immunological Review* **133**, 5–18.

Dalloul, A.H., Chmouzis, E., Ngo, K. & Fung-Leung, W.-P. (1996a) Adoptively transferred CD4+ lymphocytes from CD8 –/– mice are sufficient to mediate rejection of MHC class II or class I disparate skin grafts. *Journal of Immunology* **156**, 411–414.

Dalloul, A.H., Ngo, K. & Fung-Leing, W.-P. (1996b) CD4-negative cytotoxic T cells with a T cell receptor alpha/beta intermediate expression in CD8-deficient mice. *European Journal of Immunology* **26**, 213–218.

De Waal, R.M.W., Bogman, M.J.J., Mass, C.N. *et al.* (1983) Variable expression of Ia antigens on the vascular endothelium of mouse skin allografts. *Nature* **303**, 426–429.

Del Prete, G.F., De Carli, M., Mastromauro, C. *et al.* (1991)

Purified protein derivative of *Mycobacterium tuberculosis* and excretory-secretory antigen (s) of *Toxocara canis* expand *in vitro* human T cells with stable and opposite (type 1 T helper or type 2 T helper) profile of cytokine production. *Journal of Clinical Investigations* **88**, 346–350.

Dierich, A., Chan, S.H., Benoist, C. & Mathis, D. (1993) Graft rejection by T cells not restricted by conventional major histocompatibility complex molecules. *European Journal of Immunology* **23**, 2725–2728.

Dorling, A. & Lechler, R.I. (1996) The passenger leucocyte, dendritic cell and antigen-presenting cell (APC). In: *Transplantation Biology: Cellular and Molecular Aspects* (eds N.L. Tilney, T.B. Strom, & L.C. Paul). Lippincott-Raven, Philadelphia, USA.

Dunnill, M.S. (1984) Histopathology of rejection in renal transplantation. In: *Kidney Transplantation: Principles and Practice* (ed. P.J. Morris), 2nd edn, pp. 355–382. Grune and Stratton New York.

Dvorak, H.F., Mihm, M.C.J., Dvorak, A.M. *et al.* (1979) Rejection of first-set skin allografts in man—The microvasculature is the critical target of the immune response. *Journal of Experimental Medicine* **150**, 322–337.

Engers, H.D., Glasebrooke, A.L. & Sorenson, G.D. (1982) Allogeneic tumour rejection induced by the intravenous injection of Lyt-2+ cytolytic T lymphocyte clones. *Journal of Experimental Medicine* **156**, 1280–1285.

Fangmann, J., Dalchau, R. & Fabre, J.W. (1992) Rejection of skin allografts by indirect allorecognition of donor class I major histocompatibility complex peptides. *Journal of Experimental Medicine* **175**, 1521–1529.

Farges, O., Morris, P.J. & Dallman, M.J. (1994) Spontaneous acceptance of liver allografts in the rat: analysis of the immune response. *Transplantation* **57**, 171–177.

Farges, O., Morris, P.J. & Dallman, M.J. (1995) Spontaneous acceptance of rat liver allografts is associated with an early down regulation of intragraft IL-4 mRNA expression. *Hepatology* **21**, 767–775.

Fellous, M., Nir, U., Wallach, D. *et al.* (1982) Interferon-dependent induction of mRNA for the major histocompatibility antigens in human fibroblasts and lymphoblastoid cells. *Proceedings of the National Academy of Science (USA)* **79**, 3082–3086.

Florey, H.W. & Jennings, M.A. (1970) In: *General Pathology*. (ed. H.W. Florey), 4th edn, pp. 124–174. Lloyd-Luke, London.

Freeman, G.J., Boussiotis, V.A., Anumanthan, A. *et al.* (1995) B7–1 and B7–2 do not deliver identical costimulatory signals, since B7–2 but not B7–1 preferentially costimulates the initial production of IL-4. *Immunity* **2**, 523–532.

Fuggle, S., McWhinnie, D.L., Chapman, J.R., Taylor, H.M. & Morris, P.J. (1986) Sequential analysis of HLA-Class II

antigen expression in human renal allografts. *Transplantation* **42**, 144–150.

Gajewski, T.F. & Fitch, F.W. (1988) Anti-proliferative effect of IFN-γ in immune regulation I. IFN-γ inhibits the proliferation of TH2 but not TH1 murine helper T lymphocyte clones. *Journal of Immunology* **140**, 4245–4252.

Gajewski, T.F., Schell, S.R., Nau, G. & Fitch, F.W. (1989) Regulation of T cell activation: differences among T-cell subsets. *Immunological Reviews* **111**, 79–110.

Galili, U., Rachmilewitz, E.A., Peleg, A. & Flechner, I. (1984) A unique natural human IgG antibody with anti α-galactosyl specificity. *Journal of Experimental Medicine* **160**, 1519–1531.

Galili, U., Macher, B.A., Buchler, J. & Shohet, S.B. (1985) Human natural anti-a-galactosyl IgG II. The specific recognition of α (1–3) -linked galactosyl residues. *Journal of Experimental Medicine* **162**, 573–582.

Garcia, K.C., Degano, M., Stanfield, R.L. *et al.* (1996) An αβ T cell receptor structure at 2.5A and its orientation in the TCR-MHC complex. *Science* **274**, 209–219.

Germain, R.N. & Margulies, D.H. (1993) The biochemistry and cell biology of antigen processing and presentation. *Annual Review of Immunology* **11**, 403–450.

Gibson, J.M. & Medawar, P.B. (1943) The fate of skin homografts in man. *Journal of Anatomy* **77**, 299–310.

Golding, H. & Singer, A. (1984) Role of accessory cell processing and presentation of shed H-2 alloantigens in allospecific cytotoxic T lymphocyte responses. *Journal of Immunology* **133**, 597–605.

Gorczynski, R.M. (1992) Immunosuppression induced by hepatic portal venous immunization spares reactivity in IL-4 producing T lymphocytes. *Immunology Letters* **33**, 67–78.

Goulmy, E. (1985) Class I restricted human cytotoxic T lymphocytes directed against minor transplantation antigens and their role in organ transplantation. *Progress in Allergy* **36**, 44–72.

Gowans, J.L. (1959) The recirculation of lymphocytes from blood to lymph in the rat. *Journal of Physiology* **146**, 54–68.

Gracie, J.A., Bolton, E.M., Porteous, C. & Bradley, J.A. (1990) T cell requirements for the rejection of renal allografts bearing an isolated class I disparity. *Journal of Experimental Medicine* **172**, 1547–1557.

Grandaliano, G., Gesualdo, L., Ranieri, E. *et al.* (1997) Monocyte chemotactic peptide-1 expression and monocyte infiltration in acute renal transplant rejection. *Transplantation* **63**, 414–420.

Greenfield, A., Scott, D., Pennisi, D. *et al.* (1996) An H-YDb epitope is encoded by a novel mouse Y chromosome gene. *Natural Genetics* **14**, 474–478.

Grey, H.M. & Chestnut, R. (1985) Antigen processing and presentation to T cells. *Immunology Today* **6**, 101–106.

Gurley, K.E., Lowry, R.P. & Clarke-Forbes, R.D. (1983) Immune mechanisms in organ allograft rejection: II. T helper cells, delayed type hypersensitivity and rejection of renal allografts. *Transplantation* **36**, 401–405.

Hall, B.M., Dorsch, S. & Roser, B. (1978) The cellular basis of allograft rejection *in vivo*. *Journal of Experimental Medicine* **148**, 878–889.

Hall, B.M., DeSaxe, I. & Dorsch, S.E. (1983) The cellular basis of allograft rejection *in vivo*: restoration of first set rejection of heart grafts by T helper cells in irradiated rats. *Transplantation* **36**, 700–705.

Halloran, P.F., Broski, A.P., Batiuk, T.D. & Madrenas, J. (1993) The molecular immunology of acute rejection: an overview. *Transplant Immunology* **1**, 3–27.

Harding, F.A., McArthur, J.G., Gross, J.A., Raulet, D.H. & Allison, J.P. (1992) CD28-mediated signalling co-stimulates T cells and prevents induction of anergy in T-cell clones. *Nature* **356**, 607–609.

Hart, D.N. & Fabre, J.W. (1981) Demonstration and characterisation of Ia positive dendritic cells in the interstitial connective tissues of the rat heart and other tissues, but not brain. *Journal of Experimental Medicine* **154**, 347–361.

Haug, C.E., Colvin, R.B., Delmonico, F. & Lea. (1993) A phase I trial of immunosuppression with anti-ICAM-1 (CD54) mAb in renal allograft recipients. *Transplantation* **55**, 766–773.

Hayry, P. & Defendi, V. (1970) Mixed lymphocyte cultures produce effector cells: model *in vitro* for allograft rejection. *Science* **168**, 133–135.

Hayry, P., Mennander, A., Raisanen-Sokolowski, A. *et al.* (1993) Pathophysiology of vascular wall changes in chronic allograft rejection. *Transplantation Reviews* **7**, 1–20.

Heagy, W., Waltenbaugh, C. & Martz, E. (1984) Potent ability of anti-LFA-1 monoclonal antibody to prolong allograft survival. *Transplantation* **37**, 520–523.

Hedrick, S.M., Nielsen, E.A., Kavalar, J., Cohen, D.I. & Davis, M.M. (1984) Sequence relationships between putative T-cell receptor polypetides and immunoglobulins. *Nature* **308**, 153–158.

Henretta, J., Araneda, D., Pittman, K. & Thomas, F. (1995) Marked prolongation of incompatible class I deficient heart allografts: paradoxical effects between primarily and secondarily vascularized allografts. *Transplantation Proceedings* **27**, 1303–1304.

Herberman, R.B., Djeu, J.Y., Kay, H.D. *et al.* (1979) Natural killer cells: characteristics and regulation of activity. *Immunological Reviews* **44**, 43–70.

Hodes, R.J. & Svedmyr, E.A.J. (1970) Specific cytotoxicity of H-2-incompatible mouse lymphocytes following mixed culture *in vitro*. *Transplantation* **9**, 470–477.

Hourmant, M., Bedrossian, J., Durand, D. *et al.* (1996) A randomized multicenter trial comparing leukocyte function-associated antigen-1 monoclonal antibody with rabbit antithymocyte globulin as induction treatment in first kidney transplantations. *Transplantation* **62**, 1565–1570.

Hsieh, C.-S., Heimberger, A.B., Gold, J.S., O'Garra, A. & Murphy, K.M. (1992) Differential regulation of T helper phenotype development by interleukins 4 and 10 in an αβ T-cell-receptor transgenic system. *Proceedings of the National Academy of Sciences (USA)* **89**, 6065–6069.

Hsieh, C.S., Macatonia, S.E., Tripp, C.S. *et al.* (1993) Development of Th1, CD4+ T cells through IL-12 produced by *Listeria*-induced macrophages. *Science* **260**, 547–548.

Hughes, C.C., Savage, C.O. & Pober, J.S. (1990) The endothelial cell as a regulator of T-cell function. *Immunological Reviews* **117**, 85–102.

Hurme, M., Hetherington, C.M., Chandler, P.R. & Simpson, E. (1978a) Cytotoxic T cell responses to H-Y: mapping of the Ir genes. *Journal of Experimental Medicine* **147**, 758–767.

Hurme, M., Chandler, P.R., Hetherington, C.M. & E.S. (1978b) Cytotoxic T cell responses to H-Y: Correlation with the rejection of syngeneic male skin grafts. *Journal of Experimental Medicine* **147**, 768–775.

Imagawa, D.K., Millis, J.M., Olthoff, K.M. *et al.* (1990) The role of tumor necrosis factor in allograft rejection. II Evidence that antibody therapy against tumor necrosis factor-alpha and lymphotoxin enhances cardiac survival in rats. *Transplantation* **50**, 189–193.

Imagawa, D.K., Millis, J.M., Seu, P. *et al.* (1991) The role of tumor necrosis factor in allograft rejection III. Evidence that anti-TNF antibody therapy prolongs allograft survival in rats with acute rejection. *Transplantation* **51**, 57–62.

Ingham-Clark, C.L., Cunningham, A.J., Crane, P.W., Wood, R.F. & Lear, P.A. (1990) Lymphocyte infiltration patterns in rat small-bowel transplants. *Transplantation Proceedings* **22**, 2460.

Iwata, T., Kamei, Y., Esaki, S. *et al.* (1996) Immunosuppression by anti-ICAM-1 and anti-LFA-1 monoclonal antibodies of free and vascularized skin allograft rejection. *Immunobiology* **195**, 160–171.

Janeway, C.A. & Travers, P. (1996) *Immunobiology: The Immune System in Health and Disease*, 2nd edn. Current Biology, UK/Garland Publishing, USA.

Jenkins, M.K. & Schwartz, R.H. (1987) Antigen presentation by chemically modified splenocytes induces antigen-specific T cell unresponsiveness *in vitro* and *in vivo*. *Journal of Experimental Medicine* **165**, 302–319.

Jenkins, M.K., Pardoll, D.M., Mizuguchi, J., Chused, T.M. & Schwartz, R.H. (1987) Molecular events in the induction of a nonresponsive state in interleukin2-producing helper T-lymphocyte clones. *Proceedings of the National Academy of Sciences (USA)* **84**, 5409–5413.

Josien, R., Pannetier, C., Douillard, P. *et al.* (1995) Graft infiltrating T helper cells CD45RC phenotype and TH1/TH2-related cytokines in donor specific transfusion-induced tolerance in adult rats. *Transplantation* 60, 1131–1139.

June, C.H., Ledbetter, J.A., Gillespie, M.M., Lindsten, T. & Thompson, C.B. (1987) T cell proliferation involving the CD28 pathway is associated with cyclosporine-resistant interleukin 2 gene expression. *Molecular Cell Biology* 7, 4472–4478.

Kagi, D., Seiler, P., Pavlovic, J. *et al.* (1995) The roles of perforin- and Fas-dependent cytotoxicity in protection against cytopathic and non-cytopathic viruses. *European Journal of Immunology* 25, 3256–3262.

Kamada, N. & Wight, D.G.D. (1984) Antigen-specific immunosuppression induced by liver transplantation in the rat. *Transplantation* 38, 217–222.

Kamada, N., Davies, H. & Roser, B. (1981) Reversal of transplantation of immunity by liver grafting. *Nature* 292, 840–842.

Karandiker, N., Vanderlugt, C.L., Walunas, T.L., Miller, S.D. & Bluestone, J.A. (1996) CTLA-4: a negative regulator in autoimmune disease. *Journal of Experimental Medicine* 184, 783–788.

Katsura, Y. (1977) Cell-mediated and humoral immune responses in mice. III Dynamic balance between delayed-type hypersensitivity and antibody response. *Immunology* 32, 227–235.

Kauntz, S.L., Williams, M.A., Williams, P.L., Kapros, C. & Dempster, W.J. (1963) Mechanism of rejection of homotransplantated kidneys. *Nature* 199, 257–260.

Kawai, K., Shahinian, A., Mak, T.W. & Ohashi, P.S. (1996) Skin allograft rejection in CD28-deficient mice. *Transplantation* 61, 352–355.

Kelso, A. (1995) Th1 and Th2 subsets: paradigms lost? *Immunology Today* 16, 374–379.

Kim, P.C., Levy, G.A., Koh, I. & Cohen, Z. (1991) Immunologic basis of small intestinal allograft rejection. *Transplantation Proceedings* 23, 830.

Kirby, J.A. (1996) Function of leucocyte adhesion molecules during allograft rejection. In: *Transplantation Biology: Cellular and Molecular Aspects* (eds N.L.Tilney, T.B. Strom & L.C.Paul). Lippincott-Raven, Philadelphia.

Kirkman, R.L., Colvin, R.B., Flye, M.W., Williams, G.M. & Sachs, D.H. (1979) Transplantation in miniature swine. *Transplantation* 28, 24–30.

Kissmeyer-Nielsen, F., Olsen, S., Peterson, V.P. & Fjeldborg, O. (1966) Hyperacute rejection of kidney allografts associated with pre-existing humoral antibodies against donor cells. *Lancet* 2, 662–665.

Klein, J.A.J., Baxevanis, C.N. & Nagy, Z.A. (1981) The traditional and a new version of the mouse H-2 complex. *Nature* 291, 455–460.

Konieczny, B.T., Saleem, S., Lowry, R.P. & Lakkis, F.G.

(1996) Vigorous cardiac allograft rejection in IFN gamma knockout mice. In: *Proceedings of the 15th Annual Meeting of the American Society of Transplant Physicians.* p.170

Kreiger, N.R., Yin, D.-P. & Fathman, C.G. (1996) CD4+ but not CD8+ cells are essential for allorejection. *Journal of Experimental Medicine* 184, 2013.

Kuchroo, V.K., Das, M.P., Brown, J.A. *et al.* (1995) B7.1 and B7.2 costimulatory molecules activate differentially the Th1/Th2 developmental pathways: application to autoimmune disease. *Cell* 80, 707–718.

Kudig, T., Shahinian, A., Kawai, K. *et al.* (1996) Duration of TCR stimulation determines co-stimulatory requirement of T cells. *Immunity* 5, 41–52.

Laden, A.M.K. & Sinclair, R.A. (1971) Thickening of arterial intima in rat cardiac allografts. *American Journal of Pathology* 63, 69–84.

Lafferty, K.J., Bootes, A., Dart, G. & Talmage, D.W. (1976) Effect of organ culture on the survival of thyroid allografts in mice. *Transplantation* 22, 138–149.

Lakkis, F.G., Konieczny, B.T., Saleem, S. *et al.* (1997) Blocking the CD28–B7 T cell costimulation pathway induces long term cardiac allograft acceptance in the absence of IL-4. *Journal of Immunology* 158, 2443–2448.

Lamouse-Smith, E., Clements, V.K. & Ostrand-Rosenberg, S. (1993) Beta 2M –/– knockout mice contain low levels of CD8+ cytotoxic T lymphocyte that mediate specific tumor rejection. *Journal of Immunology* 151, 6283–6290.

Lampert, I.A., Suitters, A.J. & Chisholm, P.M. (1981) Expression of Ia antigen on epidermal keratinocytes in graft-versus-host disease. *Nature* 293, 149–150.

Larsen, C.P., Morris, P.J. & Austyn, J.M. (1990a) Migration of dendritic leucocytes from cardiac allografts into host spleens: a novel pathway for iniation of rejection. *Journal of Experimental Medicine* 171, 307–314.

Larsen, C.P., Steinman, R.M., Witmer-Pack, M. *et al.* (1990b) Migration and maturation of Langerhans cells in skin transplants and explants. *Journal of Experimental Medicine* 172, 1483–1493.

Larsen, C.P., Ritchie, S.C., Hendrix, R. *et al.* (1994) Regulation of immunostimulatory function and costimulatory molecule (B7–1 and B7–2) expression on murine dendritic cells. *Journal of Immunology* 152, 5208–5219.

Larsen, C.P., Alexander, D.Z., Hollenbaugh, D. *et al.* (1996a) CD40–gp39 interactions play a critical role during allograft rejection: suppression of allograft rejection by blockade of the CD40–gp39 pathway. *Transplantation* 61, 4–9.

Larsen, C.P., Elwood, E.T., Alexander, D.Z. *et al.* (1996b) Long term acceptance of skin and cardiac allografts after blocking CD40 and CD28 pathways. *Nature* 381, 434–438.

Lechler, R.I. & Batchelor, J.R. (1982) Restoration of immunogenicity to passenger cell-depleted kidney allografts by the addition of donor strain dendritic cells. *Journal of Experimental Medicine* **155**, 31–41.

Lee, R.S., Grusby, M.J., Glimcher, L.H., Winn, H.J. & Auchincloss, H.J. (1994) Indirect recognition by helper cells can induce donor-specific cytotoxic T lymphocytes *in vivo*. *Journal of Experimental Medicine* **179**, 865–872.

Lee, R.S., Grusby, M.J., Laufer, T.M. *et al.* (1997) CD8+ effector cells responding to residual class I antigens, with help from CD4+ cells stimulated indirectly cause rejection of 'major histocompatibility complex-deficient' skin grafts. *Transplantation* **63**, 1123–1133.

Leibson, P.J. (1995) MHC-recognising receptors: they're not just for T cells anymore. *Immunity* **3**, 5–8.

Lenschow, D.J., Zeng, Y., Thistlethwaite, J.R. *et al.* (1992) Long-term survival of xenogeneic panreatic islet grafts induced by CTLA4Ig. *Science* **257**, 789–792.

Lenschow, D.J., Sperling, A.I., Cooke, M.P. *et al.* (1994) Differential up-regulation of the B7–1 and B7–2 costimulatory molecules after Ig receptor engagement by antigen. *Journal of Immunology* **153**, 1990–1997.

Lenschow, D.J., Herold, K.C., Rhee, L. *et al.* (1996a) CD28/B7 regulation of Th1 and Th2 subsets in the development of autoimmune diabetes. *Immunity* **5**, 285–293.

Lenschow, D.J., Walunas, T.L. & Bluestone, J.A. (1996b) CD28/B7 system of T cell co-stimulation. *Annual Review of Immunology* **14**, 233–258.

Li, X. & Faustman, D. (1993) Use of donor beta 2-microglobulin-deficient transgenic mouse liver cells for isografts, allografts and xenografts. *Transplantation* **55**, 940–946.

Liew, F.Y. & Simpson, E. (1980) Delayed type hypersensitivity to H-Y: characterisation and mapping of Ir genes. *Immunogenetics* **11**, 255–266.

Lindsten, T., June, C.H., Ledbetter, J.A., Stella, G. & Thompson, C.B. (1989) Regulation of lymphokine messenger RNA stability by a surface-mediated T cell activation pathway. *Science* **244**, 339–343.

Linsley, P.S., Greene, J.L., Brady, W. *et al.* (1994) Human B7–1 (CD80) and B7–2 (CD86): bind with similar avidities but distinct kinetics to CD28 and CTLA-4 receptors. *Immunity* **1**, 793–801.

Little, C.C. & Tyzer, E.E. (1916) Further experimental studies on the inheritance of susceptibility to a transplantable tumour carcinoma (JWA) of the Japanese Waltzing mouse. *Journal of Medical Research* **33**, 393–453.

Liu, Z., Braunstein, N.S. & Suciu, F.N. (1992) T cell recognition of allopeptides in context of self MHC. *Journal of Immunology* **148**, 35–48.

Lombardi, G., Sidhu, S., Batchelor, R. & Lechler, R. (1994) Anergic T cells as suppressor cells *in vitro*. *Science* **264**, 1587–1589.

Long, E.O. & Wagtmann, N. (1997) Natural killer cell receptors. *Current Opinion in Immunology* **9**, 344–350.

Loveland, B.E. & McKenzie, I.F.C. (1982) Cells mediating graft rejection in the mouse. *Immunology* **46**, 313–320.

Loveland, B.E., Hogarth, P.M., Ceredig, R. & McKenzie, I.F.C. (1981) Delayed type hypersensitivity and allograft rejection in the mouse: correlation of effector cell phenotype. *Journal of Experimental Medicine* **153**, 1044–1057.

Lowry, R.P., Gurley, K.E. & Clarke-Forbes, R.D. (1983) Immune mechanisms in organ allograft rejection: 1. Delayed type hypersensitivity and lymphocytotoxicity in heart graft rejection. *Transplantation* **36**, 391–401.

Macatonia, S.E., Doherty, T., Knight, S.C. & O'Garra, A. (1993a) Differential effect of IL-10 on dendritic cell-induced T cell proliferation and IFNg production. *Journal of Immunology* **150**, 3755–3765.

Macatonia, S.E., Hsieh, C.-S., O'Garra, A. & Murphy, K.M. (1993b) Dendritic cells and macrophages are required for Th1 development of CD4+ T cells from alpha beta TCR transgenic mice: IL-12 substitution for macrophages to stimulate IFN-gamma production is IFN-gamma-dependent. *International Immunology* **5**, 1119–1128.

Mackay, C.R. (1993) Immunological memory. *Advances in Immunology* **53**, 217–265.

McKnight, A.J., Barclay, A.N. & Mason, D.W. (1991) Molecular cloning of rat interleukin 4 cDNA and anlaysis of the cytokine repertoire of subsets of CD4+ T cells. *European Journal of Immunology* **21**, 1187–1194.

McLean, A.G., Hughes, D., Welsh, K.I. *et al.* (1997) Patterns of graft infiltration and cytokine gene expression during the first 10 days of kidney transplantion. *Transplantation* **63**, 374–380.

Madsen, J.C., Peugh, W.N., Wood, K.J. & Morris, P.J. (1987) The effect of anti-L3T4 monoclonal antibody treatment on first set rejection of murine cardiac allografts. *Transplantation* **44**, 849–852.

Madsen, J.C., Superina, R.A., Wood, K.J. & Morris, P.J. (1988) Induction of immunological unresponsiveness using recipient cells transfected with donor MHC genes. *Nature*, **332**, 161–164.

Malaviya, R., Twesten, N.J., Ross, E.A., Abraham, S.N. & Pfeifer, J.D. (1996) Mast cells process bacterial Ags through a phagocytic route for class I MHC presentation to T cells. *Journal of Immunology* **156**, 1490–1496.

Mandrup-Poulsen, T., Bendtzen, K., Nerup, J. *et al.* (1986) Affinity-purified human interleukin I is cytotoxic to isolated islets of Langerhans. *Diabetologia* **29**, 63–67.

Mandrup-Poulsen, T., Helqvist, S., Molvig, J., Wogensen,

L.D. & Nerup, J. (1989) Cytokines as immune effector molecules in autoimmune endocrine diseases with special reference to insulin-dependent diabetes mellitus. *Autoimmunity* 4, 191–218.

Mannon, R.B., Nataraj, C., Kotzin, B.L. *et al.* (1995) Rejection of kidney allografts by MHC class 1-deficient mice. *Transplantation* 59, 746–755.

Markmann, J.F., Bassiri, H., Desai, N.M. *et al.* (1992) Indefinite survival of MHC class I-deficient murine pancreatic islet allografts. *Transplantation* 54, 1085–1089.

Mason, D.W. & Morris, P.J. (1984) Inhibition of the accumulation, in rat kidney allografts, of specific- but not nonspecific-cytotoxic cells by cyclosporine. *Transplantation* 37, 46–51.

Mason, D.W., Dallman, M.J. & Barclay, A.N. (1981) Graft-versus-host disease induces expression of Ia antigen in rat epidermal cells and gut epithelium. *Nature* 293, 150–151.

Medawar, P.B. (1944) Behaviour and fate of skin autografts and skin homografts in rabbits. *Journal of Anatomy* 78, 176–199.

Medawar, P.B. (1945) A second study of the behaviour and fate of skin homografts in rabbits. *Journal of Anatomy* 79, 157–176.

Mintz, B. & Silvers, W.K. (1967) 'Intrinsic' immunological tolerance in allophenic mice. *Science* 158, 1484–1486.

Mintz, B. & Silvers, W.K. (1970) Histocompatibility antigens on melanoblasts and hair follicle cells. *Transplantation* 9, 497–505.

Mohler, K.M. & Streilein, J.W. (1989) Differential expression of helper versus effector activity in mice rendered neonatally tolerant of class II MHC antigens. *Transplantation* 47, 633–640.

Monaco, J.J. (1992) Major histocompatibility complex-linked transport proteins and antigen processing. *Immunological Research* 11, 125–132.

Monaco, J.J. (1993) Structure and function of genes in the MHC class II region. *Current Opinion in Immunology* 5, 17–20.

Monaco, J.J. (1995) Pathways for the processing and presentation of antigens to T cells. *Journal of Leukocyte Biology* 57, 543–547.

Morikawa, M., Tamatani, T., Miyasaka, M. & Uede, T. (1994) Cardiac allografts in rat recipients with simultaneous use of anti-ICAM-1 and anti-LFA-1 monoclonal antibodies leads to accelerated graft loss. *Immunopharmacology* 28, 171–182.

Morris, P.J. & Ting, A. (1982) Studies of HLA-DR with relevance to renal transplantation. *Immunological Reviews* 66, 103–131.

Morris, R.E. (1991) Rapamycin: FK506's fraternal twin or distant cousin? *Immunology Today* 12, 137–142.

Morris, R.E. (1993) New small molecule immunosuppressants for transplantation: review of essential concepts. *Journal of Heart and Lung Transplantation* 12, S275–S286.

Morton, P.A., Fu, X.-T., Stewart, J.A. *et al.* (1996) Differential effects of CTLA-4 substitutions on the binding of human CD80 (B7–1) and CD86 (B7–2). *Journal of Immunology* 156, 1047–1054.

Mosmann, T.R. & Coffman, R.L. (1989) TH1 and TH2 cells: Different patterns of lymphokine secretion lead to different functional properties. *Annual Review of Immunology* 7, 145–173.

Mosmann, T.R. & Moore, K.W. (1991) The role of IL-10 in crossregulation of TH1 and TH2 responses. *Immunoparasitology Today* 12, A49–A53.

Mosmann, T.R., Cherwinski, H., Bond, M.W., Giedlin, M.A. & Coffman, R.L. (1986) Two types of murine helper T cell clone. 1. Definition according to profiles of lymphokine activities and secreted proteins. *Journal of Immunology* 136, 2348–2357.

Murphy, W.J., Kumar, V. & Bennett, M. (1987a) Acute rejection of murine bone marrow allografts by natural killer cells and T cells. Differences in kinetics and target antigens recognized. *Journal of Experimental Medicine* 166, 1499–1509.

Murphy, W.J., Kumar, V. & Bennett, M. (1987b) Rejection of bone marrow allografts by mice with severe combined immune deficiency (SCID): Evidence that NK cells can mediate the specificity of marrow graft rejection. *Journal of Experimental Medicine* 165, 1212–1217.

Nickerson, P., Steurer, W., Steiger, J. *et al.* (1994) Cytokines and the Th1/Th2 paradigm in transplantation. *Current Opinion in Immunology* 6, 757–764.

Nickerson, P., Zheng, X.-X., Steiger, J. *et al.* (1996) Prolonged islet allograft acceptance in the absence of interleukin 4 expression. *Transplant Immunology* 4, 81–85.

O'Brien, S.J., Roelke, M.E., Marker, L. *et al.* (1985) Genetic basis for species vulnerability in the cheetah. *Science* 227, 1428–1434.

Oppenheim, J., Zacharie, C.O.C., Mukaida, N. & Matsushima, K. (1991) Properties of the proinflammatory supergene 'intercrine' cytokine family. *Annual Review of Immunology* 9, 617–648.

Oppenheim, J.J., Wang, J.M., Chertov, O., Taub, D.D. & Ben-Baruch, A. (1996) The role of chemokines in transplantation. In: *Transplantation Biology: Cellular and Molecular Aspects* (eds N.L. Tilney, T.B. Strom & L.C. Paul), pp. 187–200. Lippincott-Raven, Philadelphia.

Osorio, R.W., Ascher, N.L., Jaenisch, R. *et al.* (1993) Major histocompatibility complex class 1 deficiency prolongs islet allograft survival. *Diabetes* 42, 1520–1527.

Page, C.S., Thompson, C., Yacoub, M. & Rose, M. (1994a)

Human endothelial stimulation of allogeneic T cells via a CTLA-4 independent pathway. *Transplant Immunology* 2, 342–347.

Page, C.S., Holloway, N., Smith, H., Yacoub, M. & Rose, M.L. (1994b) Alloproliferative responses of purified CD4+ and CD8+ T cells to endothelial cells in the absence of contaminating accessory cells. *Transplantation* 57, 1628–1637.

Parham, P., Clayberger, C., Zorn, S.L. *et al.* (1987) Inhibition of alloreactive cytotoxic T lymphocytes by peptides from the OL2 domain of HLA-A2. *Nature* 325, 625–628.

Parish, C. (1972) The relationship between humoral and cell-mediated immunity. *Transplantation Reviews* 13, 35–66.

Parker, W., Bruno, D., Holzknecht, Z.E. & Platt, J.L. (1994) Characterization and affinity isolation of xenoreactive human natural antibodies. *Journal of Immunology* 153, 3791–3803.

Patel, R. & Terasaki, P.I. (1969) Significance of the positive crossmatch test in kidney transplantation. *New England Journal of Medicine* 280, 735–739.

Paul, L.C. & Benediktsson, H. (1993) Chronic transplant rejection: magnitude of the problem and pathogenetic mechanism. *Transplantation Reviews* 7, 96–113.

Paul, L.C., Saito, K., Davidoff, A. & Benediktsson, H. (1996) Growth factor transcripts in rat renal transplants. *American Journal of Kidney Disease* 28, 441–450.

Pearson, T.C., Alexander, D.Z., Winn, K.J. *et al.* (1994) Transplantation tolerance induced by CTLA-4 Ig. *Transplantation* 57, 1701–1706.

Perlmann, P. & Holm, G. (1969) Cytotoxic effects of lymphoid cells *in vitro. Advances in Immunology* 11, 117–193.

Peugh, W.N., Superina, R.A., Wood, K.J. & Morris, P.J. (1986) The role of H-2 and non-H-2 antigens and genes in the rejection of murine cardiac allografts. *Immunogenetics* 23, 30–37.

Pfeiffer, C., Stein, J., Southwood, S. *et al.* (1995) Altered peptide ligands can control CD4 T lymphocyte differentiation *in vivo. Journal of Experimental Medicine* 181, 1569–1574.

Picker, L.J. & Butcher, E.C. (1992) Physiological and molecular mechanisms of lymphocyte homing. *Annual Review of Immunology* 10, 561–591.

Platt, J.L. & Bach, F.H. (1991) The barrier to xenotransplantation. *Transplantation* 52, 937–947.

Platt, J.L., Fischel, R.J., Matas, A.J. *et al.* (1991) Immunopathology of hyperacute xenograft rejection in swine-to-human primate model. *Transplantation* 52, 214–220.

Pober, J.S. & Cotran, R.S. (1991) Immunologic interactions of T lymphocytes with vascular endothelium. *Advances in Immunology* 50, 261–302.

Pober, J.S., Gimbrone, M.A., Jr. Lapierre, L.A. *et al.* (1986) Overlapping patterns of activation of human endothelial cells by interleukin 1, tumour necrosis factor and immune interferon. *Journal of Immunology* 137, 1893–1896.

Porter, K.A., Calne, R.Y. & Zukoski, C.F. (1964) Vascular and other changes in 200 renal homotransplants treated with immunosuppressive drugs. *Laboratory Investigations* 13, 810–824.

Rabinovitch, A., Pukel, C. & Baquerizo, H. (1988) Interleukin-1 inhibits glucose-modulated insulin and glucagon secretion in rat islet monolayer cultures. *Endocrinology* 122, 2393–2398.

Ranger, A.M., Das, M.P., Kuchroo, V.K. & Glimcher, L.H. (1996) B7–2 (CD86) is essential for the development of IL-4 producing cells. *International Immunology* 8 (10), 1549–1560.

Reis e Sousa, C., Stahl, P.D. & Austyn, J.M. (1993) Phagocytosis of antigens by Langerhans cells *in vitro. Journal of Experimental Medicine* 178, 509–519.

Roche, P.A. (1995) HLA-DM: an *in vivo* facilitator of MHC class II peptide loading. *Immunity* 3, 259–262.

Rock, K.L., Barnes, M.C., Germain, R.N. & Benacerraf, B. (1983) The role of Ia molecules in the activation of T lymphocytes. II Ia-restricted recognition of allo-K/D antigens is required for class I MHC-stimulated mixed lymphocyte responses. *Journal of Immunology* 130, 457–462.

Rolstad, B. & Ford, W.L. (1974) Immune responses of rats deficient in thymus-derived lymphocytes to strong transplantation antigens. *Transplantation* 17, 405–415.

Rosenberg, A.S. (1993) The T cell populations mediating rejection of MHC class I disparate skin grafts in mice. *Transplant Immunology* 2, 93–99.

Rosenberg, A.S. & Singer, A. (1992) Cellular basis of skin allograft rejection: an *in vivo* model of immune-mediated tissue destruction. *Annual Review of Immunology* 10, 333–358.

Rosenberg, A.S., Mizuochi, T. & Singer, A. (1986) Analysis of T cell subsets in rejection of K$^b$ mutant skin allograft differing at class I MHC. *Nature* 322, 829–831.

Rosenberg, A.S., Mizuochi, T., Sharrow, S.O. & Singer, A. (1987) Phenotype, specificity and function of T cell subsets and T cell interactions involved in skin allograft rejection. *Journal of Experimental Medicine* 165, 1296–1315.

Rotzschke, O., Falk, K., Faath, S. & Rammensee, H.G. (1991) On the nature of peptides involved in T cell alloreactivity. *Journal of Experimental Medicine* 174, 1059–1071.

Rudd, C.E. (1996) Upstream–downstream: CD28 cosignalling pathways and T cell function. *Immunity* 4, 527–534.

Rudd, C.E., Janssen, O., Cai, Y.-C. *et al.* (1994) Two-step TCRζ/CD3–CD4 and CD28 signalling in T cells: SH2/SH3 domains, protein-tyrosine and lipid kinases. *Immunology Today* 15, 225–234.

Rygaard, J. (1974) Skin grafts in nude mice. *Acta Pathologica Microbiologica Scandinavica* **82**, 93–104.

Saleem, S., Konieczny, B.T., Lowry, R.P., Baddoura, F.K. & Lakkis, F.G. (1996) Acute rejection of vascularized heart allografts in the absence of IFNγ. *Transplantation* **62**, 1908–1911.

Sandrin, M.S., Vaughan, H.A., Dabkrowski, P.L. & McKenzie, I. (1993) Anti-pig IgM antibodies in human serum react predominantly with Gal (α1–3) Gal epitopes. *Proceedings of the National Academy of Sciences (USA)* **90**, 11391–11395.

Schilham, M.W., Fung-Leung, W.P., Rahemtulla, A. *et al.* (1993) Alloreactive cytotoxic T cells can develop and function in mice lacking both CD4 and CD8. *European Journal of Immunology* **23**, 1299–1304.

Schulz, M., Schuurman, H.-J., Joergensen, J. *et al.* (1995) Acute rejection of vascular heart allografts by perforin-deficient mice. *European Journal of Immunology* **25**, 474–480.

Schwartz, R.H. (1990) A cell culture model for T lymphocyte clonal anergy. *Science* **248**, 1349–1356.

Schwartz, R.H. (1997) T cell clonal anergy. *Current Opinion in Immunology* **9**, 351–357.

Scott, D.M., Ehrmann, I.E., Ellis, P.S. *et al.* (1995) Identification of a mouse male-specific transplantation antigen, H-Y. *Nature* **376**, 695–698.

Scott, D.M., Ehrmann, I.E., Ellis, P.S., Chandler, P.R. & Simpson, E. (1997) Why do some females reject males? The molecular basis for male-specific graft rejection. *Journal of Molecular Medicine* **75**, 103–114.

Selvaggi, G., Ricordi, C., Podack, E.R. & Inverardi, L. (1996) The role of the perforin and Fas pathways of cytotoxicity in skin graft rejection. *Transplantation* **62**, 1912–1915.

Sherwood, R.A., Brent, L. & Rayfield, L.S. (1986) Presentation of allo-antigens by host cells. *European Journal of Immunology* **16**, 569–574.

Snider, M.E. & Steinmuller, D. (1987) Non-specific tissue destruction as a consequence of cytotoxic T lymphocyte interaction with antigen-specific target cells. *Transplantation Proceedings* **19**, 421–423.

Sprent, J., Schaeffer, M., Lo, D. & Korngold, R. (1986) Properties of purified T cell subsets II. *In vivo* class I vs class II H-2 differences. *Journal of Experimental Medicine* **163**, 998–1011.

Steiger, J., Nickerson, P.W., Steurer, W., Moscovitch-Lopatin, M. & Strom, T.B. (1995) IL-2 knockout recipient mice reject islet cell allografts. *Journal of Immunology* **155**, 489–498.

Steinman, R.M. (1991) The dendritic cell system and its role in immunogenicity. *Annual Review of Immunology* **9**, 271–296.

Steinman, R.M. & Witmer, M.D. (1978) Lymphoid dendritic cells are potent stimulators of the primary mixed leucocyte reaction in mice. *Proceedings of the National Academy of Sciences (USA)* **75**, 5132–5136.

Steinman, R.M., Gutchinov, B., Witmer, M.D. & Nussenzweig, M. (1983) Dendritic cells are the peripheral stimulators of the primary mixed leukocyte reaction in mice. *Journal of Experimental Medicine* **157**, 613–627.

Strom, T.B., Roy-Chadhury, P., Manfro, R. *et al.* (1996) The Th1/Th2 paradigm and the allograft response. *Current Opinion in Immunology* **8**, 688.

Swain, S.L., Weinberg, A.D., English, M. & Huston, G. (1990) IL-4 directs the development of TH2-like helper effectors. *Journal of Immunology* **145**, 3796–3806.

Swain, S.L., Huston, G., Tonkonogy, S. & Weinberg, A.D. (1991) Transforming growth factor-β and IL-4 cause helper T cell precursors to develop into distinct effector helper cells that differ in lymphokine secretion pattern and cell surface phenotype. *Journal of Immunology* **147**, 2991–3000.

Takeuchi, T., Lowry, R.P. & Konieczny, B. (1992) Heart allografts in murine systems. *Transplantation* **53**, 1281–1294.

Thompson, C.B., Lindsten, T., Ledbetter, J.A. *et al.* (1989) CD28 activation pathway regulates the production of multiple T-cell-derived lymphokines/cytokines. *Proceedings of the National Academy of Sciences (USA)* **86**, 1333–1337.

Tilney, N.L., Strom, T.B., MacPherson, S.G. & Carpenter, C.B. (1975) Surface properties and functional characteristics of filtrating cells harvested from acutely rejecting cardiac allografts in inbred rats. *Transplantation* **20**, 323–330.

Tilney, N.L., Kupiec-Weglinski, J.W., Heidecke, C.D., Lear, P.A. & Strom, T.B. (1984) Mechanisms of rejection and prolongation of vascularised organ allografts. *Immunological Reviews* **77**, 185–216.

Ting, A. & Morris, P.J. (1977) Renal transplantation and B cell crossmatches with autoantibodies and alloantibodies. *Lancet* **2**, 1095–1097.

Ting, A. & Morris, P.J. (1978) Reactivity of autolymphocytotoxic antibodies from dialysis patients with lymphocytes from chronic lymphocytic leukemia (CLL) patients. *Transplantation* **25**, 31–33.

Ting, A. & Morris, P.J. (1981) Positive-crossmatch transplants—safe or not. *Transplantation Proceedings* **13**, 1544–1546.

Tivol, E.A., Borriello, F., Schweitzer, A.N. *et al.* (1995) Loss of CTLA-4 leads to massive lymphoproliferation and fatal multiorgan tissue destruction, revealing a critical negative regulatory role of CTLA-4. *Immunity* **3**, 541–547.

Tono, T., Moden, M., Yoshizaki, K. *et al.* (1992) Biliary interleukin 6 levels as indicators of hepatic allograft rejection in rats. *Transplantation* **53**, 1195–1201.

Toogood, G.J., Rankin, A.M., Tam, P.K.H., Morris, P.J. & Dallman, M.J. (1997) The immune response following small bowel transplantation II: a very early cytokine response in the gut associated lymphoid tissue. *Transplantation* **63**, 1118–1123.

Turka, L.A., Linsley, P.S., Lin, H. *et al.* (1992) T-cell activation by the CD28 ligand B7 is required for cardiac allograft rejection *in vivo. Proceedings of the National Academy of Sciences (USA)* **89**, 1102–1105.

Tyler, J.D., Galli, S.J., Snider, M.E., Dvorak, A.M. & Steinmuller, D. (1984) Cloned LyT-2+ cytolytic T lymphocytes destroy allogeneic tissue *in vivo. Journal of Experimental Medicine* **159**, 234–243.

Van der Merwe, P.A., Bodian, D.L., Daenke, S., Linsley, P. & Davis, S.J. (1997) CD80 (B7–1) binds both CD28 and CTLA-4 with a low affinity and very fast kinetics. *Journal of Experimental Medicine* **185**, 393–403.

Walsh, C.M., Hayashi, F., Saffron, D.C. *et al.* (1996) Cell-mediated cytotoxicity results from, but may not be crtical for, primary allograft rejection. *Journal of Immunology* **156**, 1436–1441.

Wang, W., Meadows, L.R., den Haan, J.M.M. *et al.* (1995) Human H-Y: a male-specific histocompatibility antigen derived from the SMCY protein. *Science* **269**, 1588–1590.

Weiss, A., Imboden, J., Hardy, K. *et al.* (1986) The role of the T3/antigen receptor complex in T-cell activation. *Annual Review of Immunology* **4**, 593–619.

Williams, G.M., Hume, D.M., Hudson, R.P.J. *et al.* (1968) 'Hyperacute' renal homograft rejection in man. *New England Journal of Medicine* **279**, 611–618.

Wolf, B.A., Hughes, J.H., Florholmen, J., Turk, J. & McDaniel, M.L. (1989) Interleukin-1 inhibits glucose-induced Ca2+ uptake by islets of Langerhans. *FEBS Letters* **248**, 35.

Wong, G.H.W., Clark-Lewis, I., Harris, A.W. & Schrader, J.W. (1984) Effect of cloned interferon-γ on expression of H-2 and Ia antigens on cell lines of hemopoietic, lymphoid, epithelial, fibroblastic and neuronal origin. *European Journal of Immunology* **14**, 52–56.

Yang, H., Issekutz, T.B. & Wright, J.R. Jr. (1995) Prolongation of rat islet allograft survival by treatment with monoclonal antibodies against VLA-4 and LFA-1. *Transplantation* **60**, 71–76.

Yilmaz, S., Taskninen, E., Paavonen, T., Mennander, A. & Hayry, P. (1992) Chronic rejection of rat renal allograft. I Histological differentiation between chronic rejection and cyclosporin nephrotoxicity. *Transplant International* **5**, 85–95.

Zimmerman, C., Seiler, P., Lane, P. & Zinkernagel, R.M. (1997) Antiviral immune responses in CTLA4 transgenic mice. *Journal of Virology* **71**, 1802–1807.

# Chapter 2/Major and minor histocompatibility antigens

SHERYL L. FULLER-ESPIE, ELIZABETH SIMPSON &
ROBERT I. LECHLER

## Function of MHC molecules

### Discovery of histocompatibility antigens

Tissues transplanted from an unrelated donor are usually destroyed by the recipient's immune system because the donor cells in the tissue express cell surface molecules that differ from those present in the recipient. The immunological compatibility between donor and recipient is dictated by these cell surface molecules, some of which are encoded in the major histocompatibility complex (MHC). MHC antigens usually elicit rapid graft rejection while the more numerous minor histocompatibility antigens, which are not encoded in the MHC, tend to stimulate a slower rejection response.

Although MHC molecules were discovered in the context of transplantation, and were initially referred to as transplantation antigens, their influence in allograft rejection merely reflects the central role that they have in the presentation of antigens to T lymphocytes. The earliest observation of discrimination between self and foreign tissues was reported using skin and tumour grafts of mice in the pioneering studies of Gorer *et al.*

The major stimulus to rejection of non-self tissues was mapped to the MHC region, known as H-2 in mice, on chromosome 17. Characterization of the cell surface molecules encoded in the MHC and responsible for graft rejection has been aided by the use of alloantibodies (produced in inbred strains of mice immunized with cells from MHC-disparate strains), protein chemistry and molecular biological techniques. Similar techniques have also been employed to characterize the human MHC, known as the human leucocyte antigen (HLA) system, which is encoded on the short arm of chromosome 6 at 6p21.3.

The MHC consists of three major linked gene clusters in both the HLA system in humans and the H-2 region in the mouse. These include the following.

1 *The class I region.* This encodes three classical MHC class I molecules (termed H-2K, H-2D and H-2L in the mouse, and HLA-A, B and C in humans). Class I molecules are expressed on most nucleated cells. Other non-classical class I genes in the mouse map telometric to the H-2K, D and L loci are known as Qa2, 3 and Tla. An equivalent cluster of genes is also present in man. Three additional non-classical class I molecules, HLA-E, F and G are encoded in the HLA class I region and have distinct patterns of tissue expression. The products of these loci, however, do not provoke strong alloimmune responses.

2 *The class II region.* This encodes MHC class II molecules, including H-2A and H-2E in the mouse and HLA-DR, DQ and DP in humans. Class II molecules have a much more limited distribution and are only expressed constitutively on B cells, macrophages, dendritic cells, thymic epithelial cells and some vascular endothelial cells. A cluster of genes whose products are involved in the processing and presentation of antigens with MHC molecules are also found within the class II region.

3 *The class III region.* This comprises a diverse collection of loci including the genes encoding complement components (C4, C2 and factor B), the cytochrome P450 enzyme steroid 21-hydroxylase, tumour necrosis factors (TNF) α and β, and the 70 kilodalton (kDa) heat shock proteins. A large number of other genes have been discovered in this region, although their functions have yet to be defined.

## T cell recognition of antigen is MHC-restricted

The central part played by MHC molecules in T cell immunity reflects the manner in which T cells recognize antigens. Unlike B cells that recognize antigen in its native form, T cells are specific for short peptide fragments, derived by proteolytic cleavage of intact antigens, physically complexed to an MHC molecule (Bevan 1975a). Thus, the T cell's antigen receptor (TCR) has dual specificity for a peptide fragment of an antigen and for the MHC molecule to which it is bound, as shown schematically in Fig. 2.1. The derivation of peptide fragments from an intact protein antigen occurs within the cell, and is discussed in detail in a later section.

T cell receptors are two-chain heterodimers encoded by genes which, like Ig molecules (Yancopoulos *et al.* 1986), rearrange to give rise to a multitude of specificities. The TCR exists in two forms. The large majority (~95% in mice and humans) of peripheral T cells express a TCR composed of a disulphide-linked αβ heterodimer non-covalently associated with the CD3 complex. A minority (~5%) of T cells, often associated

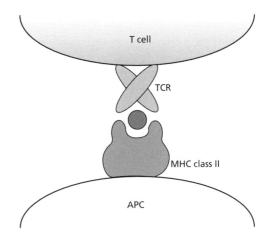

**Fig. 2.1** Schematic diagram of the tri-molecular complex. The three elements of the complex that are at the heart of T cell recognition are shown, namely the dimeric T cell receptor, an MHC molecule and a bound peptide. The simultaneous interaction of the T cell's receptor with the MHC molecule and with the MHC-bound peptide is illustrated.

with epithelial tissues, express a γδ heterodimer (Takagaki *et al.* 1989) which is also associated with CD3. The γδ TCR-expressing subset of T cells are thought to provide a first line of defence at epithelial and mucosal surfaces, possibly involving the recognition of conserved microbial antigens, although the details of their specificity and function remain obscure. A great deal more is known about the specificity and functions of αβ TCR-bearing T cells that are restricted by MHC class I and II molecules. The remainder of this discussion will therefore focus on TCR αβ T cells in antigen- and allo-specific responses.

Mature T cells can be divided into two non-overlapping populations, according to their surface expression of CD4 or CD8 molecules. The CD4/CD8 phenotype of a T cell correlates closely with the class of MHC molecule by which it is restricted. Almost invariably CD4+ T cells are MHC class II-restricted and CD8+ T cells are MHC class I-restricted. There is a loose correlation between CD4/8 phenotype and T cell function in that most CD4+ T cells function as cytokine-secreting helper cells, and most CD8+ T cells as cytotoxic effector cells, However, CD4+ T cells can have cytotoxic function (Shinohara *et al.* 1986) and some CD8+ T cells can act as helper cells (Swain 1981).

## Generation of T cell receptor diversity

The T cell repertoire is required to be enormously diverse in order to be capable of dealing with the myriad of different antigens that are encountered during a normal lifespan. This diversity is generated, as for immunoglobulins, by recombining single variable, diversity and junctional elements from a pool of germline segments (combinatorial diversity). This diversity is greatly amplified by the random loss of small numbers of nucleotides from the recombining ends of these segments, and by the simultaneous random addition of nucleotides at these junctions (junctional diversity). This gives rise to variable domains with three hypervariable regions when the molecule folds into an immunoglobulin-like domain. The predicted model of how the TCR interacts with peptide:MHC complexes has been reviewed by Davis and Bjorkman (1988) and subsequently confirmed by

Garcia *et al.* (1996) and Garboczi *et al.* (1996), who resolved the αβ TCR crystal structure and the TCR/class I crystal structure associated with peptide (see p. 36).

## Structure of MHC products

Pivotal to our understanding of the function of MHC gene products in immune responses is a detailed knowledge of their structure. Hypothetical models of MHC molecular structure had been developed over the decade following the definition of the primary sequence of MHC genes and proteins by nucleotide and amino acid sequencing. However, the next major landmark arose in 1987 when the three-dimensional structure of an HLA class I molecule was solved by crystallography. Subsequently, the structures of several HLA and H-2 (mouse) class I and II molecules have been solved by the same approach. This has provided numerous insights into MHC-restricted recognition of antigen by T cells, and into the nature of alloimmune responses.

### MHC class I structure

HLA class I molecules are heterodimeric membrane-bound glycoproteins consisting of an MHC-encoded 46 kDa heavy chain and a non-covalently associated, non-MHC-encoded 12 kDa invariant light chain called β2 microglobulin (β2m). The β2m protein is encoded on chromosome 15q21 and is found in substantial levels in normal serum. The heavy chain is composed of extracellular α1, α2 and α3 domains followed by transmembrane and cytoplasmic regions, each encoded by separate exons (Sodoyer *et al.* 1984; Strachan *et al.* 1984). The α1 domain contains a single N-linked glycan and the α2 and α3 domains are stabilized by intradomain disulphide bonds between cysteine residues. There is extensive allelic polymorphism of the HLA-A, B and C genes that is almost entirely located in the α1 and α2 domains (Parham *et al.* 1988), the functional significance of which became clear when the three-dimensional structure of the HLA-A2.1 molecule was first solved (Bjorkman *et al.* 1987a,b).

X-ray diffraction techniques have been applied in

order to obtain the crystal structure of several class I molecules. The first three to be subjected to this analysis were HLA-A2.1, HLA-Aw68.1 and HLA-B27 (Bjorkman *et al.* 1987a,b; Garrett *et al.* 1989; Madden *et al.* 1991). These data have provided a detailed three-dimensional view of class I molecules confirming a four-domain extracellular structure consisting of membrane-proximal α3 and β2m domains and membrane-distal α1 and α2 domains. The α3 and β2m domains resemble classical immunoglobulin-like domains. In contrast, the α1 and α2 domains have a unique structure that is elegantly tailored to the function of the molecule. Each consists of four antiparallel β-pleated strands, which are connected at their C-terminal ends to an α-helix that has an arched configuration. The α1 and α2 domains are arranged symmetrically, giving rise to a platform of eight β-strands which support the two α-helices. This arrangement gives rise to a peptide-binding cleft, ~25 angstroms long and 10 angstroms wide, the floor of which is formed by the β-pleated strands and the walls by the α-helices of the α1 and α2 domains.

It was observed in the course of the crystallographic studies that the cleft formed by the α1 and α2 domains contained electron-dense material which could not be attributed to amino acid residues encoded by the HLA molecule itself. This material was composed of heterogeneous peptide fragments associated with the cleft which copurified with class I during crystallization, and represented naturally processed peptides derived from the array of proteins in the host cell. A computer-generated model of the structure of an MHC class I molecule occupied by a viral peptide is shown in Plate 2.1 (facing p. 342).

The nature of a β-pleated sheet means that the side chains of alternate amino acids in the floor of the peptide-binding groove point up and are likely to make contact with bound peptide. Similarly, the side chains of amino acid residues on the inner walls of the α-helices are likely to contact bound peptide. In contrast, residues of the α-helices that point up are candidates for TCR contact. Importantly, almost all of the polymorphic residues in class I are localized in the peptide-binding groove on the β-strands comprising the floor, the sides of the α-helices, and the upper, TCR-contacting face, of the α-helices. Sixteen of 20 of the most variable positions are found in this region (Bjorkman & Parham 1990). Site-directed mutagenesis studies involving a number of these polymorphic positions have been shown to affect T cell responses (McMichael *et al.* 1988; Santos-Aguado *et al.* 1989).

When comparing the outcome of the three crystallographic studies on HLA-A2, Aw68 and B27 molecules several noteworthy features became apparent. Although all three molecules share a very similar overall structure, differences are seen in the shape of the peptide-binding groove, particularly the conformation of 'pockets', spaces in the floor of the peptide-binding groove that are lined by polymorphic residues and accommodate the side chains of bound peptide. For instance, in HLA-Aw68, a deep negatively charged pocket is formed by the presence of an aspartic acid at position 74, compared to histidine in HLA-A2. This pocket in Aw68 accommodates the side chains of positively charged amino acids, as seen in the crystallography data. In HLA-B27, a cysteine at position 67 resides near the entry of pocket 45 (Taurog & El-Zaatari 1988). Access to pocket 45 can be blocked by amino acids with large side chains linked via a disulphide bond to cysteine 67, affecting drastically the shape of the groove in HLA-B27. These high-definition X-ray crystallographic studies help to explain how class I molecules that are closely related can bind to discrete sets of peptides (see p. 39).

## MHC class II structure

HLA class II molecules are membrane-bound heterodimeric glycoproteins consisting of 35 kDa (α) and 27 kDa (β) chains (Cresswell & Geier 1975) that are both encoded by genes in the class II region of the MHC. The non-covalently associated α and β chains each contain two extracellular domains (α1, α2 and β1, β2), a transmembrane region and a cytoplasmic domain. The β chain contains two intradomain disulphide bonds, one in the β1 and one in the β2 domain, while the α chain contains only one, in the α2 domain. The disulphide bond residing in the β1 domain of class II corresponds to that found in the α2 domain of class I. Similarly the glycosylation site found in the α1 domain of class II parallels the glycosylation site in the $\alpha 1$ domain of class I.

Based on these, and other, structural similarities, and despite the little overall sequence homology between class I and class II, Brown *et al.* (1988) proposed that the structures of the class II amino-terminal $\alpha 1$ and $\beta 1$ domains would be analogous to the class I $\alpha 1$ and $\alpha 2$ domains. Their hypothetical model was built on sequence alignments and comparisons of 26 class I and 54 class II amino acid sequences. Common patterns of variability were identified; highly polymorphic residues appeared every third or fourth position in the $\alpha$-helices corresponding (according to the model) to positions facing into the peptide-binding groove of class II. Taken together with the observed alternate spacing of polymorphic residues in the N-terminal halves of the $\alpha 1$ and $\beta 1$ domains of class II, corresponding to the sequences in the floor of the peptide-binding groove of class I, they suggested that the class II structure would be analogous to class I. Mutagenesis studies (Ronchese *et al.* 1987; Kwok *et al.* 1990; Lombardi *et al.* 1991b) and monoclonal antibody epitope mapping studies (Mellins *et al.* 1990a) supported the hypothetical model. These predictions were confirmed by the subsequent crystallographic analysis of numerous human and mouse class II molecules (Brown *et al.* 1993; Stern *et al.* 1994; Ghosh *et al.* 1995; Fremont *et al.* 1996, 1998; Jardetzky *et al.* 1996; Dessen *et al.* 1997; Scott *et al.* 1998a,b).

An additional level of individual variation in the expressed array of cell surface class II molecules is created by variations in $\alpha\beta$ chain paring, particularly in MHC heterozygotes. Several transfection studies have demonstrated that the pairing of $\alpha$ and $\beta$ chains within the isotypes that have polymorphic $\alpha$ and $\beta$ chains, namely H-2A in mouse, HLA-DQ and DP in humans, is under allelic control. Braunstein and Germain (1987) using three alleles of Ab and Aa, showed that the *cis*, haplotype-matched pairs were always expressed with the highest efficiency, but the expression of haplotype-mismatched $\alpha\beta$ dimers showed substantial variation that was under allelic control. For example, cotransfection of Aa$^k$ with Ab$^b$ and Aa$^b$ with Ab$^k$ gave rise to high levels of the corresponding haplotype-mismatched dimers. In contrast, no surface expression of $A_\alpha{}^k A_\beta{}^d$

could be detected after transfection of the appropriate genes.

These results correlate with the findings of Beck *et al.* (1982), who demonstrated several years earlier that some of their alloreactive mouse T cell clones obtained from a mixed-lymphocyte reaction (MLR) of A/J anti-(C57/BL6×A/J)F$_1$ had specificity for two hybrid H-2A molecules, namely $A_\alpha{}^k A_\beta{}^b$ and $A_\alpha{}^b A_\beta{}^k$. They showed both functionally and biochemically that these hybrid F$_1$ H-2A molecules existed on (C57/BL6×A/J)F$_1$ splenocytes and that both pairs were recognized specifically by T cells. Zamvil *et al.* (1985) also demonstrated that haplotype-mismatched pairs exist in mice. Ten out of 16 T cell clones isolated from (PL/J× SJL/J)F$_1$ mice sensitized to rat myelin basic protein responded to the amino-terminal peptide in the context of the restriction element $A_\alpha{}^s A_\beta{}^u$.

Transfection studies involving human class II genes carried out by Kwok *et al.* (1993) demonstrated that DQ$_\alpha$ and DQ$_\beta$ heterodimer surface expression appears to follow similar rules in that not all DQ$_\alpha$ and DQ$_\beta$ dimers are expressed with equal efficiency at the cell surface. There appear to be allele-specific constraints on DQ heterodimer formation, limiting the possible haplotype-mismatched combinations. For instance, the DQ1β chain, encoded by DQB1*0101 (WHO nomenclature described on p. 47), failed to form stable cell surface dimers with either DQA1*0201-, *0301-, *0401- or *0501-encoded gene products. Also DQ3.2β chains (encoded by DQB1*0302) did not form stable dimers with DQA1*0101-, *0102- or *0103-encoded gene products. The formation of haplotype-mismatched pairs is illustrated schematically in Fig. 2.2.

During the course of the transfection studies using mouse class II genes a surprising result was obtained in that expression of an isotype-mismatched dimer was detected, namely $E_\alpha A_\beta{}^d$. Subsequent studies showed that expression of isotype-mismatched dimers was also under allelic control in that, although $E_\alpha A_\beta{}^d$ was readily expressed, no surface expression of $E_\alpha$ with $A_\beta{}^k$ or $A_\beta{}^b$ could be detected (Germain & Quill 1986). Comparison of the expression of $E_\alpha A_\beta{}^d$ with $A_\alpha{}^d A_\beta{}^d$ suggested that the isotype-matched dimer was assembled and expressed 20-fold more efficiently. None the

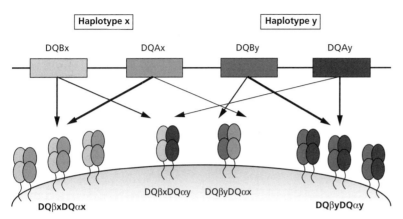

**Fig. 2.2** Haplotype-mismatched MHC class II heterodimers. The four possible DQ heterodimers that can be expressed at the cell surface of a DQ heterozygous class II-positive cell are represented. As indicated by the bold arrows, and the larger number of class II dimers, *cis* pairing is favoured over *trans* pairing. As discussed in the text, the extent of haplotype-mismatched assembly and expression is determined by the class II alleles carried by the two haplotypes.

less, the $E_\alpha A_\beta{}^d$ heterodimer was detected on splenocytes from a mouse strain defective in $E_\beta$ expression (Anderson & David 1989) and in mice expressing an $E_\alpha$ transgene (Anderson & David 1989; Matsunaga *et al.* 1990), where they served as restriction elements for both allo- (Kimoto *et al.* 1989) and antigen- (Matsunaga *et al.* 1990) specific T cell responses. Most strikingly, in normal H-2$^d$ mice Ruberti *et al.* (1992) demonstrated that the $E_\alpha A_\beta{}^d$ mixed-isotype heterodimer served as a major restriction element for a peptide of sperm whale myoglobin.

Naturally occurring expression of the isotype-mismatched pair $DR_\alpha DQ_\beta$ (the human homologue of $E_\alpha A_\beta$) was detected in human B cell lines using immunoprecipitation and isoelectric focusing on two-dimensional polyacrylamide gels (Lotteau *et al.* 1987). Kwok *et al.* (1993), while examining the limited surface heterodimer formation among allelic $DQ_\alpha$ and $DQ_\beta$ chains, sought to determine whether $DQ_\beta$ allelic variation affected the efficiency of dimer formation with $DR_\alpha$ chains in transfected cells. Cells were cotransfected with cDNAs encoding DRA and DQB1*0501 (DQ1$_\beta$) or DRA and DQB1*0302 (DQ3.2$_\beta$) and, although similar levels of mRNA transcripts for DQ1$_\beta$ and DQ3.2$_\beta$ were detected by Northern blot analysis, only the $DR_\alpha DQ1_\beta$ heterodimer could be detected by cell surface immunofluorescence. Whether or not $DR_\alpha DQ_\beta$ mixed-isotype pairs are expressed naturally at the cell surface at levels that

influence the T cell repertoire has yet to be determined. However, it is clear from the above studies that haplotype- and isotype-mismatched class II dimers can act as restriction elements for T cell recognition, and thus may contribute to the alloimmune response following transplantation.

## Peptide as an integral part of MHC class I and II molecular structure

### ROLE OF PEPTIDE IN STABILIZING MHC CLASS I MOLECULES

The interaction of peptide with MHC class I is a prerequisite for efficient folding of the heavy chain, binding to β2m and subsequent transport of stable class I–peptide complexes to the cell surface. Many of these conclusions have been based on studies of mutant cell lines that are defective in peptide loading of class I molecules (Townsend *et al.* 1989; Ljunggren *et al.* 1990; Cerendolo *et al.* 1991; Elliott *et al.* 1992). One such cell line is RMA-S, a murine tumour cell line that escapes immunological recognition across a minor histocompatibility barrier *in vivo* and expressses only 5% of normal levels of H-2D$^b$, K$^b$ and β2m at the cell surface. Townsend *et al.* (1989) noted that cell surface expression of H-2D$^b$ and H-2K$^b$ increased substantially when RMA-S was cultured in the presence of peptides known to bind to these class I molecules. This

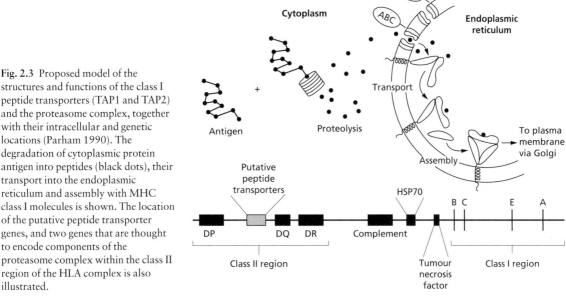

**Fig. 2.3** Proposed model of the structures and functions of the class I peptide transporters (TAP1 and TAP2) and the proteasome complex, together with their intracellular and genetic locations (Parham 1990). The degradation of cytoplasmic protein antigen into peptides (black dots), their transport into the endoplasmic reticulum and assembly with MHC class I molecules is shown. The location of the putative peptide transporter genes, and two genes that are thought to encode components of the proteasome complex within the class II region of the HLA complex is also illustrated.

is the consequence of peptide binding to empty D$^b$ or K$^b$ molecules as they reach the surface of the cell. In the absence of bound peptide the empty class I molecules are highly unstable and are either degraded or internalized very rapidly. Added peptide stabilizes these empty molecules and renders them serologically detectable. If RMA-S is cultured at 26°C in the absence of peptide, cell surface class I expression increases similarly owing to the increased stability of 'empty' class I molecules at this lower temperature. Returning the cells to 37°C results in a rapid decrease in cell surface expression of class I. These experiments demonstrate the dependence of class I molecules on peptides for efficient assembly and transport. Peptide-free, or empty, complexes can form and reach the cell surface, albeit with a much reduced efficiency, but they are highly unstable.

The mutant phenotype of RMA-S was subsequently shown to be caused by a defect in TAP2, one of the genes responsible for transport of peptides from the cytosol of the cell into the endoplasmic reticulum (ER), thereby limiting the access of peptides to class I molecules. TAP1 and TAP2 gene products, which assemble

to form a heterodimeric complex (Kelly *et al.* 1992), are required for efficient class I expression on the cell surface and are involved in transporting peptides from the cytosol into the endoplasmic reticulum (ER) for association with class I molecules (Howard 1995; Lehner & Cresswell 1996). Complementation studies have demonstrated the critical importance of both of these genes in class I assembly and antigen presentation by transfecting various class I-deficient cell lines with the TAP genes, including the murine RMA-S (Powis *et al.* 1991) and the human 134 and BM36.1 cell lines (Attaya *et al.* 1992; Kelly *et al.* 1992; Spies *et al.* 1992).

The source of cytosolic peptides available for transport by TAP1 and TAP2 is believed to be generated through the associated proteolytic activity of the large multifunctional proteases 2 and 7 (LMP2 and LMP7), which make up ATP-dependent proteasomes in the cytosol (Neefjes & Momburg 1993; Rock *et al.* 1994; Kuckelhorn *et al.* 1995). Two subunits of the proteasome, LMP2 and 7, are encoded adjacent to the TAP genes within the MHC class II region. The roles of the proteasome and TAP complexes are illustrated in Fig. 2.3.

The influence of peptide binding on the conformation and stability of MHC class II molecules has also been illustrated by the study of mutant cell lines. Mellins *et al.* (1990b) described a series of mutant human B cell lines which are unable to present intact exogenous antigens, but are fully able to present synthetic peptides that require no further processing. The HLA-DR molecules expressed by these mutant cells are conformationally altered, as detected by loss of an antibody-defined epitope, and are highly unstable such that they dissociate in non-denaturing SDS gels. Parallel studies of another cell line, T2, which has a large deletion in the HLA class II region, have mapped the genetic defect to this chromosomal region, in that transfection of T2 cells with HLA-DR genes gives rise to cell surface DR molecules with the same features as those seen in the mutant B cell lines. The gene locus responsible for this phenotype was identified as HLA-DM, a locus encoding an α chain and a β chain (HLA-DMA and HLA-DMB, respectively) which loosely resemble other class II molecules (Denzin *et al.* 1994; Morris *et al.* 1994). They are not, however, expressed at the cell surface. HLA-DM catalyses the loading of peptides on to class II molecules and thus aids in their stabilization (Fling *et al.* 1994; Weber *et al.* 1996).

## The role of CD4 and CD8 in T cell development and activation

A trimolecular complex involving the association of the TCR with MHC and its bound, processed peptide constitutes the key antigen-specific, cognate interaction in the generation of an immune response. The crystal structure of the αβ TCR heterodimer and TCR complexed to class I MHC plus peptide was reported by Garcia *et al.* (1996) and Garboczi *et al.* (1996), allowing the first detailed analyses of how TCR interacts with MHC. Garcia *et al.* (1996) discussed the importance of structural plasticity in the interaction between TCR, MHC and peptide (TCR-pMHC) and the accommodation of a variety of different peptide antigens by the same TCR. They suggested that this plastic-

ity enables the TCR recognition repertoire to interact with multiple peptide ligands bound by MHC molecules. Teng *et al.* (1998) proposed that the TCR utilizes a general docking mode whereby Vα and Vβ of the TCR interact with the α2 and α1 domains, respectively, of MHC class I. In the absence of structural data for class II, inferences for docking orientation are drawn from studies involving variant peptide immunization of single-chain transgenic mice (Jorgensen *et al.* 1992; Sant-Angelo *et al.* 1996). A similar docking orientation has been suggested with TCR Vα and Vβ overlying the helices of MHC class II β1 and α1 domains, respectively. Aggregates of TCR-pMHC may play an important part in signal transduction. Several studies have proposed that dimerization or oligomerization of TCR-pMHC complexes may contribute to the extent and nature of T cell activation upon encounter with antigenic peptide (Brown *et al.* 1993; Fields *et al.* 1995; Reich *et al.* 1997).

In addition to TCR-pMHC associations, there exist numerous non-antigen-specific, non-cognate cell surface interactions which contribute to and help to focus specific immune responses. Included in these non-cognate interactions are the molecules involved in intercellular adhesion, e.g. the ligand–receptor complexes of LFA-3 with CD2 and LFA-1 with ICAM-1, and the 'coreceptor' molecules CD8 and CD4, whose ligands are the MHC class I and II molecules themselves, respectively (Fig. 2.4).

The major role of the CD4 and CD8 molecules is in the transduction of signals across the T cell membrane, in cooperation with signals transduced via the TCR-associated CD3 complex. Because of this cooperativity these molecules are sometimes referred to as coreceptors (Janeway 1989). Consistent with this role is the fact that CD4 and CD8 are physically associated with the TCR in the T cell membrane (Saizawa *et al.* 1987). The cytoplasmic tails of both of these coreceptor molecules are associated with a tyrosine kinase, p56[lck] (Veillette *et al.* 1988). The consequence of CD4 or CD8 ligation by MHC molecules at the cell surface is activation of this kinase, which, in turn, phosphorylates a variety of substrates, including the ζ chain of the CD3 complex.

Several groups have implicated the importance of the

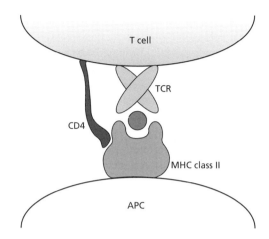

**Fig. 2.4** Schematic representation of the quaternary molecular complex. The CD4 T cell coreceptor is shown interacting with the same MHC class II molecule as the T cell's antigen receptor, at a site distant from the peptide-binding and TCR contact sites on the MHC molecule.

CD4/CD8 coreceptor function in the critical events involved in intrathymic T cell development (Kisielow *et al.* 1988; MacDonald *et al.* 1988; Sha *et al.* 1988). The specificity of the TCR for MHC class I or II ligands in association with CD8 or CD4, respectively, appears to result from these molecules serving as coreceptors during T cell development. T cells are positively selected for recognition of self MHC class I or II by the association of TCR with one of these MHC restriction elements on thymic cortical epithelial cells when T cells are still expressing both CD4 and CD8, i.e. at the double positive stage of thymocyte differentiation. Depending on which MHC molecule the TCR is specific for, the coreceptor associated with that MHC molecule (CD4 with class II, CD8 with class I) delivers a signal resulting in loss of expression of the coreceptor not involved in the TCR interaction. The T cell consequently matures to a single positive phenotype, i.e. CD4+CD8– or CD4–CD8+. Hence, it appears to be the specificity of the TCR for self MHC during positive selection that determines coreceptor expression. This helps to explain the strong association of MHC class I or II restriction of the TCR with CD8 or CD4 expression, respectively.

Riberdy *et al.* (1998) demonstrated that T cell repertoire formation was dramatically altered when CD4 interaction with murine class II was inhibited. They introduced two mutations in the β2 domain of I-Ab at positions 137 and 142 which disrupted class II–CD4 interaction *in vivo* (see below). The effect of this was the substantial loss of CD4+ T cells both in the thymus and the peripheral lymphoid organs owing to ineffective positive selection of CD4+ T cells in the absence of class II interaction.

Frank and Parnes (1998) reported that mice expressing reduced levels of CD4 had fewer CD4 single positive and double positive thymocytes compared to control mice. These data support the differential avidity model of positive and negative selection, implicating an important role for CD4 in contributing to the overall avidity of the interaction between developing thymocytes with MHC class II-bearing antigen presenting cells in the thymus; thymocytes with too little avidity for MHC are subjected to programmed cell death.

## Ligands for CD4 and CD8 are MHC molecules themselves

Direct evidence exists demonstrating that the ligands for CD8 and CD4 T cell coreceptors are MHC class I and II molecules, respectively. The site on the class I molecule with which CD8 interacts has been mapped to the α3 domain by several groups. Potter *et al.* (1989) reported that a single substitution of a lysine for a glutamic acid at amino acid position 227 in the α3 domain of the H-2D$^d$ class I molecule abrogated recognition by CD8-dependent primary CTL. Salter *et al.* (1990), using 48 single point mutations of HLA-A2.1, localized the CD8 interaction site between residues 223 and 229 using cell–cell adhesion assays and alloreactive CTL responses. In both reports the proposed CD8 binding site mapped to an exposed (accessible) loop of the α3 domain of the mouse (H-2D$^d$) and human (HLA-A2.1) class I molecules.

Several studies have addressed the binding site for CD4 on MHC class II molecules. The first observations that implicated the β2 domain of the class II molecule were reported by Lombardi *et al.* (1991a) and Ramesh *et al.* (1992). They noted that substitution of the β2 domain of HLA-DR1 with the β2 domain from the mouse class II molecule, H-2E, led to a marked inhibition of reactivity by anti-DR alloreactive responses of human T cell clones and peripheral blood lymphocytes. Similar results were described by Vignali *et al.* (1992) in a mouse system. These results suggested that a partial species barrier affects the interaction of human CD4 with mouse class II and vice versa. In addition to interacting with human class II molecules, human CD4 appears to be capable of a productive interaction with the mouse I-A$_\beta$ chain, but not the I-E$_\beta$ chain. Mouse CD4, in contrast, interacts inefficiently with human class II β chains. Using IA$_\beta$ mutants, König *et al.* (1992) demonstrated that residues 137–143 of the class II β2 domain, a region that is structurally analogous to the exposed α3 domain loop implicated in class I binding to CD8, are involved in the interaction between class II molecules and CD4.

Cammarota *et al.* (1992), working in the human system with soluble HLA-DR4 molecules (heterodimers and isolated β chains) synthesized by transfected insect cells and using synthetic peptides corresponding to DRβ2 domain sequences, demonstrated that binding to immobilized recombinant, soluble CD4 could be achieved. The DRβ chain peptide corresponding to residues 134–148, and to a lesser extent residues 138–152, bound specifically to soluble CD4.

Hence, in both mouse and human systems, the β2 domain of MHC class II molecules contributes significantly to the ligand for CD4. It is possible that other domains of the class II molecule may also be involved in or affect efficient CD4 binding. For instance, it has been suggested that the class II α chain contributes to the CD4 interaction (Anderson *et al.* 1988; Zhou *et al.* 1991). This could be of particular importance if the CD4 molecule contributes to the stabilization of doublets of class II molecules at the interface between the T cell and the APC. This possibility has been raised by the finding that all of the class II molecules in the crystals that have been analysed exist as doublets or 'dimer²' (Stern *et al.* 1994). Consistent with this model, it appears that CD4 interacts with sites on both the β2 and α2 membrane-proximal domains of the class II

molecule, and that both of these sites would be available to a single CD4 molecule on two adjacent class II molecules in a double dimer, thereby cross-linking TCR/CD4 complexes (König *et al.* 1995). This speculative possibility has yet to be tested. The quaternary molecular complex involving the TCR, the MHC class II, bound peptide and CD4 molecules is portrayed schematically in Fig. 2.4.

## Processing of antigenic determinants for MHC class I and II presentation to T cells

There are many similarities in the way that antigenic peptides are recognized by T cells restricted by the two classes of MHC molecule, as illustrated by the fact that the variable region genes encoding the TCR for class I- and II-restricted responses are drawn from the same V gene loci. The relatedness of TCRs on class I- and II-restricted T cells suggests that the form in which antigen is recognized by the two distinct T cell populations (CD4+ and CD8+) is structurally similar, and this is indeed the case. However, although the resulting antigenic determinant presented by class I and II MHC molecules is a short peptide fragment, the generation and loading of peptides for presentation by the two classes of restriction elements involve two distinct routes of antigen processing within the cell. In most instances, class I associated peptides are obtained from intracellular, cytoplasmic proteins, such as those derived from virus-encoded antigens in virus-infected cells. In contrast, class II associated peptides are generally derived from extracellular or membrane-bound proteins that enter the endosomal–lysosomal recycling pathway (Morrison *et al.* 1986; Reid & Watts 1990).

### Class I presentation of endogenous antigen

Loading of MHC class I molecules with antigen for presentation to CD8+ CTL requires *de novo* protein synthesis of antigen within the antigen-presenting cell (APC) (Morrison *et al.* 1986), degradation of antigen by proteolytic cleavage to generate peptide lengths capable of binding to class I (Townsend *et al.* 1988), delivery of peptides from the cytosol into the ER

(Kleijmeer *et al.* 1992) for binding to nascent class I molecules, and adequate affinity of peptide fragments for the class I molecules available in the ER (Falk *et al.* 1991).

Separation of class I from class II antigen processing pathways was originally demonstrated by Morrison *et al.* (1986) by introducing the influenza antigen haemagglutinin (HA) into target cells using a recombinant vaccinia virus expression vector system. Cells expressing HA in vaccinia- or influenza-infected cells were lysed by MHC class I-restricted, HA-specific cytotoxic T cell (CTL) clones, but not by HA-specific class II-restricted CTL clones. Target recognition by the class I-restricted clones was abolished if APCs were treated with emetine, a protein synthesis inhibitor, suggesting that *de novo* protein synthesis was required for antigen association with class I. The conclusions drawn from these results have been supported by many subsequent studies and it appears that, with a limited number of exceptions, peptides derived from cytoplasmic proteins assemble with class I molecules for presentation to CD8+ T cells.

A variety of experimental approaches have been used to address the intracellular site at which cytoplasmic proteins are proteolytically cleaved into peptides for loading on to class I molecules. Townsend *et al.* (1986a) examined the effect on CD8+ T cell recognition of removing the signal peptide-encoding sequence of HA. They observed that transfected cells presented the truncated HA antigen more efficiently than intact HA to class I-restricted, HA-specific CTL. This suggested that entry into the ER, caused by the presence of a signal sequence, resulted in impaired processing and association with class I and that the ER is not the major location for proteolytic degradation of cytoplasmic proteins.

Proteolysis occurs elsewhere in the cytosol in proteasomes, which are multisubunit, multicatalytic proteases which carry out non-lysosomal protein degradation in the cytosol of eukaryotic cells (Coux *et al.* 1996). They have a critical role in the generation of peptides that will be presented by MHC class I (Rock *et al.* 1994). The proteasome contains constitutive subunits ($\delta$, $x$ and $z$) which are replaced by three IFN-$\gamma$ inducible subunit homologues (LMP2, LMP7

and MECL1, respectively), which alters the peptidase specificity favouring cleavage at the carboxy side of basic or hydrophobic amino acids (Driscoll *et al.* 1993; Gaczynska *et al.* 1993; Foss *et al.* 1998; Griffin *et al.* 1998). Peptides generated in this manner contain preferred anchor residues that are more suitable for binding to most MHC class I molecules (Rammensee *et al.* 1993; Howard 1995; Lehner & Cresswell 1996). The delivery of peptide fragments is mediated by a specific transporter complex molecule into the ER, where they can assemble with nascent class I molecules. Peptide transporter genes (called transporters associated with antigen processing, or TAP1 and TAP2) from humans, rats and mice have been cloned and sequenced by several groups (Deverson *et al.* 1990; Spies *et al.* 1990; Trowsdale *et al.* 1990). They share features with a family of ATP-dependent peptide transporters. Their role is to direct proteolysed peptides to the ER to assemble with newly synthesized class I molecules (Howard 1995; Lehner & Cresswell 1996) (see Fig. 2.4). Recent evidence suggests that MHC class I molecules physically associate with the TAP complex, and that this is facilitated by a newly discovered glycoprotein, tapasin (Sadasivan *et al.* 1996). Interestingly, TAP1 and TAP2 expression is enhanced following activation with IFN-$\gamma$ and this up-regulation is increased further by the addition of lipopolysaccharide (LPS) (Cramer & Klemsz 1997). Clearly IFN-$\gamma$ is a cytokine of major importance during immune responses affecting the expression of multiple components of the antigen processing pathway of MHC class I.

Also important in the assembly and folding of nascent MHC class I in the ER are the chaperon molecules calnexin and calreticulin. Zhang and Salter (1998) investigated the effect of altered MHC class I N-glycosylation on interactions with these chaperons and addressed the differences reported between the assembly processes of mouse compared to human. Calnexin dissociates from human class I when $\beta$2m binds, while dissociation from mouse class I occurs in later events following peptide loading. Zhang and Salter (1998) proposed that these differences are caused by the number and location of *N*-oligosaccharides on MHC class I; human class I heavy chains contain a single site whereas mouse heavy chains contain two or three sites. Additional sites may contribute to the strength of class I heavy chain binding to calnexin following β2m association.

A series of observations, made over several years, have highlighted the existence of an alternative pathway of antigen presentation by MHC class I molecules whereby exogenous antigens gain access to the class I pathway (Jin *et al.* 1988; Yewdell *et al.* 1988; Carbone & Bevan 1990; Rock *et al.* 1990). One mechanism by which this occurs appears to involve macropinocytosis and is particularly efficiently achieved by the most highly specialized antigen-presenting cell type, the dendritic cell (Sallusto *et al.* 1995). Similar results have been reported following phagocytosis of antigens by macrophages (Harding & Song 1994). This pathway is likely to be crucially important in the priming of CD8+ T cells against viral antigens by dendritic cells.

## Class II presentation of exogenous antigen

The need for active processing of antigen for MHC class II-restricted presentation was elegantly demonstrated by the early studies of Ziegler and Unanue (1981). A period of 45–60 min was required by macrophages in order to process soluble antigen (*Listeria monocytogenes*) before T cells were able to recognize antigen-pulsed APC. After 1 h, antigen-pulsed macrophages could be fixed with aldehyde without losing their ability to present antigen to specific T cells. During the first hour antigen was taken up and metabolically processed to a form that could associate with MHC class II. In contrast, aldehyde fixation of APC before exposure to antigen abolished their ability to present to T cells. These early experiments demonstrated that a metabolically active step (processing) was required in order to render antigen recognizable by T cells.

Morrison *et al.* (1986), working with class II-restricted, influenza-specific T cell clones, demonstrated that infectious or UV-inactivated (non-infectious, non-replicating) virus could prime class II-bearing target cells. Furthermore, when infectious or non-infectious virus was incubated with target cells

that had been treated with emetine the class II-restricted CTL response was unaffected. This clearly demonstrated that *de novo* protein synthesis was not a prerequisite for MHC class II presentation of influenza antigenic determinants.

In subsequent experiments purified HA was used to pulse APC. Soluble exogenous HA was able to stimulate CD4+ T cells when presented by MHC class II-expressing APC. However, this was inhibited by the addition of chloroquine, a lysosomotropic agent that neutralizes endosomal and lysosomal pH and blocks acidic proteolysis (Ziegler & Unanue 1981).

Some of the earliest direct evidence supporting the idea that processed antigenic determinants presented to class II-restricted T cells are proteolytic fragments of the soluble protein came from the studies of Shimonkevitz *et al.* (1983) using ovalbumin (OVA)-specific T cell hybridomas. As for the *Listeria* system described above presentation of OVA was abolished by aldehyde fixation of the APC before exposure to antigen. If, however, OVA was proteolytically digested with cyanogen bromide or trypsin prior to APC pulsing, fixed APC were fully able to induce a T cell response. These results demonstrated that the active metabolic processing step involved proteolytic cleavage of antigen for presentation by MHC class II. Peptide pulsing of APC is now a method that is commonly exploited in defining T cell specificities and MHC binding.

Regarding viral infection, there is a logical basis for the immune system to have evolved two alternative pathways of antigen presentation. Most CTL are class I-restricted and it is desirable to target the attention of antiviral CTL to virus-infected host cells that are actively synthesizing viral proteins, because it is the infected cell that poses a threat to the host and must be eliminated. Presentation of viral antigens with class I molecules is the natural result of the activity of the major class I antigen presentation pathway. In contrast, the class II pathway is biased towards the presentation of exogenous, internalized antigen, is responsible for priming and activating CD4+ T cells, and does not require that MHC class II-expressing specialized APC are infected with virus in order for effective presentation to occur.

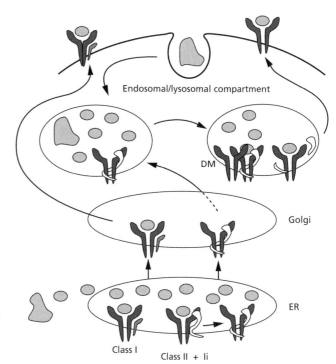

**Fig. 2.5** Major pathways of antigen presentation with MHC class I and class II molecules. A simplified version of the major antigen presentation pathways for class I and class II molecules are shown. This highlights the fact that the majority of peptides presented by class I molecules are derived from cytosolic proteins and that the major site of peptide loading for class I molecules is within the endoplasmic reticulum (ER). The role of the invariant chain in creating a separate pathway for class II molecules is illustrated, as is the function of HLA-DM (DM) in class II molecule peptide loading.

## Distinction between MHC class I and II antigen presentation pathways

An alternative pathway exists for the presentation of exogenous antigens by MHC class I molecules, as outlined above. Similarly, MHC class II molecules have access to both endogenously and exogenously derived antigens (for review see Neefjes & Ploegh 1992; Lechler *et al.* 1996). The endosomal–lysosomal compartment appears to be the major intracellular location involved in degrading class II-associated peptides and it is possible that some cytosolic proteins are delivered directly to lysosomes by translocation across lysosomal membranes (Dice 1990). In addition, endogenous proteins may be delivered to class II molecules through a process called 'autophagy', by which cytosolic proteins are entrapped in vesicles that then exchange or fuse their contents with endosomes (Yewdell & Bennink 1990). The numerous, naturally processed, class II-associated peptides that have recently been defined shed additional light on the major pathway of class II processing and presentation. Most class II-bound peptides are derived from cell surface proteins such as MHC molecules themselves, cell surface receptors and from the invariant chain (Ii). However, a limited number of the naturally processed peptides eluted from HLA-DR molecules do appear to arise from cytosolic proteins, providing further evidence that a pathway does exist for the presentation of endogenous, cytosolic proteins with class II MHC molecules. The possible contribution of the endogenous pathway to class II-restricted presentation is probably dependent upon the concentrations and the characteristics of the endogenous protein. Despite the possibility of class II presentation of cytosolic proteins, the endocytic pathway provides most class II-associated peptides and it is the Ii molecule that appears to play a major part in keeping the two pathways of antigen processing separate (Fig. 2.5).

## The role of invariant chain in MHC class II–peptide association

As mentioned above, MHC class II molecules are associated within the cell with a non-polymorphic glycoprotein called the invariant chain (Ii). The expression of MHC class II and Ii genes is coregulated both for constitutive and for cytokine-induced expression, and it is the Ii molecule that appears to be important in keeping the two pathways of antigen processing largely separate. Figure 2.5 illustrates how the Ii chain and class II associate in the ER and remain asssociated through the trans-Golgi network before intersecting the acidic endosome, where the proteolysis of Ii occurs (Lotteau *et al.* 1990). Proteolysis of Ii results in a small fragment, called the class II-associated Ii peptide, or CLIP, to remain bound to class II (Kropshofer *et al.* 1995). Its removal from class II to enable binding to peptides derived from exogenous or cell-membrane bound sources is facilitated by HLA-DM (Denzin & Cresswell 1995), a class II-like αβ heterodimer. The Ii chain thus has two functions (reviewed by Castellino *et al.* 1997). First, it inhibits the binding of peptide to MHC class II molecules until the class II molecule reaches the endosomal–lysosomal compartment of the cell. Secondly, Ii serves as a chaperon and targets class II to the endosomal compartment. This is supported by the data of Lotteau *et al.* (1990), who demonstrated the presence of three separate targeting signals in human Ii which serve to direct class II molecules to the relevant subcellular compartment. Similar conclusions were drawn from the study of Ii knockout mice, in which the level of MHC class II molecules was found to be reduced 10-fold compared to normal, and the APC from these mice were defective in presenting most of antigens tested (Bikoff *et al.* 1993; Viville *et al.* 1993).

X-ray crystallographic analysis revealed the manner in which CLIP binds to HLA-DR3 (Ghosh *et al.* 1995) and apparently CLIP assumes the same conformation as that observed with antigenic peptides (Stern *et al.* 1994).

An interesting feature of the monomorphic, intracellular Ii molecule is the phylogenetically conserved region of CLIP between amino acid residues 91 and 99, believed to have evolved to accommodate two important properties:

1 to allow exchange with antigenic peptides that will be presented to T cells; and
2 to maintain affinity for numerous polymorphic MHC class II molecules.

The first property requires that CLIP binds class II with a relatively low to intermediate affinity compared to antigenic peptides to ensure adequate chaperon occupancy and peptide exchange. Interestingly, high affinity CLIP sequences produced by introducing mutations at positions 93 and 99 inhibit not only cell surface expression of class II, but also class II antigen presentation in an allele-dependent manner (Gautam *et al.* 1997). In addition, although not proven, it is interesting to speculate that conservation of CLIP is necessary to ensure dissociation by HLA-DM. The second property requires that CLIP is able to bind to most class II alleles, accommodated not necessarily in the same binding frame (Weenink *et al.* 1997) but by employing a 'supermotif', as described by Malcherek *et al.* (1995).

It has become clear that DM has a more general role in MHC class II peptide loading and may be best regarded as a peptide editor, leading to the exchange of poorly for efficiently bound peptides to MHC class II molecules, in the MIIC compartment. This has been demonstrated by Vogt *et al.* (1996) and is further illustrated by the findings that DM physically associates with MHC class II molecules (Sanderson *et al.* 1996) and DM appears to alter peptide occupancy independently of the presence of the Ii chain (Sant-Angelo *et al.* 1996; Lightstone *et al.* 1997). Albert *et al.* (1998) suggested that HLA-DM may even have a role in altering the conformation of class II molecules, a hypothesis that, if correct, would help to explain the inability of T1.Ak (a T2 cell line deficient in HLA-DM and transfected with H-2Ak) to bind to and present the superantigen staphylococcal enterotoxin A.

## Characteristics of MHC molecule-associated naturally processed peptides

The array of peptides presented at the surface of APC is dictated by MHC class I and II molecules themselves. The polymorphic nature of the different allelic forms of class I and II molecules gives rise to a multitude of peptide fragments which are capable of associating with the peptide-binding cleft of MHC molecules.

MHC polymorphism increases the range of antigens that can potentially bind to MHC molecules, thereby leading to more effective and comprehensive immune responses. Analysis of MHC-bound, naturally processed, peptides has become possible by acid elution, high-pressure liquid chromatography and microsequencing.

The information acquired from these methods has provided a unique insight into the mechanisms of peptide generation and presentation. Allele-specific motifs revealed by sequencing of peptides eluted from MHC molecules, have been identified for class I and II products (Rammensee 1995). Different MHC alleles favour the binding of peptides that have in common from one to three conserved amino acid residues that serve to anchor the peptide to the MHC groove, often interacting with the binding pockets in an allele-specific manner.

Edman degradation of self peptides eluted from several class I proteins of mouse (H-2K$^d$, D$^b$, K$^b$) (Falk *et al*. 1991) and humans (HLA-A2.1 (Falk *et al*. 1991), B27 (Jardetzky *et al*. 1991)) have revealed a characteristic consensus motif for each class I allele. H-2K$^d$, D$^b$, HLA-A2.1 and B27 present peptides as nonamers whereas H-2K$^b$-associated peptides seem to be predominantly octamers. The peptide motifs usually consist of two anchor positions, which vary for each allele, at which a single or highly conserved set of residues is found. Anchor positions are at positions (P) 5 and P9 (D$^b$), P2 and P9 (K$^d$, A2) and P5 and P8 (K$^b$) (Falk *et al*. 1991). For B27 P2 is the most conserved, arginine being found in all of the peptide sequences analysed, followed by P1 and P9, which usually contain positively charged amino acids (Jardetzky *et al*. 1991); see Table 2.1 for some examples.

The interaction of MHC class II molecules with peptides is considerably more flexible in that the range of length is much greater and the anchor residues are defined less clearly. Naturally processed peptides occupying mouse (Hunt *et al*. 1992; Rudensky *et al*. 1992) and human (Chicz *et al*. 1992) class II molecules have been defined, and range from 13 to 25 residues in length. The class II peptide motif is not assigned a defined position with respect to the N-terminal amino acid owing to the irregular length of permitted peptides. A putative DR1-binding motif was revealed when sequence alignments of the core epitopes (minimum length) of naturally processed peptides were made. Key residues included: a positively charged group at the first position, referred to as the index position for orientation (I); a hydrogen bond donor at I+5; and a hydrophobic residue at I+9. A hydrophobic residue is also often found at I+1 and/or I−1. DR1-bound peptides are heterogeneous at both the N and C termini (Chicz *et al*. 1992), contrasting with H-2A$^b$- and H-2E$^b$-bound peptides, which contain precise N-terminal cleavages (Rudensky *et al*. 1991). In DR1, it appears that the ends of the peptide-binding cleft are conformationally open, allowing the peptide to bind centrally to the MHC peptide cleft while having its ends overhanging on either side of the peptide-binding cleft.

The differences in peptide length required for class I vs. class II binding suggest that quite different mechanisms of processing operate for the two classes of MHC molecules. Generally the loading of class I and II peptide-binding clefts occurs in different cellular compartments (reviewed by Yewdell & Bennink 1990); class I–peptide association occurs in the ER while class II–peptide association occurs in an endosomal compartment of the cell. Considerable progress has been made in defining motifs for MHC class II-bound peptides using phage display technology (Hammer 1995). This information is currently being put to use by groups interested in defining T cell epitopes in autoimmune diseases.

## Regulation of MHC class I and II expression

### Tissue distribution of MHC class I and II antigens

The two major classes of MHC molecules have very different patterns of tissue distribution. MHC class I molecules have a very wide tissue distribution, although they are not entirely ubiquitous (Daar *et al*. 1984a). Most endocrine tissues, excluding the adrenal gland, express only low levels of class I and MHC molecules are undetectable on corneal endothelium, the exocrine region of the pancreas, acinar cells of the parotid gland, neurones of the central nervous system

**Table 2.1** (a) Sequence motifs of peptides bound to HLA class I antigens.

| Class I | 1 | 2 | 3 | 4 | 5 | 6 | 7 | 8 | 9 |
|---|---|---|---|---|---|---|---|---|---|
| HLA-A2* | – | **L** | – | – | – | – | – | – | V |
|  | – | M | – | E | – | V | – | K | – |
|  | – | – | – | K | – | – | – | – | – |
| HLA-B27† | – | **R** | – | – | – | – | – | – | – |
|  | R | – | – | – | – | – | – | – | K |
|  | – | – | – | – | – | – | – | – | R |
| HLA-B53‡ | – | **P** | – | – | – | – | – | – | – |
|  | – | – | – | E | I | – | – | – | – |
| HLA-B35‡ | – | **P** | – | – | – | – | – | – | Y |
|  | – | – | F | – | – | – | – | – | – |

Amino acid sequence (single letter code) of eluted peptides from different HLA class I molecules, and the dominant motifs obtained by protein sequencing. The prevalence of particular amino acids in relation to their sequence position on the eluted peptides was determined (* Falk *et al.* 1991; † Jardetzky *et al.* 1991; ‡ Hill *et al.* 1992). Dominant residues are indicated in bold and commonly occurring residues indicated in plain text.

(b) Features of peptide binding by MHC class II molecules.

| Peptide | MHC | Association (m/s) | Dissociation (per second) | Affinity ($K_d$) | Reference |
|---|---|---|---|---|---|
| OVA 323–339 | IA$^d$(pH7) | 1.9 | $1.6 \times 10^{-5}$ | $2 \times 10^{-6}$ M | Buus *et al.* (1986) |
|  | IA$^d$(pH5) | – | – | $0.76 \times 10^{-6}$ M | Jensen (1991) |
| HA 307–319 | DR1 | 120 | $1.6 \times 10^{-6}$ | $13 \times 10^{-9}$ M | Roche & Cresswell (1990) |
| PCC 88–104 | IE$^k$ | 120 | $1.2 \times 10^{-3}$ | – | Sadegh-Nasseri & McConnell (1989) |
| HEL 46–61 | IA$^k$ | – | – | $2 \times 10^{-6}$ M | Babbitt *et al.* (1985) |

HA, influenza haemagglutinin; HEL, hen egg lysozyme; OVA, ovalbumin; PCC pigeon cytochrome c.

and cells of the villous trophoblast. Class I expression can be detected at all other sites.

The expression of MHC class II antigens is more restricted than that of class I. Class II molecules are only expressed constitutively on B lymphocytes, macrophages and dendritic cells, all of which are specialized APC for CD4+ T cells (Daar *et al.* 1984b). Other cell types express class II antigens under physiological or pathological conditions. Vascular endothelial cells (Hirschberg *et al.* 1980), Langerhans cells (Broathen 1981) and the lymphatics in most tissues (Daar *et al.* 1984b) normally express class II. Resting human T cells are class II negative but can be induced to express class II molecules by mitogen- or antigen-specific stimulation (Ko *et al.* 1979; Yu *et al.* 1980). Epithelial cells of various organs including the small intestine, trachea, tongue, tonsil, epiglottis, proximal renal tubules, urethra and epididymis can also be induced to express class II antigens (Daar *et al.* 1984b).

Under pathological conditions class II expression has been demonstrated in tissues which are otherwise class II negative. For instance, in Graves' disease and Hashimoto's thyroiditis thyroid epithelial cells bear class II antigens (Bottazzo *et al.* 1983) while in human insulin-dependent diabetes mellitus (IDDM) class II expression is observed on β-cells in pancreatic islet tissue (Bottazzo *et al.* 1985). The patterns of expression of MHC molecules are summarized in Table 2.2.

**Table 2.2** (a) HLA class I antigens and their expression.

| Antigen | Distribution |
|---------|--------------|
| *Classical* | |
| HLA-A | |
| HLA-B | Present on most nucleated cells; low expression by myocardium, and skeletal muscle. Not detected on CNS neurones and villous trophoblast |
| HLA-C | |
| *Non-classical* | |
| HLA-E | Resting peripheral T cells |
| HLA-F | Not known |
| HLA-G | Chorionic cytotrophoblast |

(b) Tissue distribution of HLA-DR antigen expression.

| Constitutive expression | Induced expression |
|-------------------------|--------------------|
| Macrophage | Vascular endothelium |
| B cell | Gut epithelium |
| Dendritic cell | Dermal fibroblasts |
| Thymic epithelium | Melanocytes, astrocytes, Schwann cells, T cells, thyroid follicular epithelium, synovial lining cells |

# Gene regulation of MHC class I and II

The expression of class I and II genes can be induced or enhanced by certain immune modulators such as the interferons (Collins *et al.* 1984; Pujol-Borrell *et al.* 1987) and TNFα (Collins *et al.* 1986; Arenzana-Seisdedos *et al.* 1988). This regulation is predominantly at the transcriptional stage. For both class I and II genes *cis*-acting DNA elements (promoters and enhancers) and *trans*-acting factors that bind to these DNA elements have been described which control the levels of mRNA transcription from these loci. The promoter region contains a TATA box, usually located 25–30 base pairs (bp) upstream (5′) of the mRNA initiation site (cap site). Its function is to direct RNA polymerase to the correct transcription start site. Upstream elements (UPE) (e.g. the CCAAT box) are located about 20–70 bp further upstream, and are involved in regulating the frequency of transcriptional initiation. Enhancer sequences are usually positioned even further upstream. Occasionally they reside within the gene and have been shown to activate transcription independently of their orientation or distance with regard to these promoters (Gluzman & Shenk 1983). The function of enhancer elements has been linked to tissue specificity (Gillies *et al.* 1984). These regulatory sequences bind to *trans*-acting protein factors which enhance the binding or activity of one or more components of the transcription complex.

In humans and mice regulatory elements located 5′ of the transcription initiation sites have been identified for class I genes. Several enhancer elements, identified by their ability to regulate expression of a reporter gene (chloramphenicol acetyltransferase) *in vitro*, have been demonstrated for human and mouse class I genes (Kimura *et al.* 1986; Ganguly *et al.* 1989). Enhancer A (−193 to −158) and enhancer B (−120 to −61) are conserved within the promoter of several classical MHC class I genes (reviewed by David-Watine *et al.* 1990). Enhancer A overlaps an interferon response sequence (−165 to −137) identified in a number of other gene promoters (Friedman & Stark 1985). In addition, enhancer activity has been localized to introns 3 and 5 of the HLA-B7 gene (Ganguly *et al.* 1989). Many nuclear binding proteins, including KBF1, KBF2, H2TF1, NF-κB, MBP-1, H-2RIIBP, PRDII-BF1 and AP2, can bind to enhancer A while enhancer B contains binding sites for CREB-ATF factor and a CCAAT binding factor called CP2 (David-Watine *et al.* 1990). These numerous DNA-binding proteins interact with multiple regulatory sequences and ultimately exert their effect by fine-tuning of MHC class I gene expression.

As with class I, the regulation of class II gene expression is controlled by multiple DNA-binding proteins which interact with specific sequences residing at the 5′ end of the gene, affecting tissue specificity and cytokine induction. The regulatory mechanisms of class II gene expression have been studied using DNA-binding assays (Reith *et al.* 1989), promoter deletion constructs linked to reporter genes (Dorn *et al.* 1987; Sherman *et al.* 1989), and transgenic mice harbouring constructs of the H-2Ea gene with defined deletions in the promoter region (van Ewijk *et al.* 1988). In addition to the

CCAAT and TATA boxes associated with most eukaryotic genes, four different regulatory sequences, W or Z (encompassing a core of 8 bp designated S or H), X, Y and O have been identified for some of the murine and human class II genes (Benoist & Mathis 1990). They reside at the 5′ end of the class II coding sequences ~180 bp upstream of the initiation of transcription.

Some important advances in our understanding of MHC class II gene regulation have been acquired from the study of families suffering from a rare form of immunodeficiency called the bare lymphocyte syndrome. These individuals lack both constitutive and inducible MHC class II expression. Different complementation groups have been defined and several independent genetic defects have been identified. The most revealing of these defects led to the absence of a transactivator, named CIITA, which is required for the expression of all MHC class II genes, both constitutive and inducible. Indeed, transfection of a CIITA cDNA in several class II-negative cells types led to MHC class II expression without any other manipulation (Steimle *et al.* 1993). Expression of CIITA is induced by IFN-γ and requires STAT1 protein (signal transducer and activator of transcription) and is attenuated by TGF-β (Lee & Benveniste 1996; Lee *et al.* 1997). Once IFN-γ has bound to its cell surface receptor, the Jak tyrosine kinases become activated and in turn activate STAT1, which then translocates to the nuclear compartment (Darnell 1997). Distinguishing IFN-γ induction of CIITA from other IFN-γ-inducible genes is the necessary binding of USF-1 to STAT1 to enable STAT1 to bind stably to the GAS element of the CIITA promoter leading the CIITA gene expression (Darnell 1997; Muhlethaler-Mottet *et al.* 1998). The regulatory sequences governing IFN-γ induction and TGF-β suppression of CIITA gene expression have been extensively analysed (Lennon *et al.* 1997; Muhlethaler-Mottet *et al.* 1997; Piskurich *et al.* 1998).

Also involved in the regulation of MHC class II genes are sequences located far upstream (−2000 to −1000) of the transcription initiation site which can influence the cell type specificity of class II expression. Transgenic mice harbouring 1.9 kilobases (kb) of 5′ flanking DNA express H-2Eα correctly, while transgenic mice containing shorter lengths of upstream regulatory sequence (1.3 or 1.2 kb) produce atypical patterns of expression. Truncated Ea transgenes give rise to little or no expression in B cells, while expression in thymus, peripheral macrophages and dendritic cells is unaffected (Widera *et al.* 1987; Dorn *et al.* 1988; van Ewijk *et al.* 1988; Burkly *et al.* 1989). The results of these transgenic studies have defined the B cell control region (BCCR) between −1900 and −1180 in the H-2Ea gene. Sequence motifs responsible for activity of the BCCR have been revealed through sequence and functional analyses (Dorn *et al.* 1988). These include copies of the X–Y and W motifs, mentioned above for the promoter–proximal region, and a copy of the B motif, found in a number of genes believed to serve as a binding site for a family of factors (Lenardo & Baltimore 1989). The DNA-binding factors that associate with class II regulatory motifs are too numerous to discuss here but are considered in detail elsewhere (Reith *et al.* 1989; Benoist & Mathis 1990; Accolla *et al.* 1991).

How DNA-binding factors contribute to the fine-tuning of MHC class I and II genes under physiological and pathological circumstances is under intensive investigation and no doubt the fundamental details of class I and II regulation will soon be unravelled.

## Genetics of the MHC

One of the most striking features of the classical MHC genes is their interallelic sequence variation, or polymorphism. These are the most polymorphic genes in the mammalian genome and multiple allelic forms have evolved by several mechanisms including point mutations, recombination, homologous but unequal crossing over and gene conversion. Throughout evolution all three major linked gene clusters of the MHC, including the class I, II and III regions, have undergone expansion and contraction. Some duplicated genes have lost their function and as a result have become pseudogenes. Others encode well-characterized protein products while some have functions yet to be defined.

Large numbers of genes within the HLA region encoding class I and II molecules and their multiple allelic forms have been and are being identified, and the nomenclature of the genes and their products is constantly updated by the WHO Nomenclature Committee for Factors of the HLA System (Bodmer *et al.* 1992a,b, 1994, 1995; Marsh 1998; Mason & Parham 1998). With new alleles being identified continuously, this list is currently under monthly revision and new additions are published in *Tissue Antigens*, *Human Immunology* and the *European Journal of Immunogenetics*. The organizing committee for the 13th International Histocompatibility Workshop and Conference (IHWC), which will take place in Seattle in June 2001, is coordinating an international repository of plasmids containing HLA class I and II DNA or cDNA clones. It is hoped by making such clones widely available that they will be utilized as research tools and standard reagents worldwide.

The different HLA class I genes are denoted by a suffix: HLA-A, B, C, E, F, G, H, J and X, while the HLA class II genes are indicated by the subregion of localization: HLA-DR, DQ, DP, DM, DN and DO. In addition, class II names indicate whether they encode the α chain (e.g. HLA-DRA) or the β chain (e.g. HLA-DRB) sequence. In accordance with WHO nomenclature, the locus is identified first, followed by the identification number of the allele. For instance, for class I HLA-A2 is designated HLA-A*02, followed by a number to indicate the subtype, e.g. HLA-A*0201, HLA-A*0202, etc.

The human MHC spans more than 3500 kb of DNA (Spies *et al.* 1989a,b; Trowsdale *et al.* 1991), as illustrated in Fig. 2.6. The orientation of the three major gene clusters on chromosome 6 was mapped using genomic cloning and pulsed-field gel electrophoresis techniques (Hardy *et al.* 1986; Dunham *et al.* 1987; Lawrance *et al.* 1987; Sargent *et al.* 1989a,b; Spies *et al.* 1989a,b). The class I and II gene families occupy distinct 1600 and 900 kb regions at the telomeric and centromeric end of the MHC, respectively, and flank the central 1000 kb class III gene family. The MHC has proved to be the region of the mammalian genome most densely populated with genes; in addition to the genes encoding MHC class I and II molecules and the complement genes of the class III region, many other genes have recently been located. Current estimates are that the total number of genes contained within the 3500 kb of DNA that encompass the HLA region in humans is 300.

## MHC class I region

At present, 86 distinct HLA-A, 185 HLA-B and 45 HLA-C classical class I alleles have been assigned allellic code numbers (Mason & Parham 1998). The frequency with which these alleles appear varies according to the ethnic group and the geographical location of the population studied. For example, HLA-A2 occurs in 45% of European caucasoid individuals, while in black African its frequency is only 20%. HLA-Bw52, conversely, is present in only 3% of caucasoids while it is present in 20.5% of the Japanese population (Baur & Danilovs 1980).

In addition to the classical class I genes, there are six non-classical, relatively non-polymorphic class I genes designated HLA-E, F, G, H, J and X which are related to the murine Qa and Tla genes (Flaherty 1976, 1980). HLA-H and J are pseudogenes (Bodmer *et al.* 1992a), which are non-functional genes that usually arise by gene duplication of an active gene and accumulate mutations during evolution. The genomic organization and pattern of expression of HLA-E have been characterized (Koller *et al.* 1988) and four alleles have been defined (Bodmer *et al.* 1995). It is located between the HLA-A and C class I loci, has a broad tissue distribution (mRNA was found in all tissues examined) and the HLA-E heavy chain associates with β2m. Although mRNA was present in all tissues analysed (Koller *et al.* 1988), translation into cell surface proteins may be restricted to a more exclusive subset of cells or expression may be restricted to different stages of differentiation (Shimizu *et al.* 1988).

HLA-F has been cloned and characterized and shown to contain an exon and domain organization similar to those of HLA-A, B and C genes (Geraghty *et al.* 1990). Transcriptional analysis revealed HLA-F mRNA in resting T cells, skin cells and in B-lymphoblastoma cell lines but not in the immature leukaemic T cell line Molt-4.

HLA-G encodes a protein similar to HLA-A, B and C genes (86% homologous) except that it lacks most of the intracellular segment, suggesting that it is a

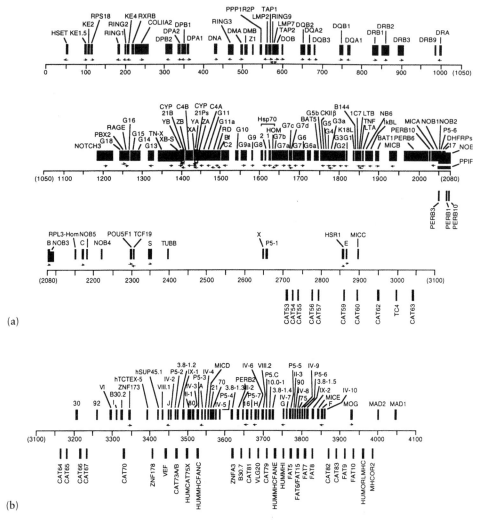

**Fig. 2.6** (a) The arrangement of the three major regions of the HLA region are shown; the distances between the loci are not to scale. (b) Map of the human major histocompatibility complex. This map is updated as new genes are identified. The most recent version (Trowsdale & Campbell 1997) has not been used as the map has become increasingly crowded; an earlier version is shown here for ease of interpretation.

structural homologue of a murine Qa-region class I gene (Geraghty *et al.* 1987). When HLA-G was transfected into a classical class I-deficient B cell line, a molecule detected by monoclonal antibody W6/32 (specific for a non-polymorphic epitope on classical class I antigens) was present on the cell surface (Orr 1989). The most unusual feature of this HLA gene is its pattern of expression, which has been detected in a choriocarcinoma cell line and in chorionic cytotrophoblast cell membranes (Ellis *et al.* 1986, 1990; Pazmany *et al.* 1996), tissues that do not express the classical class I antigens. Four allelic variants have been reported (Bodmer *et al.* 1995).

The function of the molecules encoded by the HLA-

E, F and G and the murine Qa/Tla-region genes is unclear. The fact that they are expressed in widely separate species such as humans and mouse argues that there is selective pressure for their maintenance but their precise function remains to be elucidated. Diehl *et al.* (1996) provided evidence that HLA-G can present peptide in a similar manner to that of classical HLA molecules. They reported a common peptide motif shared by peptides eluted from HLA-G, having hydrophobic amino acids in positions 2 and 9. They concluded that non-classical HLA-G more closely resembles human classical peptide receptors than murine non-classical MHC molecules, namely H2-M3, Qa-2 and Qa-1. Studies by Pazmany *et al.* (1996) suggested that HLA-G expressed on cytotrophoblast cells at the fetomaternal interface, where it may be involved in establishing maternal tolerance of the fetus, protects these cells, and presumably the fetal tissue that lies behind these cells, from maternal NK1- and NK2-cell mediated lysis. Using HLA-G-specific monoclonal antibody, Rouas-Freiss *et al.* (1997) demonstrated directly under physiological conditions that this is indeed the case. Blaschitz *et al.* (1997) using four different HLA-G-specific monoclonal antibodies investigated the expression of HLA-G in placental cell types to determine whether cell types other than extravillous cytotrophoblasts express HLA-G. They detected low-level expression on villous cytotrophoblasts previously considered to be HLA-G negative. In addition, expression of endothelial cells in the fetal capillaries of the chorionic villi was also detected. The authors proposed that soluble HLA-G may play an immunological and non-immunological part in fetal vascularization during the angiogenesis process in chorionic villi; however, functional evidence is still needed to support their hypothesis.

## MHC class II region

### THE DRB SUBREGION

The HLA class II region spans ~1000 kb with the DP loci at the centromeric end, the DR loci at the telomeric end and the DQ loci situated between them (Hardy *et al.* 1986; Trowsdale *et al.* 1991). There is one DRA and multiple DRB genes in the DR subregion. The DRA locus is almost completely invariant; only one amino acid substitution (leucine for valine at position 217) has been detected in all the DRA genes that have been sequenced (Lee *et al.* 1982; Das *et al.* 1983; Bodmer *et al.* 1995). The DRB locus, in contrast, is extremely variable, encoding one of the most polymorphic group of alleles in the human genome. In addition, there is variation in the number of loci which are expressed on different haplotypes.

There are five group haplotypes recognized by the 1991 WHO Nomenclature Committee, designated DR1, DR51, DR52, DR8 and DR53 group haplotypes (reviewed in Bodmer *et al.* 1992a). The DR alleles associated with each group haplotype are illustrated in Fig. 2.7. Within the DR1 and DR8 group haplotypes there is only one expressed DRB locus. The DR1, 10, 103 and (rarely) 15 alleles are associated with the DR1 group haplotype while the DR8 allele is associated with the DR8 group haplotype. The DR52 group haplotype contains two expressed DRB loci. At the first functional locus the following alleles have been identified: DR3, 11, 12, 13, 14, 1403 and 1404. The second expressed locus invariably contains the DR52 allele. The DR51 and DR53 group haplotypes also contain two expressible DRB loci; however, the second locus may not be expressed on certain haplotypes (Bodmer *et al.* 1992a). Included at the first locus of the DR51 group haplotype are the DR15, 16 and (rarely) 1 alleles, with the second locus containing the DR51 allele. The first locus of the DR53 group haplotype contains the DR4, 7 or 9 alleles while the second locus contains the DR53 allele. Residing within the DRB region are multiple pseudogenes (Bodmer *et al.* 1992a). The DR51 and DR53 group haplotypes contain two and three pseudogenes, respectively. The DR1 and DR52 group haplotypes contain one and possibly two pseudogenes. The DR8 group haplotype may contain one pseudogene, but this has yet to be confirmed.

The designation of HLA-DRB alleles is further complicated by the presence of additional polymorphism within each main serotype. Marsh (1998) has compiled a list of all known HLA alleles for MHC class II recognized by the WHO Nomenclature Committee for the Factors of the HLA System. The number of DRB alleles

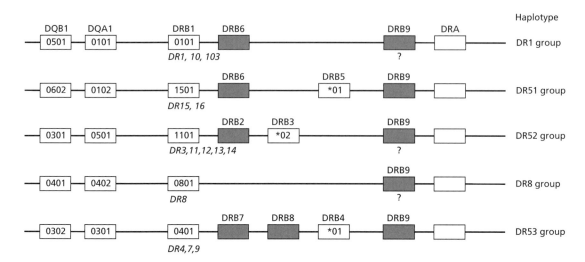

**Fig. 2.7** Common HLA haplotypes and linkage disequilibrium between HLA-DR and DQ alleles. The 1991 nomenclature of HLA alleles is used (Bodmer *et al.* 1992b). The alleles of the DRB1, DQA1 and DQB1 loci are shown within the appropriate boxes. Shaded boxes indicate pseudogenes. The alleles of the other DRB loci which are expressed on different haplotypes are shown within the appropriate boxes. The question marks under the DRB9 genes on three haplotypes indicate that its presence on these haplotypes has yet to be confirmed.

currently stands at 243, but this number is likely to change as more alleles are identified.

### THE DQ SUBREGION

There are five DQ genes present in all haplotypes analysed to date, namely DQA1, DQA2, DQB1, DQB2 and DQB3. There is no evidence for expression of DQA2, B2 (also known as DXA and DXB) or DQB3 (Bodmer *et al.* 1992a). Unlike DRA and DRB, there is polymorphism at both DQA and DQB loci, which is concentrated in the membrane-distal α1 and β1 domains of the molecule; however, they do not share the well-defined regions of allelic hypervariability that are found in DRB genes (Bell *et al.* 1989). Recently DQA1 and DQB1 loci were reported to contain 19 and 35 alleles, respectively (Marsh 1998).

### THE DP SUBREGION

There are two pairs of HLA-DP genes residing within the DP subregion. DPA1 and DPB1 are expressed with 13 and 83 alleles, respectively, reported to date (Marsh 1998). The other pair of DP genes, DPA2 and DPB2 genes, are pseudogenes owing to several coding region mutations (Servenius *et al.* 1984). In contrast to DQ, there does not appear to be a strong linkage disequilibrium (see below) between DR and DP allelic variation.

### THE DOB, DNA AND DM SUBREGIONS

Tonnelle *et al.* (1985) isolated and sequenced the DOB gene from a cDNA library generated from a B-lymphoblastoid cell line. It is highly homologous to other HLA-D region genes (DRB, DQB and DPB), containing ~70% nucleotide identity. It has been localized to the region between DQ and DP using pulsed-field gel electrophoresis. Its expression appears to be mainly confined to B cell lines, as T cell lines and IFN-γ-treated fibroblasts contained no DOB mRNA (Tonnelle *et al.* 1985). A more recent study by Douek and Altmann (1997) illustrated expression of DOB in the thymic cortex and medulla as well as dendritic cells.

The HLA-DNA gene (also known as DZA or DOA)

was cloned from a genomic library following hybridization with a HLA-DRA probe (Trowsdale & Kelly 1985). Pulsed-field gel electrophoresis analyses mapped the DNA locus 170 kb telomeric to the DPA locus (Hardy *et al.* 1986; Carroll *et al.* 1987). Cosmid walking procedures, spanning 120 kb around the DNA gene, demonstrated that DPA and DNA must be separated by a minimum of 50 kb (Blanck & Strominger 1990) and perhaps up to 110 kb if DPA and DNA are orientated as in the rabbit (Sittisombut & Knight 1986; Kuluga *et al.* 1987). It has been established that DNA and DOB gene products form a heterodimer and that the DO αβ dimer, HLA-DO, associates with DM (Liljedahl *et al.* 1996; Denzin *et al.* 1997; Douek & Altmann 1997; Jensen 1998). The function of HLA-DO remains to be fully elucidated; however, it is likely to have some role in MHC class II expression, targeting and peptide loading. Douek and Altmann (1997) demonstrated intrathymic expression of HLA-DO in epithelium surrounding Hassall's corpuscles in the thymic medulla, suggesting an important functional role for HLA-DO involving tolerance induction. Denzin *et al.* (1997) reported that HLA-DO negatively regulates class II-restricted antigen processing by inhibiting HLA-DM function (discussed below), described by Jensen (1998) as a 'hitchhiking inhibitor' of HLA-DM. These results suggest a role for HLA-DO in regulating HLA-DM-catalysed peptide loading.

Residing between DNA and DOB are two new genes, DMA and DMB, which were originally referred to as RING 6 and 7, respectively (Kelly *et al.* 1991a). They are adjacent to each other and are situated 50 kb telomeric to the DNA gene and 80 kb centromeric to the DOB locus. Although DMA and DMB share many similarities with conventional class II sequences, there are differences, particularly notable in the distinctive DMB membrane-distal domain, which contains five cysteines. These may contribute to the formation of disulphide bridges around the framework of the antigen-binding cleft, imposing a rigid conformation that restricts peptide-binding capacity. In addition, HLA-DM is not expressed on the cell surface but rather is confined to class II vesicles within the cell (Denzin *et al.* 1994; Fling *et al.* 1994; Morris *et al.* 1994).

Although distinct from other class II sequences, DMA and DMB are highly conserved between human and mouse (>70%, Cho *et al.* 1991), implying a functional role which may have antedated the duplications that gave rise to the conventional class II loci. The murine homologues of DMA and DMB are Ma and Mb. Unlike other class II β2 domains, the Mb immunoglobulin-like domain is as homologous to class I α3 domains (28–33%) and to class II α2 domains (31–36%) as it is to its own family members (33–39%) (Cho *et al.* 1991). The function of the DM molecule in the class II antigen presentation pathway was discussed on p. 36 and p. 42. Westerheide *et al.* (1997) illustrated that HLA-DMA and DMB are expressed in a similar manner involving conserved upstream regulatory elements, suggesting the coordinate regulation of the DM genes with other class II genes. Four allelic variants for HLA-DMA and five allelic variants for HLA-DMB have been identified (Marsh 1998).

## Non-MHC genes mapping to the class II subregion

Recently a group of additional genes whose products appear to be involved in the generation and loading of peptides on to class I molecules has been located in the middle of the MHC class II subregion, between DNA and DOB. This group includes TAP1, TAP2, LMP2 and LMP7 (Trowsdale *et al.* 1990; Glynne *et al.* 1991; Kelly *et al.* 1991b) and their role in class I peptide presentation is discussed on p. 31, p. 35 and p. 39. Powis *et al.* (1992a) reported sequence polymorphism in rat TAP2 (mtp2) and demonstrated that the consequence of this polymorphism was the differential loading of distinct populations of peptide on to class I, resulting in the *cim* phenomenon observed by Livingston *et al.* (1989, 1991). Polymorphism for human TAP1 and TAP2 is also observed (Powis *et al.* 1992b; Cano & Baxter-Lowe 1995). To date, five TAP1 alleles and four TAP2 alleles have been identified (Marsh 1998). Thus far there is no evidence that the polymorphism in human TAP genes has any functional consequences regarding the nature of MHC class I-presented peptides.

## MHC class III region

The class III region of the human MHC contains a large number of genes with diverse or unknown function. Among the genes residing in the centromeric region of class III, between C2 and G18, are the steroid 21-hydroxylase genes (CYP21A and B) which encode a cytochrome P450 enzyme involved in the hydroxylation of progesterone in the cortisol biosynthesis pathway. Deficiency of this enzyme results in congenital adrenal hyperplasia occurring in ~1 in 10000 births. CYP21B encodes the functional enzyme while CYP21A is a pseudogene (Higashi *et al.* 1986). Also included in this region are the C4A and C4B genes which code for the fourth component of complement (Campbell *et al.* 1990) and the Factor B (BF) and C2 genes (Campbell *et al.* 1988), which play an important part in the activation of the complement cascade.

Additionally, many genes of unknown function have been localized to this region, including G11 and RD (Sargent *et al.* 1989b; Spence *et al.* 1989), G12–G18 (Kendall *et al.* 1990; Spies *et al.* 1990) and OSG (Morel *et al.* 1989; Spence *et al.* 1989).

The telomeric end of the class III region has been studied in great detail using overlapping cosmid clones spanning a 550 kb interval between C2 and HLA-B (Spies *et al.* 1989b). This region includes functional genes encoding TNFα and β and the major heat shock proteins Hsp70-1 and Hsp70-2. Many genes of unknown function reside in this region also (Sargent *et al.* 1989a,b; Spence *et al.* 1989; Spies *et al.* 1989a,b), including G1–10, G9a, Hsp70-HOM, B144, BAT1 and BAT5. The G7a gene, which encodes valyl-tRNA synthetase (Dunham *et al.* 1990; Hsieh & Campbell 1991), has no obvious association with the immune system.

## Linkage disequilibrium and disease susceptibility

Another notable feature of the MHC is linkage disequilibrium. This term refers to the observation that some of the alleles of widely separated HLA loci occur together on the same chromosome, or haplotype, more frequently than would be expected if the assortment were totally random. In the context of a randomly breeding population at equilibrium the expected frequency with which two specificities occur together in a population is given by the product of the individual gene frequencies. For example, if 17% of the population have HLA-A1 and 11% have HLA-B8, the probability of finding the two alleles on the same chromosome is, theoretically, 1.9% (17% × 11%). However, the observed frequency in European caucasoid populations is actually 8.8% (Bodmer & Bodmer 1970), indicating a high degree of association between these two alleles; such non-random association is termed linkage disequilibrium.

It has become apparent that there are strong associations between HLA antigens and a large number of specific diseases. Ankylosing spondylitis is one of the most striking examples of an HLA and disease association (Ryder *et al.* 1981). HLA-B27 occurs in 90% of patients compared to 9.4% of controls. Other strong associations include HLA-DR3 with coeliac disease (79% vs. 26.3%), HLA-DR2 with multiple sclerosis (59% vs. 25.8%) and HLA-DR1 or DR4 with rheumatoid arthritis, to name but a few.

For some diseases, there are variations in HLA and disease associations between different racial groups. For instance, the Japanese have an HLA-DR4 association with myasthenia gravis, while in Caucasians this disease is associated with DR3 (Ryder *et al.* 1981). It is notable that most HLA-associated diseases have an autoimmune pathogenesis, and they are almost invariably associated with HLA class II loci. This is consistent with the central part played by MHC class II molecules in regulating CD4+ T cell help.

An interesting feature of these multiple HLA disease assosciations is that they often involve alleles exhibiting linkage disequilibrium with each other. For instance, the HLA-A3, B7 and DR2 haplotype is associated with multiple sclerosis, and many diseases exhibit associations between HLA-B8 and DR3 (Dausset & Svejgaard 1977). Two possibilities have been proposed to explain HLA and disease associations.

1 Disease susceptibility is the direct result of possession of a particular HLA antigen.

2 Disease association with a particular antigen(s) is the result of linkage disequilibrium between the HLA gene and an allele of a nearby gene.

Thus, the HLA gene and the molecule it encodes, which can be typed, may simply be markers for an allele of a susceptibility gene that has not yet been identified.

HLA population and family studies on susceptibility to insulin-dependent diabetes mellitus (IDDM) have demonstrated genetic associations. The earliest described associations were with HLA-B8, B18 and B15 but a more striking association was noted with the class II DR3 and DR4 antigens (Tiwari & Terasaki 1985), where 95% of Caucasian IDDM patients express either DR3 of DR4 (compared to 45–54% of healthy individuals). Furthermore, the risk of developing IDDM is enhanced in DR3/4 heterozygotes (Wolf *et al.* 1983). The HLA-DR3 and DR4 associations and the increased risk in heterozygotes have been established unequivocally in studies of HLA allele frequencies in IDDM families.

Molecular analyses using restriction fragment length polymorphisms (RFLP) have been employed to study the subtypes of DR3 and DR4 associated with IDDM susceptibility. Unexpectedly, the presence of particular allelic patterns of DQB1 restriction fragments was found to be associated more strongly with IDDM than DR3/4 heterozygosity (Michelson & Lernmark 1987). Transcomplementation has been offered as the explanation for such findings, where synergy between two haplotypes confers susceptibility greater that the summation of individual haplotype risks. Both *cis*- and *trans*-associated DQ heterodimers have been detected in IDDM patients, most notably the *trans*-associated dimer consisting of $DQ_\alpha$ (DR3) and $DQ_\beta$ (DR4) (Nepom *et al.* 1987).

Sequencing DQ genes from IDDM patients has provided the most direct evidence to date for linking HLA class II molecular structure with autoimmune disease susceptibility. Disease risk coincides with the presence of a non-charged amino acid at position 57 of DQB1 (Horn *et al.* 1988; Morel *et al.* 1988; Todd *et al.* 1988a), whereas haplotypes encoding a negatively charged aspartic acid (Asp-57) are associated with neutral or negative risk. This association extends to the non-obese diabetic (NOD) mouse (Todd *et al.* 1988b), which encodes a unique $IA_\beta$ chain in having a serine at position 57; non-diabetic mouse strains possess a protective Asp-57.

The strong association between DQB1 and susceptibility to IDDM favours the suggestion that the autoreactive effector T cells are specific for a pancreatic cell antigen in the context of particular DQ heterodimers. Based on the predicted structure of the MHC class II molecule (Brown *et al.* 1988), residue 57 of $DQ_\beta$ points in towards the antigen-binding groove. In addition, Asp-57 may form a salt bridge with the conserved arginine in $DQ_\alpha$ at position 79, serving to occlude one end of the groove. Hence, position 57 substitutions might alter the $DQ_{\alpha\beta}$ heterodimer, affecting antigen binding or T cell recognition. However, studies in other racial groups suggest that factors other than $DQ_\beta 57$ are involved in disease susceptibility (Lundin *et al.* 1989; Yamagata *et al.* 1989). The precise mechanisms underlying the HLA associations with IDDM will only become clear when the autoantigenic peptides seen by disease-inducing T cells are defined.

## T cell allorecognition of foreign MHC molecules

As mentioned at the start of this chapter, allogeneic MHC molecules are capable of stimulating uniquely strong primary immune responses. This is illustrated *in vitro* in the mixed lymphocyte reaction, and *in vivo* leads to organ graft rejection and graft versus host disease in recipients of allogeneic bone marrow grafts. This is the result of a very high frequency of T cells in the unperturbed T cell repertoire that react with MHC alloantigens. This was first observed in chickens in 1969 by Nisbet *et al.*, and was subsequently confirmed in several other species (Fischer Lindahl & Wilson, 1977).

### Two hypotheses to account for the high precursor frequency of anti-MHC alloreactive T cells — high determinant density or multiple binary complexes

Two hypotheses have been put forward to account for these observations, and are illustrated schematically in Fig. 2.8. The first is referred to as the 'high determinant density hypothesis', and envisages that the alloreactive T cell's receptor is specific for the foreign MHC struc-

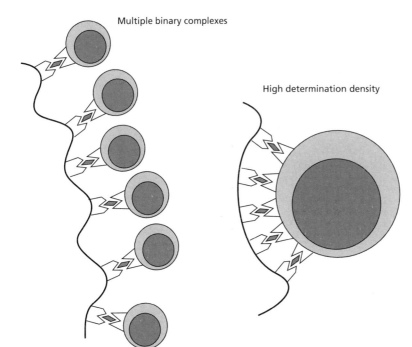

Multiple binary complexes

High determination density

**Fig. 2.8** Schematic representation of the two hypotheses that have been proposed to explain the high precursor frequency of anti-MHC alloreactive T cells.

ture, irrespective of what, if any, peptides are bound and displayed with the allogeneic MHC molecules at the cell surface (Bevan, 1984). If this was the case, all the MHC molecules of a given type on the surface of an allogeneic cell (approximately 105 class II molecules of a given isotype are expressed on the surface of a B cell) could act as ligands for the alloreactive T cell. This represents at least a 100-fold higher 'determinant density' than is available for an antigen-specific, self MHC-restricted T cell. In the latter case, it is unlikely that more than 1% of the MHC molecules of a particular type become occupied with any one individual peptide derived from a processed protein antigen. The relevance of this to the high frequency of alloreactive T cells is that, in the presence of such a high determinant density, T cells with a much lower specific affinity for their ligand could be recruited into the alloresponse, thereby expanding the frequency of alloreactive cells.

The second explanation may be referred to as the multiple binary complex hypothesis (Matzinger & Bevan, 1977). This explanation proposes that anti-MHC alloresponses are closely analogous to antigen responses, in that they are mediated by T cells that are specific for peptide:MHC complexes. In this case the peptide is a naturally processed peptide derived from a serum or cellular protein, and the MHC molecule is allogeneic. This would account for high frequencies of anti-MHC alloreactive T cells because of the wide diversity of different naturally processed peptides that are displayed with cell surface MHC molecules. It has been estimated that 2000 different species of peptides may be bound to a single type of MHC molecule at any one point in time. Thus, according to this hypothesis, a single MHC alloantigen could stimulate a large number of different T cell clones, each specific for a different peptide:MHC complex.

## Accommodating allorecognition within the context of positive selection of the T cell repertoire for self MHC restriction

During the past several years experimental data have

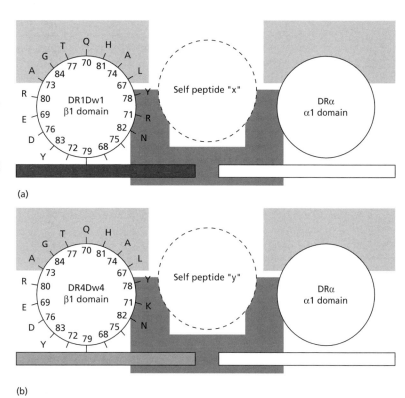

**Fig. 2.9** Schematic representation of a cross-section through the α-helices (solid circles) and the antiparallel strands (rectangles), forming the floor of the antigen-binding groove, that together constitute the amino terminal domains of (a) DR1Dw1 and (b) DR4Dw4. The orientation of individual amino acid residues of the β1 domain α-helix from positions 67 to 84 are shown as derived from Brown *et al.* (1988). The sequences of the antiparallel strands include multiple differences in the exposed regions, as indicated by the use of different patterns in the rectangular boxes. The surface of the molecules that is predicted to interact with the T cell receptor is highlighted with light shading, and the surface that is predicted to interact with bound peptides is highlighted with darker shading.

been accumulated that support both of the above hypotheses. For example, mutagenesis experiments have demonstrated the importance of exposed, TCR-contacting, residues on the surface of MHC alloantigens in T cell allorecognition (Ajitkumar *et al.*, 1988 ; Hogan *et al.*, 1989; Santos-Aguado *et al.*, 1989; Lombardi *et al.*, 1991b). Similarly, many groups have reported results that emphasize the involvement of MHC-bound peptides in T cell alloresponses (Heath *et al.*, 1989; Lombardi *et al.*, 1989; Panina-Bordignon *et al.*, 1991). Both of these hypotheses offer an explanation for the phenomenon of alloreactivity, but they fail to address a fundamental question, namely why does the unperturbed T cell repertoire, which has been selected in the thymus for self MHC restriction, contain such a high frequency of cells with specificity for allogeneic MHC molecules? Consideration of the structural relatedness of the responder and stimulator MHC molecules may provide mechanistic explana-

tions of allorecognition that can be accommodated within the framework of positive selection of the T cell repertoire for self MHC restriction. We have considered this issue in the context of allorecognition of HLA-DR molecules, and proposed that two distinct models may be necessary to resolve this conundrum (Lechler & Lombardi, 1990). The first is well illustrated by the alloresponse between a DR1 responder and a DR4Dw4 stimulator. The amino-terminal domains of these two DR types are portrayed schematically in Fig. 2.9. As can be seen, the amino acid sequences that make up the α-helical portions of these two molecules are highly conserved. Given that it is the sequences in this region that contact the TCR and impose the constraints of self MHC restriction, it is reasonable to imagine that T cells from a DR1 responder will recognize the exposed surface of DR4Dw4 as remarkably familiar, and can therefore utilize DR4Dw4 as a restriction element. Why then do DR1-

| DR consensus | 60 | 70 | 80 | 90 | | | Revised nomenclature |
|---|---|---|---|---|---|---|---|
| | RP–AE–WNSQKD–LE– | –R– | –VD–YCRHNYGV–ESFTVQRR | | | | |
| 1 w 1 | D Y | L | QR | AA | T | G | DRB1*0101 |
| 4 w 4 | D Y | L | QK | AA | T | G | DRB1*0401 |
| 4 w 14 | D Y | L | QR | AA | T | V | DBR1*0404 |
| 4 w 15 | S Y | L | QR | AA | T | G | DRB1*0105 |
| w 14 w 16 | D Y | L | QR | AA | T | G | DRB1*1401 |
| w 15 w2 | D Y | F | DR | AA | T | G | DRB5*0101 |
| w 15 w 12 | D Y | F | DR | AA | T | G | DRB5*0102 |
| w 16 w 21 | D Y | F | DR | AA | T | G | DRB5*0201 |
| w 11 w 5 | DE Y | F | DR | AA | T | G | DRB1*1101 |
| w 8 w 8.1 | S Y | F | DR | AL | T | G | DRB1*0801 |
| 4 w 10 | D Y | I | DE | AA | T | V | DRB1*0402 |
| w 11 wJVM | DE Y | I | DE | AA | T | V | DRB1*1102 |
| w 13 w 18 | D Y | I | DE | AA | T | V | DRB1*1301 |
| w 13 w 19 | D Y | I | DE | AA | T | G | DRB1*1302 |
| w 17 w 3 | D Y | L | QK | GR | N | V | DRB1*0301 |
| w 52 a | V S | L | QK | GR | N | G | DRB3*1010 |

**Fig. 2.10** Amino-terminal sequences of the carboxy-terminal half of multiple DRβ1 domains are presented. Only those residues that differ from the DR concensus sequence are shown Residues that are predicted to interact with the TCR are boxed.

restricted T cells recognize DR4Dw4 as an alloantigen? The probable explanation is provided by the fact that multiple sequence differences lie in the floor of the β1 domains of these two DR types. These differences are likely to lead to the binding and display of a significantly different array of serum and cellular peptides by DR4Dw4 compared to those displayed by DR1. Thus the alloresponse in this combination may be best explained by the recognition of multiple peptides that are bound by DR4Dw4 but not by DR1. The T cell repertoire from a DR1 individual would therefore not be tolerant to these 'novel' peptides. Furthermore, because of the conserved T cell-contacting regions of these two molecules, these novel peptides can be recognized by T cells selected for DR1 restriction in a manner that mimics self MHC restriction. This model of allorecognition can be invoked in a surprising number of responder:stimulator combinations, as illustrated by the comparison of DR β1 domain sequences, as shown in Fig. 2.10. DRβ chain sequences fall into groups that have conserved sequence in the α-helical portions of their β1 domains. This model of allorecognition envisages that the alloreactive T cells are specific for MHC-bound peptides, and has been supported by several experimental observations (as described above). This is consistent with the multiple binary complex hypothesis, outlined above.

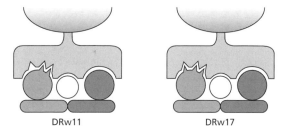

DRw11    DRw17

**Fig. 2.11** Allorecognition between responder:stimulator combinations with disparate MHC molecules may result from a chance high-affinity cross-reaction. The complex of MHC class II molecule (membrane-distal domains) and bound peptide (empty small circle) involved in DRw11-restricted and anti-DRw17 allospecific recognition by the same T cell clone are shown. The basis of this cross-reaction is explained in the text.

However, this does not account for all allore-sponses, in that strong alloresponses are observed in combinations in which multiple sequence differences exist in the TCR-contacting regions of the responder and stimulator MHC molecules. This is well illustrated by comparing the sequences of DRw17 and DRw11 (Fig. 2.11). In this kind of combination it is difficult to imagine anything resembling self MHC restriction occurring. The model that we have proposed to account for the alloresponse in this kind of combination involves specificity, by the alloreactive T cell, for the exposed MHC polymorphisms. The current model of positive selection of TCRs for self MHC restriction proposes that thymocytes are selected whose receptors have intermediate affinity for thymically expressed MHC molecules. Thymocytes whose receptors have high affinity for self MHC are deleted, to avoid autoreactivity. Thymocytes whose receptors have no useful affinity for thymically expressed MHC products fail to receive signals for further differentiation because they would serve no useful purpose in the individual's immune system (reviewed in Von Boehmer *et al.*, 1989). Within this context it can be imagined that a small fraction of T cells selected on the basis of having intermediate affinity for self MHC molecules may cross-react with higher affinity on allogeneic MHC types. This would be a chance event, and would only need to apply to 0.1% of all T cells to account for the kinds of frequencies that are observed against MHC alloantigens. This model of allorecognition is schematically represented in Fig. 2.11. One prediction that can be made, if this model applies, is that biased usage of TCR variable domains may be observed in an alloresponse between two individuals whose MHC molecules differ extensively in their TCR-contacting regions. This prediction is based on a computer-generated model of how the TCR interacts with an MHC molecule (Davis & Bjorkman, 1988). This model suggests that the portions of the TCR that make direct contact with the MHC α-helices are those that are encoded by the germline variable segments. To test this prediction, we analysed Vβ chain usage by a panel of alloreactive T cell clones generated from a DRw17 responder against a DRw11 stimulator. This revealed that five of nine clones utilized the Vβ13.1 or 13.2 family. In contrast, a panel of clones raised in a responder:stimulator combination that shared sequence identity in the β1 domain α-helix showed no biased Vβ usage (R.I. Lechler, unpublished results).

These considerations may prove to be important in the design of strategies for specific inhibition of allorecognition. For example, in the first kind of combination the administration of MHC-binding peptides that will compete for occupancy of the allogeneic MHC molecules may be advantageous; in the second, structurally dissimilar, kind of responder:stimulator combination, monoclonal antibodies or synthetic peptides will interfere directly with the interaction between the TCR and the allogeneic MHC molecule.

## Two pathways of allorecognition — direct and indirect

The above discussion has been confined to the phenomenon referred to as 'direct allorecognition', whereby T cells recognize the MHC alloantigen in an intact form on the surface of the allogeneic cell. This provides the most potent stimulus to the rejection of allogeneic tissue. However, alloimmunization by this route may be the prerogative of allogeneic cells with specialized APC function, such as dendritic cells and macrophages. This suggestion has been supported by the results of experimental models of kidney and thyroid transplantation, in which the depletion of donor-derived APC from the transplanted tissue led to greatly extended, if not indefinite, allograft survival (Lafferty *et al.*, 1975; Lechler & Batchelor, 1982).

In addition to the direct route of allorecognition, there is an alternative route by which MHC alloantigens can be recognized by T cells. MHC molecules can behave in a manner analogous to other protein antigens, in other words they can be taken up by responder APC, processed and presented in peptidic form with responder MHC molecules. This is known as 'indirect allorecognition'. It has been argued that this plays an important role in later forms of allograft rejection, once the donor-derived specialized APC have been replaced within the graft by recipient APC (Lechler & Batchelor 1982; Braun *et al.*, 1993). Evidence that allosensitization via the indirect route can accelerate graft rejection has been described by Dalchau *et al.* (1992).

## Minor histocompatibility antigens

### *In vivo* and *in vitro* definitions

All histocompatibility (H) antigens were originally identified by graft rejection (Snell 1948). Once the major histocompatibility antigens which elicited the most rapid graft rejection were defined as products of the HLA locus or complex in humans and the H2 in mice (Gorer *et al*. 1948; Ceppellini *et al*. 1969), it was clear that there were many additional loci encoding other minor histocompatibility antigens. These caused graft rejection between donor–recipient pairs matched for MHC antigens. In mice, it was possible by breeding experiments to follow the segregation of individual minor H loci and to develop congenic strains differing at single minor H loci (Bailey 1975). From studies using these mice, it was apparent that, while the antigens encoded by many single loci were indeed weak, eliciting prolonged graft rejection times, differences at multiple minor loci could stimulate almost as rapid a rejection as that against MHC antigens, i.e. their effects were additive or even synergistic. This is apparent in humans from the potential for developing severe graft vs. host disease in recipients of bone marrow transplants from HLA identical siblings (Van Els *et al*. 1990a,b). In humans matched for HLA antigens, there are always multiple minor H differences except in the case of monozygotic twins. Although kidney transplant patients receiving grafts from HLA-identical siblings do much better than recipients of HLA-mismatched grafts, they still require immunosuppression because of minor H incompatibilities.

*In vivo* host vs. graft and graft vs. host responses to histoincompatible tissue are mediated predominantly by T lymphocytes. B lymphocytes also make antibodies to MHC antigens and serological studies were of great importance in the early investigations of the genetics of the MHC and subsequently in their biochemical characterization, culminating in the crystal structure (Bjorkman *et al*. 1987a,b). T cell responses to histocompatibility antigens can also be obtained *in vitro*. Against MHC antigens, primary MLRs occur, characterized by proliferation, predominantly of CD4+ T cells stimulated by MHC class II disparities, and the development of CD8+ cytotoxic T cells specific for class I disparities. MLR against minor H antigens can also be obtained but only with responder T cells from individuals previously immunized *in vivo* by skin grafting or with spleen cells expressing the relevant antigen (Bevan 1975b; Gordon *et al*. 1975). No antibodies are

made to minor H antigens. However, both CD4+ and CD8+ T cell clones specific for components of minor H antigens can be isolated from secondary mixed lymphocyte cultures (MLC) and the minor H specificities defined by these T cell clones cosegregate with the loci encoding minor H antigens defined by *in vivo* grafting (Loveland & Simpson 1986). Minor H-specific cells, like those specific for viruses, are MHC restricted, that is they recognize the minor H antigen associated with a self MHC molecule, either class I in the case of CD8+ T cells or class II in the case of CD4+ T cells (Tomonari 1983). These T cells have been very useful in chromosomal mapping studies of the genetic regions encoding minor H antigens and tracing the segregation of minor H loci in experimental backcross or family studies (Loveland *et al*. 1985).

## Immunogenetics of responses to minor H antigens

The earliest *in vivo* studies in mice showed that minor H antigen genes were not linked to the MHC but were scattered throughout the genome. They were chromosomally mapped in congenic and recombinant inbred strains, using their linkage to previously identified markers (Bailey 1975). The development of minor H congenic strains, each differing from the parental strain by a putatively single minor locus, allowed investigations of *in vivo* and *in vitro* responses to isolated minor H antigens, as did the use of selected inbred strains in which the females were able to generate immune responses to cells and grafts from males of the same strain. These responses defined the male-specific minor H antigen, H-Y, encoded on the Y chromosome. The responses to H-Y, both *in vivo* and *in vitro*, demonstrated an asymmetry which is now apparent in responses to some other minor H antigens and endogenous T cell-recognized epitopes, such as the minor lymphocyte stimulatory (Mls) antigens (Festenstein 1973; Simpson *et al*. 1993). Female mice of H-Y responder strains (comprising mainly those of the $H2^b$ haplotype) reject syngeneic male skin grafts but males do not reject syngeneic female grafts (Eichwald & Silmser 1955; Simpson 1982). Between minor H congenic strains and their parental strain, there is also often an asymmetry in the response. For example, the H1 congenic strain B6.H1b rapidly rejects parental skin grafts from B6 mice which have the H1c allele, whereas B6 mice reject only very slowly, or fail to reject, skin grafts from B6.H1b mice (Bailey 1975).

It was originally assumed that such asymmetries were caused by differences in strengths of allelic genes located in homologous regions of the chromosome in the parental strain and its minor H congenic partner. However, recent work of Roopenian *et al.* (1993) provides an alternative explanation of some +/− alleles from the observation of a loss mutation in an inbred strain allowing it to recognize by *in vivo* graft rejection or *in vitro* CTL a minor H antigen present on the wild-type strain and a number of laboratory strains, as well as different *Mus* species. In this study, it was also reported that the chromosomal localization of several minor H antigens defined in inbred laboratory strains of mice (*Mus musculus*) was found in other mouse species such as *M. spretus* and *M. castaneous*, suggesting limited polymorphism predating speciation. Furthermore, there was an evolutionary relationship between strains or species not expressing these antigens, consistent with them inheriting a shared loss mutation. The presence of a minor H antigen may thus represent a + allele and its absence a mutation resulting in loss of expression detectable by T cells, i.e. a null allele.

This explanation could also account for the very interesting pattern of occurrence of minor H antigens defined by T cell clones in human populations (Van Els *et al.* 1992; Schreuder *et al.* 1993). Some minor H antigens appear with very high frequency (>90%), others much lower (<10%). Each is inherited in a Mendelian fashion, transmitted by parents who from analysis of their progeny are phenotypically positive for a particular minor H antigen, by being either homozygous (+/+) or heterozygous (+/−) for the encoding gene. However, more recently it has been shown that there are examples of autosomally encoded minor H antigens in mice and humans in which the two alleles are created by single amino acid substitutions (see Simpson & Roopenian 1997).

There is, however, a particular set of T cell-recognized endogenous molecules characterized by a + or − genotype. These are the endogenous superantigens encoded by mouse mammary tumour provirus (Mtv) integrations, some of which stimulate primary MLRs *in vitro* and most of which are associated with T cell receptor V-specific repertoire selection *in vivo* (Simpson *et al.* 1993). Mice having the relevant Mtv delete the appropriate Vβ+ T cells in the thymus and their spleen cells can stimulate T cells from mice not having this Mtv. However, the evidence suggests that Mtv integrations do not encode antigens that can be recognized *in vivo* by graft rejection responses. This comes from experiments in which skin grafts were exchanged between the Mlsa (Mtv-7) congenic strains BALB/c (wt) and BALB/c Mlsa (with the Mlsa derived from the DBA/2 strain): BALB/c mice do not readily reject skin from BALB/c Mlsa donors (Berumen *et al.* 1983). This finding may be related to the need for the involvement of both CD4+ and CD8+ T cells, responding to MHC class II and I presented epitopes, respectively, for graft rejection to occur (Roopenian 1992). Responses to Mtv superantigens are primarily of CD4+ T cells but an additional factor to take into account is that expression of Mtv integrants is tissue-specific and limited to B lymphocytes and thus absent on skin. Minor H antigens which are the targets of graft vs. host (gvh) and host vs. graft (hvg) responses *in vivo* must be expressed on target issues and there is evidence for ubiquitous expression on most tissues of a number of minor H antigens (Johnson *et al.* 1981) and this includes HY antigens, encoded by at least two ubiquitously expressed Y chromosome genes (Simpson *et al.* 1997).

## Two-signal requirement for rejection of minor H mismatched grafts

On close examination, it became clear that minor H loci consisted of a complex of closely linked genes (Roopenian 1992). From spleen cells of mice immunized *in vivo* by grafting with skin disparate for minor H antigens, such as H-Y, H3 or H4, can be isolated both CD4+ and CD8+ T cell clones restricted by MHC class II and I molecules, respectively (Tomonari 1983; Roopenian 1992). These clones can be used to type inbred, recombinant inbred and backcross mice

(Loveland *et al.* 1985; Fowlis *et al.* 1992; Roopenian *et al.* 1993) for the presence of the relevant minor H antigen. This has been done using a CD4+ and a CD8+ T cell clone raised following immunization between an H3 congenic pair (Roopenian & Davis 1989). A number of independently derived H3 congenic strains were typed and from the results it was clear that the CD4+ T cell clone identified an epitope encoded by a gene separate from that of the CD8+ T cell clone. This was subsequently confirmed by classic backcross analysis, in which the genes encoding the two epitopes were separated by recombination. A similar study of the H4 region produced comparable results (Davis & Roopenian 1990), as did an analogous approach to the region encoding the H-Y gene (Scott *et al.* 1991; King *et al.* 1994). These data, together with the findings from transgenic mice expressing just components of minor H antigens recognized by CD8+ T cells, whose skin grafts are not rejected by transgene negative (or wild-type) littermates (Antoniou *et al.* 1996; Hederer *et al.* 1996), argue that, to stimulate graft rejection, separate epitopes recognized by CD4+ and CD8+ T cells are both necessary.

## Molecular nature of minor H antigens

One of the earliest findings using T cells specific for minor H antigens was that their recognition was MHC-restricted (Bevan 1975b; Gordon *et al.* 1975). In this they did not differ from viral antigens (Zinkernagel & Doherty 1974), subsequently shown to be short peptides (Townsend *et al.* 1986b). The crystal structure of HLA class I molecules showed the peptide-binding groove of the presenting molecule with an electron-dense area corresponding to a peptide (Bjorkman *et al.* 1987a) and it is now clear that peptide is an essential component stabilizing the structure of MHC molecules (see Plate 2.1, facing p. 342).

Taken together these observations strongly suggested that minor H antigens were likely to be endogenous peptides bound in the peptide-binding grooves of class I and II molecules. From knowledge of allele-specific peptide-binding motifs (Falk *et al.* 1991), the relevant class I-bound peptides were predicted to be octamers to pentamers with characteristic anchor residues and found within the groove, the class II-bound peptides to be longer and protrude at either end of the groove but held within it by allele-specific anchor residues. The genetic *in vivo* and *in vitro* data suggest that both class I- and II-bound peptides are derived from endogenous proteins and become loaded into the corresponding MHC molecule during biosynthesis. For class I molecules, there is good evidence that this occurs in the ER but the route by which class II molecules acquire peptides from endogenously synthesized proteins within the cell may represent leakage of the class II pathway involving autophagy (see Fig. 2.3).

There is now direct evidence for the peptide nature of several minor histocompatibility antigen components defined by CD8+ T cells *in vitro*. The pioneering work of Rammensee in this area showed that peptides separated from membrane-bound MHC class I molecules by acid elution followed by high-performance liquid chromatography (HPLC) fractionation could subsequently be used to sensitize target cells expressing the appropriate MHC molecules (but lacking the minor H antigen in question) for lysis by minor H antigen-specific CTL clones (Rötzschke *et al.* 1990). CD8+ T cell clones specific for an HY epitope recognized in the context of $D^b$ and an H4 epitope recognized in association with $D^b$ were defined in this way (Rötzschke *et al.* 1990). A $D^b$-restricted H1 epitope recognized by CD8 cells has been similarly defined (Yin *et al.* 1993), as well as HLA class I restricted minor H epitopes recognized by human CD8 T cell clones (Sekimata *et al.* 1992). Loveland *et al.* (1990) described the identification of a peptide derived from a mitochondrial genome-encoded protein, recognized by T cells in association with a non-classic MHC class I molecule, Hmt (H2M3), and which accounted for the maternally transmitted minor transplantation antigen, Mtf. This was the first molecular identification of a minor H antigen as a specific peptide. In addition, a number of tumour-specific transplantation antigens (TSTA) defined by CD8+ T cells have also been shown to be peptides following the cloning of genes encoding them and identification of the minimal DNA sequence which could specify the peptide (De Plaen *et al.* 1988; Van den Eynde *et al.* 1991; Van der Bruggen *et al.* 1991). This has been found to be true of a number of mutagen-induced TSTA in an experimental mouse tumour (De Plaen *et al.* 1988), as well as endogenous TSTA of that same tumour (Van den Eynde *et al.* 1991) and endogenous TSTA in human melanomas (Van der Bruggen *et al.* 1991). So far there have been no reports of elution from class II molecules of minor H or TSTA recognized by CD4+ T cells.

The molecular identification of several minor H peptides has recently been achieved using a combination of peptide elution followed by sequencing, and the cloning of genes encoding them following transfection. The peptide elution and sequencing approach has relied on the presence in the DNA database of genes already identified and sequenced. The human HLA-A2 restricted HA-2 peptide was found in this way to be derived from a member of the myosin heavy chain gene family (den Haan 1995) and the human HLA-B7 restricted HY peptide the product of the *SMCY* gene (Wang *et al.* 1995), whose mouse homologue, *Smcy*, had already been identified as encoding the mouse HY/K$^k$-restricted epitope (Scott *et al.* 1995). The sequence of the HY/K$^k$ peptide epitope was determined following the identification of the encoding gene following transfection and, by comparing the DNA sequence of the Y chromosome gene, *Smcy*, with the X chromosome homologue, *Smcx*. A second quite separate gene, *Uty*, was discovered by a similar process to encode the immunodominant HY/D$^b$ peptide epitope (Greenfield *et al.* 1996). This finding illustrates at the genomic level the genetic complexity of a minor H locus, and shows it rather to be a gene complex. It is likely that there will be further genes in the same region of the Y chromosome that encode HY peptide epitopes restricted by MHC class II molecules and recognized by CD4+ cells, and the expression cloning approach is a good way to discover them as they may, like *Smcy* and *Uty*, be novel genes whose sequence is not yet in the database.

A better understanding of how to trigger activation of effector T cells directed against TSTA and of how best to prevent activation of effector cells against the minor H antigen targets of graft vs. host and host vs. graft responses is now needed. The identification of the endogenous peptide targets is an important step forward. It is very likely that CD8 recognized epitopes alone are insufficient to cause activation and may in fact induce tolerance (Antoniou *et al.* 1996); concomitant triggering of CD4+ T cells against epitopes of other TSTA or alloantigens are almost certainly necessary to obtain effector function. There is also evidence in mice and humans that certain epitopes present amongst many, as in responses to multiple minor H antigens, elicit a dominant response (Loveland & Simpson 1986; Wettstein 1986; Yin *et al.* 1993; Wolpert *et al.* 1995). The molecular basis of this potentially clinically important finding is not yet understood but the tools to unravel the questions are now to hand, with the extensive battery of T cell clones of known restriction and peptide specificity, the methods of eluting, separating and sequencing peptides, and the expression cloning systems now modified for detection using T cell clones for the identification of genes encoding the peptide epitopes (De Plaen *et al.* 1988; Rötzschke *et al.* 1990; Van den Eynde *et al.* 1991; Van der Bruggen *et al.* 1991; Hunt *et al.* 1992; Scott *et al.* 1992; Sekimata *et al.* 1992; Yin *et al.* 1993; Simpson & Roopenian 1997).

## References

Accolla, R.S., Auffray, C., Singer, D.S. & Guardiola, J. (1991) The molecular biology of MHC genes. *Immunology Today* **12**, 97–99.

Ajitkumar, P., Geier, S.S., Kesaro, L.V. *et al.* (1988) Evidence that multiple residues on both the α-helices of the class I MHC molecule are simultaneously recognized by the T cell receptor. *Cell* **54**, 47–56.

Albert, L.J., Denzin, L.K., Ghumman, B. *et al.* (1998) Quantitative defect in staphylococcal enterotoxin A binding and presentation by HLA-DM deficient T2.Ak cells corrected by transfection of HLA-DM genes. *Cell Immunology* **183**, 42–51.

Anderson, G.D. & David, C.S. (1989) In vivo expression and function of hybrid Ia dimers (EαAβ) in recombinant and transgenic mice. *Journal of Experimental Medicine* **170**, 1003–1008.

Anderson, P., Blue, M.-L. & Schlossman, S.F. (1988) Comodulation of CD3 and CD4. Evidence for a specific association between CD4 and approximately 5% of the CD3: T cell receptor complexes on helper T lymphocytes. *Journal of Immunology* **140**, 1732–1737.

Antoniou, A., McCormick, D., Scott, D. *et al.* (1996) T cell tolerance and activation to a transgene-encoded tumor antigen. *European Journal of Immunology* **26**, 1094–1102.

Arenzana-Seisdedos, F., Morgensen, S.C., Vuillier, F., Fiers, W. & Virelizier, J.L. (1988) Autocrine secretion of tumor necrosis factor under the influence interferon-gamma amplifies HLA-DR gene induction in human monocytes. *Proceedings of the National Academy of Sciences USA* 85, 6087–6091.

Attaya, M., Jameson, S., Martinez, C.K. *et al.* (1992) Ham-2 corrects the class I antigen-processing defect in RMA-S cells. *Nature* 355, 647–649.

Babbitt, B., Allen, P.M., Matsueda, G., Haber, E. & Unanue, E.R. (1985) The binding of immunogenic peptides to Ia histocompatibility molecules. *Nature* 317, 359–361.

Bailey, D.W. (1975) Genetics of histocompatibility in mice I. New loci and congenic lines. *Immunogenetics* 2, 249–256.

Baur, M.P. & Danilovs, J.A. (1980) Population analysis of HLA-A, B, C, DR and other genetic markers. In: *Histocompatibility Testing* (ed. P. I. Terasaki), pp. 955–993. UCLA Tissue Typing Laboratory, Los Angeles.

Beck, B.N., Frelinger, J.G., Shigeta, M. *et al.* (1982) T cell clones specific for hybrid I-A molecules. Discrimination with moloclonal anti-I-A$^k$ antibodies. *Journal of Experimental Medicine* 156, 1186–1194.

Bell, J.I., Todd, J.A. & McDevitt, H.O. (1989) Molecular structure of human class II antigens. In: *Immunobiology of HLA,* Vol II. (ed. B. Dupont), pp. 40–48. Springer-Verlag, New York.

Benoist, C. & Mathis, D. (1990) Regulation of major histocompatibility complex class II genes: X, Y and other letters of the alphabet. *Annual Review of Immunology* 8, 681–715.

Berumen, L., Halle-Pannenko, O. & Festenstein, H. (1983) Histocompatibility effects of the Mls locus. *Transplantation Proceedings* 15, 213–216.

Bevan, M.J. (1975a) Interaction antigens detected by cytotoxic T cells with the major histocompatibility complex as modifier. *Nature* 256, 419–421.

Bevan, M.J. (1975b) The major histocompatibility complex determines susceptibility to cytotoxic T cells directed against minor histocompatibility antigens. *Journal of Experimental Medicine* 142, 1349–1364.

Bevan, M.J. (1984) High determinant density may explain the phenomenon of alloreactivity. *Immunology Today* 5, 128–130.

Bikoff, E.K., Husng, L.Y., Episkopou, V. *et al.* (1993) Defective major histocompatibility complex class II assembly, transport, peptide acquisition, and CD4+ T cell selection in mice lacking invariant chain expression. *Journal of Experimental Medicine* 177, 1699–1712.

Bjorkman, P.J. & Parham, P. (1990) Structure, function and diversity of class I major histocompatibility molecules. *Annual Review of Biochemistry* 59, 253–288.

Bjorkman, P.J., Saper, M.A., Samraoui, B. *et al.* (1987a) Structure of the human class I histocompatibility antigen HLA-A2. *Nature* 329, 506–512.

Bjorkman, P.J.H., Saper, M.A., Samraoui, B. *et al.* (1987b) The foreign antigen binding site and T cell recognition regions of class I histocompatibility antigens. *Nature* 329, 512–518.

Blanck, G. & Strominger, J.L. (1990) Cosmid clones in the HLA-DZ and -DP subregions. *Human Immunology* 27, 265–268.

Blaschitz, A., Lenfant, F., Mallet, V. *et al.* (1997) Endothelial cells in chorionic fetal vessels of first trimester placenta express HLA-G. *European Journal of Immunology* 27, 3380–3388.

Bodmer, J.G. & Bodmer, W.F. (1970) Studies on African pygmies. (IV) A comparative study of the HLA polymorphism in the Babinga pygmies and other African and Caucasian population. *American Journal of Human Genetics* 22, 396–411.

Bodmer, J.G., Marsh, S.G.E., Albert, E.D. *et al.* (1992a) Nomenclature for factors of the HLA system, 1991. *Tissue Antigens* 39, 161–173.

Bodmer, J., Marsh, S.G.E., Albert, E.D. *et al.* (1992b) Nomenclature for factors of the HLA system 1991. *European Journal of Immunogenetics* 19, 327–344.

Bodmer, J.G., Marsh, S.G., Albert, E.D. *et al.* (1994) Nomenclature for factors of the HLA system, 1994. *Tissue Antigens* 44, 1–18.

Bodmer, J.G., Marsh, S.G.E., Albert, E.D. *et al.* (1995) Nomenclature for factors of the HLA system, 1995. *Tissue Antigens* 46, 1–18.

Bottazzo, G.F., Pujol-Borrell, R., Hanafusa, A. & Feldman, M. (1983) Role of aberrant HLA-DR expression and antigen presentation in induction of endocrine autoimmunity. *Lancet* ii, 1115–1118.

Bottazzo, G.F., Dean, B.M., McNally, J.M. *et al.* (1985) In situ characterization of autoimmune phenomena and expression of HLA molecules in the pancreas in diabetic insulitis. *New England Journal of Medicine* 313, 353–360.

Braun, M.Y., McCormack, A., Webb, G. & Batchelor, J.R. (1993) Mediation of acute but not chronic rejection of MHC-imcompatible rat kidney grafts by alloreactive CD4 T cells activated by the direct pathway of sensitization. *Transplantation* 55, 177–182.

Braunstein, N.S. & Germain, R.N. (1987) Allele-specific control of Ia molecule surface expression and conformation: implication for a general model of Ia structure-function relationships. *Proceedings of the National Academy of Sciences USA* 84, 2921–2925.

Broathen, L.R. (1981) Studies on human epidermal Langerhans cells. III. Induction of T lymphocyte response to nickel sulphate in sensitized individuals. *British Journal of Dermatology* 103, 517–526.

Brown, J.H., Jardetzky, T., Saper, M.A. *et al.* (1988) A hypothetical model of the foreign antigen binding site of class II histocompatibility molecules. *Nature* 332, 845–850.

Brown, J.H., Jardetzky, T.S., Gorga, J.C. *et al.* (1993) Three dimensional structure of the human class-II histocompatibility antigen DR-1. *Nature* **364**, 33–39.

Burkly, L.C., Lo, D., Cowing, C. *et al.* (1989) Selective expression of class II $E_\alpha^d$ gene in transgenic mice. *Journal of Immunology* **142**, 2081–2088.

Buus, S., Sette, A., Colon, S.M., Jenis, D.M. & Grey, H.M. (1986) Isolation and characterization of antigen-Ia complexes in T cell recognition. *Cell* **47**, 1071–1077.

Cammarota, G., Scheirle, A., Takacs, B. *et al.* (1992) Identification of the CD4 binding site on the β2 domain of HLA-DR molecules. *Nature* **356**, 799–801.

Campbell, R.D., Alex Law, S.K., Reid, K.B.M. & Sim, R.B. (1988) Structure, organization and regulation of the complement genes. *Annual Review of Immunology* **6**, 161–195.

Campbell, R.D., Dunham, I., Kendall, E. & Sargent, C.A. (1990) Polymorphism of the human complement component C4. *Experimental Clinical Immunogenetics* **7**, 69–84.

Cano, P. & Baxter-Lowe, L.A. (1995) Novel human TAP2*103 allele shows further polymorphism in the ATP-binding domain. *Tissue Antigens* **45**, 143–144.

Carbone, F.R. & Bevan, M.J. (1990) Class I-restricted processing and presentation of exogenous cell-associated antigen in vivo. *Journal of Experimental Medicine* **171**, 377–387.

Carroll, M.C., Katzman, P., Alicot, E.M. *et al.* (1987) Linkage map of the human major histocompatibility complex including the tumor necrosis factor genes. *Proceedings of the National Academy of Sciences USA* **84**, 8535–8539.

Castellino, F., Zhong, G. & Germain, R.N. (1997) Antigen presentation by MHC class II molecules: invariant chain function, protein trafficking, and the molecular basis of diverse determinant capture. *Human Immunology* **54**, 159–169.

Ceppellini, R., Mattiuz, P.L., Schudeller, G. & Visetti, M. (1969) Experimental allotransplantation in man I. The role of the HLA system in different genetic combinations. *Transplantation Proceedings* **1**, 385–389.

Cerendolo, V., Elliott, T., Elvin, J. *et al.* (1991) The binding affinity and dissociation rates of peptides for class I major histocompatibility complex molecules. *European Journal of Immunology* **21**, 2069–2075.

Chicz, R.M., Urban, R.G., Lane, W.S. *et al.* (1992) Predominantly naturally processed peptides bound to HLA-DR1 are derived from MHC-related molecules and are heterogeneous in size. *Nature* **358**, 764–768.

Cho, S., Attaya, M. & Monaco, J.J. (1991) New class II-like genes in the murine MHC. *Nature* **353**, 573–576.

Collins, T., Korman, A.J., Wake, C.T. *et al.* (1984) Immune interferon activates multiple class II major histocompatibility complex genes and the associated invariant chain gene in human endothelial cells and dermal fibroblasts. *Proceedings of the National Academy of Sciences USA* **81**, 4917–4921.

Collins, T., Lapierre, L., Fiers, W., Strominger, J. & Pober, J. (1986) Recombinant human tumor necrosis factor increases mRNA levels and surface expression of HLA-A,B antigens in vascular endothelial cells and dermal fibroblasts in vitro. *Proceedings of the National Academy of Sciences USA* **83**, 446–450.

Coux, O., Tanaka, K. & Goldberg, A.L. (1996) Structure and function of the 20S and 26S proteasomes. *Annual Review of Biochemistry* **65**, 801–847.

Cramer, L.A. & Klemsz, M.J. (1997) Altered kinetics of Tap-1 gene expression in macrophages following stiumulation with both IFN-γ and LPS. *Cell Immunology* **178**, 53–61.

Cresswell, P. & Geier, S.S. (1975) Antisera to human B-lymphocyte membrane glycoproteins block stimulation in mixed lymphocyte culture. *Nature* **257**, 147–149.

Cresswell, P., Turner, M.J. & Strominger, J.L. (1973) Papain-solubilized HL-A antigens from cultured human lymphocytes contain two peptide fragments. *Proceedings of the National Academy of Sciences USA* **70**, 1603–1607.

Daar, A.S., Fuggle, S.V., Fabre, J.W., Ting, A. & Morris, P.J. (1984a) The detailed distribution of HLA-A, B, C antigens in normal human organs. *Transplantation* **38**, 287–292.

Daar, A.S., Fuggle, S.V., Fabre, J.W., Ting, A. & Morris, P.J. (1984b) The detailed distribution of MHC class II antigens in normal human organs. *Transplantation* **38**, 293–298.

Dalchau, R., Fangmann, J. & Fabre, J.W. (1992) Allorecognition of isolated, denatured chains of class I and class II major histocompatibility complex molecules. Evidence for an important role for indirect allorecognition in transplantation. *European Journal of Immunology* **22**, 669–677.

Darnell, J.E. Jr (1997) STATs and gene regulation. *Science* **277**, 1630–1635.

Das, H.K., Lawrance, S.K. & Weissman, S.M. (1983) Structure and nucleotide sequence of the heavy chain gene of HLA-DR. *Proceedings of the National Academy of Sciences USA* **80**, 3543–3547.

Dausset, J. & Svejgaard, A., eds (1977) *HLA and Disease.* Munksgaard, Copenhagen.

David-Watine, B., Israel, A. & Kourilsky, P. (1990) The regulation and expression of MHC class I genes. *Immunology Today* **11**, 286–292.

Davis, A.P. & Roopenian, D.C. (1990) Complexity at the mouse minor histocompatibility locus H-4. *Immunogenetics* **31**, 7–12.

Davis, M.M. & Bjorkman, P.J. (1988) T-cell antigen receptor genes and T-cell recognition. *Nature* **334**, 395–402.

De Plaen, E., Lurquin, C., Van Pel, A. *et al.* (1988) Immunogenic (tum-) variants of mouse tumor P815:

cloning of the gene of tum- antigen P91A and identification of the tum- mutation. *Proceedings of the National Academy of Sciences USA* **85**, 2274–2278.

Den Haan, J.M., Sherman, N.E., Blokland, E. *et al.* (1995) Identification of a graft versus host disease-associated human minor histocompatibility antigen. *Science* **268**, 1476–1480.

Denzin, L.K. & Cresswell, P. (1995) HLA-DM induces CLIP dissociation from MHC class II alpha beta dimers and facilitates peptide loading. *Cell* **82**, 155–165.

Denzin, L.K., Robbins, N.F., Carboy-Newcomb, C. & Cresswell, P. (1994) Assembly and intracellular transport of the HLA-DM and correction of the class II antigen-processing defects in T2 cealls. *Immunity* **1**, 595–606.

Denzin, L.K., Sant'Angelo, D.B., Hammond, C., Surman, M.J. & Cresswell, P. (1997) Negative regulation by HLA-DO of MHC class II-restricted antigen processing. *Science* **278**, 106–109.

Dessen, A., Lawrence, C.M., Cupo, S., Zaller, D.M. & Wiley, D.C. (1997) X-ray crystal structure of HLA-DR4 (DRA*0101, DRB1*0401) complexes with a peptide from human collagen II. *Immunity* **7**, 473–481.

Deverson, E.V., Gow, I.R., Coadwell, W.J. *et al.* (1990) MHC class II region encoding proteins related to the multidrug resistance family of transmembrane transporters. *Nature* **348**, 738–741.

Dice, J.F. (1990) Peptide sequences that target cytosolic proteins for lysosomal proteolysis. *Trends in Biochemistry and Science* **15**, 305–309.

Diehl, M., Munz, C., Keiholz, W. *et al.* (1996) Nonclassical HLA-G molecules are classical peptide presenters. *Current Biology* **6**, 305–314.

Dorn, A., Durand, B., Marfing, C. *et al.* (1987) Conserved major histocompatibility complex class II boxes -X and -Y are transcriptional control elements and specifically bind nuclear proteins. *Proceedings of the National Academy of Sciences USA* **84**, 6249–6253.

Dorn, A., Fehling, H.J., Kock, W. *et al.* (1988) B-cell control region at the 5′ end of a MHC class II gene: sequences and factors. *Molecular Cell Biology* **8**, 3975–3987.

Douek, D.C. & Altmann, D.M. (1997) HLA-DO is an intracellular class II molecule with distinctive thymic expression. *International Immunology* **9**, 355–364.

Driscoll, J., Brown, M.G., Finley, D. & Monaco, J.J. (1993) MHC-linked LMP gene products specifically alter peptidase activity of the proteasome. *Nature* **365**, 262–264.

Dunham, I., Sargent, C.A., Trowsdale, J. & Campbell, R.D. (1987) Molecular mapping of the human major histocompatibility complex by pulsed-field gel electrophoresis. *Proceedings of the National Academy of Sciences USA* **84**, 7237–7241.

Dunham, I., Sargent, C.A., Kendall, E. & Campbell, R.D. (1990) Characterization of the class III region in different MHC haplotypes by pulsed-field gel electrophoresis. *Immunogenetics* **32**, 175–182.

Eichwald, E.J. & Silmser, C.R. (1955) Untitled. *Transplant Bulletin* **2**, 148.

Elliott, T., Elvin, J., Cerundolo, V., Allen, H. & Townsend, A. (1992) Structural requirements for the peptide-induced conformational change of free major histocompatibility complex class I heavy chains. *European Journal of Immunology* **22**, 2085–2091.

Ellis, S.A., Sargent, I.L., Redman, W.G. & McMichael, A.J. (1986) Evidence for a novel HLA antigen found on human extravillous trophoblast and a choriocarcinoma cell line. *Immunology* **59**, 595–601.

Ellis, S.A., Palmer, M.S. & McMichael, A.J. (1990) Human trophoblast and the choriocarcinoma cell line BeWo express a truncated HLA class I molecule. *Journal of Immunology* **144**, 731–735.

Falk, K., Rötzschke, O., Stevanovic, S., Jang, G. & Rammensee, H.-G. (1991) Allele-specific motifs revealed by sequencing of self-peptides eluted from MHC molecules. *Nature* **351**, 290–296.

Festenstein, H. (1973) Immunogenetic and biological aspects of in vitro lymphocyte allotransformation (MLR) in the mouse. *Transplantation Reviews* **15**, 62–88.

Fields, B.A., Ober, B., Malchiodi, E.L. *et al.* (1995) Crystal structure of the Vα domain of a T cell antigen receptor. *Science* **270**, 1821–1824.

Fischer Lindahl, K. & Wilson, D.B. (1977) Histocompatibility antigen-activated cytotoxic T lymphocytes. I. Estimates of the absolute frequency of killer cells generated in vitro. *Journal of Experimental Medicine* **145**, 500–507.

Flaherty, L. (1976) The Tla region of the mouse: identification of a new serologically defined locus, Qa-2. *Immunogenetics* **3**, 533.

Flaherty, L. (1980) Tla-region antigens. In: *Role of the Major Histocompatibility Complex in Immunology* (ed. M. Dorf), pp. 33–57. Garland Press, New York.

Fling, S., Arp, B. & Pious, D. (1994) HLA-DMA and -DMB genes are both required for MHC class II/peptide complex formation in antigen presenting cells. *Nature* **368**, 554–558.

Foss, G.S., Larsen, F., Solheim, J. & Prydz, H. (1998) Constitutive and interferon-g-induced expression of the human proteasome subunit multicatalytic endopeptidase complex-like 1. *Biochimica et Biophysica Acta* **1402**, 17–28.

Fowlis, G.A., Fairchild, S., Tomonari, K. & Simpson, E. (1992) Toward identification of minor histocompatibility antigens in mouse and man. *Transplantation Proceedings* **24**, 1689–1691.

Frank, G.D. & Parnes, J.R. (1998) The level of CD4 surface protein influences T cell selection in the thymus. *Journal of Immunology* **160**, 634–642.

Fremont, D.H., Hendrickson, W.A., Marrack, P. & Kappler, J.W. (1996) Structure of an MHC class II molecule with covalently bound single peptides. *Science* 272, 1001–1004.

Fremont, D.H., Monnale, D., Nelson, C.A.S., Hendrickson, W.A. & Unanue, E.R. (1998) Crystal structure of I-Ak in complex with a dominant epitope of lysozyme. *Immunity* 8, 305–317.

Friedman, R.L. & Stark, G.R. (1985) Alpha interferon induces transcription of HLA and metallothionein genes which have homologous upstream sequences. *Nature* 314, 637–639.

Gaczynska, M., Rock, K.L. & Goldberg, A.L. (1993) γ-Interferon and expression of MHC genes regulate peptide hydrolysis by proteasomes. *Nature* 365, 264–267.

Ganguly, S., Vasavada, H.A. & Weissman, S.M. (1989) Multiple enhancer-like sequences in the HLA-B7 gene. *Proceedings of the National Academy of Sciences USA* 86, 5247–5251.

Garboczi, D.N., Ghosh, P., Utz, U. *et al.* (1996) Structure of the complex between human T-cell receptor, viral peptide and HLA-A2. *Nature* 384, 134–141.

Garcia, K.C., Degano, M., Stanfield, R.L. *et al.* (1996) An αβ T cell receptor structure at 2.5 Angstroms and its orientation in the TCR-MHC complex. *Science* 274, 209–219.

Garrett, T.P., Saper, M.A., Bjorkman, P.J., Strominger, J.L. & Wiley, D.C. (1989) Specificity pockets for the side chains of peptide antigens in HLA-Aw68. *Nature* 342, 692–696.

Gautam, A.M., Yang, M., Milburn, P.J. *et al.* (1997) Identification of residues in the class II-associated Ii peptide (CLIP) region of variant chain that affect efficiency of MHC class II-mediated antigen presentation in an allele-dependent manner. *Journal of Immunology* 159, 2782–2788.

Geraghty, D.E., Koller, B.H. & Orr, H.T. (1987) A human major histocompatibility complex class I gene that encodes a protein with a shortened cytoplasmic segment. *Proceedings of the National Academy of Sciences USA* 84, 9145–9149.

Geraghty, D.E., Wei, X., Orr, H.T. & Koller, B.H. (1990) Human leukocyte antigen F (HLA-F). An expressed HLA gene composed of a class I coding sequence linked to a novel transcribed repetitive element. *Journal of Experimental Medicine* 171, 1–18.

Germain, R.N. & Quill, H. (1986) Unexpected expression of a unique mixed isotype class II MHC molecule by transfected L-cells. *Nature* 320, 72–75.

Ghosh, P., Amaya, M., Mellins, E. & Wiley, D.C. (1995) The structure of an intermediate in class II MHC maturation: CLIP bound to HLA-DR3. *Nature* 378, 457–462.

Gillies, S.D., Falsam, V. & Tonegawa, S. (1984) Cell type specific enhancer element associated with a mouse MHC gene, Eβ. *Nature* 310, 594–597.

Gluzman, Y. & Shenk, T., eds (1983) *Enhancers and Eukaryotic Expression.* Cold Spring Harbor Laboratory, New York.

Glynne, R., Powis, S.H., Beck, S. *et al.* (1991) A proteosome-related gene between the two ABC transporter loci in the class II region of the human MHC. *Nature* 353, 357–360.

Gordon, R., Simpson, E. & Samelson, L. (1975) In vitro cell-mediated immune responses to the male specific (H-Y) antigen in mice. *Journal of Experimental Medicine* 142, 1108–1120.

Gorer, P.A., Lyman, S. & Snell, G.D. (1948) Studies on the genetic and antigenic basis of tumour transplantation: linkage between a histocompatibility gene and 'fused' in mice. *Proceedings of the Royal Society of London (B)* 135, 499–505.

Greenfield, A., Scott, D., Pennisi, D. *et al.* (1996) An H-YDb epitope is encoded by a novel mouse Y chromosome gene. *Nature Genetics* 14, 474–478.

Griffin, T.A., Nandi, D., Cruz, M. *et al.* (1998) Immunoproteasome assembly: cooperative incorporation interferon g (IFN-g) -inducible subunits. *Journal of Experimental Medicine* 187, 97–104.

Hammer, J. (1995) New methods to predict MHC-binding sequences within protein antigens. *Current Opinion in Immunology* 7, 263–269.

Harding, C. & Song, R. (1994) Phagocytic processing of exogenous particulate antigens by macrophages for presentation by class I MHC molecules. *Journal of Immunology* 153, 4925–4933.

Hardy, D.A., Bell, J.I., Long, E.O., Linksten, T. & McDevitt, H.O. (1986) Mapping of the class II region of the human major histocompatibility complex by pulsed-field gel electrophoresis. *Nature* 323, 453–455.

Heath, W.R., Hurd, M.E., Carbone, F.R. & Sherman, L.A. (1989) Peptide-dependent recognition of H-2Kb by alloreactive cytotoxic T lymphocytes. *Nature* 341, 749–752.

Hederer, R.A., Chandler, P.R., Dyson, P.J. *et al.* (1996) Acceptance of skin grafts between mice bearing different allelic forms of 2-microglobulin. *Transplantation* 61, 299–304.

Higashi, Y., Yoshioka, H., Yamane, M., Gotoh, O. & Fuji-Kuriyama, Y. (1986) Complete nucleotide sequence of two steroid 21-hydroxylase genes tandemly arranged in the human chromosome: a pseudogene and a genuine gene. *Proceedings of the National Academy of Sciences USA* 83, 2841–2845.

Hill, A.V.S., Elvin, J., Willis, A. *et al.* (1992) Molecular analysis of the association of HLA-B53 and resistance to severe malaria. *Nature* 360, 434–439.

Hirschberg, H., Bergh, O.J. & Thorsby, E. (1980) Antigen presenting properties of human vascular endothelial cells. *Journal of Experimental Medicine* 152, 249S–255S.

Hogan, K.T., Clayberger, C., Bernhard, E.J. *et al.* (1989) A panel of unique HLA-A2 mutant molecules define epitopes recognized by HLA-A2-specific antibodies and cytotoxic T lymphocytes. *Journal of Immunology* **142**, 2097–2104.

Horn, G.T., Bugawan, T.L., Long, C.M. & Erlich, H.A. (1988) Allelic sequence variation of the HLA-DQ loci: relationship to serology and to insulin-dependent diabetes susceptibility. *Proceedings of the National Academy of Sciences USA* **85**, 6012–6016.

Howard, J.C. (1995) Supply and transport of peptides presented by class I MHC molecules. *Current Opinion in Immunology* **7**, 69–76.

Hsieh, S.L. & Campbell, R.D. (1991) Evidence that gene G7a in the human major histocompatibility complex encodes valyl-tRNA synthetase. *Biochemistry Journal* **278**, 809–816.

Hunt, D.F., Henderson, R.A., Shabanowitz, J. *et al.* (1992) Characterization of peptides bound to the class I MHC molecule HLA-A2.1 by mass spectrometry. *Science* **255**, 1261–1263.

Janeway, C.A. Jr (1989) The role of CD4 in T-cell activation: accessory molecule or co-receptor. *Immunology Today* **10**, 234–238.

Jardetzky, T.S., Lane, W.S., Robinson, R.A., Madden, D.R. & Wiley, D.C. (1991) Identification of self peptides bound to purified HLA-B27. *Nature* **353**, 326–329.

Jardetzky, T.S., Brown, J.H., Gorga, J.C. *et al.* (1996) Crystallographic analysis of endogenous peptides associated with HLA-DR1 suggests a common polyproline II-like conformation for bound peptides. *Proceedings of the National Academy of Sciences USA* **93**, 734–738.

Jensen, P.E. (1991) Enhanced binding of peptide antigen to purified class II major histocompatibility glycoproteins at acidic pH. *Journal of Experimental Medicine* **174**, 1111–1120.

Jensen, P.E. (1998) Antigen processing: HLA-DO – a hitchhiking inhibitor of HLA-DM. *Current Biology* **8**, R128–R131.

Jin, Y., Shih, J.W.-K. & Berkower, I. (1988) Human T cell response to the surface antigen of hepatitis B virus (HBsAg). Endosomal and non-endosomal processing pathways are accessible to both endogenous and exogenous antigen. *Journal of Experimental Medicine* **168**, 293–306.

Johnson, L.L., Bailey, D.W. & Mobraaten, L.W. (1981) Genetics of histocompatibility in mice. IV. Detection of certain minor (non-H-2) H antigens in selected organs by the popliteal node test. *Immunogenetics* **14**, 63–71.

Jorgensen, J.L., Esser, U., Fazekas de St. Groth, B., Reay, P.A. & Davis, M.M. (1992) Mapping T cell receptor-peptide contacts by variant peptide immunization of single chain transgenics. *Nature* **335**, 224–230.

Kelly, A.P., Monaco, J.J., Cho, S. & Trowsdale, J. (1991a) A new human HLA class II-related locus, DM. *Nature* **353**, 571–573.

Kelly, A., Powis, S.H., Glynne, R. *et al.* (1991b) Second proteasome-related gene in the human MHC class II region. *Nature* **353**, 667–668.

Kelly, A., Powis, S.H., Kerr, L.-A. *et al.* (1992) Assembly and function of the two ABC transporter proteins encoded in the human major histocompatibility complex. *Nature* **355**, 641–644.

Kendall, E., Sargent, C.A. & Campbell, R.D. (1990) Human major histocompatibility complex contains a new cluster of genes between the HLA-D and complement C4 loci. *Nucleic Acids Research* **18**, 7251–7257.

Kimoto, M., Seki, K., Matsunaga, M. & Mineta, T. (1989) Unique mixed lymphocyte-stimulating determinants in $E_\alpha^d$ gene-introduced C57BL/6 transgenic mice. *Immunology* **67**, 154–159.

Kimura, A., Israel, A., LeBail, O. & Kourilsky, P. (1986) Detailed analysis of the mouse H-2K$^b$ promoter: enhancer-like sequences and their role in the regulation of class I gene expression. *Cell* **44**, 261–272.

King, T.R., Christianson, G.J., Mitchell, M.J. *et al.* (1994) Deletion mapping using immunoselection for H-Y further resolves the Sxr region of the mouse Y chromosome and reveals complexity at the Hya locus. *Genomics* **24**, 159–168.

Kisielow, P., Bluthmann, H., Staerz, U.D., Steinmetz, M. & von Boehmer, H. (1988) Tolerance in T-cell receptor transgenic mice involves deletion of nonmature CD4+8+ thymocytes. *Nature* **333**, 742–746.

Kleijmeer, M.J., Kelly, A., Geuze, H.J. *et al.* (1992) Location of MHC-enoded transporters in the endoplasmic reticulum and *cis*-Golgi. *Nature* **357**, 342–344.

Ko, H.S., Fu, S.M., Winchester, R.J., Yu, D.T.Y. & Kunkel, H.G. (1979) Ia determinants on stimulated human T lymphocytes. Occurrence on mitogen and antigen activated T cells. *Journal of Experimental Medicine* **150**, 246–255.

Koller, B.H., Geraghty, D.E., Shimizu, Y., DeMars, R. & Orr, H.T. (1988) HLA-E. A novel class I gene expressed in resting T lymphocytes. *Journal of Immunology* **141**, 897–904.

König, R., Shen, X. & Germain, R.N. (1995) Involvement of both major histocompatibility complex class II alpha and beta chains in CD4 function indicates a role for ordered oligomerization in T cell activation. *Journal of Experimental Medicine* **182**, 779–787.

König, R., Huang, L.-Y. & Germain, R.N. (1992) MHC class II interaction with CD4 mediated by a region analogous to the MHC class I binding site for CD8. *Nature* **356**, 796–798.

Kropshofer, H., Vogt, A.B. & Hammerling, G.J. (1995) Structural features of the invariant chain fragment CLIP controlling rapid release from HLA-DR molecules and inhibition of peptide binding. *Proceedings of the National Academy of Sciences USA* **92**, 8313–8317.

Kuckelhorn, U., Frentzel, S., Kraft, R. *et al.* (1995) Incorporation of major histocompatibility complex-encoded subunits LMP2 and LMP 7 changes the quality of the 20S proteasome polypeptide processing products independent of interferon-γ. *European Journal of Immunology* 25, 2605–2611.

Kuluga, H., Sogn, J.A., Weissman, J.D. *et al.* (1987) Expression patterns of MHC class II genes in rabbit tissues indicate close homology to human counterparts. *Journal of Immunology* 139, 587–592.

Kwok, W.W., Mickelson, E., Masewisz, S. *et al.* (1990) Polymorphic DQα and DQβ interactions dictate HLA class II determinant of allo-recognition. *Journal of Experimental Medicine* 171, 85–89.

Kwok, W.W., Kovats, S., Thurtle, P. & Nepom, G.T. (1993) HLA-DQ allelic polymorphisms constrain patterns of class II heterodimer formation. *Journal of Immunology* 150, 2263–2272.

Lafferty, K.J., Cooley, M.A., Woolnough, J. & Walker, K.Z. (1975) Thyroid allograft immunogenicity is reduced after a period in organ culture. *Science* 188, 259–261.

Lawrance, S.K., Smith, C.L., Srivastava, R., Cantor, C. & Weissman, S.M. (1987) Megabase-scale mapping of the HLA gene complex by pulsed field gel electrophoresis. *Science* 235, 1387–1390.

Lechler, R.I. & Batchelor, J.R. (1982) Restoration of immunogenicity to passenger cell-depleted kidney allografts by the addition of donor strain dendritic cells. *Journal of Experimental Medicine* 155, 31–41.

Lechler, R.I. & Lombardi, G. (1990) The structural basis of alloreactivity. *Immunological Research* 9, 135–146.

Lechler, R.I., Aichinger, G. & Lightstone, L. (1996) The endogenous pathway of MHC class II antigen presentation. *Immunological Reviews* 151, 51–79.

Lee, J., Trowsdale, J., Travers, P.J. *et al.* (1982) Sequence of an HLA-DR α chain cDNA clone and intron-exn organization of the corresponding gene. *Nature* 299, 750–752.

Lee, Y.-J. & Benveniste, D.N. (1996) Stat 1 alpha expression is involved in IFN-gamma induction of the class II transactivator and class II MHC genes. *Journal of Immunology* 157, 1559–1568.

Lee, Y.-J., Han, Y., Lu, H.-T. *et al.* (1997) TGF-β suppresses IFN-γ induction of class II MHC gene expression by inhibiting class II transactivator messenger RNA expression. *Journal of Immunology* 158, 2065–2072.

Lehner, P.J. & Cresswell, P. (1996) Processing and delivery of peptides presented by MHC class I molecules. *Current Opinion in Immunology* 8, 59–67.

Lenardo, M.J. & Baltimore, D. (1989) NF-κB: a pleiotropic mediator of inducible and tissue-specific gene control. *Cell* 58, 227–229.

Lennon, A.M., Ottore, C., Rigaud, G. *et al.* (1997) Isolation of B-cell-specific promoter for the human class II transactivator. *Immunogenetics* 45, 266–274.

Lightstone, L., Hargreaves, R., Bobek, G. *et al.* (1997) In the absence of the invariant chain, HLA-DR molecules display a distinct array of peptides which is influenced by the presence or absence of HLA-DM. *Proceedings of the National Academy of Sciences USA* 94, 5772–5777.

Liljedahl, M., Kuwana, T., Fung-Leung, W.P. *et al.* (1996) HLA-DO is a lysosomal resident which requires association with HLA-DM for efficient intracellular transport. *EMBO Journal* 15, 4817–4824.

Livingston, A.M., Powis, S.J., Diamond, A.G., Butcher, G.W. & Howard, J.C. (1989) A *trans*-acting major histocompatibility complex-linked gene whose alleles determine gain and loss changes in the antigenic structure of classical class I molecules. *Journal of Experimental Medicine* 170, 777–795.

Livingston, A.M., Powis, S.J., Gunther, E. *et al.* (1991) *Cim*: an MHC class II-linked allelism affecting the antigenicity of a classical class I molecule for T lymphocytes. *Immunogenetics* 34, 157–163.

Ljunggren, H.-G., Stam, M.J., Ohlen, C. *et al.* (1990) Empty MHC class I molecules come out in the cold. *Nature* 346, 476–480.

Lombardi, G., Sidhu, S., Lamb, R., Batchelor, J.R. & Lechler, R.I. (1989) Co-recognition of endogenous antigens with HLA-DR1 by alloreactive human T cell clones. *Journal of Immunology* 142, 753–759.

Lombardi, G., Barber, L., Aichinger, G. *et al.* (1991a) Structural analysis of anti-DR1 allorecognition by using DR1/H-2E$^k$ hybrid molecules. Influence of the β2 domain correlates with CD4 dependence. *Journal of Immunology* 147, 2034–2040.

Lombardi, G., Barber, L., Sidhu, S., Batchelor, J.R. & Lechler, R.I. (1991b) The specificity of alloreactive T cells is determined by MHC polymorphisms which contact the T cell receptor and which influence peptide biding. *International Immunology* 3, 769–775.

Lotteau, V., Teyton, L., Burroughs, D. & Charron, D. (1987) A novel HLA class II molecule (DRα–DRβ) created by mismatched isotype pairing. *Nature* 329, 339–341.

Lotteau, V., Teyton, L., Peleraux, A. *et al.* (1990) Intracellular transport of class II MHC molecules directed by the invariant chain. *Cell* 348, 600–605.

Loveland, B.E. & Simpson, E. (1986) The non-MHC transplantation antigens reviewed: neither weak nor minor. *Immunology Today* 7, 223–229.

Loveland, B.E., Sponaas, A.-M. & Simpson, E. (1985) Mapping H-1 with the distal break point of chromosome 7 in Cattanach's insertion. *Immunogenetics* 22, 503–510.

Loveland, B.E., Wang, C.R., Yonekawa, H., Hermel, E. & Fischer Lindahl, K. (1990) Maternally transmitted histocompatibility antigen of mice: a hydrophobic peptide of a mitochondrially encoded protein. *Cell* 60, 971–980.

Lundin, K.E., Ronningen, K.S., Aono, S. *et al.* (1989) HLA-DQ antigens and DQ beta amino acid 57 of Japanese patients with insulin-dependent diabetes mellitus: detection of a DRw8DQw8 haplotype. *Tissue Antigens* **34**, 233–241.

MacDonald, H.R., Hengartner, H. & Padrazzini, T. (1988) Intrathymic deletion of self-reactive cells prevented by neonatal anti-CD4 antibody treatment. *Nature* **335**, 174–176.

McMichael, A.J., Gotcha, F.M., Santos-Aguado, J. & Strominger, J.L. (1988) Effect of mutations and variations of HLA-A2 on recognition of a virus peptide epitope by cytotoxic T lymphocytes. *Proceedings of the National Academy of Sciences USA* **85**, 9194–9198.

Madden, D.R., Gorga, J.C., Strominger, J.L. & Wiley, D.C. (1991) The structure of HLA-B27 reveals nonamer self-peptides bound in an extended conformation. *Nature* **353**, 321–325.

Malcherek, G., Gnau, V. & Jung, G. (1995) Supermotifs enable natural invariant chain-derived peptides to interact with many major histocompatibility complex class II molecules. *Journal of Experimental Medicine* **181**, 527–538.

Marsh, S.G. (1998) HLA class II region sequences, 1998. *Tissue Antigens* **51**, 467–507.

Mason, P.M. & Parham, P. (1998) HLA class I region sequences, 1998. *Tissue Antigens* **51**, 417–466.

Matsunaga, M., Seki, K., Mineta, T. & Kimoto, M. (1990) Antigen-reactive T cell clones restricted by mixed isotype $A_\beta{}^d/E_\alpha{}^d$ class II molecules. *Journal of Experimental Medicine* **171**, 577–582.

Matzinger, P. & Bevan, M.J. (1977) Why do so many lymphocytes respond to major histocompatibility antigens? *Cell* **29**, 1–5.

Mellins, E., Arp, B., Singh, D. *et al.* (1990a) Point mutations define positions in HLA-DR3 molecules that affect antigen presentation. *Proceedings of the National Academy of Sciences USA* **87**, 4785–4789.

Mellins, E., Smith, L., Arp, B. *et al.* (1990b) Defective processing and presentation of exogenous antigens in mutants with normal HLA class II genes. *Nature* **343**, 71–74.

Michelson, B. & Lernmark, A. (1987) Molecular cloning of a polymorphic DNA endonuclease fragment associates insulin dependent diabetes mellitus with HLA-DQ. *Journal of Clinical Investigations* **75**, 1144–1152.

Morel, P.A., Dorman, J.S., Todd, J.A., McDevitt, H.O. & Trucco, M. (1988) Aspartic acid at position 57 of the $DQ_\beta$ chain protects against Type 1 diabetes: a family study. *Human Immunology* **23**, 126.

Morel, Y., Bristow, J., Gitelman, S.E. & Miller, W.L. (1989) Transcript encoded on the opposite strand of the human steroid 21-hydroxylase/complement component C4 gene locus. *Proceedings of the National Academy of Sciences USA* **86**, 6582–6586.

Morris, P., Shaman, J.H., Attaya, M. *et al.* (1994) An essential role for HLA-DM in antigen presentation by class II major histocompatibility molecules. *Nature* **368**, 551–554.

Morrison, L.A., Lakacher, A.E., Braciale, V.L., Fan, D.P. & Braciale, T.J. (1986) Differences in antigen presentation to MHC class I- and class II-restricted influenza virus-specific cytolytic T lymphocyte clones. *Journal of Experimental Medicine* **163**, 903–921.

Muhlethaler-Mottet, A., Otten, L.A., Steimle, V. & Mach, B. (1997) Expression of MHC class II molecules in different cellular and functional compartments is controlled by differential usage of multiple promoters of the transactivator CIITA. *EMBO Journal* **16**, 2851–2860.

Muhlethaler-Mottet, A., Di Berardino, W., Otten, L.A. & Mach, B. (1998) Activation of the MHC class II transactivator CIITA by interferon-g requires cooperative interaction between Stat1 and USF-1. *Immunity* **8**, 157–166.

Neefjes, J.J. & Momburg, F. (1993) Cell biology of antigen presentation. *Current Opinion in Immunology* **5**, 27–34.

Neefjes, J.J. & Ploegh, H.L. (1992) Intracellular transport of MHC class II molecules. *Immunology Today* **13**, 179–183.

Nepom, B.S., Schwartz, D., Palmer, J.P. & Nepom, G.T. (1987) Transcomplementation of HLA genes in IDDM HLA DQ α and β chains produced hybrid molecules in DR3/4 heterozygotes. *Diabetes* **36**, 114–117.

Nisbet, N.W., Simonsen, M. & Jensen, E. (1969) Kidney transplantation in siblings. Is immunosuppressive treatment invariably needed? *Transplantation* **7**, 444–446.

Orr, H.T. (1989) HLA class I gene family: characterization of genes encoding non-HLA-A, B, C proteins. In: *Immunobiology of HLA*, Vol II. (ed. B. Dupont), pp. 33–39. Springer-Verlag, New York.

Panina-Bordignon, P., Corradin, G., Roosnek, E., Sette, A. & Lanzavecchia, A. (1991) Recognition by class II alloreactive T cells of processed determinants from human serum proteins. *Science* **252**, 1548–1550.

Parham, P., Lomen, C.E., Lawlor, D.A. *et al.* (1988) Nature of polymorphism in HLA-A, -B and -C molecules. *Proceedings of the National Academy of Sciences USA* **85**, 4005–4009.

Pazmany, L., Mandelboim, O., Vales-Gomex, M. *et al.* (1996) Protection from natural killer cell-mediated lysis by HLA-G expression on target cells. *Science* **274**, 792–795.

Piskurich, J.F., Wang, Y., Linhoff, M.W., White, L.C. & Ting, J.P.-Y. (1998) Identification of distinct regions of 5′ flanking DNA that mediate constitutive, IFN-g, STAT1, and TGF-b-regulated expression of the class II transactivator gene. *Journal of Immunology* **160**, 233–240.

Potter, T.A., Rajan, T.V., Dick, I.I.R.F. & Bluestone, J.A. (1989) Substitution at residue 227 of H-2 class I molecules abrogates recognition by CD8-dependent but not CD8-independent, cytotoxic T lymphocytes. *Nature* 337, 73–75.

Powis, S.J., Townsend, A.R.M., Deverson, E.V. *et al.* (1991) Restoration of antigen presentation to the mutant cell line RMA-S by an MHC-linked transporter. *Nature* 354, 528–531.

Powis, S.J., Deverson, E.V., Coadwell, W.J. *et al.* (1992a) Effect of polymorphism of an MHC-linked transporter on the peptides assembled in a class I molecule. *Nature* 357, 211–215.

Powis, S.J., Mockbridge, I., Kelly, A. *et al.* (1992b) Polymorphism in a second ABC transporter gene located within the class II region of the human MHC. *Proceedings of the National Academy of Sciences USA* 89, 1463–1467.

Pujol-Borrell, R., Todd, I., Doshi, M. *et al.* (1987) HLA class II induction in human islet cells by interferon-γ plus tumour necrosis factor or lymphotoxin. *Nature* 326, 304–306.

Ramesh, P., Barber, L., Batchelor, J.R. & Lechler, R.I. (1992) Structural analysis of human anti-mouse H-2E xenorecognition: T cell receptor bias and impaired CD4 interaction contribute to weak xenoresponses. *International Immunology* 4, 935–943.

Rammensee, H.-G. (1995) Chemistry of peptides associated with MHC class I and class II molecules. *Current Opinion in Immunology* 7, 85–96.

Rammensee, H.-G., Falk, K. & Rötzschke, O. (1993) Peptides naturally presented by MHC class I molecules. *Annual Review of Immunology* 11, 213–244.

Reich, Z., Boniface, J.J., Lyons, D.S. *et al.* (1997) Ligand-specific oligomerization of T-cell receptor molecules. *Nature* 387, 617–620.

Reid, P.A. & Watts, C. (1990) Cycling of cell-surface MHC glycoproteins through primaquine-sensitive intracellular compartments. *Nature* 346, 655–657.

Reith, W., Barras, E., Satola, S. *et al.* (1989) Cloning of the major histocompatibility complex class II promoter binding protein affected in a hereditary defect in class II gene regulation. *Proceedings of the National Academy of Sciences USA* 86, 4200–4204.

Riberdy, J.M., Mostaghel, E. & Doyle, C. (1998) Disruption of the CD4-major histocompatibility complex class II interaction blocks the development of CD4+ T cells *in vivo*. *Proceedings of the National Academy of Sciences USA* 95, 4493–4498.

Roche, P. & Cresswell, P. (1990) High affinity binding of an influenza haemagglutinin derived peptide to purified HLA-DR. *Journal of Immunology* 144, 1849–1856.

Rock, K.L., Gamble, S. & Rothstein, L. (1990) Presentation of exogenous antigen with class I major histocompatibility complex molecules. *Science* 249, 918–921.

Rock, K.L., Gramm, C., Rothstein, L. *et al.* (1994) Inhibitors of the proteasome block the degradation of most cell proteins and the generation of peptides presented on MHC class I molecules. *Cell* 79, 761–771.

Ronchese, F., Brown, M.A. & Germain, R.N. (1987) Structure-function analysis of the $A_\beta^{bm12}$ mutation using site-directed mutagenesis and DNA-mediated gene transfer. *Journal of Immunology* 139, 629–638.

Roopenian, D.C. (1992) What are minor histocompatibility loci? A new look at an old question. *Immunology Today* 13, 7–10.

Roopenian, D.C. & Davis, A.P. (1989) Responses against antigens encoded by the H-3 histocompatibility locus: antigens stimulating class I MHC- and class II MHC-restricted T cells are encoded by separate genes. *Immunogenetics* 30, 335–343.

Roopenian, D.C., Christianson, G.J., Davis, A.P., Zuberi, A.R. & Mobraaten, L.E. (1993) The genetic origin of minor histocompatibility antigens. *Immunogenetics* 38, 131–140.

Rötzschke, O., Falk, K., Wallny, H.J., Faath, S. & Rammensee, H.G. (1990) Characterisation of naturally occurring minor H peptides including H-4 and H-Y. *Science* 249, 283–287.

Rouas-Freiss, N., Marchal-Bras Goncalves, R., Manier, C., Dausset, J. & Carosella, E.D. (1997) Direct evidence to support the role of HLA-G in protecting the fetus from maternal uterine natural killer cytolysis. *Proceedings of the National Academy of Sciences USA* 94, 11520–11525.

Ruberti, G., Sellins, K.S., Hill, M. *et al.* (1992) Presentation of antigen by mixed isotype class II molecules in normal H-$2^d$ mice. *Journal of Experimental Medicine* 175, 157–162.

Rudensky, A.Y., Preston-Hurlburt, P., Hong, S.-C., Barlow, A. & Janeway, C.A. Jr (1991) Sequence analysis of peptides bound to MHC class II molecules. *Nature* 353, 622–627.

Rudensky, A.Y., Preston-Hurlburt, P., Al-Ramadi, B.K., Rothbard, J. & Janeway, C.A. Jr (1992) Truncation variants of peptides isolated from MHC class II molecules suggest sequence motifs. *Nature* 359, 429–431.

Ryder, L.P., Svejgaard, A. & Dausset, J. (1981) Genetics of HLA disease association. *Annual Review of Genetics* 15, 169–187.

Sadasivan, B., Lehner, P.J., Ortmann, B., Spies, T. & Cresswell, P. (1996) Roles for calreticulin and a novel glycoprotein, tapasin, in the interaction of MHC class I molecules with TAP. *Immunity* 5, 103–114.

Sadegh-Nasseri, S. & McConnell, H.M. (1989) A kinetic intermediate in the reaction of an antigenic peptide and I-$E^k$. *Nature* 337, 274–276.

Saizawa, K., Rojo, J. & Janeway, C.A. Jr (1987) Evidence for the physical association of CD4 and the CD3: α:β T-cell receptor. *Nature* 328, 260–263.

Sallusto, F., Cella, M., Danieli, C. & Lanzavecchia, A. (1995) Dendritic cells use macropinocytosis and the mannose receptor to concentrate macromolecules in the major histocompatibility complex class II compartment: downregulation by cytokines and bacterial products. *Journal of Experimental Medicine* 182, 389–400.

Salter, R.D., Benjamin, R.J., Wesley, P.K. *et al.* (1990) A binding site for the T-cell co-receptor CD8 on the α3 domain of HLA-A2. *Nature* **345**, 41–46.

Sanderson, F., Thomas, C., Neefjes, J. & Trowsdale, J. (1996) Association between HLA-DM and HLA-DR in vivo. *Immunity* **4**, 87–96.

Sant-Angelo, D.B., Waterburg, G., Preston-Hurlburt, P. *et al.* (1996) The specificity and orientation of a TCR to its peptide-MHC class II ligands. *Immunity* **4**, 367–376.

Santos-Aguado, J., Crimmins, M.A.V., Mentzer, S.J., Burakoff, S.J. & Strominger, J.L. (1989) Alloreactivity studies with mutants of HLA-A2. *Proceedings of the National Academy of Sciences USA* **86**, 8936–8940.

Sargent, C.A., Dunham, I., Trowsdale, J. & Campbell, R.D. (1989a) Human major histocompatibility complex contains genes for the major heat shock protein HSP70. *Proceedings of the National Academy of Sciences USA* **86**, 1968–1972.

Sargent, D.C., Dunham, I. & Campbell, R.D. (1989b) Identification of multiple HTF-island associated genes in the human major histocompatibility complex class III region. *EMBO Journal* **8**, 2305–2312.

Schreuder, G.M.T., Pool, J., Blokland, E. *et al.* (1993) A genetic analysis of human minor histocompatibility antigens demonstrating Mendelian segregation independent of HLA. *Immunogenetics* **38**, 98–105.

Scott, C.A., Garcia, K.C., Stura, E.A. *et al.* (1998a) Engineering protein for X-ray crystallography: the murine major histocompatibility complex class II molecule I-Ad. *Protein Science* **7**, 413–418.

Scott, C.A., Peterson, P.A., Teyton, L. & Wilson, I.A. (1998b) Crystal structures of two I-Ad-peptide complexes reveal that high affinity can be achieved without large anchor residues. *Immunity* **8**, 319–329.

Scott, D., McLaren, A., Dyson, P.J. & Simpson, E. (1991) Variable spread of X inactivation affecting the expression of different epitopes of the Hya gene product in mouse B cell clones. *Imunogenetics* **33**, 54–61.

Scott, D., Dyson, P.J. & Simpson, E. (1992) A new approach to the cloning of genes encoding T cell epitopes. *Immunogenetics* **36**, 86–94.

Scott, D.M., Ehrmann, I.E., Ellis, P.S. *et al.* (1995) Identification of a mouse male-specific transplantation antigen, H-Y. *Nature* **376**, 695–698.

Sekimata, M., Griem, P., Egawa, K., Rammensee, H.G. & Takiguchi, M. (1992) Isolation of human minor histocompatibility peptides. *International Immunology* **4**, 301–304.

Servenius, B., GustafssonK., Widmark, E. *et al.* (1984) Molecular map of the human HLA-SB (HLA-DP) region and sequence of an SB-alpha (DP-alpha) pseudogene. *EMBO Journal* **3**, 3209–3214.

Sha, W.C., Nelson, C.A., Newberry, R.D. *et al.* (1988) Selective expression of an antigen receptor on CD8-bearing T lymphocytes in transgenic mice. *Nature* **335**, 271–274.

Sherman, P.A., Basta, P.V., Moore, T.L., Brown, A.M. & Ting, J.P. (1989) Class II box consensus sequences in the HLA-DRA gene: transcriptional function and interaction with nuclear proteins. *Molecular Cell Biology* **9**, 50–56.

Shimizu, Y., Geraghty, D.E., Koller, B.H., Orr, H.T. & DeMars, R. (1988) Transfer and expression of three cloned human non-HLA-A, B, C class I histocompatibility complex genes in mutant lymphoblastoid cells. *Proceedings of the National Academy of Sciences USA* **85**, 227–231.

Shimonkevitz, R., Kappler, J.W., Marrack, P. & Grey, H.M. (1983) Antigen recognition by H-2 restricted T cells. I. Cell-free antigen processing. *Journal of Experimental Medicine* **158**, 303–316.

Shinohara, N., Bluestone, J.A. & Sachs, D.H. (1986) Cloned cytotoxic T lymphocytes that recognize an I-A region product in the context of a class I antigen. *Journal of Experimental Medicine* **163**, 972–980.

Simpson, E. (1982) The role of H-Y as a minor transplantation antigen. *Immunology Today* **3**, 97–106.

Simpson, E. & Roopenian, D. (1997) Minor histocompatibility antigens. *Current Opinion in Immunology* **9**, 655–661.

Simpson, E., Dyson, P.J., Knight, A.M. *et al.* (1993) T cell receptor repertoire selection by mouse mammary tumour viruses and MHC molecules. *Immunological Reviews* **131**, 93–115.

Simpson, E., Scott, D. & Chandler, P. (1997) The male-specific histocompatibility antigen, H-Y: a history of transplantation, immune response genes, sex determination and expression cloning. *Annual Review of Immunology* **15**, 39–61.

Sittisombut, N. & Knight, K. (1986) Rabbit major histocompatibility complex. I. Isolation and characterization of three subregions of class II genes. *Journal of Immunology* **136**, 1871–1875.

Snell, G.D. (1948) Methods for the study of histocompatibility genes. *Journal of Genetics* **49**, 87–103.

Sodoyer, R., Damotte, M., Delovitch, T.L. *et al.* (1984) Complete nucleotide sequence of a gene encoding a functional human class I histocompatibility antigen (HLA-Cw3). *EMBO Journal* **3**, 879.

Spence, M.A., Spurr, N.K. & Field, L.L. (1989) Report of the committee on the genetic constitution of chromosome 6. *Cytogenetics and Cell Genetics* **51**, 149–165.

Spies, T., Blanck, G., Bresnahan, M., Sands, J. & Strominger, J.L. (1989a) A new cluster of genes within the human major histocompatibility complex. *Science* **243**, 214–217.

Spies, T., Bresnahan, M. & Strominger, J.L. (1989b) Human major histocompatibility complex containing a minimum of 19 genes between the complement cluster and HLA-B. *Proceedings of the National Academy of Sciences USA* **86**, 8955–8958.

Spies, T., Bresnahan, M., Bahram, S. *et al.* (1990) A gene in the human major histocompatibility complex class II region controlling the class I antigen presentation pathway. *Nature* **348**, 744–747.

Spies, T., Cerundolo, V., Colonna, M. *et al.* (1992) Presentation of viral antigen by MHC class I molecules is dependent on a putative peptide transporter heterodimer. *Nature* **355**, 644–646.

Steimle, V., Otten, L.A., Zufferey, M. & Mach, B. (1993) Complementation cloning of an MHC class II transactivator mutated in hereditary MHC class II deficiency (or bare lymphocyte syndrome). *Cell* **75**, 135–146.

Stern, L.J., Brown, J.H., Jardetzky, T.S. *et al.* (1994) Crystal structure of the human class II MHC protein HLA-DR1 complexed with an influenza virus peptide. *Nature* **368**, 215–221.

Strachan, T., Sodoyer, R., Damotte, M. & Jordan, B.R. (1984) Complete nucleotide sequence of a functional class I HLA gene HLA-A3: implications for the evolution of HLA genes. *EMBO Journal* **3**, 887–894.

Swain, S.L. (1981) Significance of class 1 and class 2 major histocompatibility complex antigens: help to allogeneic K and D antigens does *not* involve I recognition. *Journal of Immunology* **126**, 2307–2309.

Takagaki, Y., DeCloux, A., Bonneville, M. & Tonegawa, S. (1989) Diversity of γδ T-cell receptors on murine intestinal intra-epithelial lymphocytes. *Nature* **339**, 712–714.

Taurog, J.D. & El-Zaatari, A.K. (1988) In vitro mutagenesis of HLA-B27. Substitution of unpaired cysteine residue in the α1 domain causes loss of antibody defined epitopes. *Journal of Clinical Investigations* **82**, 987–992.

Teng, M.-K., Smolyar, A., Tse, A.G.D. *et al.* (1998) Identificatiion of a common docking topology with substantial variation among different TCR-peptide-MHC complexes. *Current Biology* **8**, 409–412.

Tiwari, J.L. & Terasaki, P.I. (1985) In: *HLA and Disease Association*. Springer-Verlag, New York.

Todd, J.A., Acha-Orbea, H., Bell, J.I. *et al.* (1988a) A molecular basis for MHC class II-associated autoimmunity. *Science* **240**, 1003–1009.

Todd, J.A., Bell, J.I. & McDevitt, H.O. (1988b) A molecular basis for genetic susceptibility to insulin-dependent diabetes mellitus. *Trends in Genetics* **4**, 129–134.

Tomonari, K. (1983) Antigen and MHC restriction specificity of two types of cloned male-specific T cell lines. *Journal of Immunology* **131**, 1641–1645.

Tonnelle, C., DeMars, R. & Long, E.O. (1985) DOβ: a new β chain gene in HLA-D with a distict regulation of expression. *EMBO Journal* **4**, 2839–2847.

Townsend, A.R.M., Gould, B.K. & Brownlee, G.G. (1986a) Cytotoxic T lymphocytes recognise influenza haemagglutinin that lacks a signal sequence. *Nature* **324**, 575–577.

Townsend, A.R.M., Rothbard, J., Gotch, F.M. *et al.* (1986b) The epitopes of influenza nucleoprotein recognised by cytotoxic T lymphocytes can be defined by short synthetic peptides. *Cell* **44**, 959–968.

Townsend, A., Bastin, J., Gould, K. *et al.* (1988) Defective presentation to class I-restricted cytotoxic T lymphocytes in vaccinia-infected cells is overcome by enhanced degradation of antigen. *Journal of Experimental Medicine* **168**, 1211–1224.

Townsend, A., Ohlen, C., Bastin, J. *et al.* (1989) Association of class I major histocompatibility heavy and light chains induced by viral peptides. *Nature* **340**, 443–448.

Trowsdale, J. & Kelly, A. (1985) The human HLA class II α chain gene DZα is distinct from genes in the DP, DQ and DR subregion. *EMBO Journal* **4**, 2231–2237.

Trowsdale, J., Hanson, I., Mockbridge, I. *et al.* (1990) Sequences encoded in the class II region of the MHC related to the ABC superfamily of transporters. *Nature* **348**, 741–744.

Trowsdale, J., Ragoussis, J. & Campbell, R.D. (1991) Map of the human MHC. *Immunology Today* **12**, 443–446.

Van den Eynde, B., Lethe, B., Van Pel, A., De Plaen, E. & Boon, T. (1991) The gene coding for a major tumor rejection antigen of tumor P815 is identical to the normal gene of syngeneic DBA/2 mice. *Journal of Experimental Medicine* **173**, 1373–1384.

Van der Bruggen, P., Traversari, C., Chomez, P. *et al.* (1991) A gene encoding an antigen recognised by cytolytic T lymphocytes on a human melanoma. *Science* **254**, 1643–1647.

Van Els, C.A.C.M., Bakker, A., Zwinderman, A.H. *et al.* (1990a) Effector mechanisms in graft versus host disease in response to minor histocompatibility antigens. I. Absence of correlation with cytotoxic effector cells. *Transplantation* **50**, 62–66.

Van Els, C.A.C.M., Bakker, A., Zwinderman, A.H. *et al.* (1990b) Effector mechanisms in graft versus host disease in response to minor histocompatibility antigens. II. Evidence of a possible involvement of proliferative T cells. *Transplantation* **50**, 67–71.

Van Els, C.A.C.M., D-Amaro, J., Pool, J. *et al.* (1992) Immunogenetics of human minor histocompatibility antigens: their polymorphisms and immunodominance. *Immunogenetics* **35**, 161–165.

Van Ewijk, W., Ron, Y., Monaco, J. *et al.* (1988) Compartmentalization of MHC class II gene expression in transgenic mice. *Cell* **53**, 357–370.

Veillette, A., Bookman, M.A., Horak, E.M. & Bolen, J.B. (1988) The CD4 and CD8 T cell surface antigens are associated with the internal membrane tyrosine-protein kinase p56[lck]. *Cell* **55**, 301–308.

Vignali, D.A.A., Moreno, J., Schiller, D. & Hammerling, G.J. (1992) Species-specific binding of CD4 to the β2 domain of major histocompatibility complex class II molecules. *Journal of Experimental Medicine* **175**, 925–932.

Viville, S., Neefjes, J., Lottwau, V. *et al.* (1993) Mice lacking the MHC class II-associated invariant chain. *Cell* **72**, 635–648.

Vogt, A.B., Kropshofer, H., Moldenhaur, G. & Hammerling, G.J. (1996) Kinetic analysis of peptide loading onto HLA-DR molecules mediated by HLA-DM. *Proceedings of the National Academy of Sciences USA* **93**, 9724–9729.

Von Boehmer, H., Teh, H.S. & Kisielow, P. (1989) The thymus selects the useful, neglects the useless and destroys the harmful. *Immunology Today* **10**, 57–61.

Wang, R.F., Robbins, P.F., Kawakami, Y., Kang, X.-Q. & Rosenberg, S.A. (1995) Identification of a gene encoding a melonoma tumour antigen recognized by HLA-A31-restricted tumour-infiltrating lymphocytes. *Journal of Experimental Medicine* **181**, 799.

Weber, D.A., Evavold, B.D. & Jensen, P.E. (1996) Enhanced dissociation of HLA-DR-bound peptides in the presence of HLA-DM. *Science* **274**, 618–620.

Weenink, S.M., Milburn, P.J. & Gautam, A.M. (1997) A continuous central motif ofvariant chain peptides, CLIP, is essential for binding to various I-A MHC class II molecules. *International Immunology* **9**, 317–325.

Westerheide, S.C., Louis-Plence, P., Ping, D., He, X.F. & Boss, J.M. (1997) HLA-DMA and HLA-DMB gene expression functions through the conserved S-X-Y region. *Journal of Immunology* **158**, 4812–4821.

Wettstein, P.J. (1986) Immunodominance in the T cell response to multiple non H-Y histocompatibility antigens. II. Observation of a hierarchy among dominant antigens. *Immunogenetics* **24**, 24–31.

Widera, G., Burkly, L.C., Pinkert, C.A. *et al.* (1987) Transgenic mice selectively lacking MHC class II (I-E) antigen expression on B cells: an in vivo approach to investigate Ia gene function. *Cell* **51**, 175–187.

Wolf, E., Spencer, K. & Cudworth, A.G. (1983) The genetic susceptibility to type I (insulin-dependent) diabetes. Analysis of the HLA–DR association. *Diabetologia* **24**, 224–230.

Wolpert, E., Franksoon, L. & Karre, K. (1995) Dominant and cryptic antigens in the MHC class I restricted T cell response across a complex minor histocompatibility barrier: analysis and mapping by elution of cellular peptides. *International Immunology* **7**, 919.

Yamagata, K., Nkajima, H., Hanafusa, T. *et al.* (1989) Aspartic acid at position 57 of DQβ chain does not protect against type I (insulin-dependent) diabetes mellitus in Japanese subjects. *Diabetologia* **32**, 762–764.

Yancopoulos, G.D., Blackwell, T.K., Suh, H., Hood, L. & Alt, F.W. (1986) Introduced T cell receptor variable regions gene segments recombine in pre-B cells: evidence that B and T cells use a common mechanism. *Cell* **44**, 251–259.

Yewdell, J.W. & Bennink, J.R. (1990) The binary logic of antigen processing and presentation to T cells. *Cell* **62**, 203–206.

Yewdell, J.W., Bennink, J.R. & Hosaka, Y. (1988) Cells process exogenous proteins for recognition by cytotoxic T lymphocytes. *Science* **239**, 637–640.

Yin, L., Poirier, G., Neth, O. *et al.* (1993) Few peptides dominate CTL responses to single and multiple minor histocompatibility antigens. *International Immunology* **5**, 1003–1009.

Yu, D.T.Y., Winchester, R.J., Fu, S.M. *et al.* (1980) Peripheral blood Ia positive T cells increased in certain diseases and after immunization. *Journal of Experimental Medicine* **151**, 91–100.

Zamvil, S.S., Nelson, P.A., Mitchell, D.J. *et al.* (1985) Encephalitogenic T cell clones specific for myelin basic protein. *Journal of Experimental Medicine* **162**, 2107–2124.

Zhang, Q. & Salter, R.D. (1998) Distinct patterns of folding and interactions with calnexin and calreticulin in human class I MHC proteins with altered N-glycosylation. *Journal of Immunology* **160**, 831–837.

Zhou, P., Anderson, G.D., Savarirayan, S., Inoko, H. & David, C. (1991) Thymic deletion of Vβ11+, Vβ5+ T cells in H-2E negative, HLA-DQ β+ single transgenic mice. *Journal of Immunology* **146**, 854–859.

Ziegler, K. & Unanue, E.R. (1981) Identification of a macrophage antigen-processsing event required for I-region-restricted antigen presentation to T lymphocytes. *Journal of Immunology* **127**, 1869–1875.

Zinkernagel, R.M. & Doherty, P.C. (1974) Restriction of in vitro mediated cytotoxicity in lymphocytic choriomeningitis within a syngeneic or semi-allogeneic system. *Nature* **248**, 701–702.

# Chapter 3/New methods in tissue typing

KEN I. WELSH & MIKE BUNCE

## Introduction

The major role of the tissue typing laboratory in performing a service for transplantation has remained unchanged over the past 25 years, but the services performed have continually evolved to keep pace with continuing developments. New methods have therefore been introduced within laboratories on a very regular basis, both to keep pace with new demands and to replace existing procedures. Table 3.1, although not comprehensive, indicates the extent of this expansion and shows that in the 1980s a move away from HLA typing as the dominant procedure occurred. This trend is continuing at such a pace that in some laboratories histocompatibility tests themselves are no longer dominant. In this chapter, however, we will only discuss new methods for the three current mainstays of histocompatibility: HLA typing itself, HLA antibody screening and cross-matching. The methods discussed are molecular methods, flow cytometry, ELISA and cross-matching.

Soon after the first solid organ clinical transplants were performed it became apparent that some degree of HLA typing was prudent, originally for matching, and later as an aid to both cross-matching and antibody screening. Such typing was performed by the use of a panel of antisera specific for different antigenic products of the system in an assay that became known as the complement-dependent cytotoxicity test (CDC) (Mittal *et al.* 1968) or serology. CDC is robust and can provide results within 3 h, critical for reducing cold ischaemia times in cadaveric transplantation. The close cooperation between HLA laboratories throughout the world in terms of serum exchange kept the cost of such tests to a minimum while ever increasing the resolution. With the advent of monoclonal antibodies, CDC slowly but surely improved until it was an adequate sole method of HLA typing for all forms of transplantation except bone marrow, where other additional tests were required for non-HLA identical pairs. There are drawbacks of CDC: viable lymphocytes are required; the antibodies needed are generally non-renewable; and the technique has limited powers of resolution, particularly at HLA class II but also at HLA-C. In the 1980s many blood transfusion and transplant laboratories cut their HLA antibody screening programmes for reasons of cost. This action curtailed the free exchange of reagents and led to increased commercialization of HLA typing with a resultant cost increase for all.

Cost increases, decreasing sera availability, the problem of serological discrimination of class II antigens—arguably the most important antigens for solid organ transplantation—all encouraged the search for

**Table 3.1** Shifting trends in tissue typing methodologies from 1970 to 1975.

| Method | 1970 | 1980 | 1990 | 1995 |
|---|---|---|---|---|
| HLA serology | A then A, B then A, B, C | HLA A, B, C, DR | A, B, C, DR, DQ, DP | Decreasing |
| Cellular | A, B, D | A, B, DR, DQ, DP | A, B, C, DR, DQ, DP | Rare* |
| Electrophoresis | 1-D | 1-D + 2-D | 1-D + 2-D | Rare |
| Molecular HLA typing | No | RFLP for DR | SSO DR, DQ | A, B, C, DR, DQ, DP |
| Molecular non-HLA typing† | No | No | No | Considerable† |
| Sequencing | No | Research only | PCR sequencing | For bone marrow |
| Cytotoxic screening | No | +/− No specificity | Allele specificity | Amino acid specificity |
| Flow screening | No | No | +/− No specificity | +/− M and G |
| ELISA screening | No | No | A, B | A, B, DR |
| Flow cross-match | No | No | Rare | Routine in sensitized patients |
| Other cross-matching | No | No | Anti-epithelial/endothelial | Rare but useful |
| ATG monitoring | No | Rosette inhibition | Flow | Flow |
| CyA levels | No | Rare | Common | Common + FK506 levels |

* Medium- to high-resolution typing are replacing the need for these.
† These include HLA-HFE, TAP, DM, HSP70, TNF, LT in the MHC region and polymorphisms in adhesion molecule, cytokine, enzyme and receptor molecules throughout the genome. Other methods in use include PCR for CMV and EBV, viraemia for CMV, immunocytochemistry using a range of monoclonals, platelet (HPA) and blood grouping (ABO, rhesus, Duffy, Lewis) by SSO and many others.

alternative tissue typing methods, two-dimensional gel electrophoresis and restriction fragment length polymorphism (RFLP) being the main contenders. Neither was ideal for solid organ transplantation but both were eminently suitable for tissue typing in situations where the result was not needed within a few hours. We shall return to two-dimensional gels later, but will consider molecular development first with the pioneering work of the Petersen group in Uppsala (Andersson *et al.* 1984). Their generosity in allowing probes to be released enabled the first comprehensive molecular class II typing system using RFLP (Bidwell *et al.* 1988). RFLP, although not now the method of choice in most laboratories, is maintained in many UK centres because of its requirement in the Human Organs for Transplant Bill.

RFLP simply entails the restriction endonuclease digestion of DNA. Any polymorphism which alters the digestion site stops that particular enzyme from functioning and smaller digestion products are not therefore observed. Originally, digestion was of genomic DNA followed by electrophoretic resolution of the

endonucleolytic fragments, which are denatured *in situ* and hybridized to a nylon membrane. The membrane is then probed with homologous labelled cDNA or genomic probes which yield hybridization signals characteristic of various HLA alleles. In recent years polymerase chain reaction (PCR) amplified region of interest followed by digestion (PCR-RFLP and drop-in PCR) enabled greater specificity and sensitivity.

The relevance of RFLP was shown by Opelz *et al.* in a collaborative transplant study (Opelz *et al.* 1993) and by Mytileneos *et al.* (1990, 1992). These retrospective studies showed that RFLP-defined HLA-DR-matched renal grafts had improved survival compared to serology-defined HLA-DR-matched grafts, and that serology for class II was inadequate in many typing centres, with an overall discrepancy rate of up to 25% between serologically and RFLP-defined antigens. The main problem was the length of time from sample to results (up to 10 days) but, in addition, the resolution often depended on strong association between neighbouring sequences rather than relying on polymorphism within the DRβ1 domain. This restricted its use on mixed

**Table 3.2** Increase in number of sequenced HLA alleles, 1991–97.

| Date | HLA alleles | | | | | | | |
|---|---|---|---|---|---|---|---|---|
| | A | B | C | DRB | DQA | DQB | DPA | DPB |
| March 1991 | 26 | 35 | 14 | 56 | 13 | 17 | 4 | 21 |
| March 1995 | 59 | 122 | 35 | 152 | 16 | 25 | 8 | 62 |
| March 1997 | 85 | 188 | 42 | 221 | 18 | 32 | 10 | 76 |

ethnic populations because of differences in linkage disequilibrium values. Nevertheless, the need for molecular typing was established.

The development of PCR (Saiki *et al.* 1985), as well as improving RFLP, allowed the evolution of improved molecular HLA typing techniques. The PCR can generate specific amplified stretches of DNA sequences *in vitro*, through repeated cycles of DNA denaturation, annealing of specific primer to a single strand and nucleotide extension from primer pairs using a DNA polymerase. The PCR allowed extensive sequencing of HLA alleles from 1990 onwards, as shown in Table 3.2.

Starting with DNA, PCR can amplify an area of interest in two basic ways. In the first and most common way, generic primers are used and specificity obtained from enzymes (RFLP) or with site-specific probes (SSO). In the alternative method, site-specific amplification is used (ARMS or SSP). With the use of generic primers transplantation laboratories were for the first time able to use PCR to amplify the polymorphic regions of HLA genes, which could subsequently be analysed for polymorphism within the amplicon, thus establishing the tissue type. However, it was only the advent of the much quicker SSP technology that allowed full implementation of molecular typing into solid organ transplant laboratories. New PCR tissue typing techniques now allow histocompatibility scientists the choice of whether to use low-, medium- or high-resolution methods; low-resolution methods generally only identify broad specificities or groups of specificities. The term medium resolution is used to describe a typing system that discriminates between all serological specificities but may also give some allele-specific results, whereas high-resolution typing is a term generally used to describe a typing system that

discriminates between 90% of the alleles in the loci analysed. Thus, in solid organ transplantation medium-resolution typing is generally the method of choice whereas in unrelated bone marrow transplantation low- or medium-resolution typing is always followed up with high-resolution typing. Obviously, high-resolution methods are not used routinely as they tend to be more time consuming and more costly compared to medium-resolution methods, but they do negate the need for additional cellular tests for unrelated bone marrow transplants.

As defined above, techniques for analysing polymorphisms in DNA can be divided into two basic groups: probe hybridization and direct amplicon analysis. Currently there are many different PCR-based tissue typing assays and it is up to individual laboratories which test or combination of tests they use, and for which loci they choose to apply the tests. Most new molecular methods of tissue typing were initially developed for class II typing, particularly DQA1 and DQB1, because of the relative simplicity of these loci compared to DR and class I. However, most molecular methods are now applicable to both class I and II, the only difference being that in class I analysis exons 2, 3 and sometimes exon 4 are required for discrimination of most alleles, whereas most class II alleles can be discriminated between by analysing exon 2 only. A diagram illustrating PCR-SSOP, reverse PCR-SSOP, PCR-SSP and PCR-SSCP is shown in Fig. 3.1.

## Probe hybridization techniques

Probe hybridization techniques rely on amplification of a target DNA sequence which is generally immobilized on to a support membrane, known as dot blotting. The initial amplification is normally generic but

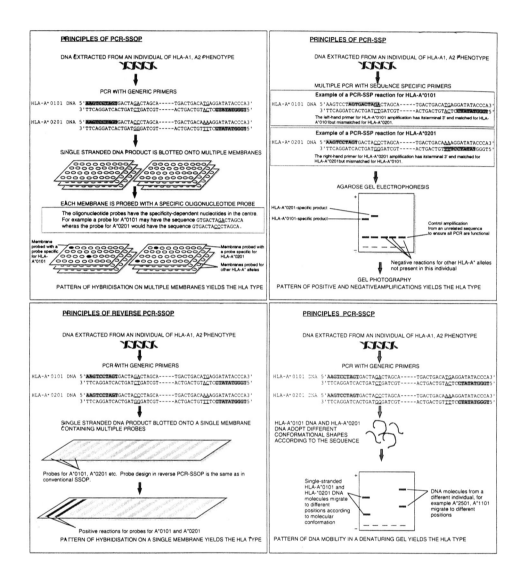

**Fig. 3.1** Principles of PCR-SSOP, reverse PCR-SSOP, PCR-SSP and PCR-SSCP.

may be a mosaic of amplifications which, when used together, amplify all possible alleles of a given locus. The polymorphisms in the immobilized amplified DNA are subsequently detected by using specific single-stranded DNA probes in combination with highly stringent washes to remove non-specifically bound probe (Saiki *et al.* 1986). In addition to the use of radioactive isotopes, hybridized probes can be detected by a variety of non-radioactive methods such as horseradish peroxidase (Saiki *et al.* 1989) or digoxygenin labelling (Gentilomi *et al.* 1989). This technique became known as PCR-SSOP (PCR followed by sequence-specific oligonucleotide probing). PCR-SSOP was first applied to histocompatibility testing in HLA-DQA1 by Saiki *et al.* (1986); subsequently PCR-SSOP was applied to HLA-DRB1 (Tiercy *et al.* 1988;

Vaughan *et al.* 1990; Scharf *et al.* 1991; Vaughan 1991; Kimura *et al.* 1992) and HLA-DQB1 (Eliaou *et al.* 1989) and a combination of DR, DQB1, DQA1, DPA1 and DPB1(Kimura & Sasazuki 1992). The assays were standardized and gained wide acceptance through the 1991 International Histocompatibility Workshop (Kimura *et al.* 1992).

In 1989 non-radioactive methods of PCR-SSOP analysis were introduced (Eliaou *et al.* 1989) which facilitated the spread of the technique to many laboratories. HLA-class I PCR-SSOP techniques were slow to develop because complete sequence data for class I alleles were not available. As more class I alleles were sequenced it became clear that serology would not be able to discriminate between certain specificities and so researchers turned their attentions to developing class I molecular techniques. The first PCR-SSOP class I dot blot techniques were described for differentiating HLA-B35 and HLA-B53 (Allsopp *et al.* 1991) and subtyping HLA-A2 and A28 (Fernandez-Vina *et al.* 1992). Complete single locus typing systems were then developed for HLA-A (Oh *et al.* 1993; Date *et al.* 1996), HLA-B (Yoshida *et al.* 1992; Oh *et al.* 1993; Fernandez-Vina *et al.* 1995; Fleischhauer *et al.* 1995; Middleton *et al.* 1995; Date *et al.* 1996) and HLA-C (Levine & Yang 1994; Kennedy *et al.* 1995), such that a combination of these techniques could be used to type completely an individual for class I.

PCR-SSOP is a generally accurate method of genotyping (Mickelson *et al.* 1993), especially suitable for large numbers of individual samples because generic amplifications from many individuals can be hybridized to a single membrane. There is, however, a problem if you wish to obtain complete results on one individual within 24 h, a problem which has led to the development of the reverse PCR-SSOP assay (Erlich *et al.* 1991). In the reverse dot blot, the SSO probes are bound to a solid support membrane via an incorporated poly (T) tail which leaves the detection end of the probe free to interact with target DNA. When labelled DNA target is applied to the reverse dot blot membrane it will only hybridize to those oligonucleotides which are complementary in sequence. Once hybridized, biotinylated products are detected by the addition of a reporter molecule, antibiotin antibody

linked to streptavidin–horseradish peroxidase complex, which induces a colour change in the substrate tetramethylbenzidine.

Reverse dot or line blot methods have been published for class II typing (Bugawan *et al.* 1990; Erlich *et al.* 1991) and HLA-A (Bugawan *et al.* 1994). HLA-B and HLA-C reverse SSOP methods are currently marketed by various commercial companies. When combined, these reverse SSOP methods should allow complete results on one individual within 4–5 h, times suitable but not ideal for genotyping cadaver donors. However, the large number of probes needed for a parallel class I and II reverse SSOP system requires considerable quality assurance input which means that these systems are most likely to be only available from commercial companies and may be too expensive for routine typing of all samples in a laboratory.

## Direct amplicon analysis techniques

Considerable impetus for rapid HLA typing comes from solid organ transplantation where HLA matching is generally regarded as being beneficial and long cold ischaemia time damaging. Current PCR-SSOP approaches cannot be completed within 5 h, double the time required for serology. There are molecular methods, which include SSP and PCR-RFLP mentioned earlier, which, while not so efficient for large sample numbers, are more suitable for rapid limited sample number throughput. Others include nested PCR-SSP, heteroduplex analysis and other conformational assays.

### PCR-RFLP

As discussed earlier, restriction endonucleases have been used to detect polymorphism with significant success on genomic DNA but the development of the PCR enabled the enzymes to be used in a much more precise way on much smaller blood samples without the necessity for detection probes. The principle of PCR-RFLP is that a precise region of target DNA is amplified and then cut. Because the sequences of the most common HLA alleles were already known, enzyme restriction sites could be defined within the PCR amplicon at sites of polymorphisms. Thus, a PCR amplicon of unknown HLA type would be digested with a variety of endonucleases, giving rise to PCR fragments of varying size depending on the alleles present. PCR-RFLP has been described for DQA1 (Maeda *et al.* 1989), DQB1 (Nomura *et al.* 1991; Mercier *et al.* 1992; Salazar *et al.* 1992), DPB1 (Hviid *et al.* 1992), DRB1 (Ota *et al.* 1991; Yunis *et al.* 1991; Mitsunaga *et al.* 1995), HLA-B44 subtyping (Varney *et al.* 1995) and HLA-C (Tatari *et al.* 1995). PCR-RFLP can rival more established class II genotyping methods for sensitivity and accuracy (Mizuki *et al.* 1992) but complex methodology interpretation and cost have prevented its widespread use. Additional problems include differential glycosylation in dialysis patients and a tendency to overestimate non-cutters because of a variety of reasons.

## PCR utilizing sequence-specific primers

In 1988–99, at least four separate groups, two in abstract form (British Society of Immunology and American Society of Histocompatibility and Immunogenetics) and two in full publication (Newton *et al.* 1989; Wu *et al.* 1989), described a system of PCR in which the specificity of the PCR reaction entailed matching the 3′ end of one primer with the target DNA sequence, allowing the identification of any point mutation to be identified within one or two PCR reactions. Newton described the detection of a single point mutation using one generic sense primer and two antisense primers: one antisense primer was specific for the 'normal' form and was refractory to PCR on 'mutant' DNA, while the other antisense primer for the 'mutant' was refractory to PCR on 'normal' DNA. This was termed the amplification refractory mutation system (ARMS). ARMS works because Taq polymerase lacks 3′ to 5′-exonucleolytic proof-reading activity (Chien *et al.* 1976; Tindall & Kunkel 1988). Such an activity would correct the mismatched terminal base of an ARMS primer in a mismatched primer–template complex and subsequently permit efficient priming with the 'repaired' primer. For efficient ARMS amplification without false priming the conditions need

to be highly stringent as it is possible for 3′-mismatch extension (Newton *et al.* 1989; Wu *et al.* 1989; Kwok *et al.* 1990). Stringency is multifactorial, relying on the concentration of all the PCR constituents such as target DNA, Taq, dNTPs, Tris and free magnesium (Bunce 1997). PCR stringency kinetics also relies on individual primer factors such as primer sequence, length and type of primer–template mismatches. An important feature of ARMS is that each individual reaction contains primers to amplify a so-called 'housekeeping' gene which detects possible PCR inhibition and thus acts as a positive control. Without this positive control it would be impossible to discriminate between a failed PCR reaction and a negative PCR reaction and hence all homozygous results would be questionable. Having the control in each well also helps with controlling for PCR product quantity variability, considered by the authors to be ±25% in our tissue types.

ARMS was predicted to be applicable to HLA analysis in 1989 (Wu *et al.* 1989) and was first applied in a limited fashion to HLA typing DPB in 1990 by Fugger *et al.* (1990), while our group utilized the 3′-mismatch concept to obtain DR4 group-specific amplification prior to DR4 SSOP subtyping (Lanchbury *et al.* 1990). The first comprehensive ARMS HLA typing system was described in 1992 by Olerup and Zetterquist for low-resolution HLA-DRB1 typing, including group-specific detection of DRB3 and DRB4 by ARMS using 19 PCR reactions (Olerup & Zetterquist 1992). Olerup and Zetterquist renamed the assay PCR-SSP (PCR using sequence-specific primers). This paper was a major breakthrough. Modern PCR-SSP features multiple PCR reactions where each reaction is specific for an allele, or more commonly a group of alleles which correspond to a serologically defined antigen. To type an individual completely at any given locus multiple PCR-SSP reactions are set up and subjected to PCR under identical conditions. The presence or absence of PCR amplification is detected in a gel electrophoresis step with visualization by ethidium bromide incorporation.

PCR-SSP was soon applied to detect polymorphisms in other class II loci such as HLA-DQB1 (Bunce *et al.* 1993; Olerup *et al.* 1993), HLA-DQA1 (Olerup *et al.* 1993) and DPB1 (Knipper *et al.* 1994). Identification of class I alleles by PCR-SSP was first reported by Browning *et al.* (1993), who described low-resolution typing of HLA-A. Thereafter, medium-resolution PCR-SSP systems were rapidly described for HLA-C (Bunce & Welsh 1994; Bunce *et al.* 1994) and HLA-B (Bunce *et al.* 1995a) with low-resolution HLA-B typing systems also being described (Sadler *et al.* 1994). We have recently developed a PCR-SSP method, known as phototyping, which allows the simultaneous detection of HLA-A, B, C, DRB1, DRB3, DRB4, DRB5 and DQB1 alleles (Bunce *et al.* 1995b). This method has a resolution and accuracy far greater than average serology and takes 3 h to complete, making it suitable for genotyping cadaver donors. More recently, improvements in DNA preparation, buffer and equipment has reduced the time necessary to under 2.5 h. The develop-

ment of automatic dispensing equipment and better electrophoresis equipment has also facilitated the use of phototyping in many laboratories and in our own—since September 1994—it has completely replaced serology. The resolution of the method is such that additional tests, such as precursor and MLC tests, are no longer necessary for unrelated bone marrow transplants.

An advantage of PCR-SSP is that it detects polymorphisms linked on an individual chromosome (*cis*) whereas PCR-SSOP detects polymorphisms on both DNA chromosomes (*cis* or *trans*). Thus PCR-SSP has greater power for discriminating between heterozygosity involving two closely related alleles, as illustrated in Fig. 3.2.

In addition, the nucleic acid substitutions present on

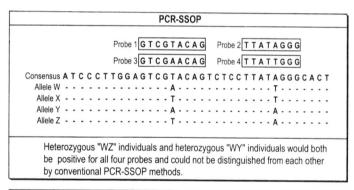

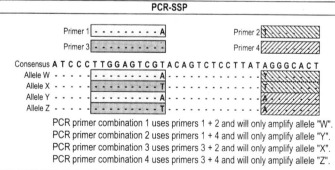

**Fig. 3.2** Comparison of PCR-SSOP and PCR-SSP for the determination of *cis*-located polymorphisms.

novel unsequenced allelic variants can be identified by PCR-mapping. With this technique, a potential new allele is mapped by using a sense primer that recognizes the allelic variant—normally from the initial molecular typing—in combination with multiple antisense primers in multiple reactions. The positive and negative reactions with these primer mixes can then be used to map out many of the allelic variants' polymorphisms. While this approach is certainly no substitute for sequencing, it has been used to identify and predict sequence of many new class I (Bunce & Welsh 1994; Bunce *et al.* 1994, 1995a,b; Krausa *et al.* 1995a) and class II alleles (Aldener & Olerup 1993; Poli *et al.* 1996), predictions which have been subsequently proved correct by sequencing.

PCR-SSP is typically used as a medium-resolution technique but recently we have described allele-specific one-step SSP for HLA-C (Bunce *et al.* 1996), while others have applied allele-specific PCR-SSP to DRB1 (Savelkoul *et al.* 1995) and to HLA-A (Krausa & Browning 1996). Allele-specific PCR-SSP is usually achieved by using a combination of group-specific amplifications coupled with some allele-specific reactions. However, while this approach to allele-specific typing is theoretically applicable to all HLA antigens, it would only be possible by using a large array of primer mixes. Therefore, to obtain allele-specific typing, techniques such as nested PCR-SSP and conformational assays have been developed to be used either as individual complete methods or methods used to supplement medium-resolution typing obtained by PCR-SSP or SSOP. The major problem with PCR-SSP is its unsuitability for large throughput of more than 12 full types (A, B, C, DR, DQ) (12×192 PCRs) per person per day. The major advantage for transplant studies is rapid results (<2 h) from blood to result. Its cost per type in consumables is around $30, while commercial prices are around $600–800, the differences reflecting the complexity of designing your own system.

## Nested PCR-SSP

Nested PCR-SSP is a two-step approach to HLA typing whereby the region of interest is amplified in the first step and this amplicon is used instead of genomic DNA for the second sequence-specific amplifications, using primers which are internal to the first pair of amplification primers. Nested PCR-SSP was first described by Bein *et al.* (1992) as a method for complete medium-resolution typing of HLA-DRB1. In Bein *et al.*'s method, exon 2 of all HLA-DRB1 alleles was amplified and subjected to a second round amplification using 18 PCR-SSP reactions which, like one-step PCR-SSP, used an internal control amplification to prove the success of each individual reaction. The results were similar to one-step PCR-SSP but it was the latter simpler quicker technique which became popular.

Nested PCR-SSP does have distinct advantages over conventional PCR-SSP in that the amount of DNA required is very small. In addition, allele-specific nested PCR-SSP is applicable to subtyping highly polymorphic alleles such as HLA-A*02 (Krausa *et al.* 1995b). For antigen-specific nested PCR-SSP only the alleles of interest are amplified, so in the case of HLA-A*02 only the A*02 alleles are amplified and these amplicons are then subjected to a second round with internal HLA-A*02 primers. This antigen-specific approach has the advantage of allowing all HLA-A*02 alleles to be detected in all combinations without the interference from closely related alleles, such as HLA-A*68, which would not be amplified in the initial reaction.

## SSP haplotyping

Conventional PCR-SSP reactions used in HLA typing utilize a pair of primers that detect just two of the many linked polymorphisms that make up a typical HLA allele. In less polymorphic systems, such as TNF, LTa and HLA-HFE, it is possible to link the polymorphisms together as a series of alleles so that all the polymorphisms are linked together to yield *cis* and *trans* information and thus haplotype information is generated (Fanning *et al.* 1997). This method can be extended to link polymorphisms on different neighbouring genes without the need for family studies. However, its potential is limited by the length over which the PCR will function and over which specificity can be obtained, at present only 3.5 kb with a potential of up to 50 kb. Although more reactions are needed than in conventional SSP the redundancy significantly reduces the need for the control amplification and hence allows very much more simple automation.

## Conformational assays

### Heteroduplex analysis

At the end of any PCR cycle the individual strands may reanneal with each other to form homoduplexes, or they may reanneal with an unrelated DNA strand to form a heteroduplex, or they may remain as single-stranded structures (Sorrentino *et al*. 1991). These different forms of PCR product have unique conformational structures which may be differentiated by their electrophoretic mobilities in a temperature or denaturing gradient gel. This PCR phenomenon has been applied to HLA to produce tissue typing methods which can theoretically not only detect existing polymorphisms but also new polymorphisms. PCR heteroduplex analysis has never gained popularity for identifying HLA polymorphisms because of the complexity of the gel analysis and the technically challenging conditions, but it has been used to match individuals for HLA-DR and HLA-DP by 'DNA cross-matching' (Clay *et al*. 1991), whereby donor and recipient DNA is mixed before the final stage of the PCR and allowing donor–recipient hetero- and homoduplexes to form, which may indicate whether the pair are indeed HLA identical.

The discrimination of heteroduplex analysis has been enhanced by the use of a universal heteroduplex generator (UHG) (Clay *et al*. 1994). The UHG is a synthetic DNA strand which is similar to the polymorphic sequence of the target gene but contains substitutions at the polymorphic sites to make the UHG different to all known alleles. By incorporating the UHG strand into the PCR the number of informative heteroduplexes, and hence discriminatory power of the technique, is increased. Heteroduplex analysis has been used for class II typing but like conventional PCR-SSOP it cannot achieve separation of single alleles. Discrimination of heterozygotes has been successfully

addressed in class I DNA typing by Arguello *et al*. using a novel method of allele separation called complementary strand analysis (CSA) (Arguello *et al*. 1996). CSA uses a biotinylated primer in the initial locus-specific amplification which labels one DNA strand. The DNA strands are then chemically dissociated and separated using streptavidin-coated magnetic beads and then allowed to anneal to a previously prepared reference DNA strand. The reference strand is generated from locus-specific amplification of an unrelated sample of known HLA type. The resulting hybridized alleles can then be separated using a two-layer gel system consisting of agarose and polyacrylamide layers. The different hybridized products migrate to different positions in the gel according to the conformational mobility of the different products. The separated allelic strands can then be excised out of the gel layer and dot blotted on to a membrane and subsequently analysed by PCR-SSOP methods. The CSA technique has two advantages: first, the alleles are separated and thus heterozygous individuals can be SSOP typed more easily than with conventional SSOP methods; and, secondly, the gel electrophoresis of the separated alleles can in itself be used as a typing system.

### Single-stranded conformational polymorphism

Single-stranded conformational polymorphism analysis (SSCP) depends on the fact that single-stranded DNA molecules of differing sequences exhibit conformational changes as a result of intrastrand complementary base pairing (Orita *et al*. 1989). The different single-stranded products exhibit different mobilities during non-denaturing polyacrylamide gel electrophoresis which can be used to ascertain the genotype of an individual. So far SSCP has been applied successfully to HLA-A typing (Blaszczyk *et al*. 1995), HLA-DRB1, DQB1 and DQA1 typing (Carrington *et al*. 1992; Lo *et al*. 1992; Clay *et al*. 1995), DPA1 and DPB1 typing (Hoshino *et al*. 1992) and HLA-DR4 subtyping (Young & Darke 1993). However, as with heteroduplex analysis, the complexity of both the technique and the interpretation has prevented the widespread application of this technique.

## Sequence-based typing

PCR-SSP and PCR-SSOP methods are limited within the context of existing sequence information; novel alleles may be missed or mistyped by both PCR methods. New alleles are often identified by PCR-SSOP and SSP by unique patterns but these always require confirmation by sequencing before a new allele is accepted by the nomenclature committee. PCR-SSOP and SSP can never identify unique polymorphisms whereas sequencing can.

The principles of sequence-based typing (SBT) are that the polymorphic regions of any given allele are amplified by flanking PCR primers. The resulting PCR product is sequenced by any one of a variety of subtly different methods and computer analysed to ascertain the type. Computer analysis is required because the sequenced product from a heterozygous individual will contain two superimposed sequences which need to be aligned with all previously known sequences in order to be identified and separated.

SBT was initially described for HLA DRB1, DQB1 and DQA1 by Santamaria *et al.* (1992) and for HLA-DPB1 by Rozemuller *et al.* (1993). SBT is admirably suited to class II typing as most of the functional polymorphism is located in exon 2. This means that a single sequencing reaction is adequate to ascertain the class II type. SBT typing of class I exons 2, 3 and 4 was first described by Santamaria *et al.* (1993); however, it is not widely used because of perceived complexity and occasional inaccuracies (Domena *et al.* 1994). Elegant alternative SBT typing approaches for class I have been developed that concentrate on exons 2 and 3 where most class I polymorphism is located (Petersdorf *et al.* 1994; Petersdorf & Hansen 1995). To alleviate the complexity of sequence-based typing of the highly polymorphic HLA-B locus, Petersdorf *et al.* have used a combination of group-specific amplification followed by SBT (Petersdorf & Hansen 1995).

The main drawbacks of SBT are the equipment costs and the time required to fully sequence one individual. A laboratory with a single automated sequencer would struggle to fully class I and II type more than five individuals per day. Offset against this is the tremendous advantage in having high-resolution typing, but the question remains of how relevant high-resolution typing is in transplantation and disease, a question which cannot now be answered without some form of extensive high-resolution typing. One cautionary note is that, like all molecular methods, sequencing is not infallible and many sequenced alleles have had to be retracted because of errors, most commonly GC inversions. In addition, even recent SBT methods do not always discriminate between all heterozygous combinations of alleles (Petersdorf *et al.* 1994).

## Other new methods in tissue typing

In most solid organ transplant-related laboratories HLA typing is not the major activity. The screening of samples for the presence or absence of antibodies—both alloantibodies and autoantibodies—is considerably more time-consuming than tissue typing itself. There is a relatively simple but not absolute way of auditing this procedure in centres performing renal allografts; simply check survival curves of grafts in sensitized and non-sensitized recipients. In centres with sophisticated screening programmes these have the potential to be, and usually are, essentially identical. Without such screening the graft survival results in sensitized recipients will be worse because, unless HLA-matched grafts are used, antibody will contribute to failure figures, especially in the first few months post-transplant.

As screening becomes more complex and as the supply of cells and expertise in CDC decrease in laboratories as a result of the implementation of DNA techniques, a keen awareness has grown that new methods for antibody screening are necessary.

The testing of each serum against antigen panels of some sort is an essential requirement for specificity determination, but most samples screened are negative. The first successful realization that a positive or negative answer would both give panel reactivity—an essential for clinical activity—and allow only those positive samples to have further time-consuming and expensive screens is the so-called Flow-Screen technology (Sutton *et al.* 1995). Here cell pools of CLL, EBV or even PBLs, usually 10–12 strong, are mixed with individual serum samples and run in conventional flow cytometry. Two pools of 12 cells have so far proved sufficient to identify all graft-damaging antibodies, often several months before conventional cytotoxic tests become positive in patients awaiting transplantation. The method is also of use for detecting platelet-reacting antibodies, but for reasons not clearly defined platelet pools are not as efficient in detecting antibodies as those utilizing CLLs, EBV cell lines or PBLs.

The reasons why Flow-Screen works are complex. Basically there are a restricted number of amino acid positions in the MHC which drive alloantibody production, this total number being considerably less than the total number of identifiable alleles. This is part of the reason why relatively few cells are necessary. A shareware program—the Sequence subtractor or Red Dot program—written by ourselves but released through the UK Transplant Support Services Authority (UKTSSA) on the Internet, is a useful teaching aid to define alloantibody drive positions. An important additional point is that for optimal complement activation an IgG antibody needs multiple proximal site occupancy. The flow cytometer, while being dependent on site occupancy, is not restricted by a need for this to be proximal. Thus on commencement of response IgG antibodies which occupy non-proximal sites are better detected, as of course are those IgG alloantibodies which are non-complement-fixing. A combination of these facts ensures that relatively few cells will pick up all HLA antibodies as they are produced. The simple replacement of the anti-Ig second layer in the Flow-Screen by an anti-C4d monoclonal will also turn the flow into a cytotoxic test, a strategy sometimes useful for the identification of some IgM antibodies and necessary if the method is to be used for cross-matching. An example of the use of anti-C4d monoclonal is shown in Fig. 3.3.

In the simplest form of the assay, cells are reacted with patient sera and a labelled monoclonal to C4d added. Only where antibody has bound to antigen will complement bind and C4d be released. No washing step is therefore necessary. In the more usual assay the serum samples analysed are not fresh and exogenous complement is needed. The assay works better for IgM and IgG because of their relative complement activat-ing capacities but, unlike conventional CDC, exoge-nous human complement works better than rabbit although this may be because of the restricted number of monoclonals available. Any normal human serum at a dilution of 1:200–500 is adequate. If no directly con-jugated anti-C4d, mouse anti-C4ds are available to use with FITC anti-mouse, the additional washing steps have very little effect on the assay. Flow-Screen itself is sufficient for identification of those antibodies which need further screening for antibody specificity; however, the C4d assay is very useful for IgM antibody detection in general and can be applied to tissue sec-tions or ELISA assays.

This realization that the detection of positivity or negativity is useful has also led commercial companies to market ELISA kits which perform this function. One of these utilizes antigen isolated from platelets and is now commercialized as GTI QuikScreen (Zaer *et al.* 1997) and although the method has flaws it is a useful prescreen in use in many centres as well as in the origi-nating centre.

A second ELISA system developed by Sangstat is more sophisticated and will detect antibodies to MHC class II. This system relies on MHC antigens secreted by cell lines. Neither assay will currently assign cyto-toxic screening to the waste-basket. Platelets are noto-rious for irregular expression of HLA class I and HLA-C in particular, and they do not express class II. Nevertheless, the speed and cost of this assay make it a competitor to Flow-Screen for the detection of positiv-ity or negativity in samples which require further screening. Here Flow-Screen has the edge in sophistica-tion because it will detect antibodies to class II but the QuikScreen GTI ELISA, for example, is faster and cheaper. Neither assay is useful for determining specificity. Here the Sangstat PRA-STAT ELISA assay has the most potential. However, there were errors in the MHC class I tissue types of the original cell lines and no MHC class II data were available. Many labo-ratories, including our own, found PRA-STAT to be incredibly reproducible but to give the wrong answers in specificity determinations. It was also excellent, indeed equivalent to Flow-Screen, in determining posi-tivity. Retyping by ourselves and others has rendered the Sangstat ELISA superior to conventional cytotoxic

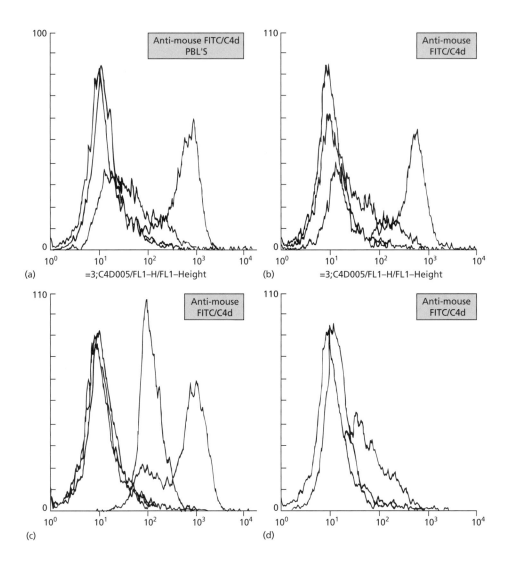

**Fig. 3.3** The C4d assay which effectively converts flow cytometry into a CDC test with human as opposed to rabbit complement.

testing in many respects and nearing the breadth necessary to be the sole method of HLA antibody screening. For financial reasons our own preferred route is Flow-Screen followed by ELISA. Flow-Screen can determine positivity or negativity on 200 samples/day and ELISA can then be performed on the positive percentage, usually around 40%.

Can good screening ever replace cross-matching? This is a complex question and the subject of both rational and irrational debate in the professions related to transplantation. The simple answer is yes—good screening can replace cross-matching. However, if we replace the question with 'Can good screening replace *all* cross-matching?' then the answer is a straight 'No' or a no accompanied by 'but it can replace some, most or almost all', dependent on the viewpoint and country.

This debate is fundamental both to transplantation and to laboratory practice and it is important therefore that the background is included with a discussion of the methods available. Imagine you have 10 potential recipients for a donor kidney and it is 2 a.m. On average each patient has been on the waiting list 3 years and there are 300 serum samples available for cross-matching. The ideal scenario would be to test all samples against donor T and B cells from the donor for IgM and IgG antibodies at two dilutions and at two temperatures and to carry out autocross-matches. Both conventional cross-matching and a method involving enhancement such as anti-immunoglobulin or flow cytometry should be used on sensitized patients or those having a past history of pregnancy or transfusion. Now you have to start finding out where the 300 samples are in your stock of thousands and begin accessing them. Several things would have happened before full testing could be completed by one or even two persons:

1 the surgeon would have proceeded anyway or given the kidney away to avoid ischaemic destruction;

2 you would be asleep or in danger of making mistakes;

3 the next kidney would have arrived and there are no more on-call staff;

4 the donor cells would be in such a bad state by the time you finish your assay that the results are uninterpretable anyway;

5 you have only tested patients who have recently come on the list and who therefore have only a few samples;

6 the samples have been out of the freezer so long they are less effective in subsequent cross-matches; and

7 you have selected, based on previous screening, only those samples from those recipients which are applicable to this donor, finished the testing and gone home.

The only option is 7; it is both scientific and common sense but it is not allowed in some countries because of standards laid down by professional or other bodies. There is no automated way of replacing the required cross-matching at present and so the more sophisticated the screening the better your definition.

The general methods now adopted by many high- or medium-throughput laboratories are as follows. Basically the format is to define a provenance for the antibody response for each recipient. Absolute rules and rules applicable to your centre and its other practices are then tailored in. Each recipient is considered as an individual on the basis of the antibody provenance plus additional factors and the rules best for that individual applied. There are, however, a series of general rules.

1 Patients who have and who have had antibodies which consistently react with cells of donor type are not considered. If, for example, a recipient has had anti-HLA-A2 antibody on monthly or bimonthly screening for the past three years he or she would not be considered for an HLA-A2-positive donor. In centres with molecular typing and amino acid level screening this is reasonable, even for those having antibodies which only react with certain A2 subtypes.

2 Samples are tested during screening at dilution where appropriate, both to aid specificity detection and to identify those which might need dilution at cross-match.

3 Conventional cytotoxicity is supplemented by Flow-Screen or ELISA for detecting which samples need specificity determination. At cross-match AHG, Flow-Screen or ELISA is used to supplement conventional cytotoxicity in those patients who are sensitized, LRD or LURD or potentially sensitized (i.e. past samples missing).

4 Samples are selected for cross-match to cover peaks in the sensitization history. Others are ignored.

5 Autoantibodies are defined before cross-match.

6 A cross-match log is kept of all unexpected reactions at cross-match.

This approach has several advantages; not least it enables realistic on-call. One unexpected advantage is in the confidence it gives to allow transplant in the face of unexpected weak cross-matches (false-positives). There are several causes of these, ranging from infected or partially viable donor cells through to recent recipient dialysis.

In our own centre, with full user permission, certain transplants are allowed to proceed without cross-match results: those transplants into patients consistently negative on Flow-Screen and where there is no transfusion or pregnancy history. In some cases the flow cytometry cross-match alone is used to confirm no recent event in such patients. No transplant must proceed if there is a current positive IgM or IgG anti-donor MHC class I and/or class II. No transplant must proceed if there is a past positive IgG antidonor class I antibody. Transplants having repeat mismatches are encouraged if there is provenance showing that the mismatch(es) have *not* been responded to. Unexpected current weak B cell positives are allowed if no event—transfusion or infection—has occurred in the past 10 days. Unexpected weak T cell reactions are also ignored after repeat with the same provisos of infection and transfusion. Frozen aliquots of the same positive antibody pool are used neat and in dilution with each flow-cytometry cross-match to control for sensitivity shift.

## Conclusions

There are many reasons for tissue typing: matching for solid organ and bone marrow transplantation, as an important aid to alloantibody definition, anthropological studies, disease association studies, drug reactions, forensic studies, cancer studies and to facilitate investigations into T-cell-mediated immunity. The tissue typing method most suited to each application is a balance of resolution, sample numbers, time, money, sample material, the method(s) used on necessary control populations and the expertise of the individuals performing the typing.

It is now possible to use molecular methods for all tissue typing applications without recourse to serology, except those involving cell type restricted loss variants, for example, surface expression of class I in tumours. For most applications a medium-resolution method is the optimum start. It allows the researcher to focus quickly on candidate loci, antigens or alleles which can then be defined further by higher-resolution techniques. It allows the transplanter to define antibody specificities, or define bone marrow panels and provide a level of discrimination easily suitable for solid organ exchange programmes. For the definition of antibodies in potential transplant recipients medium- or high-resolution typing goes hand in hand with the epitope mapping of antibody specificity. In most cases it does not matter which medium-resolution technique is used, so long as it is performed accurately. Allele-specific

typing, whether by SBT or SSOP or SSP, presents the researcher with a powerful analysis tool. In disease studies a weak association with serological antigens may become clear when individual amino acids are considered.

In transplantation the survival impact of immuno-dominant epitopes present on multiple alleles can only really be investigated by high-resolution typing of all donors and recipients. This application of high-resolution typing requires a different breed of computer analysis. Instead of correlating disease or rejection with a list of antigens the computer programs of the future will be required to correlate disease or rejection with linear *and* conformational epitopes (Barnardo *et al.* 1997). It is also expected that computer programs will be required to correlate disease or rejection with peptide presentation in either class I or II molecules. Ultimately this may lead to the discovery that certain combinations of class I and II antigens present within an individual will predispose that individual to disease or rejection given exposure to certain pathogens or transplanted antigens.

Generally, molecular typing methods used without serological backup cannot identify null alleles or expression variants which may cause problems in certain transplant situations. Most null alleles are extremely rare, although the DR53 null allele (Sutton *et al.* 1989) is common in most populations. It is important that null alleles are detected, especially in unrelated bone marrow transplantation. The photo-typing PCR-SSP method (Bunce *et al.* 1995b) incorporates a PCR-SSP reaction to identify the DR53 null allele (O'Neill *et al.* 1996) and it is theoretically possible to develop PCR-SSP reactions or PCR-SSO probes to detect the rarer null alleles such as the HLA-A2 null allele A*0215N (Ishikawa *et al.* 1996) as and when these null alleles are sequenced. In time, greater sophistication will be required so that not only null alleles are identified by molecular techniques but low- and high-expression variants are also identified.

The best current single general-purpose method for transplantation, typing all HLA loci to a medium resolution, is currently PCR-SSP. It has the advantage of flexible resolution coupled with ease of interpretation and speed of result but it is not perfect. Multiple reactions are required which require time-consuming dispensing of reagents and substantial gel electrophoresis to detect PCR products. However, it is now possible to dispense PCR mixtures and primer mixes entirely with multichannel automatic dispensing pipettes or dedicated dispensing machines, and gel electrophoresis equipment has been manufactured to allow direct loading from 96-well formats. This means that dispensing and detection of multiple reactions is as easy as dispensing multiple serological reactions. Indeed, it is now possible to automate completely PCR-SSP using Biomek workstations (Patrick Merel, personal communication). Eventually the electrophoresis step is likely to be eradicated completely as ELISA-based detection systems become commonplace (Ferencik & Grosse-Wilde 1993; Chia *et al.* 1994).

While molecular methods are here to stay they are not ideal in isolation. They do not prove that the antigen is expressed on the surface. While it is usually safer to assume expression in cases of doubt, the current situation is by no means completely satisfactory. It is true that, if we have a sequence which confers expression for an HLA molecule, e.g. for HLA-DRB4 on a DR7 haplotype, we can easily define a 'molecular' test for expression (O'Neill *et al.* 1996). However, in cases where, for example, tumour cells lose expression of individual MHC antigens the causes are varied and the loss is very much more cell-specific. It is for these and other reasons that, although we use molecular typing because its gains far outweigh its disadvantages, we are still strong supporters of serology. The use of two-dimensional gel analyses for HLA antigen recognition peaked before the advent of molecular methods and has lost favour. However, it is the only method available which gives direct information of the glycosylation and phosphorylation of proteins as well as indicating relative chain up-regulation.

For antibody screening, so necessary for renal transplantation and platelet transfusion, no single method has achieved dominance. Currently the most efficient procedure involves a prescreen for what is positive or negative; originally Flow-Screen was the only method for this but it is now rivalled by the commercial ELISA systems, GRI for class I and Sangstat for class I and II. Flow-Screen has the edge in detecting which positives

are high-titre antibodies, useful in liver and heart transplantation where low-titre antibodies are less of a problem. A recent paper, shows Flow-Screen and Sangstat ELISA to be remarkably equivalent in other respects. Such ± screens are also of use in bone marrow transplantation, where it is a very rare event for antibody to be a problem, so screening of every sample is inefficient. The identification of specificity in the positive samples after ± screening is still best achieved by CDC against panels of cells typed to medium or high resolution. However, the commercial ELISA from Sangstat is improving rapidly and new ELISA methods from other sources are now on test in various laboratories around the world.

## References

Aldener, A. & Olerup, O. (1993) Characterization of a novel DQB1 (DQB1*0609) allele by PCR amplification with sequence-specific primers (PCR-SSP) and nucleotide sequencing. *Tissue Antigens* 42, 536–538.

Allsopp, C.E., Hill, A.V., Kwiatkowski, D. *et al.* (1991) Sequence analysis of HLA-Bw53, a common West African allele, suggests an origin by gene conversion of HLA-B35. *Human Immunology* 30, 105–109.

Arguello, R., Avakian, H., Goldman, J.M. & Madrigal, J.A. (1996) A novel method for simultaneous high resolution identification of HLA-A, HLA-B and HLA-Cw alleles. *Proceedings of the National Academy of Sciences (USA)* 93, 10961–10965.

Barnardo, M.C.N.M., Bunce, M., Thursz, M. & Welsh, K.I. (1997) Analysis of the molecular epitopes of anti-HLA antibodies using a computer program, OODAS: Object Oriented Definition of Antibody Specificity. In: *Genetic Diversity of HLA: Functional and Medical Implications*. EDK, Sevres.

Bein, G., Glaser, R. & Kirchner, H. (1992) Rapid HLA-DRB1 genotyping by nested PCR amplification. *Tissue Antigens* 39, 68–73.

Bidwell, J.L., Bidwell, E.A., Savage, D.A. *et al.* (1988) A DNA-RFLP typing system that positively identifies serologically well-defined and ill-defined HLA-DR and DQ alleles, including DRw10. *Transplantation* 45, 640–646.

Blasczyk, R., Hahn, U., Wehling, J., Huhn, D. & Salama, A. (1995) Complete subtyping of the HLA-A locus by sequence-specific amplification followed by direct sequencing or single-strand conformation polymorphism analysis. *Tissue Antigens* 46, 86–95.

Browning, M.J., Krausa, P., Rowan, A. *et al.* (1993) Tissue typing the HLA-A locus from genomic DNA by sequence-specific PCR: comparison of HLA genotype and surface expression on colorectal tumor cell lines. *Proceedings of the National Academy of Sciences (USA)* 90, 2842–2845.

Bugawan, T.L., Begovich, A.B. & Erlich, H.A. (1990) Rapid HLA-DPB typing using enzymatically amplified DNA and nonradioactive sequence-specific oligonucleotide probes. *Immunogenetics* 32, 231–241. (Published erratum appears in *Immunogenetics* 34, 413.)

Bugawan, T.L., Apple, R. & Erlich, H.A. (1994) A method for typing polymorphism at the HLA-A locus using PCR amplification and immobilized oligonucleotide probes. *Tissue Antigens* 44, 137–147.

Bunce, M. (1997) *The development and applications of a single PCR-based method of genotyping.* Thesis, Nuffield Department of Surgery, Oxford Brookes University, Oxford.

Bunce, M. & Welsh, K.I. (1994) Rapid DNA typing for HLA-C using sequence-specific primers (PCR-SSP): identification of serological and non-serologically defined HLA-C alleles including several new alleles. *Tissue Antigens* 43, 7–17.

Bunce, M., Taylor, C.J. & Welsh, K.I. (1993) Rapid HLA-DQB typing by eight polymerase chain reaction amplifications with sequence-specific primers (PCR-SSP). *Human Immunology* 37, 201–206.

Bunce, M., Barnardo, M.C. & Welsh, K.I. (1994) Improvements in HLA-C typing using sequence-specific primers (PCR-SSP) including definition of HLA-Cw9 and Cw10 and a new allele HLA-'Cw7/8v'. *Tissue Antigens* 44, 200–203.

Bunce, M., Fanning, G.C. & Welsh, K.I. (1995a) Comprehensive, serologically equivalent DNA typing for HLA-B by PCR using sequence-specific primers (PCR-SSP). *Tissue Antigens* 45, 81–90.

Bunce, M., O'Neill, C.M., Barnardo, M.C.N.M. *et al.* (1995b) Phototyping: comprehensive DNA typing for HLA-A, B, C, DRB1, DRB3, DRB4, DRB5 and DQB1 by PCR with 144 primer mixes utilising sequence-specific primers (PCR-SSP). *Tissue Antigens* 46, 355–367.

Bunce, M., Barnardo, M.C.N.M., Procter, J. *et al.* (1996) High resolution HLA-C typing by PCR-SSP: identification of allelic frequencies and linkage disequilibria in 604 unrelated random UK Caucasoids and a comparison with serology. *Tissue Antigens* 48, 680–691.

Carrington, M., Miller, T., White, M. *et al.* (1992) Typing of HLA-DQA1 and DQB1 using DNA single-strand conformation polymorphism. *Human Immunology* 33, 208–214.

Chia, D., Terasaki, P., Chan, H. *et al.* (1994) A new simplified method of gene typing. *Tissue Antigens* 44, 300–305.

Chien, A., Edgar, D.B. & Trela, J.M. (1976) Deoxyribonucleic acid polymerase from the extreme thermophile *Thermus aquaticus*. *Journal of Bacteriology* 127, 1550–1557.

Clay, T.M., Bidwell, J.L., Howard, M.R. & Bradley, B.A. (1991) PCR-fingerprinting for selection of HLA matched unrelated marrow donors. Collaborating Centres in the IMUST Study. *Lancet* 337, 1049–1052.

Clay, T.M., Culpan, D., Howell, W.M. *et al.* (1994) UHG crossmatching. A comparison with PCR-SSO typing in the selection of HLA-DPB1-compatible bone marrow donors. *Transplantation* 58, 200–207.

Clay, T.M., Culpan, D., Pursall, M.C., Bradley, B.A. & Bidwell, J.L. (1995) HLA-DQB1 and DQA1 matching by ambient temperature PCR-SSCP. *European Journal of Immunogenetics* 22, 467–478.

Date, Y., Kimura, A., Kato, H. & Sasazuki, T. (1996) DNA typing of the HLA-A gene: population study and identification of four new alleles in Japanese. *Tissue Antigens* 47, 93–101.

Domena, J.D., Little, A.M., Arnett, K.L. *et al.* (1994) A small test of a sequence-based typing method: definition of the B*1520 allele. *Tissue Antigens* 44, 217–224.

Eliaou, J.F., Humbert, M., Balaguer, P. *et al.* (1989) A method of HLA class II typing using nonradioactive labelled oligonucleotides. *Tissue Antigens* 33, 475–485.

Erlich, H., Bugawan, T., Begovich, A.B. *et al.* (1991) HLA-DR, DQ and DP typing using PCR amplification and immobilized probes. *European Journal of Immunogenetics* 18, 33–55.

Fanning, G.C., Bunce, M. & Welsh, K.I. (1997) PCR-haplotyping using 3′ mismatches in the forward and reverse primers: application to the biallelic polymorphisms of TNF and LTa. *Tissue Antigens* (in press).

Ferencik, S. & Grosse-Wilde, H. (1993) A simple photometric detection method for HLA-DRB1 specific PCR-SSP products. *European Journal of Immunogenetics* 20, 123–125.

Fernandez-Vina, M.A., Falco, M., Sun, Y. & Stastny, P. (1992) DNA typing for HLA class I alleles: I. Subsets of HLA-A2: and of -A28. *Human Immunology* 33, 163–173.

Fernandez-Vina, M., Lazaro, A.M., Sun, Y. *et al.* (1995) Population diversity of B-locus alleles observed by high resolution DNA typing. *Tissue Antigens* 45, 153–168.

Fleischhauer, K., Zino, E., Bordignon, C. & Benazzi, E. (1995) Complete generic and extensive fine-specificity typing of the HLA-B locus by the PCR-SSOP method. *Tissue Antigens* 46, 281–292.

Fugger, L., Morling, N., Ryder, L.P., Odum, N. & Svejgaard, A. (1990) Technical aspects of typing for HLA-DP alleles using allele-specific DNA *in vitro* amplification and sequence-specific oligonucleotide probes. Detection of single base mismatches. *Journal of Immunological Methods* 129, 175–185.

Gentilomi, G., Musiani, M., Zerbini, M. *et al.* (1989) A hybrido-immunocytochemical assay for the *in situ* detection of cytomegalovirus DNA using digoxigenin-labeled probes. *Journal of Immunological Methods* **125**, 177–183.

Hoshino, S., Kimura, A., Fukuda, Y., Doshi, K. & Sasazuki, T. (1992) Polymerase chain reaction-single strand conformation polymorphism analysis of polymorphism in DPA1 and DPB1 genes: a simple, economical and rapid method for histocompatibility testing. *Human Immunology* **33**, 98.

Hviid, T.V., Madsen, H.O. & Morling, N. (1992) HLA-DPB1 typing with polymerase chain reaction and restriction fragment length polymorphism technique in Danes. *Tissue Antigens* **40**, 140–144.

Ishikawa, Y., Tokunaga, K., Tanaka, H. *et al.* (1996) HLA-A null allele with a stop codon, HLA-A*0215N, identified in a homozygous state in a healthy adult. *Immunogenetics* **43**, 1–5.

Kennedy, L.J., Poulton, K.V., Dyer, P.A., Ollier, W.E. & Thomson, W. (1995) Definition of HLA-C alleles using sequence-specific oligonucleotide probes (PCR-SSOP). *Tissue Antigens* **46**, 187–195.

Kimura, A. & Sasazuki, T. (1992) Eleventh International Histocompatibility Workshop reference protocol for the HLA DNA-typing technique. In: *Proceedings of the Eleventh International Histocompatibility Workshop and Conference 1991*, Vol. 1. (eds K. Tsuji, M. Aizawa & T. Sasazuki), pp. 397–419. Oxford University Press, Oxford.

Kimura, A., Dong, R.P., Harada, H. & Sasazuki, T. (1992) DNA typing of HLA class II genes in B-lymphoblastoid cell lines homozygous for HLA. *Tissue Antigens* **40**, 5–12.

Knipper, A.J., Hinney, A., Schuch, B. *et al.* (1994) Selection of unrelated bone marrow donors by PCR-SSP typing and subsequent nonradioactive sequence-based typing for HLA DRB1/3/4/5, DQB1, and DPB1 alleles. *Tissue Antigens* **44**, 275–284.

Krausa, P. & Browning, M.J. (1996) A comprehensive PCR-SSP typing system for identification of HLA-A locus alleles. *Tissue Antigens* **47**, 237–244.

Krausa, P., Barouch, D., Bodmer, J.G. & Browning, M.J. (1995a) Rapid characterization of HLA class I alleles by gene mapping using ARMS PCR. *European Journal of Immunogenetics* **22**, 283–287.

Krausa, P., Brywka, M. III, Savage, D. *et al.* (1995b) Genetic polymorphism within HLA-A*02: significant allelic variation revealed in different population. *Tissue Antigens* **45**, 223–231.

Kwok, S., Kellogg, D.E., McKinney, N. *et al.* (1990) Effects of primer-template mismatches on the polymerase chain reaction: human immunodeficiency virus type 1 model studies. *Nucleic Acids Research* **18**, 999–1005.

Lanchbury, J.S., Hall, M.A., Welsh, K.I. & Panayi, G.S. (1990) Sequence analysis of HLA-DR4B1 subtypes: additional first domain variability is detected by oligonucleotide hybridization and nucleotide sequencing. *Human Immunology* **27**, 136–144.

Levine, J.E. & Yang, S.Y. (1994) SSOP typing of the Tenth International Histocompatibility Workshop reference cell lines for HLA-C alleles. *Tissue Antigens* **44**, 174–183.

Lo, Y.M., Patel, P., Mehal, W.Z. *et al.* (1992) Analysis of complex genetic systems by ARMS-SSCP: application to HLA genotyping. *Nucleic Acids Research* **20**, 1005–1009.

Maeda, M., Murayama, N., Ishii, H. *et al.* (1989) A simple and rapid method for HLA-DQA1 genotyping by digestion of PCR-amplified DNA with allele specific restriction endonucleases. *Tissue Antigens* **34**, 290–298.

Mercier, B., Ferec, C., Dufosse, F. & Huart, J.J. (1992) Improvement in HLA-DQB typing by PCR-RFLP: introduction of a constant restriction site in one of the primers for digestion control. *Tissue Antigens* **40**, 86–89.

Mickelson, E., Smith, A., McKinney, S., Anderson, G. & Hansen, J.A. (1993) A comparative study of HLA-DRB1 typing by standard serology and hybridization of non-radioactive sequence-specific oligonucleotide probes to PCR-amplified DNA. *Tissue Antigens* **41**, 86–93.

Middleton, D., Williams, F., Cullen, C. & Mallon, E. (1995) Modification of an HLA-B PCR-SSOP typing system leading to improved allele determination. *Tissue Antigens* **45**, 232–236.

Mitsunaga, S., Oguchi, T., Tokunaga, K. *et al.* (1995) High-resolution HLA-DQB1 typing by combination of group-specific amplification and restriction fragment length polymorphism. *Human Immunology* **42**, 307–314.

Mittal, K.K., Mickey, M.R., Singal, D.P. & Terasaki, P.I. (1968) Serotyping for homotransplantation. 18. Refinement of microdroplet lymphocyte cytotoxicity test. *Transplantation* **6**, 913–927.

Mizuki, N., Ohno, S., Sugimura, K. *et al.* (1992) PCR-RFLP is as sensitive and reliable as PCR-SSO in HLA class II genotyping. *Tissue Antigens* **40**, 100–103.

Mytilineos, J., Scherer, S. & Opelz, G. (1990) Comparison of RFLP-DR beta and serological HLA-DR typing in 1500 individuals. *Transplantation* **50**, 870–873.

Mytilineos, J., Scherer, S., Trejaut, J. *et al.* (1992) Analysis of discrepancies between serologic and DNA-RFLP typing for HLA-DR in kidney graft recipients. *Transplantation Proceedings* **24**, 2478–2479.

Newton, C.R., Graham, A., Heptinstall, L.E. *et al.* (1989) Analysis of any point mutation in DNA. The amplification refractory mutation system (ARMS). *Nucleic Acids Research* **17**, 2503–2516.

Nomura, N., Ota, M., Tsuji, K. & Inoko, H. (1991) HLA-DQB1 genotyping by a modified PCR-RFLP method combined with group-specific primers. *Tissue Antigens* **38**, 53–59.

Oh, S.H., Fleischhauer, K. & Yang, S.Y. (1993) Isoelectric focusing subtypes of HLA-A can be defined by oligonucleotide typing. *Tissue Antigens* **41**, 135–142.

Olerup, O., Aldener, A. & Fogdell, A. (1993) HLA-DQB1

and -DQA1 typing by PCR amplification with sequence-specific primers (PCR-SSP) in 2 hours. *Tissue Antigens* **41**, 119–134.

Olerup, O. & Zetterquist, H. (1992) HLA-DR typing by PCR amplification with sequence-specific primers (PCR-SSP) in 2 hours: an alternative to serological DR typing in clinical practice including donor–recipient matching in cadaveric transplantation [see comments]. *Tissue Antigens* **39**, 225–235.

O'Neill, C.M., Bunce, M. & Welsh, K.I. (1996) Detection of the DRB4 null gene, DRB4*0101102N, by PCR-SSP and its distinction from other DRB4 genes. *Tissue Antigens* **47**, 245–248.

Opelz, G., Mytilineos, J., Scherer, S. *et al.* (1993) Analysis of HLA-DR matching in DNA-typed cadaver kidney transplants. *Transplantation* **55**, 782–785.

Orita, M., Iwahana, H., Kanazawa, H., Hayashi, K. & Sekiya, T. (1989) Detection of polymorphisms of human DNA by gel electrophoresis as single stranded polymorphisms. *Proceedings of theNational Academy of Sciences (USA)* **86**, 2766–2770.

Ota, M., Seki, T., Nomura, N. *et al.* (1991) Modified PCR-RFLP method for HLA-DPB1 and -DQA1 genotyping. *Tissue Antigens* **38**, 60–71.

Petersdorf, E.W. & Hansen, J.A. (1995) A comprehensive approach for typing the alleles of the HLA-B locus by automated sequencing. *Tissue Antigens* **46**, 73–85.

Petersdorf, E.W., Stanley, J.F., Martin, P.J. & Hansen, J.A. (1994) Molecular diversity of the HLA-C locus in unrelated marrow transplantation. *Tissue Antigens* **44**, 93–99.

Poli, F., Bianchi, P., Crespiatico, L. *et al.* (1996) Characterization of a new DRB5 allele (DRB5*0105) by PCR-SSP and direct sequencing. *Tissue Antigens* **47**, 338–340.

Rozemuller, E.H., Bouwens, A.G., Bast, B.E. & Tilanus, M.G. (1993) Assignment of HLA-DPB alleles by computerized matching based upon sequence data. *Human Immunology* **37**, 207–212.

Sadler, A.M., Petronzelli, F., Krausa, P. *et al.* (1994) Low-resolution DNA typing for HLA-B using sequence-specific primers in allele- or group-specific ARMS/PCR. *Tissue Antigens* **44**, 148–154.

Saiki, R.K., Scharf, S., Faloona, F. *et al.* (1985) Enzymatic amplification of beta-globin genomic sequences and restriction site analysis for diagnosis of sickle cell anemia. *Science* **230**, 1350–1354.

Saiki, R.K., Bugawan, T.L., Horn, G.T., Mullis, K.B. & Erlich, H.A. (1986) Analysis of enzymatically amplified beta-globin and HLA-DQ alpha DNA with allele-specific oligonucleotide probes. *Nature* **324**, 163–166.

Saiki, R.K., Walsh, P.S., Levenson, C.H. & Erlich, H.A. (1989) Genetic analysis of amplified DNA with immobilized sequence-specific oligonucleotide probes.

*Proceedings of the National Academy of Sciences (USA)* **86**, 6230–6234.

Salazar, M., Yunis, J.J., Delgado, M.B., Bing, D. & Yunis, E.J. (1992) HLA-DQB1 allele typing by a new PCR-RFLP method: correlation with a PCR-SSO method. *Tissue Antigens* **40**, 116–123.

Santamaria, P., Boyce, J.M., Lindstrom, A.L. *et al.* (1992) HLA class II 'typing': direct sequencing of DRB, DQB, and DQA genes. *Human Immunology* **33**, 69–81.

Santamaria, P., Lindstrom, A.L., Boyce, J.M. *et al.* (1993) HLA class I sequence-based typing. *Human Immunology* **37**, 39–50.

Savelkoul, P.H., de Bruyn-Geraets, D.P. & van den Berg-Loonen, E.M. (1995) High resolution HLA-DRB1 SSP typing for cadaveric donor transplantation. *Tissue Antigens* **45**, 41–48.

Scharf, S.J., Griffith, R.L. & Erlich, H.A. (1991) Rapid typing of DNA sequence polymorphism at the HLA-DRB1 locus using the polymerase chain reaction and nonradioactive oligonucleotide probes. *Human Immunology* **30**, 190–201.

Sorrentino, R., Iannicola, C., Costanzi, S., Chersi, A. & Tosi, R. (1991) Detection of complex alleles by direct analysis of DNA heteroduplexes. *Immunogenetics* **33**, 118–123.

Sutton, P.M., Harmer, A.H., Bayne, A.M. & Welsh, K.I. (1995) The flow cytometric detection of alloantibodies in screening for renal transplantation. *Transplant International* **8**, 360–365.

Sutton, V.R., Kienzle, B.K. & Knowles, R.W. (1989) An altered splice site is found in the DRB4 gene that is not expressed in HLA-DR7, Dw11 individuals. *Immunogenetics* **29**, 317–322.

Tatari, Z., Fortier, C., Bobrynina, V. *et al.* (1995) HLA-Cw allele analysis by PCR-restriction fragment length polymorphism: study of known and additional alleles. *Proceedings of the National Academy of Sciences (USA)* **92**, 8803–8807.

Tiercy, J.M., Gorski, J., Jeannet, M. & Mach, B. (1988) Identification and distribution of three serologically undetected alleles of HLA-DR by oligonucleotide. DNA typing analysis. *Proceedings of the National Academy of Sciences (USA)* **85**, 198–202.

Tindall, K.R. & Kunkel, T.A. (1988) Fidelity of DNA synthesis by thermus aquaticus DNA polymerase. *Biochemistry* **27**, 6008–6013.

Varney, M.D., Boyle, A.J. & Tait, B.D. (1995) Molecular typing and haplotypic associations of HLA-B*44 subtypes. *European Journal of Immunogenetics* **22**, 215–220.

Vaughan, R.W. (1991) PCR-SSO typing for HLA-DRB alleles. *European Journal of Immunogenetics* **18**, 69–80.

Vaughan, R.W., Lanchbury, J.S., Marsh, S.G. *et al.* (1990) The application of oligonucleotide probes to HLA class II typing of the DRB sub-region. *Tissue Antigens* **36**, 149–155.

Wu, D.Y., Ugozzoli, L., Pal, B.K. & Wallace, R.B. (1989) Allele-specific enzymatic amplification of beta-globin genomic DNA for diagnosis of sickle cell anemia. *Proceedings of the National Academy of Sciences (USA)* **86**, 2757–2760.

Yoshida, M., Kimura, A., Numano, F. & Sasazuki, T. (1992) Polymerase-chain-reaction-based analysis of polymorphism in the HLA-B gene. *Human Immunology* **34**, 257–266.

Young, N.T. & Darke, C. (1993) Allelic typing of the HLA-DR4 group by polymerase chain reaction-single strand conformation polymorphism analysis. *Human Immunology* **37**, 69–74.

Yunis, I., Salazar, M. & Yunis, E.J. (1991) HLA-DR generic typing by AFLP. *Tissue Antigens* **38**, 78–88.

Zaer, F., Metz, S. & Scornik, J.C. (1997) Antibody screening by enzyme-linked immunosorbent assay using pooled soluble HLA in renal transplant candidates. *Transplantation* **63**, 48–51.

# Chapter 4/The blood transfusion effect

WILLIAM J. BURLINGHAM

## Introduction

The two key immunological problems of kidney and other organ transplants are the risk of acute rejection, greatest in the early period (<1 year) after transplant, and the long-term risk of chronic rejection, a complex process initiated by host T and B lymphocytes in response to the alloantigens of the graft and perpetuated by an antigen-independent tissue remodelling process that is highly resistant to immune suppressive drug therapy (Tilney *et al.* 1991). Perhaps the greatest lesson of the clinical practice of deliberate pretransplant blood transfusions over the period 1971–88 was the discovery that pre-exposure to alloantigens is a two-edged sword: while in some cases it is clearly detrimental, it is quite often beneficial to long-term organ transplant survival.

The purpose of this chapter is to explore the mechanisms that may be involved in both the detrimental (i.e. sensitization to HLA) and beneficial (reduced incidence of acute and chronic rejection) effects of blood transfusion (BT). The hope is that the former can be more uniformly avoided and the latter exploited

more fully in clinical tolerance-induction strategies. My overview will be divided into four main parts: (i) definitions and historical perspectives; (ii) a hypothesis linking the BT effect to the semiallogeneic nature of mammalian gestation and nursing; (iii) some new data in support of this hypothesis; and (iv) models to suggest possible roles of donor leucocyte persistence and soluble donor HLA in the effects of BT treatment on the adult immune system.

## Definitions

In the interest of clarity, I will define the BT effect in two ways:

1 *Biological.* The improved graft survival seen after preconditioning of the host with blood transfusions of either graft donor or third-party origin.

2 *Clinical.* The improved graft survival seen in clinical kidney transplantation, particularly evident during the precyclosporin era (1971–86), in individuals given multiple (more than five) third-party blood transfusions or one to three donor blood transfusions prior to transplant.

## Discovery of the blood transfusion effect

The first BT effect to be described was an experiment of nature. Parabiosis, or the linking together of the circulatory systems of two genetically different individuals, occurs naturally during mammalian pregnancy in some species. For example, freemartin cattle dizygotic twins share a common placenta. The report of haematopoietic chimerism in non-identical freemartin cattle twins by Owen (1945) caused a dramatic reversal of the then prevailing view that immunological reactivity to foreign tissue and proteins was rigidly predetermined. It took little time for Owen's discovery to prompt Burnet and Fenner (1949) to postulate the existence of a cell-based immunological tolerance to 'self' that had to be induced by exposure of the developing immune system to self antigens. Owen's finding provided the explanation for the surprising discovery by Medawar and his colleagues several years later that skin grafts exchanged between adult cattle twins were not rejected as foreign but were well tolerated (Anderson *et al.* 1951). The subsequent Nobel prize-winning discovery of tolerance to skin grafts in mice following neonatal exposure to donor leucocytes by Billingham *et al.* (1953) may be thought of as the first deliberate BT experiment; tolerance to both leucocyte and tissue antigens was the direct result of a blood cell transfer. These pioneering studies of transplant tolerance focused not only on the blood exchange, but also on its consequence: the induction of stable haematopoietic chimerism in the recipient.

The classic experiments of Billingham *et al.* were performed using a mouse inbred strain combination (A/J to CBA) that later turned out to differ only for some MHC class I antigens (H-2-D and L) and various minor H antigens, and that shared both MHC class II (I-A and I-E) and some MHC class I (H-2-K) antigens. Interestingly, this situation is somewhat analogous to the natural semiallogeneic relationship between mother and fetus in outbred mammals which differ for at most one of each of the HLA class I (for example, one HLA-A, B and C antigen) and class II (HLA-DR and DQ) antigens, while sharing the other set (inherited from the mother). However, the transfer of small numbers of maternal leucocytes to the fetus may give rise to microchimerism, but does not result in the kind of robust central tolerance seen in the chimeric cattle twins and in the Medawar group's mouse experiments. This idea will be further explored in the section on 'split' tolerance to non-inherited maternal HLA antigens in adults and its relation to the BT effect.

Today immunologists and laymen alike take for granted that tissue compatibility or histocompatibility is determined largely, although not exclusively,* by antigens present both on blood cells and on the cells of the particular tissue (heart, kidney, liver, skin, etc.) to be grafted. This was not always so. Medawar was the first to demonstrate that intradermal injection of the buffy coat fraction of blood containing mainly the leucocytes was effective in inducing 'second-set' rejection of skin grafts from the leucocyte donor (Medawar 1946). His successful attempt to prove that leucocyte antigens were present on tissue allografts, together with Gorer's pioneering work on the immunogenetics of tumour allograft rejection (Gorer 1937), became the cornerstone for the discovery of the MHC of vertebrates, including the human leucocyte antigens (HLAs) (Dausset 1954). On the other hand, Medawar's failure to provoke a second-set rejection in rabbits when the leucocytes were administered intravenously as part of a whole BT (Medawar 1946) was the first hint of a BT effect in adult transplantation biology. Hasek (1954) was the first to describe a beneficial BT effect in an adult host, namely the prolongation and, in some instances, permanent acceptance of skin allografts between inbred chickens following whole BTs from the skin graft donor. Differences between rabbit and chicken responder status (high vs. low) may well account for Hasek's success in detecting a BT effect in an adult skin graft model. Because of the rapid influx of cells and serum proteins into primarily vascularized organ allografts as compared with slow diffusion into secondarily vascularized skin grafts, it remained for studies of the organ allograft later to reveal fully both

---

*The phenomenon of tissue-specific histocompatibility antigens is well established (for a review, see Steinmuller 1984). Many such phenomena may now be explained by the prominent role of tissue-derived peptides in alloreactivity.

the graft-prolonging effects of BTs (Halasz *et al.* 1964) and the rapid and damaging effects of preformed antibodies that can sometimes be induced by BTs (Kissmeyer-Nielsen *et al.* 1966). As will be considered in a later section, the early events following revascularization of the organ allograft may be critical in the prevention or inhibition of the normal acute rejection response in BT-pretreated hosts.

## The blood transfusion effect in clinical transplantation

The first clinical kidney transplants were carried out in patients who had received third-party BTs to correct anaemia resulting from chronic renal failure. A consequence of this de facto BT policy was the formation of anti-HLA antibodies in some patients. Ironically, it was the report of Kissmeyer-Nielsen *et al.* (1966) describing hyperacute rejection of renal allografts in such patients that led indirectly to the discovery of the clinical third-party BT (TBT) effect. Following that report, organ transplant centres altered their BT policies so that uraemic patients would *not* be transfused prior to kidney transplant. A drop, however, in the rate of kidney allograft survival from 1967 to 1971 led directly to the report of Opelz *et al.* (1973) that first described the better graft survival in transfused vs. non-transfused recipients.

The beneficial effect of random TBTs in uraemic patients on survival of subsequent cadaveric renal allografts led to the re-establishment of a BT policy in prospective cadaveric kidney transplant recipients. This was soon extended to deliberate donor-specific transfusions (DST) in a short-lived trial by Newton and Anderson (1973) in living-related kidney transplantation. However, DST did not become established as a clinical protocol for living-related renal transplant recipients until the report of Salvatierra *et al.* (1980) in 1980. The key finding was that early graft losses as a result of acute rejection were virtually eliminated in one HLA-haplotype mismatched combinations. These patients were recipients of sibling and parental grafts that had been proven to have HLA class II differences both by (then primitive) serological typing and by high one-way mixed lymphocyte culture (MLC) reactivity.

In fact, the 1- and 2-year graft survival in DST-treated one HLA-haplotype mismatched transplants began to approach that previously seen only in HLA-identical siblings (Salvatierra *et al.* 1980). These results were soon reproduced at other centres, and led to the impression that donor BT had made the one HLA-haplotype mismatched transplant equivalent to an HLA-identical graft (Salvatierra *et al.* 1985). In fact this was never true in terms of long-term graft outcome—the half-life (time to the loss of half the allografts) of an HLA-identical sibling donor kidney remained approximately double that of a parental donor kidney (Terasaki *et al.* 1996). However, the point was that, in this era of suboptimal immune suppression, donor BT caused a dramatic lessening in the incidence and severity of early acute rejection and led to superior graft survival in one HLA-haplotype mismatched renal allografts. This was a totally unexpected result. More predictable was the upsurge in transfusion-associated sensitization; although tempered by the concomitant use of azathioprine, donor BT consistently resulted in an 8–12% rate of anti-HLA antibody formation resulting in positive cross-matches, forcing the cancellation of the scheduled living donor kidney transplants. However, the benefits of BT on transplant survival were thought to outweigh the risk of sensitization until the late 1980s.

New immunosuppressive drugs that could specifically inhibit T cell-mediated acute rejection, especially cyclosporin A and the mouse monoclonal antibody OKT3, began to be introduced in the early 1980s, and by 1987 the difference between transfused and non-transfused patients had disappeared as a result of improved graft survival in non-transfused renal allograft recipients (Opelz 1987). A *Lancet* editorial in 1988 posed the question of abandoning pretransplant BTs, which had become a prerequisite for transplant at most major centres (Editorial 1988). Only the UCLA transplant registry continued to show a BT effect on graft survival after 1988. Interestingly, a positive effect of TBT was now found only in recipients of kidneys serologically mismatched for at least one HLA-DR allele, but recipients of fully HLA-DR matched (O DR mismatched) renal allografts showed no benefit from transfusions (Terasaki 1989).

The demise of the clinical TBT effect, as well as the risk of specific sensitization by DST, only partially mitigated by the concomitant use of azathioprine (Colombe *et al.* 1987), led many to question the value of DST protocols. To determine if there was a beneficial DST effect beyond that of TBT in the cyclosporin era, Reed *et al.* (1991) compared two non-concurrent but demographically matched groups of living-related renal transplant recipients: a group pretreated with three DST plus azathioprine (1986–88) and a third-party random BT-pretreated group (1988–90). Although the study found no difference in short-term (2-year) graft survival rates, a highly significant increase in rejection-free interval and in percentage of patients that never experienced a rejection episode was observed in the donor-specific DST group as compared with the TBT group. Thus, the 'biological' DST effect remained, even though improved graft survival at 2 years could no longer be discerned.

The BT effect, regardless of whether donor-specific or third-party blood was used, may have depended in part upon HLA-antigen sharing between blood recipient and donor; indeed this might account for the 'weaker' effect of third-party BT as opposed to DST because third-party BT will not always share HLA with the recipient. Living-related one HLA-haplotype mismatched kidney grafts, which formed the vast majority of DST cases, fall into the category of one HLA-DR matched donor–recipient combinations. Lagaaij *et al.* (1989) reported that the survival of a cadaveric kidney transplant was significantly higher (81% at 5 years) in recipients pretreated with third-party BT from a blood donor that shared one HLA-DR antigen as compared with recipients who were pretreated with a fully HLA-DR mismatched TBT (57% 5-year graft survival). HLA-DR sharing between blood donor and recipient also appeared to mitigate the production of anti-HLA antibodies (Lagaaij *et al.* 1989). Thus, the beneficial impact of DST on one HLA-haplotype mismatched living-related renal transplants appeared to be analogous to the benefit imparted by HLA-DR sharing with the transfusion donor. We will see later that the graft survival benefit imparted by a donor blood transfusion depends not only upon HLA-DR sharing with the donor, but also on the nature of the mismatched HLA antigens: i.e. whether the recipient has been pre-exposed to the antigens during development.

This brief historical review brings us to our present paradox. Abandonment of pretransplant BT—including DST—policies in organ transplant centres worldwide led initially to a resurgence in the incidence of acute rejection episodes that required potentially toxic therapeutic regimens (Reed *et al.* 1991), yet clinical outcome remained equivalent in the 'post-BT' to that in the BT era. Clinical transplantation no longer needed BT for early immunosuppression, a result of advances in the development of monoclonal antibody (OKT3) and calcineurin inhibitor (cyclosporin and tacrolimus)-based drug therapy. Late chronic rejection has now become the principal cause of immunological graft loss, and because of it long-term graft survival has improved little from the days of azathioprine and prednisone immunosuppression (Paul 1993). Overcoming chronic rejection awaits the next major advance on the horizon: induction of specific immunological tolerance to donor histocompatibility antigens in clinical transplantation.

The key question is: can tolerance to histocompatibility antigens be achieved in human beings? When a medical student asked him in 1957 about the clinical applicability of his group's classic experiments demonstrating immunological tolerance to skin transplants in neonatal mice, Medawar was said to have answered that there was absolutely none (Calne 1998). The donor BT experiment of the 1980s did little to contradict Medawar's contention: while improving graft survival and reducing rejection episodes in transplants across formidable MHC barriers, donor BT also caused a significant number of patients to become humorally sensitized to HLA antigens. Furthermore, contrary to initial claims based on short-term follow-up, donor BT did not eliminate the long-term difference in graft survival between an HLA-identical and a one HLA-haplotype mismatched living-related kidney graft. However, evidence from a multicentre analysis of living donor renal transplants (Burlingham *et al.* 1998a) suggests that neonatal tolerance to maternal HLA-antigens *can* abolish the difference in long-term graft survival between a one HLA-haplotype mismatched and an HLA-identical sibling allograft. I will also present data below which support the idea originally proposed by van Rood and Claas (1990) that the recall of the neonatal priming event by blood transfusions in the adult can potentiate maternal HLA-specific tolerance in human beings.

## 'Split' tolerance to non-inherited maternal antigens

The possibility of specific immunological tolerance to maternal histocompatibility antigens induced *in utero* was first suggested by the work of Owen *et al.* (1954) on Rh antigen sensitization and was later extended to HLA antigen sensitization by Claas *et al.* (Claas *et al.* 1988). In both of these studies the presence of an Rh or HLA antigen in the mother not inherited by the fetus, but to which the developing immune system of the child was presumably exposed during gestation and nursing, had resulted in long-lasting tolerance at the humoral level, i.e. the adult was significantly less likely to form anti-Rh or anti-HLA antibodies when challenged either by a pregnancy or by multiple blood transfusions bearing the maternal antigens not inherited by the woman or by the transfused recipient. However, unlike the central tolerance found in freemartin cattle twins (Owen 1945) and in neonatally transfused mice (Billingham *et al.* 1953), the tolerance was incomplete, or 'split'. In the case of Rh, when a neonatally Rh-exposed but Rh− woman did manage to make a response to her Rh+ fetus, the result was invariably a more severe form of erythroblastosis fetalis than that seen in Rh− women who had not been exposed to Rh during ontogeny (Owen *et al.* 1954). In the case of HLA, multiple blood transfusions in adults failed to elicit antibodies to maternal HLA antigens not inherited by the transfused recipient in 50% of the individuals tested. No such privilege was afforded to paternal HLA antigens not inherited by the same individuals. However, the mechanism of neonatal B cell tolerance was not sufficient to block antibody responses to certain highly immunogenic maternal HLA alleles (for example, HLA-A2 and HLA-B8) (Claas *et al.* 1988). In addition, no defects in the immune response to non-inherited maternal HLA could be found at the level of

primary cytotoxic T lymphocyte responses (Hadley *et al.* 1990; Roelen *et al.* 1995).

These interesting findings raise two important questions: first, of the two major types of HLA antigens, those expressed by viable migrant maternal cells and those maternal soluble HLA proteins found in serum and milk, which is the critical tolerogen *in utero*? and, secondly, do grafts expressing maternal HLA antigens not inherited by the recipient enjoy superior graft survival? As to the first question, a similar form of humoral−/CTL+ 'split' tolerance to a histocompatibility antigen has been described in normal mice given daily intraperitoneal (i.p.) injections of a soluble form of the HLA-B7 xenoantigen (Grumet *et al.* 1994) and, more recently, in mice made transgenic for a secreted form of the MHC class I alloantigen H-2 D$^d$ (Hunziker *et al.* 1997). The latter (H-2$^b$ haplotype, soluble H-2 D$^d$) transgeneic mice made normal CTL responses to cells expressing the membrane form of the antigen but failed to produce anti-D$^d$ alloantibody. Interestingly, the mice transgeneic for soluble H-2 D$^d$ also showed a delayed rejection and, in some cases, tolerance of skin grafts that differed for the H-2 D$^d$ membrane form. If the split tolerance to MHC class I in these mouse models is analogous to natural split tolerance to non-inherited maternal HLA in adult humans, then soluble HLA, rather than membrane-bound HLA on maternal cells, may be the critical tolerogen *in vivo*. However, one cannot rule out an important influence of migrant maternal cells, especially because the levels of maternal soluble HLA antigen in the fetal circulation are currently unknown and may be far less than the µg/mL levels required for humoral tolerance in the mouse studies. The second question, concerning the impact of maternally-induced split tolerance on graft survival of transplants has been recently re-examined.

## Recall of *in utero* HLA antigen exposure in the adult kidney transplant recipient

The first attempt to demonstrate a benefit of neonatal tolerance to non-inherited HLA in kidney transplants revealed a negative result. It was shown by Opelz in a study of the the Eurotransplant database (Opelz and the Collaborative Transplant Study 1990) that there was no benefit in short-term (3-year) graft survival of a maternal kidney as compared with a paternal kidney transplant. In fact, there appeared to be a slight benefit in favour of the grafts donated by fathers. This finding

is confirmed in Fig. 4.1a, which shows a Kaplan–Meier graft survival analysis of parental transplants in unmodified (no donor blood; $n = 144$ patients) recipients from a single centre (University of Wisconsin,

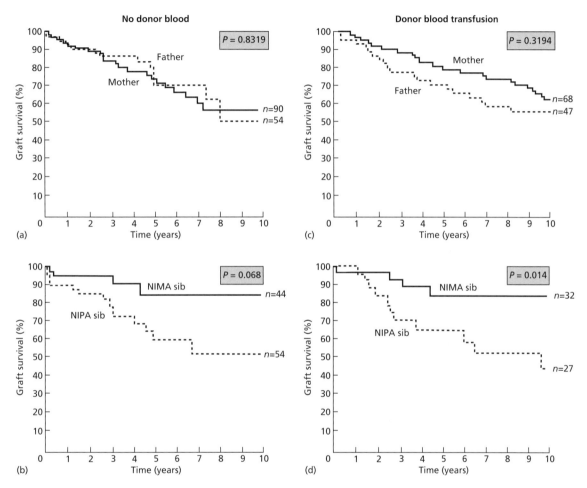

**Fig. 4.1** Effect of donor blood transfusions on 10-year graft survival of one HLA-haplotype mismatched kidney transplants from parental and sibling donors. This figure shows the Kaplan–Meier analysis of graft survival of primary kidney transplants performed between 1966 and 1996, either after pretransplant donor blood transfusions (c and d) or with no donor blood transfusions (a and b). The numbers of patients transplanted in each group are indicated. Patients at a single-centre (University of Wisconsin, Madison) were used for the analysis of recipients of parental transplants (a and c),

while patients at four different centres (OHSU, Portland, OR; Washington University, St Louis; Leiden University, Leiden, the Netherlands; and University of Wisconsin, Madison) were used for the analysis of recipients of transplants from HLA haploidentical sibling donors expressing either the non-inherited maternal (NIMA sib) or non-inherited paternal (NIPA sib) HLA antigens (b and d). The log rank P values for comparison of two groups on each graph were determined either for the 10-year period only (parental transplants) or for the entire follow-up period (sibling transplants).

Madison). The primary grafts from fathers indeed seemed to do better than grafts from mothers at certain time points, although the difference in overall graft survival at 10 years was not significant by the log rank test ($P=0.83$). Interestingly, as shown in Fig. 4.1c, there was a consistent trend toward a better survival of maternal vs. paternal kidney transplants when the recipients were given three donor BTs prior to transplant. Although the trend was not statistically significant in this small sample from a single centre ($n=115$ pt; log rank $P=0.32$), the difference from the results in non-donor blood transfused patients is striking. For example, the maternal graft survival after donor BT was 77% at 8 years, as compared with 62% for paternal kidney grafts in donor BT-treated recipients. At the very least, the preliminary data suggest that a multicentre retrospective study of a larger sample of donor-transfused patients is warranted. If proven significant in a larger series, this would provide the first evidence of a link between the BT effect and the split tolerance to non-inherited maternal antigens. None the less, with the unique exception of transplants performed on infant recipients (Neu *et al.* 1995; Cecka *et al.* 1997), the maternal kidney graft does not convincingly reveal a beneficial impact of neonatally induced tolerance to non-inherited maternal HLA antigens.

Thus it came as a surprise when the results of a multicentre study on the graft survival of one HLA-haplotype mismatched primary renal transplants from living-related sibling donors were analysed. In this retrospective analysis, the patients, their sibling donors and at least one parent had been HLA-typed, revealing the maternal and paternal origin of the familial HLA haplotypes so that each sibling transplant could be grouped according to whether the mismatched HLA haplotype consisted of non-inherited maternal HLA antigens (NIMA sibling) or non-inherited paternal HLA antigens (NIPA sibling). As shown in Fig. 4.1b, even without the use of pretransplant donor BTs, renal grafts from sibling donors expressing the NIMA HLA antigens had a 30% better graft survival at 10 years as compared with renal grafts from sibling donors expressing the NIPA HLA antigens (88 vs. 58%; $n=98$ pt; $P=0.068$). A smaller group of patients who had received pretransplant BT from the sibling donor ($n=$ 59 pt) showed an even stronger benefit of pre-exposure to maternal HLA (88 vs. 52% graft survival at 10 years; $P=0.014$). The combined data of all siblings analysed for maternal and paternal mismatched HLA in the multicentre study ($n=205$) showed a highly significant ($P<0.006$) benefit of maternal HLA pre-exposure (Burlingham *et al.* 1998a). In fact, there was no difference in long-term graft survival in one HLA-haplotype mismatched recipients of sibling transplants from a NIMA+ donor as compared with recipients of HLA-identical sibling transplants (Burlingham *et al.* 1998a). The benefit previously, but erroneously, claimed for the effect of donor BT on one HLA-haplotype mismatched kidney transplants was now found to be true for the tolerogeneic effect of maternal HLA antigen exposure. Thus, the primary BT effect in transplantation now appears to be that of the maternal BT *in utero*. As originally shown by Lagaaij *et al.* (1989), BT in the adult did not appear to help everyone — rather, those semiallogeneic BTs that specifically recalled the maternal HLA exposure of the neonate were beneficial. Such BTs included those from a one HLA-haplotype matched NIMA+ sibling, and perhaps from the mother as well.

We were curious about the basis for the strong effect of maternal HLA antigen pre-exposure on renal transplant survival in siblings: was the improved graft survival the result of an absence of acute cellular rejection episodes? The results of a study of the timing of first rejection episodes in all four types of one HLA-haplotype mismatched living related donor kidney transplants ($n=338$ pt) are shown in Fig. 4.2. All the maternal and paternal kidney transplants from the University of Wisconsin, Madison ($n=259$), as well as the subset of sibling transplants in the multicentre trial for whom first rejection information was available ($n=79$; patients from the University of Wisconsin, Madison, USA, and the University of Leiden, the Netherlands) were included in the analysis, and are subdivided into those who received no donor BTs (Fig. 4.2a), and those who received 1–3 donor BTs prior to transplant (Fig. 4.2b). Remarkably, the only group to show a significant difference in the timing of first rejection episodes was the group that received a transplant without prior donor BT from a NIMA+ sibling (log

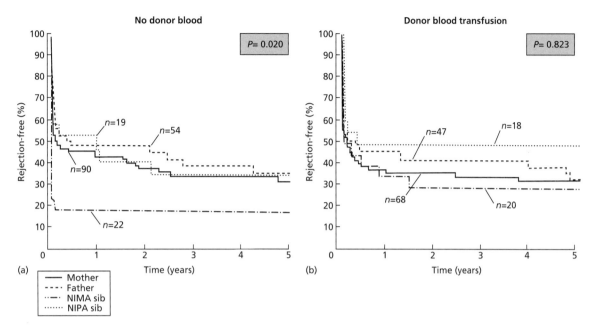

**Fig. 4.2** Effect of donor blood transfusions on the incidence and timing of first acute rejection episodes in one HLA-haplotype mismatched kidney tranplants from parental and sibling donors. This figure shows the Kaplan–Meier analysis of incidence of first acute rejection episodes in primary kidney transplants performed either after pretransplant donor blood transfusions (b) or with no blood donor transfusions (a). The numbers of patients transplanted in each group are indicated. The patient groups were the same as described in Fig. 4.1. The log rank *P* values for comparison of all four groups for the entire follow-up period are shown.

rank *P*=0.02). This subset of patients clearly showed a priming effect of neonatal exposure to the maternal HLA antigens they did not inherit: over 80% had a rejection episode within the first 6 weeks. Donor BT suppressed the accelerated tempo of early acute rejection episodes in this group, abolishing the difference between the recipients of grafts from a NIMA+ sibling and the three other groups (mother, father and NIPA+ sibling donor). Interestingly, the timecourse of first acute rejection episodes in donor-transfused patients was similar in maternal and NIMA+ sibling donor transplants (Fig. 4.2b).

Taken together, the data in Figs 4.1 and 4.2 and in Burlingham *et al.* (1998a) support the concept that the benefit of BT resides principally in the recall of prior *in utero* and nursing exposure to semiallogeneic cells of the mother, as has been previously proposed (Bean *et al.* 1990; van Rood & Claas 1990). The first report of a NIMA effect in cadaver kidney transplants (Smits *et al.* 1998) and in cord blood stem cell transplantation (Wagner 1997) lends further support to this idea.

## Presentation of HLA antigens *in utero* and in the adult: a model

The key features of direct and indirect presentation of a foreign or allo-HLA antigen are illustrated in Fig. 4.3 for the natural form of alloreactivity in the developing immune system of viviparous mammals.

### Step 1: gestation

Our model presupposes the transplacental transfer to the unborn of one HLA-haplotype mismatched leucocytes (Hall *et al.* 1995) and soluble HLA antigens of the mother. The mother's and father's diploid cells with the

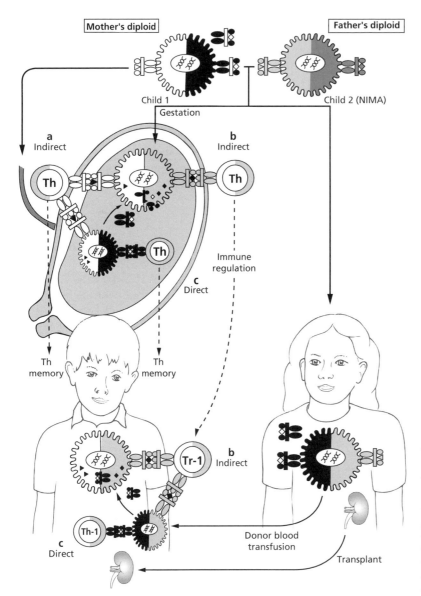

**Fig. 4.3** Proposed model for the three major pathways of alloantigen presentation to recipient T cells during fetal exposure to maternal non-inherited HLA antigens (NIMA) and during restimulation by transfusion and kidney transplant from a NIMA+ sibling donor. Each cell is divided into two halves, representing the two inherited HLA haplotypes. The two major types of *indirect* pathway T helper cells are indicated by the letters 'a' and 'b', corresponding to those recognizing maternally derived peptides presented by the maternal inherited HLA and those presented by the paternal inherited HLA antigens, respectively. The *direct* pathway T helper cells are indicated by the letter 'c'. (Courtesy Joan Kozel, University of Wisconsin, Madison.)

four parental HLA haplotypes are indicated at the top of the diagram. As the mother's cells and soluble antigens penetrate the unborn child, three distinct subsets of fetal T cells (a–c on Fig. 4.3) may be recruited to recognize maternal cells and soluble antigens. The first two subsets (a and b) are the fetal T cells that can respond via the indirect pathway to processed soluble MHC proteins present in the blood and breast milk of the mother. Only the pathway of indirect alloantigen presentation to CD4+ T helper cells which recognize processed class II-bound peptides is shown in Fig. 4.3; there is evidence that a similar indirect pathway exists for recognition of class I-bound allopeptides and CD8+ T cells (Arnold *et al.* 1990). As illustrated in Fig. 4.3, during fetal life the soluble HLA antigens of the mother may be internalized by antigen-presenting cells of either the mother or the fetus, and are then processed by the antigen-presenting cells (APCs) into:

• peptides (depicted as filled triangles) that can be bound by the class II proteins encoded by the maternal inherited HLA alleles (white); or

• peptides (depicted as filled diamonds) that can only be bound by those class II proteins encoded by the paternal inherited HLA alleles (grey).

Each set of peptides is then presented to a distinct subset of fetal T cells (a or b). Thus all indirect pathway alloreactive T cells in the offspring may be referred to as being either: (a) maternal HLA-restricted; or (b) paternal HLA-restricted. The third subset is the direct pathway T cells (c) that respond only to the intact, membrane-bound non-inherited maternal HLA antigens (shown in black) and their associated peptides on the surface of the maternal APC. Only the T helper cells are illustrated; however, the direct pathway T cells include both the T helper (CD4+) and T cytotoxic (CD8+) T cells that can recognize and respond to the maternal HLA class II and class I antigens, respectively.

## Step 2: memory T cells and blood transfusions

In the weaned child or adult, the model assumes that the maternal cells and soluble HLA antigens have been cleared, leaving behind memory T cells. The predicted frequency of memory T cells of each subset is: c >> a > b. The dominance of 'c' memory cells makes sense because direct pathway T cells to a given alloantigen are known to be present in high frequency even in the unselected T cell repertoire, and the proportion of these present as memory cells in the adult after exposure to maternal non-inherited HLA-bearing migrant maternal leucocytes is likely to be high. The lack of a difference in CTL precursor frequency specific for NIMA vs. NIPA HLA antigens in the normal adult (Hadley *et al.* 1990; Roelen *et al.* 1995) may be because standard limiting dilution and bulk culture CTL analyses are relatively insensitive to the presence of memory T cells. Perhaps a better indi-

cation of a memory response is the more rapid onset of acute rejection episodes. The observation that > 80% of non-transfused recipients of kidney grafts from a NIMA+ sibling had a rejection episode within the first 5 weeks after transplant strongly suggests a memory response to non-inherited maternal HLA antigens (Burlingham *et al.* 1998a). The absence of such a strong early acute rejection incidence in the maternal grafts may have to do with factors unique to the maternal kidney (for example, the presence of primed maternal passenger T cells capable of mediating a low-level graft vs. host response) that could interfere with the primed subset of host antidonor T memory cells.

Both types of indirect pathway T cells are predicted to be of relatively low frequency in the T cell repertoire (Liu *et al.* 1993), but those of type 'a' (white nucleus) are predicted to be substantially increased in the memory compartment resulting from the interaction with maternal 'migrant' APC; this is true because, once the maternal APCs have crossed into the fetal circulation and lymphoid tissues, they could have presented to the subset 'a' T cells the same allopeptide (triangle) bound to the inherited maternal HLA antigens as did the immature fetal APC. Finally, paternal HLA-restricted T cells (b) would be predicted to be in low frequency in the memory compartment of the adult because only fetal APCs, which are immature at birth and have a reduced stimulatory capacity (Trivedi *et al.* 1997), would have been able to present this allopeptide (diamond) to this indirect pathway T cell subset (Fig. 4.3) during fetal and early postnatal life. Indeed, the high affinity type 'b' T cell clones may be clonally deleted by this interaction, as shown, further trimming the available alloreactive T cell repertoire in the adult. Alternatively, type 'b' alloreactive memory T cells may give rise to T-regulatory (Tr-1) cells after the placement of a sibling renal allograft that shares the paternal (grey) haplotype, but differs for the maternal non-inherited antigens (black). These regulatory cells, slow to develop in unmodified hosts, may develop more rapidly following blood transfusion, thus limiting the 'recall' Th-1 memory response of type 'c' direct pathway T cells.

Transfusion with either maternal blood or with blood from a sibling donor expressing the non-inherited maternal HLA antigens (Fig. 4.3, child number 2) would be predicted to restimulate all three memory T cell subsets. Because of the tendency of antigen exposure via the intravenous route to activate Th-2 but not Th-1 responses efficiently (Takeuchi *et al.* 1992; Kearney *et al.* 1994), as well as the fact that antigen priming in the neonate generally leads to a type 2 (Th-2) memory T cell pool (Forsthuber *et al.* 1996; Singh *et al.* 1996), that the recall response to NIMA in all three T cell subsets would be predominately Th-2 rather than Th-1. Alternatively, activation by BT of Tr-1 cells may limit expression of both Th-1 (delayed-type hypersensitivity, DTH) and Th-2 (humeral immunity) recall responses. Donor APCs present in the transfused blood from either the mother or a NIMA+ sibling donor (Fig. 4.3) ought to activate subset 'c' direct pathway T memory cells equally well. Soluble non-inherited maternal HLA antigens present in the transfused blood of the mother or NIMA+ sibling donor might be expected to reactivate subset 'a' indirect pathway T memory cells specific for allopeptides presented on the maternal inherited HLA (white) of the recipient. The subset 'b' indirect pathway T memory cells are predicted to be capable of mounting an effective regulatory response to BT challenge.

### Step 3: living donor renal transplant

The living related kidney transplant was usually performed 4–6 weeks after the last donor BT according to the protocol of Salvatierra *et al.* (1980) followed at most centres from 1980 to 1988. As in the case of the maternal-to-fetal anastomosis via the placenta, the anastomosis of the donor kidney to the host circulation allows donor passenger leucocytes to enter the blood and lymph of the recipient. This initial movement of donor leucocytes to the regional lymph nodes and spleen of the host may activate a massive T cell direct pathway response of the 'c' type, leading to an early intense Th-1 cytokine response followed by clonal exhaustion, as proposed by Bishop *et al.* (1997). Alternatively, some passenger leucocytes, including tissue macrophages, lymphocytes and dendritic cells, may persist for long periods of time within the graft itself (Fung *et al.* 1985), a situation which in the case of the

lung transplant correlates strongly with a favourable graft outcome (O'Connell *et al.* 1998). Eventually, persisting donor passenger leucocytes may seed haematopoietic precursors to the recipient bone marrow, leading to long-term microchimerism (Starzl *et al.* 1992); however, the causal link between this phenomenon and tolerance is still controversial (Wood & Sachs 1998). None the less, the correlation of good graft outcome with persistence of donor passenger leucocytes within the graft suggests that the direct pathway 'c' T cells will be activated more strongly and remain a dominant component of the host response for longer periods in the grafts of patients with favourable outcome as compared with grafts of those patients who undergo acute or chronic rejection. How the dominance of direct pathway T cells is compatible with tolerance will be considered below, in considering the CTL response and its regulation by donor veto cells.

Finally, the blood transfusion model proposed in Fig. 4.3 suggests that the release of low amounts of soluble donor HLA antigens from the kidney transplant has a beneficial consequence when the donor is a NIMA+ sibling, because of the persistence of donor APCs expressing the shared paternal haplotype. This shared haplotype channels the indirect pathway toward the presentation of NIMA HLA-derived peptides (diamonds) to the regulatory paternal HLA-restricted indirect pathway 'b' memory T cells in the recipient. Thus, the long-term graft survival of the NIMA+ sibling graft may be favoured over a maternal graft, because the persisting passenger leucocytes of the latter, which would share maternal inherited HLA with the recipient, would be much more likely to activate maternal HLA-restricted indirect pathway 'a' memory T cells. The cause for the relatively poor survival of maternal grafts, in this view, is allorecognition via the indirect pathway 'a', rather than any major differences in direct pathway responses. Direct pathway 'c' cells, the model suggests, cause early acute rejection but may in fact be beneficial to long-term graft survival (Kusaka *et al.* 2000). The possible mechanisms for indirect pathway-mediated graft loss will be considered in greater detail in the sections on the CTL pathway and humoral sensitization.

## Semiallogeneic blood transfusions and natural killer cells

As we have seen, the beneficial BT effects seen in the adult kidney transplant recipient may derive from the semiallogeneic experience of the fetus in mammalian pregnancy. Studies of the BT effect in humans suggest that fully allogeneic, particularly two, HLA-DR mismatched BT are harmful, and that zero HLA-DR mismatched BT are not as beneficial as one HLA-DR mismatched BT to kidney transplant survival (Lagaaij *et al.* 1989; Lazda *et al.* 1990). What are the characteristic features of the semiallogeneic system that account for the suppressive effect of priming by maternal-to-fetal blood exchange and its recall by HLA partially matched BTs?

An important barrier to engraftment of bone marrow and bone-marrow-derived cells are the natural killer (NK) cells of the innate immunity system. The NK cells rapidly destroy cells that express either no MHC class I or HLA class I of foreign HLA type; they undergo HLA class I antigen-dependent inactivation via so-called killer inhibitory receptors (KIR) when these recognize specific class I MHC–peptide ligands present on autologous cells (Moretta & Moretta 1997). Semiallogeneic (for example, $f1 \rightarrow P$) blood leucocytes escape destruction by the NK cell system as a result of recognition of the shared HLA class I antigens, giving rise to alloantigenic cell persistence and long-term veto activity, whereas fully allogeneic cells ($A \rightarrow B$) are rapidly destroyed (Sheng-Tanner & Miller 1992). The latter can persist and yield significant veto cell activity, but only if the NK cells of the recipient are first depleted (Sheng-Tanner & Miller 1992). Thus, just as class II sharing may be advantageous for channelling the indirect pathway of allorecognition (Fig. 4.3), class I sharing may be necessary to allow for escape of blood and graft leucocytes from NK cell-mediated destruction. The rules for NK cell inhibitory receptor engagement are still being worked out, but it may be possible in the future to predict the extent of chimerism and donor passenger cell persistence following BT and organ transplantation based on analysis of key class I compatibilities.

Besides evasion of the NK system, HLA-1DR matched or semiallogeneic whole blood, especially blood that contains non-inherited maternal soluble HLA antigens previously encountered *in utero*, may evoke a novel version of the indirect pathway T cell response that can suppress direct pathway T cells. This pathway, originally proposed by van Rood and Claas (1990) involves a T–T cell instead of a T–macrophage or T–DC interaction. Essentially, any indirect pathway T memory cell can mediate T cell suppression if the peptide ligand it seeks is presented by an activated HLA class II+ T cell. Because of the high frequency of direct pathway T cells that become rapidly activated following antigen exposure, these will be induced to express HLA class II and present allopeptides to indirect pathway T cells. If this interaction leads to up-regulation of Fas-ligand on the responder T cells, these may mediate induction of apoptosis in focal infiltrates of T cells within the graft via a Fas/Fas ligand interaction.

## The CTL pathway and its regulation by donor veto cells and host regulatory T cells

Our interest in the CD8+ direct pathway cytotoxic T lymphocytes in patients that had received three pre-transplant donor-specific transfusions (DST) was kindled by the observation of a gradual loss of anti-donor CTL responsiveness in primary cultures of peripheral blood lymphocytes occurring in these patients over a period of 12 months after transplant from a living kidney donor (Grailer *et al.* 1991). This defect was caused in at least one patient by a deficient IL-2 response, i.e. the CTL deficiency was easily overcome by addition of rIL-2 to the culture (Grailer *et al.* 1991). Others, however, reported that the CTL defect could be attributed in most patients to a low apparent CTL precursor frequency, a result of either clonal deletion following recovery from ablative (e.g. OKT3) therapy or CTL precursor functional unresponsiveness or anergy (Hadley *et al.* 1992).

Beginning in 1991, my laboratory team had the opportunity to study a rare case of a patient who had

successfully withdrawn himself from all immunosuppression 2 years previously, 2 years following DST and
kidney transplantation from his mother (Burlingham *et
al*. 1995). In cases like this one (maternal donor), the
donor BT protocol may be necessary to reveal a beneficial NIMA effect (Fig. 4.1); none the less, even after BT
the probability of graft survival at 10 years is much
lower than for a NIMA+ one HLA-haplotype mismatched sibling donor and HLA-identical sibling transplants (compare Fig. 4.1c and 4.1d). We were able to
follow the progress of the patient for 5 of his 7 years of
good renal function (serum Cr 1.6–2.0 mg/dL), after
which time he lost his kidney as a result of cellular rejection. During the period of stable tolerance, the patient
turned out to have a form of donor-specific CTL anergy
that was not easily restored by IL-2 addition to his
primary antidonor MLC. This finding, coupled with
the discovery that he, like many other tolerant liver and
kidney transplant patients studied recently (Starzl *et al*.
1992, 1993), was a microchimera, prompted an investigation into the possible connection between his CTL
primary unresponsiveness to the kidney donor and the
presence of rare (<0.1%) donor-derived cells in his
blood and skin (Burlingham *et al*. 1995).

The CTL precursors specific for donor HLA class I
in the patient's peripheral blood had the following
features suggestive of anergic CD8+ direct pathway T
cells: (a) IL-2-resistant, donor-specific 1 CTL unresponsiveness, and (b) restoration of full cytotoxic
response to mismatched donor HLA class I-A and B
antigens by a 10-day 1 MLR culture *in vitro* followed
by a 2 restimulation with donor X-irradiated cells for 7
days in the presence of exogenous IL-2. Through the
use of a monoclonal antibody specific for the donor
HLA-Bw6 antigen and immunomagnetic beads, we
were able to remove the rare donor cells from the
peripheral blood as assessed by PCR analysis of both
the depleted and enriched cell population. We discovered that a profound donor-specific inhibition of this
patient's CTL response could be achieved by addition
of fresh patient peripheral blood leucocytes (PBL) or
separated donor HLA class I+ cell fractions thereof
to 3 CTL responder cultures. The effect was not seen
with control beaded cell preparations treated with an
isotype-matched control monoclonal antibody, and

was completely donor-specific, in that 3 CTL response
to a third-party stimulator was unaffected by additions
of fresh PBL or donor-enriched cell fraction thereof
(Burlingham *et al*. 1995). Our results were consistent with the hypothesis of establishment of a persistent
and powerful chimeric veto cell population following
DST and kidney transplant from an NIMA+ donor
(Burlingham 1995).

Based on our findings in this patient, as well as recent
developments in the field of CTL differentiation
(Bennett *et al*. 1998; Ridge *et al*. 1998), we have developed a new model for regulation of CD8+ direct
pathway cytotoxic T cell response by BT and subsequent kidney transplantation. Figure 4.4 shows the
proposed pathways of activation or inhibition of CTL
responses to donor HLA class I driven by specialized
donor APCs. The initial step (top) involves the persistence of immature dendritic cells (DC) derived from the
organ or tissue graft or from the donor BTs. In the case
of irreversible acute or chronic rejection, the release of
high levels of soluble donor HLA antigens from the
graft drives the presentation of allopeptides by the
shared HLA antigens present on the DC. This results in
activation of indirect pathway Th-1 cells specific for
cryptic epitopes of the donor or self MHC (Benichou
*et al*. 1998). The activated Th-1 cell then triggers CD40
signalling and costimulation in the immature DC by
interaction with CD40-ligand (Bennett *et al*. 1998;
Ridge *et al*. 1998). The mature DC can then interact
with a precursor cytotoxic T cell (pTc), which uses its
clonotypic antigen receptor (TcR) plus a CD8 coreceptor to recognize the allogeneic MHC class I protein and
its bound peptide on the surface of the DC. The activated DC is able to provide the proper costimulatory
signals to the CD8 T cell, allowing it to express a functional IL-2 receptor and to proliferate and differentiate
in an IL-2-dependent fashion to become a mature T
cytotoxic cell (CD8 Tc).

This two-stage APC-linked model of CTL differentiation provides the possibility of at least two distinct
sites of regulation of the CTL generation pathway by
BTs:

1 limitation of IL-2 production by the Th-1 cell — for
example, by CD4+ host T cell encounter with a costim-
ulator-deficient, class II+ resting donor B cell; or

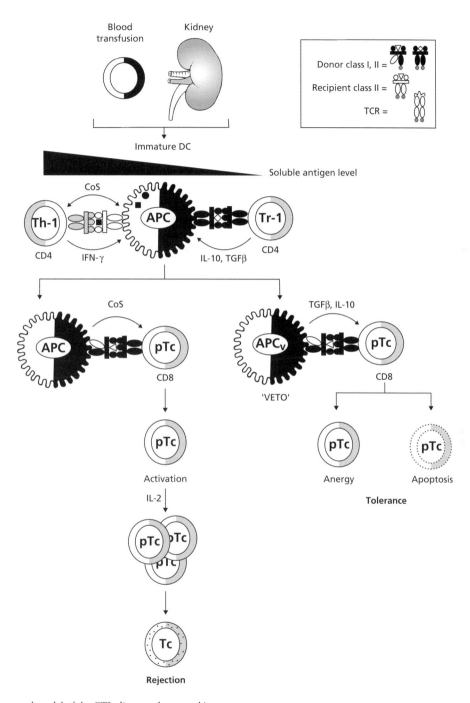

**Fig. 4.4** Proposed model of the CTL *direct* pathway and its regulation by host T helper and donor dendritic cells (DC). See text for explanation. (Courtesy Joan Kozel, University of Wisconsin, Madison.)

**2** development of a Tr-1 response leading to a different APC phenotype and veto of precursor CTL.

The former mechanism could theoretically lead to CTL unresponsiveness resulting from an insufficient generation of IL-2 for the subsequent differentiation of the pTc, as originally proposed by Fuchs and Matzinger (1992). While IL-2 insufficiency may be relevant to the early post-transplant immunosuppression in the DST-treated host (Dallman *et al.* 1991), other data indicate that CTL accumulation at the transplant site early after engraftment was unaffected in the DST-treated host, despite the curtailment of IL-2 generation (Dallman *et al.* 1987). The reversal of the DST effect by early post-transplant administration of IL-2 (Dallman *et al.* 1989) suggests that IL-2 may serve other key roles *in vivo* besides that of a limiting CD8+ T cell differentiation factor. The recent discovery (Josien *et al.* 1988a) that neutralizing antibody to TGFβ also reverses the donor BT effect in a model of rat heart allograft tolerance, adds considerable support to the regulatory T cell (Tr-1) mechanism (point 2, above). Furthermore, the establishment of the regulatory mechanism by BTs appears to require donor DC (Josien *et al.* 1988b).

The second possibility, that of CTL regulation by a veto mechanism is illustrated in the right half of Fig. 4.4. If the level of soluble donor HLA generated from the allograft remains low, the default pathway of allorecognition of the donor DC will be the direct pathway. In the case of Tr-1 responses induced *in utero* and recalled by BT, these direct pathway T cells will be unable to license the DC for activation of CTL; instead the precursor CD8+ T cell is inactivated by encounter with a class II+, class I+ but IL-10 or TGFβ-producing dendritic veto cell, leading to anergy and eventually to apoptosis (Fig. 4.4, lower right). Veto cell activity was first described by Miller and Phillips (1976). It consists of the rapid inactivation of precursor CD8+ T cells by a non-conventional allogeneic APC, either a CD8+ donor T or other donor CD8+ leucocyte (Fink *et al.* 1983; Zhang *et al.* 1994). The encounter with the veto cell is depicted in Fig. 4.4 as involving the class I-specific antigen receptor of the precursor CTL, together with an additional interaction with TGFβ or IL-10 delivered by the veto cell (Thomas *et al.* 1994). Expression of CD8 α chain by the veto cell has been found to

be of critical importance in veto effects in mice (Zhang *et al.* 1994) and in non-human primates (Thomas *et al.* 1993); CD8 α may be also be expressed by lymphoid dendritic cell lineages thought to have immunosuppressive capabilities. The model proposes that triggering of the immature DC by a Tr-1 cell directs it toward an inhibitory phenotype, just as the triggering of the immature DC by a Th-1 cell directs it to develop a CTL-stimulatory phenotype. Support for an inhibitory role of TGFβ-treated DC in modulating alloreactivity has recently been reported (Lu *et al.* 1997). Thus the induction of Tr-1 responses, or the recall of memory Tr-1 responses to non-inherited maternal class II alloantigens present in the BT, may help establish a pool of 'veto' DC that can suppress CTL direct pathway responses. As in induction of anergy in Th-1 CD4+ T cells, veto effects on CD8+ T cells appear to require an active calcineurin-dependent signal delivered through the TcR complex of the precursor CD8+ T cell (Hiruma & Gress 1992).

The persistence of veto activity derived from intravenously transferred blood cells (DST) has been correlated with the development of prolonged allograft survival in mice (Johnson 1987). In humans, the data on veto activity mediated by BTs are more controversial. One study showed that BT in which the donor shares one HLA haplotype, or at least one HLA-B and HLA-DR antigen, with the transfusion recipient results in the delayed development of CTL hyporesponsiveness to the HLA class I antigens of the transfusion donor (Arnold *et al.* 1993); however, this finding could not be repeated by other groups (F. Claas, personal communication). Alternatively, the inhibitory veto cell lineage may always be graft passenger leucocyte-derived, with the BT serving only to increase the Tr-1 response in the direct pathway, favouring deviation of graft passenger DC toward a CTL-inhibitory phenotype. The discovery of rare but powerful donor-derived veto-like cells in the peripheral blood of a DST-pretreated recipient of a maternal renal allograft during a period of stable tolerance (Burlingham *et al.* 1995) supports the model depicted in the lower right portion of Fig. 4.4. However, while donor BT enhances the development of post-transplant microchimerism in kidney transplant patients, it is not yet clear whether the persistent donor cells are always beneficial (Sivasai *et al.* 1997).

This 'two-edged sword' of microchimerism is suggested in Fig. 4.4. The donor-derived dendritic cell depicted is of maternal origin, for example, from a maternal kidney transplant. It can therefore present maternal non-inherited HLA and associated peptides to direct pathway 'c' T cells, some of which have assumed a regulatory 'Tr-1' phenotype. This interaction would lead to an inhibitory DC phenotype during the period of stable tolerance to the maternal kidney, which can last for years. However, because the graft donor—in this case, the mother—shares maternal inherited HLA, the same passenger cell can present allopeptides to *in utero*-primed indirect pathway 'a' T cells. This circumstance runs the risk of an eventual breakthrough of a Th-1 response to allopeptides as the levels of circulating soluble HLA antigen increase—for example, during activation of the graft by an opportunistic viral infection (DeVito-Haynes *et al.* 1996)—leading to epitope spreading (Clubotariu *et al.* 1998). Because HLA antigens shared with the donor permit the donor APC to present the same allopeptides as host APC, the same donor APC that had previously been induced by Tr-1 regulatory cells to block the host CTL response, by interaction with indirect pathway Th-1 cells could instead be licensed to enhance CTL development and thus contribute to eventual loss of the kidney due to rejection. Although the patient described in Burlingham *et al.* (1995) managed to maintain kidney function for 7 years without immunosuppressive drug therapy, he suddenly developed a progressive chronic rejection 9 years after transplant and lost his maternal kidney function by year 10. The effects of PBL obtained during chronic rejection strongly suggest that the phenotype of the rare donor cells can indeed change: instead of a dose-dependent veto effect seen during the tolerance phase, the donor fraction of the PBL caused an enhancement of the antidonor CTL response when added to secondary antidonor CTL cultures (W.J. Burlingham and S. Kusaka, unpublished data).

In addition to the loss of a 'veto' effect of rare donor cells, the loss of tolerance to a maternal kidney allograft involved changes in both direct and indirect pathway responses. Direct pathway T cell clonotypes (type 'c') were defined by cloning and sequencing of T cell receptor genes of NIMA-specific T cells from PBL during the period of tolerance. Clonotype analysis of mRNA amplified by polymerase chain reaction indicated that many such clones persisted at high levels in peripheral blood as late as 9.0 years post-transplant (Kusaka *et al.* 2000). However, during the loss of tolerance and onset of rejection between year 9 and 10, these 'direct pathway' T cell clonotypes were rapidly lost from both peripheral blood and from the graft (Kusaka *et al.* 2000). In contrast, over the same period of time there was a parallel recovery of antidonor DTH response, as measured by an adoptive transfer (human-to-SCID mouse footpad, Carrodeguas *et al.* 1999) assay. Because the DTH transfer assay measures the *indirect* pathway response to soluble donor alloantigens, it is possible that the loss of direct pathway *regulatory* T cells (as well as *indirect* pathway regulatory T cells that were not studied by clonotype analysis but may also have been present during the tolerance phase) permitted the recovery of indirect pathway DTH responses during the breakdown of tolerance (W.J. Burlingham *et al.*, manuscript in preparation). Indeed, the regulation of DTH response by both direct and by indirect pathway 'regulatory' T cells appears to be a characteristic feature of stable allograft tolerance in humans (VanBuskirk *et al.* 2000). The T cells that can mediate DTH are abundant during tolerance according to this view but they are prevented from destroying the graft by other T cells that generate immunosuppressive cytokines such as IL-10 and TGFβ in response to donor cells (direct pathway Tr-1) and soluble antigens (indirect pathway Tr-1).

## Humoral sensitization to HLA

The benefits of the BT effect on cell-mediated immunity to a transplant, whether in inbred rodents, outbred large animals or humans, are negated if the alloantigens of the blood evoke antidonor HLA antibodies which can lead to hyperacute rejection (Kissmeyer-Nielsen *et al.* 1966). In the first large clinical trial of DST between one HLA-haplotype mismatched individuals, 29% of recipients became sensitized to antigens of the blood donor after three whole BTs given without concomitant immunosuppression (Salvatierra *et al.* 1980). One might ask why 100% did not become sensitized? The answer appears to be that anti-HLA antibody formation, particularly of IgG isotypes, is limited by the recipients' immune response HLA class II genes (Butcher *et al.* 1982), by sex (females are more prone to sensitization than males) (Burlingham *et al.* 1988a) and, as previously noted, by exposure to maternal non-inherited HLA antigens during ontogeny (Claas *et al.* 1988). In addition, a partial HLA-DR match (Lagaaij *et al.* 1989) and the tendency of the recipient to form anti-idiotypic antibodies to anti-HLA following BT (Reed *et al.* 1987; Burlingham *et al.* 1988b; Phelan *et al.* 1991) have both been shown to counteract the sensitization process. In hosts that have not been previously sensitized to HLA antigens, a primary cytotoxic antibody response to donor HLA develops slowly in response to BT, and multiple BTs (Colombe *et al.* 1987) are usually required before any sensitization is detected by microcytotoxicity test. In contrast, patients with pre-existing anti-HLA (but *not* antidonor) antibodies had a high incidence of a rapid-onset cytotoxic antidonor HLA antibody response after a single DST; unlike the slower-onset primary response, this secondary response was resistant to prophylaxis by azathioprine (Colombe *et al.* 1987).

It is difficult to find adequate published information concerning the antibody response to deliberate immunization with leucocytes that would be useful for comparison with intravenous route (BT) data. One study of donor-specific antibody formation was carried out following deliberate immunization of women who had a history of recurrent spontaneous abortions and low or absent panel-reactive antibody (PRA). In 95 women who received intradermal injection in multiple sites on the forearm with their husband's leucocytes ($50 \times 10^6$ cells), antidonor HLA antibodies developed in 36% as measured by direct microcytotoxicity test and in 68% as measured by flow cytometry 2–3 weeks after a single treatment (Gilman-Sachs *et al.* 1989). These results, taken together with the DST experience, suggest that the intradermal injection of donor leucocytes induces a rapid and sustained IgG response to donor HLA, whereas the intravenous injection of whole blood in

recipients not previously allosensitized is relatively inefficient, requiring multiple transfusions to achieve comparable donor-specific antibody responses.

Figure 4.5 shows a hypothetical model of how the cells and soluble antigens present in a BT, or those released from activated donor cells in the host after transfusion or transplantation, can trigger the IgM and IgG primary B cell responses to an HLA class I alloantigen. The top portion of Fig. 4.5 (boxed) shows a model for a T-independent pathway that results in formation of a low-affinity IgM antibody capable of interacting with multivalent, membrane-bound HLA class I, either on the surface of the donor cell or in lipophilic vesicles shed by donor cells and present as high-MW complexes in normal blood (shed HLA, Fig. 4.5). Studies in mice have established that the primary IgM response to an allogeneic MHC class I can be stimulated in the absence of T cells by a small lymphocyte fraction that lacks classical T and B cell markers (Klein *et al.* 1974; Nakashima & Lake 1979). The B cell pool that can interact with such a donor stimulator cell is assumed to have been trimmed by elimination of certain high-affinity B cell clones by interaction with maternal cells or soluble HLA *in utero* (Fig. 4.5, top). The remaining B cells capable of responding go on to produce a relatively low-affinity but high-avidity IgM anti-HLA class I antibody that binds to multivalent complex detergent-solubilized forms of donor soluble HLA, but does not bind to secreted or monomeric forms of class I (DeVito *et al.* 1993). IgM anti-HLA antibody may not be detrimental to graft survival, but may lead to the formation of IgG anti-HLA antibodies which are harmful.

The bottom portion of Fig. 4.5 shows a model of the distinct but interacting pathway of CD4+ T helper cell-dependent IgG response. B cells that have first been activated by the direct pathway of recognition (upper boxed portion) can then be further switched into IgG production by interaction with a T helper cell that has been triggered via the indirect pathway. The model of the indirect sensitization pathway (Fig. 4.5, bottom) is supported by the finding that preimmunization with immunogeneic peptides of the rat class I protein RT1A$^a$ or with plasmid DNA encoding a water-soluble RT1A$^a$, could prime rats for the production of anti-

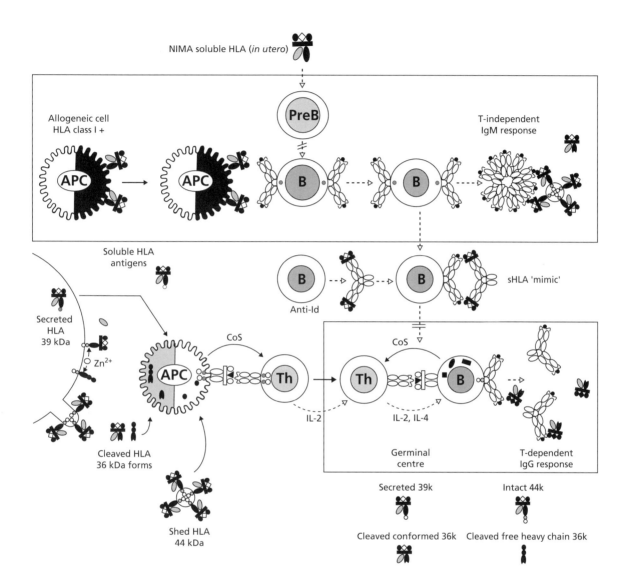

**Fig. 4.5** Proposed model of T-independent IgM and T-dependent IgG antibody responses to allogeneic HLA, and its regulation by soluble HLA antigens and anti-idiotypic 'HLA mimic' antibodies. See text for explanation. (Courtesy Joan Kozel, University of Wisconsin, Madison.)

RT1A[a] IgG following subsequent challenge with an RT1A[a+] skin or heart graft (Fangmann *et al*. 1992; Geissler *et al*. 1994; Pettigrew *et al*. 1998).

Three distinct sources of antigen for the generation of the immunogenic peptide are depicted in Fig. 4.5. One is a secreted HLA class I water-soluble monomeric protein present in the plasma (Krangel 1987) of the whole BT; this form is released without being expressed on the cell surface through RNA splicing of the full-length transcripts to produce an mRNA encoding a 39 kDa protein (Krangel 1986). Another source of donor soluble HLA pictured in Fig. 4.5, lower left, is shed HLA class I antigen, also present in plasma, which is released as a multimeric lipid–protein complex form (generally >220 kDa by gel filtration) of the full-length (44 kDa) HLA antigen (Allison *et al.* 1977). A third pathway of HLA soluble antigen release, consisting of the proteolytic cleavage of cell surface $\beta_2$m-free HLA class I heavy chains, has recently been proposed as the principal pathway of soluble classical MHC class I release by activated cells (Demaria *et al.* 1994; Zhai & Knechtle 1998). Appearance in cell supernatants of both 36 kDa $\beta_2$m-associated and $\beta_2$m-free HLA class I forms was blocked *in vitro* by inhibitors of $Zn^{2+}$-dependent metalloproteinase (DeVito-Haynes *et al.* 1998). Preliminary evidence favours a model in which some of the HLA class I retains a peptide-induced conformation when cleaved by the metalloproteinase as a $\beta_2$m-free molecule, then rapidly reassociates with $\beta_2$m in the supernatant (Zhai & Knechtle 1998).

The model shown in Fig. 4.5 proposes that all four major forms (44 kDa, 39 kDa and the two 36 kDa forms) of soluble HLA can stimulate T helper responses for IgG production *in vivo*. As illustrated in Fig. 4.5, autologous APCs (or donor APCs which share HLA-DR antigen) can process both forms of the class I antigen and can present the immunogeneic donor-HLA-derived peptide, bound to MHC class II, to a T helper cell. If the APC can provide a costimulatory signal to the precursor T helper cell — for example, by ligation of CD28 on the T helper cell by CD80 on the APC (Sayegh & Turka 1998) — then the T helper cell specific for a donor-soluable HLA-derived allopeptide becomes activated to produce IL-2 (Burlingham *et al.* 1993). It can then proliferate and migrate to the parafollicular areas of the lymph node where it provides specific lymphokines and contact-mediated signals, including CD40-ligand binding to CD40 on the antigen-specific B cell required for germinal centre formation and IgM→IgG switching (Kearney *et al.* 1994). The allospecific B cell binds and internalizes the donor soluble HLA and presents the specific peptide–HLA class II complex on its surface which is recognized by the clonotypic TcR of the CD4+ T helper cell. The result of these interactions is the secretion of an IgG that is capable of binding both lipophilic complex and hydrophilic monomer forms of HLA class I (DeVito *et al.* 1993).

In light of the importance of epitope spreading via the indirect pathway in chronic allograft rejection (Clubotariu *et al.* 1998), one could speculate that the metalloproteinase pathway, because it generates denatured donor HLA class I $\beta_2$m-free HC, would be most likely to generate the epitope spreading phenomenon. The relationship of the metalloproteinase pathway to epitope spreading remains to be explored. As the concentration of 36 kDa denatured free HC in normal blood plasma is very low relative to the conformed $\beta_2$m-associated forms (DeVito-Haynes *et al.* 1998), exposure to soluble HLA via BT would not be expected to stimulate presentation of cryptic peptides. Thus, soluble HLA exposure via BT may carry a lower risk of sensitization than does the release of HLA soluble antigens from activated donor cells within an allograft.

The selective formation of IgM–HLA lipophilic complexes depicted in Fig. 4.5 may have important implications for the generation of a regulatory idiotype network. Investigations into the formation of anti-idiotype antibodies indicate that the optimal condition for induction of anti-idiotype is the formation of immune complexes in slight antibody excess (Klaus 1978). Because IgMs are formed first, this means that, early after a BT, only the shed high-molecular-weight membrane-bound form of HLA is likely to induce the formation of immune complexes. Because the level of shed antigen is likely to diminish over time after BT, this could allow antibody excess to occur as the IgM response develops. If the CD4+ T helper cell function is limited in the recipient during this period — for example, by insufficient costimulation (Sayegh & Turka 1998) — germinal centre formation and a T helper-mediated switch to the high-affinity IgG response will not occur.

Under these circumstances, IgM interaction with donor MHC class I lipid complexes derived from the BT or from the transplant may favour the formation of anti-idiotypic antibodies rather than progression to an IgG anti-MHC response. The predicted outcome — IgM antidonor class I, failure of IgM→IgG switch and development of an anti-idiotypic Ig response — has indeed been found to occur experimentally in DST-treated rats following transplantation of an organ allograft (Downey *et al.* 1990). Recent work suggests that at least some of the anti-idiotypic antibodies formed in response to anti-HLA are themselves divalent molecular mimics of a polymorphic HLA epitope (Burlingham *et al*. 1998b). Thus they may be able to compete effectively with monovalent soluble HLA protein for binding to HLA-specific B cells and inhibit the progression to IgG formation, as shown.

If IgG responses to donor HLA do occur after transplant, the ability of water-soluble forms of HLA class I to form immune complexes with IgG (Fig. 4.5, lower right) may predispose to chronic rejection, because deposition of these complexes in the graft vascular bed could elicit macrophage activation and chronic vessel injury. Immune complex formation may also predispose to epitope spreading at the humoral level as macrophages and DC, which bind these complexes, would present these to newly recruited B cells, because the initial wave of IgG antibody would block sites recognized by the original B cell pool. Indeed, recent data indicate that the chronically rejecting heart is a source for the chronic release of donor-type soluble HLA class I antigens into serum, a necessary precondition for complex formation (Suciu-Foca *et al*. 1991; DeVito-Haynes *et al*. 1996). Preliminary data in lung transplant recipients indicate that waves of tissue activation that accompany repeated episodes of acute rejection leading to early graft loss are accompanied by cycles of release of soluble donor HLA antigen (including HLA class I free heavy chain) in the serum. Each of these cycles was followed by the formation of anti-HLA antibodies, but the specificity of the antibody changed with each cycle of antigen release (E. Jankowska-Gan, L.D. Haynes and W.J. Burlingham, unpublished observations).

## Conclusions

The beneficial BT effect can be divided into four distinct but interacting components.

1 Avoidance of sensitization—particularly IgG anti-MHC antibodies—prior to transplant and continuing suppression of anti-HLA responses after transplant, by limiting T cell indirect pathway help and by induction of anti-idiotypic antibodies which mimic soluble donor HLA.

2 Attenuation of acute rejection in the early post-transplant period by limiting IL-2 production by T helper cells and by a form of T–T cell interaction that uses the indirect pathway to down-regulate acute rejection responses mediated by direct pathway T cells.

3 Reawakening of T regulatory cell memory responses, particularly those responses to alloantigens and allopeptides encountered during *in utero* life, leading to establishment of local (intragraft) and peripheral cytokine conditions for long-term graft acceptance.

4 Facilitation of donor passenger leucocyte persistence within the graft and gradual development of peripheral microchimerism, which leads to inhibition or veto—rather than activation—of newly arising host CD8+ CTL precursors specific for donor HLA class I.

A unifying hypothesis has been proposed that the reawakening of T cell memory of neonatal exposure to semiallogeneic maternal cells and soluble HLA predisposes to all four beneficial effects of BT in organ transplantation.

A major unsolved problem is how to ensure the stability of the donor-cell-based peripheral tolerance mechanisms in transplant patients evoked by fetal–neonatal antigen exposure, followed by BT and other donor-specific strategies, such as bone marrow supplementation of chimerism in organ allografts (Fontes *et al*. 1994). More research is needed to determine how to ensure that the donor cell phenotype in microchimerism remains favourable in the long term to infectious tolerance (Bemelman *et al*. 1998) rather than to chronic rejection.

## References

Allison, J.P., Pellegrino, M.A., Ferrone, S., Callahan, G.I.V. & Reisfeld, R.A. (1977) Biologic and chemical characterization of HLA antigens in human serum. *Journal of Immunology* **118**, 1004.

Anderson, D., Billingham, R.E., Lampkin, G.H. & Medawar, P. (1951) The use of skin grafting to distinquish between monozygotic and dizygotic twins in cattle. *Heredity* **5**, 379 (Abstract).

Arnold, B., Messerle, M., Jatsch, L., Kublbeck, G. & Koszinowski, U. (1990) Transgenic mice expressing a soluble foreign H-2 class I antigen are tolerant to allogeneic fragments presented by self class I but not to the whole membrane-bound alloantigen. *Proceedings of the National Academy of Sciences (USA)* **87**, 1762.

Arnold, B., Schonrich, G. & Hammerling, G. (1993) Multiple

levels of peripheral tolerance. *Immunology Today* 14, 12.

Bean, M.A., Mickelson, E., Yanagida, J. *et al.* (1990) Suppressed antidonor MLC responses in renal transplant candidates conditioned with donor-specific transfusions that carry the recipient's noninherited maternal HLA haplotype. *Transplantation* 49, 382.

Bemelman, F., Honey, K., Adams, E., Cobbold, S. & Waldmann, H. (1998) Bone marrow transplantation induces either clonal deletion or infectious tolerance depending on the dose. *Journal of Immunology* 160, 2645.

Benichou, G., Malloy, K.M., Tam, R.C., Heeger, P.S. & Fedoseyeva, E.V. (1998) The presentation of self and allogeneic MHC peptides to T lymphocytes. *Human Immunology* 59, 540.

Bennett, S.R.M., Carbone, F.R., Karamalis, F. *et al.* (1998) Help for cytotoxic T-cell responses is mediated by CD40 signalling. *Nature* 393, 478.

Billingham, R.E., Brent, L. & Medawar, P.B. (1953) Actively acquired tolerance of foreign cells. *Nature* 172, 603.

Bishop, G.A., Sun, J., Sheil, A.G. & McCaughan, G.W. (1997) High-dose/activation-associated tolerance: a mechanism for allograft tolerance. *Transplantation* 64, 1377.

Burlingham, W.J. (1995) Chimerism and transplantation tolerance. Part 2: Case study of a functionally tolerant patient. *Transplantatie Bulletin (Dutch)* 3, 10.

Burlingham, W.J., Stratta, R.J., Mason, B. *et al.* (1988a) Multivariate analysis of risk factors for sensitization and early rejection episodes in a donor-specific transfusion plus azathioprine protocol. *Transplantation* 45, 342.

Burlingham, W.J., Pan, M.H., Mason, B., Ceman, S. & Sollinger, H.W. (1988b) Induction of antiidiotypic antibodies to donor HLA-A2: following blood transfusions in a highly sensitized HLA-A2+ recipient. *Transplantation* 45, 1066.

Burlingham, W.J., Fechner, J.H., DeVito, L.D. *et al.* (1993) Human interleukin-2 and lymphoproliferative (T-helper cell) responses to soluble HLA class I antigens in vitro: I. Specificity for polymorphic domains. *Tissue Antigens* 42, 35.

Burlingham, W.J., Grailer, A.P., Fechner, J.H. Jr *et al.* (1995) Microchimerism linked to cytotoxic T lymphocyte functional unresponsiveness (clonal anergy) in a tolerant renal transplant recipient. *Transplantation* 59, 1147.

Burlingham, W.J., Grailer, A.P., Heisey, D. *et al.* (1998a) Effect of tolerance to non-inherited maternal HLA antigens on the survival of renal transplants from sibling donors. *New England Journal of Medicine* 339, 1657–1664.

Burlingham, W.J., Jankowska-Gan, E., DeVito-Haynes, L.D. *et al.* (1998b) HLA (A*0201) mimicry by anti-idiotypic monoclonal antibodies. *Journal of Immunology* 161, 6705–6714.

Burnet, F.M. & Fenner, F. (1949) *The Production of Antibodies.* Macmillan, New York.

Butcher, G.W., Corvalan, J.W., Licence, D.R. & Howard, J.C. (1982) Immune response genes controlling responsiveness to major histocompatibility antigens: specific MHC-linked defect for antibody response to class I alloantigens. *Journal of Experimental Medicine* 155, 303.

Calne, R.Y. (1998) Panel discussion on the role of immunology in the development of clinical transplantation. *Immunology Letters* 21, 82.

Carrodeguas, L., Orosz, C.G., Waldman, W.J., Sedmak, D.D., Adams, P.W. & VanBuskirk, A.M. (1999) Trans vivo analysis of human delayed-type hypersensitivity reactivity. *Human Immunology* 60, 640–651.

Cecka, J.M., Gjertson, D.W. & Terasaki, P.I. (1997) Pediatric renal transplantation: a review of the UNOS data. *Pediatric Transplantation* 1, 55.

Claas, F.H., Gijbels, Y., van Der Velden-de Munck, J. & van Rood, J.J. (1988) Induction of B cell unresponsiveness to noninherited maternal HLA antigens during fetal life. *Science* 241, 1815.

Clubotariu, R., Zhuoru, L., Colovai, A. & Suciu-Foca, N. (1998) Persistent allopeptide reactivity and epitope spreading in chronic rejection of organ allografts. *Journal of Clinical Investigations* 101, 1.

Colombe, B.W., Lou, C.D., Salvatierra, O. Jr & Garovoy, M.R. (1987) Two patterns of sensitization demonstrated by recipients of donor-specific transfusion. Limitations to control by Imuran. *Transplantation* 44, 509.

Dallman, M.J. Wood, K.J. & Morris, P.J. (1987) Specific cytotoxic T cells are found in the nonrejected kidneys of blood-transfused rats. *Journal of Experimental Medicine* 165, 566.

Dallman, M.J., Wood, K.J. & Morris, P.J. (1989) Recombinant Interleukin-2 can reverse the blood transfusion effect. *Transplantation Proceedings* 21, 1165.

Dallman, M.J., Shiho, O., Page, T.H., Wood, K.J. & Morris, P.J. (1991) Peripheral tolerance to alloantigen results from altered regulation of the interleukin 2 pathway. *Journal of Experimental Medicine* 173, 79.

Dausset, J. (1954) Leuco-agglutinins IV. Leuco-agglutinins and blood transfusion. *Vox Sanguinis* 4, 190.

Demaria, S., Schwab, R., Gottesman, S.R.S. & Bushkin, Y. (1994) Soluble β2microglobulin-free class I heavy chains are released from the surface of activated and leukemia cells by a metalloprotease. *Journal of Biological Chemistry* 269, 6689.

DeVito, L.D., Jankowska-Gan, E. & Burlingham, W.J. (1993) IgM anti-HLA-A2: antibody binds detergent-solubilized native HLA-A2: but fails to bind secreted recombinant forms of A2. *Human Immunology* 37, 122 (Abstract).

DeVito-Haynes, L.D., Jankowska-Gan, E., Heisey, D. *et al.* (1996) Donor-derived HLA class I proteins in the serum of heart transplant recipients. *Journal of Heart and Lung Transplantation* 15, 1012.

DeVito-Haynes, L.D., Demaria, S., Bushkin, Y. & Burlingham, W.J. (1998) The metalloproteinase-mediated pathway is essential for generation of soluble HLA class I proteins by activated cells *in vitro*: proposed mechanism for soluble HLA release in transplant rejection. *Human Immunology* **59**, 426.

Downey, W.E. III, Baldwin, W.M. III & Sanfilippo, F. (1990) Association of donor-specific blood transfusion enhancement of rat renal allografts with accelerated development of antiidiotypic antibodies and reduced alloantibody responses. *Transplantation* **49**, 160.

Editorial (1988) Time to abandon pre-transplant blood transfusion? *Lancet* **8585**, 567.

Fangmann, J., Dalchan, R. & Fabre, J.W. (1992) Rejection of skin allografts by indirect allorecognition of donor class I major histocompatibility complex peptides. *Journal of Experimental Medicine* **175**, 1521.

Fink, P.J., Weissman, I.L. & Bevan, M.J. (1983) Haplotype-specific suppression of cytotoxic T cell induction by antigen inappropriately presented on T cells. *Journal of Experimental Medicine* **157**, 141.

Fontes, P., Rao, A.S., Demetris, A.J. *et al.* (1994) Bone marrow augmentation of donor-cell chimaera in kidney, liver, heart, and pacreas islet transplantation. *Lancet* **344**, 151.

Forsthuber, T., Yip, H.T. & Lehmann, P.V. (1996) Induction of Th1 and Th2 Immunity in neonatal mice. *Science* **271**, 1728.

Fuchs, E.J. & Matzinger, P. (1992) B cells turn off virgin but not memory T cells. *Science* **258**, 1156.

Fung, J.J., Zeevi, A., Kaufman, C. *et al.* (1985) Interactions between bronchoalveolar lymphocytes and macrophages in heart–lung transplant recipients. *Human Immunology* **14**, 287.

Geissler, E.K., Wang, J., Fechner, J.H., Burlingham, W.J. Jr & Knechtle, S.J. (1994) Immunity to MHC class I antigen after direct DNA transfer into skeletal muscle. *Journal of Immunology* **152**, 413.

Gilman-Sachs, A., Luo, S.P., Beer, A.E. & Beaman, K.D. (1989) Analysis of anti-lymphocyte antibodies by flow cytomery or micro-lymphocytotoxicity in women with recurrent spontaneous abortions immunized with paternal leukocytes. *Journal of Clinical and Laboratory Immunology* **30**, 53.

Gorer, P.A. (1937) The genetic and antigenic basis of tumor transplantation. *Journal of Experimental Medicine* **44**, 691.

Grailer, A.P., Sollinger, H.W., Kawamura, T. & Burlingham, W.J. (1991) Donor-specific cytotoxic T lymphocyte hyporesponsiveness following renal transplantation in patients pretreated with donor-specific transfusions. *Transplantation* **51**, 320.

Grumet, F.C., Krishnaswamy, S., See-Tho, K., Filvaroff, E. & Hiraki, D.D. (1994) Soluble form of an HLA-B7 class I

antigen specifically suppresses humoral alloimmunization. *Human Immunology* **40**, 228 (Abstract).

Hadley, G.A., Phelan, D.L., Duffy, B.F. & Mohanakumar, T. (1990) Lack of T-cell tolerance of noninherited maternal HLA antigens in normal humans. *Human Immunology* **28**, 373.

Hadley, G.A., Anderson, C.B. & Mohanakumar, T. (1992) Selective loss of functional antidonor cytolytic T cell precursors following donor-specific blood transfusions in long-term renal allograft recipients. *Transplantation* **54**, 333.

Halasz, N.A., Orloff, M.J. & Hirose, F. (1964) Increased survival of renal homografts in dogs after injection of graft donor blood. *Transplantation* **2**, 453.

Hall, J.M., Lingenfelter, P., Adams, S.L. *et al.* (1995) Detection of maternal cells in human umbilical cord blood using fluorescence *in situ* hybridization. *Blood* **86**, 2829.

Hasek, M. (1954) Manifestation of vegatative assimilation in adaptation of higher animals to foreign antigens. *Czechoslovak Biology* **3**, 327.

Hiruma, K. & Gress, R.E. (1992) Cyclosporine A and peripheral tolerance. Inhibition of veto cell-mediated clonal deletion of postthymic precursor cytotoxic T lymphocytes. *Journal of Immunology* **149**, 1539.

Hunziker, R.D., Lynch, F., Shevach, E.M. & Margulies, D.H. (1997) Split tolerance to the MHC class I molecule H-2D$^d$ in animals transgenic for its soluble analog. *Human Immunology* **52**, 82.

Johnson, L.L. (1987) Prolonged minor allograft survival in intravenously primed mice—a test of the veto hypothesis. *Transplantation* **44**, 92.

Josien, R., Douillard, P., Guillot, C. *et al.* (1998a) A critical role for transforming growth factor-beta in donor transfusion-induced allograft tolerance. *Journal of Clinical Investigation* **102** (11), 1920–1926.

Josien, R., Heslan, M., Brouard, S., Soulillou, J.P. & Cuturi, M.C. (1998b) Critical requirement for graft passenger leukocytes in allograft tolerance induced by donor blood transfusion. *Blood* **92** (12), 4539–4544.

Kearney, E.R., Pape, K.A., Loh, D.Y. & Jenkins, M.K. (1994) Visualization of peptide-specific T cell immunity and peripheral tolerance induction *in vivo*. *Immunity* **1**, 327.

Kissmeyer-Nielsen, F., Olsen, S., Petersen, V.P. & Fjeldborg, O. (1966) Hyperacute rejection of kidney allographs, associated with pre-existing humoral antibodies against donor cells. *Lancet* **2**, 662.

Klaus, G.G.B. (1978) Antigen–antibody complexes elicit anti-idiotypic antibodies to self-idiotopes. *Nature* **272**, 265.

Klein, J., Livnat, S., Hauptfeld, V., Jerabek, L. & Weissman, I. (1974) Production of anti-H-2 antibodies in thymectomized mice. *European Journal of Immunology* **4**, 41.

Krangel, M.S. (1986) Secretion of HLA-A and -B antigens via

an alternative RNA splicing pathway. *Journal of Experimental Medicine* **163**, 1173.

Krangel, M.S. (1987) Two forms of HLA Class I molecules in human plasma. *Human Immunology* **20**, 155.

Kusaka, S., Grailer, A.P., Fechner, J.H. Jr *et al.* (2000) Clonotype analysis of human alloreactive T cells: a novel approach to studying peripheral tolerance in transplant recipients. *Journal of Immunology* **164**, 2240–2247.

Lagaaij, E.L., Henneman, P.H., Ruigrok, M.B. *et al.* (1989) Effect of one HLA-DR antigen matched and completely HLA-DR mismatched blood transfusions on survival of heart and kidney allografts. *New England Journal of Medicine* **321**, 701.

Lazda, V.A., Pollak, R., Mozes, M.F., Barber, P.L. & Jonasson, O. (1990) Evidence that HLA class II disparity is required for the induction of renal allograft enhancement by donor-specific blood transfusions in man. *Transplantation* **49**, 1084.

Liu, Z., Sun, Y.K., Yu-Ping, X. *et al.* (1993) Contribution of direct and indirect recognition pathways to T cell alloreactivity. *Journal of Experimental Medicine* **177**, 1643.

Lu, L., Li, W., Fu, F. *et al.* (1997) Blockade of the CD40-CD40 ligand pathway potentiates the capacity of donor-derived dendritic cell progenitors to induce long-term cardiac allograft survival. *Transplantation* **64**, 1808–1815.

Medawar, P.B. (1946) Immunity to homologous grafted skin. II. The relationship between the antigens of blood and skin. *British Journal of Experimental Pathology* **27**, 15.

Miller, R.G. & Phillips, R.A. (1976) Reduction of the *in vitro* cytotoxic lymphocyte response produced by *in vivo* exposure to semi-allogeneic cells: recruitment or active suppression. *Journal of Immunology* **117**, 1913.

Moretta, A. & Moretta, L. (1997) HLA Class I specific inhibitory receptors. *Current Opinion in Immunology* **9**, 694.

Nakashima, I. & Lake, P. (1979) A novel subset of antigenic cells triggers B-cell responses to MHC antigens. *Nature* **279**, 716.

Neu, A., Furth, S., Zachary, A.A. & Stablein, D. (1995) Beneficial effect of non-inherited maternal antigens on graft survival in pediatric renal transplantation. *Journal of the American Society of Nephrology* **7**, 1917.

Newton, W.T. & Anderson, C.B. (1973) Planned preimmunization of renal allograft recipients. *Surgery* **74**, 430.

O'Connell, P.J., Mba-Jonas, A., Leverson, G.E. *et al.* (1998) Stable lung allograft outcome correlates with the presence of intragraft donor-derived leukocytes. *Transplantation* **66**, 1167.

Opelz, G. (1987) Improved kidney graft survival in non-transfused recipients. *Transplantation Proceedings* **19**, 149.

Opelz, G. and the Collaborative Transplant Study (1990) Analysis of the 'NIMA effect' in renal transplantaion. In: *Clinical Transplants 1990* (ed. P.I. Terasaki), 6th edn, p. 63. UCLA Tissue Typing Laboratory, Los Angeles.

Opelz, G., Sengar, G.P.S., Mickey, M.R. & Terasaki, P.I. (1973) Effect of blood transfusions on subsequent kidney transplants. *Transplantation Proceedings* **4**, 253.

Owen, R.D. (1945) Immunogenetic consequences of vascular anastomoses between bovine twins. *Science* **102**, 400.

Owen, R.D., Wood, H.R., Foord, A.G., Sturgeon, P. & Baldwin L.G. (1954) Evidence for actively acquired tolerance to Rh antigens. *Proceedings of the National Academy of Sciences (USA)* **40**, 420.

Paul, L.C. (1993) Chronic rejection of organ allografts: magnitude of the problem. *Transplantation Proceedings* **25**, 2024.

Pettigrew, G.J., Lovegrove, E., Bradley, J.A., Maclean, J. & Bolton, E.M. (1998) Indirect T cell allorecognition and alloantibody-mediated rejection of MHC class I-disparate heart grafts. *Journal of Immunology* **161**, 1292.

Phelan, D., Hadley, G., Duffy, B., Mohanam, S. & Mohanakumar, T. (1991) Antiidiotypic antibodies to HLA class I alloantibodies in normal individuals: a mechanism of tolerance to noninherited maternal HLA antigens. *Human Immunology* **31**, 1.

Reed, A., Pirsch, J., Armbrust, M.J. *et al.* (1991) Multivariate analysis of donor-specific versus random transfusion protocols in haploidentical living-related transplants. *Transplantation* **51**, 382.

Reed, E., Hardy, M.A., Benveristy, A. *et al.* (1987) Effect of antiidiotypic antibodies to HLA on graft survival in renal-allograft recipients. *New England Journal of Medicine* **316**, 1450.

Ridge, J.P., Di Rosa, F. & Matzinger, P. (1998) A conditioned dendritic cell can be a temporal bridge between a CD4+ T-helper and a T-killer cell. *Nature* **393**, 474.

Roelen, D.L., Van Bree, S.P.M.J., Van Beelen, E., van Rood, J.J. & Claas, F.H.J. (1995) No evidence of an influence of the non-inherited maternal HLA antigens on the alloreactive T cell repertoire in healthy individuals. *Transplantation* **59**, 1728.

Salvatierra, O. Jr, Vincenti, F., Amend, W. *et al.* (1980) Deliberate donor-specific blood transfusions prior to living related renal transplantation. A new approach. *Annals of Surgery* **192**, 543.

Salvatierra, O. Jr, Melzer, J., Potter, D. *et al.* (1985) A seven-year experience with donor-specific blood transfusions. Results and considerations for maximum efficacy. *Transplantation* **40**, 654.

Sayegh, M. & Turka, L.A. (1998) The role of T cell co-stimulatory activation pathways in transplant rejection. *New England Journal of Medicine* **338**, 1813.

Sheng-Tanner, X. & Miller, R.G. (1992) Correlation between lymphocyte-induced donor-specific tolerance and donor cell recirculation. *Journal of Experimental Medicine* **176**, 407.

Singh, R.R., Hahn, B.H. & Sercarz, E.E. (1996) Neonatal peptide exposure can prime T cells and, upon subsequent immunization, induce their immune deviation: implications for antibody vs. T cell mediated autoimmunity. *Journal of Experimental Medicine* **183**, 1613.

Sivasai, K.S.R., Alevy, Y.G., Duffy, B.F. *et al.* (1997) Peripheral blood microchimerism in human liver and renal transplant recipients. *Transplantation* **64**, 427.

Smits, J.M.A., Claas, F.H.J., van Houwelingen, H.C. & Persijn, G.G. (1998) Do non-inherited maternal antigens (NIMAs) enhance renal allograft survival? *Transplant International* **11**, 82.

Starzl, T.E., Demetris, A.J., Trucco, M. *et al.* (1992) Systemic chimerism in human female recipients of male livers. *Lancet* **340**, 876.

Starzl, T.E., Demetris, A.J., Trucco, M. *et al.* (1993) Cell migration and chimerism after whole-organ transplantation: the basis of graft acceptance. *Hepatology* **17**, 1127.

Steinmuller, D. (1984) Tissue-specific transplantation antigens. *Immunology Today* **5**, 234.

Suciu-Foca, N., Reed, E., Marboe, C. *et al.* (1991) The role of anti-HLA antibodies in heart transplantation. *Transplantation* **51**, 716.

Takeuchi, T., Lowry, R.P. & Koniecsny, B. (1992) Heart allografts in murine systems. The differential activation of Th-2-like effector cells in peripheral tolerance. *Transplantation* **53**, 1281.

Terasaki, P.I. (1989) Kidney transplant outcome. In: *Clinical Kidney Transplants 1989*, p. 25. UCLA Tissue Typing Laboratory, Los Angeles.

Terasaki, P.I., Cecka, J.M., Gjertson, D.W. *et al.* (1996) Risk rate and long term kidney transplant survival. In: *Clinical Transplants 1996* (eds P.I. Terasaki & J.M. Cecka), p. 443. UCLA Tissue Typing Laboratory, Los Angeles.

Thomas, J.M., Carver, F.M., Kasten-Jolly, J., Haisch, C.E. & Thomas, F.T. (1993) Transplantation tolerance in nonhuman primates: a case for veto cells. *Transplant Science* **3**, 69.

Thomas, J.M., Carver, F.M., Kasten-Jolly, J. *et al.* (1994) Further studies of veto activity in rhesus monkey bone marrow in relation to allograft tolerance and chimerism. *Transplantation* **57**, 101.

Tilney, N.L., Whitley, W.D., Diamond, J.R., Kupiec-Weglinski, J.W. & Adams, D.H. (1991) Chronic rejection—an undefined conundrum. *Transplantation* **52**, 389.

Trivedi, H.N., HayGlass, K., Gangur, V. *et al.* (1997) Analysis of neonatal T cell and antigen presenting cell functions. *Human Immunology* **57**, 69.

Van Rood, J.J. & Claas, F.H. (1990) The influence of allogeneic cells on the human T and B cell repertoire. *Science* **248**, 1388.

VanBuskirk, A.M., Burlingham, W.J., Jankowska-Gan, E. *et al.* (2000) Human allograft acceptance is associated with immune regulation. *Journal of Clinical Investigation* (submitted).

Wagner, J.E. (1997) Allogeneic umbilical cord blood transplantation. *Cancer Treatment Research* **77**, 187.

Wood, K.J. & Sachs, D.H. (1998) Chimerism and transplantation tolerance: cause and effect. *Immunology Today* **17**, 584.

Zhai, Y. & Knechtle, S.J. (1998) Two distinct forms of soluble MHC class I molecules synthesized by different mechanisms in normal rat cells *in vitro*. *Human Immunology* **59**, 404.

Zhang, L., Shannon, J., Sheldon, J. *et al.* (1994) Role of infused CD8+ cells in the induction of peripheral tolerance. *Journal of Immunology* **152**, 2222.

# Chapter 5 / Cellular and molecular basis of immunosuppression

JEAN-FRANÇOIS BACH & LUCIENNE CHATENOUD

## Introduction

A wide array of chemical and biological agents are currently used to suppress undesirable immune responses, notably rejection of allografts and autoimmune diseases. In addition, novel drugs that are presently under preclinical or early clinical development seem to hold the promise of interfering with various types of immune responses with much greater efficacy than that previously observed with more conventional immunosuppressants. The currently available compounds differ greatly in their biochemical nature, in the molecular structure of their specific targets as well as in the pattern of immunosuppression they induce.

The aim of this chapter will be to review the principal targets as well as the mode of action of the immunosuppressive drugs that are the most commonly used in clinical practice, including those that have more recently entered the clinical arena.

An immune response is a complex reaction that ensues from the interaction between various functionally distinct cell types, antigen-presenting cells, B and T lymphocytes, which communicate through an intricate network of cell receptors and soluble mediators. This cell cooperation involves a number of surface receptors interacting with their specific ligands, as well as a variety of soluble mediators, namely cytokines. Each of these 'cell actors' of immunity or their functionally relevant membrane or intracellular molecules can be targeted with the aim of suppressing the immune response.

At this stage, it is important to distinguish between two completely different modalities of action of immunosuppressive drugs:
1 the *physical destruction* or the *inhibition of proliferation* of the immune cells involved in the response;
2 the selective *neutralization* of the cell receptors and/or soluble molecules that mediate the functional capacity of these immune cells.

We shall first discuss the nature of the targets for the most commonly available immunosuppressants and then address the molecular basis of their mode of action.

## Target cells and molecules

All immune cells, including antigen-presenting cells (dendritic cells, macrophages and monocytes) and lymphocytes (B cells, T cells including CD4+—Th-1 and Th-2—and CD8+ subsets), are potential targets of immunosuppressant agents. These various cell types can be affected by altering haemopoiesis, thus preventing their production in the bone marrow, or preferably at a later stage once they are mature or, even more selectively in the case of B and T lymphocytes, after they have been committed by the antigen and once they entered the proliferation and differentiation processes. Schematically four main mechanisms can be distinguished that will promote an inhibition of immune cell responses. These are:

1 the inhibition of cell proliferation;

2 the physical elimination or depletion of a cell type or subset;

3 the inactivation or down-modulation of the cell functional capacity; and

4 the induction of antigen specific tolerance.

## Inhibition of cell proliferation

Inhibition of cell proliferation is obtained with drugs that interfere with nucleic acid synthesis (Table 5.1) by acting on one or more of the various metabolic steps involved. In this category one finds different chemicals which affect:

• *purine metabolisms*: 6-mercaptopurine (6-MP) or its imidazole derivative—azathioprine, thioguanine, mycophenolic acid (Bach & Strom 1985a; Platz *et al.* 1991; Dayton *et al.* 1992; Brazelton & Morris 1996) (Fig. 5.1);

**Table 5.1** Mode of action of 6-MP and its nucleotide forms in enzymatic reactions in nucleic acid biosynthesis. (From Bach & Strom 1985a–d.)

| Reaction catalysed | Inhibitor | $K_m$ | $K_I$ |
|---|---|---|---|
| IMP → SAMP | TIMP | $3 \times 10^{-5}$ | $3 \times 10^{-4}$ |
| IMP → XMP | TIMP | $1.4 \times 10^{-5}$ | $3.6 \times 10^{-6}$ |
| H → IMP | 6-MP | $1.1 \times 10^{-5}$ | $8.3 \times 10^{-6}$ |
| ADP → (ADP)$_n$ | TIDP | $1.7 \times 10^{-3}$ | $3.3 \times 10^{-5}$ |
| PRPP → PRA | TIMP | | $4.4 \times 10^{-5}$ |
| ATP + NMN → NAD | TITP | $7.4 \times 10^{-5}$ | $5 \times 10^{-5}$ |
| SAMP → AMP | TIMP | $2.8 \times 10^{-6}$ | $3 \times 10^{-3}$ |
| H$_4$FA $\xrightarrow{\text{ATP}}$ FH$_4$FA | 6-MP | $5 \times 10^{-4}$ | $3.3 \times 10^{-3}$ |
| | | | $2.5 \times 10^{-4}$ |

ADP, adenosine diphosphate; AMP, adenylic acid; ATP, adenosine triphosphate; GMP, guanylic acid; H, hypoxanthine; IMP, inosinic acid, the active metabolite of 6-mercaptopurine; NAD, nicotinamide adenine dinucleotide; NMN, nicotinamide mononucleotide; PRA, 5-phosphoribosylamine; PRPP, phosphoribosyl pyrophosphate; SAMP, adenylo-succinate; TIDP, thioinosine diphosphate; TIMP, thioinosinic acid; TITP, thioinosine triphosphate; XMP, xanthylic acid.

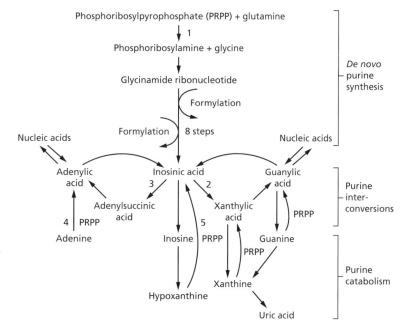

**Fig. 5.1** Pathways of purine *de novo* synthesis and purine catabolism. Enzyme activities regulated by the concentration of nucleotide end products include: (1) phosphoribosylpyrophosphate amidotransferase, (2) inosinic dehydrogenase, (3) adenylsuccinic acid synthetase, (4) adenine phosphoribosyltransferase and (5) hypoxanthine-guanine phosphoribosyltransferase. (Redrawn from Bach & Strom 1985a–d.)

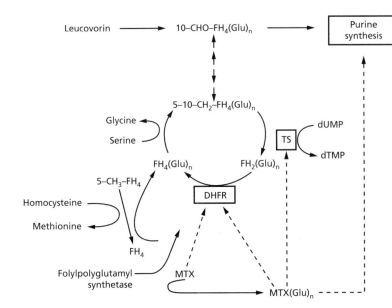

**Fig. 5.2** Major enzymatic reactions involving methotrexate and folates as cosubstrates. Broken lines indicate enzyme inhibition. MTX, methotrexate; DHFR, dihydrofolate reductase; TS, thymidylate synthetase; $FH_2$, dihydrofolate; $FH_4$, tetrahydrofolate; Glu, glutamyl; dTMP, thymidylate; dUMP, dioxyuridylate. (Modified from Jolivet *et al.* 1983.)

- *pyrimidine synthesis*: brequinar (Cramer *et al.* 1992a,b; Kahan 1992)
- *folate synthesis*: amethopterin (Endresen 1992) (Fig. 5.2); and
- *DNA replication*: irradiation (Bach & Strom 1985b), cyclophosphamide and other alkylating agents (Bach & Strom 1985c).

Obviously these agents are not specific for lymphoid cells as they interfere with the proliferation of any cell type. However, at the doses used therapeutically, these drugs will preferentially affect rapidly proliferating cells as are lymphoid cells undergoing antigen-driven differentiation (Berenbaum 1969).

## Depletion

### CYTOLYSIS AFTER BINDING TO AN INTRACYTOPLASMIC RECEPTOR

This is typically the case of high-dose corticosteroids which bind to widespread cytosol receptors (Cohen 1971). The most conspicuous lysis occurs in the thymus cortex but it is difficult to determine the relevance of this depletion in corticosteroid-mediated immunosuppression (Cohen & Claman

1971). Depletion of other cell types is not well documented and its interpretation is complicated by the cellular sequestration—notably from peripheral blood to bone marrow—that follows corticosteroid administration (Fauci & Dale 1975).

### CYTOLYSIS AFTER BINDING TO A MEMBRANE RECEPTOR

This mechanism is essentially elicited upon usage of biological immunosuppressants, namely depleting polyclonal or monoclonal anti-T cell antibodies. The immunological effects of cell depletion will depend on its degree and on its cellular selectivity. Both of these parameters will vary significantly depending on the type of antibody used. Thus, depletion may affect:

- all leucocytes, following the administration of antibodies to CD52 (Hale *et al.* 1988; Isaacs *et al.* 1992a);
- all T cells, when polyclonal anti-T cell antibodies or antibodies to CD3 antibodies are used (Cosimi *et al.* 1981; Hirsch *et al.* 1988);
- T cell subsets, when antibodies to CD4 are administered (Dialynas *et al.* 1983; Reiter *et al.* 1991). In some cases, only activated T cells may be affected as is the case with the use of antibodies to the α chain of the IL-

2 receptor (CD25) (Nashan *et al.* 1997; Vincenti *et al.* 1998).

Immunotoxins that consist of conjugates of a toxin (diphtheria toxin or ricin) coupled to an antibody or to a cytokine (Kronke *et al.* 1985, 1986) should be mentioned here. The immunotoxin is brought to the target cell by an antibody CD25 (Waldmann & O'Shea 1998), CD3 (Knechtle *et al.* 1997; Thomas *et al.* 1997) or a cytokine (IL-2 or IL-6) (Bacha *et al.* 1988; Strom *et al.* 1993) and the toxin kills the target cell after being internalized (Walz *et al.* 1989).

## Target cell inactivation

The specific targeting of numerous molecules can significantly impair the functional capacity of immune cells without the need to physically destroy them. Among these targets are intracytoplasmic receptors, membrane receptors and soluble mediators (cytokines).

Compared with depleting immunosuppressive agents, the drugs that decrease or inhibit the functional capacity of immune cells are frequently characterized by the rapid reversibility of their effect at the end of treatment.

### INTRACYTOPLASMIC RECEPTORS

#### Steroid receptors

At low or moderate dosage corticosteroids act essentially by inhibiting various cellular functions after binding to specific intracytoplasmic receptors (Bach & Strom 1985d). These receptors exist in a wide variety of cell types under an 'inactive' oligomeric form that associates the glucocorticoid receptor to a heat shock protein (hsp90) and an immunophilin. After diffusing through the cell membrane glucocorticoids bind to the receptor, a process that promotes the shedding from the complex of the hsp90 and the immunophilin, thus leading to the 'active' form of the receptor. The active steroid receptor complex is then translocated to the nucleus, where it will interact with the glucocorticoid responsive elements of different gene promoter regions and will thus up- or down-modulate gene transcrip-

tion. Thus, through its capacity to interact with the AP-1 transcription factor (the *c-fos/c-jun* heterodimer), the steroid receptor complex will down-modulate the transcription of several cytokine genes. On the other hand, among the proteins whose production is up-regulated by glucocorticoids lipocortin is a well-known anti-inflammatory agent (Blackwell *et al.* 1982). Glucocorticoids also increase the transcription of the gene encoding for the NFκB inhibitor IκB. This inhibits the translocation of NKκB to the nucleus that is essential for the transcription of several cytokine genes. Given this capacity to inhibit cytokine production, corticosteroids significantly affect cellular immune reactions.

The immunosuppressive effect of corticosteroids correlates with the concentration of the drug in the circulation. It should be realized, however, that a saturation level exists which renders the use of very high doses (e.g. 250–500 mg methylprednisolone) inappropriate except for maintaining blood levels persistently high.

#### Immunophilins

Immunophilins constitute an ever-growing group of cytosolic drug receptors that have an essential role in the transduction of activation signal pathways in lymphocytes, leading, among other consequences, to the production of key cytokines. Cyclophilin was the first immunophilin to be characterized by Handschumacher *et al.* (1984) in their search for the cytosolic receptor for cyclosporin A, a cyclic undecapeptide isolated from the fungus *Tolypocladium inflatum.* Cyclophilin is an abundant (0.1% of all cell proteins) ubiquitous 17 kDa protein present in both procaryotic and eucaryotic cells. The comparative study of cyclosporin A analogues showed that their immunosuppressive capacity correlated with their binding affinity for cyclophilin (Sigal & Dumont 1992). Cyclophilin is an enzyme expressing a peptidyl-prolyl-*cis-trans* isomerase (also called rotamase) activity implicated in protein folding which is blocked by cyclosporin binding (Fischer *et al.* 1989).

FK506, a highly immunosuppressive macrolide isolated from *Streptomyces tsukubaensis*, specifically binds and blocks the rotamase activity of another 12 kDa cytosolic immunophilin termed FK-binding protein (FKBP) (Schreiber & Crabtree 1992; Liu 1993). FKBP is also the cytosolic receptor for rapamycin, another macrolide isolated from *Streptomyces hygroscopicus*. The immunosuppressive properties of rapamycin are very interesting because, at variance with cyclosporin and FK506, it is an extremely potent inhibitor of the IL-2-mediated proliferation of activated T cells (Sigal & Dumont 1992).

The blockade of cyclophilin and FKBP rotamase activity by cyclosporin and FK506, respectively, does not explain the immunosuppressive activity of these drugs, which is mainly based on their selective capacity to inhibit the production of various cytokines—and in particular IL-2—by T lymphocytes (Granelli-Piperno *et al.* 1990). The current view assimilates cyclosporin–cyclophilin and FK506–FKBP complexes to pro-drugs which specifically bind to an intracellular complex, including calmodulin and the two subunits of calcineurin, which is a $Ca^{2+}$-dependent serine-threonine phosphatase (Liu *et al.* 1991). This phosphatase activity is blocked by the interaction with the pro-drug complexes, thus interfering with the translocation to the nucleus of a DNA-binding protein, namely, the cytosolic subunit of the nuclear factor of activated T cells (NFAT), specific for enhancer sequences located within various cytokine gene promoters, including the IL-2 gene.

As previously noted, cyclosporin and FK506 exert their immunosuppressive effect essentially by preventing lymphocyte activation through the inhibition of the transcription of genes encoding for various cytokines (Granelli-Piperno *et al.* 1990). In contrast, although rapamycin also binds FKBP, this pro-drug complex does not interact with calmodulin and calcineurin. Instead, the rapamycin–FKBP complex targets two other intracellular proteins named TOR (for targets of rapamycin) 1 and 2, which are kinases associated with G1 cell cycle progression (Lorenz & Heitman 1995; Zheng *et al.* 1995). The precise G1 effector substrate(s) of the kinase domain of TOR affecting cell cycle progression has(ve) not yet been identified. This particular point of impact of rapamycin that targets the cell cycle is well in keeping with the selective capacity of the drug

to affect activated and/or proliferating T lymphocytes (Brazelton & Morris 1996).

MEMBRANE RECEPTORS

Lymphoid cells recognize antigen and participate in cell interactions via a wide variety of membrane receptors that are all appealing potential targets for immunosuppressive agents, essentially under the form of monoclonal antibodies.

*Antigen recognition and costimulation*

B cells recognize antigens via surface Ig receptors. T cells recognize antigens that are peptides presented in the context of major histocompatibility (MHC) molecules through specialized dimeric receptors: the T cell receptor (TCR) α and β chains. TCR-mediated recognition signals are transduced to T cells via the CD3 complex (Clevers *et al.* 1988; Weiss 1991). The CD3 molecular complex consists of at least five invariant membrane proteins designated γ, δ, ε, ζ and η (Clevers *et al.* 1988). The γ, δ and ε subunits are expressed as non-covalently linked γ–δ and γ–ε dimers; the ζ and η subunits form disulphide-linked homo- ζζ and ζη heterodimers. CD4 and CD8 molecules also have a major role in signalling the corresponding T cell subsets (Rudd 1990). They were initially considered to be simple adhesion molecules interacting with their specific ligands: the MHC class II for CD4 and class I products for CD8. However, it soon became apparent that they were important for effective CD3-TCR signalling (Rudd 1990). Thus, according to Thome *et al.* (1995), CD4, through its associated tyrosine kinase p56[lck], associates with the 'activated' form of the CD3 ζ–ζ chains, thereby stabilizing the CD3-TCR/antigen/MHC interaction and amplifying the signalling process. Most of these important receptors (Ig, TCR, MHC, CD3, CD4 and CD8) have been successfully used as targets of immunosuppressive antibodies.

Although T cell activation is initiated through the CD3-TCR complex, it is well known that this signal (signal 1) is insufficient to guarantee full activation of naïve T cells. To allow sustained T cell activation upon engagement of CD3-TCR, costimulatory signals (signal 2), derived from specialized receptors, are needed. In the case of naïve T cells, CD28 has been identified as one key receptor mediating costimulation upon interaction with its specific ligands B7.1 and B7.2, which are expressed on antigen-presenting cells and B lymphocytes (Linsley *et al.* 1990; Boise *et al.* 1995). Antibodies or soluble molecules binding these cell receptors or their ligands (B7 and CD40 ligand, respectively) may strongly inhibit immune responses (Lenschow *et al.* 1992; Linsley *et al.* 1992; Lin *et al.* 1993).

### Cellular interactions

*Adhesins.* Adhesins that enhance cell contacts represent interesting targets for immunosuppressive agents (Springer *et al.* 1987; Makgoba *et al.* 1989; Springer 1990). Two major systems have been investigated: ICAM-1–LFA-1 (Fischer *et al.* 1986; Cosimi *et al.* 1990; Isobe *et al.* 1992) and CD2–LFA-3 (Bromberg *et al.* 1991; Guckel *et al.* 1991). Moreover, there is increasing evidence that, under particular circumstances, several adhesion receptor–ligand pairs can modulate an immune response not simply by enhancing adhesion but by providing additional activation signals (Clark & Ledbetter 1994). Thus, in the case of memory T cells, which possess a lower activation threshold compared to naïve T cells, adhesins may enter into play to deliver effective costimulatory signals.

*Receptors expressed on activated T cells.* Some cytokine receptors are selectively expressed by activated immune cells and are thus, for obvious reasons, suitable targets of therapeutic monoclonal antibodies. So far, efforts have been essentially devoted to the targeting of the IL-2 receptor. Both murine and humanized antibodies directed at the $\alpha$ chain of the IL-2 receptor (CD25) have been applied (Nashan *et al.* 1997; Vincenti *et al.* 1998; Waldmann & O'Shea 1998). Especially humanized antibodies to CD25 seem to express a potent therapeutic capacity when used for prophylaxis of allograft rejection (Nashan *et al.* 1997; Vincenti *et al.* 1998).

Upon activation, T lymphocytes also express a molecule termed CD40 ligand (CD40 L), which seems a very attractive immunointervention target. CD40 L is a member of the tumour necrosis factor (TNF) cytokine superfamily, which includes TNF$\alpha$, lymphotoxin $\alpha/\beta$, Fas ligand and the ligands for 41BB, CD30, CD27 and OX40. The receptor for CD40 L, CD40, is expressed on various cell types, including dendritic cells, B cells, macrophages and endothelial cells. In functional terms the CD40 pathway has a major role in all T cell-dependent immune responses and its blockade, using specific monoclonal antibodies, combined with donor antigen delivery or simultaneous CD28 blockade, has been recently proposed to promote immune tolerance to organ allografts (Van Den Eertwegh *et al.* 1993; Larsen & Pearson 1997).

### SOLUBLE MEDIATORS

Various attempts, some of which have been very successful, have been made both in experimental and clinical settings to neutralize cytokines, mainly using monoclonal antibodies or fusion proteins, including the specific receptor.

One can mention the use of antibodies for:
• TNF (Beutler *et al.* 1985; Charpentier *et al.* 1992; Elliott *et al.* 1994a,b);
• IL-6 (Klein *et al.* 1991; Lu *et al.* 1992); and
• IFN-$\gamma$ (Skoglund *et al.* 1988; Nicoletti *et al.* 1990; Bach 1993).

### THE CASE OF POLYCLONAL ANTILYMPHOCYTE SERA

Polyclonal antilymphocyte globulins (ALG), which are widely used in transplantation, represent a mixture of a wide spectrum of antibody specificities that probably include, in variable proportions, a large number—if not all—the T cell specificities mentioned above (i.e. CD2, CD3, LFA-1.). This variability in the concentration of each given specificity, added to that concerning the isotype and the affinity of antibodies, explains the differences in the batch-to-batch therapeutic potencies (Balner *et al.* 1968). Antithymocyte globulins (ATG) are enriched in anti-T cell antibodies but other antibodies, including contaminating antibodies to non-lymphoid cells, are also present.

## Antigen-directed immunointervention

This is probably the future approach for treating a wide array of immunological diseases including autoimmune diseases and the rejection of organ allografts. This strategy will imply the use of autoantigen or alloantigen-derived peptides, possibly in conjunction with some of the products mentioned above, notably some of the monoclonal antibodies.

It is fair to recognize, however, that this approach is not yet clinically applicable although the very promising data obtained in experimental models of induced or spontaneous autoimmune diseases have encouraged the launching of some pilot trials in patients (Wraith *et al.* 1989; Hurtenbach *et al.* 1993).

## Cellular mechanisms

The immunosuppressive agents we have presented above exert their therapeutic activity through four distinct but not mutually exclusive mechanisms:
1  cell depletion;
2  inhibition of proliferation;
3  inhibition of functional capacity;
4  cell signalling.

## Cell depletion

Cell depletion is characterized, compared to the three other mechanisms, by its long-lasting effect which poses the central question of the turnover of the depleted cell population. The mechanisms of depletion largely depend on the agent used.

In the case of antibodies (polyclonal or monoclonal) the depleting properties rely on the structure of the constant region, which allows the activation of the complement cascade and the interaction with Fc receptors at the surface of natural killer (NK) and phagocytic cells to trigger antibody-dependent cell cytotoxicity (ADCC). In the case of polyclonal antibodies, such as rabbit or horse anti-T cell antibodies, regularly used in clinical transplantation, cell lysis mostly occurs following direct complement-dependent lysis in the circulation or by means of cell opsonization and removal in the liver and the spleen by reticuloen-dothelial cells (Martin & Miller 1968; Greaves *et al.* 1969). The trapping in these organs of lymphoid cells preincubated with antilymphocyte antibodies has been demonstrated in various *in vitro* and *in vivo* models (Martin & Miller 1967, 1968) in the mouse and in humans. Only the C1, C4, C2 and C3 complement components are needed for effective opsonization; some data suggest that only C1 and C4 could be sufficient (Bach *et al.* 1972).

On the other hand, with cell-directed monoclonal antibodies the mechanisms involved in antibody-mediated cell destruction *in vivo* are more complex. Actually, not only the antibody isotype but also its fine specificity can influence the lytic capacity and it is not sufficient to select for the adequate antibody isotype to achieve the desired *in vivo* depleting or non-depleting effect (Bindon *et al.* 1988; Isaacs *et al.* 1992b). Moreover, the density and the distribution of the antigen on the target cell surface will also greatly influence the lytic capacity of the monoclonal antibody. Finally, among a given set of monoclonal antibodies sharing the same variable region, a hierarchy in terms of lytic capacity can be established that, in the case of monoclonal antibodies bearing a human constant region (humanized chimeric or reshaped monoclonal antibodies), is as follows: IgG1 > IgG2 > IgG3 >> IgG4.

When injected into humans mouse and rat monoclonal antibodies to cell determinants mostly expressed, in the presence of human complement, a rather poor lytic capacity. This is caused by the now well-characterized membrane-bound factors that inhibit complement activation in a species-restricted manner. Despite this, some antibody specificities, such as antibodies to CD52 (CAMPATH-1), are highly depleting. Given its potent lytic capacity, this monoclonal antibody has been extensively used to purge T cells from allogeneic bone marrow prior to transplant for prevention of graft vs. host disease (Bindon *et al.* 1988).

Other mechanisms that may also be involved in antibody-mediated depletion are redirected T cell lysis upon bridging of cytotoxic lymphocytes to the targets (Wong & Colvin 1991) and, in particular for antibodies to CD3 and CD4, the induction of apoptosis or programmed cell death. Apoptosis is a signal-dependent suicidal process associated with the activation of an endogenous endonuclease that leads to genomic DNA fragmentation. Apoptosis mediated via CD3-TCR signalling was initially demonstrated in immature thymocytes but accumulating evidence indicates that it can also be triggered in activated mature peripheral T cells (Smith *et al.* 1989; Wesselborg *et al.* 1993). Resting T cells seem insensitive to such apoptotic signals. Interestingly, this has also been described for some CD4 antibodies. In this same vein, some recent data have indicated that, when used *in vitro* at submitogenic concentrations, polyclonal antilymphocyte globulins triggered apoptosis of activated T cells. This effect was clearly dependent on the presence of antibodies to CD2 and CD3 in the polyclonal preparation (Genestier *et al.* 1998).

In the case of cyclophosphamide cell depletion is the direct consequence of the DNA lesion. The immunological effects of the depletion will closely depend on the cellular selectivity of the immunosuppressive agent and on the renewal rate of the target population. The depletion may globally affect leucocytes (CD52) or T cells (CD3) or T cell subsets (CD4, CD8). In other cases, only activated T cells will be affected, as is the case for IL-2 toxin (Walz *et al.* 1989). Irradiation and cyclophosphamide will only affect rapidly proliferating cells with a hierarchy of cell sensitivity that has been established from *in vitro* data (B lymphocytes>T helper lymphocytes>cytotoxic T lymphocytes) (Askenase *et al.* 1975).

The renewal rate varies considerably with cellular subsets. Pools of B cells and short-lived T cells will rapidly reappear after short-term depletion. Conversely, recirculating long-lived T cells will take several weeks in the mouse and several months in humans to replenish the initial cell pools. In fact it is this very slow turnover of the circulating T cells that explains the T cell selectivity of polyclonal antilymphocyte sera (Lance 1970). The case of depleting CD4 antibodies is intriguing because the depletion may last over 1 year after a single antibody injection (Moreland *et al.* 1994), opening the possibility that an active phenomenon could succeed to the initial passive depletion. In some cases the rapid disappearance of a given cell type (notably the 'natural suppressor cell') after total lym-phoid irradiation will provide an additional source of immunosuppression (Strober 1984).

## Antiproliferative effect

Many drugs can affect the complex metabolic processes leading to nucleic acid synthesis.

PURINE SYNTHESIS

*Azathioprine* (Bach & Strom 1985a)

Azathioprine is, as 6-mercaptopurine, a member of hypoxanthine analogues, which depress antibody production and delay hypersensitivity responses. Azathioprine is largely used for the prevention of allograft rejection. Azathioprine is transformed by hypoxanthine-guanine-phosphoribosyl transferase (HGPRT) into thio-inosidic acid, which is the active drug metabolite.

Azathioprine has several biochemical effects that finally mediate the inhibition of DNA and RNA synthesis, including the interference with coenzymes; the incorporation into nucleic acids; the inhibition of certain enzymes; the interference with purine interconvertion; and the inhibition of *de novo* purine synthesis. These activities well explain the azathioprine-mediated inhibition of nucleic acid synthesis. In addition, it has also been proposed that the active compound could bind amino acids constitutive of membrane proteins and interfere with adenosine metabolism.

Main side effects observed with azathioprine are bone marrow aplasia and hepatotoxocity.

*Mycophenolic acid* (Platz *et al.* 1991; Dayton *et al.* 1992; Figueroa *et al.* 1993; Brazelton & Morris 1996)

Mycophenolic acid and its ester morpholino-ethyl derivative (mycophenolate mofetil) are purine analogues that act through the inhibition of inosinomonophosphate dehydrogenase, thus inducing an irreversible inhibition of guanosine monophosphate (GMP) formation and thus of DNA synthesis. This drug shows potent immunosuppressive properties: *in vitro* it inhibits B and T cell proliferation, the generation of allospecific cytotoxic T cells and antibody production. *In vivo* it prolongs renal and liver allograft survival in dogs, cardiac allograft survival in rats and islet allograft in mice. Minimal side effects were described; mycophenolic acid is not nephrotoxic or hepatotoxic and it shows only minor toxicity on bone marrow cells. In the clinic mycophenolic acid was also shown to be effective at reducing the incidence and the intensity of acute organ allograft rejection (Sollinger 1995; Brazelton & Morris 1996).

## PYRIMIDINE SYNTHESIS

### *Brequinar* (Cramer *et al.* 1992a,b; Kahan 1992)

Brequinar is an analogue of quinoline carboxylic acid, which acts by inhibiting dihydro-orotate dehydrogenase and *de novo* pyrimidine synthesis. As a consequence, it promotes a significant reduction of both DNA and RNA precursors. *In vitro* it depresses B and T cell proliferation and *in vivo* it significantly affects allergic reactions and organ allograft rejection. There are descriptions claiming that brequinar can prolong the survival of concordant kidney xenografts (hamster to rat) and may induce liver allograft tolerance in rats. Unfortunately, important side effects were observed when the product was used in the clinic (severe thrombocytopenia) and its development has been interrupted.

## FOLATE SYNTHESIS

### *Amethopterine* (Endresen 1992)

Amethopterine (methotrexate) was initially used as an antitumoral agent. Subsequently, it was introduced with success for the treatment of psoriasis, rheumatoid arthritis and graft vs. host disease. As an analogue of folic acid, amethopterine inhibits dehydrofolate reductase which transfers folates in biologically active tetrahydrofolate. Thus, it directly interferes with the folate-dependent synthesis of purines and thymidinilic acids indispensable for DNA synthesis.

The exact mechanisms responsible for the immunosuppressive activity of amethopterine are not fully elucidated. Some reports indicate that amethopterine inhibits T cell proliferation; results suggest a lower effect on helper T cells as compared to immunoregulatory T cells. *In vivo*, patients treated with amethopterine at low doses show decreased levels of IgM rheumatoid factors without lymphopenia or clear-cut signs of aberrant T cell responses to antigens or mitogens.

The problem is further complicated by the well-established anti-inflammatory effect of amethopterine which is probably responsible for some of the clinical benefits observed, particularly in rheumatoid arthritis.

## DNA REPLICATION

### *Cyclophosphamide* (Bach & Strom 1985c)

Cyclophosphamide is one of the most potent chemical immunosuppressants available. It is an alkylating agent which significantly depresses antibody production and may induce tolerance to a wide array of antigens. Its effect on cellular immunity is well documented although less spectacular than the one on antibody production. Its use is essentially limited by the important side effects it may elicit, namely, bone marrow aplasia, haemorrhagic cystitis and bladder carcinoma, alopecia and sterility.

The cellular mode of action of cyclophosphamide seems tightly linked to the antiproliferative and cytolytic effects secondary to its dose-dependent capacity to alkylate DNA.

Lymphoid cells show a variable degree of sensitivity to the effect of cyclophosphamide. It is worth recalling the particularly high sensitivity of suppressor T cells, which explains the fact that in mice low doses of cyclophosphamide (one or two injections of 20–50 mg/kg) induce a clear-cut increase of delayed hypersensitivity responses and of the production of certain antibodies, notably IgE (Askenase *et al.* 1975).

Much work has been devoted to defining the best timing of administration of single doses of antiproliferative immunosuppressive agents (Berenbaum 1967). The best timing usually appears to be 1–2 days after antigen administration. These data suggest that cyclophosphamide essentially acts on antigen-driven lymphocyte proliferation. Paradoxically, however, the drug is no more efficient later on, when cellular prolif-eration is expected to be maximum. Perhaps the prolif-eration rate is then too high to be stopped by non-toxic doses of the agent. Alternatively, some of these drugs could have other effects, namely, binding to cell mem-branes like azathioprine (Bach & Strom 1985a) or anti-inflammatory effects like amethopterine, azathioprine or cyclophosphamide. In fact, this latter effect could relate to the decreased production of non-lymphoid mononuclear cells by the bone marrow, which is also sensitive to the antiproliferative effect (Van Putten & Relieveld 1970).

## Functional inhibition

### RECEPTOR BLOCKADE

Monoclonal and polyclonal antibodies may act by coating their target cells and preventing them from interacting with their ligand or other cell types. This steric hindrance effect (also called blindfolding) is probably operating for monoclonal antibodies that do not deplete and do not induce antigenic modulation. The coating can be visualized *ex vivo* by demonstrating the presence of the xenogeneic or human immuno-globulins on the lymphocyte surface. The case has been demonstrated for polyclonal ALG by showing that *ex vivo* trypsin treatment of lymphoid cells collected from ALG-treated mice reverses their inability to mount a graft vs. host reaction (Brent *et al.* 1967).

### ANTIGENIC MODULATION

Some antibodies, such as CD3 antibodies, induce the redistribution of the molecules which they bind on the cell surface (Chatenoud & Bach 1984). The antigen–antibody complex will ultimately cap at a cellular pole and disappear after internalization or shedding. When the antigenically modulated receptor is central for the cell function, as is the case for the CD3-TCR complex at the surface of T lymphocytes, its lack of expression will determine the functional incapacity of the target cell (Chatenoud *et al.* 1982; Hirsch *et al.* 1988).

### INHIBITION OF LYMPHOKINE TRANSCRIPTION

The inhibition of lymphokine transcription represents the molecular basis for the potent immunosuppressive effect of the two well-known immunophilin ligands, cyclosporin and FK506 (Emmel *et al.* 1989; Sigal & Dumont 1992). The principal target of the inhibi-tory action of these drugs on the immune system is the T lymphocyte and, more precisely, the cytokine-producing helper T cell (independently of the expressed CD4 or CD8 phenotype). Cyclosporin and FK506 inhibit the *in vitro* activation of T lymphocytes by antigen, antibodies to CD3-TCR, antibodies to CD2, mitogens, calcium ionophores and phorbol esters (Sigal & Dumont 1992). In contrast with their potent inhibi-tion of resting T cells, cyclosporin and FK506 are much less effective in suppressing activated T lymphocytes. This strongly suggested that the inhibitory effect of these products was primarily directed against the early phase of T lymphocyte activation. It is generally agreed that cyclosporin mediates a pretranscriptional inhibi-tion that selectively affects the expression of some cytokine genes, including IL-2, IFN-γ and IL-4 (Randak *et al.* 1990). In contrast, the expression of other cytokine genes, such as GM-CSF, IL-7, are not influenced by cyclosporin. FK506 was shown to have similar inhibitory activities. Inhibition of cytokine receptor expression generally occurs at higher concen-trations than the ones required to block cytokine production. When studying various analogues of cyclosporin A a very good correlation was found between their immunosuppressive potency and the ability to inhibit IL-2 mRNA transcription (Granelli-Piperno 1993; Thomson 1993). This inhibition is sec-ondary to an interference with proteins binding regulatory sequences of the cytokine genes. This has been particularly well dissected for the IL-2 gene, whose expression is regulated by five transcriptional segments located in the enhancer lying between − 548 and + 39 base pairs 5′ to the transcription initiation site of the gene. The identified nuclear factors binding to these sites are AP-1, NFκB, AP-3, OCT-1 and NFAT-1. NFAT-1 is composed of a nuclear and a cytoplasmic subunit and is the main candidate for dictating the tissue specificity of the IL-2 gene because it is only expressed in activated T cells (Granelli-Piperno 1993). As previously mentioned, the hypothesis proposed at present suggests that cyclosporin–cyclophilin or FK506–FKBP complexes bind to calmodulin and calcineurin, thus inhibiting the phosphatase activity of this latter enzyme (Liu *et al.* 1991). As a consequence, the dephosphorylation of the cytoplasmic component of NFAT-1, which is required for its translocation to the nucleus, is blocked, as is the transcription of the IL-2 gene. The coordinate induction of several lymphokine genes, such as IL-2 and IFN-γ, upon T cell stimulation and their similar sensitivity to cyclosporin suggest common regulatory steps.

### CYTOKINE NEUTRALIZATION

In order to neutralize the biological effect of cytokines one must effectively interfere with their binding to the specific receptors. In theory this can be achieved by different means, including anticytokine antibodies, soluble cytokine receptors (Fanslow *et al.* 1990; Jacobs *et al.* 1991; Ozmen *et al.* 1993), antagonists of cytokine receptors (Dinarello & Thompson 1991) and genetically engineered immunoadhesins, including two soluble receptor fragments linked to an immunoglobulin constant frame (Lesslauer *et al.* 1991; Peppel *et al.* 1991). In practice, because of the variable pharmacodynamic behaviour of the devised cytokine-binding molecules, it is not so simple to achieve cytokine neutralization. Thus, depending both on the protein used (antibody, soluble receptor, immunoadhesin) and on its dosage, these agents may not behave as antagonists but rather as agonists. This was typically shown in the case of anti-IL-6, anti-IL-3, anti-IL-4 and anti-IL-7 monoclonal antibodies, which, far from enhancing the clearance of the target cytokine, act as *in vivo* carrier proteins, thus prolonging the half-life and enhancing the biological effect of their ligand (Klein *et al.* 1991; Lu *et al.* 1992; Finkelman *et al.* 1993; Jones & Ziltener 1993; May *et al.* 1993).

Among the pathological conditions that may benefit from therapeutic strategies aimed at cytokine neutralization one finds two distinct situations. First, there are

diseases associated with over-production of a given cytokine; this is the case of sepsis and cytokine-dependent tumoral growth (multiple myeloma) (Klein *et al.* 1991; Dinarello 1992). Secondly, there are pathological situations involving an immunologically mediated target tissue damage, namely, autoimmune diseases and allograft rejection, in which some cytokines, such as IFN-γ and IL-12, may exert a central role.

The heterogeneity among helper T lymphocytes was first evidenced through the study of CD4+ murine T cell clones and then extended to human CD4+ cells. Following activation they were divided in two categories, Th-1 and Th-2, depending on the pattern of cytokines they produced that correlated well with the type of immune reactions in which they were implicated. Th-1 cells are essentially involved in delayed-type hypersensitivity reactions while Th-2 cells are essential for B cell differentiation and immunoglobulin production, the defence against parasitic and helminthic infections and allergy (Mosmann & Coffman 1989). The fine balance between Th-1 and Th-2 responses is well explained by the reciprocal inhibition these subsets express on each other because IFN-γ, produced by Th-1 cells, inhibits the proliferation of Th-2 cells and, conversely, IL-10, produced by Th-2 cells, inhibits the synthesis of cytokines by Th-1 cells by acting, at least in part, on antigen-presenting cells (Mosmann & Coffman 1989). Some of the data reported in rodent experimental models on different therapeutic strategies that promote specific long-term tolerance to alloantigens and/or autoantigens were interpreted as being the fate of favouring the establishment and the maintenance of a Th-2 vs. a Th-1 response. Among such immunointervention regimens one finds the treatment with anticytokine antibodies (anti-IFN-γ) (Bach 1993), anti-T cell antibodies (especially anti-CD4) (Pearson *et al.* 1992; Qin *et al.* 1993), or with the cytokines themselves, i.e. IL-4 (Rapoport *et al.* 1993).

In explaining the central role exerted by IFN-γ in the control of alloimmune and autoimmune responses, and thus the therapeutic effect of anti-IFN-γ antibodies, one should consider, in addition to its Th-2 down-regulatory effect, its well-known capacity to upregulate and/or induce the expression of MHC class I and II antigens. It has been suggested that this capacity of IFN-γ to promote an 'aberrant' expression of class II MHC antigen on cells which are usually negative (astrocytes, keratinocytes, thyroid and pancreatic islet cells) could represent a major triggering factor in autoimmune diseases (Pujol-Borrell *et al.* 1987; Sarvetnick *et al.* 1988). In human allograft recipients, acute rejection is often associated with the *de novo* expression of class II MHC antigens on cells within the allograft, such as kidney tubular cells or myocytes (Hall *et al.* 1984; Fuggle *et al.* 1987). Such *de novo* MHC class II antigen expression on normally negative target tissue cells may in theory increase the antigenicity of the graft and the susceptibility of such cells to specific cytotoxic T cell effectors.

Finally, proinflammatory cytokines may represent privileged targets in the treatment of some autoimmune diseases, well illustrated by the impressive clinical results reported in patients presenting with rheumatoid arthritis treated with a monoclonal antibody to TNF (Elliott *et al.* 1994a).

## Cell signalling

CAPACITY OF ANTIBODIES TO SIGNAL
FOR UNRESPONSIVENESS OR TOLERANCE

*Antibodies to class II MHC molecules*

*In vivo* treatment with polyclonal and monoclonal antibodies specifically directed at class II MHC products results in significant immunosuppression of humoral responses, delayed hypersensitivity responses to tumour antigens (DTH) (Perry *et al.* 1979), experimentally induced experimental allergic encephalomyelitis (EAE) (Sriram & Steinman 1983), experimental allergic thyroiditis (EAT) (Vladutiu & Steinman 1987), collagen-induced arthritis (Wooley *et al.* 1985), lupus nephritis of (NZB×NZW)F1 mice (Adelman *et al.* 1983), type I diabetes in the BB rat (Boitard *et al.* 1985) and in the NOD mouse (Boitard *et al.* 1988). Although the precise mechanisms explaining the protection mediated by antibodies to class II molecules are still ill-defined, several hypotheses have been proposed, including a direct action on antigen-

presenting cells or on autoimmune target cells. The existence of an aberrant class II antigen expression at the surface of target cells within autoimmune sites has, for example, been proposed for thyroid epithelial cells. In addition, it has also been suggested that anticlass II treatment could activate suppressor T cells. This is well supported by the data obtained in NOD mice that develop a spontaneous type I T cell-mediated autoimmune diabetes by 10–12 weeks of age. Overt diabetes is preceded by infiltration of the islets of Langerhans with mononuclear cells; adoptive transfer of disease is obtained by injection of CD4+ and CD8+ spleen cells from diabetic donors into neonates or irradiated 8-week-old adult recipients. A treatment using antibodies to class II molecules, started at 3 weeks of age, protects NOD mice from diabetes. Importantly, the injection of spleen cells from the anticlass II-treated NOD mice into irradiated recipients 24h prior to the transfer of diabetogenic T cells (spleen cells from overtly diabetic mice) significantly protects the recipients from the transfer of disease (Boitard *et al.* 1988). In the same vein, the anticlass II-mediated inhibition of antitumoral antigen DTH responses can be transferred to syngeneic animals by spleen cells from treated mice; transfer is abolished by T cell depletion and is sensitive to low doses of cyclophosphamide (Perry & Greene 1982).

*Antibodies to CD3*

Anti-CD3 are very potent immunosuppressive tools for the prevention and the treatment not only of allograft rejection but also of autoimmune conditions (Cosimi *et al.* 1981; Ortho Multicenter Transplant Study Group 1985; Chatenoud *et al.* 1994).

In NOD neonates, Hayward and Shreiber induced substantial and durable protection from the disease by injecting a single high dose (250 μg) of anti-CD3. At 10 weeks of age only 8% of treated animals had developed insulitis vs. 80% of controls and less than 10% showed overt diabetes at 8 months vs. 50% in controls (Hayward & Shreiber 1989). Perturbations of the T cell repertoire inducing long-lasting specific tolerance are probably involved in this particular model of neonatal treatment because, at this early stage, anti-

CD3 may penetrate into the thymus and interfere with thymocyte binding to cortical epithelial cells and with further lymphocyte maturation. This is not the case in adult animals, in which anti-CD3 does not reach thymic CD3+ cells: depletion, coating and antigenic modulation of medullary single-positive CD3+ thymocytes do not occur. The thymus rapidly eliminates double-positive cortical thymocytes because of the endogenous corticosteroid production associated with the anti-CD3-induced cytokine release (Ferran *et al.* 1990).

Injection of low doses (5 μg/day for five consecutive days) of anti-CD3 to 10–12-week-old NOD females reversed established insulitis but the mononuclear cell infiltration recurred within 10–15 days after stopping the treatment.

The same protocol halts the progression of overt autoimmune insulin-dependent diabetes mellitus (IDDM) as reflected by the disappearance of glycosuria and a return to normal glycaemia within 2–4 weeks of the end of the treatment in 62 and 84% of the treated mice. This remission is durable and maintained despite the presence of peripheral, but not invasive/destructive, insulitis, including CD3+, αβ+, CD4+ and CD8+ cells (Chatenoud *et al.* 1994). The various experimental data collected so far point to active T cell-mediated suppressor circuits (active or dominant tolerance) being a central mechanism leading to the establishment of such CD3-induced long-term remissions (Chatenoud *et al.* 1997).

Finally, in the rat, CD3 antibody was also shown to induce permanent engraftment of histoincompatible vascularized heart grafts and tolerance (Nicolls *et al.* 1993).

### Antibodies to CD4

More than a simple adhesion molecule specifically binding MHC class II-bearing targets, CD4 acts as a coreceptor for the TCR–CD3 complex, thus contributing to its signalling function (Anderson *et al.* 1988). Moreover, microclusters can be formed artificially by bispecific antibody constructs cross-linking CD4 and TCR–CD3 on the cell membrane, which results in a strong activating signal (Emmrich *et al.* 1988).

However, when both receptors are ligated independently, as is the case when using soluble anti-CD4 antibodies, the physiological stimulation of resting T cells is significantly inhibited. This is reflected by a decreased proliferative response and lymphokine production in response to various stimuli, including soluble antigens, alloantigens, lectins, antibodies to TCR–CD3. The simple blockade of adhesion to MHC class II does not account for the inhibition observed (Bank & Chess 1985; Emmrich *et al.* 1987). One hypothesis suggests that CD4 binding interferes with the physical proximity between CD4 and TCR–CD3 needed for optimal signal transduction. Alternatively, some authors claim that a 'negative signal' could be transduced upon anti-CD4 binding that is independent of TCR–CD3 ligation. The molecular basis of this putative anti-CD4-induced negative signalling is totally unknown.

The unique tolerogenic properties of CD4 antibodies is a well-established fact. The initial experiments were those showing that rat CD4 antibodies injected into mice did not trigger an antiglobulin response as most rodent anti-T cell monoclonals did (Cobbold *et al.* 1984; Benjamin & Waldmann 1986). Specific tolerance to soluble or tissue antigens, such as alloantigens, could also be induced by introducing them into normal adult animals under the cover of depleting or non-depleting antibodies to CD4 (Cobbold *et al.* 1984; Wofsy *et al.* 1985; Qin *et al.* 1989). Importantly, all that was needed to maintain this immune tolerance was the antigen alone, delivered at regular time intervals, in the absence of any further monoclonal antibody treatment.

In some models combinations of antibodies to CD4 and CD8 have been used to induce classical transplantation tolerance to skin grafts across partial and fully mismatched combinations (Qin *et al.* 1989). This antibody-induced tolerance can also be induced and maintained in thymectomized animals, clearly showing that it is a peripheral event; no evidence for clonal deletion of specific alloreactive T cells was found (Qin *et al.* 1993; Cobbold *et al.* 1996).

### Biological agents blocking costimulatory pathways

Very interesting data have been reported on the *in vivo* use in experimental models of antibodies or fusion proteins that interfere with costimulatory signals (Lenschow *et al.* 1992; Lin *et al.* 1993; Larsen *et al.* 1996; Larsen & Pearson 1997). Thus, in a mouse heart and skin allograft model the simultaneous but not independent blockade of the CD28 and CD40 costimulatory pathways promoted long-term, although not indefinite, allograft survival and, importantly, also inhibited the development of chronic vascular rejection in the grafted hearts (Larsen *et al.* 1996; Larsen & Pearson 1997). Chronic vascular rejection remains a major cause of long-term graft failure for which no effective therapy is available. If confirmed, these data point to selective inhibitors of costimulation as major immunosuppressive tools capable of interfering simultaneously with acute and chronic rejection.

## Relevance to therapeutic strategy

Immunosuppressive therapy can be applied to a large spectrum of pathological conditions such as allogeneic transplantation and autoimmune diseases. Three distinct immunointervention strategies may be applied, depending on the nature of the immune response under consideration.

The treatment can be essentially administered for prophylaxis to prevent the activation of immune effector mechanisms, or maintenance, when the reaction does not present a high burden. Drugs such as cyclosporin A, FK506 or, to a lesser degree, azathioprine show a remarkable therapeutic ratio in this context (therapeutic effectiveness vs. toxicity).

When the immune response is in its acute phase more aggressive strategies are needed, implying the use of drugs such as anti-T cell monoclonal antibodies (anti-CD3 or anti-CD4), polyclonal antilymphocyte antibodies or immunotoxins. These agents cannot, however, be administered for a long period of time because of the risk of overimmunosuppression.

One may also attempt to induce tolerance. This can be achieved by giving the antigen simultaneously when this antigen is known and available. In other cases the antigen is present in the implanted tissue in allogeneic transplantation or is available *in situ* in the target organ in the case of autoimmune diseases. It is then necessary to give a depleting regimen (total irradiation,

total lymphoid irradiation) (Sykes & Sachs 1990), anti-lymphocyte sera (Monaco *et al.* 1966; Thomas *et al.* 1991), depleting anti-CD4 sometimes associated with anti-CD8 (Qin *et al.* 1989, 1993; Shizuru *et al.* 1990; Pearson *et al.* 1992) or non-depleting antibodies such as anti-CD4 (Darby *et al.* 1992), anti-CD3 (Chatenoud *et al.* 1994) or anti-LFA-1–ICAM-1 (Isobe *et al.* 1992). Importantly, some recent data point to the role of T cell activation in the induction of immune tolerance using biological agents. Of particular relevance are the studies showing that cyclosporin abrogates the tolerogenic properties of antibodies to CD3 or of agents blocking the CD28 and CD40 costimulatory pathways (Larsen *et al.* 1996; Chatenoud *et al.* 1997). This, although indirectly, stresses the role of TCR–CD3 T cell activation leading to the transcription of cytokine genes that are selectively inhibited by cyclosporin and related compounds (Granelli-Piperno *et al.* 1988; Durez *et al.* 1993) in the tolerance-promoting ability of these biological agents. This is of relevance for all future clinical settings in which drug associations are indispensable—for instance, clinical transplantation—and where it will be important to adapt at best the combinations used to avoid deleterious antagonistic effects.

An important consideration that also influences the selection of an immunosuppressive agent is the nature of the immune processes involved in the pathological immune reaction, i.e. a humoral vs. a cellular immune reaction. Some agents show a selectivity for macrophages (steroids), others for B cells (cyclophosphamide), still others (more numerous) for T cells (immunophilin ligands, azathioprine, anti-T cell monoclonals, etc.).

In any case, great attention should be given to the hazards of the therapy used. These hazards can be specific to the agent used (nephrotoxicity of cyclosporin and FK506, sterility and direct carcinogenetic effect of cyclophosphamide, cytokine release syndrome of monoclonal antibodies to CD3). Other side effects are the consequence of overimmunosuppression: malignancies (eventually virus-induced cancer) and opportunistic infections. Importantly, all these complications are highly dependent on the dosage used.

A last point worth noting is the dramatic dependency

of the sensitivity of the pathological immune response to immunointervention on the intensity of the immune response. Primary immune responses are much more sensitive than secondary or lasting immune responses to most immunosuppressor agents. Hence the need for treatment as early as possible, without waiting for an overwhelmingly intense immune response. All efforts made to render possible early diagnosis of the pathogenic immune response, possibly before onset of clinical manifestations, should be encouraged.

## Conclusions

Many agents are now available to inhibit B or T cell-mediated immune responses. One may regret, though, that insufficient response is seen in a number of cases, even with the most active agents. The solution is first to select the most adapted products and, secondly, to intervene as early as possible before the immune response has reached its zenith. The other major limitation at present is the frequent relapse seen when therapy is discontinued. The obvious solution is tolerance induction, which will allow definitive control of the response without perpetuating the therapy. The final concern is that of side effects. Direct drug toxicity is no longer the major problem because drug combinations are used and there is probably little risk from less toxic analogues of currently used drugs. The problem of overimmunosuppression is more serious, at least in organ or bone marrow transplantation. The solution is again tolerance induction where the immunosuppressants are only administered for a limited period of time, too short to expose to the risk of opportunistic infections and tumours.

## References

Adelman, N.E., Watling, D.L. & McDevitt, H.O. (1983) Treatment of (NZB×NZW)F1 disease with anti-I-A monoclonal antibodies. *Journal of Experimental Medicine* **158**, 1350–1355.

Anderson, P., Blue, M.L. & Schlossman, S.F. (1988) Comodulation of CD3 and CD4. Evidence for a specific association between CD4 and approximately 5% of the CD3:T cell receptor complexes on helper T lymphocytes. *Journal of Immunology* **140**, 1732–1737.

Askenase, P.W., Hayden, B.J. & Gershon, R.K. (1975) Augmentation of delayed-type hypersensitivity by doses of cyclophosphamide which do not affect antibody responses. *Journal of Experimental Medicine* **141**, 697–702.

Bach, J.F. (1993) Anti-gamma interferon (IFN-gamma) monoclonal antibodies. In: *Monoclonal Antibodies and Peptide Therapy in Autoimmune Diseases* (ed. J.F. Bach), pp. 319–391. Marcel Dekker, New York.

Bach, J.F. & Strom, T.B. (1985a) Thiopurines (6-mercaptopurine, azathioprine, thioguanine). In: *The Mode of Action of Immunosuppressive Agents* (eds J.F. Bach & T.B. Strom), pp. 105–174. Elsevier, Amsterdam.

Bach, J.F. & Strom, T.B. (1985b) Total lymphoid irradiation. In: *The Mode of Action of Immunosuppressive Agents* (eds J.F. Bach & T.B. Strom), pp. 393–402. Elsevier, Amsterdam.

Bach, J.F. & Strom, T.B. (1985c) Alkylating agents. In: *The Mode of Action of Immunosuppressive Agents* (eds J.F. Bach & T.B. Strom), pp. 175–239. Elsevier, Amsterdam.

Bach, J.F. & Strom, T.B. (1985d) Corticosteroids. In: *The Mode of Action of Immunosuppressive Agents* (eds J.F. Bach & T.B. Strom), pp. 21– 104. Elsevier, Amsterdam.

Bach, J.F., Gigli, I., Dardenne, M. & Dormont, J. (1972) Mechanism of complement action in rosette inhibition and lymphocytotoxicity of antilymphocyte serum. *Immunology* **22**, 625–635.

Bacha, P., Williams, D.P., Waters, C. *et al.* (1988) Interleukin 2 receptor-targeted cytotoxicity. Interleukin 2 receptor-mediated action of a diphtheria toxin-related interleukin 2 fusion protein. *Journal of Experimental Medicine* **167**, 612–622.

Balner, H., Eysvoogel, V.P. & Cleton, F.J. (1968) Testing of anti-human lymphocyte sera in chimpanzees and lower primates. *Lancet* **1**, 19–22.

Bank, I. & Chess, L. (1985) Perturbation of the T4 molecule transmits a negative signal to T cells. *Journal of Experimental Medicine* **162**, 1294–1303.

Benjamin, R.J. & Waldmann, H. (1986) Induction of tolerance by monoclonal antibody therapy. *Nature* **320**, 449–451.

Berenbaum, M.C. (1967) Immunosuppressive agents and the cellular kinetics of the immune response. In: *Immunity, Cancer and Chemotherapy* (ed. E. Mihic), pp. 217–236. Academic Press, New York.

Berenbaum, M.C. (1969) Immunosuppressive agents: the design of selective therapeutic schedules. In: *The Immune Response and its Suppression* (ed. E. Sorkin), p. 155. Karger, Basel.

Beutler, B., Milsark, I.W. & Cerami, A.C. (1985) Passive immunization against cachectin/tumor necrosis factor protects mice from lethal effect of endotoxin. *Science* **229**, 869–871.

Bindon, C.I., Hale, G. & Waldmann, H. (1988) Importance of antigen specificity for complement-mediated lysis by monoclonal antibodies. *European Journal of Immunology* **18**, 1507–1514.

Blackwell, G.J., Carnuccio, R., Di Rosa, M. *et al.* (1982) Glucocorticoids induce the formation and release of anti-inflammatory and anti-phospholipase proteins into the peritoneal cavity of the rat. *British Journal of Pharmacology* **76**, 185–194.

Boise, L.H., Noel, P.J. & Thompson, C.B. (1995) CD28 and apoptosis. *Current Opinion in Immunology* **7**, 620–625.

Boitard, C., Michie, S., Serrurier, P. *et al.* (1985) *In vivo* prevention of thyroid and pancreatic autoimmunity in the BB rat by antibody to class II major histocompatibility complex gene products. *Proceedings of the National Academy of Sciences (USA)* **82**, 6627–6631.

Boitard, C., Bendelac, A., Richard, M.F., Carnaud, C. & Bach, J.F. (1988) Prevention of diabetes in non-obese diabetic mice by anti-I-A monoclonal antibodies: transfer of protection by splenic T cells. *Proceedings of the National Academy of Sciences (USA)* **85**, 9719–9723.

Brazelton, T.R. & Morris, R.E. (1996) Molecular mechanisms of action of new xenobiotic immunosuppressive drugs: tacrolimus (FK506), sirolimus (rapamycin), mycophenolate mofetil and leflunomide. *Current Opinion in Immunology* **8**, 710–720.

Brent, L., Courtenay, T. & Gowland, G. (1967) Immunological reactivity of lymphoid cells after treatment with anti-lymphocytic serum. *Nature* **215**, 1461–1464.

Bromberg, J.S., Chavin, K.D., Altevogt, P. *et al.* (1991) Anti-CD2 monoclonal antibodies alter cell-mediated immunity *in vivo*. *Transplantation* **51**, 219–225.

Charpentier, B., Hiesse, C., Lantz, O. *et al.* (1992) Evidence that antihuman tumor necrosis factor monoclonal antibody prevents OKT3-induced acute syndrome. *Transplantation* **54**, 997–1002.

Chatenoud, L. & Bach, J.F. (1984) Antigenic modulation: a major mechanism of antibody action. *Immunology Today* **5**, 20–25.

Chatenoud, L., Baudrihaye, M.F., Kreis, H. *et al.* (1982) Human *in vivo* antigenic modulation induced by the anti-T cell OKT3 monoclonal antibody. *European Journal of Immunology* **12**, 979–982.

Chatenoud, L., Thervet, E., Primo, J. & Bach, J.F. (1994) Anti-CD3 antibody induces long-term remission of overt autoimmunity in non-obese diabetic mice. *Proceedings of the National Academy of Sciences (USA)* **91**, 123–127.

Chatenoud, L., Primo, J. & Bach, J.F. (1997) CD3 antibody-induced dominant self tolerance in overtly diabetic NOD mice. *Journal of Immunology* **158**, 2947–2954.

Clark, E.A. & Ledbetter, J.A. (1994) How B and T cells talk to each other. *Nature* **367**, 425–428.

Clevers, H., Alarcon, B., Wileman, T. & Terhorst, C. (1988) The T cell receptor/CD3 complex: a dynamic protein ensemble. *Annual Review of Immunology* **6**, 629–662.

Cobbold, S.P., Jayasuriya, A., Nash, A., Prospero, T.D. &

Waldmann, H. (1984) Therapy with monoclonal antibodies by elimination of T cell subsets *in vivo*. *Nature* **312**, 548–551.

Cobbold, S.P., Adams, E., Marshall, S.E., Davies, J.D. & Waldmann, H. (1996) Mechanisms of peripheral tolerance and suppression induced by monoclonal antibodies to CD4 and CD8. *Immunological Reviews* **149**, 5–33.

Cohen, J.J. (1971) The effects of hydrocortisone on the immune response. *Annals of Allergy* **29**, 358–361.

Cohen, J.J. & Claman, H.N. (1971) Thymus-marrow immunocompetence. V. Hydrocortisone-resistant cells and processes in the hemolytic antibody response of mice. *Journal of Experimental Medicine* **133**, 1026–1034.

Cosimi, A.B., Colvin, R.B., Burton, R.C. *et al.* (1981) Use of monoclonal antibodies to T-cell subsets for immunologic monitoring and treatment in recipients of renal allografts. *New England Journal of Medicine* **305**, 308–314.

Cosimi, A.B., Conti, D., Delmonico, F.L. *et al.* (1990) *In vivo* effects of monoclonal antibody to ICAM-1 (CD54) in nonhuman primates with renal allografts. *Journal of Immunology* **144**, 4604–4612.

Cramer, D.V., Chapman, F.A., Jaffee, B.D. *et al.* (1992a) The prolongation of concordant hamster-to-rat cardiac xenografts by brequinar sodium. *Transplantation* **54**, 403–408.

Cramer, D.V., Knoop, M., Chapman, F.A. *et al.* (1992b) Prevention of liver allograft rejection in rats by a short course of therapy with brequinar sodium. *Transplantation* **54**, 752–753.

Darby, C.R., Morris, P.J. & Wood, K.J. (1992) Evidence that long-term cardiac allograft survival induced by anti-CD4 monoclonal antibody does not require depletion of CD4+ T cells. *Transplantation* **54**, 483–490.

Dayton, J.S., Turka, L.A., Thompson, C.B. & Mitchell, B.S. (1992) Comparison of the effects of mizoribine with those of azathioprine, 6-mercaptopurine, and mycophenolic acid on T lymphocyte proliferation and purine ribonucleotide metabolism. *Molecular Pharmacology* **41**, 671–676.

Dialynas, D.P., Quan, Z.S., Wall, K.A. *et al.* (1983) Characterization of the murine T cell surface molecule, designated L3T4, identified by monoclonal antibody GK1.5: similarity of L3T4 to the human Leu-3/T4 molecule. *Journal of Immunology* **131**, 2445–2451.

Dinarello, C.A. (1992) Anti-cytokine strategies. *European Cytokine Network* **3**, 7–17.

Dinarello, C.A. & Thompson, R.C. (1991) Blocking IL-1: interleukin 1 receptor antagonist *in vivo* and *in vitro*. *Immunology Today* **12**, 404–410.

Durez, P., Abramowicz, D., Gerard, C. *et al.* (1993) *In vivo* induction of interleukin 10 by anti-CD3 monoclonal antibody or bacterial lipopolysaccharide: differential modulation by cyclosporin A. *Journal of Experimental Medicine* **177**, 551–555.

Elliott, M.J., Maini, R.N., Feldmann, M. *et al.* (1994a)

Randomised double-blind comparison of chimeric monoclonal antibody to tumour necrosis factor alpha (cA2) versus placebo in rheumatoid arthritis. *Lancet* **344**, 1105–1110.

Elliott, M.J., Maini, R.N., Feldmann, M. *et al.* (1994b) Repeated therapy with monoclonal antibody to tumour necrosis factor alpha (cA2) in patients with rheumatoid arthritis. *Lancet* **344**, 1125–1127.

Emmel, E.A., Verweij, C.L., Durand, D.B. *et al.* (1989) Cyclosporin A specifically inhibits function of nuclear proteins involved in T cell activation. *Science* **246**, 1617–1620.

Emmrich, F. & Bach, J.F. (1993) Therapeutic anti-CD4 antibodies. In: *T-Cell-Directed Immunointervention* (ed. J.F. Bach), pp. 176–200. Blackwell Science, Oxford.

Emmrich, F., Kanz, L. & Eichmann, K. (1987) Cross-linking of the T cell receptor complex with the subset-specific differentiation antigen stimulates interleukin 2 receptor expression in human CD4 and CD8 T cells. *European Journal of Immunology* **17**, 529–534.

Emmrich, F., Rieber, P., Kurrle, R. & Eichmann, K. (1988) Selective stimulation of human T lymphocyte subsets by heteroconjugates of antibodies to the T cell receptor and to subset-specific differentiation antigens. *European Journal of Immunology* **18**, 645–648.

Endresen, L. (1992) Pharmacology and general therapeutic principles of methotrexate. In: *Immunopharmacology in Autoimmune Disases and Transplantation* (eds H.E. Rugstad, L. Endresen & O.Forre), pp. 127–140. Plenum Press, New York.

Fanslow, W.C., Sims, J.E., Sassenfeld, H. *et al.* (1990) Regulation of alloreactivity *in vivo* by a soluble form of the interleukin-1 receptor. *Science* **248**, 739–742.

Fauci, A.S. & Dale, D.C. (1975) The effect of hydrocortisone on the kinetics of normal human lymphocytes. *Blood* **46**, 235–243.

Ferran, C., Dy, M., Merite, S. *et al.* (1990) Reduction of morbidity and cytokine release in anti-CD3 MoAb-treated mice by corticosteroids. *Transplantation* **50**, 642–648.

Figueroa, J., Fuad, S.A., Kunjummen, B.D., Platt, J.L. & Bach, F.H. (1993) Suppression of synthesis of natural antibodies by mycophenolate mofetil (RS-61443). Its potential use in discordant xenografting. *Transplantation* **55**, 1371–1374.

Finkelman, F.D., Madden, K.B., Morris, S.C. *et al.* (1993) Anti-cytokine antibodies as carrier proteins. Prolongation of *in vivo* effects of exogenous cytokines by injection of cytokine–anti-cytokine antibody complexes. *Journal of Immunology* **151**, 1235–1244.

Fischer, A., Griscelli, C., Blanche, S. *et al.* (1986) Prevention of graft failure by an anti-LFA-1 monoclonal antibody in HLA-mismatched bone-marrow transplantation. *Lancet* **2**, 1058–1061.

Fischer, G., Wittmann-Liebold, B., Lang, K., Kiefhaber, T. & Schmid, F.X. (1989) Cyclophilin and peptidyl-prolyl cis-trans isomerase are probably identical proteins. *Nature* **337**, 476–478.

Fuggle, S.V., McWhinnie, D.L. & Morris, P.J. (1987) Precise specificity of induced tubular HLA-class II antigens in renal allografts. *Transplantation* **44**, 214–220.

Genestier, L., Fournel, S., Flacher, M. *et al.* (1998) Induction of Fas (Apo-1, CD95)-mediated apoptosis of activated lymphocytes by polyclonal antithymocyte globulins. *Blood* **91**, 2360–2368.

Granelli-Piperno, A. (1993) Cellular mode of action of cyclosporin A. In: *T-Cell Directed Immunointervention* (ed. J.F. Bach), pp. 3–25. Blackwell Science, Oxford.

Granelli-Piperno, A., Keane, M. & Steinman, R.M. (1988) Evidence that cyclosporine inhibits cell-mediated immunity primarily at the level of the T lymphocyte rather than the accessory cell. *Transplantation* **46**, 53S–60S.

Granelli-Piperno, A., Nolan, P., Inaba, K. & Steinman, R.M. (1990) The effect of immunosuppressive agents on the induction of nuclear factors that bind to sites on the interleukin 2 promoter. *Journal of Experimental Medicine* **172**, 1869–1872.

Greaves, M.F., Tursi, A., Playfair, J.H. *et al.* (1969) Immunosuppressive potency and *in vitro* activity of antilymphocyte globulin. *Lancet* **1**, 68–72.

Guckel, B., Berek, C., Lutz, M. *et al.* (1991) Anti-CD2 antibodies induce T cell unresponsiveness *in vivo*. *Journal of Experimental Medicine* **174**, 957–967.

Hale, G., Dyer, M.J., Clark, M.R. *et al.* (1988) Remission induction in non-Hodgkin lymphoma with reshaped human monoclonal antibody CAMPATH-1H. *Lancet* **2**, 1394–1399.

Hall, B.M., Bishop, G.A., Duggin, G.G. *et al.* (1984) Increased expression of HLA-DR antigens on renal tubular cells in renal transplants: relevance to the rejection response. *Lancet* **2**, 247–251.

Handschumacher, R.E., Harding, M.W., Rice, J., Drugge, R.J. & Speicher, D.W. (1984) Cyclophilin: a specific cytosolic binding protein for cyclosporin A. *Science* **226**, 544–547.

Hayward, A.R. & Shreiber, M. (1989) Neonatal injection of CD3 antibody into nonobese diabetic mice reduces the incidence of insulitis and diabetes. *Journal of Immunology* **143**, 1555–1559.

Hirsch, R., Eckhaus, M., Auchincloss, H.J.R., Sachs, D.H. & Bluestone, J.A. (1988) Effects of *in vivo* administration of anti-T3 monoclonal antibody on T cell function in mice. I. Immunosuppression of transplantation responses. *Journal of Immunology* **140**, 3766–3772.

Hurtenbach, U., Lier, E., Adorini, L. & Nagy, Z.A. (1993) Prevention of autoimmune diabetes in non-obese diabetic mice by treatment with a class II major histocompatibility complex-blocking peptide. *Journal of Experimental Medicine* 177, 1499–1504.

Isaacs, J.D., Watts, R.A., Hazleman, B.L. *et al.* (1992a) Humanised monoclonal antibody therapy for rheumatoid arthritis. *Lancet* 340, 748–752.

Isaacs, J.D., Clark, M.R., Greenwood, J. & Waldmann, H. (1992b) Therapy with monoclonal antibodies. An *in vivo* model for the assessment of therapeutic potential. *Journal of Immunology* 148, 3062–3071.

Isobe, M., Yagita, H., Okumura, K. & Ihara, A. (1992) Specific acceptance of cardiac allograft after treatment with antibodies to ICAM-1 and LFA-1. *Science* 255, 1125–1127.

Jacobs, C.A., Lynch, D.H., Roux, E.R. *et al.* (1991) Characterization and pharmacokinetic parameters of recombinant soluble interleukin-4 receptor. *Blood* 77, 2396–2403.

Jolivet, J., Cowan, K.H., Curt, G.A., Clendeninn, N.J. & Chabner, B.A. (1983) The pharmacology and clinical use of methotrexate. *New England Journal of Medicine* 309, 1094–1104.

Jones, A.T. & Ziltener, H.J. (1993) Enhancement of the biologic effects of interleukin-3 *in vivo* by anti-interleukin-3 antibodies. *Blood* 82, 1133–1141.

Kahan, B.D. (1992) Immunosuppressive therapy. *Current Opinion in Immunology* 4, 553–560.

Klein, B., Wijdenes, J., Zhang, X.G. *et al.* (1991) Murine anti-interleukin-6 monoclonal antibody therapy for a patient with plasma cell leukemia. *Blood* 78, 1198–1204.

Knechtle, S.J., Vargo, D., Fechner, J. *et al.* (1997) FN18-CRM9 immunotoxin promotes tolerance in primate renal allografts. *Transplantation* 63, 1–6.

Kronke, M., Depper, J.M., Leonard, W.J. *et al.* (1985) Adult T cell leukemia: a potential target for ricin A chain immunotoxins. *Blood* 65, 1416–1421.

Kronke, M., Schlick, E., Waldmann, T.A., Vitetta, E.S. & Greene, W.C. (1986) Selective killing of human T-lymphotropic virus-I infected leukemic T-cells by monoclonal anti-interleukin 2 receptor antibody-ricin A chain conjugates: potentiation by ammonium chloride and monensin. *Cancer Research* 46, 3295–3298.

Lance, E.M. (1970) The selective action of antilymphocyte serum on recirculating lymphocytes: a review of the evidence and alternatives. *Clinical and Experimental Immunology* 6, 789–802.

Larsen, C.P. & Pearson, T.C. (1997) The CD40 pathway in allograft rejection, acceptance, and tolerance. (Review.) *Current Opinion in Immunology* 9, 641–647.

Larsen, C.P., Elwood, E.T., Alexander, D.Z. *et al.* (1996) Long-term acceptance of skin and cardiac allografts after blocking CD40 and CD28 pathways. *Nature* 381, 434–438.

Lenschow, D.J., Zeng, Y., Thistlethwaite, J.R. *et al.* (1992)

Long-term survival of xenogeneic pancreatic islet grafts induced by CTLA4Ig. *Science* 257, 789–792.

Lesslauer, W., Tabuchi, H., Gentz, R. *et al.* (1991) Recombinant soluble tumor necrosis factor receptor proteins protect mice from lipopolysaccharide-induced lethality. *European Journal of Immunology* 21, 2883–2886.

Lin, H., Bolling, S.F., Linsley, P.S. *et al.* (1993) Long-term acceptance of major histocompatibility complex mismatched cardiac allografts induced by CTLA4Ig plus donor-specific transfusion. *Journal of Experimental Medicine* 178, 1801–1806.

Linsley, P.S., Clark, E.A. & Ledbetter, J.A. (1990) T-cell antigen CD28 mediates adhesion with B cells by interacting with activation antigen B7/BB-1. *Proceedings of the National Academy of Sciences (USA)* 87, 5031–5035.

Linsley, P.S., Wallace, P.M., Johnson, J. *et al.* (1992) Immunosuppression *in vivo* by a soluble form of the CTLA-4 T cell activation molecule. *Science* 257, 792–795.

Liu, J. (1993) FK506 and cyclosporin, molecular probes for studying intracellular signal transduction. *Immunology Today* 14, 290–295.

Liu, J., Farmer, J.D., Lane, W.S. *et al.* (1991) Calcineurin is a common target of cyclophilin–cyclosporin A and FKBP-FK506 complexes. *Cell* 66, 807–815.

Lorenz, M.C. & Heitman, J. (1995) TOR mutations confer rapamycin resistance by preventing interaction with FKBP12-rapamycin. *Journal of Biological Chemistry* 270, 27531–27537.

Lu, Z.Y., Brochier, J., Wijdenes, J. *et al.* (1992) High amounts of circulating interleukin (IL)-6 in the form of monomeric immune complexes during anti-IL-6 therapy. Towards a new methodology for measuring overall cytokine production in human *in vivo*. *European Journal of Immunology* 22, 2819–2824.

Makgoba, M.W., Sanders, M.E. & Shaw, S. (1989) The CD2-LFA-3 and LFA-1-ICAM pathways: relevance to T-cell recognition. *Immunology Today* 10, 417–422.

Martin, W.J. & Miller, J.F. (1967) Site of action of antilymphocyte globulin. *Lancet* 2, 1285–1287.

Martin, W.J. & Miller, J.F. (1968) Cell to cell interaction in the immune response. IV. Site of action of antilymphocyte globulin. *Journal of Experimental Medicine* 128, 855–874.

May, L.T., Neta, R., Moldawer, L.L. *et al.* (1993) Antibodies chaperone circulating IL-6. Paradoxical effects of anti-IL-6 'neutralizing' antibodies *in vivo*. *Journal of Immunology* 151, 3225–3236.

Monaco, A.P., Wood, M.L. & Russell, P.S. (1966) Studies on heterologous antilymphocyte serum in mice. III. Immunological tolerance and chimerism produced across the H2-locus with adult thymectomy and antilymphocyte serum. *Annals of the New York Academy of Sciences* **129**, 190–209.

Moreland, L.W., Pratt, P.W., Bucy, R.P. *et al.* (1994) Treatment of refractory rheumatoid arthritis with a chimeric anti-CD4 monoclonal antibody. Long-term followup of CD4+ T cell counts. *Arthritis and Rheumatism* **37**, 834–838.

Mosmann, T.R. & Coffman, R.L. (1989) TH1 and TH2 cells: different patterns of lymphokine secretion lead to different functional properties. *Annual Review of Immunology* **7**, 145–173.

Nashan, B., Moore, R., Amlot, P. *et al.* (1997) Randomised trial of basiliximab versus placebo for control of acute cellular rejection in renal allograft recipients. CHIB 201 International Study Group. *Lancet* **350**, 1193–1198. (Published erratum appears in *Lancet* **350**, 1484.)

Nicoletti, F., Meroni, P.L., Landolfo, S. *et al.* (1990) Prevention of diabetes in BB/Wor rats treated with monoclonal antibodies to interferon-gamma. *Lancet* **336**, 319.

Nicolls, M.R., Aversa, G.G., Pearce, N.W. *et al.* (1993) Induction of long-term specific tolerance to allografts in rats by therapy with an anti-CD3-like monoclonal antibody. *Transplantation* **55**, 459–468.

Ortho Multicenter Transplant Study Group (1985) A randomized clinical trial of OKT3 monoclonal antibody for acute rejection of cadaveric renal transplants. *New England Journal of Medicine* **313**, 337–342.

Ozmen, L., Gribaudo, G., Fountoulakis, M. *et al.* (1993) Mouse soluble IFN gamma receptor as IFN gamma inhibitor. Distribution, antigenicity, and activity after injection in mice. *Journal of Immunology* **150**, 2698–2705.

Pearson, T.C., Madsen, J.C., Larsen, C.P., Morris, P.J. & Wood, K.J. (1992) Induction of transplantation tolerance in adults using donor antigen and anti-CD4 monoclonal antibody. *Transplantation* **54**, 475–483.

Peppel, K., Crawford, D. & Beutler, B. (1991) A tumor necrosis factor (TNF) receptor-IgG heavy chain chimeric protein as a bivalent antagonist of TNF activity. *Journal of Experimental Medicine* **174**, 1483–1489.

Perry, L.L. & Greene, M.I. (1982) Conversion of immunity to suppression by *in vivo* administration of I-A subregion-specific antibodies. *Journal of Experimental Medicine* **156**, 480–491.

Perry, L.L., Dorf, M.E., Benacerraf, B. & Greene, M.I. (1979) Regulation of immune response to tumor antigen: interference with syngeneic tumor immunity by anti-IA alloantisera. *Proceedings of the National Academy of Sciences (USA)* **76**, 920–924.

Platz, K.P., Sollinger, H.W., Hullett, D.A. *et al.* (1991) RS-61443—a new, potent immunosuppressive agent. *Transplantation* **51**, 27–31.

Pujol-Borrell, R., Todd, I., Doshi, M. *et al.* (1987) HLA class

II induction in human islet cells by interferon-gamma plus tumour necrosis factor or lymphotoxin. *Nature* **326**, 304–306.

Qin, S.X., Cobbold, S., Benjamin, R. & Waldmann, H. (1989) Induction of classical transplantation tolerance in the adult. *Journal of Experimental Medicine* **169**, 779–794.

Qin, S., Cobbold, S.P., Pope, H. *et al.* (1993) 'Infectious' transplantation tolerance. *Science* **259**, 974–977.

Randak, C., Brabletz, T., Hergenrother, M., Sobotta, I. & Serfling, E. (1990) Cyclosporin A suppresses the expression of the interleukin 2 gene by inhibiting the binding of lymphocyte-specific factors to the IL-2 enhancer. *EMBO Journal* **9**, 2529–2536.

Rapoport, M.J., Jaramillo, A., Zipris, D. *et al.* (1993) Interleukin 4 reverses T cell proliferative unresponsiveness and prevents the onset of diabetes in nonobese diabetic mice. *Journal of Experimental Medicine* **178**, 87–99.

Reiter, C., Kakavand, B., Rieber, E.P. *et al.* (1991) Treatment of rheumatoid arthritis with monoclonal CD4 antibody M-T151. Clinical results and immunopharmacologic effects in an open study, including repeated administration. *Arthritis and Rheumatism* **34**, 525–536.

Rudd, C.E. (1990) CD4, CD8 and the TCR–CD3 complex: a novel class of protein–tyrosine kinase receptor. *Immunology Today* **11**, 400–406.

Sarvetnick, N., Liggitt, D., Pitts, S.L., Hansen, S.E. & Stewart, T.A. (1988) Insulin-dependent diabetes mellitus induced in transgenic mice by ectopic expression of class II MHC and interferon-gamma. *Cell* **52**, 773–782.

Schreiber, S.L. & Crabtree, G.R. (1992) The mechanism of action of cyclosporin A and FK506. *Immunology Today* **13**, 136–142.

Shizuru, J.A., Seydel, K.B., Flavin, T.F. *et al.* (1990) Induction of donor-specific unresponsiveness to cardiac allografts in rats by pretransplant anti-CD4 monoclonal antibody therapy. *Transplantation* **50**, 366–373.

Sigal, N.H. & Dumont, F.J. (1992) Cyclosporin A, FK-506, and rapamycin: pharmacologic probes of lymphocyte signal transduction. *Annual Review of Immunology* **10**, 519–560.

Skoglund, C., Scheynius, A., Holmdahl, R. & Van Der Meide, P.H. (1988) Enhancement of DTH reaction and inhibition of the expression of class II transplantation antigens by *in vivo* treatment with antibodies against gamma-interferon. *Clinical and Experimental Immunology* **71**, 428–432.

Smith, C.A., Williams, G.T., Kingston, R., Jenkinson, E.J. & Owen, J.J. (1989) Antibodies to CD3/T-cell receptor complex induce death by apoptosis in immature T cells in thymic cultures. *Nature* **337**, 181–184.

Sollinger, H.W. (1995) Mycophenolate mofetil for the prevention of acute rejection in primary cadaveric renal allograft recipients. *Transplantation* **60**, 225–232.

Springer, T.A. (1990) Adhesion receptors of the immune system. *Nature* 346, 425–434.

Springer, T.A., Dustin, M.L., Kishimoto, T.K. & Marlin, S.D. (1987) The lymphocyte function-associated LFA-1, CD2, and LFA-3 molecules: cell adhesion receptors of the immune system. *Annual Review of Immunology* 5, 223–252.

Sriram, S. & Steinman, L. (1983) Anti I-A antibody suppresses active encephalomyelitis: treatment model for diseases linked to IR genes. *Journal of Experimental Medicine* 158, 1362–1367.

Strober, S. (1984) Natural suppressor (NS) cells, neonatal tolerance, and total lymphoid irradiation: exploring obscure relationships. *Annual Review of Immunology* 2, 219–237.

Strom, T.B., Kelley, V.R., Murphy, J.R., Nichols, J. & Woodworth, T.G. (1993) Interleukin-2 receptor-directed therapies: antibody- or cytokine-based targeting molecules (Review). *Annual Review of Medicine* 44, 343–353.

Sykes, M. & Sachs, D.H. (1990) Bone marrow transplantation as a means of inducing tolerance. *Seminars in Immunology* 2, 401–417.

Thomas, J.M., Carver, F.M., Cunningham, P.R., Olson, L.C. & Thomas, F.T. (1991) Kidney allograft tolerance in primates without chronic immunosuppression—the role of veto cells. *Transplantation* 51, 198–207.

Thomas, J.M., Neville, D.M., Contreras, J.L. *et al.* (1997) Preclinical studies of allograft tolerance in rhesus monkeys: a novel anti-CD3-immunotoxin given peritransplant with donor bone marrow induces operational tolerance to kidney allografts. *Transplantation* 64, 124–135.

Thome, M., Duplay, P., Guttinger, M. & Acuto, O. (1995) Syk and ZAP-70 mediate recruitment of p56lck/CD4 to the activated T cell receptor/CD3/zeta complex. *Journal of Experimental Medicine* 181, 1997–2006.

Thomson, A.W. (1993) Immunological effects of cyclosporin A. In: *T-Cell Directed Immunointervention* (ed. J.F. Bach), pp. 26–50. Blackwell Science, Oxford.

Van Den Eertwegh, A.J., Noelle, R.J., Roy, M. *et al.* (1993) *In vivo* CD40–gp39 interactions are essential for thymus-dependent humoral immunity. I. *In vivo* expression of CD40 ligand, cytokines, and antibody production delineates sites of cognate T–B cell interactions. *Journal of Experimental Medicine* 178, 1555–1565.

Van Putten, L.M. & Relieveld, P. (1970) Factors determining cell killing by chemotherapeutic agents *in vivo*. I.

Cyclophosphamide. *European Journal of Cancer* 6, 313–321.

Vincenti, F., Kirkman, R., Light, S. *et al.* (1998) Interleukin-2-receptor blockade with daclizumab to prevent acute rejection in renal transplantation. Daclizumab Triple Therapy Study Group (see comments). *New England Journal of Medicine* 338, 161–165.

Vladutiu, A.O. & Steinman, L. (1987) Inhibition of experimental autoimmune thyroiditis in mice by anti-I-A antibodies. *Cellular Immunology* 109, 169–180.

Waldmann, T.A. & O'Shea, J. (1998) The use of antibodies against the IL-2 receptor in transplantation (Review). *Current Opinion in Immunology* 10, 507–512.

Walz, G., Zanker, B., Brand, K. *et al.* (1989) Sequential effects of interleukin 2–diphtheria toxin fusion protein on T-cell activation. *Proceedings of the National Academy of Sciences (USA)* 86, 9485–9488.

Weiss, A. (1991) Molecular and genetic insights into T cell antigen receptor structure and function. *Annual Review of Genetics* 25, 487–510.

Wesselborg, S., Janssen, O. & Kabelitz, D. (1993) Induction of activation-driven death (apoptosis) in activated but not resting peripheral blood T cells. *Journal of Immunology* 150, 4338–4345.

Wofsy, D., Mayes, D.C., Woodcock, J. & Seaman, W.E. (1985) Inhibition of humoral immunity *in vivo* by monoclonal antibody to L3T4: studies with soluble antigens in intact mice. *Journal of Immunology* 135, 1698–1701.

Wong, J.T. & Colvin, R.B. (1991) Selective reduction and proliferation of the CD4+ and CD8+ T cell subsets with bispecific monoclonal antibodies: evidence for inter-T cell-mediated cytolysis. *Clinical Immunology and Immunopathology* 58, 236–250.

Wooley, P.H., Luthra, H.S., Lafuse, W.P. *et al.* (1985) Type II collagen-induced arthritis in mice. III. Suppression of arthritis by using monoclonal and polyclonal anti-Ia antisera. *Journal of Immunology* 134, 2366–2374.

Wraith, D.C., Smilek, D.E., Mitchell, D.J., Steinman, L. & McDevitt, H.O. (1989) Antigen recognition in autoimmune encephalomyelitis and the potential for peptide-mediated immunotherapy. *Cell* 59, 247–255.

Zheng, X.F., Florentino, D., Chen, J., Crabtree, G.R. & Schreiber, S.L. (1995) TOR kinase domains are required for two distinct functions, only one of which is inhibited by rapamycin. *Cell* 82, 121–130.

# Chapter 6/Xenotransplantation

ANTHONY DORLING & ROBERT I. LECHLER

## The need for xenografts

Clinical transplantation has evolved rapidly over the last 40 years from the first successes in the early 1950s to the stage where today organ allografts have become a routine treatment for end-stage kidney, heart, lung and liver disease. Continuing improvements in patient and graft survival rates (Table 6.1) illustrate the increasing success of transplantation medicine.

However, there is a growing problem that these achievements only serve to highlight; there are simply not enough cadaveric organs to meet the present clinical demand. In the UK the disparity between the supply and demand for organs is particularly apparent for

kidneys (Fig. 6.1), but the shortfall affects all organs and every year a significant number of patients with heart, lung or liver disease die while awaiting a transplant. In the USA the problem is similar but on a larger scale. In 1993 the total number of patients awaiting a cadaveric organ increased over the year by 35%, but the number of donors rose by only 11% (Cooper 1993) and more than 2000 potential recipients died while on transplant waiting lists.

Increasing the supply of donors from present sources may not be enough to solve the problem. For example, a 1992 study from Seattle, USA (Evans *et al.* 1992), identified an annual maximum of only 7000 brain-dead donors in the USA. Assuming 100% consent and

**Table 6.1** The increasing success of renal transplantation (data from the UK Transplant Support Services Anthority).

| Year of transplant | Post-transplant survival (%) | |
| --- | --- | --- |
| | 1 year | 5 year |
| 1985–86 | 74.2 | 57.4 |
| 1987–88 | 78.8 | 60.5 |
| 1989–90 | 80.4 | 64.6 |
| 1991–92 | 83.3 | 67.9 |

suitability, these 14 000 potential kidney grafts would still not satisfy the needs of the 36 000 American patients starting dialysis for the first time each year. Similar calculations have been made in the UK (Gore 1993). The clear implication is that an alternative source of organs is required.

Increasing the supply of allografts from sources other than brain-dead cadavers is one option, but the socially acceptable and technically feasible ways of doing this are limited. Using mechanical or bioengineered organs is another option, but the technology to 'manufacture' organs as complex and compact as the kidney or liver, for example, is at an extremely premature stage. It is in this context that the use of organs from an animal donor, or xenotransplantation, is particularly attractive.

## Xenotransplantation

Although the history of xenotransplantation is as long as that of allografting, the scientific interest in cross-species transplantation was focused until recently on xenografts as models to explore the mechanisms of allograft rejection. The last decade has seen a resurgence of interest in clinical xenotransplantation with the realization that this may solve the problem of allograft shortage. The benefits of xenotransplantation are illustrated in Table 6.2.

An unlimited inexhaustible supply of organs will not only allow current waiting lists to be cleared, but will also expand the opportunity for all patients with end-stage disease to receive a new organ. Moreover, readily

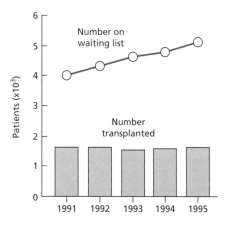

**Fig. 6.1** The number of kidney transplants in the UK over 5 years, compared to the number of patients awaiting transplantation, illustrating the growing discrepancy between supply and demand for organs. (Data from the UK Transplant Support Services Authority.)

**Table 6.2** The advantages and disadvantages of xenografting compared to allografting.

**Perceived benefits of xenografting over allografts**

Inexhaustible supply if rapidly breeding donors with large litters are used. Organs available for people currently excluded from waiting lists

Extend the therapeutic possibilities of transplantation (for example, diabetes mellitus)

Opportunity for genetic manipulation of donor organ to influence recipient rejection responses

Planned unhurried operations

Species differences in susceptibilities to disease may make xenografts useful for transplants in specific patient groups (e.g. HIV or hepatitis B+ patients)

**Problems with xenotransplantation**

Ethical: animal rights and speciesism

Transmission of donor pathogens to human host

Emergence of recombinant viral strains of unknown pathogenicity

Transmission of human pathogens to xenograft

Physiological incompatibilities, including the potential for differential ageing of xenograft and recipient

Immunological: vascular and cellular rejection

available xenogeneic tissues may allow effective treatment of other diseases; for example, diabetes mellitus and Parkinson's disease.

Xenotransplantation also offers opportunities to

develop and refine strategies for pretransplant manipulation of donor organs so that recipient rejection responses can be modified. For example, human DAF-expressing transgenic pigs have already been generated to help deal with the problem of hyperacute rejection (HAR) but the same technology could be applied to prevent other aspects of rejection (see below). This type of pretransplant intervention is impossible with clinical allografting.

Assuming that manoeuvres such as these help overcome recipient rejection responses, there are a number of other potential problems, listed in Table 6.2, that may limit the widespread application of xenotransplantation. Of these, the threat of transmissible disease was the major concern expressed recently in two formal reports on the subject of xenotransplantation (Nuffield Council on Bioethics 1996; Advisory Group on the Ethics of Xenotransplantation 1997). The ethical concerns regarding the use of animal organ donors very much depend on the species being considered (see below).

## Clinical experience with solid organ xenografts from primates

At the beginning of this century, tissue slices from a rabbit kidney were implanted into a child with renal insufficiency in France and case reports describing transplantation of whole kidneys from pigs, goats, lambs and non-human primates can be found in the literature from the early 1900s (reviewed in Reemtsma 1991). Needless to say, all of these very early attempts at xenotransplantation were unsuccessful.

However, in the early 1960s at the stage when clinical transplantation was still in its infancy and the concept of brain death was not widely accepted, several attempts were made by investigators in the USA to transplant kidneys from chimpanzees and baboons into humans (Reemtsma *et al.* 1964a,b,c; Starzl *et al.* 1964). Although none of these attempts achieved long-term patient survival, in one case a chimpanzee kidney functioned without rejection for 9 months (Reemtsma *et al.* 1964b). Since then there have been several well-publicized baboon-to-human solid organ transplants performed in the USA, including a baboon heart that

survived for 20 days in a baby in 1984 (Bailey *et al.* 1985). Most recently, baboon livers were transplanted into two patients in Pittsburgh (Starzl *et al.* 1993) who survived for 70 and 26 days, respectively.

Each of these cases has demonstrated the potential use of xenografts in clinical transplantation. The total experience with primate organs is illustrated in Table 6.3.

## Problems with primates as organ donors for humans

There are several fundamental reasons why primates are unsuitable for routine use as organs donors. First, although chimpanzees are closest to humans in phylogenetic terms—and therefore the most suitable donors on immunological grounds (see next section)—they breed very slowly, have never been 'farmed' or undergone intensive captive breeding and are already endangered as a species. Similarly, baboons breed relatively slowly and have never been extensively farmed, although they are not yet endangered.

Secondly, the concern about the transmission of infectious disease from primates is of greater concern than the risk from other species. This is probably because of the recent experience with HIV, which is now believed to have originated when the simian counterpart virus, SIV, was transmitted from primates to humans (Chapman *et al.* 1995).

Thirdly, there are very difficult ethical problems with the use of highly intelligent and social animals, like primates, as organ donors. All these considerations have led to the recommendation that primates not be used in the UK for xenotransplantation.

**Table 6.3** The clinical experience with solid organ xenografts from primates, 1964–96.

| Primate | Organ | | |
| --- | --- | --- | --- |
| | Heart | Liver | Kidney |
| Baboon | 2 | 2 | 7 |
| Chimpanzee | 2 | 3 | 12 |
| Monkey | – | – | 1 |

## Use of porcine organs for xenotransplantation

It is difficult to define who first suggested that the pig might be the most suitable animal for use as an organ donor in humans, but the idea has been widespread for more than 30 years (Calne 1970). Their breeding characteristics are those of an ideal donor; they reach sexual maturity in 9 months, gestate for 3.5 months and produce litters of 6–16 piglets.

Pigs are also a more ethically acceptable choice of xenogeneic donor than primates (Nuffield Council on Bioethics 1996). Besides displaying fewer human-like qualities than primates, pigs have been captively reared and extensively farmed for generations. On an annual basis, millions of pigs are slaughtered worldwide for food and clothing.

The concerns about disease transmission from pig to humans have not yet been addressed in great detail. However, the transmission of endogenous retroviruses or herpesviruses has aroused especial concern, with the demonstration that human cells can be infected *in vitro* by porcine retroviruses (Patience *et al.* 1997). However, two recent clinical studies involving patients with limited exposure to xenogeneic tissue have indicated that viral transmission may not be an immediate or common event (Heneine *et al.* 1998; Patience *et al.* 1998), although further experiments are needed to address this issue in greater depth. Overall, there is a widespread perception that pigs will be safer than primates in this respect. Nevertheless, it has been recommended that specific pathogen-free herds be established for the purpose of xenotransplantation (Nuffield Council on Bioethics 1996).

There are also uncertainties about the physiological suitability of porcine organs in humans. It is difficult to address these directly, but several lines of evidence indicate that pig organs may adequately support human life. For example, comparison of physiological profiles (Table 6.4) suggests that porcine organs function in an environment similar to that of human organs. Also, porcine livers have been perfused *ex vivo* to support the lives of several patients in hepatic coma, sometimes with dramatic short-term improvements in patient well-being (Burdick & Fair 1994).

All these factors indicate that there are reasonable

**Table 6.4** Limited comparison of pig and human physiological values.

|  | Porcine | Human |
|---|---|---|
| Core temperature (°C) | 38.6–39.5 | 36.5–37.5 |
| Respiratory rate (/min) | 8–18 | 14–18 |
| Heart rate (/min) | 65–85 | 50–100 |
| Mean systolic blood pressure* (mmHg) | 170 | 120 |
| Mean diastolic blood pressure* (mmHg) | 108 | 75 |
| Haemoglobin (g/dL) | 10–16 | 11.5–18 |
| Whole blood cells ($\times 10^9$/L) | 11–22 | 4–11 |
| Platelets ($\times 10^9$/L) | 300–700 | 150–400 |
| Packed cell volume (%) | 32–50 | 37–54 |
| $Na^+$ (mmol/L) | 135–142 | 135–145 |
| $K^+$ (mmol/L) | 4.9–7.1 | 3.5–5.0 |
| $Cl^-$ (mmol/L) | 94–106 | 95–105 |
| Glucose (mmol/L) | 3.3–7.5 | 4.0–6.0 |
| Urea (mmol/L) | 6–17 | 2.5–6.7 |

* Susceptible to age variation in humans.

grounds for optimism about the suitability of pigs as xenograft organ donors. But one other factor, the problem of rejection, has inhibited their use so far.

## Rejection of xenografts

### Concordant and discordant combinations

In general, organs transplanted between closely related species, such as humans and chimpanzees or rats and mice, are not rejected as aggressively as those transplanted between more distantly related species, such as pigs and humans or pigs and primates. In these cases xenografts are rejected within hours and in some cases minutes after transplantation, a process called hyperacute rejection (HAR). Calne coined the terms concordant and discordant in 1970 (Calne 1970) to distinguish between these two clinically defined species combinations, concordant referring to 'first-set cross-species grafts which are rejected at a tempo and with morphological characteristics similar to first-set allografts' and discordant referring to 'first-set cross-species grafts which are hyperacutely rejected with vas-

| Donor | Recipient | Organs | Discordant/concordant |
|-------|-----------|--------|----------------------|
| Pig | Human (*ex vivo* perfusion) | Kidney/heart | Discordant |
| Pig | Primate (rhesus and cynomolgus monkey, baboon) | Kidney/heart | Discordant |
| Guinea pig | Rat | Heart | Discordant |
| Hamster | Rat | Heart | Concordant |
| Mouse | Rat | Heart | Concordant |

**Table 6.5** The major experimental models of vascularized organ xenotransplantation (models of skin or islet xenograft rejection are not included).

cular lesions similar to those observed in second-set allografts in sensitized animals'.

While only implied in Calne's original definitions, the terms concordant and discordant are now commonly used to refer to closely and distantly related species, respectively, although there are factors other than phylogenetic disparity that determine whether an organ will be hyperacutely rejected. For instance, baboon organs transplanted into the concordant species, humans, will be hyperacutely rejected if unmatched for blood group. Similarly, the tempo with which rat organs are rejected by hamsters would lead to this species combination being labelled as discordant. However, the results of transplantation in the reverse direction suggest that this should be called a concordant combination (Auchincloss 1988). Furthermore, different organs show differing degrees of susceptibility to HAR. A heart graft may be rejected at a different tempo from a liver or lung graft between the same species combinations (Settaf *et al.* 1987; Kaplon *et al.* 1995).

Several species combinations have been more commonly employed than others in xenotransplantation research and these are listed in Table 6.5. Each of these experimental systems has provided, and continues to provide, valuable information about the nature of xenograft rejection.

### Hyperacute rejection of discordant xenografts

The rapid rejection of organs, which may occur within several minutes of revascularization, is the hallmark of rejection in discordant species combinations. Understanding HAR assumed a critical importance with the realization that any large-scale clinical programme would have to rely on the use of organs from a species discordant to our own (i.e. the pig).

The pathology of hyperacutely rejected organs in all species combinations is typical of vascular rejection, the prominent features being haemorrhage, oedema and infarction of interstitial tissues with thrombosis of xenogeneic vessels (Perper & Najarian 1966; Platt *et al.* 1990a). The factors that initiate and sustain this rejection process have been described in several experimental models. Activation of complement upon graft endothelium is responsible for the vigour and rapidity of HAR in all models. However, in the clinically relevant models—pig organs into primates—it is clear that the initiators of HAR are naturally occurring xenoreactive natural antibodies (XNA), which bind to the xenograft endothelium and without which complement is not activated. Accordingly, major efforts are under way to target these events and prevent HAR (see below).

The principal paradigm of HAR (see Fig. 6.2), first proposed by Platt *et al.* (1990a) and now widely accepted, also places the activation of xenograft endothelium at the centre of the rejection process, the third component of a triad of factors contributing to HAR, the other two being XNA and complement. There is ample evidence to support the hypothesis that endothelial cells have a prominent role in rejection, not just by being the front-line target of recipient effector systems, but also by actively promoting pathological changes leading to acute graft failure. The individual

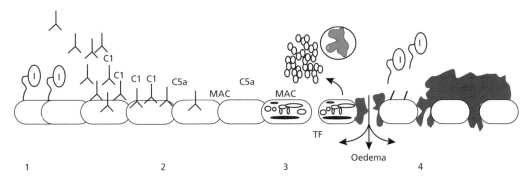

**Fig. 6.2** The four sequential phases of hyperacute rejection (HAR). 1, Normal endothelium. Two important functions of normal endothelium are provision of a tight seal and maintenance of an anticoagulant environment within the vessel lumen. Anticoagulation is achieved by expression of thrombomodulin and by the tethering of coagulation inhibitors such as antithrombin III and tissue factor pathway inhibitor to surface glycosaminoglycan (represented as 'I' on the diagram). 2, After revascularization, HAR is initiated by binding of xenoreactive natural antibodies which activate complement by the classical pathway through C1. Of the effector molecules generated on the xenogeneic endothelial cell surface, the two most important are C5a and C5b-9 (membrane attack complex, MAC), both of which directly interact with endothelium to initiate 'endothelial cell activation'. 3 and 4, Endothelial cell activation and vascular thrombosis. Several changes which compromise the normal functioning of endothelium occur immediately upon activation by complement. Retraction of individual cells leads to a loss of vascular integrity and egress of serum components into the tissues. Weibel–Palade bodies, containing von Willebrand factor and P-selectin, fuse with the cell membrane leading to expression of these two molecules. Circulating leukocytes and platelets are attracted and activated, tissue factor (TF), expressed on adventitial layers of endothelium, is exposed and coagulation is initiated. Thrombosis proceeds in an uncontrolled manner partly because luminal coagulation inhibitors are lost as thrombomodulin and glycosaminoglycan chains are cleaved from endothelial cells as part of the activation process.

components of the HAR process will be discussed in detail, below.

## Xenoreactive natural antibodies

Naturally occurring antibodies can lead to HAR in the context of allotransplantation if organs are transplanted across an ABO incompatibility (Paul *et al.* 1978). That anti-A and anti-B antibodies are responsible for this process has been demonstrated, albeit indirectly, by Cooper *et al.* (1993), who have shown that the process can be prevented by infusion of synthetic oligosaccharides that block the binding of these antibodies before transplantation.

The role of antibodies in HAR in many xenograft models has been established using several approaches. First, examination of hyperacutely rejected organs by immunofluorescence reveals deposition of xenoreactive antibodies along the endothelium (Platt *et al.*

1991a) in conjunction with complement deposition. Secondly, depletion of antibodies in these models by a variety of methods (discussed below) generally leads to prolongation of graft survival and delayed HAR (Fischel *et al.* 1990).

There has been controversy about the isotype of XNA that initiates HAR. In the pig to rhesus monkey model, the pattern of antibody deposition revealed by immunofluorescence studies of renal grafts implies a prominent role for IgM but not IgG in HAR (Platt *et al.* 1991a). While the IgM is found bound to the endothelium, IgG, like albumin and $\alpha_2$-macroglobulin, is found within the interstitium. However, *ex vivo* perfusion of porcine organs with human blood is associated with deposition of both isotypes on vascular endothelium (Tuso *et al.* 1993a). Naturally occurring IgG and IgA antibodies against non-vascular pig tissue have been documented (Schaapherder *et al.* 1993) but such antibodies would have a questionable role in HAR of vascularized organs. In other models, though, for instance the mini-pig to rabbit kidney model, IgG and IgA, but not IgM, have been found deposited along the endothelium of rejecting kidneys (Marino *et al.* 1991).

Confusion about the nature of XNAs may have arisen in the past because a variety of different assay systems for their detection have been used, including red blood cell agglutination and lymphocyte cytotoxicity assays. Platt *et al.* (1990b) argued that using cultured porcine endothelial cells to detect endothelial specific antibodies by ELISA was the most logical test for xenoreactive antibody, and it appears that both IgM and IgG isotypes can be detected in human serum by this method. However, while IgM is found in all humans tested, IgG XNA are found in only two-thirds of individuals (Parker *et al.* 1996a).

Much of the evidence obtained within the last few years indicates that in primates, including humans, IgM, but not IgG antipig, XNA initiate HAR. Most *in vitro* studies have demonstrated that only IgM XNA initiate complement activation and cause lysis of cultured porcine endothelial cells. Thus, serum treated with 2-mercapto-ethanol or DL-penicillamine, both of which inhibit IgM but not IgG, causes loss of lytic activity (Xu *et al.* 1994). Similarly, serum depleted of or naturally lacking IgM (Xu *et al.* 1995) is noncytotoxic. Finally, in experiments using purified preparations of human antipig antibodies, only the IgM fraction mediates endothelial cell lysis (Borche *et al.* 1994; d'Apice & Pearse 1996).

*In vivo* studies also support this conclusion. Most of the IgG deposited in porcine organs after perfusion with human blood is of the IgG2 subclass, which only activates complement weakly (Ross, R. *et al.* 1993). Also, in cynomolgus monkeys transplanted with porcine hearts, infusion of IgG delays rather than hastens rejection, the opposite of what might be expected if IgG initiated HAR (Magee *et al.* 1995).

### IgM xenoreactive antibodies

IgM XNA, which constitute 0.1% of circulating IgM (Vanhove & Bach 1993), appear to be polyreactive antibodies generated by CD5+ B cells (Turman *et al.* 1991), sharing many common features with naturally occurring anti-A and anti-B isohaemagglutinins (Parker *et al.* 1996a).

A number of studies have shown that these antibodies react with the unfucosylated terminal non-reducing disaccharide of the αGal linear B epitope Galα1 → 3Galβ1 → 4GlcNAc-R,* commonly known as the galα(1–3) gal epitope. This epitope corresponds to that recognized by human natural anti-αGal antibodies first described by Galili (Galili 1993). Naturally occurring anti-αGal and XNA are therefore one and the same.

This was initially determined by eluting IgM from pig organs that had been perfused with human serum and testing their specificity against synthetic carbohydrates (Good et al. 1992). MacKenzie and colleagues (Sandrin et al. 1993) repeated these experiments and showed that the binding of antipig antibodies to porcine erythrocytes could be blocked by mono- or disaccharides containing the α-galactose linkage. They then cloned cDNA encoding the murine enzyme α1,3-galactosyltransferase, which is responsible for introducing the galα(1–3) gal linkage into carbohydrate chains. COS cells transfected with this cDNA clone developed the ability to absorb antipig IgM from human serum. The same group have cloned the cDNA encoding the porcine α1,3-galactosyltransferase and found it to have significant homology to the murine clone (Sandrin et al. 1994).

Confirmatory evidence of the importance of galα(1–3) gal has been provided by Platt's group, who have shown that treatment of porcine endothelial cells with an enzyme, α-galactosidase, which cleaves α-gal groups, abolishes the binding of 80% of the human IgM XNA (Collins *et al.* 1994). This also confirmed what others have shown, that ~20% of the human antipig IgM binding to cultured porcine endothelial cells appears not to be specific for galα(1–3) gal. However, this fraction is not absorbed from human serum by perfusion through porcine kidneys, and its binding can be blocked by preincubating pig cells with pig serum (Parker *et al.* 1996a). This indicates that binding by this fraction is an *in vitro* artefact and

---

* Abbreviations: Gal, galactose; GlcNAc, *N*-acetyl glucosamine; R, core structure.

implies that all of the antipig IgM may be specific for galα(1–3) gal.

The α1,3-galactosyl enzyme is present in most mammalian species but not in Old World monkeys, apes and humans, who therefore do not express the galα(1–3) gal epitope. IgM XNA in these species are probably produced after exposure to gastrointestinal bacteria expressing similar carbohydrate structures and their role in serum is probably as a defence against invasion by these organisms (Galili *et al.* 1988). Unfortunately, from the point of view of xenotransplantation, tissue from any non-primate mammal or New World monkey that expresses the αGal linear B carbohydrate epitope will also be recognized by these antibodies. In pigs, galα(1–3) gal is expressed at high levels throughout all vascular beds (Oriol *et al.* 1993).

Several groups have identified a variety of glycoproteins on endothelial cells that carry the epitope and bind human antipig antibodies (Platt *et al.* 1990c; Tuso *et al.* 1993b). Platt's group have further characterized three of these glycoproteins, the gp115–135 triad, and found them to have sequence homology to human integrin chains (Platt & Holzknecht 1994). Other groups are pursuing similar methodologies to identify other target glycoproteins on pig endothelial cells. As yet, the functions of these important molecules in pigs are unknown, but such information may give insights into ways that the antipig antibodies interact with graft endothelium, and allow predictions to be made of the effects that deleting such molecules may have on pig physiology.

## The role of complement in hyperacute rejection

On contact with xenogeneic endothelium, IgM XNA trigger complement activation. The significance of this in the pathogenesis of HAR is demonstrated by the lack of HAR in models utilizing animals with complement deficiency, in cobra venom factor-treated animals (Leventhal *et al.* 1993a) or in animals treated with other anticomplement agents (Miyagawa *et al.* 1993a).

IgM activates the classical pathway, producing C3b and thereby triggering an amplification loop involving the alternative pathway. The complement system is illustrated in a simplified form in Fig. 6.3.

There has been considerable debate about the role of the alternative pathway in the initiation of HAR.

**Fig. 6.3** Diagrammatic representation of the complement system.

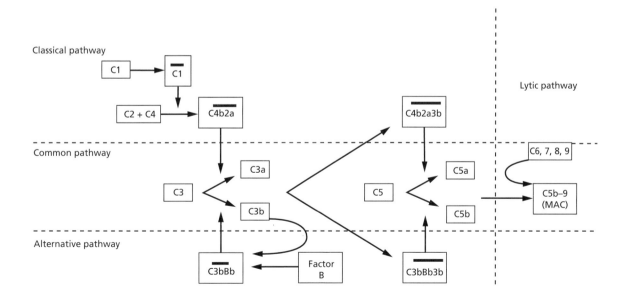

Several important points are clear. In the pig to rhesus monkey model, although C4b, C3b and the membrane attack complex (MAC) are deposited on the endothelium of rejecting organs, no components of the alternative pathway such as factor B and properdin are detected. In the same model, depletion of natural antibodies prevents HAR and prolongs graft survival in animals with intact classical and alternative complement systems (Platt & Bach 1991), implying no significant role for antibody-independent complement activation. Evidence from a study showing that C1 inhibitor, which acts purely on the classical pathway, can prevent the lysis of porcine endothelial cells by human serum, also argues against a role for the alternative pathway in HAR (Dalmasso & Platt 1993).

However, another group using similar *in vitro* studies to assess human complement-mediated lysis of porcine endothelial cells has presented evidence that contradicts this view, showing that alternative pathway activation does occur *in vitro* on the surface of porcine endothelial cells (Zhao *et al.* 1994). The precise involvement of the two pathways in pig to human grafts therefore remains controversial.

In other models, the alternative pathway is a major route of complement activation and the major initiator of HAR. Thus, in the guinea pig to rat model, despite the presence of circulating xenoreactive antibodies, the alternative pathway contributes significantly (Leventhal *et al.* 1993b). In the rabbit to presuckling-pig model (Johnston *et al.* 1992), in which the recipients have no circulating immunoglobulin, and in the cat to rabbit model (Zhow *et al.* 1990), the alternative pathway is the main initiator of HAR. Direct activation of the alternative pathway in the absence of antibody has also been described in a large number of other situations. Indeed, the alternative pathway was first described in the 1950s as a result of its activation by the yeast wall polysaccharide, zymosan (Pilemer *et al.* 1954).

Alternative pathway activation results from the binding of C3b, activated continuously at a low level by the enzyme plasmin, to the cell surface. C3b binding is the first critical step in the generation of an active alternative pathway, C3 convertase enzyme. Thus, even in those models where initiation of complement activation is via the classical pathway, amplification of the response via the alternative pathway may be an important feature of HAR. The debate about initiation of HAR is of relevance because of the need to design strategies for future intervention. The evidence suggests that the most therapeutically useful complement inhibitor may be one that inhibits the activation of both pathways.

Once activated, the mechanism by which complement acts to promote HAR is still poorly understood. Experiments using human blood to perfuse porcine hearts *ex vivo* have indicated that inhibiting C5 cleavage, thereby preventing the formation of C5a and MAC, can effectively prevent HAR (Kroshus *et al.* 1995; Rollins *et al.* 1995). The implication is that complement components formed proximal to C5 cleavage are not important in the pathogenesis of HAR.

*In vivo* experiments in C6-deficient animals (Hattori *et al.* 1989; Zhow *et al.* 1990) demonstrating prolonged survival and absence of HAR similarly imply that only terminal complement components beyond C6 are important in the pathogenesis of HAR. However, interpretation of these data is complicated by the fact that these animals may suffer associated C5 deficiency.

While endothelial MAC deposition is a feature of HAR, as shown by the immunofluorescence studies mentioned earlier, endothelial cell lysis is not a feature, indicating that the MAC is possibly acting to promote endothelial cell activation, along with other complement components (see below). It is clear that human endothelial cells can be 'activated' *in vitro* by sublytic amounts of surface MAC deposition, in a process that involves a rapid calcium influx leading to fusion of Weibel–Palade bodies with the cell membrane and immediate expression of von Willebrand's factor and P-selectin (Hattori *et al.* 1989). At the same time, thrombogenic vesiculations of endothelial cell membrane are released from the cell surface. All these changes promote platelet activation, attract neutrophils and promote a procoagulant environment. It may be that MAC acts on porcine endothelium in a similar way during HAR.

Another complement protein, C5a, has been shown to directly mediate, independently of other components, some of the changes associated with porcine endothelial cell activation *in vitro* (see below).

Products of the complement pathway may also contribute to HAR indirectly. For example, C3a formation may attract neutrophils (Vercellotti *et al.* 1991), which could then bind to C3bi deposited on the endothelial cell surface. C5a can also activate leucocytes and has anaphylotoxin and chemotactin properties, all of which may be important in the pathogenesis of HAR.

## The role of xenograft endothelium in hyperacute rejection

Platt and Bach were the first to suggest that activation of endothelial cells was a key event in HAR (Platt *et al.* 1990a). As it is difficult to separate the many events that occur *in vivo*, definitive proof of their hypothesis is still awaited, but there is accumulating evidence from *in vitro* studies for the active participation of endothelial cells in HAR.

It is clear that vascular endothelium plays a crucial part in a variety of physiological and pathological processes, including trafficking of leucocytes, secretion of cytokines and regulation of the coagulation cascade system. Many of these functions are dependent on alterations in the display, by endothelial cells, of certain proteins. The term activation refers to these changes in phenotype, which can be caused by a number of defined stimuli, although most *in vitro* studies that have defined endothelial cell activation have used cytokines such as interleukin 1 (IL-1) and tumour necrosis factor (TNF) (Pober & Cotran 1990).

Many of the changes that characterize endothelial cell activation involve transcription of novel genes and consequently occur relatively slowly compared, for example, to the tempo of HAR. However, a number of stimuli relevant to xenograft rejection have been dis-covered to cause almost immediate changes in endothelial cell physiology. Bach and Pober have called this type of immediate endothelial cell activation type 1 activation (Bach *et al.* 1993) to differentiate it from that which depends on gene transcription, which they have called type 2 activation. It is likely that type 1 activation contributes towards the pathophysiology of HAR (see Fig. 6.2), whereas type 2 changes may be significant beyond the hyperacute phase during later stages of rejection (see below). Table 6.6 lists the changes in porcine endothelial cells hypothesized to be important in HAR.

*In vitro*, a rapid change in the shape of porcine endothelial cells can be observed by phase contrast microscopy after incubation with human serum, leading to the appearance of gaps in endothelial cell monolayers. These changes appear to be dependent on activated complement factors C5b6 and MAC (Saadi & Platt 1995). It is postulated that the formation of such gaps *in vivo* after the perfusion of an organ xenograft could, in part, be responsible for the rapid oedema and haemorrhage that characterize HAR. The formation of gaps within endothelium will also expose tissue factor expressed on adventitial layers and initiate coagulation.

XNA and complement together have been shown to cause a rapid and substantial loss of two surface molecules, heparan sulphate and thrombomodulin, from cultured porcine endothelial cells (Platt *et al.* 1990d). Loss of heparan sulphate, shown to result from the generation of C5a (Platt *et al.* 1991b), has been assumed to be important in HAR because it normally anchors certain biologically active molecules, including antithrombin III (ATIII), tissue factor pathway

**Table 6.6** Type 1 endothelial cell activation. Changes in porcine endothelium that are probably important in the pathogenesis of hyperacute rejection.

| Changes known to occur | | Changes postulated to occur |
|---|---|---|
| *In vivo* | *In vitro* | |
| Loss of vascular integrity | Endothelial shape change | Exposure of adventitial tissue factor |
| Loss of heparan sulphate | Loss of heparan sulphate | P selectin expression |
| Platelet-activating factor secretion | Loss of thrombomodulin | Vesiculation of thrombogenic endothelial cell membrane |
| | | Von Willebrand factor secretion |

inhibitor (TFPI) and superoxide dismutase (SOD), to the surface of endothelial cells. Loss of cell surface ATIII, thrombomodulin and TFPI may contribute significantly to the procoagulant environment generated early in HAR. However, evidence from experiments with human endothelial cells has indicated that up to 50% of the surface ATIII can be lost without significant impairment of anticoagulant activity (Kobayashi *et al.* 1990). Along with the fact that porcine TFPI may not be fully interactive with human tissue factor–Xa complexes (Kopp *et al.* 1997), this calls into question the significance of heparan sulphate loss *in vivo*.

*In vivo* evidence from several models of HAR supports the hypothesis that endothelial cell factors, particularly platelet activating factor (PAF), play a crucial part in rejection. One group (Forty *et al.* 1992) showed that perfusion of rabbit hearts with human blood led to thrombosis within 1 min caused by the release of PAF, possibly from endothelial cells lining the graft. Another group (Saumweber *et al.* 1994) also demonstrated the importance of this factor using *ex vivo* perfusion of porcine kidneys with human blood, during which HAR was associated with a rapid rise in inflammatory prostaglandin and TNF levels. A specific PAF antagonist attenuated and delayed these changes and prevented HAR. Similar delayed HAR after administration of a specific PAF antagonist was reported by O'Hair *et al.* (1992) in a guinea-pig heart to rat model.

## Hyperacute rejection: conclusions

Hyperacute rejection is the major problem to be overcome before transplantation of organs into humans from a species such as the pig can be carried out successfully. It is clear that, in clinically relevant models, XNA bind to endothelial cell carbohydrate epitopes and activate complement by the classical pathway. This initiates changes in the xenogeneic endothelium which rapidly cause thrombosis, haemorrhage, oedema and infarction of the transplanted organ. The pathophysiology of HAR is becoming clear, with an understanding of the role that endothelial cell activation may have and the appreciation that rejection is the result of a complex interplay between donor organ-derived and recipient factors. The information so far available on the pathogenesis of HAR, while by no means complete, has enabled the evolution of a number of strategies for overcoming HAR. These will be discussed in the next section.

## Overcoming hyperacute rejection

In recent years great efforts have been devoted to investigating ways to overcome HAR. Increasing knowledge of the mechanisms involved in rejection, especially in clinically relevant animal models, has enabled various strategies to emerge. There are two broad approaches to overcoming HAR. The first involves manipulation of the recipient systems responsible for rejection, while the second involves manipulating the donor organs, using transgenic or other techniques, to modify the susceptibility of donor tissues to damage by the recipient immune response.

Donor manipulation has already been mentioned as one of the advantages of xenotransplantation over allografting. The recent successful transgenic manipulation of donor pigs to express human regulators of complement activity (RCAs) has aroused much excitement, but the successful prevention of HAR is likely to depend on manipulation of both donor and recipient.

## Influencing xenoreactive antibodies–galα(1–3) gal interactions

MANIPULATION OF THE RECIPIENT

In experimental models in which XNA are the prime initiators of HAR, depletion delays the rejection process (Fischel *et al.* 1990). A number of methods have been used. Perfusion of excised organs derived from the same species as the graft seems to be an effective way of removing circulating antibodies (Platt *et al.* 1991a), but the depletion obtained is temporary and as antibody levels return to normal rejection has been observed (Platt *et al.* 1990a). There is evidence to suggest that different organs may have different capacities to absorb antibodies. For example, spleen and liver perfusion appear to be more efficient than kidney perfusion (Brewer *et al.* 1993; Tuso *et al.* 1993a). However, it is unlikely that such 'disposable organ' immunoadsorption techniques will be appropriate for widespread application for both ethical and financial reasons.

Other methods used to deplete xenoantibody temporarily include repeated rounds of immunoadsorption or plasmaphaeresis (Figueroa *et al.* 1993) and perfusion of extracorporeal circuits containing xenogeneic cells (Watkins *et al.* 1991), but whether these methods are any more appropriate for large-scale transplantation programmes is unclear.

Alternative strategies based on the use of anti-idiotype monoclonal antibodies (Geller *et al.* 1993) or anti-IgM monoclonals (Soares *et al.* 1993) may be possible, taking advantage of the fact that only IgM causes HAR.

Cooper's group have shown that immunoadsorption through columns containing carbohydrates may be a cheap and therefore widely applicable way of depleting XNA (Good *et al.* 1992). In a similar vein, and following on from their work with infusions of synthetic carbohydrate in ABO mismatched allografts, they have also shown that intravenous infusions of melibiose and arabinogalactan can significantly modify the cytotoxic actions of baboon and human serum on cultured porcine kidney (PK15) cells (Neethling *et al.* 1994) and prevent HAR of porcine hearts in baboon recipients (Ye *et al.* 1994), apparently without the theoretical complication of immune complex deposition. Large quantities of synthetic carbohydrate containing the galα(1–3) gal linkage are now available (Cooper, D.K.C. *et al.* 1996) and both these approaches may be clinically applicable. Alternatively, peptide analogues that mimic galα(1–3) gal, identified by screening a bacteriophage display library with XNA (Kooyman *et al.* 1996), could be used in a similar way.

The length of time for which XNA need to be depleted is not clear, but the aim of many early investigators was to try and prevent HAR for long enough to allow accommodation to occur (Bach 1991). The methods just described will certainly achieve a short-term reduction in XNA titres (i.e. a few days) but repeated treatments may be required if longer-term depletion is necessary, and it may be more appropriate then to employ other techniques to suppress or inhibit antibody production.

Splenectomy clearly leads to a significant reduction in serum levels of antibody (Figueroa *et al.* 1993) but is very unlikely to be adopted for clinical transplantation. Drugs, either singly or in combination, have been extensively investigated in concordant models but little work on their use in HAR has been reported. Short-term cyclophosphamide given to rats together with specific xenoantigen causes the suppression of natural IgM xenoantibodies as well as preventing the induction of specific IgG antibodies (Breitkreuz *et al.* 1993). The new agent mycophenolate mofetil (RS-61443), a mycophenolic acid derivative that inhibits *de novo* synthesis of guanine nucleotides, when given to rats after a depletion procedure inhibits the return of IgM antibodies (Figueroa *et al.* 1993).

MANIPULATION OF THE DONOR

Hyperacute rejection of transplanted guinea-pig hearts in rat recipients has been delayed by pretransplantation perfusion of the graft with rat IgM Fab fragments (Fabμ), which were shown to bind to endothelial cell surfaces and prevent the binding of rat antiglycoprotein antibodies (Gambiez *et al.* 1992). The modest, though significant, delay reported in this experiment (13 min survival in control animals extended to 26 min in Fabμ-treated animals), reflects the modest though important contribution to HAR made by circulating antibodies in this species combination, and is similar to the results obtained by depletion of IgM from the recipient (Leventhal *et al.* 1993b). It appears that masking or disguising the ligands for natural antibody may be an effective way of inhibiting the effects of natural antibodies.

Another approach would be to remove the antigenic carbohydrate ligands by perfusion of grafts prior to transplantation with α-galactosidase. *In vitro* data suggest that this may be feasible (Collins *et al.* 1994; LaVecchio *et al.* 1995) although the effect might only be temporary.

Galα(1–3) gal epitopes could also be manipulated by transgenic approaches. MacKenzie and colleagues have shown that coexpression of α1,2-fucosyltransferase together with α1,3-galactosyltransferase results in a reduction in the expression of the galα(1–3) gal epitopes caused by intracellular competition for *N*-acetyl lactosamine acceptor substrate. The fucosyltransferase catalyses addition of non-antigenic fucosyl linkages, and pig cells expressing both enzymes bind less human antipig XNA and are less susceptible to lysis in human serum than normal controls (Sandrin *et al.* 1995). Similarly, cells from transgenic mice expressing fucosyltransferase bind less antigal-specific XNA than non-transgenic littermate controls. Transgenic pigs expressing α1,2-fucosyltransferase have been recently generated; cells from these pigs are resistant to lysis by human serum, implying that organs from these pigs may be resistant to HAR (Koike *et al.* 1996). An alternative approach would be to reduce the expression of α1,3-galactosyl transferase using antisense techniques (Galili 1993), although this has proven unreliable in the past.

A third approach, disrupting the α1,3-galactosyltransferase gene by homologous recombination, has been shown to be effective in mice. Cells from these α-1,3-galactosyltransferase 'knockouts' bind little human XNA and consequently activate human complement less efficiently than cells from wild-type mice (Tearle *et al.* 1996). These mice are otherwise healthy. A similar approach in pigs is not yet possible, as porcine embryonic stem cells, necessary for the generation of knockouts, have proven difficult to isolate.

### Inhibiting the activation of complement

#### MANIPULATION OF THE RECIPIENT

Soluble complement receptor 1 (sCR1) has been shown to extend survival of guinea-pig cardiac grafts transplanted into rats from 15–20 min to over 10 h (Xia *et al.* 1993). Cobra venom factor (CVF), a reptilian protein which stabilizes the C3 convertase C3bBb and exhausts serum of C3, has the same effect in this model (Leventhal *et al.* 1993b) and in the rabbit heart to suckling-pig model (Johnston *et al.* 1992).

In these two models, complement activation via the alternative pathway is the main initiator of HAR. CVF can also delay HAR from 1.5 h to 3 days in the pig heart to baboon model (Leventhal *et al.* 1993a), and sCR1 has been shown to prolong graft survival in a pig heart to cynomolgus monkey model from a mean of 1 h up to a maximum of 4 days. Rejection of pig hearts perfused *ex vivo* by human blood is also delayed by sCR1

(Pruitt *et al.* 1994). These findings are significant because of the demonstrated importance of XNA-initiated complement activation in these species combinations and because the effects were noticed without any manipulation of XNA. Of the two agents, sCR1, with low immunogenicity, is the most likely to be used clinically, although CVF now exists in a highly purified form and may find some use. Another promising anti-complement agent is C1-inhibitor, which at high concentrations has been shown to prevent the lysis of porcine endothelial cells exposed to human serum *in vitro* (Dalmasso & Platt 1993) but has yet to be tested in an *in vivo* model.

The synthetic anticomplement drugs K76COOH and FUT 175, which inhibit the alternative pathway, have also had significant effects on HAR in the guinea-pig heart to rat model (Miyagawa *et al.* 1993a), indicating that pharmacological control of complement activation may hold promise for the future.

As with antibody depletion, the duration of anticomplement therapy that will be necessary after xenografting is not clear. Because the major drawback with systemic inhibition of complement is the risk of serious bacterial infection, most of these agents may have only a limited place in clinical practice if long periods of treatment are needed.

#### MANIPULATION OF THE DONOR

The complement system is normally kept in check by a number of regulatory proteins (regulators of complement activity: RCAs), some which are illustrated in Fig. 6.4. Despite possessing structures which have been highly conserved through evolution, the membrane-bound inhibitory proteins are relatively species-specific (Dalmasso *et al.* 1991; Zhao *et al.* 1991). This is postulated to be the main reason why complement activation proceeds apparently unhindered on the surface on porcine cells once XNA are bound (Parker *et al.* 1996b). The idea of expressing human RCAs on xenogeneic cells to prevent HAR arose out of this hypothesis. The advantages of this approach are that high levels of RCA expression within a xenograft would be expected to inhibit complement control only locally, so avoiding the risks of systemic complement inhibition.

*In vitro* studies have demonstrated the ability of

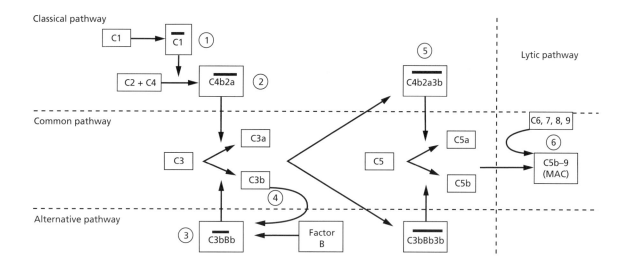

**Fig. 6.4** The sites of action of some of the human regulators of complement activity. C1 inh, C1 inhibitor; C4bp, C4 binding protein; CR1, complement receptor 1; DAF, decay accelerating factor (CD55); MAC, membrance attack complex; MCP, membrane cofactor protein (CD46).

human membrane-bound RCAs, such as CD55 (decay-accelerating factor: DAF), CD46 (membrane cofactor protein: MCP) and CD59, to prevent complement-mediated lysis of xenogeneic cells when expressed on the surface of transfected cells, or introduced by passive transfer in the case of phosphatidylinositol-linked DAF or CD59 (Dalmasso *et al.* 1991; Akami *et al.* 1993; Loveland *et al.* 1993; Miyagawa *et al.* 1993b).

Transgenic mice expressing human DAF and CD59 have also been generated (Somerville *et al.* 1994; Byrne *et al.* 1995; McCurry *et al.* 1995a; van Denderen *et al.* 1996) and although tissues from these animals bind XNA normally they are protected from complement-mediated lysis.

More recently, transgenic pigs expressing DAF, CD59 or both molecules together have been generated by a number of different groups (Fodor *et al.* 1994; Cozzi & White 1995; McCurry *et al.* 1995b; Rosengard *et al.* 1995; Diamond *et al.* 1996). Organs from these pigs, as expected, are resistant to HAR in baboons and after *ex vivo* perfusion with human blood (McCurry *et al.* 1995b; Kroshus *et al.* 1996; Schmoeckel *et al.* 1996, 1998; Byrne *et al.* 1997).

### Alternative targets for intervention

It may be beneficial to target some of the other processes involved in HAR besides binding of XNA and complement. For example, inhibiting coagulation may be particularly fruitful (Hunt & Rosenberg 1993).

Administration of intravenous heparin, in non-anticoagulant doses, in one model inhibited cleavage and release of radiolabelled heparan sulphate from xenograft endothelium and led to prolonged graft survival (Stevens *et al.* 1993). *In vitro* inhibition of heparan sulphate release was observed by the same group when porcine endothelial cells were treated with heparinized human serum. The assumption in these studies is that the two effects of heparin—graft prolongation and inhibition of heparan sulphate release from endothelial cells—are connected. This is the only evidence so far that proteoglycan loss from endothelial cells after activation may be important in the pathogenesis of HAR.

Another potential target is PAF; pharmacological antagonists have been shown to prolong graft survival in a number of models, including an *ex vivo* model of pig kidneys perfused by human blood (Saumweber *et al.* 1994). Similarly, the intense vasoconstriction that occurs early in HAR, possibly contributing to the pathology of rejected grafts, might be beneficially inhibited by vasodilator therapy.

Several anticoagulant molecules would be excellent candidates for expression in transgenic pigs. Amongst these, human TFPI, a natural inhibitor of tissue factor (Riesbeck *et al.* 1997), human thrombomodulin, which activates protein C activator (Kopp *et al.* 1998) and human CD39 (Koyamada *et al.* 1996) are particularly suitable as the porcine homologues of these either inefficiently interact with their human ligands or are lost rapidly during endothelial cell activation (Kopp *et al.* 1997; Robson *et al.* 1997).

### Beyond hyperacute rejection

There is a realistic chance that some of the strategies outlined in the previous section, perhaps in combination, will prevent HAR and enable xenografts to survive beyond 1 or 2 days. However, there are several other immunological barriers beyond HAR. These are illustrated in Fig. 6.5.

Xenografts may be rejected by an acute vascular rejection histologically indistinguishable from HAR, if serum complement levels return to baseline after a period of inhibition (Pruitt *et al.* 1994). Similarly, after XNA depletion, in the face of normal complement levels, xenografts undergo acute vascular rejection once IgM reappears in the circulation (Fischel *et al.* 1990; Platt *et al.* 1991a; Leventhal *et al.* 1994). These were all systems in which xenograft 'accommodation' did not occur (see below). The implication of studies showing that elicited antibodies have a similar specificity to XNA (Satake *et al.* 1994; Cotterell *et al.* 1995) is that these antibodies will also predispose to vascular rejection in the presence of complement.

Temporary complement inhibition or XNA depletion in isolation therefore appears to postpone, rather

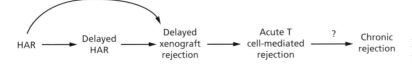

**Fig. 6.5** The immunological barriers to hyperacute rejection (HAR).

than prevent, acute vascular rejection of xenografts. In light of this, the strategies to manipulate donor xenograft organs to express human RCAs or fucosyl carbohydrate groups, both of which would be permanent, seem particularly attractive.

However, even in combination, both may not be enough to prevent vascular rejection; one group (Leventhal *et al.* 1994) has reported rejection of a porcine graft by microvascular thrombosis in a baboon treated with splenectomy, plasmaphaeresis, anti-B cell agents and CVF, along with conventional immunosuppressive agents, implying that some of the alternative approaches outlined earlier may also be necessary.

## Delayed xenograft rejection

This distinct form of xenograft rejection is also called acute vascular rejection (AVR) by some investigators, although delayed xenograft rejection (DXR) was proposed recently as the preferred term to use (see Rogers *et al.* 1998 for report on Fourth International Congress on Xenotransplantation). DXR has been documented in the guinea pig to rat model (Leventhal *et al.* 1993b; Blakely *et al.* 1994) and the pig to primate model (Leventhal *et al.* 1994), although it is from work in the former that most of the information on DXR has been derived.

The pathophysiology is still poorly understood. Histological studies show IgG and IgM XNA deposited along graft endothelium, fibrin deposition platelet aggregation and a prominent infiltration of inflammatory cells, most commonly polymorphonuclear cells, monocytes and natural killer cells.

Several lines of evidence indicate that three factors are involved in the development of DXR: binding by XNA, activation of graft endothelium and intrinsic natural killer cell activity against xenogeneic tissues.

### The role of antibody in delayed xenograft rejection

It is clear from several experiments by different groups that when XNA are depleted, either alone or in combination with complement inhibition, DXR tends not to occur. However, until recently, only one study had directly addressed whether XNA were important in DXR (Scheringa *et al.* 1995). Splenectomy was used to reduce pretransplant IgM XNA titres in rats by over 80% compared to levels in control rats. In spite of this, these animals rejected guinea pig heart grafts in under 30 min, as did controls, whereas grafts survived for nearly 2 days in CVF-treated rats before rejection by DXR. These results were anticipated because complement activation via the alternative pathway is important in this model and XNA contribute little to HAR. However, a role for XNA in DXR was suggested by the observation that graft survival in splenectomized animals treated with CVF was extended to 3.3 days. Recently, with the development of human RCA-expressing transgenic pigs, this question has been addressed in a pig heart to baboon model (Lin, S.S. *et al.* 1998). In this study, all animals survived HAR but underwent DXR within several days. However, five out of six organs transplanted into XNA-depleted baboons survived without DXR, strongly supporting the notion that XNA binding to xenograft endothelium initiate DXR.

Antibodies may act in at least two independent ways to promote DXR. Bach's group have shown that IgM XNA can directly activate porcine endothelial cells *in vitro* (Vanhove *et al.* 1994). After incubation with IgM for 2 or more hours, the cells up-regulated expression of several molecules, including IL-8, that are predicted to have a proinflammatory effect on whole endothelium. *In vivo*, it is postulated that XNA could contribute signals to activate endothelial cells.

Independently of this, IgG XNA may promote Fc receptor-mediated transmigration of inflammatory cells into the graft. Inverardi *et al.* (1992), by removing IgG from human serum, have shown that this is the main mechanism by which natural killer cells bind to the endothelium of rat xenografts.

### The role of the endothelium in delayed xenograft rejection

The postulated role of type 1 endothelial cell activation in the pathogenesis of HAR has already been reviewed. Bach *et al.* (1996) have suggested that type 2 activation could be important in DXR. Many of the phenotypic changes associated with type 2 endothelial cell activation have been documented in immunopathological studies of guinea-pig grafts rejected by rats (Blakely *et al.* 1994), although whether these changes are involved in initiating DXR or arise as a secondary phenomenon has not been addressed. What is clear is that there are multiple mechanisms by which the endothelium could be activated as the initial event in DXR.

For instance, IgM XNA can directly stimulate endothelial cells, as discussed earlier. Human natural killer cells can also directly activate porcine endothelial cell monolayers, causing gaps to appear, up-regulating expression of E-selectin and promoting the secretion of IL-8 (Goodman *et al.* 1996; Malyguine *et al.* 1996). These effects require cell–cell contact and occur independently of IgG XNA, although in the presence of antibody the activation stimulus is increased by secretion of TNFα and IFN-γ. Although human IFN-γ has no effect on porcine cells (Murray *et al.* 1994), human TNFα will stimulate pig endothelial cells to up-regulate expression of adhesion molecules and tissue factor (Batten *et al.* 1996). The two principal effects of activating xenograft endothelium will therefore be promotion of local coagulation and transmigration of inflammatory cells into the graft.

Two molecules on endothelial cells that are particularly important for transmigration of natural killer cells and monocytes are ICAM-1 and VCAM (Bianchi *et al.* 1993; Inverardi *et al.* 1993; Pinola *et al.* 1994; Takahashi *et al.* 1994) and the expression of each of these is up-regulated by TNFα. Other changes that might be important in DXR are listed in Table 6.7.

The molecular mechanisms that control the activation of porcine and human endothelial cells have been recently dissected by several groups (de Martin *et al.* 1993; Read *et al.* 1994). Many of the changes of type 2 activation are mediated by the transcription factor nuclear factor κB (NFκB), which is normally held within the cytoplasm of cells by association with an inhibitory protein IκBα. Upon endothelial cell stimulation by cytokines such as TNFα, IκB is phosphorylated and dissociates from NFκB. NFκB is then translocated to the nucleus where it binds the promoters of several genes, including those for VCAM, ICAM-1, E-selectin, IL-1 and IL-8, and initiates transcription. Expression of these is transient as NFκB also induces transcription of IκB, thus establishing a negative feedback control loop.

Using this knowledge Bach's group have developed a novel system to regulate endothelial cell activation. They originally transfected porcine endothelial cells with an adenoviral construct that resulted in high-level constitutive expression of IκB. These transfectants were resistant to activation by IL-1 and lipopolysaccarides (Bach *et al.* 1996), but were also susceptible to apoptosis. More recently, the same group has identified a number of genes which inhibit NFκB-mediated endothelial cell activation but also protect the cell against apoptosis (Bach *et al.* 1997a). These same 'survival' genes also appear to be up-regulated during the process of 'accommodation' (see below), implying that the expression of these genes might dictate whether an organ is sensitive or resistant to DXR. If confirmed, these genes would be candidates for manipulation by transgenesis, to generate animals whose organs are

| Changes known to occur | | Changes postulated to occur |
|---|---|---|
| *In vivo* | *In vitro* | |
| P- and E-selectin expression | IL-1 secretion | ICAM-1 expression |
| Loss of thrombomodulin, ATIII and ADPase | IL-8 secretion | |
| Tissue factor expression | VCAM expression | |
| Von Willebrand factor expression | | |

**Table 6.7** The porcine endothelial cell changes that accompany delayed xenograft rejection.

intrinsically resistant to DXR and conversely easy to 'accommodate' (Cooper, J.T. *et al.* 1996; Ferran *et al.* 1998; Soares *et al.* 1998).

## Natural killer cells and xenograft rejection

Definitive evidence that natural killer cells contribute directly to DXR has still to be obtained. However, there is accumulating evidence from *in vitro* studies that natural killer cell-mediated damage may be important in DXR. Most of these studies indicate that porcine cells, especially in the presence of IgG XNA, induce significant natural killer cell proliferation and cytotoxicity. For example, the extent of direct cytotoxicity by unprimed natural killer cells on porcine targets is relatively small as assessed by cultures set up in serum-free medium (Seebach *et al.* 1996), but lysis increases substantially in the presence of human serum (Chan & Auchincloss 1996), reflecting antibody-dependent cytotoxicity mediated by signals through CD16 (FcRγIII) (Goodman *et al.* 1996). During 6-day bulk culture of peripheral blood mononuclear cell (PBMC) with porcine targets, the natural killer cell population expands rapidly and mediates most of the killing (Kirk *et al.* 1993; Yamada *et al.* 1996), in contrast to allogeneic cultures, where T cell-mediated cytotoxicity is prominent.

## Accommodation of xenografts

Transplanted organs protected from HAR by XNA depletion or inhibition of complement can sometimes continue to function despite the return of antidonor antibody and complement back to pretransplant levels. This phenomenon has been termed graft 'accommodation' (Platt *et al.* 1990a; Bach *et al.* 1991). Allografts transplanted across both ABO and HLA barriers have been seen to 'accommodate' (Chopek *et al.* 1987; Alexandre *et al.* 1989, 1991; Palmer *et al.* 1989; Ross, C.N. *et al.* 1993) and there is evidence that a similar process can occur with xenografts, although the usual outcome after return of XNA is rejection. Implicit within the concept is that accommodated grafts are also resistant to DXR.

For example, a pig cardiac graft transplanted into a rhesus monkey survived 8 days, after which time the animal had to be sacrificed (Fischel *et al.* 1991). IgM antibodies were initially depleted to undetectable levels by two rounds of plasmaphaeresis followed by perfusion of pig kidneys on the day of transplantation. At necropsy only patchy IgM deposition was noticed without any evidence of rejection, despite the fact that serum IgM had rebounded to normal levels within 48 h of transplantation and IgM XNA were detected in the serum at various times. Similar experiences have been reported by another group (Alexandre *et al.* 1989).

In recent years, a reproducible model of accommodation using hamster hearts transplanted into rats has been developed by several groups (Hasan *et al.* 1992, 1994; Bach *et al.* 1997b; Brouard *et al.* 1998; Lin, Y. *et al.* 1998). Although this involves transplantation between concordant species, HAR occurs in sensitized recipients. Studies using this model have enabled the description of an 'accommodated phenotype', comprised of endothelial cell up-regulation of survival gene expression, such as Bcl-2, Bcl-xl and A20, skewing of antigraft antibody responses towards production of non-complement fixing subtypes and a Th-2-like pattern of cytokine secretion by infiltrating leucocytes—compared to the Th-1-like pattern found in rejecting grafts (Bach *et al.* 1997b), although this last feature has not been a consistent finding by all investigators (Brouard *et al.* 1998).

A strategy to prevent vascular rejection of xenografts would be to induce xenograft accommodation at the time of transplantation. This was the early objective of investigators looking for ways to achieve survival beyond HAR (Platt *et al.* 1990a; Bach 1991). Although the nature of accommodation was ill-defined, they hoped that it would occur naturally if vascular rejection could be inhibited for a suitable period, but in practice the most common scenario was graft rejection by delayed HAR or DXR.

The mechanisms that mediate accommodation are far from clear. One important factor might be the ischaemia that the graft is subject to during the period between donor and recipient; accommodation could be caused partially by recovery from these effects. However, because XNA depletion is crucial for accommodation to occur (Magee & Platt 1994), other factors are clearly involved. Platt and Bach were the first to propose three mechanisms that might explain the phenomenon (Platt *et al.* 1990a):

1 the XNA that return to the circulation after depletion might have an affinity or specificity different from those depleted;

2 the endothelial cell epitopes for XNA could somehow be altered during the time they are depleted; and

3 the graft endothelial cells could become more resistant to damage by XNA and complement.

The first of these possibilities has been effectively discounted by studying the antipig antibodies elicited in patients after *ex vivo* perfusion of porcine livers or transplantation of porcine islets. Elicited antibodies are mainly specific for galα(1–3) gal and have a similar functional avidity to XNA (Satake *et al.* 1994; Cotterell *et al.* 1995). The second possibility appears to have received little attention, perhaps because there is mounting evidence to support the third alternative that accommodation reflects a change in the physiology of xenograft endothelial cells, rendering them resistant to the effects of complement and preventing the widespread type 2 activation associated with DXR (Winkler *et al.* 1995).

   The study most often quoted to support this is from Vercellotti's group, who investigated the protective mechanisms of endothelium against exposure to oxidant stress. They incubated human umbilical vein endothelial cells and porcine endothelial cells with haem and noted that after short incubation periods the cells were more sensitive to the effects of $H_2O_2$. However, after 16 h they had acquired a resistance to damage because of transcriptional up-regulation of expression of two molecules, ferritin and haem oxygenase (Balla *et al.* 1992). These results indicated that endothelial cells could alter the way they responded to injury and that similar mechanisms operating on intact endothelium might provide the basis of xenograft accommodation. There is increasing evidence that it is XNA that provide the stimulus for accommodation to occur in xenogeneic endothelium.

## The role of IgG antigraft antibodies in accommodation

### EVIDENCE FROM A CONCORDANT MODEL

In general, hamster cardiac grafts transplanted into rats survive for 3 days before undergoing vascular rejection, a process that is dependent on elicited antihamster antibodies (AHA) and complement. Predictably, grafts transplanted into sensitized rats with an intact complement system are rejected within minutes by HAR because of the presence of preformed IgG AHA.

   The importance of these antibodies to the process of HAR was confirmed by White's group, who injected preparations of purified AHA into unsensitized rats at the time of xenografting. Instead of surviving 3 days, these grafts were rejected after 30 min (Hasan *et al.* 1992, 1994).

   In a further series of experiments by the same group, two different immunosuppressive regimes were used to achieve long-term survival of cardiac grafts (Hasan *et al.* 1992, 1994). The essentials of their experiments are illustrated in Table 6.8. Cyclosporin A was included in each regime to prevent cellular rejection, which has been documented by several other groups to occur within a week if vascular rejection is inhibited. In the first group of rats, vascular rejection was avoided by preventing the emergence of AHA with cyclophosphamide. In the second group, CVF was used for 28 days to inhibit complement activation during the period when AHA appeared in the circulation. After stopping CVF, hamster grafts were not rejected, suggesting that they had accommodated (or 'adapted', as White called it). To demonstrate that this was the case, the rats were challenged with intravenous AHA and the grafts survived. However, cardiac grafts in group 1 rats underwent HAR within minutes after challenge with intravenous AHA. To investigate whether the absence of elicited AHA was the reason why cardiac grafts in group 1 rats had not accommodated, they were challenged over a 4-week period with AHA, given under the protective cover of CVF to prevent HAR. On subsequent challenge with AHA, at a time when complement levels had returned to normal, these grafts had partially accommodated.

Table 6.8 Experiments in rats given hamster cardiac grafts to examine the role of IgG antigraft antibodies in accommodation.

|  | Group 1 | Group2 |
| --- | --- | --- |
| Immunosuppression | CyP/CyA | CVF (28 days)/CyA |
| Emergence of antibody? | No | Yes |
| Intravenous challenge with AHA | HAR (7 mins) (≥100 days)* | No rejection (≤40 days)† |
| Intravenous AHA therapy with CVF cover (4 weeks) | No rejection |  |
| Subsequent AHA challenge | No rejection (<14 days)‡ |  |

AHA, antihamster antibodies; CyA, cyclosporin A; CyP, cyclophosphamide; CVF, cobra venom factor; HAR, hyperacute rejection.
* Grafts that had survived for over 100 days still underwent HAR.
† Rats only challenged up to 40 days after transplantation.
‡ When challenged within 14 days of stopping CVF there was no rejection. At 14 days, HAR (122.5 min) was noted.

The implication of these results was that IgG AHA, prevented from mediating HAR by CVF, were able to induce changes within graft endothelium in a manner similar to that mediated *in vitro* by incubation with haem.

## IgG xenoreactive antibodies

In the original description by Galili, naturally occurring antigal antibodies were of the IgG isotype, comprising up to 1% of all circulating IgG (for review see Galili 1993). However, most IgG XNA appear not to be specific for galα(1–3) gal. This has been demonstrated in two ways. One group has treated porcine endothelial cells with α-galactosidase to remove galα(1–3) gal epitopes and observed the binding of XNA. As expected, the binding of IgM XNA was reduced by ~80%, as was the binding by IgG antigalα(1–3) gal antibodies. In contrast, the binding of non-fractionated IgG XNA was unaffected (Collins *et al.* 1994). A second group used galα(1–3) gal-containing oligosaccharides to block the binding of XNA to endothelial cells or, in separate experiments, used melibiose columns to retain IgG with specificity for galα(1–3) gal linatural killerages, before assessing XNA binding to endothelium. Neither of these procedures caused a gross reduction in binding by IgG XNA, implying that antigalα(1–3) gal IgG was a minority species (Cooke *et al.* 1995). Relatively little is known about the endothelial cell surface glycoproteins that bind IgG XNA, except that on immunoprecipitation they are different to those that bind IgM XNA.

It is now clear that these antibodies are not involved in HAR, as was discussed earlier, although they may have a prominent role in DXR by allowing FcR-mediated binding of inflammatory and natural killer cells to xenograft endothelium.

## Effect of antixenograft antibodies on endothelium: a paradox?

The evidence from discordant models of xenografting, which was reviewed earlier, supports a role for XNA in the initiation of both HAR and DXR. Yet the evidence from White's concordant model suggests that antixenograft antibody may promote accommodation. How can this apparent paradox be explained?

An attractive hypothesis is that in the concordant model antigraft antibodies appear in the circulation over the course of several days, whereas in discordant models the levels of circulating antibody are high from the moment of revascularization. Accommodation might arise because the endothelium is exposed to an initially low level of antibody. This hypothesis was first suggested in general terms (i.e. exposure to low level of stimulus) by Bach *et al.* (1991), and it might explain why accommodation is associated with XNA depletion (Magee & Platt 1994).

An alternative hypothesis is that IgM and IgG XNA each have a different effect on endothelial cell physiology. The basis of this might be signalling through different membrane glycoproteins that each isotype is thought to bind. IgM XNA have been shown to cause direct activation of porcine endothelium, a process hypothesized to be important in DXR, so a reasonable supposition to make is that IgG XNA might mediate the changes of accommodation. If this were the case, the outcome of rejection or accommodation would be determined by the relative concentrations of each during the period after transplantation.

We have attempted to investigate these two possibilities in an *in vitro* model of porcine endothelial cell accommodation (Dorling *et al.* 1996a, 1998; Dorling & Lechler 1997). Our results imply that IgG antipig antibodies can mediate the development of an accommodated phenotype that is characterized by the development of resistance to complement-mediated lysis, down-regulation of expression of molecules such as VCAM and MHC class I and expression of inducible nitric oxide synthase. However, fully accommodated cells only developed after exposure to low concentrations of IgG for at least 4 days, supporting the low-level stimulus hypothesis. The implications are that the development of accommodation *in vivo* may be crucially determined by the titre of IgG antipig antibodies in the immediate post-transplantation period. This *in vitro* model is expected to be of value in characterizing further the process of endothelial cell accommodation.

## T cell response to xenografts

Precise definition of T cell xenoresponses has been difficult in most discordant models because of the problem of prolonging survival beyond the HAR phase. In many experiments where this has been achieved, immunosuppression has usually been included to inhibit a T cell response.

Observations on the role of cellular immune responses to xenografts come from two main sources. First, experiments involving transplantation of non-vascularized skin and pancreatic islet grafts across various species barriers have allowed examination of cellular responses in the absence of HAR. Secondly, *in*

*vitro* experiments over the last three decades have provided a wealth of information about the potential for cellular rejection and the mechanisms of interaction between lymphocytes and xenogeneic cell populations.

Comparisons between allorecognition and xenorecognition have been made from the earliest days of research in this field (Widmer & Bach 1972) and knowledge of the cellular mechanisms underlying the allograft response has provided an important foundation for the investigation of xenograft rejection.

The orchestration of any successful immune response, whether against invading pathogens or transplanted organs, starts with the generation of proliferating CD4+ helper T cells, which then influence the development of antigen-specific effector mechanisms, such as the production of specific antibody by B cells, cytotoxic T lymphocyte maturation and macrophage-dependent delayed-type hypersensitivity reactions. Before any of this can begin, antigen has to be encountered by specific CD4+ T cells (Germain 1994).

Hence, the initiation of T cell-mediated graft rejection begins with the recognition of graft antigens by specific T cells (for review see Dorling & Lechler 1996). Several key events are necessary during this initial encounter for activation and proliferation of CD4+ T cells (Janeway & Bottomly 1994). These include cognate engagement of the T cell receptor (TCR) by MHC–peptide complexes and non-cognate interactions between CD4 and the membrane-proximal domains of MHC class II, adhesion molecules on the T cell and antigen-presenting cell (APC) including ICAM 1/LFA 1 and CD2/LFA 3, and delivery of crucial intercellular 'second' or 'costimulatory' signals by interactions between B7 family molecules on APC and CD28 on T cells. A similar cascade of activation signals is required for CD8+ T cells (Harding & Allison 1993; O'Rourke & Mescher 1993).

### Direct and indirect xenorecognition

Two pathways by which transplantation antigens are recognized have been described (Lechler & Batchelor 1982a; Wecker & Auchincloss 1992). In the first of these, the 'direct' pathway, appropriate MHC-expressing allo- or xenogeneic stimulators provide all

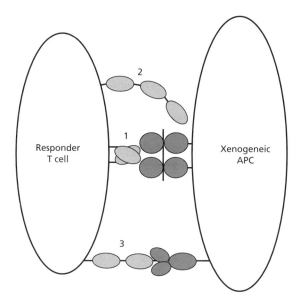

**Fig. 6.6** Diagrammatic representation of direct xenorecognition. The types of molecular interactions necessary for efficient direct xenorecognition are numbered 1–3. 1, Cognate interaction between TCR on responder T cell and MHC molecules on xenogeneic antigen-presenting cells (APC). 2, Non-cognate interaction between coreceptors CD4 and membrane proximal domains of MHC class II, and CD8 and α3 domains of MHC class I. 3, Non-cognate interactions between accessory and costimulatory molecules. Important interactions are between the B7 family (APC) and CD28 (T), LFA-3 (APC) and CD2 (T), and ICAM-1 (APC) and LFA-1 (T).

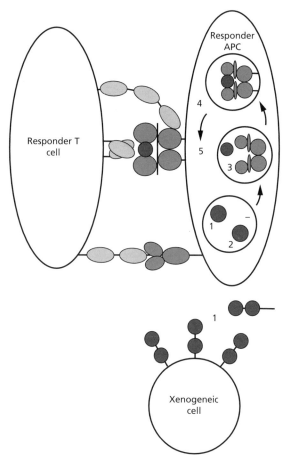

**Fig. 6.7** Diagrammatic representation of indirect xenorecognition. Xenoantigens (1), released by xenogeneic cells, are taken up and processed (2) into peptide fragments by specialized antigen-presenting cells (APC) (3) before binding to MHC class II molecules (4) and display on the cell surface (5) for presentation to xenospecific self class II MHC-restricted T cells.

the signals required for T cell activation, including that through the TCR, as illustrated in Fig. 6.6.

The second recognition pathway, used by CD4+ T cells, is called 'indirect' to reflect the necessity for processing of allo- or xenoantigens before presentation of the peptides generated on cell surface class II MHC molecules. This mechanism is illustrated in Fig. 6.7. In these responses, crucial molecular signals leading to T cell activation and proliferation, provided by recipient APCs, are always efficient and do not limit the vigour of the response.

### *In vivo* analyses of murine T cell xenoresponses

It is clear from *in vivo* studies in mice that T cells can

initiate rejection of xenogeneic skin grafts at a similar tempo to that of allografts (Pierson *et al.* 1989) by a process that is dependent on CD4+ T cells (Pierson *et al.* 1989; Wecker *et al.* 1994). Experiments with islet xenografts are in broad agreement with those using skin grafts (Simeonovic *et al.* 1990; Wolf *et al.* 1995). Accordingly, both types of graft survive indefinitely in athymic mice (Ricordi & Lacy 1987) and after treatment with anti-CD4 mAb (Simeonovic *et al.* 1990; Marchetti *et al.* 1995).

*In vitro* studies, described below, indicate that the response of murine T cells to most xenogeneic stimulators is self-MHC-restricted (i.e. indirect xenoresponses). The implication is that *in vivo*, indirect recognition of xenoantigens must be a major mechanism by which murine T cells are sensitized against xenograft antigens. In support of this, experiments in mice have shown that murine class II-restricted CD4+ T cells specific for xenogeneic peptides are sensitized during rejection of rat xenoislets (Murphy *et al.* 1996). In a different model, rat T cells with indirect xenospecificity were sensitized during rejection of MHC-deficient mouse vein grafts (Markmann *et al.* 1994). That these T cells have functional significance has been shown by Gill's group. Rat islet grafts depleted of passenger leucocytes were rapidly rejected in mice (Wolf *et al.* 1995), implying that indirect xenorecognition is capable of mediating rejection as effectively as sensitization via the direct xenorecognition pathway. Passenger leucocyte-depleted grafts in murine allograft models survive indefinitely, consistent with a minor role for indirect allograft responses (Faustman *et al.* 1981; Wolf *et al.* 1995).

Although there is evidence that a delayed-type hypersensitivity reaction may be involved in islet xenograft rejection (Simeonovic *et al.* 1990; Wecker *et al.* 1994), little is known about the precise effector mechanisms involved in either skin or islet rejection. CD4+-dependent humoral responses develop after transplantation but antibody-mediated vascular rejection is not involved (Matsumiya *et al.* 1993) and, whereas CD8+ CTL responses are important in allograft rejection and in the rejection of rat skin grafts (Click *et al.* 1994), their role in rejection of xenografts from phylogenetically distant donors is less clear-cut. Experiments with skin from porcine SLA class I transgenic mice support the conclusion that CD8+ xenoreactive effector cells are less important than their alloreactive counterparts (Auchincloss *et al.* 1990). Similarly, addition of anti-CD8 antibody to anti-CD4 prolongs survival of monkey skin grafts on mice, but anti-CD8 antibody alone has little effect on skin (Pierson *et al.* 1989) or islet xenograft survival (Wolf *et*

*al.* 1995), and SCID mice with established porcine skin grafts retain their grafts even after intravenous administration of purified CD8+ T cells, whereas purified CD4+ T cells initiate rejection (Wecker *et al.* 1994).

Another way in which T cell xenoresponses have been compared to alloresponses is by assessing how easily each can be suppressed with immunosuppressive agents. Auchincloss (1988), in a definitive review of xenotransplantation, analysed all the previous studies of cell-mediated xenograft rejection and came to the conclusion that, 'except for the most closely related species, the more divergent the species combination the harder it is to prolong xenograft survival'. He qualified his statement by pointing out that, because many of the studies included in his analysis had not defined the mechanism by which xenografts were rejected, it was difficult to conclude that cell-mediated responses to xenografts were stronger than those to allografts.

However, in his own studies of skin graft rejection in mice, Auchincloss has shown that cyclosporin A is less effective at prolonging xenograft survival than it is at prolonging allograft survival (Pierson *et al.* 1989). Using rodent models, another group has come to similar conclusions (Thomas *et al.* 1990).

The clear implication for clinical xenotransplantation is that the T cell response to porcine xenografts may be as strong as that to allografts but less easily controlled by conventional immunosuppressive agents.

## *In vitro* T cell xenoresponses

Two factors determine the vigour of 'direct' T cell responses: first, on a cell–cell level, the efficiency of interaction between the crucial molecular ligand pairs necessary for T cell activation; secondly, at the level of the whole organism, the proportion of T cells with TCR that have specificity for intact allo- or xeno-MHC.

In the case of allogeneic stimulators, efficient molecular interactions and a high frequency of specific T cells (Simonsen 1967; Lindahl & Wilson 1977; van Oers *et al.* 1978) provide the basis for significant primary *in vitro* alloresponses and strong *in vivo* cellular responses (Lechler *et al.* 1990). However, it has been established that primary direct xenoresponses are of variable vigour, as illustrated by the following discussion of experiments detailing both murine and human xenoresponses.

## *In vitro* murine T cell xenoresponses

The primary *in vitro* proliferative and CTL responses of mouse T cells to rat stimulatory cells is similar to the response to alloantigens because direct recognition occurs (Wolf *et al.* 1995). This similarity between *in vitro* xeno- and alloresponses is not unusual between species that are phylogenetically close.

However, primary proliferative responses to a variety of other xenostimulators are weak (Bargaza-Gilbert *et al.* 1992; Inamitsu *et al.* 1992) or non-existent (Viguier *et al.* 1987; Moses *et al.* 1990, 1992) and when detected they are usually recipient APC-dependent (Yoshizawa & Yano 1984), suggesting indirect xenorecognition. Many secondary proliferative responses are also dependent on the presence of recipient APC.

Similarly, the frequency of cytotoxic T lymphocytes (CTL) specific for intact HLA class I in naïve mice is undetectable (Holterman & Engelhard 1986) or very low at around 1 in $10^5$ (Kievits *et al.* 1989) and, although the frequency rises after *in vivo* priming with human cells, it remains 10–100 times lower than the frequencies documented against allogeneic targets. Priming with murine cells expressing HLA class I increases the frequency by a factor of 10 (Kievits *et al.* 1989; Le *et al.* 1989), but many of the xenospecific CTL generated in this way are self H-2-restricted (Maryanski *et al.* 1986a,b). Even after *in vivo* priming with human cells, CTL activity against HLA-transfected murine targets following restimulation *in vitro* tends to be H-2-restricted (Engelhard *et al.* 1984), indicating that human cells prime an indirect, far more efficiently than a direct, response.

So, in the absence of a significant direct response, most murine xenoresponses are mediated by indirect xenorecognition. Experiments to establish the molecular basis of weak direct xenorecognition have contributed significantly to the understanding of basic T cell physiology, by helping define the nature and importance of various T cell activation signals.

From this work it is clear that cross-species incompatibilities affecting a number of intercellular interactions are responsible for the failure of murine direct xenoresponses.

For example, T cells from human CD4-transgenic mice demonstrate enhanced xenoresponses to HLA class II-expressing human stimulators, implying that in normal mice, a relatively inefficient interaction between murine CD4 and the membrane-proximal domains of xenogeneic class II molecules contributes to poor direct xenorecognition (Bargaza-Gilbert *et al.* 1992). However, these enhanced xenoresponses still fail to match those seen against allogeneic stimulators, even when high levels of human CD4 expression are achieved on murine T cells. Furthermore, if all other non-cognate interactions are optimized, for instance by using stimulators from HLA DQ-transgenic mice, the direct anti-HLA proliferative xenoresponse is still much reduced compared to the response against an H-2A-expressing stimulator cell.

The implication is that another significant reason for weak xenoresponses is a low frequency of murine T cells with specificity for intact xenogeneic class II molecules, compared to the higher numbers specific for intact allogeneic MHC. In other words, the TCR repertoires of peripheral murine T cells appear biased away from specific interactions with α1–β1 domains of xenogeneic class II molecules. Unfortunately, no studies have directly addressed this question for CD4+ responses in the murine system; in the study quoted above, frequencies of DQ-specific T cells were not measured.

In the anti-class I response, one study, which was designed to address the question of repertoire bias, using hybrid HLA B7/H-2L$^d$ molecules expressed on a murine background, did suggest that this may contribute to weakened xenoresponses (Engelhard *et al.* 1988). Low frequencies of specific anti-HLA class I CTL against all murine stimulators expressing HLA α1–α2 domains, irrespective of the origin of the α3 domain, suggested that even after optimizing all non-cognate interactions, including that between CD8 and the α3 domain, few T cells specific for the α1–α2 domains of HLA class I could be detected.

However, most other studies contradict this result

and indicate that direct xenorecognition of MHC class I-expressing murine cells is weak because of a failure of murine CD8 to interact with the α3 domain of xenogeneic MHC class I (Moses *et al.* 1992). In a series of experiments utilizing murine transfectants expressing HLA A2 or hybrid molecules, naïve CD8+ T cells could recognize the A2 α1–α2 domains efficiently if coexpressed with the murine α3 domain. Efficient CD8–α3 interactions were crucial to the process of priming a direct xenoresponse (Samberg *et al.* 1989). Similarly, the precursor frequency of CTL against stimulators from transgenic mice expressing a hybrid HLA B27 molecule, consisting of the α1 and α2 domains of HLA B 27 and the α3 domain of H-2Kᵈ (Kalinke *et al.* 1990), was the same as that of CTL to wild-type Kᵈ, but 100 times greater than that to wild-type HLA B27. These results imply there is no bias of the TCR repertoire away from xenogeneic class I molecules.

Cross-species incompatibilities between a number of non-cognate accessory molecules have also been described and these undoubtedly contribute to reduced responses to xenogeneic cells. For example, the binding of murine LFA-1 to human ICAM-1 is much reduced compared to intraspecies binding (Johnston *et al.* 1990), although interestingly the reciprocal interaction between murine ICAM-1 and human LFA-1 is more efficient (Cowan *et al.* 1985). Other molecular interactions required for murine T cell activation, including those between LFA-3 and CD2, are also inefficiently supplied by xenogeneic stimulators (Moses *et al.* 1992).

### *In vitro* human T cell xenoresponses

Early *in vitro* experiments addressing the nature of human T cell xenoresponses used mainly murine stimulator cells, although aspects of the response to other species have been documented (Lucas *et al.* 1990). In parallel to the studies with murine T cells, the precise molecular basis of weakened direct xenoresponses has not been fully clarified.

Proliferation and IL-2 production by human CD4+ T cells in primary assays with murine stimulators are reduced or absent compared to primary alloresponses and when responses are seen they are dependent on the presence of human APC (Lindahl & Bach 1976; Alter

& Bach 1990; Haisch *et al.* 1990). Although Alter and Bach's study suggested that human IL-2 or IL-1 could substitute for responder APCs, implying that direct recognition was occurring, the others indicated that APCs were needed to process and present murine xenoantigens, as indicated by inhibition of the response with anti-HLA-DR antibodies or abolition of the response if chloroquine-treated APCs are used. These results suggest that, although direct recognition of murine class II is possible under some circumstances (in the presence of T cell growth factors), in most assays it does not occur and indirect recognition is the predominant route by which human antimurine proliferative responses are mediated. In contrast, human CD8+ T cells can interact functionally with murine class I (Swain *et al.* 1983; Lucas *et al.* 1990; Gress *et al.* 1993), although they are reliant on IL-2 produced by CD4+ T cells to initiate a CTL effector response.

Examination of the CD4+ T cell response to murine class II in isolation from accessory or costimulatory influences, using transfectants expressing high levels of human accessory ligands (Batten *et al.* 1995), has allowed some interesting observations to emerge on why direct xenorecognition is weak. The recognition of H-2E molecules by human T cells is severely impaired by a very weak interaction between human CD4 and the β2 domain of H-2E. This has been confirmed using transfectants expressing MHC class II molecules with hybrid β chains made up of domains from either HLA-DR1 or H-2E (Ramesh *et al.* 1992). In these experiments, the precursor frequency of T cells specific for H-2E is significantly increased, from undetectable levels, by the substitution of the wild-type β2 domain with that from HLA-DR1 and, conversely, the frequency of HLA-DR1-specific cells is significantly impaired by the reverse substitution.

In contrast, the interaction between human CD4 and the β2 domain of H-2A appears quite efficient (Batten *et al.* 1995), confirming observations from studies using murine T cell hybridomas (von Hoegen *et al.* 1989). Substituting the β2 domain of HLA-DR1 with that from H-2A does not impair the observed frequencies of anti-DR1-specific T cells. However, even in this system, where accessory and costimulatory signals to responding T cells were optimized, the precursor frequency of human T cells against wild-type H-2A molecules was still approximately fivefold lower than that against HLA-DR1. This may be evidence that bias of the TCR repertoire, away from interaction with murine class II α1–β1 sequences, contributes to weakened direct xenoresponses. However, the frequencies detected were still of the order of 3 in $10^4$, indicating that, if bias does occur, it is relatively slight.

What these studies suggest is that the lack of a direct xenoresponse against murine APC is likely to be caused by weak CD4 interactions with murine class II only when H-2E is predominantly expressed; when H-2A is predominant, other factors must be responsible. Alter and Bach's results are consistent with this conclusion. They found that the proliferative response of purified human T cells to BALB/c splenocytes was dependent on the presence of responder APC, but IL-1, IL-2 or an undefined 'T cell growth factor' could substitute for these APCs. The authors' interpretation was that the APCs were required to provide these cytokines, implying either that murine APCs could not supply them or that secreted murine homologues were functionless in human T cells (Alter & Bach 1990). However, these possibilities appear to have remained uninvestigated. Another explanation for these results, not considered at the time because the nature of costimulation was largely undetermined, is that human APCs are required to provide bystander costimulation for IL-2 production (Ding & Shevach 1994), a requirement bypassed in the presence of exogenous T cell growth factors (Jenkins 1992).

The implication of this interpretation is that murine APCs fail to supply adequate accessory or costimulatory interactions for human T cell activation. A little evidence exists to support this. Direct recognition, by T cell clones, of some alloantigens transfected on to various cell lines is dependent on the species origin of the cell line (Barbosa *et al.* 1984; Bernabeu *et al.* 1984); this could reflect inefficiency in cross-species provision of accessory signals, although another equally plausible explanation is that the response measured in these experiments depended on a species-specific peptide occupying the antigen-binding groove of the alloantigen (Lombardi *et al.* 1989).

In conflict with the idea that inadequate provision of

costimulation is an important consideration are the studies showing that the accessory and costimulatory signals delivered by some murine stimulators are comparable to those delivered by human cells. Thus HLA-DR-transfected murine L cells can costimulate naïve human T cell alloresponses as effectively as professional human APC (Lombardi *et al.* 1989), a property which has been exploited to allow efficient generation of human T cell clones (Warrens *et al.* 1994). Similarly, HLA class I-transfected L cells can prime an efficient *in vitro* CTL response (Maryanski *et al.* 1985).

Also, where it has been possible to examine the provision of individual non-cognate signals, the results indicate productive interactions. For example, murine B7 (CD80) costimulates the proliferative response of freshly prepared human T cells to both mitogeneic (Freeman *et al.* 1991) and allogeneic (Hargreaves *et al.* 1995) stimuli, and there is a functional interaction between murine ICAM-1 and human LFA-1 (Cowan *et al.* 1985; Achour *et al.* 1986).

These results, by appearing to refute the conclusion that murine cells provide inadequate non-cognate signals for T cell activation, leave unresolved the question about why the overall direct human antimurine response to H-2A-expressing stimulators is weak.

## Human antipig responses

Within the last few years human antipig T cell responses have been examined in some detail, with the realization that porcine organs are probably the most suitable for use in humans. Direct xenorecognition of porcine MHC antigens by human CD4+ T cells is a significant phenomenon. Thus, the primary proliferative and IL-2 responses against porcine stimulators by human PBMC are brisk (Lucas *et al.* 1990; Kirk *et al.* 1992; Murray *et al.* 1994; Rollins *et al.* 1994; Bravery *et al.* 1995; Yamada *et al.* 1995; Dorling *et al.* 1996b). Depletion of APC from human PBMC does not affect proliferation (Yamada *et al.* 1995; Dorling *et al.* 1996b) or IL-2 production (Lucas *et al.* 1990), and responses are inhibited by monoclonal antibodies specific for SLA class II (Kirk *et al.* 1993; Yamada *et al.* 1995; Dorling *et al.* 1996b), confirming true direct xenorecognition. In mixed populations of purified T cells, proliferation is predominantly by CD4+, SLA-DR-specific human T cells (Yamada *et al.* 1995; Dorling *et al.* 1996b), despite the fact that humans have a high precursor frequency of T cells specific for SLA-DQ. A similar discrepancy between high frequencies of anti-DQ-specific T cells and a relatively minor role in rejection responses has been documented in human alloresponse (Merkenschlager *et al.* 1991).

Experiments using porcine dendritic cell or PBMC stimulators suggest that CD8+ cells play no part in primary direct proliferative responses, as antibodies against SLA class I fail to inhibit proliferation despite high levels of expression of porcine MHC class I on these cells (Kirk *et al.* 1992; Yamada *et al.* 1995; Dorling *et al.* 1996c) and purified CD8+ T cells do not proliferate (Satake *et al.* 1996). However, contradictory results have been generated when porcine endothelial cells have been used as stimulators; purified CD8+ T cells do mount significant primary proliferative responses (Murray *et al.* 1994; Rollins *et al.* 1994; Bravery *et al.* 1995) and produce IL-2 (Bravery *et al.* 1995) and these are inhibited by anti-SLA class I antibodies (Murray *et al.* 1994; Rollins *et al.* 1994), indicating direct xenorecognition of porcine MHC class I rather than non-specific proliferation. The reason why porcine endothelial cells, but not PBMC or dendritic cells, should stimulate CD8+-mediated proliferation is not clear; all three express functional porcine B7 (Murray *et al.* 1994; Bravery *et al.* 1995; Dorling *et al.* 1996c) and support a B7-dependent CD4+ response (Bravery *et al.* 1995; Dorling *et al.* 1996b; Restifo *et al.* 1996), implying that inadequate provision of costimulatory signals is not to blame. The implication of one study, which detected proliferation by CD8+ T cells using porcine PBMC stimulators only if the cultures were supplemented with supernatant from allogeneic MLRs (Satake *et al.* 1996), is that porcine endothelial cells supply signals that enable CD8+ cells to proliferate independently from CD4+ T cells. These signals could be quantitatively or qualitatively different to those supplied by dendritic cells and PBMC, but the likely effect of them is to enable CD8+ cells to produce sufficient IL-2 to support autocrine proliferation.

Despite being unable to support a proliferative response, porcine PBMC can prime CD8+ T cell cyto-toxic responses from human PBMC bulk cultures (Yamada *et al.* 1995; Chan & Auchincloss 1996; Satake *et al.* 1996) that are haplotype-specific (Yamada *et al.* 1996), inhibited by anti-CD8 monoclonal antibodies (Chan & Auchincloss 1996; Yamada *et al.* 1996) and SLA class I-specific (Satake *et al.* 1996), supporting the conclusion of the proliferative studies that direct recognition of porcine class I molecules is efficient. CD4+ T cell, SLA class II-specific killing (Yamada *et al.* 1995, 1996) and non-classical MHC molecule-specific killing (Seebach *et al.* 1996) have also been described.

The implication of such prominent and easily detected direct T cell xenoresponses is that the sum total of intercellular molecular interactions between human T cells and porcine stimulators is efficient and adequate to initiate T cell activation (see Fig. 6.6). This is supported by studies that show similar proliferation and IL-2 production in antipig and allogeneic cultures (Murray *et al.* 1994; Bravery *et al.* 1995) and by studies showing that the precursor frequency of human IL-2-secreting T cells with direct antipig specificity is similar to the frequencies of T cells with direct allospecificity (Kumagai-Braesch *et al.* 1993; Murray *et al.* 1994; Dorling *et al.* 1996b).

Results of experiments to examine the provision of non-cognate costimulatory and accessory molecular signals by porcine APC to human T cells also support this general conclusion. We and others have found that porcine stimulators are as efficient as human APC at providing non-cognate interactions to support mitogenic T cell proliferation (Dorling *et al.* 1996c) and IL-2 production (Murray *et al.* 1994; Rollins *et al.* 1994) and that porcine B7 is capable of costimulating human T cell proliferative responses (Murray *et al.* 1994; Dorling *et al.* 1996c; Restifo *et al.* 1996). Functional interactions between human LFA-1 and porcine ICAM (Pleass *et al.* 1994; Rollins *et al.* 1994), human VLA-4 and porcine VCAM (Pleass *et al.* 1994; Mueller *et al.* 1995; Dorling *et al.* 1996a) and human CD2 and porcine LFA-3 (Murray *et al.* 1994; Rollins *et al.* 1994) have also been documented. Each of these interactions is a potential target for strategies to promote xenograft survival.

However, there does appears to be a relative weakness of CD4+ T cell direct antiporcine xenoresponse when compared formally with direct alloresponses. We have found that at high responder : stimulator ratios, 5–10 times more porcine dendritic cells are required to stimulate T cell proliferative responses equivalent to those stimulated by allogeneic dendritic cells. Using identical murine DAP.3 cell populations transfected either with allogeneic HLA-DR1 or xenogeneic SLA-DRc, we have documented a relative inefficiency in the interaction between human CD4+ T cells and porcine class II molecules (Dorling *et al.* 1996c), which could partially explain this phenomenon.

Although probably without any practical relevance, because the human antiporcine direct xenoresponse is appreciable despite this weakness, it is of interest that these findings are reminiscent of the inefficient interactions between human and murine cells and they illustrate the general point that intercellular signals tend to be less efficient across species barriers.

## Strength of 'indirect' T cell responses

In many allograft models, the indirect pathway makes no contribution to graft rejection. For example, depleting passenger leucocytes from murine islet allografts (Faustman *et al.* 1981) or thyroid grafts (Lafferty *et al.* 1976; Iwai *et al.* 1989) prior to transplantation prevents direct alloresponses and leads to long-term graft survival; the indirect pathway does not mediate rejection. Similarly, passenger leucocyte-depleted rat kidney allografts avoid rejection by direct allorecognition and enjoy long-term survival in some strains (Batchelor *et al.* 1979; Welsh *et al.* 1979; Lechler & Batchelor 1982b).

However, evidence from other allograft models indicates a significant role for indirect responses in graft rejection. The earliest indication of this came from rat allograft models. In some strains, acute rejection of kidney allografts occurred in spite of manoeuvres to prevent or inhibit the direct pathway of allorecognition (Hart *et al.* 1980; Lechler & Batchelor 1982a). In other strains, grafts survived but suffered a chronic low-grade graft-specific immune response (Hewitt *et al.* 1990). In other models, depletion of passenger leucocytes does not always result in long-term survival of grafts (Silvers *et al.* 1982, 1984; La Rosa & Talmage 1983, 1985; Ketchum *et al.* 1992). The implication of all these studies was that indirect allorecognition could initiate graft rejection.

Evidence in support of this conclusion comes from congenic grafts in murine and porcine models. These grafts were quickly rejected, despite differing only at minor antigeniec loci (Silvers *et al.* 1982; Sundt *et al.* 1989; Gracie *et al.* 1990). This implied that presentation of alloantigens by donor APCs which shared MHC molecules with the recipient could initiate rejection through activation of self-MHC-restricted T cells. A final piece of evidence came from experiments placing skin grafts from MHC class I and II 'knockout' mice on to normal mice. The grafts, which contained no expressed donor MHC molecules, were rejected promptly by CD4+ T cells (Dierich *et al.* 1993; Grusby *et al.* 1993). This implied that alloresponsive T cells were activated by self APCs.

Immunization with soluble MHC molecules leads to the development of self-restricted alloreactive T cells (Dalchau *et al.* 1992) and, during an allograft response, T cells primed by the indirect pathway appear in lymph nodes (Benichou *et al.* 1992; Fangmann *et al.* 1992a), implying that activation of indirect alloresponsive T cells occurs physiologically during graft rejection.

That these cells are of any functional importance has been recently shown by two groups. Priming the indirect pathway in naïve rats with soluble MHC class I or II molecules leads to accelerated rejection of skin and solid organ grafts (Dalchau *et al.* 1992; Fangmann *et al.* 1992b; Benham *et al.* 1995) and the CD4+ T cell-mediated rejection of skin grafts from MHC class II knockout mice involves MHC class II self-restricted recognition of alloantigens (Auchincloss *et al.* 1993; Lee *et al.* 1994). These results have confirmed that the indirect pathway is an important route of allosensitization which, like the direct pathway, can initiate graft rejection.

*In vitro*, it is clear that T cells which recognize processed alloantigen in a self MHC class II-restricted manner are part of the normal repertoire in rats (Parker *et al.* 1992) and in humans (Liu *et al.* 1992). Several studies have documented responder APC-dependent proliferation in the primary MLR (Via *et al.* 1990;

Sundt *et al.* 1992; Clerici *et al.* 1993). However, true indirect recognition in these experiments was never firmly established and alternative explanations for responder APC dependence, such as transcostimulation of a direct response (Liu & Janeway 1992), were not excluded.

In mice, indirect presentation of alloantigens to H-2A-restricted CD4+ T cells has been shown to provide help for a primary CD8+ T cell-mediated proliferative and CTL response (Rock *et al.* 1983; Weinberger *et al.* 1983). These observations were made using MHC class I-mismatched class II-matched responder–stimulator combinations. They showed that indirect recognition of the class I alloantigen in the context of the shared class II molecules when the stimulator cell was the allogeneic class I-mismatched cell was more efficient than when the class I alloantigen was internalized, processed and presented by the responder APC. In the first situation, the class I molecule was displayed in peptidic form as a naturally processed endogenous protein. Furthermore, proliferation by CD4+ T cells played no part in these primary responses and CD4+ Th cells were needed only when stimulator numbers were limiting, to provide IL-2 required for CTL induction.

True primary indirect alloresponses are difficult to detect *in vitro* for two reasons. First, they are usually obscured by stronger direct responses (Egner *et al.* 1993). Secondly, the precursor frequency of T cells specific for processed alloantigen is either undetectable or very low. Although the frequency increases in a secondary MLR (Liu *et al.* 1993) it remains ~100 times lower than that of T cells activated by direct allorecognition.

In xenoresponses, studies using avascular skin and islet grafts, which were mentioned in an earlier section, have clearly established that CD4+ T lymphocytes with indirect xenospecificity can mediate graft rejection and that T cell-mediated xenograft rejection is often as vigorous, or more so, than T cell-mediated allograft rejection. Along with the work showing that conventional immunosuppressive agents may be less effective at prolonging xenograft than allograft survival, these results suggest that indirect xenoresponses may be stronger than direct alloresponses.

Our studies support this conclusion. We have demonstrated that HLA-DR-restricted human CD4+ T cells mount substantial primary proliferative responses after indirect recognition of porcine antigens (Dorling *et al.* 1996b,d). The precursor frequency of IL-2-producing pig-specific self-MHC-restricted T cells, lying between $2 \times 10^4$ and $1.5 \times 10^5$, is significantly higher than the very low or undetectable frequencies documented against processed alloantigen (Liu *et al.* 1992).

Several explanations could account for strong indirect xenoresponses, two of which would advocate that indirect xenorecognition was qualitatively different to indirect allorecognition. First, the presence of xenospecific B cells, responsible for production of XNA, might act as efficient APCs for porcine antigens. The unique antigen-concentrating abilities of antigen-specific B cells have been well documented (Rock *et al.* 1984; Sallusto & Lanzavecchia 1994). Such efficient antigen presentation could contribute significantly to the strength of indirect responses. Alternatively, in a similar vein, the presence of XNA could contribute to antigen uptake and processing by conventional FcR-expressing APC. The second possibility is that T cell xenoresponses could be primed by exposure to antigens shared between environmental pathogens and xenostimulator populations or by exposure to antigens present within food. Oral priming after ingestion of antigens has been documented in some animal models (Liu & MacPherson 1993). A third possibility is that indirect xenoresponses may be stronger than allo-responses purely because of the greater number of xenoantigens compared to alloantigens. The basis for this would be the high degree of protein polymorphisms across different species compared to the small degree of polymorphism between individuals of the same species.

It is also clear from our studies that the third possibility is most likely. Pig-specific B cells are not needed for antigen processing and priming is not required, as naïve T cells, from umbilical cord specimens, mount significant indirect responses. The indirect xenoresponse to porcine antigens appears inherently strong because of the very large number of peptides processed from pig proteins by human APC.

## Conclusions drawn from T cell xenoresponses

Direct recognition of certain xenogeneic stimulator populations by human and murine T cells appears to be weak because of a number of cross-species disparities in the provision of T cell activation signals and variations in the frequency of xenogeneic MHC-specific T cells. However, direct recognition of pig stimulators by human T cells is efficient and results in significant primary proliferative and CTL responses, comparable in strength to primary alloresponses.

However, human HLA-DR-restricted T cells also mount significant indirect proliferative responses to processed porcine xenoantigens and, with the results of studies in murine models in mind, these are likely to play a major part in initiating acute cellular rejection *in vivo*. The available evidence therefore suggests that a formidable T cell response to porcine antigens will develop in recipients of pig organs.

## Prospects for clinical xenotransplantation

There is a pressing need for a solution to the problem of allograft shortage and xenotransplantation of pig organs is now a realistic possibility. It is widely predicted that the use of organs from transgenic pigs expressing human regulators of complement activity (Fodor *et al.* 1994; Cozzi & White 1995; Rosengard *et al.* 1995), coupled with strategies for the depletion of xenoreactive natural antibodies, will circumvent the problem of HAR, a process responsible for the immediate destruction of vascularized xenografts (Anonymous 1991; Clipstone 1992). Clinical evaluation of transgenic pig organs is expected in the near future, once the fears about viral transmisson have been addressed (Miller 1992; Parham 1992), and, although additional approaches, such as targeting coagulation mechanisms (Parker *et al.* 1996b; Dorling & Lechler 1994), may be required eventually for complete control of vascular rejection, successful trials of these organs will represent a major advance towards the prospect of 'routine' xenotransplantation.

However, it is evident that a number of other immunological hurdles, beyond HAR, will need to be overcome if the ultimate goal of long-term xenograft survival is to be achieved. The emerging evidence for the importance of DXR is important because natural killer cells and IgG XNA have so far been largely ignored in the strategies to prevent HAR and promote xenograft survival. None of the proposed methods to target IgM XNA or the gal$\alpha$(1–3) gal epitope, for instance, will be effective against IgG XNA, because most of them are specific for epitopes other than gal$\alpha$(1–3) gal (Cooke *et al.* 1995). The implication is that specific strategies to target both IgG and natural killer cells may be required to prevent DXR.

Similarly, for cellular responses, the relative prominence of the indirect antipig response may have important implications *in vivo*. Indirect responses are less easily suppressed by cyclosporin A *in vitro* (Johansson Borg *et al.* 1996), suggesting that the level of immunosuppression required to prevent T cell rejection of pig xenografts may be higher than that currently used routinely for allografts. Evidence from animal models of xenotransplantation supports this prediction (Auchincloss 1988).

Notwithstanding that newer pharmacological agents may be more potent than those currently in use (Thomas *et al.* 1990; Johansson Borg *et al.* 1996), there is an anxiety that systemic immunosuppressive regimes may be relatively ineffective at preventing acute xenograft rejection in clinical practice. In addition to this worry there are other strong incentives to identify and develop alternative approaches of controlling cellular xenoresponses.

So, although modern immunosuppressive regimes are successful at promoting short-term allograft survival, they have made little impact on long-term survival of allografts and are ineffective at preventing chronic rejection, a problem that may be more prominent in xenografts than allografts. Secondly, the two major complications of systemic immunosuppressives —infection and neoplasia—may both be more serious in xenograft recipients needing high levels of maintenance immunosuppression. Finally, the risk of transmission of zoonoses from xenografts (Chapman *et al.* 1995; Taylor 1995) may be greatly exacerbated in the context of generalized immunosuppression.

However, xenografts offer opportunities to develop

graft-specific immunosuppression strategies not possible in allotransplantation and these could be exploited to deal with multiple aspects of recipient immune responses. In this context, targeting and inducing tolerance in xenospecific T cells may be easier to achieve than with allospecific cells. For example, pig-specific monoclonal antibody therapy, targeting molecules involved in T cell activation, may be an effective means of inducing tolerance in graft-reactive T cells.

## References

Achour, A., Begue, B., Gomard, E. *et al.* (1986) Specific lysis of murine cells expressing HLA molecules by allospecific human and murine H-2-restricted anti-HLA T killer lymphocytes. *European Journal of Immunology* 16, 597–604.

Advisory Group on the Ethics of Xenotransplantation (1997) *Animal Tissue into Humans*. Stationery Office, London.

Akami, T., Arakawa, K., Okamoto, M. *et al.* (1993) The role of human CD59 in discordant xenotransplantation between humans and non-primates. *Transplantation Proceedings* 25, 394–395.

Alexandre, G.P.J., Gianello, P., Latinne, D. *et al.* (1989) Plasmapheresis and splenectomy in experimental renal transplantation. In: *Xenograft 25* (ed. M.A. Hardy), pp. 259–266. Elsevier Science Publishers, New York.

Alexandre, G.P.J., Latinne, D., Gianello, P. & Squifflet, J.P. (1991) Pre-formed cytotoxic antibodies and ABO-incompatible grafts. *Clinical Transplantation* 5, 583–594.

Alter, B.J. & Bach, F.H. (1990) Cellular basis of the proliferative response of human T-cells to mouse xenoantigens. *Journal of Experimental Medicine* 171, 333–338.

Anonymous. (1991) The thymus at thirty. *Lancet* 338, 788–789.

Auchincloss, H. (1988) Xenogeneic transplantation. *Transplantation* 46, 1–20.

Auchincloss, H., Moses, R., Sundt, T. *et al.* (1990) Xenograft rejection of class I-expressing transgenic skin is CD4 dependent and CD8 independent. *Transplantation Proceedings* 22, 2335–2336.

Auchincloss, H., Lee, R., Shea, S. *et al.* (1993) The role of 'indirect' recognition in initiating rejection of skin grafts from major histocompatibility complex class II-deficient mice. *Proceedings of the National Academy of Sciences (USA)* 90, 3373–3377.

Bach, F.H. (1991) Revisiting a challenge in transplantation: discordant xenografting. *Human Immunology* 30, 262–269.

Bach, F.H., Turman, M.A., Vercellotti, G.M., Platt, J.L. & Dalmasso, A.P. (1991) Accommodation: a working paradigm for progressing toward clinical discordant xenografting. *Transplantation Proceedings* 23, 205–207.

Bach, F.H., Blakely, M.L., Van der Werf, M. *et al.* (1993) Discordant xenografting: a working model of problems and issues. *Xeno* 1, 8–16.

Bach, F.H., Winkler, H., Ferran, C., Hancock, W.W. & Robson, S.C. (1996) Delayed xenograft rejection. *Immunology Today* 17, 379–384.

Bach, F.H., Hancock, W.W. & Ferran, C. (1997a) Protective genes expressed in endothelial cells: a regulatory response to injury. *Immunology Today* 18, 483–486.

Bach, F.H., Ferran, C., Hechenleitner, P. *et al.* (1997b) Accommodation of vascularized xenografts: expression of 'protective genes' by donor endothelial cells in a host Th2 cytokine environment. *Nature Medicine* 3, 196–204.

Bailey, L.L., Nehtseu-Cannarella, S.L., Concepcion, W. & Joley, W.B. (1985) Baboon to human cardiac xenotransplantation in a neonate. *Journal of the American Medical Association* 254, 3321.

Balla, G., Jacob, H.S., Balla, J. *et al.* (1992) Ferritin: a cytoprotective antioxidant stratagem of endothelium. *Journal of Biological Chemistry* 267, 18148–18153.

Barbosa, J.A., Mentzer, S.J., Minowada, G. *et al.* (1984) Recognition of HLA A2 and B7 antigens by cloned cytotoxic T lymphocytes after gene transfer into human and monkey but not mouse cells. *Proceedings of the National Academy of Sciences (USA)* 81, 7549–7553.

Bargaza-Gilbert, E., Grass, D., Lawrence, S.K. *et al.* (1992) Species specificity and augmentation of responses to class II major histocompatibility complex molecules in human CD4 transgenic mice. *Journal of Experimental Medicine* 175, 1707–1715.

Batchelor, J.R., Welsh, K.I., Maynard, A. & Burgos, H. (1979) Failure of long surviving, passively enhanced kidney allografts to provoke T-dependent alloimmunity 1. Retransplantation of (AS×Aug) F1 kidneys into secondary AS recipients. *Journal of Experimental Medicine* 150, 455–464.

Batten, P., Heaton, T., Fuller-Espie, S. & Lechler, R.I. (1995) Human anti-mouse xenorecognition. Provision of noncognate interactions reveals the plasticity of the T cell repertoire. *Journal of Immunology* 155, 1057–1065.

Batten, P., Yacoub, M.H. & Rose, M.L. (1996) Effect of human cytokines (IFNγ, TNF-α, IL-1β, IL-4) on porcine endothelial cells: induction of MHC and adhesion molecules and functional significance of these changes. *Immunology* 87, 127–133.

Benham, A.M., Sawyer, G.J. & Fabre, J.W. (1995) Indirect T cell allorecognition of donor antigens contributes to the rejection of vascularized kidney allografts. *Transplantation* 59, 1028–1032.

Benichou, G., Takizawa, P.A., Olson, C.A., McMillan, M. &

Sercarz, E.E. (1992) Donor MHC peptides are presented by recipient MHC molecules during graft rejection. *Journal of Experimental Medicine* 175, 305–308.

Bernabeu, C., Maziarz, R., Spits, H. *et al.* (1984) Co-expression of the human HLA-A2 or HLA-B7 heavy chain gene and human $\beta_2$-microglobulin gene in L-cells. *Journal of Immunology* 133, 3188–3194.

Bianchi, G., Sironi, M., Ghibaudi, E. *et al.* (1993) Migration of natural killer cells across endothelial cell monolayers. *Journal of Immunology* 151, 5135–5144.

Blakely, M.L., Van der Werf, W.J., Berndt, M.C. *et al.* (1994) Activation of graft endothelial and mononuclear cells during discordant xenograft rejection. *Transplantation* 58, 1059–1066.

Borche, L., Thibaudeau, K., Navenot, J.M. & Blanchard, D. (1994) Cytolytic effect of human anti-Gal IgM and complement on porcine endothelial cells: a kinetic analysis. *Xenotransplantation* 1, 125–131.

Bravery, C.A., Batten, P., Yacoub, M.H. & Rose, M.L. (1995) Direct recognition of SLA- and HLA-like class II antigens on porcine endothelium by human T cells results in T cell activation and release of interleukin-2. *Transplantation* 60, 1024–1033.

Breitkreuz, A., Ulrichs, K., Eckstein, V. & Müller-Ruchholtz, W. (1993) Long term suppression of natural and graft induced xenophile antibodies by short term antigen-cyclophosphamide treatment. *Transplantation Proceedings* 25, 416–418.

Brewer, R.J., Del Rio, M.J., Roslin, M.S. *et al.* (1993) Depletion of preformed antibody in primates for discordant xenotransplantation by continuous donor organ plasma perfusion. *Transplantation Proceedings* 25, 385–386.

Brouard, S., Blancho, G., Moreau, A. *et al.* (1998) Long-term survival of hamster-to-rat cardiac xenografts in the absence of a Th2 shift. *Transplantation* 65, 1555–1563.

Burdick, J.F. & Fair, J.H. (1994) Xenoperfusion: the pig liver as a bridge. *Xeno* 2, 3–5.

Byrne, G.W., McCurry, K.R., Kagan, D. *et al.* (1995) Protection of xenogeneic cardiac endothelium from human complement by expression of CD59 or DAF in transgenic mice. *Transplantation* 60, 1149–1156.

Byrne, G.W., McCurry, K.R., Martin, M.J. *et al.* (1997) Transgenic pigs expressing human CD59 and decay-accelerating factor produce an intrinsic barrier to complement-mediated damage. *Transplantation* 63, 149–155.

Calne, R.Y. (1970) Organ transplantation between widely disparate species. *Transplantation Proceedings* 2, 550–553.

Chan, D.V. & Auchincloss, H. (1996) Human anti-pig cell-mediated cytotoxicity *in vitro* involves non-T as well as T cell components. *Xenotransplantation* 3, 158–165.

Chapman, L.E., Folks, T.M., Salomon, D.R. *et al.* (1995) Xenotransplantation and xenogeneic infections. *New England Journal of Medicine* 333, 1498–1501.

Chopek, M.W., Simmons, R.L. & Platt, J.L. (1987) ABO-incompatible kidney transplantation: initial immunopathologic evaluation. *Transplantation Proceedings* 19, 4553–4557.

Clerici, M., DePalma, L., Rollides, E., Baker, R. & Shearer, G.M. (1993) Analysis of T helper and antigen-presenting cell functions in cord blood and peripheral blood leukocytes from healthy children of different ages. *Journal of Clinical Investigations* 91, 2829–2836.

Click, R.E., Weisberg, D., White, J., Reicenbach, D. & Jamieson, S.W. (1994) Rejection of rat skin xenografts by either murine CD4 or CD8 T cells. *Transplantation* 58, 1020–1026.

Clipstone, N.A.C.G. (1992) Identification of calcineurin as a key signalling enzyme in T-lymphocyte activation. *Nature* 357, 695–697.

Collins, B.H., Parker, W. & Platt, J.L. (1994) Characterization of porcine endothelial cell determinants recognized by human natural antibodies. *Xenotransplantation* 1, 36–46.

Cooke, S.P., Hederer, R.A., Pearson, J.D. & Savage, C.O.S. (1995) Characterization of human IgG-binding xenoantigens expressed by porcine aortic endothelial cells. *Transplantation* 60, 1274–1284.

Cooper, D.K.C. (1993) Xenografting: how great is the clinical need? *Xeno* 1, 25–26.

Cooper, D.K.C., Ye, Y., Niekrasz, M. *et al.* (1993) Specific intravenous carbohydrate therapy. A new concept in inhibiting antibody-mediated rejection—experience with ABO-incompatible cardiac allografting in the baboon. *Transplantation* 56, 769–777.

Cooper, D.K.C., Koren, E. & Oriol, R. (1996) Manipulation of the anti-αgal antibody-αgal epitope system in experimental discordant xenotransplantation. *Xenotransplantation* 3, 102–111.

Cooper, J.T., Stroka, D.M., Brostjan, C. *et al.* (1996) A20 blocks endothelial cell activation through a NF-kappaB-dependent mechanism. *Journal of Biological Chemistry* 271, 18068–18073.

Cotterell, A.H., Collins, B.H., Parker, W., Harland, R.C. & Platt, J.L. (1995) The humoral immune response in human following cross-perfusion of porcine organs. *Transplantation* 60, 861–868.

Cowan, E.P., Coligan, J.E. & Biddison, W.E. (1985) Human cytotoxic T-lymphocyte recognition of an HLA A3 gene product expressed on murine L-cells: the only human gene product required on the target cells for lysis is the class I heavy chain. *Proceedings of the National Academy of Sciences (USA)* 82, 4490–4494.

Cozzi, E. & White, D.J.G. (1995) The generation of transgenic pigs as potential organ donors for humans. *Nature Medicine* 1, 964–966.

Dalchau, R., Fangmann, J. & Fabre, J.W. (1992) Allorecognition of isolated, denatured chains of class I and class II MHC molecules. Evidence for an important role for indirect allorecognition in transplantation. *European Journal of Immunology* **22**, 669–677.

Dalmasso, A.P. & Platt, J.L. (1993) Prevention of complement-mediated activation of xenogeneic endothelial cells in an *in vitro* model of xenograft hyperacute rejection by C1 inhibitor. *Transplantation* **56**, 1171–1176.

Dalmasso, A.P., Vercellotti, G.M., Platt, J.L. & Bach, F.H. (1991) Inhibition of complement-mediated endothelial cell cytotoxicity by decay-accelerating factor. *Transplantation* **52**, 530–533.

d'Apice, A.J. & Pearse, M.J. (1996) Xenotransplantation. In: *Transplantation Biology; Cellular and Molecular Aspects* (eds N.L. Tilney, T.B. Strom & L.C. Paul), pp. 701–716. Lippincott-Raven, Philadelphia.

De Martin, R., Vanhove, B., Cheng, Q. *et al.* (1993) Cytokine-inducible expression in endothelial cells of an IκBα-like gene is regulated by NFκB. *EMBO Journal* **12**, 2773–2779.

Diamond, L.E., McCurry, K.R., Martin, M.J. *et al.* (1996) Characterization of transgenic pigs expressing functionally active human CD59 on cardiac endothelium. *Transplantation* **61**, 1241–1249.

Dierich, A., Chan, S.H., Benoist, C. & Mathis, D. (1993) Graft rejection by T cells not restricted by conventional major histocompatibility molecules. *European Journal of Immunology* **23**, 2725–2728.

Ding, L. & Shevach, E.M. (1994) Activation of CD4+ T cells by delivery of the B7 costimulatory signal on bystander antigen-presenting cells (transcostimulation). *European Journal of Immunology* **24**, 859–866.

Dorling, A. & Lechler, R.I. (1994) Prospects for xenografting. *Current Opinion in Immunology* **6**, 765–769.

Dorling, A. & Lechler, R.I. (1996) The passenger leukocyte, dendritic cell and antigen-presenting cells (APC). In: *Transplantation Biology; Cellular and Molecular Aspects* (eds N.L. Tilney, T.B. Strom & L.C. Paul), pp. 355–379. Lippincott-Raven, Philadelphia.

Dorling, A. & Lechler, R.I. (1997) Glaxo/MRS Young Investigator Prize. Xenotransplantation: immune barriers beyond hyperacute rejection. *Clinical Science* **93**, 493–505.

Dorling, A., Stocker, C., Tsao, T., Haskard, D.O. & Lechler, R.I. (1996a) *In vitro* accommodation of immortalized porcine endothelial cells: resistance to complement mediated lysis and down-regulation of VCAM expression induced by low concentrations of polyclonal human IgG antipig antibodies. *Transplantation* **62**, 1127–1136.

Dorling, A., Lombardi, G., Binns, R. & Lechler, R.I. (1996b) Detection of primary direct and indirect human anti-porcine T cell responses using a porcine dendritic cell population. *European Journal of Immunology* **26**, 1378–1387.

Dorling, A., Binns, R. & Lechler, R.I. (1996c) Cellular xenoresponses: although vigorous, direct human T cell anti-pig primary xenoresponses are significantly weaker than equivalent alloresponses. *Xenotransplantation* **3**, 149–157.

Dorling, A., Binns, R. & Lechler, R.I. (1996d) Cellular xenoresponses: observation of significant primary indirect human T cell anti-pig xenoresponses using co-stimulator-deficient or SLA class II-negative porcine stimulators. *Xenotransplantation* **3**, 112–119.

Dorling, A., Delikouras, A., Nohadani, A.M., Polak, J. & Lechler, R.I. (1998) *In vitro* accommodation of porcine endothelial cells by low dose human anti-pig antibody: reduced binding of human lymphocytes by accommodated cells associated with increased nitric oxide production. *Xenotransplantation* **5**, 84–92.

Egner, W., Andreesen, R. & Hart, D.N. (1993) Allostimulatory cells in fresh human blood: heterogeneity in antigen-presenting cell populations. *Transplantation* **56**, 945–950.

Engelhard, V.H., Powers, G.A., Moore, L.C., Holterman, M.J. & Correa-Freire, M.C. (1984) Cytotoxic T lymphocyte recognition of HLA-A/B antigens introduced into EL4 cells by liposome fusion. *Journal of Immunology* **132**, 76–80.

Engelhard, V.H., Le, A.X.T. & Holterman, M.J. (1988) Species-specific structural differences in the α1 and α2 domains determine the frequency of murine cytotoxic T cell precursors stimulated by human and murine class I molecules. *Journal of Immunology* **141**, 1835–1839.

Evans, R.W., Orians, C.E. & Ascher, N.L. (1992) The potential supply of organ donors. An assessment of the efficacy of organ procurement efforts in the United States. *Journal of the American Medical Association* **267**, 239–246.

Fangmann, J., Dalchau, R., Sawyer, G.J., Priestly, C.A. & Fabre, J.W. (1992a) T cell recognition of donor major histocompatibility complex class I peptides during allograft rejection. *European Journal of Immunology* **22**, 1525–1530.

Fangmann, J., Dalchau, R. & Fabre, J.W. (1992b) Rejection of skin allografts by indirect allorecognition of donor class I major histocompatibility complex products. *Journal of Experimental Medicine* **175**, 1521–1529.

Faustman, D., Hauptfeld, V., Lacy, P. & Davie, J. (1981) Prolongation of murine islet allograft survival by pretreatment of islets with antibody directed to Ia determinants. *Proceedings of the National Academy of Sciences (USA)* **78**, 5156–5159.

Ferran, C., Stroka, D.M., Badrichani, A.Z. *et al.* (1998) A20 inhibits NF-kappaB activation in endothelial cells without sensitizing to tumor necrosis factor-mediated apoptosis. *Blood* **91**, 2249–2258.

Figueroa, J., Fuad, S.A., Kmjummen, B.D., Platt, J.L. & Bach, F.H. (1993) Suppression of synthesis of natural antibodies by mycophenolate mofetil (RS-61443). *Transplantation* **55**, 1371–1374.

Fischel, R.J., Bolman, R.M., Platt, J.L. *et al.* (1990) Removal of IgM anti-endothelial antibodies results in prolonged cardiac xenograft survival. *Transplantation Proceedings* **22**, 1077–1078.

Fischel, R.J., Platt, J.L., Matas, A.J. *et al.* (1991) Prolonged survival of a discordant cardiac xenograft in a rhesus monkey. *Transplantation Proceedings* **23**, 589–590.

Fodor, W.L., Williams, B.L., Matis, L.A. *et al.* (1994) Expression of a functional human complement inhibitor in a transgenic pig as a model for the prevention of xenogeneic hyperacute organ rejection. *Proceedings the National Academy of Sciences (USA)* **91**, 11153–11157.

Forty, J., Hasan, R., Lacy, N., White, D.J.G. & Wallwork, J. (1992) Perfusion of rabbit hearts with human blood results in immediate graft thrombosis, which is temporally distinct from hyperacute rejection. *Transplantation Proceedings* **24**, 610–611.

Freeman, G.J., Gray, G.S., Gimmi, C.D. *et al.* (1991) Structure, expression and T cell costimulatory activity of the murine homologue of the human B lymphocyte activation antigen B7. *Journal of Experimental Medicine* **174**, 625–631.

Galili, U. (1993) Interaction of the natural anti-gal antibody with α-galactosyl epitopes: a major obstacle for xenotransplantation in humans. *Immunology Today* **14**, 480–482.

Galili, U., Shobet, S., Kobrin, E., Stults, C. & Macjer, B. (1988) Man, apes and old world monkeys differ from other mammals in the expression of α-galactosyl epitopes on nucleated cells. *Journal of Biological Chemistry* **263**, 17755–17762.

Gambiez, L., Salanne, E., Chereau, C. *et al.* (1992) The role of natural IgM in the hyperacute rejection of discordant heart xenografts. *Transplantation* **54**, 577–583.

Geller, R.L., Bach, F.H., Turman, M.A., Casali, P. & Platt, J.L. (1993) Evidence that polyreactive antibodies are deposited in rejected discordant xenografts. *Transplantation* **55**, 168–172.

Germain, R.N. (1994) MHC-dependent antigen processing and peptide presentation: providing ligands for T lymphocyte activation. *Cell* **76**, 287–299.

Good, A.H., Cooper, D.K.C., Malcolm, A.J. *et al.* (1992) Identification of carbohydrate structures that bind human anti-porcine antibodies: implications for discordant xenografting in humans. *Transplantation Proceedings* **24**, 559.

Goodman, D.J., Von Albertini, M., Willson, A., Millan, M.T.

& Bach, F.H. (1996) Direct activation of porcine endothelial cells by human natural killer cells. *Transplantation* **61**, 763–771.

Gore, S. (1993) The shortage of donor organs: whither, not whether. *Xeno* **1**, 23–24.

Gracie, J.A., Bolton, E.M., Porteous, C. & Bradley, J.A. (1990) T cell requirements for the rejection of renal allografts bearing an isolated class I MHC disparity. *Journal of Experimental Medicine* **172**, 1547–1557.

Gress, R.E., Katz, S.I. & Lucas, P.J. (1993) Human CD8+ xenoreactive T cells mediate tissue injury *in vivo*. *Transplantation* **56**, 484–486.

Grusby, M.J., Auchincloss, H., Lee, R. *et al.* (1993) Mice lacking major histocompatibility complex class I and II molecules. *Proceedings of the National Academy of Sciences (USA)* **90**, 3913–3917.

Haisch, C.E., Lodge, P.A., Huber, S.A. & Thomas, F.T. (1990) *In vitro* human versus murine xenogeneic reactions. *Transplantation* **50**, 528–530.

Harding, F.A. & Allison, J.P. (1993) CD28–B7 Interactions allow the induction of CD8+ cytotoxic T lymphocytes in the absence of exogenous help. *Journal of Experimental Medicine* **177**, 1791–1796.

Hargreaves, R., Logiou, V. & Lechler, R. (1995) The primary alloresponse of human CD4+ T cells is dependent on B7 (CD80), augmented by CD58, but relatively uninfluenced by CD54 expression. *International Immunology* **7**, 1505–1513.

Hart, D.N.J., Winearls, C.G. & Fabre, J.W. (1980) Graft adaptation: studies on possible mechanisms in long term surviving rat renal allografts. *Transplantation* **30**, 73–80.

Hasan, R., Van den Bogaerde, J., Forty, J. *et al.* (1992) Xenograft adaptation is dependent on the presence of antispecies antibody, not prolonged residence in the recipient. *Transplantation Proceedings* **24**, 531–532.

Hasan, R.I.R., Sriwatanawangosa, V., Wallwork, J. & White, D.J.G. (1994) Graft adaptation in hamster-to-rat cardiac xenografts. *Transplantation Proceedings* **23**, 1282–1283.

Hattori, R., Hamilton, K.H., McEver, R.P. & Sims, P.J. (1989) Complement proteins C5b-9 induce secretion of high molecular weight multimers of endothelial von Willebrand factor and translocation of granule membrane protein GMP-140 to the cell surface. *Journal of Biological Chemistry* **264**, 9053–9060.

Heneine, W., Tibell, A., Switzer, W.M. *et al.* (1998) No evidence of infection with porcine endogenous retrovirus in recipients of porcine islet-cell xenografts (see comments). *Lancet* **352**, 695–699.

Hewitt, C.W., Black, K.S., Harman, J.C. *et al.* (1990) Partial tolerance in rat renal allograft recipients following multiple blood transfusions and concomitant cyclosporine. *Transplantation* **49**, 194–198.

Holterman, M.J. & Engelhard, V.H. (1986) HLA antigens

expressed on murine cells are preferentially recognized by murine cytotoxic T cells in the context of the H-2 major histocompatibility complex. *Proceedings of the National Academy of Sciences (USA)* 83, 9699–9703.

Hunt, B.J. & Rosenberg, R.D. (1993) The essential role of haemostasis in hyperacute rejection. *Xeno* 1, 16–19.

Inamitsu, T., Nishimma, Y. & Sasazuki, T. (1992) Different recognition of transgenic HLA DQw6 molecules by mouse CD4+ and CD8+ T cells. *Immunogenetics* 35, 46–50.

Inverardi, L., Samaja, M., Motterini, R. *et al.* (1992) Early recognition of a discordant xenogeneic organ by circulating lymphocytes. *Journal of Immunology* 149, 1416–1423.

Inverardi, L., Socci, C. & Pardi, R. (1993) Leucocyte adhesion molecules in graft recognition and rejection. *Xeno* 1, 35–39.

Iwai, H., Kuma, S.-I., Inaba, M.M. *et al.* (1989) Acceptance of murine thyroid allografts by pretreatment of anti-Ia antibody or anti-dendritic cell antibody *in vitro*. *Transplantation* 47, 45–49.

Janeway, C.A. & Bottomly, K. (1994) Signals and signs for lymphocyte responses. *Cell* 76, 275–285.

Jenkins, M.K. (1992) The role of cell division in the induction of clonal anergy. *Immunology Today* 13, 69–73.

Johansson Borg, A., Kumagai-Braesch, M. & Möller, E. (1996) Effect of DSG on xenogeneic immune reactivity with special emphasis on human anti-pig cellular reactions *in vitro*. *Xenotransplantation* 3, 171–178.

Johnston, P.S., Wang, M.W., Lim, S., Wright, L.J. & White, D.J.G. (1992) Discordant xenograft rejection in an antibody free model. *Transplantation* 54, 573–576.

Johnston, S.C., Dustin, M.L., Hibbs, M.L. & Springer, T.A. (1990) On the species specificity of the interaction of LFA-1 with intercellular adhesion molecules. *Journal of Immunology* 145, 1181–1187.

Kalinke, U., Arnold, B. & Hammerling, G.J. (1990) Strong xenogeneic HLA response in transgenic mice after introducing an α3 domain into HLA B27. *Nature* 348, 642–644.

Kaplon, R.J., Platt, J.L., Kwiatkowski, P.A. *et al.* (1995) Absence of hyperacute rejection in pig-to-primate orthotopic pulmonary xenografts. *Transplantation* 59, 410–416.

Ketchum, R.J., Moore, W.V. & Hegre, O.D. (1992) Increased islet allograft survival after extended culture by a mechanism other than depletion of donor APCs. Lack of correlation between the elimination of donor MHC class II-positive accessory cells and increased transplantability. *Transplantation* 54, 347–351.

Kievits, F., Waffels, J., Lokhorst, W. & Ivanyi, P. (1989) Recognition of xeno (HLA, SLA) MHC antigens by mouse cytotoxic T-cells is not H-2 restricted. A study with transgenic mice. *Proceedings of the National Academy of Sciences (USA)* 86, 617–620.

Kirk, A.D., Hall, B.L., Finn, O.J. & Bollinger, R.R. (1992) *In vitro* analysis of the human anti-porcine T-cell repertoire. *Transplantation Proceedings* 24, 602.

Kirk, A.D., Li, R.A., Kirch, M.S. *et al.* (1993) The human antiporcine cellular repertoire. *Transplantation* 55, 924–931.

Kobayashi, M., Shimada, K. & Ozawa, T. (1990) Human recombinant IL-1β and TNF α-mediated suppression of heparin-like compounds on cultured porcine aortic endothelial cells. *Journal of Cellular Physiology* 144, 383–390.

Koike, C., Kannagi, R., Takuma, Y. *et al.* (1996) Introduction of α(1-2)-fucosyltransferase and its effect on a-gal epitopes in transgenic pig. *Xenotransplantation* 3, 81–86.

Kooyman, D.L., McClellan, S.B., Parker, W. *et al.* (1996) Identification and characterization of a galactosyl peptide mimetic. *Transplantation* 61, 851–855.

Kopp, C.W., Siegel, J.B., Hancock, W.W. *et al.* (1997) Effect of porcine endothelial tissue factor pathway inhibitor on human coagulation factors. *Transplantation* 63, 749–758.

Kopp, C.W., Grey, S.T., Siegel, J.B. *et al.* (1998) Expression of human thrombomodulin cofactor activity in porcine endothelial cells. *Transplantation* 66, 244–251.

Koyamada, N., Miyatake, T., Candinas, D. *et al.* (1996) Apyrase administration prolongs discordant xenograft survival. *Transplantation* 62, 1739–1743.

Kroshus, T.J., Rollins, S.A., Dalmasso, A.P. *et al.* (1995) Complement inhibition with an anti-C5 monoclonal antibody prevents acute cardiac tissue injury in an *ex vivo* model of pig-to-human xenotransplantation. *Transplantation* 60, 1194–1202.

Kroshus, T.J., Bolman, R.I., Dalmasso, A.P. *et al.* (1996) Expression of human CD59 in transgenic pig organs enhances organ survival in an *ex vivo* xenogeneic perfusion model. *Transplantation* 61, 1513–1521.

Kumagai-Braesch, M., Satake, M., Korsgren, O., Andersson, A. & Möller, E. (1993) Characterisation of cellular human anti-porcine xenoreactivity. *Clinical Transplantation* 7, 273.

La Rosa, F.G. & Talmage, D.W. (1983) The failure of a major histocompatibility antigen to stimulate a thyroid allograft reaction after culture in oxygen. *Journal of Experimental Medicine* 157, 898–906.

La Rosa, F.G. & Talmage, D.W. (1985) Synergism between minor and major histocompatibility antigens in the rejection of cultured allografts. *Transplantation* 39, 480–485.

LaVecchio, J.A., Dunne, A.D. & Edge, A.S.B. (1995) Enzymatic removal of alpha-galactosyl epitopes from porcine endothelial cells diminishes the cytotoxic effect of natural antibodies. *Transplantation* 60, 841–847.

Lafferty, K.J., Bootes, A., Dart, G. & Talmage, D.W. (1976) Effect of organ culture on the survival of thyroid allografts in mice. *Transplantation* 22, 138–149.

Le, A.X.T., Bernhard, E.J., Holterman, M.J. *et al.* (1989) Cytotoxic T cell responses in HLA A2.1 transgenic mice. Recognition of HLA alloantigens: utilization of HLA A2.1 as restriction element. *Journal of Immunology* **142**, 1366–1371.

Lechler, R.I. & Batchelor, J.R. (1982a) Immunogenicity of retransplanted rat kidney allografts. *Journal of Experimental Medicine* **156**, 1835–1841.

Lechler, R.I. & Batchelor, J.R. (1982b) Restoration of immunogenicity to passenger cell-depleted kidney allografts by the addition of donor strain dendritic cells. *Journal of Experimental Medicine* **155**, 31–41.

Lechler, R.I., Lombardi, G., Batchelor, J.R., Reinsmoen, N. & Bach, F.H. (1990) The molecular basis of alloreactivity. *Immunology Today* **11**, 83–88.

Lee, R.S., Grusby, M.J., Glimcher, L.H., Winn, H.J. & Auchincloss, H. (1994) Indirect recognition by helper cells can induce donor-specific cytotoxic T lymphocytes *in vivo*. *Journal of Experimental Medicine* **179**, 865–872.

Leventhal, J.R., Dalmasso, A.P., Cranwell, J.W. *et al.* (1993a) Prolongation of cardiac xenograft survival by depletion of complement. *Transplantation* **55**, 857–866.

Leventhal, J.R., Matas, A.J., Sun, L.H. *et al.* (1993b) The immunopathology of cardiac xenograft rejection in the guinea pig-to-rat model. *Transplantation* **56**, 1–8.

Leventhal, J.R., Sakiyalak, P., Witson, J. *et al.* (1994) The synergistic effect of combined antibody and complement depletion on discordant cardiac xenograft survival in nonhuman primates. *Transplantation* **57**, 974–977.

Lin, S.S., Weidner, B.C., Byrne, G.W. *et al.* (1998) The role of antibodies in acute vascular rejection of pig-to-baboon cardiac transplants. *Journal of Clinical Investigations* **101**, 1745–1756.

Lin, Y., Vandeputte, M. & Waer, M. (1998) Accommodation and T-independent B cell tolerance in rats with long term surviving hamster heart xenografts. *Journal of Immunology* **160**, 369–375.

Lindahl, K.F. & Bach, F.H. (1976) Genetic and cellular aspects of xenogeneic mixed lymphocyte culture reaction. *Journal of Experimental Medicine* **144**, 305–318.

Lindahl, K.F. & Wilson, D.B. (1977) Histocompatibility antigen-activated cytotoxic T lymphocytes. I: Estimates of the absolute frequency of killer cells generated *in vitro*. *Journal of Experimental Medicine* **145**, 500–507.

Liu, L.M. & MacPherson, G.G. (1993) Antigen acquisition by dendritic cells: intestinal dendritic cells acquire antigen administered orally and can prime T cells. *Journal of Experimental Medicine* **177**, 1299–1307.

Liu, Y. & Janeway, C.A.J. (1992) Cells that present both specific ligand costimulatory activity are the most efficient inducers of clonal expansion of normal CD4 T cells. *Proceedings of the National Academy of Sciences (USA)* **89**, 3845–3849.

Liu, Z., Braunstein, N.S. & Suciu-Foca, N. (1992) T cell recognition of allopeptides in context of syngeneic MHC. *Journal of Immunology* **148**, 35–40.

Liu, Z., Sun, Y.K., Xi, Y.P. *et al.* (1993) Contribution of direct and indirect recognition pathways to T cell alloreactivity. *Journal of Experimental Medicine* **177**, 1643–1650.

Lombardi, G., Sidhu, S., Lamb, J.R., Batchelor, J.R. & Lechler, R.I. (1989) Co-recognition of endogenous antigens with HLA-DR1 by alloreactive human T cell clones. *Journal of Immunology* **142**, 753–759.

Loveland, B.E., Johnstone, R.W., Russel, S.M., Thorley, B.R. & McKenzie, T.F.C. (1993) CD46 (MCP) confers protection from lysis by xenogeneic antibodies. *Transplantation Proceedings* **25**, 396–397.

Lucas, P.J., Shearer, G.M., Neudorf, S. & Gress, R.E. (1990) The human antimurine xenogeneic cytotoxic response. I: Dependence on responder APC. *Journal of Immunology* **144**, 4548–4554.

McCurry, K.R., Kooyman, D.L., Diamond, L.E. *et al.* (1995a) Transgenic expression of human complement regulatory proteins in mice results in diminished complement deposition during organ xenoperfusion. *Transplantation* **59**, 1177–1182.

McCurry, K.R., Kooyman, D.L., Alvarado, C.G. *et al.* (1995b) Human complement regulatory proteins protect swine-to-primate cardiac xenografts from humoral injury. *Nature Medicine* **1**, 423–427.

Magee, J.C. & Platt, J.L. (1994) Xenograft rejection – molecular mechanisms and therapeutic implications. *Therapeutic Immunology* **1**, 45–58.

Magee, J.C., Collins, B.H., Harland, R.C. *et al.* (1995) Immunoglobulin prevents complement-mediated hyperacute rejection in swine-to-primate xenotransplantation. *Journal of Clinical Investigations* **96**, 2404–2412.

Malyguine, A.M., Saadi, S., Platt, J.L. & Dawson, J.R. (1996) Human natural killer cells induce morphologic changes in porcine endothelial cell monolayers. *Transplantation* **61**, 161–164.

Marchetti, P., Scharp, D.W., Lacy, P.E. & Navalesi, R. (1995) Long term survival of pig-to-mouse islet xenografts. *Xenotransplantation* **2**, 154–156.

Marino, I.R., Ferla, G., Celli, S. *et al.* (1991) *In vivo* and *in vitro* study of hyperacute rejection mechanism of renal discordant xenograft. *Transplantation Proceedings* **23**, 620–622.

Markmann, J.F., Campos, L., Bhandoola, A. *et al.* (1994) Genetically engineered grafts to study xenoimmunity: a role for indirect antigen presentation in the destruction of major histocompatibility complex antigen deficient xenografts. *Surgery* **116**, 242–249.

Maryanski, J.L., Moretta, A., Jordan, B. *et al.* (1985) Human T cell-recognition of cloned HLA class I gene products expressed on DNA transfectants of mouse mastocytoma P815. *European Journal of Immunology* **15**, 1111–1117.

Maryanski, J.L., Pala, P., Corradin, G., Jordan, B.R. & Cerotini, J.C. (1986a) H-2 restricted cytolytic T-cells specific for HLA can recognise a synthetic HLA peptide. *Nature* 324, 378–379.

Maryanski, J.L., Accoll, R.S. & Jordan, B. (1986b) H-2-restricted recognition of cloned HLA class I gene products expressed in mouse cells. *Journal of Immunology* 136, 4340–4347.

Matsumiya, G., Shirakura, R., Miyagawa, S. *et al.* (1993) Inhibitory effect of the complement receptor specific monoclonal antibody on the induced antibody response and the role of CD4+ and CD8+ T cells in the rat to mouse xenotransplantation. *Transplantation Proceedings* 25, 402–404.

Merkenschlager, M., Ikeda, H., Wilkinson, D. *et al.* (1991) Allorecognition of HLA-DR and -DQ transfectants by human CD45RA and CD45RO CD4 T cells: repertoire analysis and activation requirements. *European Journal of Immunology* 21, 79–88.

Miller, A.D. (1992) Human gene therapy comes of age. *Nature* 357, 455.

Miyagawa, S., Shirakura, R., Matsumiya, G. *et al.* (1993a) Prolonging discordant xenograft survival with anticomplement reagents K76COOH and FUT 175. *Transplantation* 55, 709–713.

Miyagawa, S., Shirakura, R., Matsumiya, G. *et al.* (1993b) Test for ability of DAF and CD59 to alleviate complement-mediated damage of xeno erythrocytes. *Scandinavian Journal of Immunology* 38, 37–44.

Moses, R.D., Pierson, R.N., Winn, H.J. & Auchincloss, H. (1990) Xenogeneic proliferation and lymphokine production are dependent on CD4+ helper T-cells and self antigen presenting cells in mouse. *Journal of Experimental Medicine* 172, 567–575.

Moses, R.D., Winn, H.J. & Auchincloss, H. (1992) Multiple defects in cell surface molecule interactions across species differences are responsible for diminished xenogeneic T-cell responses. *Transplantation* 53, 203–209.

Mueller, J.P., Evans, M.J., Cofiell, R. *et al.* (1995) Porcine vascular cell adhesion molecule (VCAM) mediates endothelial cell adhesion to human T cells. Development of blocking antibodies specific for porcine VCAM. *Transplantation* 60, 1299–1306.

Murphy, B., Auchincloss, H., Carpenter, C.B. & Sayegh, M.H. (1996) T cell recognition of xeno-MHC peptides during concordant xenograft rejection. *Transplantation* 61, 1133–1137.

Murray, A.G., Khodadoust, M.M., Pober, J.S. & Bothwell, A.L.M. (1994) Porcine aortic endothelial cells activate human T cells: direct presentation of MHC antigens and costimulation by ligands for human CD2 and CD28. *Immunity* 1, 57–63.

Neethling, F.A., Koren, E., Ye, Y. *et al.* (1994) Protection of

pig kidney (PK15) cells from the cytotoxic effect of anti-pig antibodies by α-galactosyl oligosaccharides. *Transplantation* 57, 959–963.

Nuffield Council on Bioethics (1996) *Animal-to-Human Transplants*. Nuffield Foundation, London.

O'Hair, D.P., Roza, A.M., Pieper, G.M. *et al.* (1992) Platelet activating factor antagonist RP-59227 reduces vascular injury in discordant cardiac xenograft rejection. *Transplantation Proceedings* 24, 702–703.

Oriol, R.Y.E.Y., Koren, E. & Cooper, D.K.C. (1993) Carbohydrate antigens of pig tissues reacting with human natural antibodies as potential targets for hyperacute vascular rejection in pig-to-man organ xenotransplantation. *Transplantation* 56, 1433–1442.

O'Rourke, A.M. & Mescher, M.F. (1993) The roles of CD8 in cytotoxic T lymphocyte function. *Immunology Today* 14, 183–188.

Palmer, A., Welsh, K., Gjorstup, P. *et al.* (1989) Removal of anti-HLA antibodies by extracorporeal immunoadsorption to enable renal transplantation. *Lancet* i, 10–12.

Parham, P. (1992) The box and the rod. *Nature* 357, 538–539.

Parker, K.E., Dalchau, R., Fowler, V.J. *et al.* (1992) Stimulation of CD4+ T lymphocytes by allogeneic MHC peptides presented on autologous antigen-presenting cells. Evidence of the indirect pathway of allorecognition in some strain combinations. *Transplantation* 53, 918–924.

Parker, W., Lundberg-Swanson, K., Holzknecht, Z.E. *et al.* (1996a) Isohemagglutinins and xenoreactive antibodies. Members of a distinct family of natural antibodies. *Human Immunology* 45, 94–104.

Parker, W., Saadi, S., Lin, S.S. *et al.* (1996b) Transplantation of discordant xenografts: a challenge revisited. *Immunology Today* 17, 373–378.

Patience, C., Takeuchi, Y. & Weiss, R.A. (1997) Infection of human cells by an endogenous retrovirus of pigs (see comments). *Nature Medicine* 3, 282–286.

Patience, C., Patton, G.S., Takeuchi, Y. *et al.* (1998) No evidence of pig DNA or retroviral infection in patients with short-term extracorporeal connection to pig kidneys (see comments). *Lancet* 352, 699–701.

Paul, L., van Els, L. & la Riviera, G. (1978) Blood group B antigen on renal endothelium as the target for rejection in an ABO-incompatible recipient. *Transplantation* 26, 268–271.

Perper, R.J. & Najarian, J.S. (1966) Experimental renal heterotransplantation. 1: In widely divergent species. *Transplantation* 4, 377.

Pierson, R.N., Winn, H.J., Russell, P.S. & Auchincloss, H. (1989) Xenogeneic skin graft rejection is especially dependent on CD4+ T cells. *Journal of Experimental Medicine* 170, 991–996.

Pilemer, L., Blum, L., Lepow, I. *et al.* (1954) The properdin system and immunology. 1: Demonstration and isolation of a new serum protein properdin and its role in immune phenomena. *Science* 120, 279–285.

Pinola, M., Saksela, E., Tiisala, S. & Renkonen, R. (1994) Human NK cells expressing α4β1/β7 adhere to VCAM-1 without pre-activation. *Scandinavian Journal of Immunology* 39, 131–136.

Platt, J.L. & Bach, F.H. (1991) The barrier to xenotransplantation. *Transplantation* 52, 937–947.

Platt, J.L. & Holzknecht, Z.E. (1994) Porcine platelet antigens recognized by human xenoreactive natural antibodies. *Transplantation* 57, 327–335.

Platt, J.L., Vercellotti, G.M., Dalmasso, A.P. *et al.* (1990a) Transplantation of discordant xenografts: a review of progress. *Immunology Today* 11, 450–456.

Platt, J.L., Turman, M.A., Noreen, H.J. *et al.* (1990b) An ELISA assay for xenoreactive natural antibodies. *Transplantation* 49, 1000.

Platt, J.L., Lindman, B.J., Chen, H., Spitalnik, S.L. & Bach, F.H. (1990c) Endothelial cell antigens recognized by xenoreactive human natural antibodies. *Transplantation* 50, 817–822.

Platt, J.L., Vercellotti, G.M., Lindman, B.J. *et al.* (1990d) Release of heparan sulphate from endothelial cells—implications for pathogenesis of hyperacute rejection. *Journal of Experimental Medicine* 171, 1363–1368.

Platt, J.L., Fischel, R.J., Matas, A.J. *et al.* (1991a) Immunopathology of hyperacute xenograft rejection in a swine-to-primate model. *Transplantation* 52, 214–220.

Platt, J.L., Dalmasso, A.P., Lindman, B.J., Ihrcke, N.S. & Bach, F.H. (1991b) The role of C5a and antibody in the release of heparan sulfate from endothelial cells. *European Journal of Immunology* 21, 2887–2890.

Pleass, H.C.C., Forsythe, J.L.R., Proud, G., Taylor, R.M.R. & Kirby, J.A. (1994) Xenotransplantation: an examination of the adhesive interactions between human lymphocytes and porcine renal epithelial cells. *Transplant Immunology* 2, 225–230.

Pober, J.S. & Cotran, R.S. (1990) Cytokines and endothelial cell biology. *Physiological Reviews* 70, 427.

Pruitt, S.K., Kirk, A.D., Bollinger, R.R. *et al.* (1994) The effect of soluble complement receptor type 1 on hyperacute rejection of porcine xenografts. *Transplantation* 57, 363–370.

Ramesh, P., Barber, L., Batchelor, J.R. & Lechler, R.I. (1992) Structural analysis of human anti-mouse H-2E xenorecognition: T cell receptor bias and impaired CD4 interaction contribute to weak xenoresponses. *International Immunology* 4, 935–943.

Read, M.A., Whitley, M.Z., Williams, A.J. & Collins, T. (1994) NFκB and IκBα: an inducible regulatory system in endothelial activation. *Journal of Experimental Medicine* 179, 503–512.

Reemtsma, K. (1991) Xenotransplantation—a brief history of clinical experience: 1900–1965. In: *Xenotransplantation The Transplantation of Organs and Tissues Between Species* (eds D.K.C. Cooper, E. Kemp, K. Reemtsma & D.J.G. White), pp. 9–22. Springer-Verlag, Heidelberg.

Reemtsma, K., McCracken, B., Schlegel, J. & Pearl, M. (1964a) Heterotransplantation of the kidney: two clinical experiences. *Science* 143, 700–702.

Reemtsma, K., McCracken, B., Schlegel, J. *et al.* (1964b) Renal heterotransplantation in man. *Annals of Surgery* 160, 384–410.

Reemtsma, K., McCracken, B., Schlegel, J. *et al.* (1964c) Reversal of early graft rejection after renal heterotransplantation in man. *Journal of the American Medical Association* 187, 691–696.

Restifo, A.C., Ivis-Woodward, M.A., Tran, H.M. *et al.* (1996) The potential role of xenogeneic antigen-presenting cells in T cell co-stimulation. *Xenotransplantation* 3, 141–148.

Ricordi, C. & Lacy, P.E. (1987) Renal subcapsular xenotransplantation of purified porcine islets. *Transplantation* 44, 721–723.

Riesbeck, K., Dorling, A., Kemball, C.G. *et al.* (1997) Human tissue factor pathway inhibitor fused to CD4 binds both FXa and TF/FVIIa at the cell surface. *Thrombosis and Haemostasis* 78, 1488–1494.

Robson, S.C., Kaczmarek, E., Siegel, J.B. *et al.* (1997) Loss of ATP diphosphohydrolase activity with endothelial cell activation. *Journal of Experimental Medicine* 185, 153–163.

Rock, K.L., Barnes, M.C., Germain, R.N. & Benacerraf, B. (1983) The role of Ia molecules in the activation of T lymphocytes. II: Ia-restricted recognition of allo K/D antigens is required for class I MHC-stimulated mixed lymphocyte responses. *Journal of Immunology* 130, 457–462.

Rock, K.L., Benacerraf, B.J. & Abbas, A.K. (1984) Antigen presentation by hapten-specific B lymphocytes. I. Role of surface immunoglobulin receptors. *Journal of Experimental Medicine* 160, 1102–1113.

Rogers, N.J., Dorling, A. & Moore, M. (1998) Xenotransplantation: steps towards a clinical reality. *Immunology Today* 19, 206–208.

Rollins, S.A., Kennedy, S.P., Chodera, A.J. *et al.* (1994) Evidence that activation of human T cells by porcine endothelium involves direct recognition of porcine SLA and costimulation by porcine ligands for LFA-1 and CD2. *Transplantation* 57, 1709–1716.

Rollins, S.A., Matis, L.A., Springhorn, J.P., Setter, E. & Wolff, D.W. (1995) Monoclonal antibodies directed against human C5 and C8 block complement-mediated damage of xenogeneic cells and organs. *Transplantation* 60, 1284–1292.

Rosengard, A.M., Cary, N.R.B., Langford, G.A. *et al.* (1995) Tissue expression of human complement inhibitor, decay-accelerating factor, in transgenic pigs. *Transplantation* 59, 1325–1333.

Ross, C.N., Gaskin, G., Gregor-Macgregor, S. *et al.* (1993) Renal transplantation following immunoadsorption in highly sensitized recipients. *Transplantation* 55, 785–789.

Ross, R., Kirk, A.D., Ibrahim, S.E. *et al.* (1993) Characterization of human anti-porcine 'natural antibodies' recovered from *ex vivo* perfused hearts: predominance of IgM and IgG2. *Transplantation* 55, 1144–1150.

Saadi, S. & Platt, J.L. (1995) Transient perturbation of endothelial integrity induced by natural antibodies and complement. *Journal of Experimental Medicine* 181, 21–31.

Sallusto, F. & Lanzavecchia, A. (1994) Efficient presentation of soluble antigen by cultured human dendritic cells is maintained by granulocyte/macrophage colony-stimulating factor plus interleukin 4 and downregulated by tumor necrosis factor alpha. *Journal of Experimental Medicine* 179, 1109–1118.

Samberg, N.L., Scarlett, E.C. & Stauss, H.J. (1989) The $\alpha$-3 domain of MHC complex class I molecules plays a critical role on cytotoxic T lymphocyte stimulation. *European Journal of Immunology* 19, 2349–2354.

Sandrin, M.S., Vaughan, H.A., Dabkowski, P.L. & McKenzie, I.F.C. (1993) Anti-pig IgM antibodies in human serum react predominantly with gal$\alpha$ (1–3) gal epitopes. *Proceedings of the National Academy of Sciences (USA)* 90, 11391–11395.

Sandrin, M.S., Dabkowski, P.L., Henning, M.M., Mouhtouris, E. & MacKenzie, I.F.C. (1994) Characterization of cDNA clones for porcine $\alpha$ (1,3) galactosyl transferase: the enzyme generating the Gal$\alpha$ (1–3) Gal epitope. *Xenotransplantation* 1, 81–88.

Sandrin, M.S., Fodor, W.L., Mouhtouris, E. *et al.* (1995) Enzymatic remodelling of the carbohydrate surface of a xenogeneic cell substantially reduces human antibody binding and complement-mediated cytolysis. *Nature Medicine* 1, 1261–1267.

Satake, M., Kawagishi, N., Rydberg, L. *et al.* (1994) Limited specificity of xenoantibodies in diabetic patients transplanted with fetal porcine islet cell clusters. Main antibody reactivity against $\alpha$-linked galactose containing epitopes. *Xenotransplantation* 1, 89–101.

Satake, M., Kawagishi, N. & Möller, E. (1996) Direct activation of human responder T cells by porcine stimulator cells leads to T cell proliferation and cytotoxic T cell development. *Xenotransplantation* 3, 198–206.

Saumweber, D.M., Bergman, R., Gokel, M. & Hammer, C. (1994) Hyperacute rejection in an *ex vivo* model of renal xenografting. *Transplantation* 57, 358–363.

Schaapherder, A.F.M., Daha, M.R., van der Woode, F.J., Bruijn, J.A. & Gooszen, H.G. (1993) IgM, IgG, IgA antibodies in human sera directed against porcine islets of Langerhans. *Transplantation* 56, 739–741.

Scheringa, M., Schraa, E.O., Bouwman, E. *et al.* (1995) Prolongation of survival of guinea pig heart grafts in cobra venom factor-treated rats by splenectomy. *Transplantation* 60, 1350–1353.

Schmoeckel, M., Nollert, G., Shahmohammadi, M. *et al.* (1996) Prevention of hyperacute rejection by human decay accelerating factor in xenogeneic perfused working hearts. *Transplantation* 62, 729–734.

Schmoeckel, M., Bhatti, F.N., Zaidi, A. *et al.* (1998) Orthotopic heart transplantation in a transgenic pig-to-primate model. *Transplantation* 65, 1570–1577.

Seebach, J.D., Yamada, K., McMorrow, I.M., Sachs, D.H. & DerSimonian, H. (1996) Xenogeneic human anti-pig cytotoxicity mediated by activated natural killer cells. *Xenotransplantation* 3, 188–197.

Settaf, A., Merrigi, F., Van de Stadt, J. *et al.* (1987) Delayed hyperacute rejection of liver xenografts compared to heart xenografts in rats. *Transplantation Proceedings* 19, 1155–1157.

Silvers, W.K., Fleming, H.L., Naji, A. & Barker, C.F. (1982) Evidence for major histocompatibility complex restriction in transplantation immunity. *Proceedings of the National Academy of Sciences (USA)* 79, 171–174.

Silvers, W.K., Bartlett, S.T., Chen, H.-D. *et al.* (1984) Major histocompatibility complex restriction and transplantation immunity. A possible solution to the allograft problem. *Transplantation* 37, 28–32.

Simeonovic, C.J., Ceredig, R. & Wilson, J.D. (1990) Effect of GKI-5 monoclonal antibody dosage on survival of pig proislet xenografts in CD4+ T cell depleted mice. *Transplantation* 49, 849–856.

Simonsen, M. (1967) The clonal selection hypothesis evaluated by grafted cells reacting against their hosts. *Cold Spring Harbor Symposium on Quantitative Biology* 32, 517.

Soares, M.P., Latinne, D., Elsen, M. *et al.* (1993) *In vivo* depletion of xenoreactive natural antibodies with an anti-μ monoclonal antibody. *Transplantation* 56, 1427–1433.

Soares, M.P., Lin, Y., Anrather, J. *et al.* (1998) Expression of heme oxygenase-1 can determine cardiac xenograft survival. *Nature Medicine* 4, 1073–1077.

Somerville, C.A., Kyriazis, A.G., McKenzie, A. *et al.* (1994) Functional expression of human CD59 in transgenic mice. *Transplantation* 58, 1430–1435.

Starzl, T., Marcioro, T., Peters, G. *et al.* (1964) Renal heterotransplantation from baboon to man: experience with six cases. *Transplantation* 2, 752–776.

Starzl, T.E., Fung, J., Tsakis, A. *et al.* (1993) Baboon-to-human liver transplantation. *Lancet* 341, 65.

Stevens, R.B., Wang, Y.L., Kaji, H. *et al.* (1993) Administration of nonanticoagulant heparin inhibits the loss of glycosaminoglycans from xenogeneic cardiac grafts and prolongs graft survival. *Transplantation Proceedings* **25**, 382.

Sundt, T.M., Guzzetta, P.C., Suzuki, T., Rosengard, B.R. & Sachs, D.H. (1989) Influence of bone marrow derived elements on renal allograft rejection. *Surgery Forum* **40**, 375–378.

Sundt, T.M., Arn, J.S. & Sachs, D.H. (1992) Patterns of T cell–accessory cell interaction in the generation of primary alloresponses in the pig. *Transplantation* **54**, 911–916.

Swain, S.L., Dutton, R.W., Scwab, R. & Yamamoto, J. (1983) Xenogeneic human anti-mouse T cell responses are due to the activity of the same functional T cell subsets responsible for allospecific and MHC-restricted responses. *Journal of Experimental Medicine* **157**, 720–729.

Takahashi, M., Ikeda, U., Masuyama, J.-I. *et al.* (1994) Involvement of adhesion molecules in human monocyte adhesion to and transmigration through endothelial cells *in vitro*. *Atherosclerosis* **108**, 73–81.

Taylor, R. (1995) A pig in a poke? Xenotransplants and infectious disease. *Nature Medicine* **1**, 728–729.

Tearle, R.G., Tange, M.J., Zannettino, Z.L. *et al.* (1996) The α-1,3-galactosyltransferase knockout mouse. *Transplantation* **61**, 13–19.

Thomas, F.T., DeMasi, R.J., Araneda, D. *et al.* (1990) Comparative efficacy of immunosuppressive drugs in xenografting. *Transplantation Proceedings* **22**, 1083–1085.

Turman, M.A., Casali, P., Notkins, A.L., Bach, F.H. & Platt, J.L. (1991) Polyreactivity and antigen specificity of human xenoreactive monoclonal and serum natural antibodies. *Transplantation* **52**, 710–717.

Tuso, P.J., Cramer, D.V., Yasunaga, C. *et al.* (1993a) Removal of natural human xenoantibodies to pig vascular endothelium by perfusion of blood through pig kidneys and livers. *Transplantation* **55**, 1375–1378.

Tuso, P.J., Cramer, D.V., Middleton, Y.D. *et al.* (1993b) Pig aortic endothelial cell antigens recognized by human IgM natural antibodies. *Transplantation* **56**, 651–655.

Van Denderen, B.J.W., Pearse, M.J., Katerelos, M. *et al.* (1996) Expression of functional decay-accelerating factor (CD55) in transgenic mice protects against human complement-mediated attack. *Transplantation* **61**, 582–588.

Van Oers, M.H.J., Pinkster, J. & Zeijlemaker, W.P. (1978) Quantification of antigen-reactive cells among human T lymphocytes. *European Journal of Immunology* **8**, 477.

Vanhove, B. & Bach, F.H. (1993) Human xenoreactive natural antibodies—avidity and targets on porcine endothelial cells. *Transplantation* **56**, 1251–1292.

Vanhove, B., de Martin, R., Lipp, J. & Bach, F.H. (1994)

Human xenoreactive natural antibodies of the IgM isotype activate pig endothelial cells. *Xenotransplantation* **1**, 17–23.

Vercellotti, G.M., Platt, J.L., Bach, F.H. & Dalmasso, A.P. (1991) Neutrophil adhesion to xenogeneic endothelium via iC3b. *Journal of Immunology* **146**, 730–734.

Via, C.S., Tsokos, G.C., Stocks, N.I., Clericic, M. & Shearer, G.M. (1990) Human *in vitro* allogeneic responses. Demonstration of three pathways of T helper cell activation. *Journal of Immunology* **144**, 2524–2528.

Viguier, M., Lotteari, V., Charron, D. & Debre, P. (1987) Xenogeneic recognition of soluble and cell surface HLA class II antigens by proliferative murine T cells. *European Journal of Immunology* **17**, 1540–1546.

Von Hoegen, P., Miceli, M.C., Tourvielle, B., Schilham, M. & Parnes, J.R. (1989) Equivalence of human and mouse CD4 in enhancing antigen responses by a mouse class II-restricted T cell hybridoma. *Journal of Experimental Medicine* **170**, 1879–1886.

Warrens, A.N., Heaton, T., Sidhu, S., Lombardi, G. & Lechler, R.I. (1994) Transfected murine cells expressing HLA class II can be used to generate alloreactive human T cell clones. *Journal of Immunological Methods* **169**, 25–33.

Watkins, J.F., Edwards, N.M., Sanchez, J.A. *et al.* (1991) Specific elimination of preformed antibody activity against xenogeneic antigens by use of an extracorporeal immunoadsorptive circuit. *Transplantation Proceedings* **23**, 360–364.

Wecker, H. & Auchincloss, H. (1992) Cellular mechanisms of rejection. *Current Opinion in Immunology* **4**, 561–566.

Wecker, H., Winn, H.J. & Auchincloss, H. (1994) CD4+ T cells, without CD8+ or B lymphocytes, can reject xenogeneic skin grafts. *Xenotransplantation* **1**, 8–16.

Weinberger, O., Germain, R.N. & Burakoff, S.J. (1983) Responses to the H-2K$^{ba}$ mutant involve recognition of syngeneic Ia molecules. *Nature* **302**, 429–431.

Welsh, K.I., Batchelor, J.R., Maynard, A. & Burgos, H. (1979) Failure of long surviving, passively enhanced kidney allografts to provoke T-dependent alloimmunity 2. Retransplantation of (AS×Aug) F1 kidneys from As primary recipients into (AS×WF) F1 secondary hosts. *Journal of Experimental Medicine* **150**, 465–470.

Widmer, M.B. & Bach, F.H. (1972) Allogeneic and xenogeneic response in mixed lymphocyte cultures. *Journal of Experimental Medicine* **135**, 1204–1208.

Winkler, H., Ferran, C. & Bach, F.H. (1995) Review: accommodation of xenografts: a concept revisited. *Xenotransplantation* **2**, 53–57.

Wolf, L.A., Coulombe, M. & Gill, R.G. (1995) Donor antigen-presenting cell-independent rejection of islet xenografts. *Transplantation* **60**, 1164–1170.

Xia, W., Fearon, D.T. & Kirkman, R.L. (1993) Effect of repetitive doses of soluble human complement receptor type 1 on survival of discordant xenografts. *Transplantation Proceedings* **25**, 410–411.

Xu, H., Kwiatkowski, P., Chen, J.M. *et al.* (1994) Abrogation of baboon natural xenoantibody to pig splenocytes by DL-penicillamine. *Transplantation* **58**, 1299–1303.

Xu, H., Edwards, N.M., Chen, J.M. *et al.* (1995) Newborn baboon serum lacks natural anti-pig xenoantibody. *Transplantation* **59**, 1189–1194.

Yamada, K., Sachs, D.H. & DerSimonian, H. (1995) Human anti-porcine xenogeneic T cell response. Evidence for allelic specificity of mixed leukocyte reaction and for both direct and indirect pathways. *Journal of Immunology* **155**, 5249–5256.

Yamada, K., Seebach, J.D., DerSimonian, H. & Sachs, D.H. (1996) Human anti-pig T-cell mediated cytotoxicity. *Xenotransplantation* **3**, 179–187.

Ye, Y., Neethling, F.A., Niekrasz, M. *et al.* (1994) Evidence that intravenously administered alpha-galactosyl carbohydrates reduce baboon serum cytotoxicity to pig

kidney cells (PK15) and transplanted pig hearts. *Transplantation* **58**, 330–337.

Yoshizawa, K. & Yano, A. (1984) Mouse T lymphocytes proliferative responses specific for human MHC products in mouse anti-human xenogeneic MLR. *Journal of Immunology* **132**, 2820–2829.

Zhao, J., Rollins, S.A., Maher, J.E., Bothwell, A.L.M. & Sims, P.J. (1991) Amplified gene expression in CD59-transfected chinese hamster ovary cells confers protection against the membrane attack complex of human complement. *Journal of Biological Chemistry* **266**, 13418–13422.

Zhao, Z., Termignon, J.-L., Cardoso, J. *et al.* (1994) Hyperacute xenograft rejection in the swine-to-human donor-recipient combination. *Transplantation* **57**, 245–249.

Zhow, X.J., Niesen, N., Pawlowski, J. *et al.* (1990) Prolongation of survival of discordant kidney xenografts by C6 deficiency. *Transplantation* **50**, 896–898.

# Chapter 7/Clinical immunosuppression in renal transplantation

STEVEN J. CHADBAN, JOHN R. BRADLEY & KENNETH G.C. SMITH

## Introduction

Renal transplantation is the treatment of choice for most patients in or approaching end-stage renal failure. A sound working knowledge of transplantation medicine is therefore essential for the practice of modern nephrology. The aim of this chapter is to review current approaches to immunosuppression in the management of the renal transplant recipient. An overview of the immunological basis of renal transplantation will be given, followed by a detailed review of the pharmacology of individual immunosuppressive agents in current clinical use. Immunosuppressive regimens specific to each phase of the transplantation process will be discussed. Emphasis will be given to the side-effect profiles and clinical problems encountered in using immunosuppressants in transplant recipients. We will conclude by highlighting promising experimental developments and directions for the future in immunosuppressive therapy and by briefly outlining differences between

immunosuppression in renal transplantation and that of other solid organs.

## Immunological basis of renal transplantation

In current practice renal transplantation is performed by implanting a donor kidney into an allogeneic recipient—a kidney is transferred between two genetically non-identical individuals of the same species (with the exception of transplantation between identical twins). Xenotransplantation, the transfer of an organ from a member of one species into a recipient of another species, at present remains a procedure restricted to experimental animals and will not be discussed in this chapter.

Transplantation of an allogeneic kidney stimulates the recipient's immune system to mount a response which, in the absence of substantial immunosuppression, rejects the allograft. Allograft rejection can be classified immunologically and clinically as hyper-acute, acute or chronic. Hyperacute rejection occurs if the recipient possesses preformed antibodies to donor antigens which are expressed on vascular endothelium, such as human leucocyte antigen (HLA) or ABO antigens. Following insertion of the allograft, such antibodies adhere to recipient endothelium, fix complement and initiate coagulation, resulting in catastrophic and irreversible rejection within minutes (Sanfilippo *et al.* 1982). In contrast, cellular immunity appears to have the dominant role in acute rejection. Donor antigens, particularly HLA, are recognized by specific T cells, which either induce direct cytotoxicity (CD8+ cytotoxic T cells) or mediate allograft damage via a delayed-type hypersensitivity response (DTH). Acute rejection episodes (AREs) are most frequent within the first 6 months and are the major cause of graft loss during the first 3 years post-transplant (Gulanicar *et al.* 1992). Chronic rejection is a process which remains incompletely understood. Both immunological and non-immunological factors contribute to its pathogenesis. It appears likely that humoral immunity participates via the process of antibody-dependent cell-mediated cytotoxicity (ADCC) (Trpkov *et al.* 1996). Cellular immunity may also contribute via the indirect pathway. Chronic rejection is the main cause of allograft failure beyond 3 years post-transplantation (Naimark & Cole 1994). The role of immune cells in the processes of rejection will be discussed below, while the pathology of allograft rejection is detailed elsewhere in the book.

## Alloimmune sensitization

The type of immune response initiated by the allograft will vary depending on whether the recipient has been sensitized to donor antigens. Sensitization of the recipient to donor HLA specificities may result in hyperacute rejection of the graft if preformed specific antibodies are present or, in severe early acute rejection, when memory T and B cells are activated (Sanfilipo *et al.* 1982; Paul *et al.* 1997). Patients awaiting renal transplantation are therefore screened to assess their degree of non-specific sensitization with a panel-reactive antibody test (Dyer *et al.* 1995), in which leucocytes from a panel of blood donors are incubated with patients' serum. Reactivity with over 50% of panel cells indicates a high degree of sensitization and is a poor prognostic indicator for transplant acceptance (Dyer *et al.* 1995). Highly sensitized patients may benefit from the use of specific immunosuppressive induction regimens at the time of transplantation (see the section on donor preconditioning and sensitization below). Specific sensitization is assessed immediately prior to transplantation with a lymphocytotoxic cross-match, performed by incubating donor B and T cells in recipient serum plus rabbit complement (Martin & Class 1993). The presence of preformed donor-specific anti-T cell antibodies indicates a high probability of hyperacute rejection and is therefore a contraindication to carrying out the transplant procedure.

## Direct and indirect pathways of T cell activation

The initial immune response to a transplanted kidney in the non-presensitized recipient is a T cell-dependent process which involves recipient CD4+ T cells, CD8+ cytotoxic T cells, B cells, macrophages and dendritic cells, as well as antigen-presenting cells (APCs) of donor origin.

The classical alloimmune response involves recipient CD8+ or CD4+ T cell recognition of polymorphic differences in intact donor MHC class I or II molecules, respectively, with or without donor peptide (Strom 1992). This 'direct recognition' of donor MHC by recipient T cells then results in T cell activation with subsequent cytotoxicity (mediated by CD8+ cells) or the development of a CD4+ cell-mediated immune response (Shoskes & Wood 1994). The direct pathway of T cell activation is probably the dominant mechanism resulting in acute allograft rejection (Lechler & Batchelor 1982), but may become less important over time as donor MHC class II+ cells are progressively lost from vascularized allografts (Larsen *et al.* 1990; Braun *et al.* 1993). This appears to be the case in mice, where T cells which directly recognized donor MHC class II molecules were found to induce allograft rejection at early but not at late time points (Emerson & Cone 1982).

Alloimmune responses may also be directed against

polymorphic differences in peptide fragments of donor MHC class I or II molecules which have been processed by recipient APCs and presented to recipient CD4+ T cells via the 'indirect pathway' (Shoskes & Wood 1994). Donor MHC molecules are progressively shed by transplanted organs and taken up by recipient APCs (Via *et al.* 1990), which can in turn stimulate specific CD4+ T cells to produce IL-2 (Golding & Singer 1984) and generate T cell help for T and B cells (Welsh *et al.* 1979; Bradley *et al.* 1992; Sawyer *et al.* 1993). Less commonly, peptides derived from polymorphic molecules other than the MHC can also generate an indirect alloimmune response. Indirect presentation of alloantigen may be important in mediating delayed acute rejection episodes and chronic rejection (Shoskes & Wood 1994; Bradley 1996).

The mechanisms activated by indirect pathway stimulation differ from those involved in the direct pathway. Both pathways of activation may result in T cell proliferation and cytokine release; however, different calcium-dependent (direct pathway) or independent (indirect pathway) activation cascades may be utilized (Lafferty *et al.* 1983; Crabtree 1989; Sawyer *et al.* 1993). On this basis, direct pathway activation appears to be relatively sensitive to cyclosporin and FK506, whereas responses mediated by indirect pathway activation appear to be less so (Sawyer *et al.* 1993). A more complete understanding of the relative importance of direct vs. indirect T cell activation, including changes in this balance which occur over time, may be crucial to future developments in immunosuppression.

## Cytokines and alloimmunity: the Th-1/Th-2 paradigm

The concept that undifferentiated CD4+ T cells may evolve into two divisions, those which dominantly produce γ-interferon (IFN-γ) and IL-2 and are known as Th-1 cells, or those producing IL-4 and IL-10 and which are labelled Th-2 cells, was originally described in the mouse (Mosmann *et al.* 1986). The two populations are cross-inhibitory, as Th-1 cell products (e.g. IFN-γ) inhibit the development and activation of Th-2 cells, and Th-2 cytokines (e.g. IL-10) similarly inhibit Th-1 cells (Mosmann & Sad 1996). This paradigm may have relevance to human immune responses (Romagnani 1991); however, its applicability to organ transplantation has been much debated (Gimsa & Mitchison 1997). Th-1 responses are characterized by the DTH response in which T cells orchestrate macrophage-mediated inflammation. Acute allograft rejection has been likened to a Th-1-type response.

Several studies in rodent models of acute allograft rejection have found that Th-1 cytokines are predominantly generated within rejecting grafts, and have also shown that treatment strategies which suppress Th-1 activity or enhance Th-2 activity have been protective (Akalin *et al.* 1995; Sayegh *et al.* 1995). However, evidence obtained from other experimental animals and from human biopsy studies has been far less convincing (reviewed in Gimsa & Mitchison 1997). Great complexity is apparent and predictable in the *in vivo* setting of organ transplantation. T cell cytokines may be produced by leucocytes other than T cells (Nikolic-Paterson *et al.* 1997) and by intrinsic kidney cells (Tesch *et al.* 1997). Cytokine secretion may vary with time and with the phase of the immune response and may be altered by concurrent conditions, such as sepsis and by medication (McHugh *et al.* 1995). Overlap within the cytokine networks is also apparent, exemplified by sharing of the γ-chain subunit between several T cell growth factor receptors. This may explain the observation that T cell-dependent rejection may proceed in IL-2 knockout mice, despite the absence of this seemingly essential T cell growth factor (reviewed in Yon Su Kim *et al.* 1997). Thus, the interpretation of cytokine profiles detected in serum or in biopsies obtained from allograft recipients is fraught with difficulty and at present seems unlikely to yield answers which are clinically useful.

## The importance of antigen-presenting cells

Antigen-presenting cells, in particular dendritic cells, macrophages and B cells, constitutively express cell surface MHC class II and the costimulatory molecules CD40, B7-1 and B7-2. They are capable of receiving an antigen and processing it into a peptide fragment which the cell presents, in the groove of the MHC class II molecule, to a specific T helper cell. Antigen presentation by these APCs is accompanied by binding of the co-stimulatory molecules to their T cell receptors, CD40 ligand and CD28. Costimulatory signals appear to be critical. Adequate costimulatory signalling promotes activation of the T cell response to antigen, whereas an inadequate or absent costimulatory signal may result in antigen-specific T cell anergy (Jenkins & Schwartz 1987). Furthermore, the pattern of costimulation may determine whether the T helper cell differentiates into a Th-1 or Th-2 type of cell (Constant & Bottomly 1997). Costimulatory molecule expression and function may be altered by cytokines (Buelens *et al.* 1995) or by therapeutic agents, such as CTLA4–Ig and anti-CD40 ligand, which block the B7–CD28 and CD40–CD40L interactions, respectively, and are currently undergoing clinical trials in renal transplantation (Kirk *et al.* 1997).

Parenchymal cells, such as endothelial, mesangial and tubular cells, can be induced to express MHC class II and may thereby present antigen to T cells. The extent and significance of antigen presentation by parenchymal APCs is at present unclear. Theoretically, ineffective costimulatory signalling by parenchymal APCs may contribute to T cell anergy.

## B cells in rejection

The B cell has a number of important roles in transplant rejection. The most obvious is the production of preformed alloantibodies which mediate hyperacute rejection. It is the presence of these antibodies which make pretransplant ABO blood group matching and the performance of cross-matching critical. gal$\alpha$(1–3) gal is an antigen found ubiquitously in non-primates but not in higher primates, and preformed antibodies against it (and other antigens) mediate hyperacute rejection and pose a major obstacle to the successful performance of xenotransplantation from, for example, pigs to humans (Galili 1993; Sandrin *et al.* 1993).

Indirect antigen presentation, which is increasingly thought to be of importance in acute allograft rejection, provides T cell help enabling the production of alloantibodies (Bradley 1996). These alloantibodies

act as a marker of such presentation and there is evidence that they may be directly involved in the pathogenesis of graft rejection (Bradley 1996). There is also strongly suggestive, but inconclusive, evidence that alloantibody may have a direct role in mediating graft damage caused by chronic rejection (Paul *et al.* 1997). Given the association between alloantibody production and indirect antigen presentation, and the possible role of this mechanism in potentiating chronic rejection, it is of interest to note that the indirect pathway may be resistant to suppression by cyclosporin, perhaps explaining the lack of impact of the introduction of cyclosporin on chronic rejection rates (Sawyer *et al.* 1993).

The final part which may be played by B cells in transplant rejection is antigen presentation. While there is evidence that dendritic cells are the dominant APC, the part played by other APCs, such as macrophages and B cells, in transplant rejection is less well defined. It is of interest to note that it has recently been demonstrated that B cells play a critical part in initiation of immune injury leading to autoimmune diabetes, thought to be a prototypic 'T cell disease' (Falcone *et al.* 1998), and the same may also be true of allograft rejection (Brandle *et al.* 1998).

## Role of macrophages

In addition to serving as APCs in the initiation phase of the allograft response, there is now evidence in an experimental model of acute allograft rejection to show that macrophages mediate graft destruction by direct killing of allograft cells (Yamamoto *et al.* 1998). Activated macrophages also appear to have a pathogenic role in chronic rejection (Azuma *et al.* 1995). Killing by macrophages may be directed by a Th-1 cell response, particularly during acute rejection, or by ADCC. Proliferating stem cells give rise to monocytes which are recruited into the allograft to become graft infiltrating macrophages and these cells may undergo further proliferation *in situ* (Kerr *et al.* 1994). Given their role in the rejection process, selective targeting of macrophages is therapeutically desirable but has proven difficult in animal models and is currently not feasible in humans. To date, they are non-specifically targeted by antiproliferative agents, including mycophenolate and azathioprine, and inhibited directly by corticosteroids and indirectly by agents such as cyclosporin, rapamycin and tacrolimus, which inhibit T cell help.

## Tolerance

The phenomenon of neonatal tolerance, predicted by Burnet and Fenner in Melbourne (Burnet & Fenner 1949), was first demonstrated in 1953 by Billingham *et al.* (Billingham *et al.* 1953). Since then the application of tolerance to organ transplantation has been a holy grail of transplant immunologists. While much early work focused on B cell tolerance (reviewed by Nossal 1983), tolerance in the T cell compartment is the most important in preventing allograft rejection. It can be brought about by deletion of clones with high affinity for antigen in the thymus, which is thought to be a major mechanism of achieving self-tolerance. Peripheral T cells can be tolerized by clonal exhaustion, in which constant exposure to antigen results in activation-induced cell death, often mediated by Fas–Fas ligand interaction. Clonal ignorance, where the antigen is inaccessible to the immune system (e.g. intracellular or in 'immunologically privileged' sites, such as the eye or testis), ensures tolerance. Finally, there is increasing evidence that, in some models, induction of populations of specific regulatory T cells can maintain peripheral T cell tolerance (Groux *et al.* 1998).

These mechanisms of tolerance induction have been well described in experimental systems though their roles in models of whole-organ allograft tolerance are less clear. A large number of manipulations have led to the induction of donor-specific tolerance in the rodent models of transplantation; these include administration of donor-specific antigen with various immunosuppressive agents, such as anti-CD4 monoclonal antibody treatment (Darby *et al.* 1992; Morris 1998). Tolerance has been more difficult to achieve in large animal models, though some approaches have proven promising. The first involves the blockade of the CD40 and CD28 costimulatory pathways. This approach produced tolerance not only to vascularized organs but also to skin allografts in mice (Larsen *et al.* 1996),

though in a large animal model promising prolonged graft survival is not accompanied by formal tolerance (Kirk *et al.* 1997). Use of an immunotoxin comprising diptheria toxin targeted to CD3 with a monoclonal antibody, along with the administration of donor antigen, resulted in prolonged graft survival and apparent tolerance in large animal models (Knechtle *et al.* 1997). Induction of tolerance in human allograft systems has been less successful, though the application of knowledge derived from animal models is beginning.

A correlation between graft survival and microchimerism (the detection of persistent donor antigen in the recipient after transplantation, for example in the form of donor peripheral leucocytes) has been noted, and some feel that the persistent interaction between donor antigen and the recipient immune system which this microchimerism permits allows the maintenance of clonal exhaustion and therefore of tolerance in the recipient (Starzl 1998). Attempts to induce tolerance in humans have included the induction of microchimerism via the infusion of donor bone marrow at the time of transplantation (Rao *et al.* 1998). The production of soluble MHC by liver grafts might maintain clonal exhaustion and induce occasional tolerance, by maintaining clonal exhaustion in a similar way to that proposed for microchimerism (Geissler *et al.* 1997). On the other hand, others feel that the existence of microchimerism is an epiphenomenon, and that those more likely to be tolerant to their graft are also more likely to be tolerant to the existence of donor lymphocytes, resulting in correlation between microchimerism and graft survival without needing to invoke a role for microchimerism in maintaining that survival (Hamano *et al.* 1996). More recently Calne *et al.* (1998, 1999) have used an anti-CD52 antibody to deplete peripheral lymphocytes at the time of transplantation, allowing their subsequent recovery with only minimal immunosuppression, in the hope of inducing tolerance. Preliminary results with this technique indicate good graft survival with relatively few rejection episodes in patients maintained on only half-dose cyclosporin, though tolerance has not been demonstrated. Our understanding of the mechanism of tolerance in animal models of transplantation is increasing, and studies applying this knowledge to the human transplant situation are beginning. It appears, then, that the holy grail, if not in reach, is now at least in sight.

## Immunosuppressants: pharmacology

### Glucocorticoids

Prednisolone and methylprednisolone are more potent and longer-acting derivatives of the endogenous human glucocorticoids, cortisol and cortisone. These analogues are used extensively in renal transplantation for maintenance immunosuppression and for the treatment of acute rejection episodes. Deflazacort is a recently tested derivative of prednisolone which appears to exert equivalent immunosuppressive effects to its predecessors, but may incur less toxicity, particularly in the paediatric population (Ferraris *et al.* 1996).

#### PHARMACOKINETICS

Glucocorticoids may be administered intravenously (methylprednisolone) or orally, with similar bioavailability. Glucocorticoids exist in the circulation in an equilibrium; the majority of drug is bound to plasma proteins while the remaining unbound fraction is bioactive. Plasma concentrations of glucocorticoids correlate poorly with their biological activities. Both prednisolone and methylprednisolone have biological half-lives of approximately 24 h in adults and may therefore be administered once daily. Clearance of prednisolone is increased in children (Rose *et al.* 1981) and in the obese (Jusko & Ludwig 1992) but reduced in the elderly and in females by around 20%, making dosage adjustment appropriate (Jusko & Ludwig 1992). In contrast, methylprednisolone dosages are best calculated on the basis of lean body mass. The clearance of both drugs may be altered by the coadministration of drugs which affect hepatic p450 enzyme function; phenytoin and other enzyme inducers may increase glucocorticoid clearance and decrease bioactivity (Gambertoglio *et al.* 1982) while enzyme inhibitors, such as erythromycin, may prolong glucocorticoid activity (Table 7.1).

#### MODE OF ACTION

Free glucocorticoid diffuses easily across cell membranes and binds to a specific intracellular receptor to form a heterodimer, which is translocated to the nucleus (Miesfeld 1990; Karin *et al.* 1993). The glucocorticoid–receptor dimer then modulates proinflammatory gene expression and translation, with several transcription factors vital for the proinflammatory activities of leucocytes appearing to be the most important targets. The glucocorticoid–receptor dimer may interfere with transcription factor activity through protein–protein interactions, as in the case of AP-1 (Schule *et al.* 1990; Yang-Yen *et al.* 1990; Karin *et al.* 1993). Alternatively, NF-κB is maintained in an inactive state as the glucocorticoid–receptor dimer promotes the generation of excess I-κB (Auphan *et al.* 1995; Scheinman *et al.* 1995). Additionally, transcription factor binding to promoter regions in DNA may be displaced by dimer binding to specific glucocorticoid-responsive elements within nearby DNA sequences. By these mechanisms glucocorticoids exert potent inhibitory effects on the generation of proinflammatory cytokines, growth factors, receptors, chemokines, adhesion molecules and enzymes, including IL-1, IL-2, IL-4, IL-6, insulin-like growth factor-1, tumour necrosis factor, IFN-γ, the interleukin-2 receptor, IL-8, RANTES, ICAM-1, collagenases and elastases (Schule *et al.* 1990; Yang-Yen *et al.* 1990; Ray & Sehgal 1992). Further anti-inflammatory effects of glucocorticoids on both leucocytes and tissue cells, such as mesangial cells, are likely to be mediated by inhibition of local arachidonic acid production through blockade of phospholipase A2 activity (Coyne *et al.* 1992). The acute administration of high-dose glucocorticoid (e.g. 500 mg methylprednisolone stat.) also leads to a decrease in the numbers of all circulating leucocytes apart from neutrophils, as a result of both cell lysis and tissue sequestration (Schleimer 1993).

#### SIDE EFFECTS

The broad range of side effects associated with the use of glucocorticoids are well known to most clinicians,

**Table 7.1** Interactions of immunosuppressants with other drugs.

| Interacting drug | | Immunosuppressant drug | | | | | |
|---|---|---|---|---|---|---|---|
| Drug class | Example | Corticosteroids | Cyclosporin | Tacrolimus | Rapamycin | Azathioprine | MMF |
| Cytochrome p450 inhibitors | Erythromycin Fluconazole Verapamil/diltiazem Danazole Cimetidine Grapefruit juice | Modestly ↑ levels, immunosuppression and toxicity | ↑ Levels, immunosuppression and toxicity | ↑ Levels, immunosuppression and toxicity | ↑ Levels, immunosuppression and toxicity | | |
| Cytochrome p450 inducers | Rifampicin Phenobarbital Dexamethasone | Modestly ↓ levels | ↓ Levels, immunosuppression and toxicity | ↓ Levels, immunosuppression and toxicity | ↓ Levels, immunosuppression and toxicity | | |
| Nephrotoxic drugs | Amphotericin Cyclosporin NSAIDs | – | ↑ Nephrotoxicity | ↑ Nephrotoxicity | – | – | – |
| Immunosuppressant | Cyclosporin | ↑ Lipids ↑ Blood pressure | – | ↑ Immunosuppression | ↑ Immunosuppression with possible synergy | | ↑ MMF levels 50% |
| | Tacrolimus | – | ↑ Immunosuppression | – | ↑ Immunosuppression with possible synergy | | – |
| Others | Allopurinol Nifedipine, Phenytoin | – – | Increased gum hypertrophy | Increased gum hypertrophy | – – | ↑↑ Levels and toxicity – | No interaction – |

↑, increase; ↑↑, large increase; ↓, decrease; MMF, mycophenolate mofetil.

and are summarized in Table 7.2. Issues of most concern in the field of transplantation are the effects of steroids on cardiovascular risk factors, predisposition to infection and bone disease. Glucocorticoids promote hypertension, hyperlipidaemia and hyperglycaemia and are thereby likely to contribute to the high prevalence of cardiovascular disease in this population (Ingulli *et al.* 1993; Ong *et al.* 1994). Steroids may induce avascular necrosis, childhood growth retardation and osteoporosis. Steroid-induced bone loss occurs as a result of negative calcium balance and other unidentified mechanisms (Lukert & Raisz 1990). Osteoporosis occurs early after the commencement of glucocorticoids, afflicts both genders equally and particularly affects trabecular bone in vertebral bodies, neck of femur and humerus (Lukert & Raisz 1990). Coexistent hyperparathyroidism, immobility and steroid myopathy may contribute (Lukert & Raisz 1990). While no agent has been shown to prevent ostoeporosis or fracture risk in renal transplant recipients, the use of dihydroxy vitamin D and, more recently, biphosphonates and hormone replacement therapy in postmenopausal women has been found beneficial in other patient populations and extrapolation of these results appears to be justified. In the paediatric group, deflazacort may be less potent in retarding linear growth (Ferraris *et al.* 1996).

USE IN RENAL TRANSPLANTATION

Glucocorticoids have always been an important component of immunosuppressive regimens used for maintenance and antirejection therapy in renal transplantation. With the introduction of cyclosporin and other adjunctive immunosuppressants during the last 30 years, the use of glucocorticoids has been modified in order to minimize the toxicity associated with their use.

GLUCOCORTICOIDS AS A COMPONENT OF MAINTENANCE THERAPY

*Steroid regimens and timing*

Steroids should be commenced prior to the transplant procedure (Fricke *et al.* 1996). Studies performed prior to the introduction of cyclosporin showed that for patients receiving prednisolone and azathioprine maintenance therapy, those given low-dose steroid (20 mg prednisolone from the day of transplantation) showed equal graft and patient survival to those given higher doses (up to 200 mg prednisolone at transplantation, tapered to 0.25–0.5 mg/kg/day over 3–6 months). Some studies suggested a slight increase in AREs, but most reported a significant reduction in side effects (Buckels *et al.* 1981; Morris *et al.* 1982; D'Apice *et al.* 1984). Conversion to alternate daily dosage 3 months after transplantation was also examined by several groups who reported a slight increase in AREs, most of which were reversible but required resumption of daily steroids, no effect on patient or graft survival and a reduction in side effects, including retardation of growth and sexual development in children (Bell *et al.* 1972; McEnery *et al.* 1973).

*Steroid avoidance*

With the introduction of cyclosporin, the use of steroid-free maintenance regimens was examined. Three large prospective trials concluded that treatment with cyclosporin and prednisolone showed no advantage over cyclosporin alone in terms of patient and graft survival at 2 years (Griffin *et al.* 1987; MacDonald *et al.* 1987; Johnson *et al.* 1989); however, an increased incidence of cyclosporin nephrotoxicity has become apparent with longer follow-up (Sinclair 1992). Furthermore, up to 80% of patients treated with cyclosporin monotherapy have subsequently required the addition of prednisolone following AREs. Similarly, trials examining the utility of cyclosporin combined with azathioprine from the time of transplantation have shown that around 50% of patients have required the addition of prednisolone, subsequent to AREs (Bry *et al.* 1991).

*Steroid withdrawal*

Many studies have examined the issue of steroid withdrawal in the setting of standard triple or quadruple therapy (cyclosporin, prednisolone and azathioprine,

**Table 7.2** Summary of side effects of the immunosuppressant drugs currently used in transplantation.

| Side effect | Corticosteroids | Cyclosporin | Tacrolimus | Azathioprine | MMF | OKT3 | ATG and ALG | IL-2R mAbs |
|---|---|---|---|---|---|---|---|---|
| Nephrotoxicity | – | +++ | + | – | – | – | – | – |
| Hypertension | ++ | +++ | + | Pancreatitis | – | – | – | – |
| Dyslipidaemia | +++ | +++ | ++ | – | – | – | – | – |
| Diabetogenesis | ++ | + | +++ | – | – | – | – | – |
| Bone disease | Osteoporosis, necrosis | Bone pain | Bone pain | – | – | – | – | – |
| Neurotoxicity | Mood changes | Tremor | Headache, tremor, seizures | – | – | Headache, aseptic meningitis | Headache | – |
| Leucopenia | – | – | – | +++ | +++ | ++++ | ++++ | – |
| Thrombocytopenia | – | Haemolytic uraemic syndrome | – | ++ | ++ | – | ++ | – |
| Anaemia | – | – | – | + | + | – | – | – |
| GI toxicity | + | Hepatotoxic | Hepatotoxic | Hepatotoxic N,V&D + | Hepatotoxic, N,V&D +++ | N,V&D ++ | N,V&D + | – |
| Pulmonary toxicity | + | – | – | Fibrosis (rare) | Fibrosis (rare) | Pulmonary oedema | Wheeze | – |
| Cytokine releases | – | – | – | – | – | ++++ | ++ | – |
| Infection risk | ++ | ++ | +++ | ++ | +++ | ++++ | ++++ | – |
| Cancer risk | + | ++ | +++ | ++ | +++ | ++++ | ++++ | – |
| Other | Cataracts, ↑ appetite, fat redistribution, etc. | ↑K, ↓Mg, hirsutism | – | Safe for pregnancy | Unsafe for pregnancy | Neutralizing Ab +++ | Neutralizing Ab + | Similar to placebo |

↑, increase; ↓, decrease; + to ++++, mild to major effect; ALG, antilymphocyte globulin; ATG, antithymocyte globulin; GI, gastrointestinal; MMF, mycophenolate mofetil; N,V&D, nausea, vomiting and diarrhoea; OKT3, orthoclone OKT3 monoclonal antibody.

plus antibody induction therapy for quadruple regimens). The timing and speed of withdrawal have varied widely. In general, steroid withdrawal commencing after the first 3 months post-transplantation, tapering the dosage to zero over several months appears prudent as rapid and early withdrawals have been associated with a high incidence of AREs, which may be related to a rebound effect on T cell proliferation (Hricik *et al.* 1994).

A meta-analysis of seven randomized prospective trials of steroid withdrawal reported a significant increase in AREs but no effect on patient or graft survival (Hricik *et al.* 1993). In a randomized controlled trial, late steroid withdrawal (1–6 years post-transplantation) was found to be achievable in 86% of patients (Ratcliffe *et al.* 1996). Late steroid withdrawal caused no significant increase in the incidence of AREs, but was associated with an insidious increase in serum creatinine of at least 25% of baseline in 53% of cases, as compared to 18% of controls, in the first year post-withdrawal. This effect was significant and was sustained at 3 years of follow-up. The mechanism was not clear, with no evidence of an increased incidence of rejection on biopsy in a subgroup of patients. Factors identifying patients at higher risk of renal impairment following steroid withdrawal could not be identified. Similar results have been reported from an uncontrolled trial (Hricik *et al.* 1992). Thus, steroid inclusion in the first 3–12 months post-transplantation appears warranted. Withdrawal after this period appears to be achievable and safe in most patients receiving triple therapy with a stable transplant. Later, more gradual steroid withdrawal appears most effective. Advantages have been reported in terms of reductions in vascular risk factors, including hypercholesterolaemia (Pirsch *et al.* 1991), hypertension (Hricik *et al.* 1991; Pirsch *et al.* 1991) and glucose intolerance (Cantarovich *et al.* 1990; Hricik *et al.* 1991; Moniemi 1991), although no data on the effects of steroid withdrawal on the incidence of vascular events and mortality have been reported. Other side effects of steroids, particularly osteoporosis, may not be diminished. Uncertainty also persists over the effects of steroid withdrawal on long-term graft function and the development of chronic

rejection. The issue of complete steroid withdrawal vs. low-dose or alternate-day steroids has not been conclusively addressed.

## GLUCOCORTICOIDS IN THE TREATMENT OF ACUTE ALLOGRAFT REJECTION

Glucocorticoids have been, and in most institutions remain, the first-line antirejection therapy. Intravenous 'pulse' therapy with methylprednisolone has been preferred to similar regimens of oral prednisolone in the treatment of AREs on the theoretical grounds of achieving a higher peak blood level, resulting in a rapid onset of immunosuppression and lymphocyte lysis yet more rapid clearance of the steroid with less potential for side effects (Silverman 1981). In comparative trials, the two routes of administration have shown little difference in therapeutic efficacy but an increased incidence of adverse events with oral prednisolone has been noted (Woods *et al.* 1973; Mussche *et al.* 1976; Gray *et al.* 1978). Dosage is largely empirical, although no apparent difference in efficacy or adverse effects were detected between regimens of 250 mg and 1 g of methylprednisolone daily for 3 days (Kauffman *et al.* 1979; Park *et al.* 1984).

Antilymphocyte antibodies and the newer immunosuppressants, mycophenolate mofetil and tacrolimus, now provide alternative treatment options for the patient with acute rejection. The role of steroids in the current treatment of AREs will be discussed in the section on maintenance below.

## Cyclosporin A

Cyclosporin A has been the cornerstone of immunosuppression in solid organ transplantation since its introduction in Cambridge in 1978 (Calne *et al.* 1978, 1979) and has been responsible for the dramatic improvement in short-term graft survival rates observed since that time. Its introduction has had no impact, however, on graft attrition beyond 1 year after engraftment, which is largely a result of chronic rejection.

## PHARMACOKINETICS

Cyclosporin may be administered intravenously or orally. Absorption after oral administration is slow, variable and incomplete, averaging 30% bioavailability (Yee & Salomon 1992). This may be partially caused by metabolism of the drug by p450 cytochromes present within the small-intestinal mucosa (Lake 1991; Yee & Salomon 1992). Consequently, the intravenous dose should be approximately 30% of the oral dose. Absorption after oral administration is dependent on the presence of bile and may be affected by concomitant ingestion of food, drugs which affect gut emptying or bile content, and coexistent gut or cholestatic liver disease (Lake 1991; Yee & Salomon 1992). Blood levels peak 2–6 h after ingestion in the fasted state, though a second peak may occur when cyclosporin is taken with food, possibly as a result of enterohepatic recirculation (Lake 1991; Yee & Salomon 1992). When ingested as a microemulsion (Neoral, Sandoz), the absorption of cyclosporin appears to be less erratic and more complete with less intra- and interpatient variability, resulting in more predictable kinetics (Taesch *et al.* 1994). Following several weeks of therapy, cyclosporin absorption appears to be inducible with increases of over 200% in bioavailability being reported, requiring commensurate dosage reduction (Lake 1991; Yee & Salomon 1992). As cyclosporin activity and toxicity appear to be related to blood levels, frequent monitoring is essential, particularly during the first few months of therapy.

Cyclosporin is extremely fat-soluble and consequently is widely distributed throughout body tissues. The volume of distribution ranges from 3.5 to 13 L/kg and is generally higher in women than in men. In whole blood, approximately 60% of cyclosporin is cell-bound (predominantly to red cells), 35% is bound to plasma proteins (particularly low-density lipoprotein) and less than 5% remains free and biologically active. Notably, hypercholesterolaemia may reduce the proportion of free drug and thereby impair bioactivity (Lake 1991). As the intravascular distribution is variable, monitoring of whole-blood levels is the most reliable and preferred method of dosage monitoring.

Cyclosporin is extensively metabolized by the hepatic cytochrome p450 microsomal enzyme system to form several metabolites, some of which may be biologically active and toxic (Lake 1991; Yee & Salomon 1992). Metabolism is sensitive to inducers and suppressors of p450 microsomal enzymes and cyclosporin appears to diminish its own metabolism over time (Lake 1991; Yee & Salomon 1992). Less than 1% of the parent compound is excreted unchanged in the urine; however, most metabolites undergo renal excretion and dosage reduction is therefore necessary for patients with impaired renal function. The clearance of cyclosporin is age-dependent, being much more rapid in children under 10 years of age and twice as rapid in adults less than 25 years of age as compared to older individuals (Lake 1991; Yee & Salomon 1992).

## MODE OF ACTION

The dominant immunosuppressive effect of cyclosporin is caused by disruption of the calcium-dependent cascade of intracellular events which follow antigen-specific T cell activation through the T cell receptor complex (Fig. 7.1). Cyclosporin entry into the T cell, binding to cyclophilins and subsequent formation of a cyclosporin–cyclophilin–calcineurin complex inhibit the phosphatase activity of calcineurin. Inhibition of this phosphatase activity prevents the intracellular signalling which would normally follow T cell receptor stimulation and result in T cell activation and proliferation (reviewed in Kahan 1989). In particular, dephosphorylation of the nuclear factor of activated T lymphocytes (NFAT) is inhibited, thereby preventing the translocation of NFAT to the nucleus, binding to its recognition sequence in the IL-2 promoter region and subsequent promotion of IL-2 gene transcription (Kahan 1989; Henderson *et al.* 1991). Similarly, cyclosporin inhibits the transcription of other genes involved in the early activation of T cells, such as *c-myc*, cytokines including IL-3, IL-4, IL-5 and IFN-γ, and cytokine receptors such as IL-2 receptor. Cyclosporin up-regulates transcription of transforming growth factor (TGFβ1). This feature may contribute to the immunosuppres-

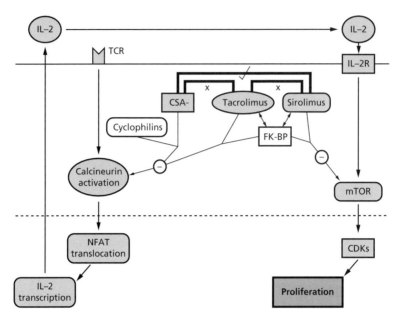

**Fig. 7.1** Mechanism of action of cyclosporin, tacrolimus and sirolimus. Cyclosporin (CSA) combines with the cyclophilins to inhibit calcineurin-dependent activation downstream of the T cell receptor (TCR). Tacrolimus binds to FK-BP and inhibits the same step as cyclosporin. Sirolimus also binds to FK-BP but has a distinct action, inhibiting the function of mTOR and thus T cell proliferation. Both cyclosporin and tacrolimus act on calcineurin activation and are therefore not used together. Cyclosporin and sirolimus, however, have distinct molecular interactions and interfere with quite separate steps in the T cell activation pathway, explaining their synergy both *in vivo* and *in vitro*. Despite sirolimus and tacrolimus both binding to FK-BP12 there appears to be an excess of this protein in the cells and the two agents appear to be able to be used together.

sive properties of cyclosporin, as TGFβ1 is an inhibitor of T cell growth and activation, but also to its adverse effects, including renal fibrosis (Khanna *et al.* 1995).

Cyclosporin has immunosuppressive effects on cells in addition to T lymphocytes. Cyclosporin retards B cell activation both directly, inhibiting calcium flux in response to surface Ig ligation, and indirectly by impairing T cell help (Thomson 1992). Antigen presenting cells appear little affected, whereas polymorph degranulation is inhibited (Forrest *et al.* 1991). Mesangial cell production of prostaglandins and inducible nitric oxide in response to IL-1 is blunted by cyclosporin, which may contribute to the propensity of cyclosporin to induce renal vasoconstriction and fibrosis (Martin *et al.* 1994).

### SIDE EFFECTS AND DRUG INTERACTIONS

Cyclosporin has numerous side effects (see Table 7.2). Nephrotoxicity and the promotion of atherogenesis are of particular concern in transplantation. Nephrotoxicity may result from the effects of cyclosporin on intrinsic renal cells and the renal vasculature (reviewed in Bennett 1995). While many mechanisms are implicated, it is apparent that nephrotoxicity is, at least partly, mediated by inhibition of calcineurin activity (Sigal *et al.* 1991). The vascular effects of cyclosporin, which include inhibition of endothelial production of endothelin-1 and nitric oxide and an enhancement of sympathomimetic responsiveness, promote vasoconstriction and probably contribute to renal ischaemia. Clinically, nephrotoxicity may present in several settings. Acute toxicity often presents with an asymptomatic reduction of glomerular filtration rate (GFR) and consequent increase in creatinine, but may also present with hypertension, fluid retention, hyperkalaemia, hyperuricaemia, hyperchloraemic metabolic acidosis or, rarely, with acute renal failure and haemolytic anaemia caused by the haemolytic–uraemic syndrome (Bennett 1995). Acute toxicity may also present as primary non-function as a result of the potentiation of renal ischaemia by cyclosporin and, for this reason, cyclosporin therapy is commonly withheld until allograft function is established (Kahan 1989). The urinary sediment in acute toxicity is typically benign and proteinuria is minimal. Differentiation of acute cyclosporin toxicity from rejection usually requires renal biopsy (Kahan 1989; Bennett 1995).

Chronic cyclosporin nephrotoxicity typically presents after at least several months of therapy with an elevation in serum creatinine, often accompanied by hyperkalaemia, metabolic acidosis, hypertension and non-nephrotic range proteinuria (Kahan 1989; Bennett 1995). The main differential diagnosis is chronic rejection. As opposed to acute toxicity, cyclosporin blood levels correlate poorly with the development of chronic toxicity.

Biopsy features of cyclosporin toxicity are relatively non-specific and include proximal tubular vacuolization with giant mitochondria and, in the more chronic setting, afferent arteriolar hyalinosis and 'striped' interstitial fibrosis (Mihatsch *et al.* 1994). Most importantly, evidence of coexistent rejection should also be sought on biopsy as cyclosporin toxicity may coexist with rejection (Mihatsch *et al.* 1994; Bennett 1995). Acute cyclosporin nephrotoxicity should be reversible within 1 week upon appropriate reduction in dosage; however, irreversible and progressive changes are seen in cases of chronic toxicity.

Hypertension frequently complicates cyclosporin therapy, even when blood levels are maintained within the therapeutic range (Curtiss 1986; Textor *et al.* 1993; Bennett *et al.* 1994). Cyclosporin alters the balance of local vasoconstrictor:vasodilator substances, enhances sympathomimetic responsiveness and promotes platelet activation at the endothelial surface, resulting in an increase in renal and peripheral vascular resistance (Curtiss *et al.* 1986). In addition to promoting hyperlipidaemia (Castelao *et al.* 1992; Webb *et al.* 1993; Kuster *et al.* 1994), cyclosporin promotes the oxidation of low-density lipoproteins (LDLs) and increases the atherogenicity of these molecules (Apanay *et al.* 1994). Platelet activation and aggregation is also enhanced. Thus, cyclosporin is a potent atherogenic agent, particularly when used in renal transplant recipients, who are commonly receiving steroids and have pre-existing cardiac risk factors and disease. Hirsutism may be problematic in female and paediatric patients. Gingival hyperplasia is frequent (10–50%) and may be accentuated in patients receiving phenytoin or dihydropyridine calcium channel blockers (Pan *et al.* 1992; Thomason *et al.* 1993).

Cyclosporin has many significant drug interactions. Potentiation of the immunosuppressive actions of cyclosporin and a possible reduction in nephrotoxicity may result from the coadministration of diltiazem (Kunzendorf *et al.* 1991; Chrysostomou *et al.* 1993). Synergism between cyclosporin and rapamycin in achieving immunosuppression has been identified (Kimball *et al.* 1991). Other drug interactions are listed in Table 7.1.

### USE IN RENAL TRANSPLANTATION

Cyclosporin is used in mono-, double and triple therapy maintenance regimens. Cyclosporin remains the principal agent for maintenance therapy, although its position is currently challenged by newer agents, such as tacrolimus and rapamycin. Cyclosporin is not of value in the treatment of established AREs.

Cyclosporin was introduced in renal transplantation in 1972 and had a dramatic effect in reducing the incidence of AREs and prolonging early graft and patient survival (Calne & White 1982). High-dose cyclosporin monotherapy was associated with excess patient morbidity (Canadian Multicentre Transplant Group 1981); however, the use of lower dosage in combination with prednisolone elicited synergy between the two compounds and yielded improvements in graft and patient outcome (reviewed in Kahan 1989). Combination maintenance therapies incorporating cyclosporin have subsequently been utilized for the past 20 years and have been largely responsible for the success of renal transplantation over this period of time (Kahan 1989). The various cyclosporin-based maintenance regimens are discussed in the section on maintenance below.

## Tacrolimus

Tacrolimus (FK506) is a newer, more potent alternative to cyclosporin, which may be used as a maintenance immunosuppressant or as a rescue agent for the treatment of refractory or recurrent allograft rejection.

### PHARMACOKINETICS

Like cyclosporin, tacrolimus is erratically and incompletely absorbed from the gut. Bioavailability averages 20% and is reduced by concurrent food intake but not by hepatic dysfunction, as opposed to cyclosporin (Venkataramanan *et al.* 1991). Blood levels peak from 0.5 to 8h after ingestion. The drug is highly bound to red cells and plasma proteins and levels are therefore best monitored in whole blood (Jusko & D'Ambrosio 1991). Metabolism is via the hepatic cytochrome p450 microsomal enzyme system and, as in the case of cyclosporin, metabolism is sensitive to inducers and suppressors of p450 microsomal enzymes (see Table 7.1).

### MODE OF ACTION

Tacrolimus binds to high-affinity FK-binding protein (FK-BP) receptors within the cytoplasm. The resulting complex disables the same calcium–calcineurin-dependent phosphatase activities that are targeted by cyclosporin, thereby inhibiting transcription of early T cell activation genes, including IL-2, IL-3, IL-4, TNFα and IFN-γ (Henderson *et al.* 1991; Peters *et al.* 1993) (see Fig. 7.1). Tacrolimus also inhibits neutrophil degranulation *in vitro* (Forrest *et al.* 1991).

### SIDE EFFECTS AND DRUG INTERACTIONS

Tacrolimus again shares many similarities with cyclosporin. Nephrotoxicity produced by tacrolimus is indistinguishable from that produced by cyclosporin, both clinically and pathologically (Fung *et al.* 1991; Connolly *et al.* 1994; Pirsch *et al.* 1997), with the exception of a lesser incidence of hypertension in patients receiving tacrolimus. Drug levels correlate only loosely with its incidence. Neurotoxicity is a more frequent sequela of tacrolimus, with headache, seizures and tremor seen at therapeutic doses. The incidence of hirsutism and gingival hyperplasia appears to be less than with cyclosporin (Fung *et al.* 1991; Pirsch *et al.* 1997). Post-transplant diabetes mellitus (PTDM) is seen far more frequently in patients treated with tacrolimus than in those treated with cyclosporin (Scantlebury *et al.* 1991; Tanabe *et al.* 1996). Risk factors for the development of PTDM have been identified and include impaired glucose tolerance pretransplant, non-white race, steroid dose (prednisolone >25mg/day), high tacrolimus trough levels and, possibly, older age (Tanabe *et al.* 1996). Of interest, PTDM has not been apparent in recipients of simultaneous pancreas–kidney allografts (Gruessner *et al.* 1996).

Drug interactions, as with cyclosporin, are numerous (see Table 7.1). Given the shared mechanisms of action and side-effect profiles of tacrolimus and cyclosporin, these agents are not used simultaneously. Tacrolimus does inhibit the metabolism of mycophenolate mofetil (MMF) such that MMF blood levels and bioactivity are effectively 50% greater than when used with cyclosporin, so that lower doses of MMF may provide adequate immunosuppression when used in combination with tacrolimus (Zucker *et al.* 1997).

### USE IN TRANSPLANTATION

*Maintenance therapy*

Tacrolimus has been compared to cyclosporin as part of quadruple therapy for patients receiving a cadaveric kidney (Pirsch *et al.* 1997). Patients were randomized to receive either cyclosporin or tacrolimus, commencing once renal function was established by a postoperative fall in serum creatinine below 4mg/dL. Tacrolimus was administered at a dose of 0.2mg/kg/day and titrated to achieve levels between 5 and 15ng/dL.

Patient and graft survival at 12 months did not differ significantly, although the incidence of AREs (30.7% vs. 46.4%) and the use of antilymphocyte antibody therapy for rejection (10.7 vs. 25.1%) were significantly reduced in the tacrolimus group. Tacrolimus was associated with a higher incidence of PTDM (20% vs. 4%, $P<0.001$) and neurological side effects, both of which were frequently reversible with dosage reduction (Pirsch *et al.* 1997). Long-term follow-up data are awaited to allow comparison of the effects of tacrolimus and cyclosporin on graft and patient survival and on the development of chronic rejection. Hypercholesterolaemia appears to be less severe in patients treated with tacrolimus rather than cyclosporin; however, the long-term effects of this on vascular disease are unknown.

### Rescue therapy

An uncontrolled multicentre trial of conversion from cyclosporin- to tacrolimus-based immunosuppression in 73 patients with acute rejection, refractory to previous therapy with pulse steroids and/or antilymphocyte antibodies (81% of patients), has shown much improved graft function and survival in comparison to historical controls (Woodle *et al.* 1996). Graft function was improved in 78% and stabilized in 11% of patients. Actuarial graft and patient survival rates were 93% and 75%, respectively. The main side effects were gastrointestinal and neurological toxicity and a single case of post-transplant lymphoproliferative disorder (PTLD), which cumulatively resulted in the cessation of tacrolimus in only 8% of patients. Thus, tacrolimus appears to be an effective agent for the treatment of refractory acute rejection.

## Sirolimus

Sirolimus (rapamycin) is a new drug likely to find a role in maintenance immunosuppression. It is a macrolide antibiotic isolated from *Streptomyces hygroscopicus*, a fungus found on Easter Island. It has been shown to reduce markedly allograft rejection in a number of animal models and phase III studies are now being carried out in humans.

PHARMACOKINETICS

Sirolimus is rapidly orally absorbed, sequestered in erythrocytes (so whole-blood levels are considerably higher than plasma levels) and has a half-life of approximately 3 days. Alterations in dosage therefore take up to 2 weeks to reach a new steady state unless a loading dose is used (Trepanier *et al.* 1998). Sirolimus, like cyclosporin and tacrolimus, is metabolized by the cytochrome P450-3A enzyme system (Trepanier *et al.* 1998), resulting in changes in drug level when drugs which inhibit or potentiate this system are used (see Table 7.1).

MODE OF ACTION

Sirolimus binds to FK-BP, as does tacrolimus. Despite the fact that both sirolimus and tacrolimus compete for binding to FK-BP, the complexes each of them form with that protein have distinct modes of action. As mentioned above, the complex of tacrolimus with FK-BP disables the calcineurin-dependent pathway of T cell activation. The complex of sirolimus with FK-BP, on the other hand, inhibits the activity of mTOR (target of rapamycin). This in turn reduces the activity of a number of the cyclin-dependent kinases (in particular the phosphorylation of ribosomal protein S17 by p70S6 kinase; Patel *et al.* 1996), which results in a reduction in the synthesis of cell cycle proteins such as CDC2 and cyclin A, and in a subsequent arrest of cell division in the late G1 phase of the cell cycle preventing entry into the S phase (see Fig. 7.1) (Sehgal 1998). Thus sirolimus inhibits T cell proliferation at a point distal to that inhibited by both cyclosporin and tacrolimus.

The fact that cyclosporin and sirolimus have different intracellular targets (cyclophilins and FK-BP, respectively), and also act on different points in the T cell activation and proliferation pathway, means that they exhibit potent synergy both *in vitro* and *in vivo*. Despite sirolimus and tacrolimus both binding to FK-BP12 there appears to be an excess of this protein in the cells and the two agents appear to be able to be used together (see Fig. 7.1).

## SIDE EFFECTS AND DRUG INTERACTIONS

Sirolimus is reasonably well tolerated though it displays the side effects inherent in all non-specific immunosuppressive drugs. In addition, it is associated with hyperlipidaemia, particularly when used with cyclosporin, and also with occasional reduction in platelet count. Despite its synergy with cyclosporin in reducing T cell activation, its side-effect profile does not overlap with or add to that of cyclosporin, with the exception of an increase in hyperlipidaemia (Brattstrom *et al.* 1998) and a possible increase in the incidence of cyclosporin-induced haemolytic–uraemic syndrome.

## USE IN TRANSPLANTATION

Phase II studies examining the use of sirolimus as a maintenance agent in renal transplantation have been performed. One study compared patients receiving cyclosporin, corticosteroids and placebo to those receiving cyclosporin, corticosteroids and sirolimus. Acute renal allograft rejection episodes were significantly reduced in the sirolimus group up to 6 months after transplantation (Kahan *et al.* 1998). Large multicentre phase III trials are now being carried out to establish the role of sirolimus more firmly in maintenance immunosuppression in renal transplantation. The phase II studies suggest, however, that its efficacy will be at least similar to that of cyclosporin and the possibility remains that there will be significant advantages with respect to toxicity, tolerability and, possibly, long-term graft survival.

## Azathioprine

Azathioprine is used as a component of triple therapy maintenance immunosuppression in many centres worldwide, although its role has recently been challenged by the introduction of mycophenolate (see section on the role of macrophages above).

## PHARMACOKINETICS

Azathioprine is a precursor of 6-mercaptopurine, with a more favourable therapeutic index than its parent compound (Chan *et al.* 1987). Oral regimens produce rapid absorption, peak blood levels after 2 h and bioavailability of approximately 60%. Azathioprine is hepatically metabolized to several active and inactive metabolites. Drug activity correlates best with tissue rather than serum levels of the metabolites and blood level monitoring is therefore not helpful. Final excretion is via the kidney. Dosage reduction may be necessary in the presence of liver disease, as a result of the accumulation of metabolites, but is not required in the presence of impaired renal function (Chan *et al.* 1987).

## MODE OF ACTION

Azathioprine inhibits purine metabolism and thereby inhibits cellular proliferation. Azathioprine also appears to interact with some cell membrane-bound molecules and may interfere with antigen recognition, adherence and cell-mediated cytotoxicity (Elion 1993).

## SIDE EFFECTS AND DRUG INTERACTIONS

Bone marrow suppression is the major adverse effect of azathioprine use. Neutropenia is most frequent; however, pure red cell aplasia, thrombocytopenia and, rarely, complete myelosuppression have all been reported (DeClerk *et al.* 1980; Pollak *et al.* 1980). Asians in particular are genetically predisposed to bone marrow suppression, caused by poor metabolism of azathioprine. Cytopenias are reversible with dosage reduction; however, this may occur at the expense of reduced allograft survival (Pollak *et al.* 1980). Azathioprine may induce liver and lung abnormalities. Reversible acute cholestasis has been most frequently reported; however, progressive veno-occlusive liver disease, which is often fatal, has also been associated with azathioprine use (Ware *et al.* 1979). Reversible interstitial pneumonitis has been reported, as has an increase in the frequency of lung malignancies (Bedrossian *et al.* 1984).

Azathioprine remains a favoured immunosuppressant for use during pregnancy as there is little evidence of fetal harm, possibly as a result of the fetal absence of the enzyme hypoxanthine-guanine phosphorybosyl transferase which is required to produce the active metabolites of 6-mercaptopurine (Lu *et al.* 1993).

The interaction of allopurinol with azathioprine is of critical clinical importance and is a frequent clinical consideration, given the high prevalence of gout in patients with renal failure. Allopurinol inhibits the enzyme xanthine oxidase, which is largely responsible for the metabolism of 6-mercaptopurine to inactive metabolites. Thus, the bioactivity and toxicity of azathioprine are markedly increased in its presence. In general, a reduction in the dosage of azathioprine of 75% is appropriate when used with allopurinol. An alternative approach is to substitute mycophenolate for azathioprine in patients who require concurrent allopurinol administration (Jacobs *et al.* 1997).

### USE IN TRANSPLANTATION

The introduction of azathioprine enabled the first successful renal transplant procedures to be performed in the 1960s (Hitchings & Elion 1963). Double therapy with prednisolone and azathioprine became standard maintenance therapy in renal transplantation until the introduction of cyclosporin in 1978. The current role of azathioprine in maintenance immuno-suppression is controversial and is discussed in the sections on mycophenolate mofetil and on maintenance below.

## Mycophenolate mofetil

Mycophenolate mofetil (MMF) is a potent immuno-suppressant now in widespread use in the USA and Australia as a first-line component of maintenance therapy, although it is less commonly employed in the UK. It is also a valuable agent for rescue therapy in the management of refractory rejection.

### PHARMACOKINETICS

Mycophenolate mofetil is well absorbed following oral administration, with a bioavailability exceeding 90%. Absorption is little affected by food. It is de-esterified to the active moiety, mycophenolic acid, which circulates in the plasma fraction of blood (not the cellular compartment), where it is approximately 90% protein-bound, regardless of plasma protein concentrations (Bullingham *et al.* 1996). Free mycophenolic acid is active via tissue receptors. Mycophenolate is hepatically metabolized to inactive conjugates which are excreted in the urine. A significant proportion of MMF undergoes enterohepatic recirculation, leading to high concentrations in the intestine which may be associated with its gastrointestinal toxicity. Dosage adjustment does not appear to be necessary in the presence of renal dysfunction (Bullingham *et al.* 1996).

### MODE OF ACTION

Mycophenolate is a potent, non-competitive inhibitor of the enzyme inosine-monophosphate dehydrogenase (IMPDH), which is pivotal in the *de novo* pathway of purine nucleotide synthesis upon which activated lymphocytes are dependent (Allison *et al.* 1993; Eugui & Allison 1993). The resulting depletion of guanosine triphosphate in particular appears to interfere with lymphocyte secondary messenger systems and nucleotide availability, thereby inhibiting DNA synthesis and causing cell cycle arrest at G1 (Eugui & Allison 1993). The early events in T cell activation, including IL-2 and IL-2R gene expression and synthesis, are not inhibited by MMF (Allison *et al.* 1993), providing a rational basis for synergies with cyclosporin or tacrolimus and also anti-CD25 (IL-2 receptor) monoclonal antibodies. The selectivity of MMF for lymphocytes relates to the reliance of these cells on *de novo* purine synthesis as, in contrast to other nucleated cells, they are unable to engage the salvage pathway. Furthermore, activated lymphocytes predominantly express the inducible type II isoform of IMPDH, which is five times more susceptible to inhibition by MMF than the constitutive type I isoform expressed on other tissues (Eugui & Allison 1993). In addition to the T cell effects of MMF, antibody production is markedly impaired both *in vitro* and *in vivo* following immunization (Smith *et al.* 1998). Mycophenolate mofetil appears to inhibit the proliferation of cytotoxic T cells and also human smooth muscle cells *in vitro* (Eugui & Allison 1993) and *in vivo* (Steele *et al.* 1993; O'Hair *et al.* 1994), which, along with its effect on B cells (Smith *et al.* 1998), raises the possibility that it may have some beneficial effect against chronic graft rejection.

### SIDE EFFECTS AND DRUG INTERACTIONS

The most common adverse effects attributed to MMF have been gastrointestinal, particularly at higher doses, involving abdominal pain and bloating, anorexia, nausea, vomiting and diarrhoea. Occasional patients have been withdrawn from therapy because of haemorrhagic gastritis (Sollinger 1995). Despite the theoretical prediction of lymphocyte selectivity, leucopenia appears at least as frequently in patients given MMF as compared to azathioprine (European Mycophenolate Mofetil Cooperative Study Group 1995; Sollinger 1995; Tricontinental Mycophenolate Mofetil Renal Transplantation Study Group 1996; Mathew 1998). Infection, particularly tissue-invasive cytomegalovirus (CMV), may also be more frequent with MMF (Sollinger 1995; Mathew 1998). As opposed to azathioprine, MMF shows no significant interaction with allopurinol, and may therefore be the agent of choice for use in patients with gout (Jacobs *et al.* 1997).

### USE IN RENAL TRANSPLANTATION

#### Maintenance therapy

Phase I trials, examining a dosage range of MMF 200 mg/day to 3.5 g/day in addition to cyclosporin and prednisolone, demonstrated a direct correlation between the dosage of MMF and prevention of acute rejection episodes (Deierhoi *et al.* 1993). Three major randomized controlled phase III trials examining the efficacy of MMF as a component of maintenance therapy in patients receiving cadaveric renal allografts have been undertaken. A European-based trial examined the efficacy of MMF vs. placebo when combined with cyclosporin and prednisolone, without antibody induction therapy (European Mycophenolate Mofetil Cooperative Study Group 1995). In the two other simultaneously performed trials, MMF was compared with azathioprine in addition to cyclosporin and prednisolone in patients who did (Sollinger 1995) or did

not (Tricontinental Mycophenolate Mofetil Renal Transplantation Study Group 1996) receive antibody induction therapy. All studies examined two regimens of MMF, 2 g or 3 g/day. Importantly, all trials were designed primarily to examine the impact of MMF on the incidence of biopsy-proven AREs during the first 6 months post-transplantation. Patient survival, graft loss, number of courses of antibody and/or high-dose steroids for the treatment of AREs, side effects and a composite measure termed overall treatment failure (percentage of patients with biopsy-proven rejection, death, graft loss or premature withdrawal from the study, analysed on an intention-to-treat basis) (Sollinger & Rayhill 1997; Mathew 1998) were secondary measures.

Overall, MMF was found beneficial in the prevention of AREs. The incidence of biopsy-proven acute rejection was reduced to 14–17% from 46% by MMF vs. placebo in the European trial (European Mycophenolate Mofetil Cooperative Study Group 1995) and to 17–20% from 37% by MMF vs. azathioprine in the US (Sollinger 1995) and Tricontinental (Tricontinental Mycophenolate Mofetil Renal Transplantation Study Group 1996) studies. There was no significant difference between a regimen of 2 g and 3 g per day. Analysis of secondary end-points revealed an overall increase in the incidence of adverse effects with MMF-based regimens vs. placebo or azathioprine in terms of gastrointestinal symptoms, leucopenia and tissue-invasive CMV infections (Sollinger & Rayhill 1997; Mathew 1998). Treatment failure was significantly less common with MMF-based regimens (average 33%) than with placebo (56%) or azathioprine (49%). Analysis of graft survival at 6 months was no different between the groups (Sollinger & Rayhill 1997; Mathew 1998). Thus, in the short term it appears that MMF as a component of maintenance therapy provides more potent immunosuppression, hence less acute rejection episodes, at a cost of a slightly higher incidence of side effects and a greater initial financial outlay as compared to two-drug (cyclosporin and prednisolone) or triple drug regimens using azathioprine.

Long-term consequences, in terms of both graft function and adverse effects, were not addressed by the short-term trials of MMF. Of particular interest is whether MMF may retard the progressive loss of allografts over time as a result of chronic rejection. It has been predicted that MMF may attenuate chronic rejection by several mechanisms:

1 reduced incidence and severity of acute rejection episodes which may be a predisposing factor for chronic rejection (Almond *et al.* 1993; Vereerstraeten *et al.* 1997);

2 suppression of humoral responses which may be important in mediating chronic rejection (Trpkov *et al.* 1996); and

3 direct inhibition of smooth muscle proliferation and consequent arteriopathy (Eugui & Allison 1993; Steele *et al.* 1993; O'Hair *et al.* 1994).

In a bid to address these issues, 3 years' follow-up data from the Tricontinental study have been reported (Mathew 1998). No difference in graft survival or function (serum creatinine and proteinuria) was found between treatment groups and rejection remained the most common cause of graft loss in all groups. An increase in the incidence of gastrointestinal toxicity, leucopenia and tissue-invasive CMV remained apparent in patients receiving MMF. A non-significant trend toward an increase in post-transplant lymphoproliferative disorders and non-cutaneous malignancies was evident in patients receiving MMF 3 g/day, as compared to those receiving azathioprine or MMF 2 g/day. There was no difference in patient survival at 3 years between the groups. Thus, this study was unable to show that the suppression of AREs by MMF would be translated into a reduction in the incidence of chronic rejection. This finding must, however, be tempered by the fact that this study was underpowered to detect small but potentially significant differences in graft and patient survival at 3 years (Mathew 1998).

### Antirejection and rescue therapy

The use of MMF in the treatment of acute rejection and refractory rejection has been reported. In a double blind, randomized, controlled trial of 221 renal allograft recipients experiencing a first acute rejection episode during the first 6 months post-transplant,

treatment with intravenous corticosteroids and MMF 3 g/day was compared with intravenous corticosteroids and azathioprine 1–2 mg/kg/day. The MMF group showed a 44% reduction in treatment failure (29.2% vs. 51.9%, $P = 0.0006$) and a 40% non-significant reduction in graft loss or death after 12 months' follow-up (Mycophenolate Mofetil Acute Renal Rejection Study Group 1998). In the treatment of acute rejection following previous treatment with either high-dose steroids or antilymphocyte antibodies, rescue therapy with MMF 2–3 g/day resulted in a stabilization or improvement in graft function in an impressive 69% of patients and a 45% reduction in graft loss or death after 6 months of follow-up (Mycophenolate Mofetil Renal Refractory Rejection Study Group 1996), representing a major improvement for a group with a previously acknowledged poor prognosis.

The place of MMF in renal transplantation is much debated. Many centres in North America and Australia have adopted MMF 2 g/day as a standard component of triple maintenance therapy, on the rationale that MMF, as a more potent immunosuppressant, can reduce the incidence of AREs and may thereby reduce the incidence of chronic rejection and improve long-term graft survival (Almond *et al.* 1993). This remains to be demonstrated. In contrast, many other centres throughout the world have elected to persist with standard triple therapy (cyclosporin, prednisolone and azathioprine), arguing that MMF usage has not demonstrated a benefit in graft or patient survival, is significantly more expensive and may incur a higher risk of adverse effects in the short and long term. Additionally, it may be argued that the potential to use MMF for the treatment of AREs or refractory rejection may be forfeit by its inclusion in standard maintenance therapy.

## Cyclophosphamide

Cyclophosphamide and other alkylating agents are infrequently used in transplant recipients because of the accumulative risk of carcinogenicity and toxicity to bone marrow, gonads and bladder that is associated with their usage in the long term (Ho *et al.* 1994). As a potent inhibitor of humoral responses, cyclophosphamide has been used in patients who are highly sensitized prior to receiving an allograft, or in whom strong evidence of antibody-mediated rejection is found (see the section on glucocorticoids above). Transplant recipients with active vasculitis, which may recur in the transplanted kidney, may also be given cyclophosphamide as part of their immunosuppressive regimen (Nyberg *et al*. 1997).

Cyclophosphamide is activated by the hepatic cytochrome p450 system to active compounds which then undergo renal excretion. The active metabolites exert cytotoxic and antiproliferative effects by binding to nucleotides and inducing their alkylation, with resultant miscoding, breaks and transcription arrest (Calabresi & Chabner 1990). Adverse effects of cyclophosphamide include cystitis, gastrointestinal upset, alopecia, gonadal toxicity (where cumulative regimens exceed 200 mg/kg) and carcinogenicity (total dose > 1 g/kg) (Ho *et al*. 1994). The risk of acute cystitis can be minimized by morning dosing and ensuring adequate hydration; however, its occurrence in renal transplant recipients may be problematic and must be distinguished from other causes of haemorrhagic cystitis in this setting, including viral cystitis.

## Deoxyspergualin

Deoxyspergualin is a potent immunosuppressant which, to date, is only available as an intravenous preparation. Its use in transplantation has been largely restricted to Japan, where it is used for induction therapy and for the treatment of resistant acute rejection. An analogue of deoxyspergualin suitable for subcutaneous administration has been developed and is undergoing clinical trials.

### MODE OF ACTION

The precise mechanism of action of deoxyspergualin is unknown. Antibody production by B cells is strongly inhibited (Tepper 1993). Cellular immunity is also inhibited through down-regulation of MHC class II expression by macrophages and also non-professional APCs, including mesangial cells (Tesch *et al*. 1997),

inhibition of T cell activation as indicated by IL-2 receptor expression (Kerr & Atkins 1989), blockade of cytotoxic T cell generation (Kerr & Atkins 1991) and inhibition of local macrophage proliferation (Kerr *et al*. 1994).

### USE IN RENAL TRANSPLANTATION

A large series of ABO-incompatible live donor kidney transplants has been reported from a single centre in Japan in which deoxyspergualin was used as a component of an induction regimen which combined plasmapheresis, splenectomy and immunosuppressant drugs (Tanabe *et al*. 1998). Patient and graft survival were 91% and 73%, respectively, after 8 years of follow-up, which is similar to the local ABO-compatible survival rates and remarkably superior to published outcomes in ABO-incompatible transplantation (Cook *et al*. 1987). The extent to which deoxyspergualin contributed to this success is not clear. Deoxyspergualin has also been used for the treatment of steroid-resistant acute rejection and was found to be as efficacious as OKT3 (Okubo *et al*. 1993).

## Immunosuppressive antibody preparations

Antilymphocyte antibodies, both polyclonal (antilymphocyte globulin (ALG) and antithymocyte globulin (ATG)) and monoclonal (murine antihuman CD3 (OKT3)), have been used extensively in induction and antirejection regimens in renal transplantation. These agents have proven to be effective immunosuppressants; however, their use in transplant recipients has been complicated by cytokine release phenomena, cytopenias, infection, loss of bioactivity as a result of the development of neutralizing antibodies and, of most concern, an increased susceptibility to malignancy in the short and long term (Penn 1990; London *et al*. 1995). In an attempt to overcome these shortfalls, newer antibody preparations have been developed with enhanced target selectivity and specificity. Antibodies have also been 'humanized' or made chimeric in order to avoid stimulating a neutralizing host antibody response. Early trials with such agents have shown great promise.

## MODE OF ACTION

The antilymphocyte antibodies induce lymphocyte depletion. Antibody binds rapidly to the target cell population, complement is activated and cells are either lysed directly or opsonized and cleared from circulation by the reticuloendothelial system (Todd & Brogden 1989). Antibody-dependent cell-mediated cytotoxicity may also contribute to cell lysis. The extent and specificity of immune suppression achieved are therefore largely determined by the cell populations which are recognized by the different antibody preparations. Antilymphocyte globulin and ATG are polyclonal antibodies, generated by the injection of human lymphocytes into horses or rabbits with subsequent retrieval of the gamma globulin fraction. These antibodies recognize a relatively broad spectrum of cells and, in addition to inducing lymphocytopenia, can cause thrombocytopenia and, less commonly, neutropenia. OKT3 is a mouse antihuman CD3 IgG2a monoclonal antibody which binds exclusively to T cells and induces profound and selective depletion of these cells within 1 h of administration of a 5-mg dose (Todd & Brogden 1989). A newer antibody preparation, Campath (anti-CD52) removes all CD52+ cells including T and B lymphocytes, natural killer cells and macrophages (Calne *et al.* 1998, 1999). Profound lymphopenia persists with daily regimens of ALG, ATG and OKT3 until therapy is ceased or, particularly in the case of OKT3, neutralizing anti-idiotype or human antimouse antibodies develop. Neutralizing antibodies develop in 25–75% of cases following a 10–14-day course of OKT3, though less frequently following polyclonal antibody therapy, and may be suppressed by the concurrent usage of other immunosuppressants (Kimball *et al.* 1995). In contrast, Campath administration results in prolonged cytopenias, possibly because of an effect on stem cells (Calne *et al.* 1998, 1999). The immunosuppression induced by the depleting antibodies appears to extend well beyond the duration of lymphocytopenia, suggesting that additional mechanisms are active. Furthermore, differential regeneration of lymphocyte subpopulations appears to occur following antibody therapy. Antithymocyte globulin may result in a sustained reduction in the CD4:CD8 ratio (Muller *et al.* 1997) while OKT3 has been reported to retard selectively Th-1 cell regeneration (Reinke *et al.* 1997).

More recent developments in antibody therapeutics have sought to produce long-acting narrow-spectrum immunosuppressants. It has been demonstrated that non-complement-fixing non-cytolytic antibody isotypes may produce selective immunosuppression by targeting and blocking specific cell surface antigens, rather than inducing lymphocyte depletion (Motoyama *et al.* 1997; Nashan *et al.* 1997). It is hoped that more selective immunosuppression will diminish the morbidity and mortality that are currently associated with the use of lymphocyte-depleting antibodies. The problem of therapy-limiting neutralizing antibodies developing in patients treated with antibody preparations raised in mouse or other animals has been addressed by the development of less immunogeneic chimeric and humanized antibodies. Chimeric and humanized antibodies targeting the IL-2 receptor, CD25, have recently been found effective as induction therapy in human renal transplantation. Two infusions of a chimeric anti-CD25 preparation were sufficient to provide sustained immunosuppression, which, in combination with prednisolone and cyclosporin, reduced the rate of AREs occurring within the first 6 months post-transplantation by one-third, as compared to placebo (30% vs. 44%, $P=0.012$) (Nashan *et al.* 1997). In contrast to the effects of lymphocyte-depleting antibodies, side effects were no different to placebo. The role of anti-CD25 induction in high-risk allograft recipients is currently the subject of clinical trials. Thus, anti-CD25 holds great promise as a relatively non-toxic induction agent, although longer-term follow-up studies are required before its use can be broadly recommended.

## USE IN RENAL TRANSPLANTATION

### Induction therapy with antilymphocyte antibodies

Antibody induction is used in standard cadaveric donor transplant protocols by many centres in the USA, but only in protocols for specific high-risk recipient groups in Europe and Australasia (Morris 1996).

Evidence for and against the use of antibody induction in renal transplantation in general, as well as in selected subgroups, is discussed in the section on cyclosporin A above.

*Polyclonal vs. monoclonal antilymphocyte antibodies*

Controversy exists as to the superiority of polyclonal (ALG and ATG) vs. monoclonal (OKT3) antibody therapies. On balance, a slightly higher risk of delayed graft function and early adverse effects, principally because of the acute cytokine release phenomenon, accompanies the use of OKT3 for induction therapy, with little difference in the incidence of AREs, graft or patient survival (Bock *et al.* 1995; Hariharan *et al.* 1996). The development of neutralizing host anti-OKT3 antibodies (human antimouse antibodies) may prevent effective reuse of OKT3 should acute rejection develop subsequently, whereas this is less of a problem with polyclonal antibodies. The overall costs of induction with the depleting antibody preparations are similar (Shield *et al.* 1996; Brennan *et al.* 1997). The newer non-depleting antibody preparations may prove to be cheaper because of their longer half-life with consequent less frequent dosage requirement, combined with a probable reduction in side effects requiring intervention and hospitalization (see also the section on cyclosporin A above).

*Antirejection therapy*

Both polyclonal and monoclonal antilymphocyte antibodies are highly effective in the treatment of acute allograft rejection, whereas preliminary data suggest anti-CD25 therapy is not. The treatment of AREs is discussed in detail in the section on the treatment of acute rejection below.

## Immunotoxins

Immunotoxins provide a means for targeted cell lysis, by coupling a toxic molecule to a monoclonal antibody. Preclinical studies in a primate renal allograft model showed that a T cell-targeted, mutant diptheria toxin (FN18-CRM9) promoted tolerance (Knechtle *et*

*al.* 1997); however, the use of immunotoxins in humans has been hampered by toxicity. The concept remains viable for the future (reviewed in Knechtle 1997).

## Immunosuppressive regimens in renal transplantation

## Donor preconditioning and sensitization

Potential allograft recipients may be immunologically modified in order to improve their chances of attaining stable and lasting engraftment. Prior recipient exposure to donor antigens may promote advantagous or disadvantageous immunological sequelae, contingent on the antigen and the setting.

### DONOR-SPECIFIC TRANSFUSION

Prior recipient exposure to donor antigens may enhance immunological tolerance, albeit by ill-defined means. In the precyclosporin era, donor-specific blood transfusions (DST) administered to recipients prior to transplantation were found to improve graft acceptance and survival (Morris *et al.* 1968). This benefit is not evident when cyclosporin-based immunosuppression is used and consequently DST is seldom practised.

### MANAGEMENT OF THE HIGHLY SENSITIZED PATIENT

Patient exposure to non-self HLA molecules prior to transplantation may stimulate the development of anti-HLA antibodies. Patients who have been exposed to foreign HLA and are thereby highly sensitized, as indicated by panel reactive antibodies (PRA) exceeding 50%, are more likely than non-sensitized recipients to exhibit a positive pretransplant donor-specific cross-match and thereby be refused transplantation. Highly sensitized patients also experience relatively poor graft survival once transplanted (Thorogood *et al.* 1991). For these reasons, sensitized patients accumulate on transplant waiting lists (Thorogood *et al.* 1991; Charpentier *et al.* 1992). To combat these problems, strategies have been developed to remove anti-HLA antibodies and suppress ongoing antibody generation in sensitized patients, prior to attempting transplantation (Taube *et al.* 1984; Charpentier *et al.* 1992; Reisaeter *et al.* 1995).

In theory, optimal therapy involves immunoadsorption, performed by plasma extraction, removal of recipient IgG against a protein A column and subsequent return of residual plasma components to the patient, although plasmapheresis is more commonly used for practical reasons. This has been coupled with cyclophosphamide 1–2.5 mg/kg/day orally, prednisolone 0.5 mg/kg/day and IgG infusion pretransplant, followed by triple (Taube *et al.* 1984) or quadruple (Reisaeter *et al.* 1995) immunosuppression. PRA positivity was significantly reduced, permitting live donor and cadaveric donor transplantation with 1-year graft survival rates of 77% and 61–70%, respectively. Graft survival remains reduced in comparison to non-sensitized recipients and the reduction in sensitization achieved varies considerably from patient to patient (Charpentier *et al.* 1992; Reisaeter *et al.* 1995). However, this may be an acceptable price for improving the access of this group to transplantation. Furthermore, the effects of MMF, which is a more potent supressor of humoral immunity than azathioprine (Smith *et al.* 1998), have not yet been reported but may provide further benefit.

## Induction therapy

Most transplant rejection occurs in the first months after transplantation. Induction therapy aims to deplete maximally the alloimmune response in the short term and thereby enable stable engraftment. Once this state is achieved, the risk of acute rejection is diminished and the amount of immunosuppression provided may be tapered in order to minimize long-term immunosuppression-related morbidity (Penn 1990; London *et al.* 1995). Factors which should be considered in planning induction therapy are the effects it may have on early and late graft function, acute and long-term patient morbidity and mortality, overall cost and the implications it may have for subsequent therapy during the maintenance phase.

The use of perioperative and, most effectively,

preoperative (Fricke *et al.* 1996) methylprednisolone is almost universal. Other maintenance immunosuppressants are commenced immediately post-transplantation, with the exception of cyclosporin, which is commonly withheld or given at low dosage until allograft function becomes evident, as the vasospastic and nephrotoxic actions of this drug have been shown to contribute to delayed graft function (Curtiss *et al.* 1986; Bennett *et al.* 1994). If cyclosporin is withheld there may be a window of inadequate immunosuppression and susceptibility to rejection and thus many centres advocate the use of antibody induction therapy to ensure high-grade suppression during this time, allowing for a delayed introduction of cyclosporin in a so-called 'sequential regimen'. Some studies have suggested a cost–benefit in favour of antibody induction over no induction on the basis of a lower requirement for subsequent hospital readmission for the treatment of AREs (Shield *et al.* 1996; Brennan *et al.* 1997), although this remains controversial (Morris 1996).

The use of antibody induction varies across the world, with antibodies frequently used in US centres, infrequently in Europe and rarely in Australasia and the UK (Okubo *et al.* 1993). Some evidence exists to support the uniform use of such induction (Opelz 1995; Shield *et al.* 1996); however, the lack of a clear graft and patient survival benefit from sequential quadruple therapy (antibody induction plus prednisolone, azathioprine (or MMF) and cyclosporin; Fig. 7.2b) as compared to standard triple therapy (no antibody induction; Fig. 7.2a), together with the increased cost of antibody induction in terms of adverse effects and expense, provides an acceptable rationale for antibody avoidance in uncomplicated cases of cadaveric and living related renal transplantation (Morris 1996). Furthermore, as antibody therapy is required for the treatment of AREs in 15–45% of allograft recipients, prior use during induction in these patients may render a subsequent course either ineffective, because of the prior development of neutralizing antibodies, or dangerous, because of the cumulative risks of such profound long-term immunosuppression, such as the development of malignancy (Penn 1990; London *et al.* 1995). Less controversy exists over the

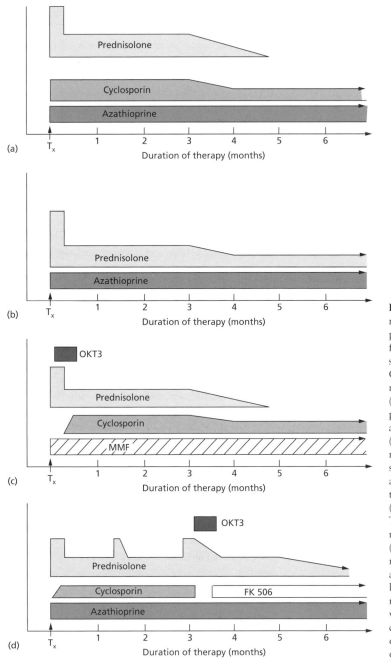

**Fig. 7.2** Immunosuppressive regimens in renal transplantation. The authors proposed immunsuppressive regimens for use in renal allograft recipients stratified for risk and clinical course. (a) Conventional triple therapy recommended for average-risk recipients. (b) Suggested therapy for low-risk patients, an example of whom would be a full match living related renal recipient. (c) A suggested course for a high-risk recipient, who may, for example, be sensitized or have lost previous grafts to acute rejection. Antibody induction therapy is used and mycophenolate (MMF) replaces azathioprine. Tacrolimus is held in reserve in case it is needed for rescue therapy after rejection. (d) Possible approaches to acute rejection. Inital episodes are treated with a pulse of high-dose steroid followed by a brief tapering. Recurrent, severe or refractory rejection is initally treated with steroids but subsequently with a course of intravenous antibody therapy or with rescue with either mycophenolate or tacrolimus (FK 506).

use of antibody induction in defined settings involving recipients stratified into high-risk categories.

1 Delayed graft function or prolonged cold ischaemia time. In patients requiring dialysis for delayed graft function, antibody therapy was found to improve 1-year graft survival by over 50% and to reduce the incidence of AREs and the duration of dialysis required (Benvenisty *et al.* 1990). In cases of prolonged cold ischaemia (>24h), OKT3 induction therapy has been associated with a reduction in AREs and a 20% increase in graft survival at 2 years post-transplantation (Abramowicz *et al.* 1996). It is unclear whether these benefits are a result of the delayed use of cyclosporin in antibody-containing protocols, which may allow the allograft to establish perfusion without the complication of cyclosporin-induced vasospasm and nephrotoxicity, or result from a different mechanism.

2 Paediatric or black recipients. Reductions in graft failure and in the incidence of acute tubular necrosis were reported in the North American Paediatric Renal Transplant Cooperative Study (Kohaut & Tejani 1996). Similarly, improved early graft survival has been noted in black patients with antibody induction (Diethelm *et al.* 1995; Opelz 1995; Kohaut & Tejani 1996).

3 Sensitized recipients and retransplants. As a subgroup of all transplant recipients, these patients have a worse outcome in terms of graft and patient survival, which can be improved by antibody induction (Opelz 1995; Takemoto 1996) (see the section on donor preconditioning and sensitization above).

4 Combined kidney–pancreas transplantation.

## Maintenance regimens in renal transplantation

The aim of providing maintenance immunosuppression is to prevent allograft rejection while exposing the recipient to minimal risks of drug toxicity, opportunistic infection and malignancy. Acute rejection remains the most frequent cause of graft loss in the first 3 years post-transplantation (Mathew 1998) and are predictive of subsequent graft loss through chronic rejection, the major cause of graft loss after the first 3 years (Moeller 1993). The prevention of acute rejection is

therefore a priority, yet excessive immunosuppression carries well-defined risks of opportunistic infection and malignancy (Penn 1990; London *et al.* 1995). Thus maintenance immunosuppression is designed to be sufficient to prevent rejection episodes but is minimized to reduce the risks of side effects. The risk of rejection varies from individual to individual, as well as within the one individual over time, and maintenance therapy therefore requires continuous review and adjustment.

In general, relatively high levels of immunosuppression are provided during the first 3–6 months post-transplantation, to cover the period during which the risk of acute rejection is greatest, then gradually tapered to the minimum required to prevent rejection (Koene & Hilbrands 1998). Additional considerations in designing maintenance regimens are simplicity and convenience, to maximize patient compliance, and the costs of drugs and monitoring.

A wide and increasing variety of agents are available for use in maintenance regimens. The existing published literature is insufficient to allow comparisons to be made between all reasonable combinations of these agents. Thus the choice of agent(s) is guided by a combination of published evidence, local experience, availability and cost, together with stratification of recipients by donor status, matching and comorbidity status.

In the case of HLA-identical sibling transplantation, patient and graft survival with cyclosporin-containing regimens has been found to be no better than with prednisolone and azathioprine double therapy (Opelz *et al.* 1991). An advantage of this regimen is the elimination of the risk of cyclosporin nephrotoxicity. In the presence of a contraindication to either of these agents, however, a cyclosporin-based regimen is a reasonable alternative.

The introduction of cyclosporin in 1972 produced a dramatic improvement in short- and long-term graft survival for recipients of cadaveric and living related (one haplotype matched) and unrelated allografts (Calne *et al.* 1978; Kahan 1989). Consequently, in 1993, 95% of units surveyed in the USA and Europe were found to be using cyclosporin-based maintenance regimens, most commonly cyclosporin-based triple therapy with prednisolone and azathioprine. The withdrawal of cyclosporin from this regimen has been associated with an increase in the incidence of AREs, though no reduction in graft survival at 26 months (Kasiske *et al.* 1993). A small meta-analysis examining azathioprine withdrawal found a trend towards increased rejection, but no effect on long-term survival (Kunz & Neumeyer 1997). Prednisolone can be successfully withdrawn in around 50% of patients, although an increase in AREs and a reduction in long-term allograft function, though not allograft survival, has been demonstrated (Ratcliffe *et al.* 1996) (see the section on alloimmune sensitization above). Cyclosporin monotherapy has been associated with worse long-term graft function (Sinclair 1992). Thus, in the 1980s, and arguably in the 1990s, cyclosporin-based triple therapy remains the gold standard providing predicted 10-year graft survival rates of 74, 51 and 40% for patients receiving first kidney allografts from HLA-identical siblings, HLA 1 haplotype living related donors and cadaver donors, respectively (Opelz *et al.* 1991). Steroids may be weaned slowly after 3 months and eliminated within 6 months in most cases, but reinstated and continued at low dosage should rejection or a significant (15% over baseline) increment in serum creatinine occur (Ratcliffe *et al.* 1996).

Several newer agents have been adopted by many centres as replacements for either cyclosporin (tacrolimus and rapamycin) or azathioprine (MMF) in their standard triple therapy maintenance regimens. Tacrolimus was found to be superior to cyclosporin in preventing AREs and reducing the number of AREs requiring antibody therapy, when used as a component of triple therapy with prednisolone and azathioprine (Scantlebury *et al.* 1991). In this short-term study, no difference in patient or graft survival was detected, while tacrolimus usage was more frequently complicated by post-transplant diabetes and neurotoxicity. Should the reduction in AREs and antirejection therapy result in improved long-term patient and/or graft survival, then a strong case could be made to use tacrolimus in preference to cyclosporin. Such long-term follow-up data are eagerly awaited.

Mycophenolate mofetil also appears to be a more potent immunosuppressant than its predecessor, azathioprine, in particular in its capacity to prevent AREs (European Mycophenolate Mofetil Cooperative Study Group 1995; Sollinger 1995; Tricontinental Mycophenolate Mofetil Renal Transplantation Study Group 1996). Again, however, short-term reductions in AREs and in the usage of antibody antirejection therapy have not been shown to confer a long-term survival advantage, despite patient follow-up for 3 years post-transplant (Deierhoi et al. 1993; Sollinger & Rayhill 1997; Mathew 1998). As MMF is more expensive than azathioprine and incurs a higher incidence of gastrointestinal toxicity, viral infection and probably malignancy, its substitution for azathioprine in standard triple therapy is difficult to justify at this time. Additionally, both tacrolimus (Woodle *et al.* 1996) and MMF (Mycophenolate Mofetil Renal Refractory Rejection Study Group 1996) are effective as rescue agents for refractory rejection. Their inclusion in standard therapy limits their utility to be added in cases of refractory rejection.

Rapamycin may have some unique advantages. Preliminary trials suggest synergy may be achieved with cyclosporin (Kimball *et al.* 1991). The capacity to substitute rapamycin for prednisolone and azathioprine would have clear advantages of simplifying the maintenance regimen and reducing the burden of drug side effects. If the synergistic action of rapamycin allowed a reduction in the dosage of cyclosporin required, reductions in long-term nephrotoxicity may be realized. Finally, rapamycin may have specific activity against chronic rejection (Sawyer *et al.* 1993). Larger clinical trials of rapamycin-based maintenance immunosuppression looking at short- and long-term efficacy are in progress. The authors' approach to immunosuppression for renal transplant recipients is provided in Fig. 7.2.

### Treatment of acute rejection episodes

Acute rejection episodes (AREs) occur in 20–45% of renal transplant recipients and confer short- and long-term risks for both graft and patient survival (Thorogood *et al.* 1991; Mathew 1998). Unsuccessfully treated acute rejection is the most frequent cause of allograft loss within the first 6 months post-transplantation. Acute rejection episodes are also a predictor of poor long-term graft function and graft survival (Almond *et al.* 1993; Mathew 1998). Minor AREs which are rapidly diagnosed and successfully treated do not appear to confer risk of long-term graft dysfunction (Vereerstraeten *et al.* 1997). However, severe AREs, during which renal function is permanently and irreversibly lost, predispose the patient to the development of chronic rejection and premature graft loss (Almond *et al.* 1993; Vereerstraeten *et al.* 1997). Thus, prompt detection and treatment of rejection are of paramount importance in optimizing transplant outcomes. At the same time, however, the risks inherent in administering antirejection therapies must be borne in mind. The most potent antirejection agents also carry the greatest risks of promoting iatrogenic infection and malignancy (Penn 1990; London *et al.* 1995). Thus, a rational approach to providing antirejection therapy is required. The severity and type of rejection, based on clinical and biopsy criteria (Solez *et al.* 1993), the current and past immunosuppressive regimens received by the patient, patient comorbidity status and the local familiarity with and availability of antirejection agents should all be considered.

Intravenous pulses of methylprednisolone, 250–1000 mg/day for 3 consecutive days, are effective in reversing 60–80% of episodes of acute cellular rejection. Given the availability, low cost and general familiarity with steroid use, this remains first-choice treatment for acute cellular rejection at most institutions. Several studies have documented the superiority of OKT3 over pulse steroids in this setting (Ortho Multicenter Transplant Study Group 1985; Deierhoi *et al.* 1998). Steroids were found to reverse 63–75% of AREs, compared to 82–94% with OKT3. When patients with resistant rejection were crossed over to receive the alternative treatment, methylprednisolone and OKT3 were found to be of equal value. The advantage of OKT3 over steroids appears to be in its greater efficacy in treating severe cellular and vascular rejection. Polyclonal lymphocyte-depleting antibodies

appear to have similar efficacy to OKT3 with less toxicity (Bock *et al.* 1995; Brennan *et al.* 1997). Thus, many units use pulse steroids as first-line treatment for acute cellular rejection, OKT3 or a polyclonal antibody as first choice for severe cellular or vascular rejection or for AREs which fail to respond to steroids.

Recent trials have demonstrated the effectiveness of both MMF and tacrolimus in the treatment of acute rejection and resistant rejection. Mycophenolate mofetil was shown to be superior to pulse steroids for the treatment of recurrent acute rejection in terms of graft and patient survival at 6 months, albeit with a higher incidence of gastrointestinal and bone marrow side effects (Mycophenolate Mofetil Renal Refractory Rejection Study Group 1996). Similarly, tacrolimus has been found highly effective in the management of recurrent and resistant rejection (Woodle *et al.* 1996). These results now provide alternatives to the use of antibody therapies for severe or resistant rejection episodes. This is particularly relevant to patients who have had previous antibody therapy for induction or rejection therapy. Antibody reuse is problematic—the efficacy of antibody therapy may wane as a result of neutralizing antibody formation and the risks of iatrogenic infection and malignacy are cumulative (Penn 1990; London *et al.* 1995). Changing antibodies, such as ATG induction then OKT3 for rejection therapy, negates the risk of antibody neutralization but is unlikely to diminish the risk of malignancy. Thus, repeated courses of depleting antibodies should be avoided if possible. Both MMF and tacrolimus provide alternatives. Whether either of these agents will expose recipients to the same risks of infection and malignancy in the long term is uncertain. As MMF and tacrolimus have not been directly compared with each other in the treatment of rejection, it appears reasonable to use either of these agents for the treatment of rejection in the following circumstances:

1 as a third-line agent after steroid and antibody therapy in recipients who had not previously received antibodies;

2 as a second-line agent after steroids, particularly for those with previous antibody exposure; and

**3** for the treatment of severe cellular or vascular rejection, particularly for those previously exposed to antibody therapy.

## Management of chronic rejection

A number of risk factors are associated with the development of chronic rejection, and initial attempts to prevent and treat chronic rejection have therefore been aimed at these factors. There appears to be a significant immunological component causing chronic rejection. The single most important risk factor is the number and severity of acute rejection episodes (Almond *et al.* 1993; Diethelm *et al.* 1995; Vereerstraeten *et al.* 1997). Immunological hyporesponsiveness to the allograft, measured by a low level of cytotoxic T lymphocyte (CTL) precursors and alloantibody, is associated with a decreased risk of chronic rejection. In addition to immune factors, a number of non-immune factors have been implicated, most of which appear to be involved in the acceleration of the vasculopathy associated with chronic rejection (Diethelm *et al.* 1995).

Measures aimed at reducing the number of acute rejection episodes have not yet been demonstrated to reduce the incidence or severity of chronic rejection. It should be emphasized, however, that studies on a number of newer immunosuppressants have either not had appropriate statistical power (e.g. those with mycophenolate; Mathew 1998) or not been followed for long enough (Brattstrom *et al.* 1998) to exclude an effect on chronic rejection. Efforts are also being made to stratify patients according to immunological risk, to allow those at higher risk of acute rejection episodes and thus subsequent chronic rejection to have intensified immunosuppression from the time of transplantation, though results of these studies are not yet available.

As attempts to modulate the immune predisposition to chronic rejection have not yet been successful, the mainstay of current management of this problem addresses the non-immune factors. Careful control of lipid profiles and of hypertension is important in reducing the rate of decline of renal function in patients with chronic rejection, and it is also important to minimize the possibility of cyclosporin toxicity which may accel-erate this process. Once chronic rejection occurs, no intervention has been clearly demonstrated to reverse its course, though the above attention to non-immunological risk factors should be intensified. Studies replacing cyclosporin with other immunosuppressive agents, such as mycophenolate and tacrolimus, in this setting are being carried out, though conclusive results are not yet available.

## Transplantation of other solid organs

### HEART

HLA matching of heart (and lung) allografts is not routinely performed because of the limited time available. In these cases, restricting the total allograft ischaemic time (time from harvest to implantation) is the main priority. Immunosuppressive regimens tend to employ considerably higher dosages of cyclosporin than are used in renal transplantation, and the more potent newer immunosuppressants, such as mycophenolate and tacrolimus, have been more rapidly taken up. As a result of increased immunosuppression, the incidence of infection and malignancy is higher in cardiac than in renal transplantation (Penn 1990). Coronary occlusive disease, a manifestation of both allograft vasculopathy associated with chronic rejection and donor atherosclerotic vascular disease, is the most common cause of graft failure. Differentiating the relative roles of these two causes of arterial disease is difficult, and management is aimed at the control of risk factors for both conditions (Nair & Morris 1995).

### LUNG

Transplantation of the lung also involves more intense immunosuppression than does renal transplantation. The major long-term problem in pulmonary transplantation is the development of obliterative bronchiolitis, which may well be the pathological expression of chronic rejection in the lungs (Heng *et al.* 1998). As for chronic rejection in other transplanted organs, prevention and treatment are currently largely ineffective (Briffa & Morris 1997).

## LIVER

Transplantation of the liver represents a special case in solid organ transplantation. Acute rejection is less common than with other organs and HLA matching is considered unnecessary. Liver transplant patients usually receive considerably less immunosuppression than patients receiving other organ allografts, and maintenance on cyclosporin monotherapy is often achievable. A proportion of liver transplant patients will, in fact, maintain their graft in the absence of any immunosuppression, having become functionally tolerant (Wall & Ghent 1995).

## PANCREAS

Pancreatic allografts are increasingly being performed, usually in association with renal allografts. Immunosuppressive regimens are similar to those used for the transplantation of the kidney alone, though there is a tendency for somewhat more intense immunosuppression to be used, with, for example, the almost universal use of antibody induction therapy (Stratta 1998).

## SMALL BOWEL

Transplantation of the small intestine is becoming increasingly common, though results are still inferior to those of solid organs. The small bowel is a particularly immunogeneic organ, containing much lymphoid tissue. Immunosuppressive regimens are therefore particularly intense, and invariably include antibody induction therapy in addition to use of the more potent recent immunosuppressive agents, such as tacrolimus and MMF. The transplantation of such a large amount of lymphoid tissue can, on occasion, lead to the development of graft vs. host disease in those undergoing small-bowel transplantation, a problem rarely seen in other vascularized allografts (Goulet *et al.* 1997).

## Future directions in immunosuppressive therapy for transplantation

Current regimens seek to promote allograft survival and long-term function while minimizing the adverse effects of immunosuppression on other aspects of bodily function. Rather than using a single agent at high dose, with consequent high risks of toxicity, several drugs at lower doses are frequently utilized. Agents with complementary immunosuppressive actions but different side-effect profiles are employed in order to maximize immunosuppression and minimize the risks of toxicity. Recent advances have resulted in the availability of more potent agents with heightened capacities to prevent acute rejection episodes and to reverse refractory, acute rejection (MMF and tacrolimus), such that AREs which cannot be prevented or controlled by currently available immunosuppressants are uncommon. Advances in potency have, unfortunately, not been equally matched by reductions in drug-associated morbidity and mortality — a reduction in these remains the major goal in the development of new immunosuppressants for transplantation. Most efforts will be directed at agents which specifically target functions of T cells, B cells or macrophages to minimize generalized immunosuppression. Use of agents in current usage may also be improved by risk stratification of graft recipients to minimize immunosuppression for those at low risk of rejection.

Currently used immunosuppressants show potency in the prevention of acute allograft rejection, but have had little discernible impact on graft survival beyond 6 months (Kahan 1989; Mathew 1998). Chronic rejection, the major cause of graft loss after the first 6 month post-transplant, remains poorly understood in terms of aetiology and pathogenesis (Diethelm *et al.* 1995). A more complete understanding of this condition may enable us to determine whether and to what extent immune factors are involved and therefore whether immunosuppressants may have a role in its prevention. Ultimately, we hope to develop strategies to facilitate tolerance of allografts and, eventually, xenografts and much work in this direction is being carried out.

## References

Abramowicz, D., Norman, D.J. & Vereerstreaten, P. (1996) OKT3 prophylaxis in renal grafts with prolonged ischaemia times: associated with improvement in long-term survival. *Kidney International* **49**, 768–772.

Akalin, E., Hancock, W.W., Perico, N. *et al.* (1995) Blocking cell microtubule assembly inhibits the alloimmune response *in vitro* and prolongs renal allograft survival by inhibition of Th1 and sparing of Th2 cell function *in vivo*. *Journal of the American Society of Nephrology* 5, 1418–1425.

Allison, A.C., Eugui, E.M. & Sollinger, H.W. (1993) Mycophenolate mofetil (RS-61443): mechanisms of action and effects in transplantation. *Transplantation Reviews* 7, 129–139.

Almond, P.S., Matas, A., Gillingham, K. *et al.* (1993) Risk factors for chronic rejection in renal allograft recipients. *Transplantation* 55, 752.

Apanay, D.C., Neylan, J.F., Ragab, M.S. & Sgoutas, D.S. (1994) Cyclosporin increases the oxidizability of low-density lipoproteins in renal transplant recipients. *Transplantation* 58, 663–669.

Auphan, N., DiDonato, J.A., Rosette, C., Helmberg, A. & Karin, M. (1995) Immunosuppression by glucocorticoids: inhibition of NF-κB activity through induction of IkB synthesis. *Science* 270, 286–290.

Azuma, H., Nadeau, K.C., Ishibashi, M. & Tilney, N.L. (1995) Prevention of functional, structural, and molecular changes of chronic rejection of rat renal allografts by a specific macrophage inhibitor. *Transplantation* 60, 1577–1582.

Bedrossian, C.W., Sussman, J., Conklin, R.H. & Kahan, B.D. (1984) Azathioprine associated interstitial pneumonitis. *American Journal of Clinical Pathology* 82, 148–154.

Bell, M.J., Martin, L.W., Gonzales, L.L., McEnery, P.T. & West, C.D. (1972) Alternate-day single-dose prednisone therapy: a method of reducing steroid toxicity. *Journal of Pediatric Surgery* 7, 223.

Bennett, W.M. (1995) The nephrotoxicity of immunosuppressive drugs. *Clinical Nephrology* 43 (Suppl. 1), 53–57.

Bennett, W.M., Burdmann, E.A., Andoh, T.F. *et al.* (1994) Nephrotoxicity of immunosuppressive drugs. *Nephrology, Dialysis and Transplantation* 9, 141–145.

Benvenisty, A. *et al.* (1990) Improved results using OKT3 as induction immunosuppression in renal allograft recipients with delayed graft function. *Transplantation* 49, 321–327.

Billingham, R.E., Brent, L. & Medawar, P.B. (1953) Actively acquired tolerance of foreign cells. *Nature* 172, 603–606.

Bock, H.A., Gallati, H., Zurcher, R.M. *et al.* (1995) A randomised prospective trial of prophylactic immunosuppression with ATG fresenius versus OKT3 after renal transplantation. *Transplantation* 59, 830–840.

Bradley, J.A. (1996) Indirect T cell recognition in allograft rejection. *International Review of Immunology* 13 (3), 245–255.

Bradley, J.A., Mowat, A.M. & Bolton, E.M. (1992) Processed MHC class I alloantigen as the stimulus for CD4+ T-cell dependent antibody-mediated graft rejection. *Immunology Today* 13, 434–438.

Brandle, D., Joergensen, J., Zenke, G., Burki, K. & Hof, R.P. (1998) Contribution of donor-specific antibodies to acute allograft rejection: evidence from B cell-deficient mice. *Transplantation* 65, 1489–1493.

Brattstrom, C., Wilczek, H., Tyden, G. *et al.* (1998) Hyperlipidemia in renal transplant recipients treated with sirolimus (rapamycin). *Transplantation* 65, 1272–1274.

Braun, M.Y., McCormack, A., Webb, G. & Batchelor, J.R. (1993) Mediation of acute but not chronic rejection of MHC-incompatible rat kidney grafts by alloreactive CD4 T cells activated by the direct pathway of sensitization. *Transplantation* 55, 177–182.

Brennan, D.C., Schnitzler, M.A., Baty, J.D. *et al.* (1997) A pharmacoeconomic comparison of antithymocyte globulin and muromonab CD3 induction therapy in renal transplant recipients. *Pharmacoeconomics* 11, 237–245.

Briffa, N. & Morris, R.E. (1997) New immunosuppressive regimens in lung transplantation. *European Respiration Journal* 10, 2630–2637.

Bry, W., Warvariv, V., Bohannon, L. *et al.* (1991) Cadaveric renal transplant without prophylactic prednisone therapy. *Transplantation Proceedings* 23, 994.

Buckels, J.A.C., Mackintosh, P. & Barnes, A.D. (1981) Controlled trial of low versus high dose oral steroid therapy in 100 cadaveric renal transplants. *Proceedings of the EDTA* 18, 394.

Buelens, C., Willems, F., Delvaux, A. *et al.* (1995) Interleukin-10 differentially regulates B7-1 (CD80) and B7-2 (CD86) expression on human peripheral blood dendritic cells. *European Journal of Immunology* 25, 2668–2672.

Bullingham, R.E.S., Nicholls, A. & Hale, M. (1996) Pharmacokinetics of mycophenolate mofetil (RS61443): a short review. *Transplantation Proceedings* 28, 925–929.

Burnet, F.M. & Fenner, F. (1949) *The Production of Antibodies*, 2nd edn. Macmillan, London.

Calabresi, P. & Chabner, B.A. (1990) Antineoplastic agents. In: *Goodman and Gilman's Pharmacological Basis of Therapeutics* (eds A.G. Gilman, T.W. Rall, A.S. Niew *et al*), pp. 1209–1236. Pergamon, New York.

Calne, R. & White, D. (1982) The use of cyclosporin A in clinical organ grafting. *Annals of Surgery* 196, 330–337.

Calne, R.Y., White, D.J., Thiru, S. *et al.* (1978) Cyclosporin A in patients receiving renal allografts from cadaver donors. *Lancet* ii, 1323–1327.

Calne, R., Rolles, K., White, D. *et al.* (1979) Cyclosporin A initially as the only immunosuppressant in 36 recipients of cadaveric organs. *Lancet* ii, 1033–1036.

Calne, R., Friend, P.J., Moffatt, S. *et al.* (1998) Prope tolerance, peri-operative campath 1H, and low-dose cyclosporin monotherapy in renal allograft recipients. *Lancet* 351, 1701–1702.

Calne, R.Y., Friend, P.J., Moffatt, S. *et al.* (1999) Campath 1H allows low-dose cyclosporin monotherapy in 31 cadaveric renal allograft recipients. *Transplantation* 68(10), 1613–1616.

Canadian Multicentre Transplant Group (1981) A randomised clinical trial of cyclosporin in cadaveric renal transplantation. *New England Journal of Medicine* 305, 266–269.

Cantarovich, D., Dantal, J., Murat, A. & Soulillou, J.P. (1990) Normal glucose metabolism and insulin secretion in CyA-treated nondiabetic renal allograft patients not receiving steroids. *Transplantation Proceedings* 22, 643.

Castelao, A.M., Barber, M.J., Blanco, A. *et al.* (1992) Lipid metabolic abnormalities after renal transplantation under cyclosporin and prednisone immunosuppression. *Transplantation Proceedings* 24, 96–98.

Chan, G.L.C., Canafax, D.M. & Johnson, C.A. (1987) The therapeutic use of azathioprine in renal transplantation. *Pharmacotherapy* 7, 165–177.

Charpentier, B.M., Hiesse, C., Kriaa, F. *et al.* (1992) How to deal with hyperimmunised potential recipients. *Kidney International* 38, S176–S181.

Chrysostomou, A., Walker, R.G., Russ, G.R. *et al.* (1993) Diltiazem in renal allograft recipients receiving cyclosporin. *Transplantation* 55, 300–304.

Connolly, J.O., Gane, E., Higgins, R.M. *et al.* (1994) Renal arteriopathy associated with FK506 therapy following liver transplantation. *Nephrology, Dialysis and Transplantation* 9, 834–836.

Constant, S.L. & Bottomly, K. (1997) Induction of Th1 and Th2, CD4+ T cell responses: the alternative approaches. *Annual Reviews in Immunology* 15, 297–322.

Cook, D.J., Graver, B. & Terasaki, P.I. (1987) ABO compatability in cadaver donor kidney allografts. *Transplantation Proceedings* 19, 4549–4552.

Coyne, D.W., Nickols, M., Bertrand, W. & Morrison, A.R. (1992) Regulation of mesangial cell cyclooxyhenase synthesis by cytokines and glucocorticoids. *American Journal of Physiology* 263, F97–F102.

Crabtree, G.R. (1989) Contingent genetic regulatory events in T-cell activation. *Science* 243, 355.

Curtiss, J.J. (1986) Hypertension and kidney transplantation. *American Journal of Kidney Disease* 7, 181–196.

Curtiss, J.J., Dubovsky, E., Whelchel, J.D. *et al.* (1986) Cyclosporin in therapeutic doses increases renal allograft vascular resistance. *Lancet* ii, 477–479.

D'Apice, A.J.F., Becker, G.J., Kincaid-Smith, P. *et al.* (1984) A prospective randomized trial of low-dose versus high-dose steroids in cadaveric renal transplantation. *Transplantation* 37, 373.

Darby, C.R., Morris, P.J. & Wood, K.J. (1992) Evidence that long-term cardiac allograft survival induced by anti-CD4 monoclonal antibody does not require depletion of CD4+ T cells. *Transplantation* 54, 483–490.

DeClerk, Y.A., Ettinger, R.B., Ortega, J.A. & Pennisi, A.J. (1980) Macrocytosis and pure RBC anemia caused by aziothioprine. *American Journal of Diseases of Children* 134, 377–379.

Deierhoi, M.H., Barber, W.H., Curtis, J.J. *et al.* (1988) Treatment of acute rejection by monoclonals. A comparison of OKT3 monoclonal antibody and corticosteroids in the treatment of acute renal allograft rejection. *American Journal of Kidney Disease* 11, 86.

Deierhoi, M.H., Sollinger, H.W., Diethelm, A.G., Belzer, F.O. & Kauffman, R.S. (1993) One-year follow-up results of phase I trial of mycophenolate mofetil (RS61443) in cadaveric renal transplantation. *Transplantation Proceedings* 25, 693–694.

Diethelm, A.G., Deierhoi, M.H., Hudson, S.L. *et al.* (1995) Progress in renal transplantation: a single centre study of 3359 patients over 25 years. *Annals of Surgery* 221, 446–458.

Dyer, P.A., Martin, S. & Sinnott, P. (1995) Histocompatability testing for kidney transplantation: an update. *Nephrology, Dialysis and Transplantation* 10 (Suppl. 1), 23–28.

Elion, G.N. (1993) The pharmacology of azathioprine. *Annals of the New York Academy of Sciences* 685, 401–407.

Emerson, S.G. & Cone, R.E. (1982) Absorption of shed I-Ak and H-2Kk antigens by lymphoid cells. *Transplantation* 33, 36–40.

Eugui, E.M. & Allison, A.C. (1993) Immunosuppressive activity of mycophenolate mofetil. *Annals of the New York Academy of Sciences* 685, 309–329.

European Mycophenolate Mofetil Cooperative Study Group (1995) Placebo-controlled study of mycophenolate mofetil combined with cyclosporin and corticosteroids for prevention of acute rejection. *Lancet* 345, 1321–1325.

Falcone, M., Lee, J., Patstone, G., Yeung, B. & Sarvetnick, N. (1998) B lymphocytes are crucial antigen-presenting cells in the pathogenic autoimmune response to GAD65 antigen in non-obese diabetic mice. *Journal of Immunology* 161, 1163–1168.

Ferraris, J.R., Tambutti, M.L., Redal, M. *et al.* (1996) Immunosuppressive activity of deflazacort in paediatric renal transplantation. *Transplantation* 62, 417–420.

Forrest, M.J., Jewell, M.E., Koo, G.C. & Sigal, N.H. (1991) FK506 and cyclosporin A: selective inhibition of calcium ionophore-induced polymorphonuclear leukocyte degranulation. *Biochemistry and Pharmacology* 42, 1221–1228.

Fricke, L., Kluter, H., Feddersen, A. *et al.* (1996) Pre-operative application of glucocorticosteroids efficaciously reduces the primary immunological response in kidney transplantation. *Clinical Transplantation* 10, 432–436.

Fung, J.J., Alessiani, M., Abu-Elmagd, K. *et al.* (1991)

Adverse effects associated with the use of FK506. *Transplantation Proceedings* **23**, 3105–3108.

Galili, U. (1993) Interaction of the natural anti-Gal antibody with alpha-galactosyl epitopes: a major obstacle for xenotransplantation in humans. *Immunology Today* **14**, 480–482.

Gambertoglio, T., Frey, F., Holford, N. *et al.* (1982) Prednisone and prednisolone bioavailability in renal transplant patients. *Kidney International* **21**, 621–626.

Geissler, E.K., Korzun, W.J. & Graeb, C. (1997) Secreted donor-MHC class I antigen prolongs liver allograft survival and inhibits recipient anti-donor cytotoxic T lymphocyte responses. *Transplantation* **64**, 782–786.

Gimsa, U. & Mitchison, A. (1997) New perspectives on the Th1/Th2 paradigm. *Current Opinion in Organ Transplantation* **2**, 18–22.

Golding, H. & Singer, A. (1984) Role of accessory cell processing and presentation of shed H-2 alloantigens in allospecific cytotoxic T lymphocyte responses. *Journal of Immunology* **133**, 597–605.

Goulet, O., January, D., Brousse, N., Revillon, Y. & Ricour, C. (1997) Small-intestinal transplantation. *Baillière's Clinical Gastroenterology* **11**, 573–592.

Gray, D., Shepherd, H., Darr, A., Oliver, D.O. & Morris, P.J. (1978) Oral versus intravenous high-dose steroid treatment of renal allograft rejection. *Lancet* i, 117.

Griffin, P.J., Da Costa, C.A., Salaman, J.R. *et al.* (1987) A controlled trial of steroids in cyclosporin-treatred renal transplant recipients. *Transplantation* **43**, 505.

Groux, H., O'Garra, A., Bigler, M. *et al.* (1998) A CD4+ T-cell subset inhibits antigen-specific T-cell responses and prevents colitis. *Nature* **389**, 737–741.

Gruessner, R.W.G., Burke, G., Stratta, R. *et al.* (1996) A multicenter analysis of the first experience with FK506 for induction and rescue therapy after pancreas transplantation. *Transplantation* **61**, 261–273.

Gulanicar, A.C., MacDonald, A.S., Sungurtekin, U. & Belitsky, P. (1992) The incidence and impact of early rejection episodes on graft outcome in recipients of first cadaver kidney transplants. *Transplantation* **53**, 323.

Hamano, K., Rawsthorne, M.A., Bushell, A.R., Morris, P.J. & Wood, K.J. (1996) Evidence that the continued presence of the organ graft and not peripheral donor microchimerism is essential for maintenance of tolerance to alloantigen *in vivo* in anti-CD4 treated recipients. *Transplantation* **62**, 856–860.

Hariharan, S., Alexander, J.W., Schroeder, T.J. & First, M.R. (1996) Outcome of cadaveric renal transplantation by induction treatment in the cyclosporin era. *Clinical Transplantation* **10**, 186–190.

Henderson, D.J., Naya, I. & Bundick, R.V. (1991) Comparison of the effects of FK506, cyclosporine-A and rapamycin on IL-2 production. *Immunology* **73**, 316–321.

Heng, D., Sharples, L.D., McNeil, K. *et al.* (1998) Bronchiolitis obliterans syndrome: incidence, natural history, prognosis, and risk factors. *Journal of Heart and Lung Transplantation* **17**, 1255–1263.

Hitchings, G.H. & Elion, G.B. (1963) Chemical immunosuppression of the immune response. *Pharmacological Reviews* **15**, 365–401.

Ho, W.K., Robertson, M.R., MacDonald, G.J. *et al.* (1994) Association of acute leukaemia with chlorambucil after renal transplantation. *Lancet* **343**, 1298–1299.

Hricik, D.E., Bartucci, M.R., Moir, E.J., Mayes, J.T. & Schulak, J.A. (1991) Effects of steroid withdrawal on posttransplant diabetes mellitus in cyclosporin-treated renal transplant recipients. *Transplantation* **51**, 374.

Hricik, D.E., Whalen, C.C., Lautman, J. *et al.* (1992) Withdrawal of steroids after renal transplantation— clinical predictors of outcome. *Transplantation* **53**, 41.

Hricik, D.E., O'Toole, M., Schulak, J.A. & Herson, J. (1993) Steroid-free, cyclosporin-based immunosuppression after renal transplantation: a meta-analysis of controlled trials. *Journal of the American Society of Nephrology* **4**, 1300.

Hricik, D.E., Almawi, W.Y. & Strom, T.B. (1994) Trends in the use of glucocorticoids in renal transplantation. *Transplantation* **57**, 979–989.

Ingulli, E., Tefani, A. & Markell, M. (1993) The beneficial effects of steroid withdrawal on blood pressure and lipid profile in children posttransplantation in the cyclosporin era. *Transplantation* **55**, 1029–1033.

Jacobs, F., Mamzer-Bruneel, M.F., Skhiri, H. *et al.* (1997) Safety of the mycophenolate mofetil–allopurinol combination in kidney transplant patients with gout. *Transplantation* **64**, 1087–1088.

Jenkins, M.K. & Schwartz, R.H. (1987) Antigen presentation by chemically modified splenocytes induces antigen-specific T-cell unresponsiveness *in vitro* and *in vivo*. *Journal of Experimental Medicine* **165**, 302–319.

Johnson, R.W., Mallick, N.P., Backram, A. *et al.* (1989) Cadaver renal transplantation without maintenance steroids. *Transplantation Proceedings* **21**, 1581.

Jusko, W.J. & D'Ambrosio, R. (1991) Monitoring FK506 concentrations in plasma and whole blood. *Transplantation Proceedings* **23**, 2732–2735.

Jusko, W.J. & Ludwig, E.A. (1992) Corticosteroids. In: *Applied Pharmacokinetics—Principles of Therapeutic Drug Monitoring* (eds W.E. Evans, J.J. Schentag & W.J. Jusko), 3rd edn, pp. 27.21–27.34. Applied Therapeutics, Vancouver.

Kahan, B.D. (1989) Cyclosporin. *New England Journal of Medicine* **321**, 1725–1738.

Kahan, B.D., Podbielski, J., Napoli, K.L. *et al.* (1998) Immunosuppressive effects and safety of a sirolimus–cyclosporin combination regimen for renal transplantation. *Transplantation* **66**, 1040–1046.

Karin, M., Yang-Yen, H.-F., Chambard, J.-C., Deng, T. & Saatcioglu, F. (1993) Various modes of gene regulation by nuclear receptors for steroid and thyroid hormones. *European Journal of Clinical Pharmacology* **45**, S9–S15.

Kasiske, B.L., Heim-Duthoy, K. & Ma, J.Z. (1993) Elective cyclosporin withdrawal after renal transplantation: a meta-analysis. *Journal of the American Medical Association* **296**, 395–400.

Kauffman, H.M. Jr, Stromstad, S.A., Sampson, D. & Stawicki, A.T. (1979) Randomized steroid therapy of human kidney transplant rejection. *Transplantation Proceedings* **11**, 36.

Kerr, P.G. & Atkins, R.C. (1989) The effects of deoxyspergualin on lymphocytes and monocytes *in vitro* and *in vivo*. *Transplantation* **48**, 1048–1052.

Kerr, P.G. & Atkins, R.C. (1991) Deoxyspergualin inhibits cytotoxic T lymphocytes but not NK or LAK cells. *Immunology and Cell Biology* **69**, 177–183.

Kerr, P.G., Nikolic-Paterson, D.J., Lan, H.Y. *et al.* (1994) Deoxyspergualin suppresses local macrophage proliferation in rat renal allograft rejection. *Transplantation* **58**, 596–601.

Khanna, A., Li, B., Sehajpal, P.K., Sharma, V.K. & Suthanthiran, M. (1995) Mechanism of action of cyclosporin: a new hypothesis implicating transforming growth factor-B. *Transplantation Reviews* **9**, 41–48.

Kimball, J.A., Pescovite, M.D., Book, B.K. & Norman, D.J. (1995) Reduced human IgG anti-ATGAM antibody formation in renal transplant recipients receiving mycophenolate mofetil. *Transplantation* **60**, 1379–1383.

Kimball, P.M., Kerman, R.H. & Kahan, B.D. (1991) Production of synergistic but nonidentical mechanisms of immunosuppression by rapamycin and cyclosporin. *Transplantation* **51**, 486–490.

Kirk, A.D., Harlan, D.M., Armstrong, N.N. *et al.* (1997) CTLA4-Ig and anti-CD40 ligand prevent renal allograft rejection in primates. *Proceedings of the National Academy of Sciences of the USA* **94**, 8789–8794.

Knechtle, S.J. (1997) Immunotoxins in organ transplantation. *Current Opinion in Organ Transplantation* **2**, 97–100.

Knechtle, S.J., Vargo, D., Fechner, J. *et al.* (1997) FN18-CRM9 immunotoxin promotes tolerance in primate renal allografts. *Transplantation* **63**, 1–6.

Koene, A.P. & Hilbrands, L.B. (1998) Choices of long term immunosuppression in renal transplantation: balancing the benefits and risks. *Nephrology, Dialysis and Transplantation* **13**, 844–846.

Kohaut, E.C. & Tejani, A. (1996) The 1994 annual report of the North American Paediatric Renal Transplant Cooperative Study. *Paediatric Nephrology* **10**, 422–434.

Kunz, R. & Neumeyer, H.H. (1997) Maintenance therapy with triple versus double immunosuppressive regimen in renal transplantation: a meta-analysis. *Transplantation* **63**, 386–392.

Kunzendorf, U., Walz, G., Brockmoeller, J. *et al.* (1991) Effects of diltiazem upon metabolism and immunosuppressive action of cyclosporin in kidney graft recipients. *Transplantation* **52**, 280–284.

Kuster, G.M., Drexel, H., Bleisch, J.A. *et al.* (1994) Relation of cyclosporin blood levels to adverse effects on lipoproteins. *Transplantation* **57**, 1479–1483.

Lafferty, K.J., Prowse, S.J., Simeonovic, C.J. & Warren, H.S. (1983) Immunobiology of tissue transplantation: a return to the passenger leukocyte concept. *Annual Review of Immunology* **1**, 143–173.

Lake, K.D. (1991) Management of drug interactions with cyclosporin. *Pharmacotherapy* **11**, 110S–118S.

Larsen, C.P., Morris, P.J. & Austyn, J.M. (1990) Migration of dendritic leukocytes from cardiac allografts into host spleens: a novel pathway for initiation of rejection. *Journal of Experimental Medicine* **171**, 307–314.

Larsen, C.P., Elwood, E.T., Alexander, D.Z. *et al.* (1996) Long-term acceptance of skin and cardiac allografts after blocking CD40 and CD28 pathways. *Nature* **381**, 434–438.

Lechler, R.I. & Batchelor, J.R. (1982) Restoration of immunogenicity to passenger cell-depleted kidney allografts by the addition of donor strain dendritic cells. *Journal of Experimental Medicine* **155**, 31–41.

London, N.J., Farmery, S.N., Will, E.J. *et al.* (1995) Risk of neoplasia in renal transplant patients. *Lancet* **346**, 403–406.

Lu, C.Y., Sicher, S.C. & Vazquez, M.A. (1993) Prevention and treatment of renal allograft refection: new therapeutic approaches and new insights into established therapies. *Journal of the American Society of Nephrology* **4**, 1239–1256.

Lukert, B.P. & Raisz, L.G. (1990) Glucocorticoid-induced osteoporosis: pathogenesis and management. *Annals of Internal Medicine* **112**, 352–364.

MacDonald, A.S., Daloze, P., Dandavino, R. *et al.* (1987) A randomised study of cyclosporin with and without prednisone in renal allograft recipients. *Transplantation Proceedings* **19**, 1865.

McEnery, P.T., Gonzalez, L.L., Martin, L.W. & West, C.D. (1973) Growth and development of children with renal transplants: use of alternate-day steroid therapy. *Journal of Pediatrics* **83**, 806.

McHugh, S.M., Rifkin, I.R., Deighton, J. *et al.* (1995) The immunosuppressive drug thalidomide induces Th2 and concommitantly inhibits Th2 cytokine production in mitogen and antigen stimulated human PBMC cultures. *Clinical and Experimental Immunology* **99**, 160–167.

Martin, M., Neumann, D., Hoff, T. *et al.* (1994) Interleukin-I-induced cyclooxygenase 2 expression is suppressed by cyclosporin A in rat mesangial cells. *Kidney International* **45**, 150–158.

Martin, S. & Class, F. (1993) Antibodies and crossmatching for transplantation. In: *Histocompatability Testing: a*

*Practical Approach* (eds P.A. Dyer & D. Middleton), p. 81. Oxford University Press, Oxford.

Mathew, T.H. (1998) A blinded, long-term, randomized multicenter study of mycophenolate mofetil in cadaveric renal transplantation (results at 3 years). *Transplantation* **65**, 1450–1454.

Miesfeld, R.L. (1990) Molecular genetics of corticosteroid action. *American Review of Respiratory Disease* **141**, S11–S17.

Mihatsch, M.J., Antonovych, T., Bohman, S.O. *et al.* (1994) Cyclosporin A nephropathy: standardization of the evaluation of kidney biopsies. *Clinical Nephrology* **41**, 23–32.

Moeller, G. (1993) Chronic graft rejection. *Immunological Reviews* **134**, 1–116.

Moniemi, H. (1991) Renal allograft immunosuppression V: glucose intolerance occurring in different immunosuppressive treatments. *Clinical Transplantation* **5**, 263.

Morris, P.J. (1996) A critical review of immunosuppressive regimens. *Transplantation Proceedings* **28** (Suppl. 1), 37–40.

Morris, P.J. (1998) Progress in the induction of tolerance to allografts. *Transplantation Proceedings* **30**, 2427–2429.

Morris, P.J., Ting, A. & Stocker, J. (1968) Leukocyte antigens in renal transplantation.1: The paradox of blood transfusions in renal transplantation. *Medical Journal of Australia* **2**, 1088.

Morris, P.J., Chan, L., French, M.E. & Ting, A. (1982) Low dose oral prednisolone in renal transplantation. *Lancet* i, 525.

Mosmann, T.R. & Sad, S. (1996) T-cell subsets, Th1, Th2 and more. *Immunology Today* **17**, 138–146.

Mosmann, T.R., Cherwinski, H., Boud, M.W. *et al.* (1986) Two types of murine T helper cell clone, 1. *Journal of Immunology* **136**, 2348–2357.

Motoyama, K., Arima, T., Lehmann, M. & Flye, M.W. (1997) Tolerance to heart and kidney grafts induced by non-depleting anti-CD4 monoclonal antibody versus depleting anti-CD4 monoclonal antibody with donor antigen administration. *Surgery* **12**, 213–219.

Muller, T.F., Grebe, S.O., Neumann, M.C. *et al.* (1997) Persistent long-term changes in lymphocyte subsets induced by polyclonal antibodies. *Transplantation* **64**, 1432–1437.

Mussche, M.M., Ringoir, S.M.G. & Lameire, N.N. (1976) High intravenous doses of methylprednisolone for acute cadaveric renal allograft rejection. *Nephron* **16**, 287.

Mycophenolate Mofetil Acute Renal Rejection Study Group (1998) Mycophenolate mofetil for the treatment of a first acute renal allograft rejection. *Transplantation* **65**, 235–241.

Mycophenolate Mofetil Renal Refractory Rejection Study Group (1996) Mycophenolate mofetil for the treatment of

refractory, acute cellular renal transplant rejection. *Transplantation* **61**, 722–729.

Naimark, D.M.J. & Cole, E. (1994) Determinants of long term renal allograft survival. *Transplantation Review* **8**, 93.

Nair, R.V. & Morris, R.E. (1995) Immunosuppression in cardiac transplantation: a new era in immunopharmacology. *Current Opinion in Cardiology* **10**, 207–217.

Nashan, B., Moore, R., Amlot, P. *et al.* (1997) Randomised trial of Basiliximab versus placebo for control of acute cellular rejection in renal allograft recipients. *Lancet* **350**, 1193–1198.

Nikolic-Paterson, D.J., Lan, H.Y. & Atkins, R.C. (1997) Macrophages in immune renal injury. In: *Immunologic Renal Diseases* (eds E.G. Neilson & W.G. Couser), pp. 575–592. Lippincott-Raven, Philadelphia.

Nossal, G.J.V. (1983) Cellular mechanisms of immunologic tolerance. *Annual Review of Immunology* **1**, 33–62.

Nyberg, G., Akesson, P., Norden, G. & Wieslander, J. (1997) Systemic vasculitis in a kidney transplant population. *Transplantation* **63**, 1273–1277.

O'Hair, D.P., McMaus, R.P. & Komorowski, R. (1994) Inhibition of chronic vascular rejection in primate cardiac xenografts using mycophenolate mofetil. *Annals of Thoracic Surgery* **58**, 1311.

Okubo, M., Tamura, K., Kamata, K. *et al.* (1993) 15-Deoxyspergualin rescue therapy for methyl-prednisolone resistant rejection of renal transplants as compared with OKT3. *Transplantation* **55**, 505–508.

Ong, C.S., Pollock, C.A., Caterson, R.J. *et al.* (1994) Hyperlipidemia in renal transplant recipients: natural history and response to treatment. *Medicine* **73**, 215–223.

Opelz, G.F. (1995) Efficacy of rejection prophylaxis with OKT3 in renal transplantation. *Transplantation* **60**, 1220–1224.

Opelz, G., Schwartz, V., Englemann, A. *et al.* (1991) Long term impact of HLA matching on kidney graft survival in cyclosporin-treated patients. *Transplantation Proceedings* **23**, 373–375.

Ortho Multicenter Transplant Study Group (1985) A randomized clinical trial of OKT3 monoclonal antibody for acute rejection of cadaveric renal transplants. *New England Journal of Medicine* **313**, 337.

Pan, W.-L., Chan, C.-P., Huang, C.-C. & Lai, M.-K. (1992) Cyclosporin-induced gingival overgrowth. *Transplantation Proceedings* **24**, 1393–1394.

Park, G.D., Bartucci, M. & Smith, M.C. (1984) High- versus low-dose methylprednisolone for acute rejection episodes in renal transplantation. *Nephron* **36**, 80.

Patel, H.R., Terada, N. & Gelfand, E.W. (1996) Rapamycin-sensitive phosphorylation of ribosomal protein S17 by P70, S6 kinase. *Biochemical and Biophysical Research Communications* **227**, 507–512.

Paul, L.C., Valentin, J.F., Muzaffar, S. & Kashgarian, M. (1997) Post-transplant antibody response and chronic rejection. *Transplantation Proceedings* 29, 2529–2530.

Penn, I. (1990) Cancers complicating organ transplantation. *New England Journal of Medicine* 23, 1767–1769.

Peters, D.H., Fitton, A., Plosker, G.L. & Faulds, D. (1993) Tacrolimus: a review of its pharmacology, and therapeutic potential in hepatic and renal transplantation. *Drugs* 46, 746–794.

Pirsch, J.D., Armbrust, M.J., Knechtle, S.J. *et al.* (1991) Effect of steroid withdrawal on hypertension and cholesterol levels in living related donors. *Transplantation Proceedings* 23, 1363.

Pirsch, J.D., Miller, J., Deierhoi, M.H. *et al.* (1997) A comparison of tacrolimus and cyclosporin for immunosuppression after cadaveric renal transplantation. *Transplantation* 63, 977–983.

Pollak, R., Nishikawa, R.A., Mozes, M. & Johasson, O. (1980) Asathioprine-induced leukopenia: clinical significance in renal transplantation. *Journal of Surgical Research* 29, 258–264.

Rao, A.S., Shapiro, R., Corry, R. *et al.* (1998) Adjuvant bone marrow infusion in clinical organ transplant recipients. *Transplantation Proceedings* 30, 1367–1368.

Ratcliffe, P.J., Dudley, C.R.K., Higgins, R.M. *et al.* (1996) Randomised controlled trial of steroid withdrawal in renal transplant recipients receiving triple immunosuppression. *Lancet* 348, 643–648.

Ray, A. & Sehgal, P.B. (1992) Cytokines and their receptors: molecular mechanism of interleukin-6 gene repression by glucocorticosteroids. *Journal of the American Society of Nephrology* 2, S214–S221.

Reinke, P., Schwinzer, H., Hoflich, C. *et al.* (1997) Selective *in vivo* deletion of alloactivated Th1 cells by OKT3 monoclonal antibody in acute rejection. *Immunology Letters* 57, 151–153.

Reisaeter, A.V., Leivestad, T., Albrechtsen, D. *et al.* (1995) Pre-transplant plasma exchange or immunoadsorption facilitates renal transplantation in immunised patients. *Transplantation* 60, 242–248.

Romagnani, S. (1991) Human TH1 and TH2 subsets. *Immunology Today* 12, 256–257.

Rose, J.Q., Nickelsen, J.A., Ellis, E.F., Middleton, E. & Jusko, W.J. (1981) Prednisolone disposition in steroid-dependent asthmatic children. *Journal of Allergy and Clinical Immunology* 67, 188–193.

Sandrin, M.S., Vaughan, H.A., Dabkowski, P.L. & McKenzie, I.F.C. (1993) Anti-pig IgM antibodies in human serum react predominantly with Gal(alpha 1–3)Gal epitopes. *Proceedings of the National Academy of Sciences of the USA* 90, 11391–11395.

Sanfilippo, F., Vaughn, W.K., Bollinger, R.R. *et al.* (1982) The comparative effects of pregnancy, transfusions and prior graft rejection on sensitisation and renal transplant results. *Transplantation* 34, 360.

Sawyer, G.J., Dalchau, R., Fabre, J.W. & Indirect, T. (1993) Cell allorecognition: a cyclosporin A resistant pathway for T cell help for antibody production to donor MHC antigens. *Transplant Immunology* 1, 77–81.

Sayegh, M.H., Akalin, E., Hancock, W.W. *et al.* (1995) CD28–B7 blockade after alloantigenic challenge *in vivo* inhibits Th1 cytokines but spares Th2. *Journal of Experimental Medicine* 181, 1869–1874.

Scantlebury, V., Shapiro, R., Fung, J. *et al.* (1991) New onset diabetes in FK506 vs cyclosporin treated kidney transplant recipients. *Transplantation Proceedings* 23, 3169.

Scheinman, R.I., Cogswell, P.C., Lofquist, A.K. & Baldwin, A.S. Jr (1995) Role of transcriptional activation of IkB in mediation of immunosuppression of glucocorticoids. *Science* 270, 283–286.

Schleimer, R.P. (1993) An overview of glucocorticoid anti-inflammatory actions. *European Journal of Clinical Pharmacology* 45, S3–S7.

Schule, R., Rangarajan, P., Kliewer, S. *et al.* (1990) Functional antagonism between oncoprotein C-Jun and the glucocorticoid receptor. *Cell* 62, 1217–1226.

Sehgal, S.N. (1998) Rapamune (RAPA, rapamycin, sirolimus): mechanism of action and immunosuppressive effect results from blockade of signal transduction and inhibition of cell cycle progression. *Clinical Biochemistry* 31, 335–340.

Shield, C.F. III, Jacobs, R.J., Wyant, S. & Das, A. (1996) A cost-effectiveness analysis of OKT3 induction therapy in cadaveric kidney transplantation. *American Journal of Kidney Disease* 27, 855–864.

Shoskes, D.A. & Wood, K.J. (1994) Indirect presentation of MHC antigens in transplantation. *Immunology Today* 15, 32–38.

Sigal, N.H., Dumont, F., Durette, P. *et al.* (1991) Is cyclophilin involved in the immunosuppressive and nephrotoxic mechanism of action of cyclosporin A? *Journal of Experimental Medicine* 172, 619–628.

Silverman, H. (1981) Dosage of corticosteroids in renal allograft rejection. *American Journal of Surgery* 142, 413.

Sinclair, N.R.StC. (1992) Low-dose steroid therapy in cyclosporin-treated renal transplant recipients with well-functioning grafts. *Canadian Medical Association Journal* 147, 645–657.

Smith, K.G.C., Isbel, N.M., Catton, M.G. *et al.* (1998) Suppression of the humoral immune response by mycophenolate mofetil. *Nephrology, Dialysis and Transplantation* 13, 160–164.

Solez, K., Axelson, R.A., Benediktsson, H. *et al.* (1993) International standardisation of criteria for the histologic diagnosis of renal allograft rejection: the Banff working classification of kidney transplant pathology. *Kidney International* 44, 411–422.

Sollinger, H.W. & Rayhill, S.C. (1997) Mycophenolate mofetil. *Current Opinion in Organ Transplantation* 2, 54–61.

Sollinger, H.W. (1995) US renal transplant mycophenolate mofetil study group: mycophenolate mofetil for the prevention of acute rejection in primary cadaveric renal allograft recipients. *Transplantation* 60, 225–232.

Starzl, T.E. (1998) The art of tolerance. *Nature Medicine* 4, 1006–1008.

Steele, D.M., Hullett, D.A., Bechstein, W.O. *et al.* (1993) Effects of immunosuppressive therapy on the rat aortic allograft model. *Transplantation Proceedings* 25, 754.

Stratta, R.J. (1998) Immunosuppression in pancreas transplantation: progress, problems and perspective. *Transplant Immunology* 6, 69–77.

Strom, T.B. (1992) Molecular immunology and immunopharmacology of allograft rejection. *Kidney International* 42, S182–S187.

Taesch, S., Niese, D. & Mueller, E.A. (1994) Sandimmun neoral, a new oral formulation of cyclosporin A with improved pharmacokinetic characteristics: safety and tolerability in renal transplant patients. *Transplantation Proceedings* 26, 3147–3149.

Takemoto, S. (1996) Sensitization and crossmatch. In: *Clinical Transplants 1995* (eds J.M. Cecka & P.I. Terasaki), pp. 417–424. UCLA Tissue Typing Laboratory, Los Angeles.

Tanabe, K., Koga, S., Takahashi, K. *et al.* (1996) Diabetes mellitus after renal transplantation under FK506 as primary immunosuppression. *Transplantation Proceedings* 28, 1304–1305.

Tanabe, K., Takahashi, K., Sonda, K. *et al.* (1998) Long-term results of ABO-incompatible living kidney transplantation: a single center experience. *Transplantation* 65, 224–228.

Taube, D.H., Williams, D.G., Cameron, J.S. *et al.* (1984) Renal transplantation after removal and prevention of resynthesis of HLA antibodies. *Lancet* i, 824–828.

Tepper, M.A. (1993) Deoxyspergualin; mechanism of action studies of a novel immunosuppressive drug. *Annals of the New York Academy of Sciences* 696, 123–132.

Tesch, G.H., Yang, N., Yu, H. *et al.* (1997) Intrinsic renal cells are the major source of IL-1b synthesis in normal and diseased kidney. *Nephrology, Dialysis and Transplantation* 12, 1109–1115.

Textor, S.C., Wiesner, R., Wilson, D.J. *et al.* (1993) Systemic and renal hemodynamic differences between FK506 and cyclosporin in liver transplant recipients. *Transplantation* 55, 1332–1339.

Thomason, J.M., Seymour, R.A. & Rice, N. (1993) The prevalence and severity of cyclosporin and nifedipine-induced gingival overgrowth. *Journal of Clinical Periodontology* 20, 37–40.

Thomson, A.W. (1992) The effects of cyclosprin A on non-T

cell components of the immune system. *Journal of Autoimmunity* 5, 167–176.

Thorogood, J., Houwelingen, J.C., Persijn, G.G. *et al.* (1991) Prognostic indicies to predict survival of first and second renal allografts. *Transplantation* 52, 831.

Todd, P.A. & Brogden, R.N. (1989) Muromonab CD3: a review of its pharmacology and therapeutic potential. *Drugs* 37, 871–899.

Trepanier, D.J., Gallant, H., Legatt, D.F. & Yatscoff, R.W. (1998) Rapamycin: distribution, pharmacokinetics and therapeutic range investigations: an update. *Clinical Biochemistry* 31, 345–351.

Tricontinental Mycophenolate Mofetil Renal Transplantation Study Group (1996) A blinded, randomized clinical trial of mycophenolate mofetil for the prevention of acute rejection in cadaveric renal transplantation. *Transplantation* 61, 1029–1037.

Trpkov, K., Campbell, P., Pazderka, F. *et al.* (1996) Pathologic features of acute renal allograft rejection associated with donor-specific antibody: analysis using the Banff grading schema. *Transplantation* 61, 1586–1592.

Venkataramanan, R., Jain, A., Warty, V.W. *et al.* (1991) Pharmacokinetics of FK506 following oral administration: a comparison of FK506 and cyclosporin. *Transplantation Proceedings* 23, 931–933.

Vereerstraeten, P., Abramowiez, D., De Pauw, L. & Kinnaert, P. (1997) Absence of deleterious effect on long-term kidney graft survival of rejection episodes with complete functional recovery. *Transplantation* 63, 1739–1743.

Via, C.S., Tsokos, G.C., Stocks, N.I., Clerici, M. & Shearer, G.M. (1990) Human *in vitro* allogeneic responses: demonstration of three pathways of T helper cell activation. *Journal of Immunology* 144, 2524–2528.

Wall, W.J. & Ghent, C.N. (1995) Immunosuppression in liver transplantation: monitoring, dose adjustment, reduction, and withdrawal. *Liver Transplant Surgery* 1 (Suppl.), 3–10.

Ware, A.J., Luby, J.P., Hollinger, B. *et al.* (1979) Etiology of liver diseases in renal transplantation patients. *Annals of Internal Medicine* 91, 364–371.

Webb, A.T., Reaveley, D.A., O'Donnell, M. *et al.* (1993) Does cyclosporin increase lipoprotein (a) concentrations in renal transplant recipients? *Lancet* 341, 268–270.

Welsh, K.I., Batchelor, J.R., Maynard, A. & Burgos, H. (1979) Failure of long surviving, passively enhanced kidney allografts to provoke T-dependent alloimmunity. II. Retransplantation of (AS×AUG) F1 kidneys from AS primary recipients into (AS×WF) F1 secondary hosts. *Journal of Experimental Medicine* 150, 465–470.

Woodle, E.S., Thistlethwaite, R., Gordon, J.H. *et al.* (1996) A multi-centre trial of FK506 therapy in refractory acute renal allograft rejection. *Transplantation* 62, 594–599.

Woods, J.E., Anderson, C.F., De Weerd, J.H. *et al.* (1973)

High dosage intravenously administered methylprednisolone in renal transplantation: a preliminary report. *Journal of the American Medical Association* **223**, 896.

Yamamoto, N., Einaga-Naito, K., Kuriyama, M., Kawada, Y. & Yoshida, R. (1998) Cellular basis of skin allograft rejection in mice. *Transplantation* **65**, 818–825.

Yang-Yen, H.-F., Chambard, J.-C., Sun, Y.-L. *et al.* (1990) Transcriptional interference between C-Jun and the glucorticoid receptor: mutual inhibition of DNA binding due to direct protein–protein interaction. *Cell* **62**, 1205–1215.

Yee, G.C. & Salomon, D.R. (1992) Cyclosporin. In: *Applied Pharmacokinetics — Principles of Therapeutic Drug Monitoring* (eds W.E. Evans, J.J. Schentag & W.J. Jusko), 3rd edn, pp. 28.21–28.40. Applied Therapeutics, Vancouver.

Yon Su Kim, *et al.* (1997) The role of novel T-cell growth factors in rejection. *Current Opinion in Organ Transplantation* **2**, 13–17.

Zucker, K., Rosen, A., Tsaroucha, A. *et al.* (1997) Unexpected augmentation of mycophenolic acid pharmacokinetics in renal transplant patients receiving tacrolimus and MMF in combination therapy, and analogous *in vitro* findings. *Transplant Immunology* **5**, 225–232.

# Chapter 8/Renal transplantation

SATHIA THIRU

## Introduction

Kidney transplantation is established as an accepted mode of treatment for end-stage renal disease. It began at the turn of the 20th century with the development, by Alexis Carrel, Nobel Prize Winner 1912, of vascular surgical techniques required for the anastomosis of the donor organ to the recipient (Hamilton 1994). The first humans received renal transplants in 1906 when Jabouloay transplanted pig and goat xenografts into two patients with chronic renal failure; neither worked for any length of time. Subsequent attempts at transplantation were all unsuccessful and the recognition of 'tissue biochemical barriers' to successful transplantation was established. Voronoy, a Soviet surgeon, transplanted the first cadaveric kidney in 1933. His work with transfusions and blood group antigens made him recognize these were related to the tissue barriers encountered in organ transplantation (Voronoy 1936). In 1954 Hume and colleagues successfully transplanted a kidney from an identical twin and demonstrated that when there was tissue identity between donor and recipient rejection did not occur (Hume et al. 1955; Murray 1992).

Immunosuppressive agents in the form of corticosteroids and total body irradiation were first used in 1953 (Murray et al. 1960). Since then there has been continuing research into developing more powerful and specific agents which could suppress graft immune response and induce tolerance. Medawar and colleagues demonstrated beyond any doubt that allograft rejection is a specific immune response provoked by antigenic components in the foreign tissue (Medawar 1944). These studies outlined and defined several cardinal points in transplantation biology including the demonstration of highly specific *second set* rejection in which animals rejected the second of two sequentially placed grafts more rapidly than the first. Carl Williamson published the first histopathological pictures of allograft rejection in 1926. He described 'marked lymphocytic infiltration' and 'intense glomerulitis' and attributed graft loss to the 'atypical glomerulonephritis' (Williamson 1926). Since then the events that lead to the destruction of *first set* grafts have been well worked out by observations made in untreated animals (Medawar 1944; Porter & Calne 1960; Porter *et al.* 1965). The pathology of rejection in human renal transplants modified by immunosuppression has been extensively studied and the terminology and classification derived by Porter widely adopted (Porter 1965, 1967).

It must be remembered that, although the most important single factor in renal graft rejection is the antigenic similarities and differences between donor and recipient, the structure and function of the graft also depend on many other antigen-independent 'non-specific' factors. These include preservation and 'quality' of the donor organ, ischaemia time prior to transplantation, integrity of the vascular and ureteric anastomoses, toxicity of immunosuppressive and other drugs used, development of urinary tract or systemic infections and the recurrence of patients' original renal disease in the allograft.

## Results of renal transplantation

Over the past two decades the development of new immunosuppressive drugs, with improved efficacy and decreased side effects and toxicity, together with better understanding of using combinations of drugs, has led to marked improvement in patient survival and short-term graft survival. The greatest improvement is in the first year post-transplant, with lower incidence of rejection and fewer infectious complications caused by over-immunosuppression. The 1-year survival of cadaveric renal allografts in the pre-cyclosporin era was 65% whereas it now exceeds 80–85% (Cecka 1996). Despite this improvement in short-term results, the long-term survival of functioning cadaveric grafts continues to be unsatisfactory, graft half-life at present being 9.5 years. The half-life of HLA-identical sibling live donor grafts is 26.5 years, one haplotype identical sibling, parent–child and unrelated live donor grafts 14.2, 11.5 and 12.6 years, respectively (Cecka 1996). The cause of this late graft loss is chronic rejection, a poorly understood process that is probably mediated by both alloantigen-dependent immune mechanisms and alloantigen-independent inflammatory mechanisms (Paul & Tilney 1996; Tilney & Paul 1996).

## Rejection reaction

The immunobiology of rejection, together with the cellular and molecular events involved, are discussed elsewhere. This chapter will concentrate predominantly on the effector mechanisms of rejection and on the histopathological features they produce within the kidney.

In order to evaluate the morphological changes of rejection in clinical renal transplants, it is necessary to have knowledge of the type, severity and time course of lesions in rejection of experimental grafts unmodified by immunosuppression. Such grafts show both cellular and antibody-mediated rejection but, depending on the species, the proportion of each type can vary. Except under very exceptional circumstances, allograft rejection in unmodified non-immunosuppressed recipients is a continuous process resulting in destruction of the graft within 1–2 weeks (Fig. 8.1). A prominent feature of all *first set* allografts in animals is the mononuclear cell infiltration, which starts within a few hours of transplantation (Pederson & Morris 1970) and is well established in a few days. There is substantial morphological heterogeneity of these cells, which consist of small and large lymphocytes, immunoblasts, macrophages, eosinophils and plasma cells. The bulk of the early lymphocytes are T cells, predominantly of CD4 phenotype. Early researchers working on unmodified dog renal allografts concluded that the infiltrating cells were derived from the donor organ and were reacting to the recipient's circulating antigens, rather similar to a graft vs. host reaction (Dempster 1953; Simonsen *et al.* 1953). Porter and Calne (1960), using autoradiographic labelling techniques, showed that the majority of the infiltrating cells are of recipient origin and carried to the graft in the circulation. In the absence of immunosuppression there is progressive accumulation of inflammatory cells, with necrosis, haemorrhage and destruction of the graft.

Dvorak *et al.* (1979) and McCluskey (1980) concluded that the specifically sensitized T lymphocytes initiate *first set* rejection by at least two mechanisms which are not mutually exclusive: (i) cytotoxic T cells, which mount a direct attack on cells of the graft; and (ii) sensitized T helper cells, which initiate a delayed-

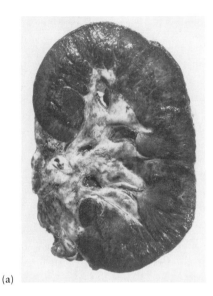

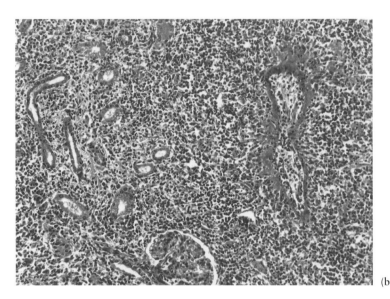

(a)                                                                                                              (b)

**Fig. 8.1** Unmodified rejection: (a) dog kidney allograft, 10 days. Enlarged, oedematous, haemorrhagic kidney with foci of haemorrhage in calyceal mucosa. (b) Section from above kidney. A diffuse infiltrate of mononuclear cells with extensive obliteration of tubules. An interlobular artery shows endotheliitis and fibrinoid necrosis of the wall.

type hypersensitivity reaction, recruiting non-specific lymphocytes and monocytes, which cause vascular damage that secondarily destroys the graft. The basic premise of this theory still holds true and there is increasing evidence that rejection of renal allografts is principally by delayed-type hypersensitivity mechanisms. The role of antibody in *first set* rejection reactions is less clear although there is no doubt that *preformed antibodies* to graft antigens produce almost instantaneous hyperacute rejection similar to the *second set* reactions that occur in experimental skin grafts (Medawar 1944).

The following forms a general discussion of the pathogenesis and morphology of acute cellular rejection, antibody-mediated humoral rejection and the progression to established chronic rejection. Although these three will be discussed separately, it is important to emphasize that in reality they are not strictly com-

partmentalized and more often than not all three processes may overlap or occur simultaneously within a rejecting graft.

## Cellular rejection

As discussed in previous chapters, the sensitized CD4 T cell has a pivotal role in the pathogenesis of allograft rejection. It orchestrates, via cytokines, the entire rejection reaction. Th-1 cells secrete IL-2 and IFN-γ inducing delayed-type hypersensitivity reactions and Th-2 cells produce IL-4, 5, 6 and 10 providing B cell help and antibody production (Mosman & Coffman 1989). IL-5 is probably involved in the induction of both peripheral blood and graft eosinophilia. IFN-γ is a powerful up-regulator of class II antigens in the graft, thus increasing the immunogenicity of the graft and perpetuating the rejection reaction. As a result of these events the initial phase of rejection, dominated by lymphocytes, progresses to a mixed inflammatory infiltrate with substantial morphological heterogeneity and containing CD4 cells, CD8 cells, macrophages, B cells, eosinophils and natural killer (NK) cells. Experimental studies on rat kidney grafts have shown that even at the peak of inflammation only a small minority of all inflammatory cells in the transplant are donor-specific (Manca *et al.* 1987).

The molecules or messengers involved in rejection include a variety of cytokines, chemokines, adhesion molecules, growth factors, complement and the coagulation system. The adhesion molecules concerned are not only those that are involved in antigen presentation and activation of T cells, but also those that promote trafficking of lymphocytes into the graft parenchyma. These adhesion molecules include LFA-1 (CD11a) and its counterligand on endothelial cells, intercellular adhesion molecule-1 (ICAM-1) (CD54), E-selectin and vascular cell adhesion molecule-1 (VCAM-1) and their counter-receptors, Sialyl Lewis X and VLA-4, respectively. The cytokines IL-1 and TNFα induce E-selectin, ICAM-1 and VCAM-1 on vascular endothelium. Anti-ICAM-1 antibody inhibits renal allograft rejection in the monkey (Cosimi *et al.* 1990), demonstrating that ICAM-1 is of importance in graft rejection. This intertwined network of activated T cells and macrophages, the cytokines they produce and the effects of cytokines on adhesion molecules, complement system, coagulation cascade and on both the specific and non-specific cells of the rejection reaction demonstrates the complexity of the reaction. It is clear that the effector events of rejection are twofold: (i) a *specific* immune response and (ii) a *non-specific* inflammatory response, the intensity of which is regulated by the immune response. The specific targets of acute rejection are primarily the vascular endothelial cells, which form the interface between donor and host, and the tubular epithelium.

### MORPHOLOGY AND PATHOGENESIS OF CELLULAR REJECTION

For the sake of clarity the microscopic appearances of the different compartments of the kidney are discussed separately although, in reality, rejection is a dynamic process involving vessels, glomeruli, tubules and interstitium more or less simultaneously. It must not be forgotten that the donor ureter is also a target of rejection and almost invariably has morphological features that reflect those occurring in the kidney. Rejection in the ureter may lead to dehiscence and leakage of urine or cause fibrosis and stricture. Macroscopically, a kidney undergoing severe rejection is enlarged, up to three times its normal size, secondary to varying degrees of vascular congestion, oedema and interstitial inflammation. The graft may be pale, with a slightly congested medulla and haemorrhagic streaks in the cortex, to a dark red cyanotic organ, often containing multiple infarcts (see Fig. 8.1).

*Vessels*

Within the first 24h of transplantation there is peritubular capillary and venous dilatation with adherence of lymphocytes to the endothelial surface. Over the next 48–72h large pyroninophilic lymphoid cells and activated immunoblasts collect within vessels and also migrate into the interstitium (Fig. 8.2). They are invariably accompanied by a number of macrophages and eosinophils as rejection reaches a peak at 7–10 days post-transplant. Initially these events tend to be particularly prominent at the corticomedullary junction, but with progression of rejection there is diffuse involvement of vessels throughout the kidney. Mononuclear cells initially adherent to the endothelium migrate into the intima, lifting it from the underlying media, and eventually extend through the full thickness of the vessel wall (Fig. 8.3). This adherence and infiltration of cells under the endothelium is

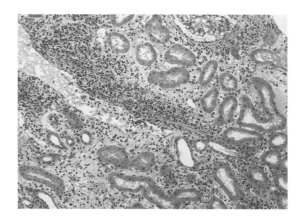

**Fig. 8.2** Cellular rejection: perivascular infiltrate of lymphocytes extending into the oedematous interstitium.

known as endothelialitis, endotheliitis or endovasculitis and is pathognomonic of acute cellular rejection. It is seen much more frequently in small arteries, often at branching points, than in arterioles (Nickeleit *et al.* 1998). The intima is widened by endothelial cell swelling, oedema and infiltrating cells, resulting in luminal narrowing. The damage to the intima encourages the deposition of platelets and fibrin but thrombi

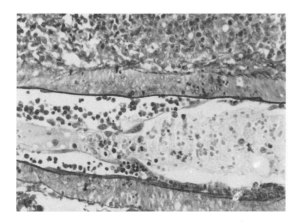

**Fig. 8.3** Cellular rejection: the endothelium is lifted from the media by infiltrating cells—endotheliitis.

are seldom seen. In severe rejection with transmural infiltration of cells, there may be foci of myocyte necrosis, but this should not be confused with the fibrinoid necrosis of antibody-meditated rejection (Fig. 8.4).

### Glomeruli

In early and mild rejection glomeruli are essentially unremarkable, but in severe rejection there is hypercellularity and an active glomerulitis. Immunohistochemical stains reveal that the hypercellularity is predominantly secondary to infiltrating T cells and macrophages (Fig. 8.5) although there is also mesangial cell proliferation. When severe glomerular changes with marked hypercellularity, endothelial cell swelling, mesangiolysis and mesangial interpositioning are present, some other pathology, such as infection—in particular cytomegalovirus (CMV)—or haemolytic uraemic syndrome, should be suspected.

### Tubules

More or less simultaneously with the development of cellular infiltrate, the interstitial tissue becomes oedematous and there is prominent tubulitis with lympho-

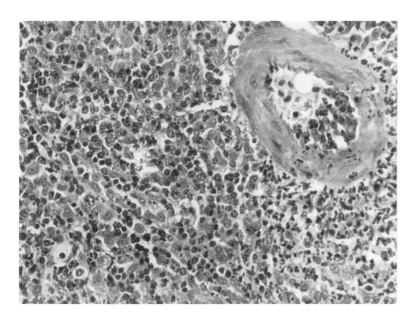

**Fig. 8.4** Cellular rejection: endotheliitis of small artery with transmural infiltration of cells and focal myocyte necrosis—nuclear fragments within media. The surrounding parenchyma is obliterated by an intense interstitial infiltrate.

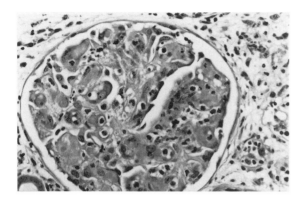

**Fig. 8.5** Cellular rejection: glomerular hypercellularity secondary to infiltrating lymphocytes and macrophages. Note the mononuclear cells within the capillary lumina.

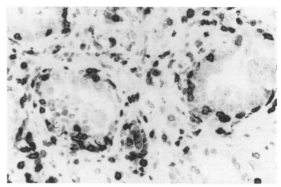

**Fig. 8.6** Cellular rejection: Tubulitis with lymphocytes and macrophages infiltraing tubular epithelium (immunohistochemical stain for leucocyte common antigen, CD45).

cytes and macrophages invading the basement membrane and insinuating between the epithelial cells (Fig. 8.6). All cortical and medullary tubules can be involved, the distal tubules particularly so. In severe cases there are extensive tubular epithelial cell necrosis, cellular casts and disruption of the basement membrane, with leakage of Tamm–Horsfall protein. There is increased tubular HLA-DR antigen expression in acute rejection, presumably a response to the IFN-γ produced by the adjacent interstitial lymphocytes (Fuggle *et al.* 1985). IFN-γ-sensitized tubular cells produce the chemotactic peptide, monocyte chemotactic peptide-1, which attracts lymphocytes and monocytes into the tubular epithelium (Schmouder *et al.* 1993). Tubular cells also make IL-8 in response to IL-1 and TNFα (Schmouder *et al.* 1992) and increase traffic of eosinophils and lymphocytes into the epithelium. In established unmodified rejection there is an intense and diffuse infiltrate of cells by 10 days post-transplant with almost complete obliteration of the tubules (Fig. 8.7).

*Interstitium*

The vascular injury produced by the rejection reaction causes interstitial oedema and, in severe cases, there are varying amounts of interstitial haemorrhage secondary to rupture of capillaries and vessels. The most charac-

teristic feature, however, is the pleomorphic infiltrate of lymphocytes and macrophages, with varying numbers of eosinophils, in a perivascular distribution around arcuate and interlobular arteries and between tubules in the vicinity of peritubular capillaries (Fig. 8.8). Immunohistochemical stains reveal the lymphocytes to be almost exclusively T cells, with the majority of CD4 phenotype and a minor component of CD8 cells. The T cells are activated, with large nuclei, prominent nucleoli, abundant cytoplasm and occasional mitoses. Eosinophils within the interstitial infiltrate are highly predictive of rejection although they often form less than 5% of the infiltrating cells (Kormendi & Amend 1988). Neutrophils are uncommon in the rejection reaction and, if present in significant numbers, raise the possibility of incipient or frank infarction or urinary tract infection.

Macrophages are always present in rejecting grafts, often in surprisingly large numbers when stained with macrophage markers (Dooper *et al.* 1992; S. Thiru, personal observation) (Fig. 8.9). They are important participants of the inflammatory component of rejection as they secrete a number of proinflammatory mediators (platelet-activating factor, prostaglandins, leucotrienes), cytokines (TNF, IL-1, IL-6) and growth factors (platelet-derived growth factor, PDGF, and transforming growth factor, TGFβ), which are potent

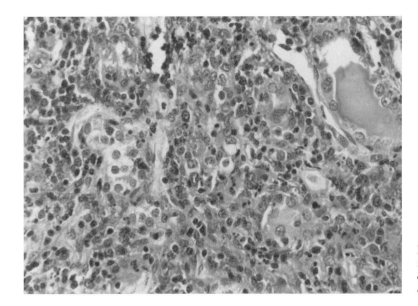

**Fig. 8.7** Unmodified cellular rejection: intense tubulitis and interstitial cellular infiltrate with almost total obliteration of tubules.

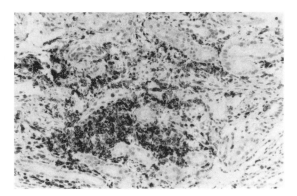

**Fig. 8.8** Cellular rejection: early rejection showing an interstitial infiltrate in a periarterial distribution and between tubules in the vicinity of peritubular capillaries. Imunoperoxidase stain for leucocyte common antigen CD45.

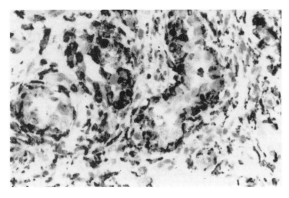

**Fig. 8.9** Cellular rejection: diffuse infiltration of tubular epithelium, arterial wall and interstitium by macrophages, many with cytoplasmic processes. Immunoperoxidase stain, CD68.

stimulators of fibroblast proliferation and collagen synthesis. Macrophages also induce tissue damage by release of proteases and free oxygen radicals, and can cause direct cytotoxicity via Fc receptors. The macrophage is thus seen to have the capacity to cause major graft injury (Sanfilippo *et al.* 1985).

In acute cellular rejection *immunofluorescent* stains for complement and immunoglobulins are essentially non-specific, inconsistent and certainly non-diagnostic. Flecks of positivity for IgG, IgM and C3 may be present within glomerular capillary walls, tubular basement membrane, peritubular capillaries, arteriolar and arterial endothelium (Feucht *et al.* 1991). Deposition of fibrin may be seen within vessels without any evidence of humoral rejection; these deposits are usually present within the intima and are probably secondary to the endothelial damage caused by infiltrating cells.

*Immunohistochemical* studies for typing the infiltrating cells and the detection of cytokines and adhesion molecules are extremely useful, not necessarily for diagnosing rejection but in understanding the pathophysiology of rejection. T cells—both CD4 and CD8 phenotype—and CD68/CD14+ macrophages are present in abundance within an actively rejecting graft (Platt *et al.* 1982; Harry *et al.* 1984; Hancock & Atkins 1985; Bishop *et al.* 1986; McWhinnie *et al.* 1986). B cells are few in number and are incidental, forming part of the inactive infiltrates. T cells and macrophages are present within endovasculitic lesions, glomeruli, tubular epithelium and interstitium (Fig. 8.10). Significant numbers (10–15%) are activated and are positive for the proliferation marker MIB-1 (Robertson *et al.* 1995) and also IL-2 (Noronha *et al.* 1993) and its receptors (CD25) (Noronha *et al.* 1992). Approximately 50–70% of the infiltrating cells are CD3+ T cells, but the proportion of CD4+ and CD8+ cells can be variable. CD4 cells are dominant in the early phase and, with time, CD8 cells are more prominent, indicating that class I antigens are the principal targets

(Tuazon *et al.* 1987). The sites of infiltration by these cells can also be variable, with CD4 cells predominantly in a perivascular distribution and CD8 cells in a more diffuse distribution throughout the interstitium (Sanfilippo *et al.* 1985). Markers for cytotoxic granules, granzymes, perforins and GMP-17 are present in about 30% of the infiltrating T cells (Meehan *et al.* 1997). Most of the GMP-17+ cells are of CD8 phenotype with a smaller proportion, approximately 10%, CD4+. Tubular damage during rejection is, in part, dependent on apoptosis possibly induced by the infiltrating mononuclear cells via the perforin–granzyme or the Fas–Fas ligand pathway (Boonstra *et al.* 1997).

Macrophage infiltration is a common histopathological feature of both acute and chronic renal graft rejection. In some cases it can be the dominant infiltrating cell (Dooper *et al.* 1992; S. Thiru, personal observation). Macrophages are CD14+ and CD68+. CD14 is the receptor for endotoxin-binding protein and is more specific than CD68, which, however, has the advantage of working on paraffin sections. Macrophages also stain for CD4, but the staining tends to be diffuse and not crisp as in T cells. In grafts with significant rejection macrophages are present throughout the parenchyma, within the interstitium—especially around tubules—within tubular epithelium and tubular lumina and within endovasculitic lesions. Tubular lumina can contain 'casts' of macrophages (Fig. 8.11). Infiltrating macrophages display activation markers VLA-4, GMP-17 (Meehan *et al.* 1997), TNFα (Noronha *et al.* 1992) and the chemokine MCP-1, which is also

**Fig. 8.10** Cellular rejection: (a) small artery with marked intimal endotheliitis showing an infiltrate of T cells within the intima and media. Imunoperoxidase stain, CD3. (b) Infiltrating T cells in glomerulus (top, centre) tubules and interstitium. Imunoperoxidase stain, CD3.

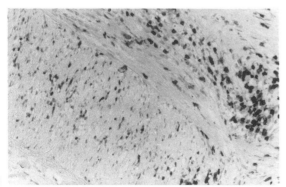

(a)

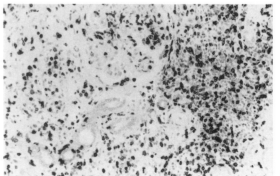

(b)

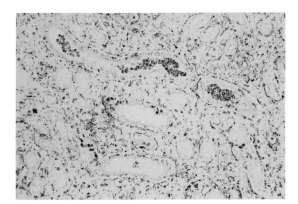

**Fig. 8.11** Cellular rejection: diffuse infiltration of macrophages with casts of macrophages within tubular lumina. Immunoperoxidase stain, CD68.

present in proximal tubular cells of rejecting grafts (Grandaliano *et al.* 1997). Compared to healthy volunteers and patients with non-rejecting grafts, urinary excretion of MCP-1 is significantly increased in patients with rejecting grafts (Prodjosudjadi *et al.* 1996). The increased urinary MCP-1 is most probably produced by the tubular epithelial cells and macrophages within tubules. Macrophages in rejecting grafts also display thromboxane synthase, which catalyses the formation of thromboxane. As thromboxane induces vasoconstriction and platelet aggregation it may play a part in graft dysfunction. Ramos *et al.* (1995) demonstrated significant increase in thromboxane synthase staining in rejecting grafts compared to normal kidneys and on 6 months' follow-up grafts with higher grades of thromboxane staining had a more rapid decline in renal function.

The role of NK cells in graft rejection is difficult to evaluate as they do not have specific markers (Gibson *et al.* 1996). CD56 and CD57 are regarded as markers for NK cells but CD57 can also be present on subsets of monocytes, B cells and T cells of CD4 and CD8 phenotype. CD56 (isoform of neural cell adhesion molecule, NCAM) is also present in subsets of T cells possibly involved in MHC non-restricted cytotoxicity. Studies using a panel of markers have observed NK cells to be uncommon in acute rejection (Anderson *et al.* 1994).

Similarly, B cells are not present in significant numbers in acutely rejecting grafts.

Immunohistochemical staining for cytokines and adhesion molecules in rejecting grafts is still in its infancy as most have to be performed on frozen tissues, with the availability of suitable and sufficient material being a significant handicap. Vascular endothelium in healthy kidneys shows variable constitutive expression of MHC class II antigen expression, depending on their site of origin. Peritubular capillary endothelial cells express intense positivity for HLA-DR, CD31 (PECAM), CD34 (ligand for CD62L—L selectin—and involved in adhesion interactions), factor VIII-related antigen and low levels of ICAM-1 and 2 (Fuggle *et al.* 1993; Anderson *et al.* 1994). Up-regulation of these molecules during rejection episodes therefore cannot be commented on, although loss of staining can be observed when there is destruction of the endothelial cell. Arterial endothelial cells, on the other hand, express very little ICAM-1 and hardly any HLA-DR although they are both markedly increased during acute rejection. Glomerular capillary endothelial staining patterns are essentially similar to peritubular capillary endothelium.

Enhanced expression of HLA-DR antigens on the tubular epithelium is almost routine in acute cellular rejection but is not diagnostic as it can also be seen in other forms of interstitial nephritis, in particular drug-induced forms (Boucher *et al.* 1986). However, an important observation is that in similar grades of rejection patients treated with cyclosporin A have less staining of tubular HLA-DR compared to patients on classical immunosuppression of azathioprine and steroids (Fuggle *et al.* 1985).

## Humoral rejection

Elaboration of serum antibodies in response to allografts is now regarded as routine, but their role in influencing the outcome of the graft is not well understood. There is no doubt that *preformed* cytotoxic antibodies have a major role in the immediate rejection of grafts, as seen in experimental second-set allografts and in patients presensitized by previous pregnancies, blood transfusions or transplants (Kissmeyer-Neilsen *et al.*

1966). The effects of antibodies formed *after* transplantation is less clear; they contribute to acute rejection in some patients and, in others, may promote chronic vascular rejection, have no obvious effect or lead to enhanced graft survival.

MORPHOLOGY AND PATHOGENESIS
OF HYPERACUTE/ACCELERATED
ACUTE REJECTION

Kissmeyer-Neilson *et al.* described hyperacute rejection in two multiparous female recipients who had received many blood transfusions. Soon after the establishment of the circulation the allografts in both patients became dark red, cyanotic, flaccid and did not produce any urine. Similar reactions have occurred when renal transplants have been performed with the donor and recipient mismatched for major blood groups (Dempster 1953; Starzl *et al.* 1968). In all these patients the tempo of graft rejection is greatly accelerated and the term 'hyperacute rejection' is applied as the destruction of the graft occurs within a few minutes to a few hours. Although hyperacute rejection is very rarely seen at present, because of the requirement of ABO compatibility and pretransplant screening by lymphotoxicity tests which prevent grafting into recipients with preformed antibodies, it has not been totally eradicated (Patel & Terasaki 1969). This is attributed to the presence in the recipient's serum of antibodies to non-HLA antigens on donor B cells, macrophages or endothelial cells (Paul *et al.* 1979a). Unlike classic hyperacute rejection, some of these cases take longer to be established—a few days instead of a few hours—presumably because the circulating antibodies have to reach a critical level. The terms 'accelerated acute rejection' and 'early acute rejection' are applied in this situation (Jordan *et al.* 1980). Macroscopically, the grafts are enlarged, soft and deeply cyanotic with numerous foci of haemorrhage.

The abnormalities in hyperacute and accelerated acute rejection are essentially similar and the microscopic appearance reflects the pathogenesis. There is binding of preformed circulating antibodies to the surface of endothelial cells with fixation of complement, chemotaxis of neutrophils, lysozomal enzyme release, lysis of endothelial cells and exposure of the underlying basement membrane, with formation of intravascular platelet aggregates and activation of the coagulation cascade, with thrombosis (Starzl *et al.* 1970). The lesions are initially in glomerular and peritubular capillaries and venules, but very rapidly involve arterioles and small arteries (Fig. 8.12). There is margination of neutrophils and the vessels are stuffed with platelets and neutrophils; intravascular coagulation is present with widespread microthrombi. Frank fibrinoid necrosis may be present in arterioles and

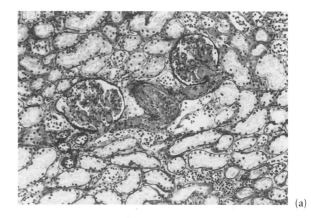

(a)

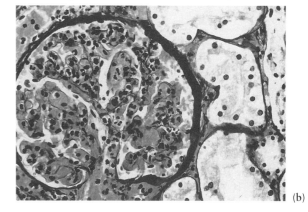

(b)

**Fig. 8.12** Accelerated acute rejection. (a) An interlobular artery, the arteriolar branches and two glomeruli showing vascular lumina filled with platelets and marginating neutrophils. (b) High-power view of a glomerulus with capillary lumina filled with neutrophils and platelet 'thrombi'.

small arteries but this is not a dominant feature. Tubules show varying degrees of acute tubular necrosis secondary to the acute ischaemia. Interstitium becomes oedematous and there is abundant interstitial haemorrhage with disruption of capillaries. There is very little, if any, mononuclear cell infiltration. Subcapsular cortical infarcts occur within 24 h and the entire kidney very rapidly becomes necrotic.

In hyperacute rejection, immunohistochemical stains reveal finely granular–linear deposition of IgG, IgM, fibrin and complement components in glomerular and peritubular capillaries. In the case of ABO blood group incompatibilities there is positive IgM staining in all vasculature. When there are class II antibodies involved there is IgG and IgM staining on glomerular and peritubular capillaries and, in the case of rejection caused by endothelial–monocyte antibodies, positivity is predominantly on peritubular capillaries (Paul *et al.* 1979b).

## MORPHOLOGY AND PATHOGENESIS OF ACUTE HUMORAL REJECTION

In addition to the intense cellular infiltration, in unmodified allografts, immunoglobulins may be found in arterial walls within a few days of transplantation. In some species, especially dogs, fibrinoid necrosis of interlobular arteries and glomerular arterioles develops with extensive foci of parenchymal necrosis (Fig. 8.13). Once parenchymal infarction occurs, neutrophils invade in large numbers, with inevitable destruction of the graft within 1–2 weeks (Simonsen 1953). Macroscopically, the graft is enlarged, swollen and congested, often with streaks of haemorrhage within the cortex. In severe cases the entire organ will be haemorrhagic with wedge-shaped cortical infarcts. The mucosa of the calyces, pelvis and allograft ureter is oedematous and contains varying numbers of haemorrhagic foci. The renal vessels may contain thrombi.

Unlike hyperacute or accelerated acute rejection, the hallmark of acute humoral rejection in the clinical situation is fibrinoid necrosis of arterioles and small arteries. Necrosis can be focal and segmental, at or near branching points or affect the entire length of the vessels. In some, only isolated smooth muscle fibres in

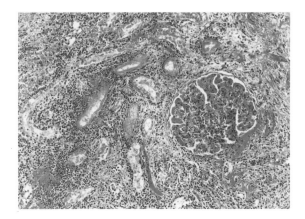

**Fig. 8.13** Acute humoral rejection: fibrinoid necrosis of glomerulus and its hilar arteriole. Infarction of parenchyma with necrotic tubules, interstitial haemorrhage and diffuse infiltrate of neutrophils.

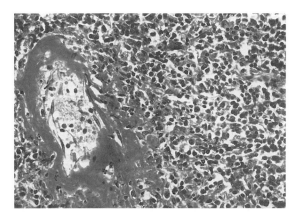

**Fig. 8.14** Acute humoral rejection: circumferential fibrinoid necrosis of interlobular artery with complete loss of structural integrity. There is also accompanying cellular rejection with a diffuse infiltrate of interstitial mononuclear cells.

the media display necrosis; in others, vascular endothelium may show varying combinations of lysis and necrosis with accumulation of fibrin in the subintimal regions and dissolution of the internal elastic lamina; in still others, there is complete loss of structural integrity with the vascular walls replaced by intensely eosinophilic material which stains similar to fibrin–fibrinoid necrosis (Fig. 8.14). Neutrophils are often present within these lesions and thrombosis is a common complication. When the necrotic process involves glomerular arterioles, there is extension into the glomeruli, with fibrin and neutrophils within capillary loops or frank necrosis and thrombosis. Peritubular capillaries are congested and have adherent neutrophils. There is variable interstitial oedema with haemorrhage and tubules show evidence of acute necrosis of the epithelium or zonal areas of infarction. Immunohistochemical stains reveal variable amounts of IgG, IgM, fibrin and complement components within the vasculitic lesions. Extensive fibrinoid necrosis implies irreversible damage and results in infarction of the graft. The graft ureter may have similar vasculitic lesions.

As distinct from hyperacute or accelerated acute rejection, acute humoral rejection occurs 1 to several weeks post-transplantation following initial good function. It often coexists with cellular rejection and, if the lesions are small and focal, they can easily be missed. Severe vasculitic lesions were present in 7% of biopsies in the pre-cyclosporin A era and the incidence has been reduced to 1–3% in the cyclosporin A period (Matas *et al.* 1983). Most patients with acute humoral rejection have antibodies to MHC class I antigens (Halloran *et al.* 1990, 1992) though some have antibodies to class II antigens (Scornik *et al.* 1992) and vascular endothelial cell antigens (Yard *et al.* 1993).

The pathogenesis of humoral rejection is presumed to be alloantibodies to donor MHC class I and II antigens and endothelial cell–monocyte alloantigens. The appearance of post-transplant serum alloantibodies has been reported in 56% of first renal graft recipients (Yard *et al.* 1993; Davenport *et al.* 1994). However, immunohistochemical studies of renal biopsies and nephrectomy specimens with rejection rarely demonstrate consistent and significant staining for immunoglobulin deposits. Does this mean that the serum antibodies have simply been induced by the rejection response and are of no significance, or that the deposition of the antibody on the target antigen is not demonstrated because it has been removed? The detection of antibodies depends on the turnover of the antigen, and low-turnover antigens retain the antibody for longer periods, e.g. persistent anti-glomerular base-

ment membrane (GBM) staining in anti-GBM nephritis. Alloantibodies, on the other hand, are directed against surface antigens of endothelial cells, which have a rapid turnover and also the capacity to remove immunoglobulins deposited on the surface by shedding and internalization (Barba *et al.* 1983). In addition, inhibition of the classical complement pathway and rapid degradation of complement proteins by membrane-bound, e.g. decay-accelerating factor (DAF), and circulating control proteins prevents permanent deposition on the cell surface (Cosio *et al.* 1989; Hamilton *et al.* 1990). Complement and antibodies binding to endothelial surface antigens will therefore be detectable only transiently and in the very early period post-transplant, predating clinical signs of rejection. Immunohistochemical evidence of humoral rejection could therefore be missed in biopsies carried out after clinical signs of rejection have developed. A stable marker of complement activation via antibody-induced classical pathway is the fragment C4d that binds covalently to tissues, resists shedding and is persistent in capillary endothelium. This is unlike the transient C4c component, which is the usual component examined. Prominent vascular deposition of C4d was found in 45% of otherwise unremarkable grafts affected by early dysfunction. The 1-year survival of grafts with capillary C4d was 57%, whereas for C4d-negative grafts the survival was 90% (Feucht *et al.* 1991, 1993). These data indicate that prevalence of lesser forms of humoral rejection is underestimated. Presumably, even though the antibody deposition is transient, they can react with surface Fc-receptors on circulating mononuclear cells, with adhesion of leucocytes that induce cell-mediated cytotoxic reactions and activate the complement and coagulation cascades and thus contribute to the development of occlusive vascular abnormalities of acute and chronic rejection (Feucht & Opelz 1996).

Humoral rejection reactions are difficult to treat as the commonly used immunosuppressive agents, such as steroids, cyclosporin and azathioprine, are directed at the T cell and only indirectly affect B cell responses via inhibition of T cell help. This low efficiency of current immunosuppressive agents may be a reason for the inevitable development of chronic rejection and poor long-term survival of most grafts. The prognosis in well-established humoral rejection is poor. Severe humoral rejection with fibrinoid necrosis was present in 7% of biopsies in the pre-cyclosporin period and 1–3% since the introduction of cyclosporin (Matas *et al*. 1983). Functional recovery is approximately 50% (Salmela *et al*. 1992) compared to 96% for acute cellular rejection. However, the long-term outcome of grafts that survive the acute humoral rejection episode is no different, indicating that the antibody response is transient (Trpkov *et al*. 1996).

## Chronic rejection

As acute rejection episodes are controlled and damped down by successful immunosuppression, chronic changes become more evident. The transition between acute and chronic rejection is indistinct, but the balance shifts from a predominance of cellular infiltrates and fibrinoid vasculitic lesions to a dominance of proliferative stenosing vascular lesions. Clinically, these patients have proteinuria of varying degrees and some are nephrotic. There is a progressive fall in creatine clearance, a rise in serum creatinine and hypertension may be a feature. Chronic rejection manifests itself, both clinically and morphologically, at any time 3–4 months after transplantation.

### MORPHOLOGY AND PATHOGENESIS OF CHRONIC REJECTION

The macroscopic appearances of grafts removed for chronic rejection can be variable. Hypertrophy is a feature of all grafts functioning for more than 3 months. In early chronic rejection the kidney is of normal size or enlarged and pale, with a rubbery and oedematous cut surface and unremarkable intrarenal vessels. With progressive rejection and resulting ischaemia the kidney becomes small, with pale firm parenchyma, loss of corticomedullary distinction and prominent thick-walled vessels visible to the naked eye. The ureter is often firm and thick with luminal narrowing.

Microscopically, the hallmark lesions of chronic rejection are in arteries of all sizes, with many of the tubulointerstitial abnormalities being secondary to the ischaemia produced by the vascular narrowing. Glomerular abnormalities are complex, with some features secondary to ischaemia and others caused by allograft nephropathy.

*Vessels*

Depending on the level of rejection activity, the intrarenal vessels present a spectrum of abnormalities ranging from hyperplasia of the intimal cells to proliferation and massive thickening of the intima with luminal narrowing and obliteration (Fig. 8.15). In early or more active lesions, the endothelial cells are oedematous and large, with basophilic cytoplasm, prominent nuclei and occasional mitoses. The intima is thickened both by oedema and by infiltrating mononuclear cells, predominantly T lymphocytes and macrophages. This is followed by loose myxoid proliferation of the intima, the matrix containing abundant acid mucopolysaccharides and hyaluronic acid. Fibrin, either as flecks or as larger deposits, may be present in the lumen, adherent to the endothelium or in a subendothelial location. Foamy lipid-laden macrophages are often present within the intima, either in small clusters or forming a band-like subendothelial zone. The internal elastic lamina may remain intact, be disrupted and fragmented or show reduplication. As the lesions progress there is fibromuscular proliferation, which may be focal, but more often than not is circumferential and causes marked narrowing of the lumen. Varying degrees of medial scarring and fibrosis are also present. These vascular abnormalities are seen predominantly in interlobular and arcuate arteries but can also involve the larger branches or even the renal artery itself. Acute lesions of rejection, in the form of endotheliitis, infiltration of lymphocytes and macrophages and fibrin deposition, may be superimposed on the established chronic lesions. Although chronic vascular rejection has been termed 'graft atherosclerosis' and 'accelerated atherosclerosis', there are distinct differences between rejection and atherosclerosis. The lesions of chronic rejection are circumferential, do not contain extracellular lipid, often have accompanying endotheliitis with infiltration of activated mononuclear cells and

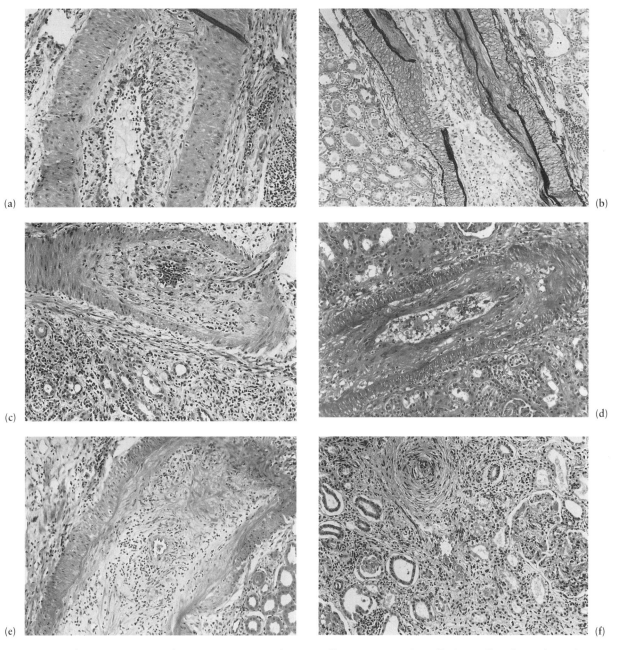

**Fig. 8.15** Chronic rejection: vessels. (a) Arcuate artery with intimal thickening secondary to oedema, infiltrating mononuclear cells and smooth muscle (upper right) proliferation. (b) Arcuate artery with lumen compromised by infiltrating mononuclear cells and foam cells. There are disruption and reduplication of the internal elastic lamina. (c) Interlobular artery showing marked intimal widening secondary to infiltrating mononuclear cells and myxoid stroma. Note the extreme narrowing of the lumen. (d) Interlobular artery with widening of intima secondary to infiltrating mononuclear cells, foam cells and smooth muscle cells. The lumen is virtually occluded by foam cells. (e) Arcuate artery with a narrow lumen and the intima widened by infiltrating cells, myxoid stroma and proliferating fibroblasts (upper right) with collagen deposition. Note the focal scarring (lower right) of the media. (f) Interlobular artery showing marked concentric, 'onion skin'-like proliferation of smooth muscle cells with extreme luminal narrowing.

tend to have prominent concentric smooth muscle proliferation.

Arterioles have only minor degrees of intimal proliferation and more often than not have hyaline sclerosis of the media. This abnormality is non-specific and can be seen in arteriolar sclerosis of age, hypertension, diabetes, chronic cyclosporin A toxicity as well as in chronically rejecting kidneys of the pre-cyclosporin era. Unless there has been substantial venous thrombosis, veins do not show any significant abnormalities.

### Glomeruli

Glomeruli in chronic allograft rejection do not show a consistent pattern of injury. They may be entirely normal or have a spectrum of ischaemic features with atrophy and shrinkage of the glomerular tufts, variable thickening and wrinkling of the glomerular capillary walls and mesangial increase with segmental sclerosis and hyalinization. Some of these abnormalities, in particular focal and segmental sclerosis, have been attributed to hyperfiltration injury (Brenner *et al.* 1992). A change not typical of ischaemia and distinctive for chronic rejection is the pronounced lobular appearance of glomeruli with increase in mesangial matrix, together with widening and reduplication of the capil-

lary basement membrane, giving the glomerulus a lacy appearance rather reminiscent of type I mesangiocapillary glomerulonephritis (Fig. 8.16). However, the absence of marked proliferative changes, including epithelial cell crescents, the lack of uniformity between the abnormal glomeruli and the absence of immune deposits on electron microscopy help to distinguish these features, designated 'allograft glomerulopathy', from mesangiocapillary glomerulonephritis. Differential diagnosis can be difficult, especially as recipients with allograft glomerulopathy often develop proteinuria, very like patients with type I mesangiocapillary glomerulonephritis (Cameron & Turner 1977); the situation is made even more complex as mesangiocapillary glomerulonephritis type I can recur in transplants.

### Tubules

Tubular damage and atrophy are variable and are in proportion to the degree of vascular narrowing and interstitial scarring. Low-grade slowly advancing damage to the tubules is evidenced by degeneration of the epithelium, basement membrane thickening and the presence of lymphocytes and macrophages between tubular cells and within the lumina. Eosinophilic and necrotic debris is often present within tubules. The

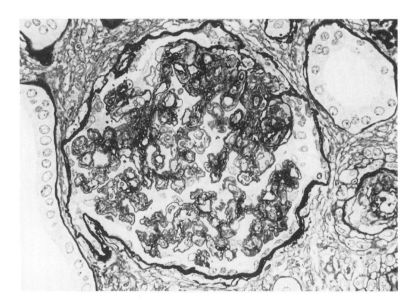

**Fig. 8.16** Chronic rejection: glomerulopathy. Silver stain of glomerulus showing reduplication of the capillary basement membrane.

tubular changes are patchy and interspersed with collections of either normal or hypertrophied tubules. Eventually there is extensive diffuse tubular atrophy with apparent crowding of glomeruli or scattered glomeruli in a background of a dense fibrous interstitium (Fig. 8.17).

### Interstitium

Interstitial cellular infiltration may persist but tends to be rather sparse and is often present as focal aggregates around tubules and larger vessels. The cells are composed of an admixture of small lymphocytes, prominent numbers of plasma cells and macrophages. Initially, the interstitium is oedematous followed by delicate fibrous strands in an oedematous background. In the later phase it is composed of compact, rather acellular fibrous tissue with extensive destruction of tubules and peritubular capillaries.

Episodes of acute rejection can be superimposed on a background of chronic rejection and can occur months to years after transplantation (Reinke *et al.* 1994; Shoker *et al.* 1994). The features of acute rejection in such cases are essentially similar to those seen in the early phase. Chronically rejecting grafts removed after immunosuppression has been withdrawn show

superimposed severe acute changes including fibrinoid vasculitis, interstitial haemorrhage, parenchymal infarction and a florid mononuclear cell infiltrate of macrophages and activated lymphocytes in the interstitium, within tubules and vessel walls on a background of chronic rejection (Fig. 8.18).

In chronic rejection there is no set pattern of immunofluorescence and a variable quantity and pattern of fibrinogen, immunoglobulins and complement components may be seen in the different components of the kidney. There may be granular or linear C3, IgM and IgG in glomerular capillary walls, focal IgM and C3 staining of tubular basement membrane and vessels with intimal thickening may show fibrin, IgM and complement components.

Immunohistochemical studies show variable numbers of CD3+, CD4+ and CD8+ lymphocytes and CD68+ macrophages within glomeruli, tubules, interstitium and endovasculitic lesions. Smooth muscle actin-positive myofibroblasts are present in prominent numbers in the interstitium and within the abnormal vessel walls. Staining for class II antigen can be very prominent in tubular epithelium and vascular endothelium. CD31 staining for endothelial cells often reveals a marked decrease in peritubular capillaries, whereas there are increased ICAM-1 and VCAM-1 on the

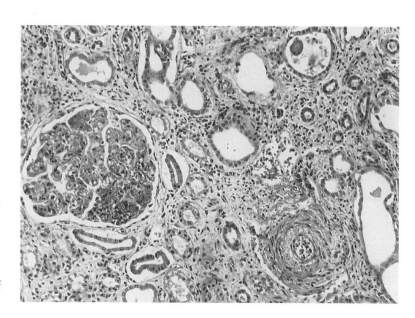

**Fig. 8.17** Chronic rejection: parenchymal atrophy. There is diffuse tubular atrophy with loss of tubules, surviving proximal tubules lined by simplified cuboidal epithelium, interstitial fibrosis and a mild mononuclear cell infiltrate. Note also the glomerular and arterial features of chronic rejection.

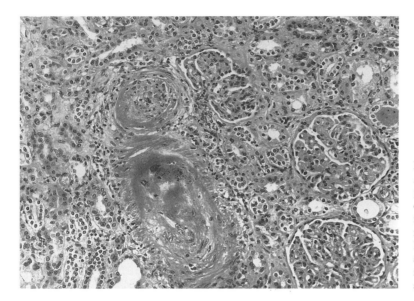

**Fig. 8.18** Acute on chronic rejection. An interlobular artery with extreme proliferative endartititis typical of chronic rejection shows superimposed fibrinoid necrosis with karyorrhectic nuclear debris (dark staining area of lower vessel). There is also tubular atrohpy, tubulitis and an infiltrate of mononuclear cells in the interstitium and glomeruli.

endothelium of larger arteries (Fig. 8.19). A number of growth factors, including PDGF and fibroblast growth factor (FGF), are present within the interstitium and abnormal vessels (Alpers *et al*. 1996; Kerby *et al*. 1996).

The pathogenesis of chronic rejection is quite complex, but both cellular and humoral immune reactions are involved in the initiation and establishment of the lesions, with non-immunological alloantigen-independent mechanisms contributing to the progression of the lesions. The most significant lesion of chronic rejection, both morphologically and functionally, is the gradual relentless compromise and obliteration of the vascular bed from arteries down to the capillaries. The tubular and glomerular abnormalities are secondary to immune injury, as well as the ischaemic effects of these vascular lesions. The lesions of chronic rejection are not seen in isografts or in animal models with syngeneic grafts, thereby indicating that they are immunologically mediated. The target antigens are most probably either major or minor histocompatibility antigens and the target tissue is primarily the endothelium. The prevalence of chronic rejection increases with time after transplantation. The incidence of vascular lesions is 2.4% within the first year (Burke *et*

*al*. 1995), 3.6% in the second year (Isoniemi *et al*. 1992) and, by 10 years, functional graft loss caused by vascular lesions is 16% (Schweitzer *et al*. 1991). Graft loss at 10 years in the pre-cyclosporin era was 18%, thus showing that prevalence has not changed significantly in the era of cyclosporin A. Transplant glomerulopathy is less common than transplant vasculopathy and when it does occur is invariably accompanied by vascular lesions. Profound vascular narrowing leads to ischaemic atrophy of glomeruli and tubules, with parenchymal destruction and fibrosis. Clinically, chronic rejection is characterized by a slow but progressive decline in glomerular filtration rate (GFR) associated with proteinuria and hypertension.

Although the fundamental pathophysiology of transplant vasculopathy is not well understood, the preferential involvement of engrafted vessels with sparing of the recipients' own vessels is a clear indication that alloantigen-dependent immunological mechanisms involving donor–recipient incompatibilities must underlie the development of chronic rejection. Although this may be the crucial component, other alloantigen-independent non-immunological factors may also play a part. These include endothelial damage caused by antigen-independent processes, such as

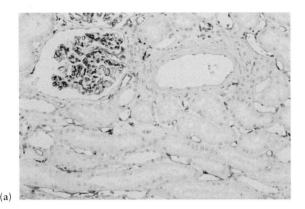

(a)

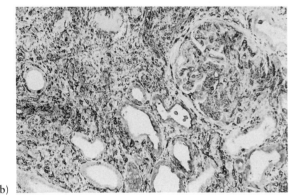

(b)

**Fig. 8.19** Acute on chronic rejection: MHC class II Ag. (a) Immunoperoxidase stain of control kidney for HLA DR. Positive staining of endothelial cells of glomerular and peritubular capillaries. Arterial endothelium is negative. (b) Immunoperoxidase stain of rejecting kidney for HLA DR. Intense positive staining of endothelial cells, tubular epithelium and infiltrating cells.

ischaemia at the time of transplantation, hypertension, CMV infection, cyclosporin A toxicity and alteration of lipid metabolism by the immunosuppressive agents cyclosporin A and prednisone. It is now quite clear that once endothelial damage has been caused, whatever the mechanism of injury, there are the same cellular and molecular mediators of tissue injury, repair and remodelling. The importance of alloantigen-dependent mechanisms is demonstrated by the fact that zero mismatched grafts have a 79% 5-year survival and a half-life of 13.2 years compared with 51% and 7.8 years,

respectively, in complete mismatch combinations (Thorogood *et al.* 1992). The half-life of allografts transplanted between HLA-identical siblings is 20 years, compared to less than 10 years for one haplotype matched sibling transplants and 7–8 years for completely mismatched cadaveric grafts (Tersaki *et al.* 1993). Acute rejection episodes have a strong correlation with the development of late graft dysfunction and the average half-life of a graft decreases from $12.8 \pm 2$ years for grafts with no rejection episodes to 6 years or less for grafts with multiple acute rejection episodes (Matas *et al.* 1994).

The development of chronic rejection is controlled by both cellular and antibody-mediated mechanisms. The evidence in favour of a humoral pathogenesis in chronic rejection is largely circumstantial: patients with chronic rejection have increased levels of IgG and IgM directed against non-HLA antigens expressed by monocytes, epithelial and endothelial cells (Al Hussein *et al.* 1995); circulating antibodies to class I and II antibodies were present in most patients who lost grafts to chronic rejection when compared to those with intact grafts (Davenport *et al.* 1994); antibodies can be eluted from chronically rejected kidneys and these react with class I, II or non-MHC antigens on endothelial and renal epithelial cells (Soulillou *et al.* 1981); immunoglobulins, complement and antiendothelial antibodies can be demonstrated in the abnormal vessel walls (Taylor *et al.* 1991). The available evidence can mean that the antibodies are pathogenic and the cause of chronic rejection *or* that the antibodies are secondary and the result of rejection. The presence of immune reactants in vessel walls can be non-specific or simply reflect altered vascular permeability. However, definite evidence for the role of antibodies in chronic rejection is available from animal studies. Mice with severe combined immunodeficiency given repeated doses of anti-class I alloantibody develop 'graft atherosclerosis' in long-standing cardiac allografts (Russell *et al.* 1994a). The mechanism of antibody action is unknown but probably involves complement activation and platelet deposition with release of growth factors PDGF and FGF (Benzaquen *et al.* 1994).

There is much evidence to indicate that cellular mechanisms have an important role in the development of chronic rejection. Host CD4 cells that recognize alloantigen are activated, with secretion of IFN-α and IL-2. IFN-α up-regulates leucocyte adhesion molecules ICAM-1 and VCAM-1 on endothelial cells and there is leucocyte adherence and transmigration into the vascular walls, where they elaborate cytokines TNF, IL-1, IFN-α, growth factors PDGF, TGFβ and chemokines MCP-1 and RANTES, which favour further entry of lymphocytes and macrophages. There is migration of smooth muscle cells into the intima, with proliferation and production of extracellular matrix (Hancock *et al.* 1993). The final result is thickening of the intima with accumulation of smooth muscle cells, leucocytes, extracellular matrix and fibrosis. Macrophages in particular are very prominent in chronic rejection and, with their ability to produce cytokines, chemokines, growth factors and degradative enzymes, probably have a crucial role in the development of the vascular lesions. The Lewis to F-344 rat cardiac allograft model transplanted across minor histocompatibility barriers is a reproducible animal model of chronic rejection (Adams *et al.* 1993). By day 120, the allograft vessels have well-developed diffuse intimal fibrotic thickening, smooth muscle proliferation and foci of cellularity, very similar to the lesions seen in chronically rejected human cardiac grafts. Detailed immunohistochemical studies revealed lymphocytes and macrophages adherent to the endothelial surface at day 15, with prominent numbers of these cells within the intima at day 45 and 75 and by day 120 variable numbers of macrophages and only rare lymphocytes. Smooth muscle cells, on the other hand, were absent in the intima on day 15, few in number on day 45, the most common intimal cell, especially within the deep intima, on day 75 and the predominant cell type by day 120. Control Lewis isografts had only occasional mild intimal thickening, composed predominantly of smooth muscle cells.

The importance of cytokines in the development of arteriopathy has been shown by injecting antibodies to IFN-γ into cardiac allograft recipient mice; the antibodies did not prevent MHC induction but did inhibit the vascular lesions, most probably by down-grading macrophage activation (Russell *et al.* 1994b). Antibod-

ies to ICAM-1 also inhibit the development of chronic vasculopathy in mice (Russell *et al.* 1995).

The selective involvement of the grafted vessels with sparing of the recipient's arteries has naturally led to the obvious conclusion that alloantigen-dependent mechanisms are crucial in the pathogenesis of chronic rejection. However, alloantigen-independent differences do exist between vessels of the donor and recipient. For example, ischaemia during harvest, or during cold or warm ischaemic periods before re-establishing blood flow could produce endothelial injury with desquamation, platelet deposition and production of PDGF, or induce up-regulation of adhesion molecules with increased adherence and transmigration of leucocytes which produce cytokines and growth factors. Cyclosporin A toxicity, hyperlipidaemia, hypertension, smoking, hyperfiltration caused by loss of critical renal mass and infections, particularly CMV (Koskinen *et al.* 1993), could cause endothelial damage and trigger responses which in essence are similar, though not as severe, to those induced by the rejection reaction. Endothelial injury, whether caused by alloantigen-dependent or alloantigen-independent causes, leads to a final common pathway in which there is production of cytokines and growth factors. The injury these systemic factors cause to the recipient's own vessels will be less severe than their additive effect on graft endothelium which is subjected to the effects of rejection. It is apparent that chronic rejection is the end result of endothelial injury caused by recurrent episodes of clinical acute rejection and/or ongoing or repeated episodes of subclinical rejection with or without superimposed alloantigen-independent injury. Repeated episodes of endothelial activation and injury followed by repair, smooth muscle cell proliferation and deposition of extracellular matrix result in the proliferative stenosing vascular lesions which are the hallmark of chronic rejection.

## Technical complications

Technical complications involve the vascular and ureteric anastomoses. Arterial anastomotic problems tend to occur when there are multiple renal arteries.

This may result in infarction in part of the kidney sup-plied by the smaller vessels. Diagnosing an arterial infarct on biopsy tissue is straightforward: the parenchyma is very pale, with ghostly outlines of cells, loss of nuclei and an acute inflammatory infiltrate at the edge of the infarct. The extent of the infarct can be assessed only by radiological studies. Renal vein thrombosis can occur early in the post-transplant period and biopsy of the graft may show early changes of interstitial oedema, peritubular capillary dilatation with congestion and adherence of neutrophils in glomerular capillaries. With progression, there are more severe abnormalities, including extreme capillary congestion, interstitial haemorrhage, engorgement of glomerular capillaries and infarction (Fig. 8.20). These abnormalities can be similar to those seen in acceler-ated acute humoral rejection. Careful examination of small arteries and arterioles for the presence of acute fibrinoid necrotizing vasculitis is essential and the absence of such lesions will indicate a diagnosis of venous occlusion. The differential diagnosis, however, can be very difficult as, on occasion, vascular lesions of acute rejection can be complicated by thrombosis, and

renal vein thrombosis can occur as a complication of severe rejection.

Ureteric anastomotic complications include kinking, ureteric fistula, stenosis and breakdown of the anasto-mosis. Any of these may be complicated by infection of the graft and, on occasion, by acute hydronephrosis. In allografts with outflow problems there is lymphatic and capillary dilatation, especially of the medulla, followed by tubular dilatation, epithelial cell degenera-tion and atrophy. The interstitium contains a sprin-kling of mononuclear cells and occasional neutrophils, which become much more prominent if infection supervenes. Ureteric complications causing renal dys-function may be suspected on renal biopsy but a defini-tive diagnosis requires imaging studies.

## Peroperative baseline biopsy

Biopsy—either a subcapsular wedge or needle core—after graft blood flow is restored is a very useful base-line of the transplanted kidney. Though small, it can give a surprising amount of information. It may indi-cate the presence or absence of pre-existing disease in

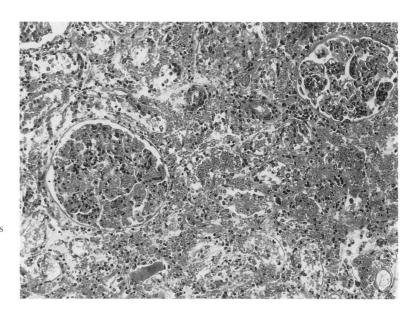

**Fig. 8.20** Renal vein thrombosis. Extreme congestion of peritubular capillaries, some ruptured, with haemorrhage into interstitium and destruction of tubules. The glomerulus on the right shows adherence of neutrophils to capillary endothelium whereas the one on the left shows additional red cell engorgement and rupture of capillary loops.

the donor, including ischaemic age changes of subcapsular glomerular shrinkage and sclerosis, arteriolar hyaline sclerosis and foci of tubular atrophy with accompanying interstitial fibrosis. Grafts with prolonged ischaemia time, particularly warm ischaemia, and machine-perfused cadaver kidneys can undergo endothelial damage, with up-regulation of adhesion molecules and liberation of reactive oxygen species. When the circulation is restored, there is evidence of flecks of fibrin, platelets and neutrophils adherent to glomerular capillaries. The tubules are often lined by poorly preserved degenerate epithelium. The capillary lesions are similar to but not as widespread or as severe as hyperacute rejection; but, unlike in hyperacute rejection, arteriolar/arterial abnormalities are minimal. It is important to distinguish between the two conditions as perfusion/preservation-related injury is usually self-limited and the allograft can recover without residual effects. However, if there is severe and extreme damage, the recovery rate is poor, with graft loss or persistent poor function. Peroperative biopsies can therefore give useful information regarding the state of the graft and some indication of how soon the graft will start to function. Pre-existing arteriolar sclerosis in the donor may be confused with chronic cyclosporin toxicity in a later biopsy if the pathologist is unaware of its existence; a baseline biopsy helps avoid this problem (Fig. 8.21).

## Primary non-function and delayed graft function

All grafts undergo some degree of ischaemia during harvesting, transportation, preparation of the recipient—including tissue typing—and transplanting. If the donor has cardiovascular problems—in particular, hypotension—it is inevitable that the graft would suffer ischaemic damage even before the transplantation procedure is set in motion. Warm ischaemia is tolerated much less well than cold ischaemia because of the higher metabolic rate of the tissue at body or room temperature. Ischaemia and reperfusion injury is the most common cause of primary non-function/delayed function. Recovery is rapid after 10 min of warm ischaemia but can take a week or longer after 30 min of

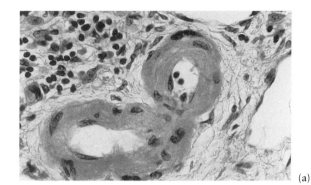

(a)

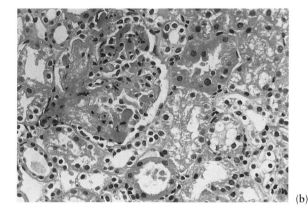

(b)

**Fig. 8.21** (a) Peroperative biopsy: donor arteriolar sclerosis. Peroperative biopsy of allograft from a road traffic accident victim donor aged 56 years. Incidental acellular hyaline sclerosis of arteriolar wall. (b) Peroperative biopsy: preservation-related injury. Peroperative biopsy of graft with prolonged ischaemia time. Fibrin and neutrophils within glomerular capillaries together with disruption of some capillary loops at the glomerular hilum. Many of the tubules are lined by coarsely vaculoated, degenerate epithelium.

warm ischaemia (Florack *et al.* 1986). On the other hand, cold ischaemia times of 24–72 h are well tolerated with no long-term effects, even though there may be a 23% incidence of delayed graft function (Troppmann *et al.* 1996).

In addition to ischaemic injury other causes of early graft dysfunction within the first week include mechanical anastomotic complications of the renal artery, vein and ureter, nephrosclerotic donor kidney, hyperacute/accelerated acute rejection and cyclosporin A toxicity.

Acute tubular necrosis (ATN) is the hallmark of

ischaemic injury. There are degeneration, vacuolation and necrosis of a proportion of cells lining the proximal tubules, which are dilated and contain eosinophilic debris within the lumina. Many of the viable proximal tubular cells show loss of brush border. Proteinaceous casts are present in scattered tubules and microcalcification of the necrotic epithelium may be present. In severe cases there is interstitial oedema together with a mild infiltrate of mononuclear cells. When epithelial cell necrosis is extensive, neutrophils are present around the tubules and within the lumina (Fig. 8.22). If the donor kidney has age-related vascular sclerosis with thickened and narrowed hyaline arterioles, the pretransplant ischaemic damage can be compounded by poor perfusion through the sclerotic vessels.

Ischaemic injury promotes induction of HLA class II antigens and cytokines on tubular epithelium and thereby can predispose to rejection within the graft (Goes *et al.* 1995). Grafts with both ATN and rejection often have cold ischaemia times longer than 24 h and rejection occurs in 57% of grafts with ATN compared to 40% without ATN (Troppmann *et al.* 1992). Acute tubular necrosis in conjunction with rejection significantly reduces graft survival, 1-year survival with no ATN and no episodes of rejection being 88% compared with 51% when both ATN and rejection were present (Lim & Terasaki 1991). Troppmann *et al.* (1992) in a study of 323 consecutive cadaver transplants found that ATN alone had no effects on long-term graft survival when there were no rejection episodes. When ATN is accompanied by a significant interstitial mononuclear cell infiltrate, the differential diagnosis from rejection can be difficult, especially as oedema and tubulitis can occur in both conditions. Eosinophils within the interstitial infiltrate are indicative of rejection, as is endothelitis of arterioles and small arteries; neither of these is seen in pure ATN.

Cyclosporin A nephrotoxicity is enhanced by ATN and patients with primary non-function or delayed graft function should have cyclosporin withdrawn. The drug increases the incidence and duration of delayed graft function caused by cold ischaemia time (Dunn *et al.* 1990). Cyclosporin is an important cause of early graft dysfunction and must be differentiated from rejection and ischaemia (see below).

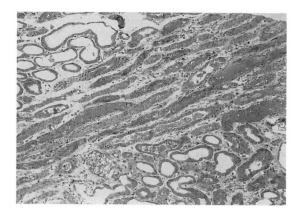

**Fig. 8.22** Acute tubular necrosis. Biopsy after 5 days' primary non-function. Groups of proximal tubules are irregularly dilated and lined by flat to cuboidal degenerate epithelium. Other tubules contain proteinaceous casts and necrotic epithelial debris. There is mild interstitial oedema.

## Nephrotoxicity

The recipient of a graft is, of necessity, given immunosuppressive agents and antibiotics, which may be nephrotoxic and also possibly injure the liver and marrow. Although nephrotoxicity of individual drugs is well recognized, the interactions between them are poorly understood. In the immediate post-transplant period the potentially toxic role of the various therapeutic agents is reduced by dialysis. Cyclosporin A is the most common and most important nephrotoxic drug, followed by other immunosuppressive agents, tacrolimus (FK506), rapamycin and azathioprine. Antibiotics and non-steroidal anti-inflammatory drugs (NSAIDs) can produce direct tubular toxicity or an allergic-type tubulointerstitial nephritis essentially similar to that seen in native kidneys.

### Cyclosporin A nephrotoxicity

The toxic effects of cyclosporin A (CsA) therapy can be caused by the drug alone, by its interaction with other drugs or by CsA enhancing and exacerbating pathological injury caused by prolonged ischaemia time, hypertension, rejection and infection. In their original report Calne *et al.* (1978) stated: 'It seems likely that cyclosporin A has direct toxic effect on renal tubules or on the blood supply of the tubules and that patients vary in their susceptibility to these toxic reactions although nephrotoxicity is probably dose dependent.' It is now clear that nephrotoxicity is manifest not only as acute dose-dependent reversible toxicity in the early post-transplant period but also as chronic and permanent damage in the years following successful transplantation. Nephrotoxicity is not confined to renal grafts but can also occur in native kidneys of recipients with bone marrow, liver, heart and lung grafts and also in patients treated for a number of autoimmune/immunologically mediated diseases (Bennett *et al.* 1996).

The clinical features and mechanisms of CsA toxicity are discussed in Chapters 5 and 7. Pathophysiologically, CsA toxicity can be divided into three phases—prolonged delayed function, acute toxicity and chronic toxicity—which may imperceptibly merge into each other. It must be stated at the very outset that there are *no* specific diagnostic pathological features that can be attributed to CsA toxicity. All the abnormalities that have been described so far are entirely non-specific and can be seen in the kidney of transplant recipients and other patients who have never received CsA. These lesions can be caused by a variety of injurious agents, such as ischaemia, hypertension, infection, sepsis and the rejection reaction itself. However, though non-specific, there are certain morphological features that are seen more frequently in CsA-treated patients with poor function and therefore, by inference, are associated with CsA nephrotoxicity. In renal allografts the major difficulty in defining the pathological abnormalities that could be associated with CsA toxicity is the problem of sorting out the concomitant changes of rejection. There is no doubt that rejection and CsA toxicity can occur at the same time and the diagnosis of nephrotoxicity can be made with confidence only when significant rejection is absent, i.e. the diagnosis is one of exclusion. No such problems are encountered in patients with healthy kidneys receiving CsA for autoimmune disorders or recipients of other organ grafts. Biopsies from such patients have helped in sorting out some of the problems of CsA-associated morphological abnormalities.

PROLONGED DELAYED FUNCTION

This is seen almost exclusively in recipients of cadaver renal allografts, especially when the quality of the donor organ has been compromised by prolonged ischaemia time, donor hypotension, age-related ischaemic disease and operative technical problems in the recipient. Primary anuria is seen frequently in centres that have organs transported from long distances and in institutions where absence of brain death legislation permits cadaveric kidneys to be harvested only after the donor's heart has stopped beating. The incidence of prolonged anuria requiring dialysis can vary between 30 and 50%. Hall *et al.* (1985) reported establishment of good graft function by an average of 2 weeks in patients treated with azathioprine and steroids and 3–14 weeks in 72% of patients treated with CsA; graft failure requiring nephrectomy occurred in 2%. The effect of cyclosporin nephrotoxicity on an ischaemic kidney has promoted protocols that delay administration of CsA until adequate renal function is established.

Biopsies of CsA grafts with prolonged delayed function can show a spectrum of changes from 'normal' appearance to tubular vacuolization, tubular epithelial cell degeneration and necrosis. Flecks of fibrin and occasional neutrophils may be seen adherent to the endothelium of glomerular capillaries and arterioles. The interstitium is unremarkable or may have mild oedema. It is clear from this description that the abnormalities seen with CsA toxicity are essentially similar to those seen with prolonged ischaemia and it would be impossible to differentiate one from the other. It is therefore essential that the clinician and pathologist have a high index of suspicion and be aware of the risks of CsA nephrotoxicity in grafts with significant ischaemia. Unless ischaemic injury is severe, reduction or withdrawal of CsA promotes improvement in graft function within a few days. This rapid recovery in function is compatible with the concept of renal vasoconstriction (Perico & Remuzzi 1991); see below.

ACUTE NEPHROTOXICITY

Acute toxicity is seen 2–3 weeks post-transplantation

and should be suspected when, after initial satisfactory function, there is deteriorating renal function with elevation of serum creatinine and fall in GFR. It is usually, but not always, associated with high serum or blood levels of CsA. This imperfect correlation is because patients vary in their sensitivity to the toxic effects of CsA and the assays detect metabolites as well. Furthermore, rejection itself raises CsA blood levels (Nankivell *et al.* 1994). Clinically, acute CsA toxicity can be almost impossible to differentiate from acute rejection as patients often do not have the characteristic features of pyrexia, graft enlargement and tenderness associated with classical rejection. Moreover, although high trough levels of serum CsA are more likely to cause toxicity, nephrotoxicity can occur with CsA at therapeutic levels or even low levels. If graft dysfunction is caused by CsA toxicity, reduction in dosage produces improvement in function by 24–48 h, thereby giving retrospective proof of toxicity. More often than not a biopsy of the graft is required to arrive at a definite diagnosis. Histologically, the diagnosis is made by the absence of evidence for rejection rather than by any specific features of CsA toxicity. However, rejection and nephrotoxicity are not mutually exclusive, especially as the vascular damage caused by rejection can be enhanced by the effect of CsA on the endothelium. When the two conditions coexist, interpretation of the biopsy can be difficult. In spite of these reservations a number of morphological abnormalities have been reported to be associated with acute CsA nephrotoxicity and these could be divided into two broad groups: *glomeruloarteriolar* and *tubulointerstitial*. Detailed and comprehensive reports of the morphological features associated with CsA toxicity have been published by Mihatsch *et al.* (1983, 1995).

The *glomerular* and *vascular* abnormalities associated with CsA are platelet–fibrin thrombi within the glomerular capillary and arteriolar lumina, intimal mucoid thickening with a microangiopathic picture of arterioles and small arteries, medial smooth muscle cell degeneration and apoptosis with replacement by nodular acellular protein deposits (Fig. 8.23). The deposits are intensely eosinophilic, stain bright magenta with PAS stain, bright red with trichrome stains and are positive for IgM and C3. They are the

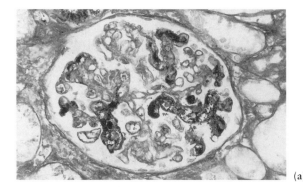

(a)

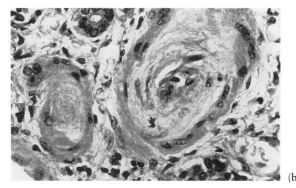

(b)

**Fig. 8.23** (a) Acute cyclosporin toxicity. Glomerular capillary loops containing platelet–fibrin aggregates and lined by swollen endothelial cells. Immunoperoxidase stain for fibrin. (b) Acute cyclosporin toxicity. Microangiopathy of interlobular artery with marked intimal mucoid thickening and almost total loss of the lumen.

early phase of chronic arteriolar hyalinosis. Glomerular thrombi with a microangiopathic picture were initially reported in CsA-treated bone marrow recipients who had poor renal function (Shulman *et al.* 1981). It was postulated these patients had a form of haemolytic uraemic syndrome (HUS) as a consequence of CsA toxicity. The patients also had active graft vs. host disease (GVHD) and systemic infections, making it doubtful if CsA was the sole contributor to the HUS. Subsequently, HUS-like pathology has been reported in patients treated with CsA for renal allografts (Neild *et al.* 1985) and liver transplants (Bonser *et al.* 1984). Although there is no doubt that thrombotic microangiopathy does occur in CsA-treated patients, it can also

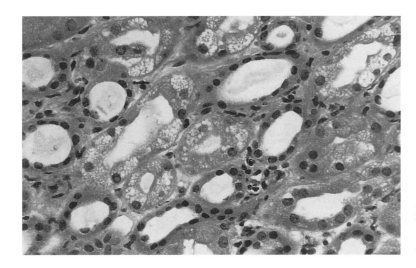

**Fig. 8.24** Cyclosporin toxicity. Uniform, fine, circumferential isometric vacuolization of proximal tubular epithelium.

occur with acute humoral rejection, sepsis, GVHD, radiation and chemotherapy. *De novo* thrombotic microangiopathy has been reported in 0.5% of 225 renal allograft patients not on CsA and 0% of 358 patients on CsA (Schwarz *et al.* 1991a). All the evidence seems to indicate that microangiopathy, in the absence of any other complicating factor, can be attributed to CsA toxicity but, when it is accompanied by the other complicating factors that can also cause endothelial injury, the finding should be interpreted with caution.

*Tubulointerstitial* abnormalities reported to be associated with CsA toxicity are isometric vacuolization, microcalcification, giant mitochondria, peritubular capillary congestion, interstitial oedema and tubular atrophy with interstitial fibrosis (Fig. 8.24). None of these abnormalities are specific or diagnostic of CsA toxicity. Giant mitochondria can be seen in a number of conditions in native kidneys and also in renal grafts not treated with CsA (Thiru & Calne 1981). Microcalcification is caused by dystrophic calcification of degenerate tubular epithelial cells and occurs in any condition causing tubular damage. Mihatsch *et al.* (1983) introduced the term 'isometric vacuolization' to describe the formation of numerous fine uniform small vacuoles within the cytoplasm of epithelial cells. The vacuolization involves the entire circumference of the tubule and tends to occur predominantly in the

descending straight portion of the proximal tubule. By electron microscopy the vacuoles are empty and represent dilated endoplasmic reticulum. Similar abnormalities can be seen in osmotic diuresis secondary to hyperosmolar solutions. Ischaemia also produces vacuolization, which can be fine and uniform or, more frequently, tends to be coarse and irregular (Fig. 8.25). Although there is correlation between the presence of isometric vacuolization, renal dysfunction and high CsA trough levels, as it can occur in other causes of ischaemic tubular damage, such as poor preservation and rejection, vacuolization is not always a helpful feature in diagnosis of nephrotoxicity. Peritubular capillary congestion indicates prominent numbers of mononuclear cells in dilated capillaries. It can be seen in ATN and early cellular rejection of both CsA and non-CsA-treated allografts and therefore is not a reliable feature in the diagnosis of nephrotoxicity.

Sibley *et al.* (1983) reported a detailed morphological study of 132 biopsies from 54 patients treated with CsA. There were 105 episodes of increase in serum creatinine and some patients had two or more biopsies. Nine parameters were examined: vasculitis, interstitial oedema, glomerulitis, tubular ectasia, tubular necrosis, tubulitis, distribution and intensity of mononuclear cell interstitial infiltrate and ratio of mononuclear cells in interstitium and peritubular capillaries (I : C ratio).

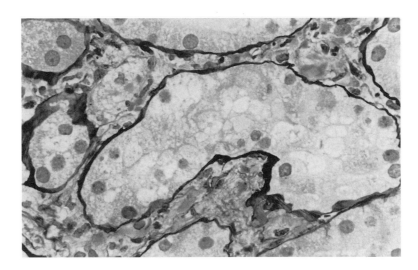

**Fig. 8.25** Ischaemic vacuolization. Predominantly coarse vacuoles of tubular epithelium together with fine vacuolization of occasional cells.

Acute rejection was defined as steroid-responsive tubulointerstitial nephritis in which steroid therapy resulted in return of serum creatinine to normal levels. CsA nephrotoxicity was defined as failure to respond to steroid therapy and fall in serum creatinine level following subsequent decrease of CsA dosage. In CsA nephrotoxicity there was mild cellular infiltrate in 85% and moderate to severe in 15%. In rejection there was a severe infiltrate in 70%. However, the degree of overlap made this an unreliable criterion. The same applied with tubular ectasia and necrosis. Glomerulitis was present in 27% of nephrotoxicity and 77% of acute rejection, and with tubulitis the figures were 35.8% of nephrotoxicity and 80% of acute rejection cases. The I : C ratio was ≥ 3 : 1 in rejection and ≤ 1 : 3 in nephrotoxicity. Endovasculitis or endotheliitis was almost exclusively present in acute rejection and was the only feature that permitted the diagnosis of rejection with any certainty. Marker studies with mononuclear antibodies were again not specific although T-cytotoxic cells were markedly increased in acute rejection, whereas the cytotoxic : helper ratio was less than 2 : 1 in CsA nephrotoxicity. Expression of cytokines, adhesion molecules and HLA class II antigens is increased in acute rejection, whereas in nephrotoxicity there is no such increase (Kyo *et al.* 1992; Gibbs *et al.* 1993). Immunohistochemical staining of

biopsy material is, however, not a useful tool for immediate diagnostic purposes.

Clearly, the presence or absence of rejection can be ascertained on most biopsies. Nephrotoxicity, on the other hand, is not so straightforward; it can be diagnosed with certainty when rejection is *not* present, but when rejection is present it can be almost impossible to assess histological evidence of CsA toxicity. The only reliable criterion for differentiating acute rejection from nephrotoxicity is the retrospective one of patient's response to increased steroid or reduction in CsA dosage.

CHRONIC NEPHROTOXICITY

Chronic toxicity presents as an insidious and progressive renal dysfunction over a period of months to years. Reports of 'recovery' from acute nephrotoxicity seldom indicate resolution to normal function and even in patients who do not have acute episodes of nephrotoxicity the renal function is often not completely normal. It is likely that all kidneys, grafts and native organs, are subjected to some degree of background nephrotoxicity which is mild and compatible with sufficient or even normal renal function in the initial phase. With time this may progress to more severe, permanent and irreversible dysfunction. With the lower dosage of CsA used in current triple therapy regimens the risk of CsA toxicity is much lower. Morphologically, many of the features of chronic CsA toxicity resemble chronic rejection. The best morphological studies, therefore, are from non-renal transplant patients and patients treated for autoimmune disorders, such as uveitis.

Glomerular lesions are of segmental to global sclerosis and most studies show that after 1–2 years on CsA increasing numbers of glomeruli are sclerotic (Nizze *et al.* 1988). Glomerular sclerosis correlated well with arteriolar hyaline sclerosis. The arteriolar lesions were first described by Mihatsch *et al.* (1983), who observed nodular circumferential acellular deposits within the media of arterioles associated with loss of myocytes. The lesions are, at first glance, similar to the arteriolar sclerosis seen in diabetic or hypertensive arteriolopathy. The nodular deposits are markedly eosinophilic and are positive for IgM and C3. The distinctive feature of CsA-associated arteriolopathy (CAA) is the nodular beaded pattern of the hyaline deposits replacing individual necrotic smooth muscle cells of the media. Karyorrhectic nuclear debris indicates that apoptosis may be present, but fibrinoid necrosis or acute inflammation is absent (Fig. 8.26). The frequency of CAA is less than 15% and the lesions can be easily

missed, especially when there is tubular atrophy with thickened basement membranes (Strom *et al.* 1994). The myocyte degeneration can be seen in the acute phase as early as 1–2 weeks post-transplant and with progressive toxicity the lesions become more frequent and more confluent. Strom *et al.* (1994) in a detailed analysis of renal transplants reported afferent arteriolar involvement to be 0% at 15 days, 5% at 6 months, 9% at 1 year and 12% at 2 years. In an autopsy study of heart and bone marrow transplant patients, Nizze *et al.* (1988) noted a significant 55% association of CAA with CsA therapy compared to 0% in patients not on CsA. However, analysis of renal biopsies from patients treated with CsA for autoimmune diseases conclude that, although tubular atrophy, interstitial fibrosis and arteriolar hyalinosis were attributable to CsA therapy, the reproducibility and diagnostic reliability were low for arteriolar lesions (Mihatsch *et al.* 1994). Although hyaline arteriolar change was present in renal biopsies of uveitis patients treated with CsA, it was not significantly increased compared to controls (Palestine *et al.* 1986). Hyaline deposits in hypertension, diabetes or 'age changes' are subendothelial and concentric rather than within the media and nodular involving individual smooth muscle cells, but this is not a universal observation and therefore not helpful in differentiating

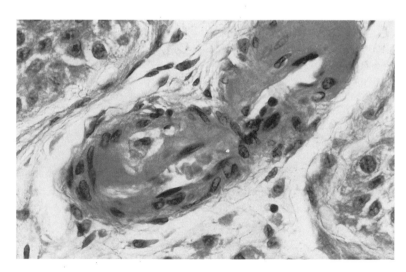

**Fig. 8.26** Cyclosporin-associated arteriolopathy. Arteriolar wall showing foci of myocyte loss with replacement by eosinophilic hyaline material. Similar abnormalities can also be seen in diabetes mellitus, hypertension or vascular sclerosis of age.

from CAA. Moreover, kidneys with focal segmental glomerular sclerosis (FSGS) or those with reduced renal mass and hyperfiltration effects often have a nodular type of arteriolar sclerosis. Differentiating chronic rejection from chronic CsA toxicity can be difficult both clinically and morphologically. Long before CsA was on the scene Porter *et al.* (1966) reported thickening of arteriolar walls by hyaline deposits containing immunoglobulin and complement; in a series of biopsies 1.75–2.5 years post-transplant this change was encountered in 48%. The significance of hyaline arteriolar lesions should be interpreted with caution and not automatically attributed to CsA toxicity. This is especially so if the peroperative baseline biopsy showed evidence of arteriolar hyalinosis in the donor kidney.

It must be remembered that chronic rejection and CsA toxicity can coexist and in such cases differentiating one from the other can be very difficult. It is even probable that chronic rejection and CsA toxicity enhance each other's injurious effects on the graft (Pascual *et al.* 1998).

Features that are helpful in differentiating CAA from chronic rejection are:

1 CAA is predominantly an arteriolar lesion while chronic rejection involves arteries;
2 CAA commonly involves the media with myocyte loss and replacement by hyaline deposits, whereas chronic rejection is primarily a proliferative intimal disorder with cellular infiltration;
3 allograft glomerulopathy lesions of chronic rejection are quite distinctive from the non-specific glomerular sclerosis of CsA toxicity; and
4 although both chronic rejection and CsA toxicity have tubular atrophy and interstitial fibrosis, in rejection there is often accompanying interstitial inflammation of lymphocytes, macrophages and plasma cells.

Tubular atrophy was a prominent feature, affecting 30% of the cortex in initial studies of CsA (Thiru *et al.* 1983). This occurred quite early, 6–8 months post-transplant, often without significant associated interstitial fibrosis, perhaps reflecting the very high dosage of CsA used at that time and early direct tubular toxicity. The incidence of tubular atrophy in CsA-treated

bone marrow graft patients is 66%, compared to 0% in the non-CsA group (Nizze *et al.* 1988). This difference between the two groups is not so well illustrated in cardiac transplant patients, perhaps because these patients are older and have intrinsic native vascular sclerosis and nephrosclerosis, with consequent ischaemic tubular damage. Tubular atrophy is accompanied by patchy, often linear, fibrosis with minimal interstitial inflammation.

Interstitial fibrosis (Nizze *et al.* 1988) again has a higher incidence in the younger population of bone marrow graft recipients (66% with CsA compared to 8% without CsA) than in cardiac graft recipients (78% with CsA compared to 86% without CsA). Tubulo-interstitial damage has also been reported in patients treated with CsA for psoriasis (Messana *et al.* 1995), uveitis (Palestine *et al.* 1986) and type I diabetes mellitus (Mihatsch *et al.* 1991). Although in some reports tubulointerstitial fibrosis is described as having a linear striped pattern, indicating a vascular distribution, others have reported a more diffuse pattern.

The pathogenesis and mechanism of CsA toxicity have not yet been completely clarified. Acute and chronic nephrotoxicity are dosage-dependent and toxicity, especially in the acute phase, is reversible by reduction of the dosage. There is no doubt that factors in addition to dosage level may contribute to nephrotoxicity: concomitant use of other drugs which act synergistically to increase the toxic effects of CsA, infection, hypertension and, in the case of renal grafts, pretransplant ischaemia, nephrosclerosis in older donor kidneys and concomitant rejection episodes. Although nephrotoxicity of CsA is readily observed in clinical practice, there is no equivalent experimental animal model.

Two theories of pathogenesis, which may not be mutually exclusive, have been offered so far: a *tubular toxic effect* and a *vasoconstrictive effect*. Myers *et al.* (1984), in their report of CsA-associated chronic nephropathy, suggested the tubule as the primary site of the injury, with subsequent nephron destruction leading to loss of filtration surface area and adaptive increase in glomerular capillary pressure. This would enhance further development of glomerulosclerosis and a vicious circle would be set up, with progressive decrease in functioning nephrons and acceleration of glomerulosclerosis. Other studies have indicated that CsA alters renal haemodynamics, thereby causing proximal tubular hypoxia and a fall in GFR (Baxter *et al.* 1982).

A number of clinical and experimental studies have demonstrated that CsA reduces effective renal blood flow and increases renal vascular resistance at the level of the glomerular afferent arteriole (Perico & Remuzzi 1991; Remuzzi & Perico 1995). The rapid improvement in renal function following reduction of CsA is further corroborative evidence of involvement of a vasomotor mechanism (Chapman *et al.* 1985). The haemodynamic disturbances produced by CsA are caused by its stimulatory effects on the renin–angiotensin system, inhibition of prostaglandin-mediated vasodilatation (Neild *et al.* 1983) and increased production of the vasoconstrictors thromboxane (Brown & Neild 1987) and endothelin (Perico & Remuzzi 1991). It is clear that even low-dose 'non-toxic' administration of CsA is associated with vaso-constriction, causing reduction in renal blood flow and fall in GFR. This would cause the mild increase in serum creatinine seen almost universally in all CsA-treated patients: so-called 'functional nephrotoxicity'. Superimposed on this 'background toxicity' there could be episodes of dosage-associated further falls in renal blood flow, leading to reversible episodes of further renal dysfunction. Vasoconstriction in the early phase is reversible, as evidenced by the return to normal function when CsA is withdrawn. With continued therapy, however, there is development of irreversible renal injury, probably secondary to vascular morphological injury and consequent nephron loss, leading to compensatory hyperfiltration. There are, in addition, coexistent CsA-induced hypertension, episodes of acute rejection and, perhaps, developing chronic rejection, further enhancing the renal damage.

## Tacrolimus (FK506) nephrotoxicity

FK506 is a fairly new immunosuppressive agent used as an alternative to CsA. Although the drugs are structurally unrelated, FK506 nephrotoxicity produces morphological abnormalities very similar to that of CsA. These include isometric vacuolization of proximal tubular epithelium, microangiopathy and arteriolar hyalinosis (Randhawa *et al.* 1993).

## Antibiotic toxicity

Aminoglycoside antibiotics and amphotericin B are powerful antimicrobial agents which are used in transplant recipients because of the infections these patients are prone to acquire. Both cause acute tubular epithelial cell necrosis, predominantly involving the proximal tubules. However, the more common antibiotic-induced toxicity is an allergic-type tubulointerstitial nephritis which is morphologically no different from that seen in native kidneys. Sulphonamides, synthetic penicillins, methicillin, ampicillin and rifampin are the antibiotics usually involved. Clinically, there is sudden deterioration in renal function, fever and perhaps a peripheral blood eosinophilia, and the differentiation from acute rejection can be almost impossible. Biopsy can also cause problems in diagnosis. Both acute rejection and drug-induced nephritis are characterized by a heavy interstitial infiltrate of lymphocytes, macrophages and variable numbers of eosinophils. There are accompanying interstitial oedema, tubulitis and varying degrees of tubular epithelial cell necrosis (Fig. 8.27). Glomeruli are usually normal or, in the case of acute rejection, may have varying degrees of hyper-cellularity. The cardinal feature that differentiates between the two conditions is the presence of endotheliitis of small arteries in rejection. NSAIDS, thiazide diuretics and miscellaneous drugs, such as pheninidione and cimetidine, can also cause an acute tubulointerstitial nephritis.

## Non-steroidal anti-inflammatory drug toxicity

Non-steroidal anti-inflammatory drugs produce several forms of renal injury, which are similar to those occurring in native kidneys. They are in common use and patients often self-medicate with these drugs. They can cause haemodynamically induced acute renal failure secondary to inhibition of vasodilatory prostaglandin synthesis, acute hypersensitivity intersti-

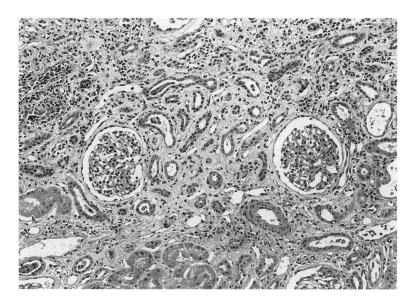

**Fig. 8.27** Drug (methicillin)-induced nephritis. Interstitial oedema with infiltration of lymphocytes, macrophages and eosinophils, together with tubulitis and tubular epithelial cell necrosis. Note that the vein and small artery in the lower part of the field do not show evidence of endotheliitis, a helpful feature in differentiating from acute cellular rejection.

tial nephritis or interstitial nephritis associated with the nephrotic syndrome.

## Infections

The association between organ transplantation, immunosuppression and bacterial, viral and fungal infections is well known. Although many of these infections are systemic, the renal graft may also be involved by the infectious process or may reflect non-specific features caused by septicaemia. Clearly it is of great therapeutic importance to distinguish between rejection and infection. Clinically, both conditions may give a similar picture, with pyrexia, graft tenderness, oliguria and a fall in renal function.

### Septicaemia

Patients with a generalized infection and septicaemia may have a spectrum of changes, including normal morphology, moderate degrees of acute tubular necrosis, prominent numbers of neutrophils within glomerular and peritubular capillaries or evidence of disseminated intravascular coagulation. The histological features of disseminated intravascular coagulation are fibrinoid necrosis and thrombi within capillaries, in particular glomerular capillaries; these abnormalities are very similar to the vascular lesions of acute humoral rejection (Fig. 8.28). Silent unsuspected fungal infections in particular can present in this way, and these patients may not have clinical or laboratory evidence of disseminated intravascular coagulation until much later in their course. Unless the possibility of infection is constantly kept in mind, it is quite easy to fall into the trap of diagnosing the allograft biopsy of such a patient as acute humoral rejection.

### Urinary tract infections

In pyelonephritis, organisms are very rarely demonstrated in the biopsy. The features to look for are linear streaks of tubules containing abundant neutrophils and neutrophil casts within the lumina and also in the surrounding interstitium (Fig. 8.29). There are accompanying tubular epithelial degeneration and necrosis, interstitial oedema and vascular congestion. The features helpful to distinguish urinary tract infections from rejection are the lack of a mononuclear interstitial infiltrate of lymphocytes and immunoblasts and the absence of endovasculitis.

However, it must be emphasized that rejection and acute pyelonephritis can coexist on occasion.

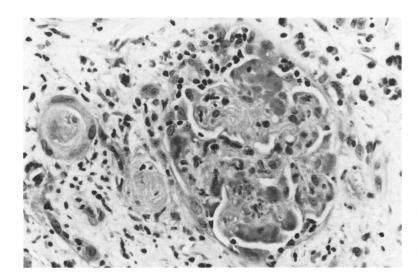

**Fig. 8.28** Disseminated intravascular coagulation. Glomerulus showing capillary thrombi, infiltrating neutrophils and necrosis of segmental capillaries. Note the microangiopathy of a small artery at the left of the field.

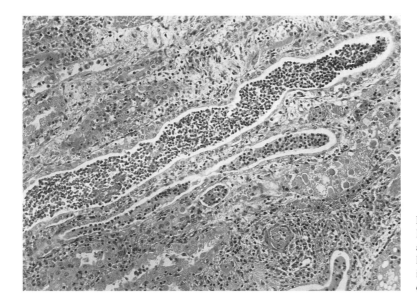

**Fig. 8.29** Urinary tract infection. Linear streaks of tubules containing aggregates of neutrophils within the lumina (white cell casts in urine). The interstitium is oedematous and contains an infiltrate of neutrophils.

Pyelonephritis can occur at any time post-transplant, from the first week to years later. The presence of ureteric narrowing, obstruction or vesicoureteric reflux is a significant risk factor for the development of pyelonephritis, as are patients whose primary renal disease was reflux nephropathy (Hamshere *et al.* 1974). In a large study of 1100 consecutive renal transplants the incidence of pyelonephritis was 1.6%, with the majority (93%) being female and 80% of the episodes arising a year or more after transplantation (Pearson *et al.* 1980).

## Viral infections

The numerous viral infections transplant patients are prone to develop do not, in general, seem to have a detrimental effect on renal function unless there are severe systemic effects. The most notable exceptions are cytomegalovirus (CMV) and Epstein–Barr virus (EBV) infections.

Cytomegalovirus infection is frequent among renal allograft recipients and is discussed in detail in Chapter 16. As far as the allograft is concerned, CMV infection can be incidental and asymptomatic with typical cytopathic changes in the tubular epithelium or produce a significant acute tubulointerstitial nephritis and/or a proliferative glomerulopathy (Fig. 8.30). When clinical signs of infection are accompanied by a decrease in renal function, it is debatable as to whether this is a result of a specific manifestation of the infection or its indirect effect on the graft and activation of rejection. Richardson *et al.* (1981) reported a proliferative glomerulonephritis characterized by foci of necrosis, infiltration of mononuclear cells and deposition of fibrin. No viral particles were detected by electromicroscopy and the glomerular mononuclear cells were shown to be CD8+ T cells. Other groups have reported similar findings (Herrera *et al.* 1986; Battegay *et al.* 1988) and also shown that such glomerular lesions did not occur in patients with CMV viraemia who did not have a renal allograft. Moreover, similar glomerular abnormalities can be seen in rejecting grafts of patients not infected with CMV. The conclusion is that the glomerular lesions are a manifestation of acute rejection triggered by the infection. Similarly, lesions of acute and chronic vascular rejection can also be seen in patients with CMV infection (Herrera *et al.* 1986; Battegay *et al.* 1988). It is postulated that CMV infection induces endothelial activation, release of cytokines, up-regulation of MHC antigens and activation of cytotoxic T cells, thus precipitating the rejection reaction.

Patients with hepatitis C virus infections may develop a mesangiocapillary-type glomerulonephritis, essentially similar to that seen in native kidneys. The consequences of EBV infection are discussed below.

## Recurrent disease

Glomerular changes in long-term allografts can be complex and it is not always possible to be certain whether they represent recurrent disease, *de novo* glomerulonephritis or chronic allograft glomerulopathy. This is especially so when the primary pathology in the patient is unknown. In spite of these difficulties, certain forms of glomerulonephritis have been documented to recur in allografts (Mathew 1991). Strict criteria are required to make a diagnosis of recurrent disease and, in addition to the clinical details, include light microscopy, immunofluorescence and electron-

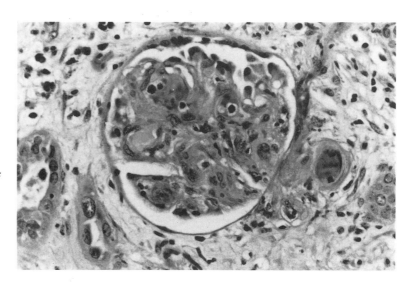

**Fig. 8.30** CMV infection. Proliferative glomerulopathy with infiltrating mononuclear cells. Note the thrombus in the hilar arteriole. Cytopathic changes of CMV infection are not shown but were present in glomeruli, tubules and arteriolar endothelium elsewhere.

microscopy examination. The frequency and clinical significance of recurrence vary with the disease. There is a 5–10% overall incidence of recurrence and approximately 2% result in graft failure. Systemic metabolic disorders, such as diabetes mellitus type I, oxalosis, amyloidosis and light-chain nephropathy, invariably recur over a variable period of time (Mauer *et al.* 1976; Scheinman *et al.* 1984; Pasternack *et al.* 1986; Alpers *et al.* 1989). Recurrence of glomerulonephritis after transplantation has been described in all the common histological types, with a wide variation in incidence. There is a high incidence in focal segmental glomerulosclerosis, IgA nephropathy, Henoch–Schönlein purpura, mesangiocapillary glomerulonephritis types I and II, anti-GBM nephritis and HUS. These are all diseases with a systemic or circulatory pathogenic disorder and are not caused by an intrinsic abnormality of the kidney. On the other hand, the unexpected rarity of recurrent lupus nephritis raises interesting speculation regarding the pathogenesis of lupus nephritis. Overall, recurrence is more likely if the initial glomerulonephritis was aggressive with a short period between presentation and end-stage renal failure, if transplantation is performed too soon after end-stage is reached—e.g. anti-GBM nephritis, Henoch–Schönlein purpura—and if living related donor grafts are used in conditions such as focal segmental glomerulosclerosis, IgA nephropathy and HUS.

Focal segmental glomerulosclerosis has an overall recurrence rate of 30%, with 9% graft loss (Cameron 1991; Mathew 1991). In a high-risk subgroup of young patients with massive proteinuria, diffuse mesangial hypercellularity and a short interval between presentation and renal failure, the recurrence rate can be as high as 70%. The average time for clinical evidence of recurrence is less than 1 year in adults (Artero *et al.* 1992) and 2 weeks in children (Tejani & Stablein 1992). Children have a higher recurrence rate than adults and there is a higher risk of recurrence with living related donor grafts. In some cases of recurrent FSGS, heavy proteinuria can be almost instantaneous and is a strong argument favouring a circulatory factor in the pathogenesis of this condition. When examining biopsy material from a patient suspected to have recurrent FSGS, it must be kept in mind that the morpholog-

ical lesions are essentially similar to those seen in hyperfiltration and also in many forms of advanced renal disease. Strict criteria must therefore be used in interpreting the biopsy findings and always in the context of the clinical history. Recurrence occurs early, usually within 1 year post-transplant, and is invariably accompanied by heavy proteinuria, with or without the nephrotic syndrome. Hyperfiltration injury, on the other hand, tends to occur later and although there is proteinuria it is only rarely in the nephrotic range.

Recurrence of mesangiocapillary glomerulonephritis (MCGN) type I is well recognized, with an overall incidence of 27% and graft loss of 9% (Schwarz *et al.* 1991b). A diagnosis of recurrence should be made only after electron-microscopic and immunohistochemical examination of biopsy material (Fig. 8.31). This is because MCGN type I can be morphologically and clinically difficult to differentiate from chronic allograft glomerulopathy. Both conditions have increased lobularity of the glomeruli with mesangial proliferation and reduplication of the glomerular capillary basement membrane. Mesangial and subendothelial deposits are prominent and numerous in MCGN type I, whereas in allograft glomerulopathy deposits are absent or sparse and the widened GBM contains finely granular flocculent electron-lucent material.

Mesangiocapillary glomerulonephritis type II (dense deposit disease) has a high (90–100%) rate of histological recurrence but, unlike the primary disease, is associated with a relatively benign course (Cameron 1982). Graft loss occurs in 10–15% and tends to occur in patients with primary aggressive disease of a crescentic glomerulonephritis and rapid renal failure.

IgA nephropathy has a high morphological recurrence rate (45–50%), but haematuria and proteinuria are mild and graft loss is 2% (Odum *et al.* 1994). The prevalence of recurrence increases with time. The recurrence rate of Henoch–Schönlein nephritis is variable (30–70%). Most of these are subclinical forms with morphological evidence of IgA deposition but a benign clinical course. Recurrence can be confined to the kidney or be systemic and, similar to IgA nephropathy, the risk for recurrence is increased with living related donor grafts.

Recurrence of anti-GBM nephritis can be kept low if

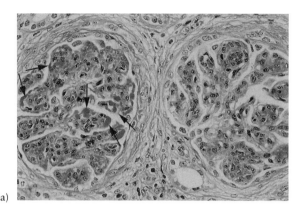
(a)

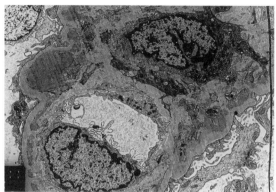
(b)

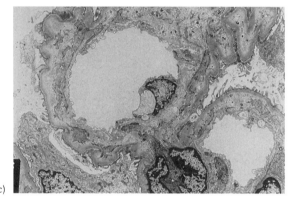
(c)

**Fig. 8.31** Recurrent mesangiocapillary GN. (a) Hypercellular glomeruli with a lobular appearance. Numerous mesangial and subendothelial immune deposits can be identified even by light microscopy (arrows). One-year allograft biopsy from a 16-year-old male who developed heavy proteinuria within 6 months of transplantation. Graft function failed over the following year. (b) Electron micrograph of biopsy shown in (a). The glomerular capillary walls are widened by numerous electron-dense subendothelial immune deposits. (c) Allograft glomerulopathy in which capillary loops are widened by electron-lucent, flocculent material.

transplantation is performed at least 1 year after the anti-GBM antibody titres have become negative. The incidence in recent series is 5% (Schwarz *et al.* 1991b) compared to 56% with 25% graft failure in earlier reports (Wilson & Dixon 1973).

Recurrent membranous glomerulonephritis (MGN) occurs early in the post-transplant period, most within the first year. In a large series of over 1500 consecutive transplants the incidence of recurrence was 25% (Couchoud *et al.* 1995). When MGN occurs late in a transplant, recurrence cannot be reliably distinguished from *de novo* disease. Recurrent MGN is much less common than *de novo* MGN, is more likely to occur in HLA-matched living related donor grafts and has a worse prognosis than *de novo* MGN (Berger *et al.* 1983).

Documented recurrence of lupus nephritis has been uncommon in most series and there is widespread agreement that patients with systemic lupus erythe-matosus (SLE) are suitable for transplantation. Even positive serology is not considered a contraindication (Goss *et al.* 1991). There is a tendency for the disease to enter an inactive 'burnt out' phase after the development of renal failure, thought to be partly a result of the immunosuppressive effect of uraemia (Mojcik & Klippel 1996), and this may be the explanation for the low rate of recurrence.

### *De novo* glomerulonephritis

*De novo* glomerulonephritis can be diagnosed with absolute confidence only when the primary disease that caused the renal failure is known. The two most important *de novo* disorders are MGN and FSGS. Anti-GBM antibodies in transplant patients with Alport's syndrome is not surprising, given that these patients lack the non-collagenous domain of type IV collagen.

However, in most large series only about 10% develop the antibodies and none had significant nephritis (Gobel *et al.* 1992; Nyberg *et al.* 1995). Any glomerular disorder can occur *de novo*, as in a native kidney, but this is extremely rare and almost invariably associated with a clear-cut causative mechanism, e.g. hepatitis C infection causing MCGN type I, IgA nephropathy associated with liver disease caused by viral hepatitis, diabetic nephropathy as a result of steroid-induced diabetes mellitus.

Membranous glomerulonephritis presents 2 years or longer after transplantation. Though most have significant proteinuria, some are picked up in incidental biopsies. Most cases of MGN in renal transplants are *de novo* rather than recurrent disease (Schwarz *et al.* 1991b). Morphologically, there is essentially no distinct difference between MGN in native kidneys and recurrent or *de novo* disease in allograft kidneys. The incidence of *de novo* MGN is between 1 and 2% at about 2 years post-transplantation but increases to 5.3% at 8 years. It may or may not be accompanied by features of chronic rejection. There is no correlation between the initial cause of renal failure and the development of *de novo* MGN. The pathogenesis remains speculative and includes antibodies generated to endogenous antigens released by the rejection process and/or antibodies developed to exogenous antigens from infections.

Focal segmental glomerulosclerosis is a frequent abnormality in long-standing grafts and is most probably caused by hyperfiltration injury secondary to reduced renal mass. It is often accompanied by other evidence of renal injury, such as chronic rejection and CsA nephrotoxicity. Unlike the primary form of FSGS seen in native kidneys or in cases of documented recurrent allograft FSGS, most allograft recipients with morphological features of *de novo* FSGS do not have heavy proteinuria or the nephrotic syndrome. This is evidence that the FSGS lesions in these grafts have a different pathogenesis, the most likely being hyperfiltration injury compounded by chronic rejection. In addition, true recurrent FSGS occurs early in the post-transplant period, whereas so-called *de novo* FSGS occurs much later, presumably because hyperfiltration injury is a chronic process related to loss of critical renal mass. The differential diagnosis of the morphological lesions

of FSGS can be difficult and confusing unless they are interpreted in conjunction with the clinical history, laboratory data and, of course, the *entire* appearance of the allograft biopsy, not simply the glomerular changes. In particular, vascular lesions of chronic rejection, hypertension and chronic CsA toxicity should be sought and if these are present the glomerular lesions are most probably secondary to ischaemia or hyperfiltration rather than true FSGS.

## Non-lymphoid post-transplant malignancies

One of the long-term consequences of immunosuppression is the evolution of malignant tumours. Several different pathogenetic mechanisms may contribute to this greater risk of cancer, including impaired immune surveillance, oncogenic viruses, chronic antigenic stimulation and genetic predisposition. The most frequent types of tumours are squamous cell carcinomas of the skin, lips, cervix, vagina, vulva and perineum, Kaposi's sarcoma and non-Hodgkin's lymphomas. All of these tumours are associated with viral infections (papillomavirus, herpesvirus, EBV) or ultraviolet radiation. Other tumours that have an increased incidence include carcinomas of the oesophagus, liver and urinary tract. The distribution of malignancies in transplant recipients differs from that of age-matched controls in the general population. The more common tumours, such as carcinoma of the breast, lung, prostate and colon, do not have a significantly higher incidence. The increase in renal cell carcinomas could be a result of renal transplant patients with native end-stage kidneys *in situ* developing tumours in the atrophic kidneys, which are predisposed to this malignancy.

### Skin cancers

The most common malignancy in allograft recipients is carcinoma of the skin and this is particularly marked in high-risk areas such as Australia and New Zealand. Squamous cell carcinomas (SCCs) are more common than basal cell carcinomas (BCCs) (1.8 vs. 1), which is in contrast to the general population, where BCCs outnumber SCCs by 5 : 1 (Penn 1989). The SCCs in transplant recipients are frequently multiple, more aggressive and occur in patients whose average age is 30 years less than their counterparts in the general population. In a review of 5879 patients with cadaveric renal transplants with a follow-up period of 24 years, Sheil *et al.* (1991) reported a skin cancer incidence of 18% with a mean time of diagnosis of 6.4 years. Of all skin cancers, SCCs occurred in 75%, BCCs in 50%, keratoacanthoma in 26%, Bowen's disease in 22% and malignant melanoma in 3%. The tumours were often multiple and patients had a variety of lesions, either concurrently or consecutively. Metastases occurred in 7% of SCCs and 4% died of the disease. Approximately 40% of transplant recipients also develop warts and most of these patients have a history of warts in childhood, suggesting reactivation of latent virus rather than primary infection.

The pathogenesis of these tumours is multifactorial and complex. Primary risk factors in the development of SCCs are genetic susceptibility, exposure to sunlight and perhaps viral infection. Ultraviolet light causes damage to DNA, with associated mutagenicity. The effects of ultraviolet light are enhanced by antimetabolite immunosuppressive agents such as azathioprine which inhibit DNA synthesis and repair. Immunosuppression also reduces the numbers of Langerhans' cells in the skin, thereby suppressing their normal surveillance function. There is now increasing evidence of an added viral pathogenesis in these tumours. DNA of human papillomavirus (HPV) types 2, 5 and 16 and several unknown HPV types have been detected within the spectrum of post-transplant skin lesions (Arends *et al.* 1997).

## Kaposi's sarcoma

Kaposi's sarcoma (KS) is a neoplasm characterized by vascular and fibroblastic proliferation and is often multicentric in origin. It accounts for 5.7% of *de novo* malignancies in transplant recipients (Penn 1995). Approximately 60% have non-invasive KS confined to the skin, conjunctiva or oropharynx and 40% have visceral disease affecting mainly the lungs and gastrointestinal tract. Within the general population KS is rare in the West but endemic in certain parts of Africa, the Mediterranean and Saudi Arabia. Ethnic origin is a major risk factor in post-transplant KS. In Saudi Arabia, for example, it is the most common post-transplant malignancy (88%) and the frequency is 5.3% of renal allograft recipients compared to 0.38% in the general population. According to the Cincinnati Transplant Tumor Registry, reduction or cessation of immunosuppressive therapy resulted in complete remission in 53% of cases restricted to the skin and 27% of those involving viscera (Penn 1995).

The pathogenesis of KS is uncertain but current evidence favours a viral-associated neoplasm of primitive mesenchymal and endothelial cells whose course is influenced by the immune status of the individual. The genomic sequences of a novel herpesvirus, known as KS herpesvirus (KSHV) or human herpesvirus type 8 (HHV8), are found in virtually all KS lesions. Approximately 50% of the circulating B cells in patients with KS also harbour the KSHV. The viral genes of KSHV encode homologues of human genes that participate in cell proliferation and include IL-6, the chemokine MIP-1$\alpha$, a G-protein-coupled chemokine receptor, cyclin D and *bcl*-2. The virally encoded IL-6 is mitogenic for spindle cells in the lesion and the chemokine receptor encoded by the virus binds to IL-8, which is mitogenic for endothelial cells and promotes angiogenesis (Murphy 1997; Boshoff 1998). In addition, KS cells produce a variety of cytokines, including TNF-$\alpha$, IL-1, IL-6, GM-CSF and basic fibroblast growth factor, which stimulate the growth of spindle cells in an autocrine and paracrine fashion.

## Post-transplant lymphoproliferative disorders

Post-transplant lymphoproliferative disorders (PTLD) include both benign and malignant lymphoid proliferations arising in transplant recipients (Fig. 8.32). These lesions develop as a consequence of powerful immunosuppression and those at the benign end of the spectrum, regarded as extreme lymphoproliferation rather than true neoplasms, may regress with reduction of immunosuppressive therapy (Starzl *et al.* 1984). The majority, 86% of the post-transplant lymphomas, are

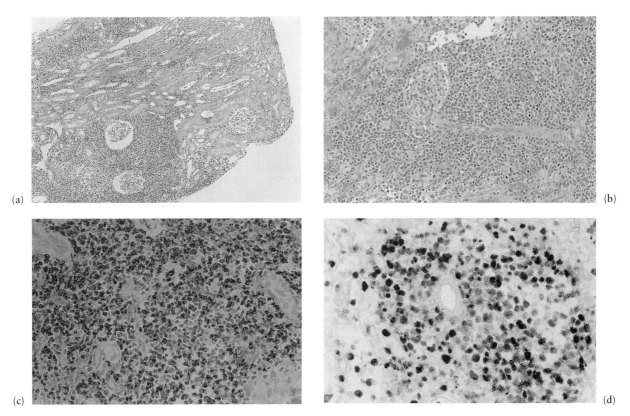

(a)

(b)

(c)

(d)

**Fig. 8.32** PTLD – allograft biopsy 6 months post-transplant. (a) Low-power view showing interstitial aggregates of mononuclear cells; the appearance can be mistaken for cellular rejection. (b) Higher-power view showing 'wipe out' of tubules by the infiltrate. The cells are large and pleomorphic with numerous mitoses. (c) Immunoperoxidase stain for CD79. The majority of infiltrating cells are B cells, in contrast to rejection, in which the cells are predominantly of T phenotype. (The tumour cells were also positive for lambda light chain.) (d) Immunoperoxidase stain with EBV antibody. Many of the large tumour cells are clearly positive.

of B cell origin, and 14% are of T cell origin (Penn 1991). The incidence of PTLD among transplant patients ranges from less than 2% up to 10%, depending on the type of transplant and degree of immunosuppression (Thiru *et al.* 1981; Nalesnik *et al.* 1988; Stephanian *et al.* 1991). Categorization of PTLD is based on morphological distinctions with ancillary studies of immunophenotyping, molecular genetic studies and EBV studies. Using these criteria a recent workshop recognized the categories of PTLD shown in Table 8.1 (Harris *et al.* 1997).

Most post-transplant lymphomas are non-Hodgkin's lymphomas and, unlike in the general popu-lation, Hodgkin's lymphoma is much less common in the transplant population: 34% compared to 2% (Penn 1981). The incidence of lymphomas is much higher in recipients treated with CsA and prednisone (26%) compared to those with prednisone, azathio-prine or cyclophosphamide (11%); the same is true of Kaposi's sarcoma (10% vs. 3%) (Penn 1989). Lymphomas in the CsA group tend to occur much earlier, 15 months vs. 48 months post-transplantation, with approximately one-third of the cases occurring within 4 months. On the other hand, the incidence of skin cancers, carcinomas of the cervix, vulva and perineum are lower in the CsA group.

**Table 8.1** Categories of post-transplant lymphoproliferative disorders (PTLD).

| | |
|---|---|
| Early lesions | Plasmacytic hyperplasia, infectious mononucleosis like PTLD |
| Polymorphic PTLD | Destructive lesions with full range of B cell maturation, immunoblasts to plasma cells; surface and cytoplasmic Ig either polytypic or monotypic; Epstein–Barr virus (EBV) present. Reduction in immunosuppression leads to regression in some and others require lymphoma treatment |
| Monomorphic PTLD | Either B or T cell type; sheets of large blastic cells, no evidence of maturation; sufficient atypia and monomorphism to be recognized as lymphoma; *B cell type* positive for B cell-associated Ags, monotypic Ig, EBV-associated Ags. Clonal Ig gene rearrangement, clonal EBV genomes, mutations in *ras* and p53 oncogenes; *T cell type* positive for T cell-associated Ags, clonal T cell receptor gene rearrangement, EBV-associated Ags positive or negative |
| Rare types of PTLD | Includes T cell-rich B-PTLD rather like Hodgkin's lymphoma and plasmacytoma-like PTLD |

Compared to non-transplant lymphomas PTLD are more likely to involve extranodal sites. They often affect the central nervous system (up to 28%) and in those with central nervous system involvement in 63% the lesions are confined only to the brain (Penn 1991). Another notable feature is that the allograft kidney or heart is involved in 18–36%, indicating that the immunological reaction in the graft could be a pathogenetic factor (Opelz & Henderson 1993). When the PTLD is confined to the graft, data also suggest it is likely to be of donor origin and these patients remain disease-free when treated with nephrectomy or graft irradiation (Randhawa *et al.* 1996). When the renal graft is involved, patients present with failing function and renal biopsy in such cases can cause differential diagnostic problems with cellular rejection. In both cases there is an interstitial infiltrate of large activated lymphoid cells, tubulitis, interstitial oedema and even endovasculitis. Differentiating between the two can be extremely difficult, particularly when the PTLD is an early lesion or of polymorphic type with a mixed population of cells in different stages of maturation. Immunotyping and stains for EBV would be helpful in the differential diagnosis. Most lymphomas involving the allograft are of B cell origin whereas the cells in the rejection reaction are predominantly T lymphocytes and macrophages.

Post-transplant lymphoproliferative disorders are an inevitable consequence of effective immunosuppressive therapy and EBV infections have been implicated in their pathogenesis (Purtilo *et al.* 1992; Su 1997). Epstein–Barr virus infects epithelial cells of the oropharynx and B lymphocytes. It gains entry into the cells via the CD21 molecule. The infection of B cells is latent, there is no replication of the virus and the infection is controlled by effective immune responses directed against viral antigens expressed on the cell membranes. Most infected individuals remain asymptomatic or develop self-limited infectious mononucleosis. The effect of immunosuppression on the cytotoxic T cell population results in failure to check the proliferation of EBV-infected B cells. The actively dividing B cell population results in polyclonal proliferation and is at increased risk of developing mutations, e.g. t(8;14) translocation, of one or more clones. Subsequently there is outgrowth of the mutant clones, leading to monoclonal or oligoclonal B cell lymphomas. Epstein–Barr virus itself is not directly oncogenic, but acts as a polyclonal B cell mitogen, providing an opportunity for mutations which release the cells from normal growth regulation. The growth of these EBV-driven cells, at least in the early polyclonal phase, is sensitive to immunoregulation, as reduction of immunosuppression results in regression of the 'tumours'.

## Monitoring graft outcome

Careful and meticulous management of recipients during the early days and months after transplantation is essential for maintaining good long-term graft function. The first 3 months after transplantation are the most critical period as this is the time when the graft is mostly likely to be lost as a result of technical problems, rejection, infections or drug-induced injury. A

**Table 8.2** Causes of early graft dysfunction.

| Immediate | Following initial good function |
|---|---|
| *Donor factors* | *Rejection* |
| Hypotension | Accelerated acute rejection |
| Nephrosclerosis | Acute cellular/humoral rejection |
| *Preservation injury* | *Mechanical factors* |
| | Renal artery stenosis |
| *Mechanical factors* | Renal vein thrombosis |
| Ureteric leak | Ureteric stenosis |
| Ureteric stenosis | |
| Renal artery thrombosis/ | *Infections* |
| stenosis | Urinary tract infections |
| Renal vein thrombosis | Septicaemia |
| *Rejection* | *Drug toxicity* |
| Hyperacute rejection | Acute CsA toxicity |
| Accelerated rejection | Antibiotics |
| | NSAIDs |
| *Drug toxicity* | |
| CsA-induced delayed | |
| function | |

**Table 8.3** Causes of late graft dysfunction.

| Sudden | Slow and progressive |
|---|---|
| Acute rejection | Chronic rejection |
| Infections | Chronic CsA toxicity |
| Urinary tract infections | Recurrent |
| Septicaemia | glomerulonephritis |
| Viral infections—CMV | *De novo* glomerulonephritis |
| Drug toxicity | Hyperfiltration/loss of |
| Antibiotics | critical mass |
| NSAIDs | Patient non-compliance |
| Lymphoproliferative disorder | |
| Patient non-compliance | |

graft that is functioning well at 3 months is very likely to continue to function for many years. In the early post-transplant period graft dysfunction can present as initial non-function or poor function, sudden deterioration of a previously well-functioning graft or initial impaired function with progressive deterioration. In the later period of months or years after transplantation graft dysfunction can be sudden or be slowly progressive (Tables 8.2 and 8.3). Evaluation and treatment of graft dysfunction requires clinical judgement, laboratory investigations, imaging studies and biopsy of the graft. Acute rejection occurs most frequently in the first 4 weeks after transplantation but can occur at any time between 3 days and many years. Chronic rejection can occur at any time after 3 months post-transplant, but the vascular lesions can on occasion be seen as early as 1 month post-transplant.

## Value of graft biopsy

Episodes of graft dysfunction in the early post-transplant period occur in approximately 50% of recipients.

The percutaneous renal allograft biopsy is the single most important tool in finding the cause of graft dysfunction and remains the gold standard. The biopsy provides one or two cores of tissue which can be processed rapidly within 2–3 h. In our laboratory, 60 serial sections are produced at 2–3 μm with three sections per slide. Slides from the two ends and middle of the serial are stained with haematoxylin and eosin, and others with periodic acid–Schiff silver methanamine and one of the trichrome methods. Unstained spare slides are reserved for further stains or subsequent immunocytochemical investigations that may be needed. Further serials are obtained if the initial sections are unhelpful. Immunofluorescence stains for immunoglobulins and complement components are only of value in the diagnosis of recurrent or *de novo* glomerulonephritis; they are not of value in the immediate post-transplant period when the differential diagnosis is predominantly between rejection, preservation injury, CsA toxicity and mechanical problems. Electron microscopy is again much more useful in the diagnosis of transplant glomerulopathy, recurrent disease and *de novo* glomerulonephritis.

The biopsy is invaluable in indicating the cause of primary non-function, in the differential diagnosis of acute rejection from acute tubular necrosis, infection or CsA toxicity, and in the differential diagnosis of chronic rejection from recurrent or *de novo* glomerulonephritis. In a study of 263 biopsies the results of the biopsy influenced change in therapy in 55% of cases (Kon *et al.* 1997).

An adequate biopsy should be from the deep cortex and contain 7–10 glomeruli and one or two small arteries. Rejection, especially in the early stages, is a focal process and can therefore be missed in a small biopsy. Superficial biopsies with predominantly subcapsular cortex can be misleading as this zone often has nephrosclerotic changes of donor origin. The deep medulla alone is unsatisfactory as it has a lower sensitivity for rejection. However, the outer medulla, particularly in the region of the corticomedullary junction, is extremely useful in assessing rejection as this is one of the earliest sites of the rejection reaction. Two cores of tissue are certainly better than one: a study of paired biopsy cores showed that sensitivity of a single core is 90% and that of two cores is approximately 99% (Sorof *et al.* 1995).

Examination of biopsy material must be meticulous and systematic. *Glomeruli* should be assessed for hypercellularity, neutrophils, fibrin or thrombi within capillaries, capillary wall abnormalities with or without mesangial matrical increase, necrosis and sclerosis. *Tubules* may be lined by degenerate and necrotic epithelium, have isometric vacuolization, tubulitis, cellular casts or cytopathic changes of CMV infection. *Interstitium* may have oedema, haemorrhage, inflammatory infiltrate of lymphocytes with activated forms, macrophages, eosinophils or neutrophils. *Arterioles* should be examined for hyaline sclerosis of the walls — with comparison to the peroperative baseline biopsy — medical smooth muscle cell necrosis with nodular hyaline change, luminal thrombi, endovasculitis, intimal proliferation, cytopathic changes of CMV and frank fibrinoid necrosis. *Arteries* may have all the changes mentioned for arterioles and also proliferative endarteritis, transmural infiltration of lymphocytes and macrophages.

## Differential diagnosis of rejection

It is the function of the pathologist to determine the presence or absence of rejection and, if present, the severity of rejection and the presence or absence of other non-immunological injuries. Differentiating rejection from the latter can pose problems as most of these disorders are marked by varying degrees of inflammatory cells and parenchymal damage. It is therefore of paramount importance that *transplant biopsies should be reported only in conjunction with all available clinical information*. In the early post-transplant period the more important differential diagnoses include preservation-related injury, ischaemic acute tubular necrosis, rejection acute CsA toxicity, drug-induced tubulointerstitial nephritis and urinary tract infections. Features helpful in the differential diagnoses of these conditions have been discussed in earlier sections of this chapter. Although many of the abnormal features are not specific and overlap between the various conditions, the cardinal feature diagnostic of acute rejection is *endovasculitis* with endothelial adherence and migration of mononuclear cells through the intima. Even greater diagnostic difficulties can arise when acute rejection coexists with other causes of early graft dysfunction. Unless this possibility is constantly kept in mind, it is quite possible to diagnose acute rejection and miss, for example, coexistent infection or drug toxicity.

Graft biopsies carried out for late graft dysfunction can cause great diagnostic problems, as many of the abnormalities of tubular atrophy, interstitial and glomerular sclerosis are non-specific and often secondary to chronic ischaemia. The important and more common differential diagnoses are chronic rejection, chronic CsA toxicity and hyperfiltration injury; glomerulonephritis, recurrent or *de novo*, is a less common problem. Helpful features in the differential diagnosis have been discussed in earlier sections. The vascular lesions of chronic rejection tend to involve, at least in the initial phase, the deeper vessels in the cortex–arcuate arteries rather than interlobular arteries and arterioles. The glomerular lesions of chronic rejection are less common than the arterial lesions and are also less specific. Chronic rejection can therefore be missed if the biopsy sample is unrepresentative and lacks diagnostic arterial lesions. It must also be remembered that the boundary between acute and chronic rejection is indistinct and biopsies can have features of both conditions.

## Grading of rejection

In reporting graft biopsies it is mandatory to assess the severity of rejection. This helps in the management of the patient and also may give some indication of the likely future course of the graft. The features of acute rejection that are sought, in increasing order of severity, include lymphocyte adherence to peritubular capillaries, interstitial mononuclear inflammation, interstitial oedema, tubulitis, tubular necrosis, endotheliitis, transmural inflammation of arteries, fibrinoid necrosis and thrombosis of arteries, arterioles and glomeruli, interstitial haemorrhage and frank parenchymal necrosis.

In *mild rejection* there is perivascular interstitial mononuclear cell infiltrates, including activated blast forms, moderate interstitial oedema and foci of tubulitis. The interstitial infiltrate occupies between 5 and 10% of the biopsy. In *moderate rejection* the interstitial oedema is pronounced, tubulitis is more extensive with evidence of tubular epithelial cell injury and necrosis, the interstitial cellular infiltrate is more intense and diffuse with increasing numbers of blast forms and scattered eosinophils. The most significant abnormality is that arteries, and to a lesser extent arterioles, show evidence of endotheliitis with infiltrating cells lifting the endothelium and accumulating in the subendothelial space. In *severe rejection*, in addition to the above features being more extensive and severe, there is transmural inflammation of arteries, small foci of subendothelial fibrin, medial necrosis in occasional vessels or frank fibrinoid necrosis of vessels and glomeruli with interstitial haemorrhage and parenchymal infarction. On occasion the biopsy may have the severe arterial lesions of fibrinoid necrosis without significant tubulointerstitial inflammation. This would also fall into the category of severe rejection and usually implies predominant humoral rejection. Herbertson *et al.* (1977) noted that transmural mononuclear cell infiltration of arteries, fibrinoid necrosis of vessels and interstitial haemorrhage were all ominous signs; any of these features occurring either separately or together in the initial 3-month post-transplant period were indicators of early graft failure.

A semiquantitative analysis of acute rejection was brought forward by Kim Solez in the form of the Banff classification (Solez *et al.* 1993). It was hoped that such a scheme would give a uniform standard of assessing rejection, be reproducible and make it easier to compare biopsies from different centres and could be applied to multicentre trials. In this scheme glomerular, interstitial, tubular and vascular lesions are graded 0–3 depending on whether they are absent (0), mild (1), moderate (2) or severe (3). A total score of 1 or less would be normal or borderline; 1–3 would be grade I, 4–6 would be grade II and more than 6 would be grade III rejection. Though such a scoring system was hoped to be reproducible, the criteria for grading are subjective and this produces less than ideal interobserver reproducibility. Moreover, the criteria for grading are quite complex, making the scheme too cumbersome for routine diagnostic work. It is, however, useful for multicentre drug trials.

The Cooperative Clinical Trials in Transplantation (CCTT) were developed to overcome the difficulties of the Banff scheme (Colvin *et al.* 1997). Three categories of acute rejection were defined: type I has interstitial infiltrate of activated lymphoblasts involving at least 5% of cortex, oedema and tubular degeneration. In type II there is arterial endotheliitis with or without features of type I, and type III shows arterial fibrinoid necrosis or transmural inflammation, which may be accompanied by haemorrhage, thrombosis or infarction. This scheme is much simpler with satisfactory interobserver reproducibility and correlates with clinical severity. The Banff classification has been revised, incorporating the simplicity of the CCTT classification but at the same time grading the individual features within the three broad categories.

Grading chronic rejection is even more problematic than acute rejection. The Banff scheme has a similar grading system to acute rejection, giving scores of 0–3 for transplant glomerulopathy, tubular atrophy, interstitial fibrosis and arterial fibrous thickening (Solez *et al.* 1993). Severity of chronic rejection is graded I–III depending on the final score. This system assumes that all the lesions are caused by chronic rejection and other pathogenetic factors, such as hyperfiltration injury, hypertension and donor vascular disease, are not taken into consideration. The criteria for grading are subjective and observer reproducibility is unsatisfactory. A refined and reproducible grading system will, no doubt, be developed in the near future.

## Conclusions

The morphological appearances of renal transplants are variable and can be complex. The important abnormalities are rejection—both acute and chronic—drug toxicity, infections and hyperfiltration injury. These conditions are not mutually exclusive and it is important to keep in mind that a biopsy may have more than one pathology, e.g. acute rejection may coexist with infection or CsA toxicity. Developments in effective immunosuppressive therapy have reduced acute rejection episodes and graft loss caused by acute rejection. Chronic rejection, however, remains a major problem. A fundamental understanding of the pathophysiology of chronic rejection would give insights into preventing and treating these lesions; it is to be hoped that this will occur in the near future. Adhesion molecules, chemokines and cytokines are now in the forefront of transplantation biology. Research has concentrated on the possibility that expression of these molecules may provide an early indication of graft rejection and that therapies centred on these molecules may add to existing immunosuppressive strategies.

## References

Adams, D.H., Wyner, L.R. & Karnovsky, M.J. (1993) Experimental graft arteriosclerosis. II. Immunocytochemical analysis of lesion development. *Transplantation* 56, 794–799.

Al Hussein, K.A., Talbot, D., Proud, G., Taylor, R.M. & Shenton, B.K. (1995) The clinical significance of post-transplantation non-HLA antibodies in renal transplantation. *Transplant International* 8, 214–216.

Alpers, C.E., Marchioro, T.L. & Johnson, R.J. (1989) Monoclonal immunoglobulin deposition disease in a renal allograft: probable recurrent disease in a patient without myeloma. *American Journal of Kidney Disease* 13, 418–423.

Alpers, C.E., Davis, C.L., Barr, D., Marsh, C.L. & Hudkins,

K.L. (1996) Identification of platelet-derived growth factor A and B chains in human renal vascular rejection. *American Journal of Pathology* 148, 439–445.

Anderson, C.B., Ladefoged, S.D. & Larsen, S. (1994) Acute kidney graft rejection: a morphological and immunohistological study on 'zero-hour' and follow-up biopsies with special emphasis on cellular infiltrates and adhesion molecules. *APIMIS* 102, 23–25.

Arends, M.J., Benton, E.C., McLaren, K.M. *et al.* (1997) Renal allograft recipients with high susceptibility to cutaneous malignancy have an increased prevalence of human papillomavirus DNA in skin tumours and a greater risk of anogenital malignancy. *British Journal of Cancer* 75, 722–728.

Artero, M., Biava, C., Amend, W., Tomlanovich, S. & Vincenti, F. (1992) Recurrent focal glomerulosclerosis: natural history and response to therapy. *American Journal of Medicine* 92, 375–377.

Barba, L.M., Caldwell, P.R., Downie, G.H. *et al.* (1983) Lung injury mediated by antibodies to endothelium. I. *Journal of Experimental Medicine* 158, 2141–2158.

Battegay, E.J., Mihatsch, M.J., Mazzucchelli, L. *et al.* (1988) Cytomegalovirus and kidney. *Clinical Nephrology* 30, 239–243.

Baxter, C.R., Duggin, G.G., Willis, N.S. *et al.* (1982) Cyclosporin A-induced increases in renin storage and release. *Research Communications in Chemical Pathology and Pharmacology* 37, 305–309.

Bennett, W.M., DeMattos, A., Meyer, M.M., Andoh, T. & Barry, J.M. (1996) Chronic cyclosporine nephropathy: the Achilles' heel of immunosuppressive therapy. *Kidney International* 50, 1089–1100.

Benzaquen, L.R., Nicholson-Weller, A. & Halperin, J.A. (1994) Terminal complement proteins C5b-9 release basic fibroblast growth factor and platelet-derived growth factor from endothelial cells. *Journal of Experimental Medicine* 179, 985–990.

Berger, B.E., Vincenti, F., Biava, C. *et al.* (1983) *De novo* and recurrent membranous glomerulopathy following kidney transplantation. *Transplantation* 35, 315–318.

Bishop, G.A., Hall, B.M., Duggin, G.G. *et al.* (1986) Immunopathology of renal allograft rejection analysed with monoclonal antibodies to mononuclear cell markers. *Kidney International* 29, 708–711.

Bonser, R.S., Adu, D., Franklin, I. & McMaster, P. (1984) Cyclosporin-induced haemolytic uraemic syndrome in liver allograft recipient. *Lancet* 2, 1337–1340.

Boonstra, J.G., Van-der Woude, F.J., Wever, P.C. *et al.* (1997) Expression and function of Fas (CD95) on human renal tubular epithelial cells. *Journal of the American Society of Nephrology* 8, 1517–1524.

Boshoff, C. (1998) Kaposi's sarcoma: coupling herpesvirus to angiogenesis. *Nature* 391, 24–27.

Boucher, A., Droz, D., Adafer, E. & Noel, L.H. (1986)

Characterisation of mononuclear cell subsets in renal cellular interstitial infiltrates. *Kidney International* 29, 1043–1049.

Brenner, B.M., Cohen, R.A. & Milford, E.L. (1992) In renal transplantation, one size may not fit all. *Journal of the American Society of Nephrology* 3, 162. [Published erratum appears in *Journal of the American Society of Nephrology* (1992) 3, 1038–1041.]

Brown, Z. & Neild, G.H. (1987) Cyclosporine inhibits prostacyclin production by cultured human endothelial cells. *Transplantation Proceedings* 19, 1178–1180.

Burke, B.A., Chavers, B.M., Gillingham, K.J. *et al.* (1995) Chronic renal allograft rejection in the first 6 months posttransplant. *Transplantation* 60, 1413–1416.

Calne, R.Y., White, D.J., Thiru, S. *et al.* (1978) Cyclosporin A in patients receiving renal allografts from cadaver donors. *Lancet* 2, 1323–1325.

Cameron, J.S. (1982) Glomerulonephritis in renal transplants. *Transplantation* 34, 237–245.

Cameron, J.S. (1991) Recurrent primary disease and *de novo* nephritis following renal transplantation. *Pediatric Nephrology* 5, 412–416.

Cameron, J.S. & Turner, D.R. (1977) Recurrent glomerulonephritis in allografted kidneys. *Clinical Nephrology* 7, 47–53.

Cecka, J.M. (1996) The UNOs scientific renal transplant registry. In: *Clinical Transplants* (eds J.M. Cecka & P.I. Terasaki), pp. 1–14. UCLA Tissue Typing Laboratory, Los Angeles.

Chapman, J.R., Griffiths, D., Harding, N.G. & Morris, P.J. (1985) Reversibility of cyclosporin nephrotoxicity after three months' treatment. *Lancet* 1, 128–130.

Colvin, R.B., Cohen, A.H., Saiontz, C. *et al.* (1997) Evaluation of pathologic criteria for acute renal allograft rejection: reproducibility, sensitivity, and clinical correlation. *Journal of the American Society of Nephrology* 8, 1930–1932.

Cosimi, A.B., Conti, D., Delmonico, F.L. *et al.* (1990) *In vivo* effects of monoclonal antibody to ICAM-1 (CD54) in nonhuman primates with renal allografts. *Journal of Immunology* 144, 1990–1994.

Cosio, F.G., Sedmak, D.D., Mahan, J.D. & Nahman, N.S. (1989) Localization of decay accelerating factor in normal and diseased kidneys. *Kidney International* 36, 100–107.

Couchoud, C., Pouteil-Noble, C., Colon, S. & Touraine, J.L. (1995) Recurrence of membranous nephropathy after renal transplantation: incidence and risk factors in 1614 patients. *Transplantation* 59, 1275.

Davenport, A., Younie, M.E., Parsons, J.E. & Klouda, P.T. (1994) Development of cytotoxic antibodies following renal allograft transplantation is associated with reduced graft survival due to chronic vascular rejection. *Nephrology, Dialysis and Transplantation* 9, 1315–1319.

Dempster, W.J. (1953) Kidney homotransplantation. *British Journal of Surgery* 40, 447–465.

Dooper, I.M., Bogman, M.J., Hoitsma, A.J. *et al.* (1992) Detection of interstitial increase in macrophages, characteristic of acute interstitial rejection, in routinely processed renal allografts biopsies using the monoclonal antibody KP1. *Transplant International* 5, 209.

Dunn, J., Grevel, J., Napoli, K. *et al.* (1990) The impact of steady-state cyclosporine concentrations on renal allograft outcome. *Transplantation* 49, 30–34.

Dvorak, H.F., Mihm, M.C. Jr, Dvorak, A.M. *et al.* (1979) Rejection of first set skin allografts in man. *Journal of Experimental Medicine* 150, 322.

Feucht, H.E. & Opelz, G. (1996) The humoral immune response towards HLA class II determinants in renal transplantation [Editorial]. *Kidney International* 50, 1464–1475.

Feucht, H.E., Felber, E., Gokel, M.J. *et al.* (1991) Vascular deposition of complement-split products in kidney allografts with cell-mediated rejection. *Clinical and Experimental Immunology* 86, 464–470.

Feucht, H.E., Schneeberger, H., Hillebrand, G. *et al.* (1993) Capillary deposition of C4d complement fragment and early renal graft loss. *Kidney International* 43, 1333–1338.

Florack, G., Sutherland, D.E., Ascherl, R. *et al.* (1986) Definition of normothermic ischemia limits for kidney and pancreas grafts. *Journal of Surgical Research* 40, 550–556.

Fuggle, S.V., McWhinnie, D.L., Chapman, J.R., Taylor, H.M. & Morris, P.J. (1985) Sequential analysis of HLA Class II antigen expression in human renal allografts: induction of tubular Class II antigens and correlation with clinical parameters. *Transplantation* 42, 144–147.

Fuggle, S.V., Sanderson, J.B., Gray, D.W., Richardson, A. & Morris, P.J. (1993) Variation in expression of endothelial adhesion molecules in pretransplant and transplanted kidneys: correlation with intergraft events. *Transplantation* 55, 117–119.

Gibbs, P., Berkley, L.M., Bolton, E.M., Briggs, J.D. & Bradley, J.A. (1993) Adhesion molecule expression (ICAM-1, VCAM-1, E-selectin and PECAM) in human kidney allografts. *Transplant Immunology* 1, 109–112.

Gibson, I.W., Marcussen, N., Brown, R.W., Solez, K. & Truong, L.D. (1996) The use of immunocytochemistry (LCA and LEU-7) in diagnosis of renal allograft rejection. *Transplantation Proceedings* 28, 457–460.

Gobel, J., Olbricht, C.J., Offner, G. *et al.* (1992) Kidney transplantation in Alport's syndrome: long-term outcome and allograft anti-GBM nephritis. *Clinical Nephrology* 38, 299–303.

Goes, N., Urmson, J., Ramassar, V. & Halloran, P.F. (1995) Ischemic acute tubular necrosis induces an extensive local cytokine response: evidence for induction of interferon-γ, transforming growth factor-β 1, granulocyte-macrophage colony-stimulating factor, interleukin-2, and interleukin-10. *Transplantation* 59, 565–572.

Goss, J.A., Cole, B.R., Jendrisak, M.D. *et al.* (1991) Renal transplantation for systemic lupus erythematosus and recurrent lupus nephritis: a single-center experience and a review of the literature. *Transplantation* 52, 805–807.

Grandaliano, G., Gesualdo, L., Ranieri, E. *et al.* (1997) Monocyte chemotactic peptide-1 expression and monocyte infiltration in acute renal transplant rejection. *Transplantation* 63, 414–420.

Hall, B.M., Tiller, D.J., Duggin, G.G. *et al.* (1985) Post-transplant acute renal failure in cadaver renal recipients treated with cyclosporine. *Kidney International* 28, 178–182.

Halloran, P.F., Wadgymar, A., Ritchie, S. *et al.* (1990) The significance of the anti-class I antibody response. I. Clinical and pathologic features of anti-class I-mediated rejection. *Transplantation* 49, 85–88.

Halloran, P.F., Schlaut, J., Solez, K. & Srinivasa, N.S. (1992) The significance of the anti-class I response. II. Clinical and pathologic features of renal transplants with anti-class I-like antibody. *Transplantation* 53, 550–555.

Hamilton, D. (1994) Kidney transplantation: a history. In: *Kidney Transplantation: Principles and Practice* (ed. P.J. Morris), pp. 1–21. W.B. Saunders, Philadelphia.

Hamilton, K.K., Ji, Z., Rollins, S., Stewart, B.H. & Sims, P.J. (1990) Regulatory control of the terminal complement proteins at the surface of human endothelial cells: neutralization of a C5b-9 inhibitor by antibody to CD59. *Blood* 76, 2572–2577.

Hamshere, R.J., Chisholm, G.D. & Shackman, R. (1974) Late urinary-tract infection after renal transplantation. *Lancet* 2, 793–794.

Hancock, W.W. & Atkins, R.C. (1985) Immunohistological analysis of sequential renal biopsies from patients with acute renal rejection. *Journal of Immunology* 136, 2416–2419.

Hancock, W.W., Whitley, D.W., Tullius, S.G. *et al.* (1993) Cytokines, adhesion molecules, and the pathogenesis of chronic rejection of rat renal allografts. *Transplantation* 56, 643–650.

Harris, N.L., Ferry, J.A. & Swerdlow, S.H. (1997) Posttransplant lymphoproliferative disorders: summary of Society for Hematopathology Workshop. *Seminars in Diagnostic Pathology* 14, 8–14.

Harry, T.R., Coles, G.A., Davies, M. *et al.* (1984) The significant of monocytes in glomeruli of human renal transplants. *Transplantation* 37, 70–73.

Herbertson, B.M., Evans, D.B., Calne, R.Y. & Banerjee, A.K. (1977) Percutaneous needle biopsies of renal allografts: the relationship between morphological changes present in biopsies and subsequent allograft function. *Histopathology* 1, 161–164.

Herrera, G.A., Alexander, R.W., Cooley, C.F. *et al.* (1986) Cytomegalovirus glomerulopathy: a controversial lesion. *Kidney International* 29, 725.

Hume, D.M., Merrill, J.P., Miller, B.F. & Thorn, G.W. (1955) Experiences with renal homotransplantation in the human: report of nine cases. *Journal of Clinical Investigations* 34, 327–382.

Isoniemi, H.M., Krogerus, L., von Willebrand, E. *et al.* (1992) Histopathological findings in well-functioning, long-term renal allografts. *Kidney International* 41, 155–160.

Jordan, S.C., Maleskzadeh, M.H., Pennisi, A.J. *et al.* (1980) Accelerated acute rejection of primary renal allografts in paediatric patients. *Transplantation* 30, 5–8.

Kerby, J.D., Verran, D.J., Luo, K.L. *et al.* (1996) Immunolocalization of FGF-1 and receptors in human renal allograft vasculopathy associated with chronic rejection. *Transplantation* 62, 467–470.

Kissmeyer-Neilsen, F., Olsen, S., Petersen, V. & Fjeldborg, O. (1966) Hyperacute rejection of kidney allografts associated with pre-existing humoral antibodies against donor cells. *Lancet* ii, 662–665.

Kon, S.P., Templar, J., Dodd, S.M., Rudge, C.J. & Raftery, M.J. (1997) Diagnostic contribution of renal allograft biopsies at various intervals after transplantation. *Transplantation* 63, 547–550.

Kormendi, F. & Amend, W. (1988) The importance of eosinophil cells in kidney allograft rejection. *Transplantation* 45, 537–539.

Koskinen, P.K., Nieminen, M.S., Krogerus, L.A. *et al.* (1993) Cytomegalovirus infection accelerates cardiac allograft vasculopathy: correlation between angiographic and endomyocardial biopsy findings in heart transplant patients. *Transplant International* 6, 341–345.

Kyo, M., Mihatsch, M.J., Gudat, F. *et al.* (1992) Renal graft rejection or cyclosporin toxicity? Early diagnosis by a combination of Papanicolaou and immunocytochemical staining of urinary cytology specimens. *Transplant International* 5, 71–75.

Lim, E.C. & Terasaki, P.I. (1991) Early graft function. *Clinical Transplantation* 5, 401–406.

McCluskey, R.T. (1980) Comments on targets in rejecting allografts. *Transplantation Proceedings* 12 (Suppl. 1), 22–25.

McWhinnie, D.L., Thompson, J.F., Taylor, H.M. *et al.* (1986) Morphometric analysis of cellular infiltration assessed by monoclonal antibody labelling in sequential human renal allograft biopsies. *Transplantation* 2, 352–355.

Manca, F., Ferry, B., Jaakkola, M. *et al.* (1987) Frequency of functional characterisation of specific T helper cells infiltrating rat kidney allografts during acute rejection. *Scandinavian Journal of Immunology* 25, 255–264.

Matas, A.J., Sibley, R., Mauer, M. *et al.* (1983) The value of needle renal allograft biopsy. I. A retrospective study of biopsies performed during putative rejection episodes. *Annals of Surgery* **197**, 226–230.

Matas, A.J., Gillingham, K.J., Payne, W.D. & Najarian, J.S. (1994) The impact of an acute rejection episode on long-term renal allograft survival. *Transplantation* **57**, 857–859.

Mathew, T.H. (1991) Recurrent disease after transplantation. *Transplantation Reviews* **5**, 31–35.

Mauer, S.M., Barbosa, J., Vernier, R.L. *et al.* (1976) Development of diabetic vascular lesions in normal kidneys transplanted into patients with diabetes mellitus. *New England Journal of Medicine* **295**, 916–921.

Medawar, P.B. (1944) The behaviour and fate of skin autografts and skin homografts in rabbits. *Journal of Anatomy (London)* **78**, 176–199.

Meehan, S., McCluskey, R., Pascual, M. *et al.* (1997) Cytotoxicity and apoptosis in human renal allografts: identification, distribution and quantitation of cells with TIA-1 (GMP-17) cytotoxic granule protein and fragmented nuclear DNA. *Laboratory Investigations* **76**, 639–643.

Messana, J.M., Johnson, K.J. & Mihatsch, M.J. (1995) Renal structure and function effects after low dose cyclosporine in psoriasis patients: a preliminary report. *Clinical Nephrology* **43**, 150–154.

Mihatsch, M.J., Theil, G., Spichtin, H.P. *et al.* (1983) Morphological findings in kidney transplants after treatment with cyclosprine. *Transplantation Proceedings* **15** (Suppl. 1), 2821–2826.

Mihatsch, M.J., Helmchen, U., Casanova, P. *et al.* (1991) Kidney biopsy findings in cyclosporine-treated patients with insulin-dependent diabetes mellitus. *Klinische Wochenschrift* **69**, 354–361.

Mihatsch, M.J., Antonovych, T., Bohman, S.O. *et al.* (1994) Cyclosporin A nephropathy: standardization of the evaluation of kidney biopsies. *Clinical Nephrology* **41**, 23–32.

Mihatsch, M.J., Ryffel, B. & Gudat, F. (1995) The differential diagnosis between rejection and cyclosporine toxicity. *Kidney International Supplement* **52**, S63–69.

Mojcik, C.F. & Klippel, J.H. (1996) End-stage renal disease and systemic lupus. *American Journal of Medicine* **101**, 100–103.

Mosman, T.R. & Coffman, R.L. (1989) TH1 and TH2 cells: different patterns of lymphokine secretion lead to different functional properties. *Journal of Immunology* **143**, 798–802.

Murphy, P.M. (1997) Pirated genes in Kaposi's sarcoma. *Nature* **385**, 296–300.

Murray, J.E. (1992) Human organ transplantation: background and consequences. *Science* **256**, 1411–1416.

Murray, J.E., Merrill, J.P., Dammin, G.J. *et al.* (1960) Study on transplantation immunity after total body irradiation: clinical and experimental investigation. *Surgery* **48**, 272–284.

Myers, B.D., Ross, J., Newton, L., Luetscher, J. & Perlroth, M. (1984) Cyclosporine-associated chronic nephropathy. *New England Journal of Medicine* **311**, 699.

Nalesnik, M.A., Jaffe, R., Starzl, T.E. *et al.* (1988) The pathology of posttransplant lymphoproliferative disorders occurring in the setting of cyclosporine A–prednisone immunosuppression. *American Journal of Pathology* **133**, 173–192.

Nankivell, B.J., Hibbins, M. & Chapman, J.R. (1994) Diagnostic utility of whole blood cyclosporine measurements in renal transplantation using triple therapy. *Transplantation* **58**, 989–992.

Neild, G.H., Rocchi, G., Imberti, L. *et al.* (1983) Effect of Cyclosporin A on prostacyclin synthesis by vascular tissue. *Thrombosis Research* **32**, 373–376.

Neild, G.H., Reuben, R., Hartley, R.B. & Cameron, J.S. (1985) Glomerular thrombi in renal allografts associated with cyclosporin treatment. *Journal of Clinical Pathology* **38**, 253–257.

Nickeleit, V., Vamvakas, E.C., Pasual, M., Polletti, B.J. & Colvin, R.B. (1998) The prognostic significance of specific arterial lesions in acute allograft rejection. *Journal of the American Society of Nephrology* **9**, 121–125.

Nizze, H., Mihatsch, M.J., Zollinger, H.U. *et al.* (1988) Cyclosporine-associated nephropathy in patients with heart and bone marrow transplants. *Clinical Nephrology* **30**, 248–251.

Noronha, I.L., Eberlein-Gonska, M., Hartley, B. *et al.* (1992) *In situ* expression on tumour necrosis factor–alpha interferon-gamma, and interleukin-2 receptors in renal allograft biopsies. *Transplantation* **54**, 1017–1021.

Noronha, I.L., Hartley, B., Cameron, J.S. & Waldherr, R. (1993) Detection of IL-1 beta and TNF-alpha message and protein in renal allograft biopsies. *Transplantation* **56**, 1026–1030.

Nyberg, G., Friman, S., Svalander, C. & Norden, G. (1995) Spectrum of hereditary renal disease in a kidney transplant population. *Nephrology, Dialysis and Transplantation* **10**, 859–863.

Odum, J., Peh, C.A., Clarkson, A.R. *et al.* (1994) Recurrent mesangial IgA nephritis following renal transplantation. *Nephrology, Dialysis and Transplantation* **9**, 309–313.

Opelz, G. & Henderson, R. (1993) Incidence of non-Hodgkin lymphoma in kidney and heart transplant recipients. *Lancet* **342**, 1514–1518.

Palestine, A.G., Austin, H.A., Balow, J.E. *et al.* (1986) Renal histopathologic alterations in patients treated with cyclosporine for uveitis. *New England Journal of Medicine* **314**, 1293–1296.

Pascual, M., Swinford, R.D., Ingelfinger, J.R. *et al.* (1998) Chronic rejection and chronic cyclosporin toxicity in renal allografts. *Immunology Today* **19**, 514–518.

Pasternack, A., Ahonen, J. & Kuhlback, B. (1986) Renal transplantation in 45 patients with amyloidosis. *Transplantation* **42**, 598–602.

Patel, R. & Terasaki, P.I. (1969) Significance of the positive crossmatch test in kidney transplantation. *New England Journal of Medicine* **280**, 735–739.

Paul, L.C. & Tilney, N.L. (1996) Alloantigen-dependent events in chronic rejection. In: *Transplantation Biology: Cellular and Molecular Aspects* (eds N.L. Tilney, T.B. Strom & L.C. Paul), pp. 567–575. Lipincott-Raven, Philadelphia.

Paul, L., Class, F., Van-Es, L., Kalff, M. & de Graeff, J. (1979a) Accelerated rejection of a renal allograft associated with pretransplantation antibodies directed against donor antigens on endothelium and monocytes. *New England Journal of Medicine* **300**, 1258–1260.

Paul, L.C., van Es, L.A., van Rood, J.J. *et al.* (1979b) Antibodies directed against antigens on the endothelium of peritubular capillaries in patients with rejecting renal allografts. *Transplantation* **27**, 175–179.

Pearson, J.C., Amend, W.J. Jr, Vincenti, F.G., Feduska, N.J. & Salvatierra, O. Jr (1980) Post-transplantation pyelonephritis: factors producing low patient and transplant morbidity. *Journal of Urology* **123**, 153–157.

Pederson, N.C. & Morris, B. (1970) The role of the lymphatic system in the rejection of homografts: a study of lymph from renal transplants. *Journal of Experimental Medicine* **131**, 936–942.

Penn, I. (1981) Malignant lymphomas in organ transplant recipients. *Transplantation Proceedings* **13**, 736.

Penn, I. (1989) In: *CRC Critical Reviews in Oncogenesis* (ed. E. Pimental), pp. 27–52. CRC Press, Boca Raton.

Penn, I. (1991) The changing pattern of posttransplant malignancies. *Transplantation Proceedings* **23**, 1101–1103.

Penn, I. (1995) Sarcomas in organ allograft recipients. *Transplantation* **60**, 1485–1486.

Perico, N. & Remuzzi, G. (1991) Cyclosporine induced renal dysfunction in experimental animals and humans. *Transplantation Reviews* **5**, 63–66.

Platt, J.L., Le Bien, T.W. & Michael, A.F. (1982) Interstitial mononuclear cell population in renal graft rejection: identification by monoclonal antibodies in tissue sections. *Journal of Experimental Medicine* **155**, 17–22.

Porter, K.A. (1965) Morphological aspects of renal homograft rejection. *British Medical Bulletin* **21**, 171–175.

Porter, K.A. (1967) Rejection in treated renal allografts. *Journal of Clinical Pathology* **20**, 518–534.

Porter, K.A. & Calne, R.Y. (1960) Origin of the infiltrating cells in skin and kidney homografts. *Transplant Bulletin* **26**, 458–464.

Porter, K.A., Marchioro, T.L. & Starzl, T.E. (1965) Pathological changes in 37 human renal homotransplants treated with immunosuppressive drugs. *British Journal of Urology* **37**, 250–255.

Porter, K.A., Rendall, J.M., Stolinski, C. *et al.* (1966) Light and electron microscopic study of biopsies from 33 human renal allografts and an isograft $1^3/_4$–$2^1/_2$ years after transplantation. *Annals of the New York Academy of Sciences* **129**, 615–619.

Prodjosudjadi, W., Daha, M.R., Gerritsma, J.S. *et al.* (1996) Increased urinary excretion of monocyte chemoattractant protein-1 during acute renal allograft rejection. *Nephrology, Dialysis and Transplantation* **11**, 1096–1103.

Purtilo, D.T., Strobach, R.S., Okano, M. & Davis, J.R. (1992) Epstein–Barr virus-associated lymphoproliferative disorders. *Laboratory Investigations* **67**, 5–12.

Ramos, E.L., Barri, Y.M., Croker, B.P. *et al.* (1995) Thromboxane synthase expression in renal transplant patients with rejection. *Transplantation* **59**, 490–494.

Randhawa, P.S., Shapiro, R., Jordan, M.L., Starzl, T.E. & Demetris, A.J. (1993) The histopathological changes associated with allograft rejection and drug toxicity in renal transplant recipients maintained on FK506: clinical significance and comparison with cyclosporine. *American Journal of Surgical Pathology* **17**, 60–64.

Randhawa, P.S., Magnone, M., Jordan, M. *et al.* (1996) Renal allograft involvement by Epstein–Barr virus associated post-transplant lymphoproliferative disease. *American Journal of Surgical Pathology* **20**, 563–569.

Reinke, P., Fietze, E., Docke, W.D. *et al.* (1994) Late acute rejection in long-term renal allograft recipients: diagnostic and predictive value of circulating activated T cells. *Transplantation* **58**, 35–41.

Remuzzi, G. & Perico, N. (1995) Cyclosporine-induced renal dysfunction in experimental animals and humans. *Kidney International Supplement* **52**, S70–73.

Richardson, W.P., Colvin, R.B., Cheeseman, S.H. *et al.* (1981) Glomerulopathy associated with cytomegalovirus viremia in renal allografts. *New England Journal of Medicine* **305**, 57.

Robertson, H., Wheeler, J., Thompson, V. *et al.* (1995) *In situ* lymphoproliferation in renal transplant biopsies. *Histochemistry and Cell Biology* **104**, 331–335.

Russell, P.S., Chase, C.M., Winn, H.J. & Colvin, R.B. (1994a) Coronary atherosclerosis in transplanted mouse hearts. II. Importance of humoral immunity. *Journal of Immunology* **152**, 5135–5140.

Russell, P.S., Chase, C.M., Winn, H.J. & Colvin, R.B. (1994b) Coronary atherosclerosis in transplanted mouse hearts. III. Effects of recipient treatment with a monoclonal antibody to interferon-gamma. *Transplantation* **57**, 1367–1371.

Russell, P.S., Chase, C.M. & Colvin, R.B. (1995) Coronary atherosclerosis in transplanted mouse hearts. IV. Effects of treatment with monoclonal antibodies to intercellular adhesion molecule-1 and leukocyte function-associated antigen-1. *Transplantation* **60**, 724–725.

Salmela, K.T., von Willebrand, E.O., Kyllonen, L.E. *et al.*

(1992) Acute vascular rejection in renal transplantation—diagnosis and outcome. *Transplantation* **54**, 858–862.

Sanfilippo, F., Kolbeck, P.C., Vaughn, W.K. & Bollinger, R.R. (1985) Renal allograft cell infiltrates associated with irreversible rejection. *Transplantation* **40**, 679–685.

Scheinman, J.I., Najarian, J.S. & Mauer, S.M. (1984) Successful strategies for renal transplantation in primary oxalosis. *Kidney International* **25**, 804–810.

Schmouder, R.L., Streiter, R.M., Wiggins, R.C., Chensue, W.W. & Lunkel, S.L. (1992) *In vitro* and *in vivo* production of interleukin-8 (IL-8) in renal cortical epithelium. *Kidney International* **41**, 191–195.

Schmouder, R.L., Streiter, R.M. & Kunkel, S.L. (1993) Interferon-γ regulation of human cortical epithelial cell derived monocyte chemotactic peptide-1. *Kidney International* **44**, 43–48.

Schwarz, A., Krause, P.H., Offermann, G. & Keller, F. (1991a) Recurrent and *de novo* renal disease after kidney transplantation with or without cyclosporine A. *American Journal of Kidney Disease* **17**, 524–528.

Schwarz, A., Krause, P.H., Offermann, G. & Keller, F. (1991b) Recurrent diseases in the renal allograft. *Journal of the American Society of Nephrology* **2**, 109–113.

Schweitzer, E.J., Matas, A.J., Gillingham, K.J. *et al.* (1991) Causes of renal allograft loss: progress in the 1980s, challenges for the 1990s. *Annals of Surgery* **214**, 679–683.

Scornik, J.C., LeFor, W.M., Cicciarelli, J.C. *et al.* (1992) Hyperacute and acute kidney graft rejection due to antibodies against B cells. *Transplantation* **54**, 61–64.

Sheil, A.G., Disney, A.P., Mathew, T.H., Amiss, N. & Excell, L. (1991) Cancer development in cadaveric donor renal allograft recipients treated with azathioprine (AZA) or cyclosporine (CyA) or AZA/CyA. *Transplantation Proceedings* **23**, 1111–1112.

Shoker, A.S., Genesis, R., George, D.H., Baltzan, R.B. & Baltzan, M.A. (1994) Can acute cellular rejection occur 27 years after a successful renal transplant? *Transplantation* **58**, 1131–1135.

Shulman, H., Striker, G., Deeg, H.J. *et al.* (1981) Nephrotoxicity of cyclosporin A after allogeneic marrow transplantation: glomerular thromboses and tubular injury. *New England Journal of Medicine* **305**, 1392–1396.

Sibley, R.K., Rynasiewicz, J., Ferguson, R.M. *et al.* (1983) Morphology of cyclosporine nephrotoxicity and acute rejection in patients immunosuppressed with cyclosporine and prednisone. *Surgery* **94**, 225–229.

Simonsen, M. (1953) Biological incompatibility in kidney transplantation in dogs. II. Serological investigations. *Acta Pathologica Microbiologica Scandinavia* **32**, 36–42.

Simonsen, M., Buemann, J., Gammeltoft, A., Jensen, F.J. & Jørgensen, K. (1953) Biological incompatibility in kidney transplantation in dogs. I. Experimental and morphological investigations. *Acta Pathologica, Microbiologica et Immunologica Scandinavica* **32**, 1–8.

Solez, K., Axelsen, R.A., Benediktsson, H. *et al.* (1993) International standardization of criteria for the histologic diagnosis of renal allograft rejection: the Banff working classification of kidney transplant pathology. *Kidney International* **44**, 411–422.

Sorof, J.M., Vartanian, R.K., Olson, J.L. *et al.* (1995) Histopathological concordance of paired renal allograft biopsy cores: effect on the diagnosis and management of acute rejection. *Transplantation* **60**, 1215–1220.

Soulillou, J.P., de Mouzon-Cambon, A., Dubois, C. *et al.* (1981) Immunological studies of eluates of 83 rejected kidneys: screening of antibodies directed against T and B lymphocytes, glomerular and tubular basement membranes, DNA, and IgG. *Transplantation* **32**, 368–374.

Starzl, T.E., Lerner, R.A., Dixon, F.J. & Groth, C.G. (1968) Shwartzman reaction after human renal homo-transplantation. *New England Journal of Medicine* **278**, 1968–1972.

Starzl, T.E., Boehmig, H.J., Amemiya, H. *et al.* (1970) Clotting changes, including disseminated intravascular coagulation, during rapid renal–homograft rejection. *New England Journal of Medicine* **283**, 383–388.

Starzl, T.E., Nalesnik, M.A., Porter, K.A. *et al.* (1984) Reversibility of lymphomas and lymphoproliferative lesions developing under cyclosporin–steroid therapy. *Lancet* **1**, 583–585.

Stephanian, E., Gruber, S.A., Dunn, D.L. & Matas, A.J. (1991) Post-transplant lymphoproliferative disorders. *Transplantation Reviews* **5**, 120–129.

Strom, E.H., Thiel, G. & Mihatsch, M.J. (1994) Prevalence of cyclosporine-associated arteriolopathy in renal transplant biopsies from 1981 to 1992. *Transplantation Proceedings* **26**, 2585–2587.

Su, I.-J. (1997) The role of Epstein–Barr virus in lymphoid malignancies. *Critical Reviews in Oncology/Hematology* **26**, 25–29.

Taylor, D.O., Ibrahim, H.M., Tolman, D.R. & Hess, M.L. (1991) Accelerated coronary arteriosclerosis in cardiac transplantation. *Transplantation Reviews* **5**, 165–174.

Tejani, A. & Stablein, D.H. (1992) Recurrence of focal segmental glomerulosclerosis posttransplantation: a special report of the North American Pediatric Renal Transplant Cooperative Study. *Journal of the American Society of Nephrology* **2**, S258–262.

Terasaki, P.I., Cecka, J.M., Gjerston, D.W. *et al.* (1993) A ten year prediction for kidney transplant survival. In: *Clinical Transplants* (eds P.I. Terasaki & J.M. Cecka), pp. 501–512. UCLA Tissue Typing Laboratory, Los Angeles.

Thiru, S. & Calne, R.Y. (1981) Giant mitochondria, renal transplant biopsy and cyclosporin A. *Lancet* **2**, 147.

Thiru, S., Calne, R.Y. & Nagington, J. (1981) Lymphoma in renal allograft patients treated with cyclosporin-A as one of the immunosuppressive agents. *Transplantation Proceedings* **13**, 359–361.

Thiru, S., Maher, E.R., Hamilton, D.V., Evans, D.B. & Calne, R.Y. (1983) Tubular changes in renal transplant recipients on cyclosporine. *Transplantation Proceedings* 15, 2846–2847.

Thorogood, J., Van Houwelinger, H.C., Van Rood, J.J. *et al.* (1992) Long-term results of kidney transplantation in Eurotransplant. In: *Organ Transplantation: Long-Term Results* (eds L.C. Paul & K. Solez), pp. 33–56. Marcel Dekker, New York.

Tilney, N.L. & Paul, L.C. (1996) Antigen-independent events leading to chronic graft dysfunction. In: *Transplantation Biology: Cellular and Molecular Aspects* (eds N.L. Tilney, T.B. Strom & L.C. Paul), pp. 629–637. Lipincott-Raven, Philadelphia.

Troppmann, C., Almond, P.S., Matas, A.J. & Najarian, J.S. (1992) Does acute tubular necrosis affect renal transplant outcome? The impact of rejection episodes. *XIV International Congress of the Transplant Society (Paris)* pp. 766–772.

Troppmann, C., Gillingham, K.J., Gruessner, R.W. *et al.* (1996) Delayed graft function in the absence of rejection has no long-term impact: a study of cadaver kidney recipients with good graft function at 1 year after transplantation. *Transplantation* 61, 1331–1336.

Trpkov, K., Campbell, P., Pazderka, F. *et al.* (1996) Pathologic features of acute renal allograft rejection associated with donor-specific antibody: analysis using the Banff grading schema. *Transplantation* 61, 1586–1590.

Tuazon, T.V., Schneeberger, E.E., Bhan, A.K. *et al.* (1987) Mononuclear cells in acute allograft glomerulopathy. *American Journal of Pathology* 129, 119–123.

Voronoy, Y.Y. (1936) Sobre el bloqueo de aparato reticulo-endothelial. *El Siglo Medicine* 97, 296–298 [in Spanish].

Williamson, C.S. (1926) Further studies on the transplantation of the kidney. *Journal of Urology* 16, 231.

Wilson, C.B. & Dixon, F.J. (1973) Anti-glomerular basement membrane antibody-induced glomerulonephritis. *Kidney International* 3, 74–80.

Yard, B.A., Spruyt-Gerritse, M. & Class, F. (1993) The clinical significance of allospecific antibodies against endothelial cells detected with an antibody-dependent cellular cytotoxicity assay for vascular rejection and graft loss after renal transplantation. *Transplantation* 55, 1287–1290.

# Chapter 9/Liver transplantation

DEREK WIGHT

## Introduction

The landmarks in liver transplantation are shown in Table 9.1. Moore and Starzl had already embarked upon an experimental programme with hepatic allografts in the dog by the time of Calne's discovery of an effective immunosuppressive agent. Moore et al. (1959) were the first to show that the operation was feasible and that the transplanted liver could maintain liver function until it was rejected. Starzl et al. (1965) then went on to produce long-term survival in dogs treated with azathioprine. They performed their first human liver transplant in 1963 (Starzl et al. 1963) and, in Europe, Calne started his own clinical programme in 1968. The next major landmark was the acceptance of the concept of brainstem death (Conference of Medical Royal Colleges and the Faculties in the United Kingdom 1976). This allowed the use of heart-beating donors and thus shortened considerably the period of warm ischaemia at the time of donor hepatectomy. The concept has now been accepted throughout the developed world. The other major advances have been the introduction into clinical transplantation, in 1979, of the fungal products cyclosporin A (Calne et al. 1979) and, more recently, FK506 (tacrolimus) (Demetris et al. 1990a), which have resulted in much improved control of the rejection process. Since then, a number of other newer agents have been used in both experimental and clinical transplantation, including mycophenolate mofetil (McDiarmid 1996; Klupp et al. 1997; Simmons et al. 1997), rapamycin (sirolimus) (Murgia et al. 1996), brequinar sodium (Cramer 1995) and gusperimus (Mignat 1997). Although results with many of these agents are promising, overall experience remains limited to date.

In 1983 an international meeting was convened to assess whether liver transplantation had developed sufficiently to be encouraged more widely (National Institutes of Health 1984). The conclusion was unequivocally in favour and worldwide interest in liver transplantation then increased dramatically so that now some 200 programmes in all parts of the world have performed over 40 000 operations (Terasaki & Cecka 1995), at a current rate of about 7000 per year (Ringe 1994). There have been a number of recent reviews of liver transplant pathology (Jaffe & Yunis 1989; Demetris 1990; Snover 1993; Hübscher 1994; Wight 1994a,c; Ludwig & Batts 1995).

## Results of transplantation

The procedure, in which the liver is inserted orthotopically—that is, into the normal site for the organ, with end-to-end anastomosis of vessels and common bile-

**Table 9.1** Liver transplant landmarks (Wight 1994c).

| Date | Development |
|------|-------------|
| 1960 | Introduction of azathioprine (Calne) |
| 1963 | First human liver graft (Starzl) |
| 1968 | First Cambridge graft (Calne) |
| 1976 | Acceptance of brainstem death |
| 1979 | Introduction of cyclosporin |
| 1983 | UK television campaign in support of child donors |
| 1984 | NIH consensus conference (USA) |
| 1986 | Special government funding (UK) |
| 1988 | UW (University of Wisconsin) preservation solution |
| 1990 | Introduction of FK506 |

duct—is now an almost routine worldwide treatment for a whole range of liver diseases (Starzl *et al.* 1989b; Ringe 1994). One-year survival has improved from less than 50% 15 years ago to more than 90% for certain low-risk groups (Bismuth *et al.* 1987; Otte 1991), while remaining lower for high-risk patients such as those in acute liver failure (Emond *et al.* 1989). Excellent results are also obtainable with reduced-size grafts when there is donor–recipient size mismatch (Bismuth & Houssin 1984; Broelsch *et al.* 1988) and even with living related partial liver grafts, almost always from parent to child (Kawarasaki *et al.* 1994; Tanaka *et al.* 1994b).

## Indications for transplantation

Virtually all kinds of parenchymal liver disease are regarded as indications for liver transplantation (Bismuth 1994). However, there has been a gradual move away from tumours, because of the unacceptably high rate of recurrence (see p. 279), towards parenchymal disease, primary biliary cirrhosis, cirrhosis as a result of chronic hepatitis C and cryptogenic cirrhosis being the most common indications. More recently, patients with fulminant hepatic failure have been transplanted (Williams & Wendon 1994), although there has been some debate about the validity of the use of historical controls as a yardstick of success in the treatment of the latter (Editorial 1990). A full controlled trial is probably overdue (Chapman *et al.* 1990). Incurable metabolic diseases form a small but significant

proportion of the patients in most series. Finally, a failed liver transplant is itself a good indication for repeating the procedure.

## Monitoring graft outcome

In clinical practice, blind core biopsy and fine needle aspiration biopsy (see below) can be used to monitor the progress of the graft (Williams *et al.* 1992); both have their place. In our series (Wight 1984), biopsy is performed routinely at the end of the transplantation operation ('time zero'), and thereafter when clinically indicated, especially before modifying immunosuppressive therapy.

### Core biopsy

The interpretation of transplant biopsies is not always straightforward. In contrast to routine biopsy practice, where one expects to find a unifying single disease to explain the patient's illness, more than one diagnosis is extremely common in transplant material (Wight 1994c). Because it is so common, there may often, for example, be evidence of rejection together with some other condition, such as bacterial or viral infection. These difficulties often magnify with increasing time after the operation (Nakhleh *et al.* 1990; Pappo *et al.* 1995). Also, abnormalities may be very focal and so it is most important to examine all the stained sections. Nevertheless, biopsy is one of the most important and useful tools available in the investigation of post-transplant liver dysfunction (Williams *et al.* 1985; Snover *et al.* 1987; Wight & Portmann 1987; Demetris 1990; Riely & Vera 1990; Colina *et al.* 1991; Kubota *et al.* 1991).

### Fine needle aspiration biopsy

Fine needle aspiration biopsy (FNAB) was first developed in Helsinki in the context of renal grafts (Häyry & von Willebrand 1984) and then subsequently applied to liver transplants (Lautenschlager *et al.* 1988, 1991, 1994). To eliminate the problem of contamination of the aspirate by blood, white cell differential counts are performed simultaneously on FNAB and blood smears and the count on the latter is then subtracted from the former. The technique has the advantage that it can be frequently repeated, even more than once daily if necessary, because of the low risks associated with the fine calibre of needle used. It is particularly useful for monitoring the quality of the infiltrate in acute cellular rejection because, especially with the help of monoclonal or polyclonal antibodies, the identification of individual cell types may be easier than in histological preparations (Schlitt *et al.* 1991; Schlitt & Nashan 1993), and for monitoring the response to treatment. Limited information can also be obtained on parenchymal changes as hepatocytes are also aspirated. Tissue biopsy is, however, essential when an assessment of architectural changes is needed, especially when irreversible lesions are suspected, for example (Kubota *et al.* 1991; Lautenschlager *et al.* 1991). Accuracy of FNAB diagnosis diminishes sharply later than 2 months after transplantation (Kirby *et al.* 1988), with no less than 40% of samples then giving inaccurate information, mainly because of the reduced proportion of abnormalities attributable to acute rejection (see below).

## Complications of liver transplantation

Because of the complexity of the procedure, complications of liver transplantation are quite common (Portmann & Wight 1987; Wight 1994c) (Table 9.2). These may damage the graft or the patient as a whole, or both. The most important complications affecting the graft are rejection and technical factors related to liver preservation or to the surgical procedure itself; the most important complications affecting the patient as a whole are bacterial and viral infections.

Table 9.2 Complications of liver transplantation.

| Complications affecting the graft | Complications affecting the host |
| --- | --- |
| Technical | Infection |
| Rejection | Graft vs. host disease |
| Disease recurrence | New tumours |
| Drug toxicity | Other medical complications |

## Rejection

Organ grafts differ from the classic skin grafts in that they are vascularized from the time of insertion, allowing the processes both of sensitization and subsequently of rejection to occur promptly. Much of the early work defining patterns of liver rejection, both with and without immunosuppressive treatment, was done with experimental animals (Wight 1984; Wight & Portmann 1987). Initially, large outbred animals such as the dog and the pig were used but now, following Kamada's development of a simplified technique (Kamada & Calne 1979), most animal experiments are performed on the laboratory rat. Although there are some differences of emphasis, the morphological changes of rejection of the liver are similar in all species so far studied. Nor are any real differences apparent in the patterns of rejection seen following the various combinations of immunosuppressive agents (Gouw *et al.* 1988a).

### CLASSIFICATION OF REJECTION

Rejection can be defined as graft damage caused by an immunological response by the recipient. In the kidney it is traditionally classified as hyperacute, acute and chronic, when the speed of onset may be measured in minutes with hyperacute, days with acute and weeks or months with chronic. In the case of the liver these terms, while generally understood, are not wholly appropriate because, as discussed below, the timing may be very different from the classic descriptions of renal grafts (Ludwig 1989). In the light of these problems, a standardized terminology was recently agreed by an international working party (Ludwig 1994; International Working Party 1995), in which humoral, cellular and chronic rejection were the preferred terms.

### Humoral rejection

Hyperacute rejection, a term coined by Kissmeyer-Nielsen *et al.* (1966), and accelerated rejection (see below) result from the presence of preformed circulating antibodies directed against donor-specific antigens within the graft and thus are more properly called humoral rejection. The antibodies of the ABO blood groups are of course innate, while presensitization to HLA antigens can occur not only from a previous graft, but also as a result of blood transfusion or pregnancy. Humoral rejection is rare in liver grafts, even when grafts are performed across ABO blood group barriers (Gordon *et al.* 1986b), an observation which has led to the widely held belief that the liver is relatively resistant to such antibody-mediated injury (Gordon *et al.* 1986a; Duquesnoy 1989). This belief was supported by the early experiments with rat liver graft models, where sensitization was followed by tolerance induction rather than hyperacute rejection (Kamada *et al.* 1981). However, Knechtle *et al.* (1987) were able to induce hyperacute rejection by presensitizing Lewis rats (RT-1[1]) with three successive 2 cm skin grafts at 14 day intervals from ACI animals (RT-1[a]). Histological studies of such livers revealed severe microvascular injury with destruction of endothelial cells, oedema, haemorrhage and hepatocyte necrosis, with bound IgG, IgM and complement demonstrable immunochemically (Knechtle *et al.* 1987). The principal target antigen in this model was subsequently shown to be the major class I antigen, RT-1[a] (Knechtle *et al.* 1989). Humoral rejection has also been induced in rhesus monkeys and pigs by a similar process of presensitization with donor-specific skin grafts and blood transfusions (Gubernatis *et al.* 1987; Colletti *et al.* 1994).

Although humoral rejection was suspected in one of the first clinical attempts at liver transplantation (Starzl 1969), its existence subsequently came to be doubted, mainly because of the success of liver transplants performed across ABO barriers. However, although individual livers might survive grafting across ABO barriers, it has been clearly shown (Demetris *et al.* 1989; Gugenheim *et al.* 1990; Sanchez-Urdazpal *et al.* 1993) that the risk of graft loss is substantially higher following mismatch than in ABO-matched controls. Similarly, lymphocytotoxic antibodies may cause graft failure in some, but not all, patients (Demetris *et al.* 1992a,b; Mañez *et al.* 1993). It is probable that many cases of vascular thrombosis may properly be attributable to severe rejection rather than to technical factors (Samuel *et al.* 1989; Yanaga *et al.* 1989). Other reports

of apparently well-documented antibody-mediated rejection (Hanto *et al.* 1987; Bird *et al.* 1989; Gubernatis *et al.* 1989; Starzl *et al.* 1989a) confirm that, in general, as well as being much rarer than following kidney grafts, the speed of onset in liver grafts is also slower. The risk of graft loss can be reduced by preoperative removal of isohaemagglutinins (Tanaka *et al.* 1994a).

The appearance of the human liver is similar to that observed in experimental animals with proven antibody-mediated rejection (Fig. 9.1) (Gubernatis *et al.* 1987; Knechtle *et al.* 1987; Colletti *et al.* 1994). The liver is swollen, dark in colour and increased in weight. The major vessels are generally patent yet microscopically the appearance closely resembles acute ischaemic damage caused by major vessel occlusion, with eosinophilic necrosis of both parenchyma and portal tracts accompanied by haemorrhage and a light neutrophilic infiltrate (Fig. 9.2) (Bird *et al.* 1989; Gugenheim *et al.* 1989). In the earliest cases sampled histologically, Demetris *et al.* (1988a, 1989) saw clusters of neutrophil polymorphs with fibrin deposition and red blood cell sludging in sinusoids, followed on

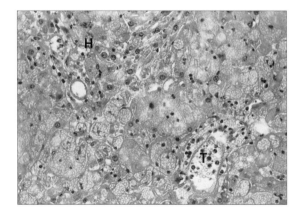

**Fig. 9.1** Humoural rejection: Lewis to BN rat liver transplant following three presensitizing Lewis skin grafts. The liver was removed 5 h after transplantation and already shows complete loss of zone III (centrilobular) liver cells and replacement by distended sinusoids filled with red blood cells. Note also necrosis of the wall of the terminal hepatic venule (T). A few residual hepatocytes (H) can be seen. H & E stain.

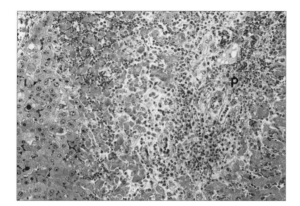

**Fig. 9.2** Humoural rejection: ABO incompatible human orthotopic liver transplant removed after 6 days. View showing a haemorrhagic portal tract (P) surrounded by necrotic hepatocytes. Canalicular cholestasis can also be seen in the surviving hepatocytes on the left. H & E stain.

the subsequent days by the appearance of hepatocyte necrosis. In contrast to the findings in kidneys, fibrinoid necrosis of arteries was unusual but focal masses of fibrin attached to a partly disrupted vessel wall, usually of veins, were quite commonly seen. Distinction from severe preservation injury or from ischaemic damage may not be easy (Demetris *et al.* 1989). Immunofluorescent studies, however, should detect immunoglobulin, C1q and C3, in arterial walls (Olson *et al.* 1988; Demetris *et al.* 1989), although the distribution of positive staining may be very focal compared to the picture in the kidney, and eluate from the failed graft contains donor-specific antibody (Demetris *et al.* 1990b).

The mechanism of the relative resistance of the liver to antibody-mediated rejection is not entirely understood (Demetris *et al.* 1992a). However, in contrast to other solid organs, the liver has no true end-arteries. Instead, the major part of the hepatic microvasculature consists of sinusoids, which are themselves fenestrated and without a basement membrane (Wight 1994b), and which derive their blood from two sources. When either the hepatic artery or portal vein flow is compromised the other vessel can probably compensate by an increased flow, although the mechanism by which this is controlled is not known. In addition, the sinusoids are lined by a vast number of macrophages, the

Kupffer's cells, which have a great capacity for removing complexes. Thus for both anatomical and functional reasons the liver might be expected to be relatively resistant to antibody-mediated damage.

*Acute cellular rejection*

Ludwig (1989) stresses that a condition which is defined morphologically should not have a name which implies speed of onset and suggests that this form of rejection should be designated cellular rather than acute, a view accepted by the international working party (Ludwig 1994). Nevertheless, the term acute rejection is well understood and widely used. Acute rejection is relatively easily defined and quantified in experimental grafts, particularly when using pure inbred strains of known HLA status, and using appropriate controls (Wight 1984; Wight & Portmann 1987). Initially, rejection was diagnosed mainly by exclusion (Demetris *et al.* 1985a) of other conditions clinically and histologically by analogy with the picture in experimental grafts. Another factor regarded as significant by some groups is a documented response to a boost of immunosuppression, usually three or more intravenous injections of methylprednisolone in the first instance. However, because the histological features of rejection are clearly self-limiting in some animal models (Wight & Portmann 1987) and possibly also in patients (Kemnitz & Cohnert 1987; Klintmalm *et al.* 1989; Dousset *et al.* 1993), on the one hand, and otherwise typical rejection may fail to respond, on the other, a response to treatment cannot be an absolute criterion. Despite these difficulties, there is now sufficient experience for there to be general diagnostic agreement as to the morphological features of acute cellular rejection, which are reproducible (Demetris *et al.* 1991, 1995; Thung & Gerber 1991; Hübscher 1994; Wight 1994a; Gupta *et al.* 1995).

Clinically, acute rejection presents with fever, malaise, graft tenderness and jaundice (Calne 1980). There may be a lymphocytosis (Munn *et al.* 1988) or, more specifically, evidence of spontaneous proliferation of peripheral blood lymphocytes measured by the incorporation of ($^3$H) thymidine *in vitro* (Kiuchi *et al.* 1994). An absolute eosinophilia may precede the other indicators of acute rejection by up to 2 days

(Lautenschlager *et al.* 1985; Foster *et al.* 1989; Manzarbeitia *et al.* 1995). Less specific findings include a variable degree of cholestasis (rise in serum bilirubin and alkaline phosphatase), abnormalities of synthetic function and elevations of enzymes that denote liver cell necrosis or injury (Starzl *et al.* 1989b). Other newer, but indirect, markers of acute rejection include increased levels in the serum of interleukin-6 (Ohzato *et al.* 1993), interleukin-2 receptors (Perkins *et al.* 1989a), serum hyaluronic acid (Adams *et al.* 1989b), γ-glutamyl transferase (Hickman *et al.* 1994) or α-glutathione S-transferase (Trull *et al.* 1994) and reduced clearance of indocyanine green (Clements *et al.* 1988), as well as various nuclear medicine techniques (Brunot *et al.* 1994).

Liver biopsy is still, however, regarded as the gold standard for the diagnosis of acute rejection and, indeed, of all types of hepatic dysfunction in transplant patients (Colina *et al.* 1991) against which other parameters are measured (Riely & Vera 1990). Snover *et al.* (1984a) defined the three cardinal features of acute rejection: mixed portal tract inflammation, bile-duct damage and attachment of lymphocytes to the endothelium of portal and/or hepatic venules, or endotheliitis (Ludwig 1988).

The earliest change seen is generally an inflammatory cell infiltration of portal tracts (Fig. 9.3). Frequently, the intensity is quite variable from one part of the liver to another and thus interpretation can be misleading unless a series of levels is examined from each biopsy. The cells are mostly lymphocytes but always include significant numbers of activated or blast cells (Plate 9.1, facing p. 342). These are large cells with large open nuclei with one or more prominent nucleoli, occasionally in mitosis, and they correspond to the pyroninophilic cells which are described in the older literature (Williams *et al.* 1973) but more recently had received scant attention until the cytologists demonstrated their true significance in the diagnosis of acute rejection (Lautenschlager *et al.* 1991). In addition, there are macrophages and often eosinophils (see Plate 9.1, facing p. 342) (Gupta *et al.* 1995) and neutrophils. Liver graft eosinophilia (defined as more than 7% of the portal inflammatory cells) was found to have 92% sensitivity and no less than 98% specificity for acute rejection of the liver (Foster *et al.* 1989), suggesting that eosinophils may be important effector cells (Krams *et al.* 1993; De Groen *et al.* 1994). Neutrophils are also commonly seen around bile-ductules in acute rejection in the absence of infection (Fig. 9.4)

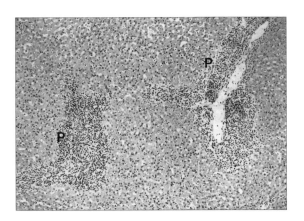

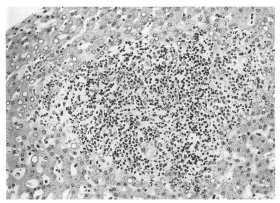

**Fig. 9.3** Acute cellular rejection: ABO compatible human liver graft. Biopsy taken at 7 days for minor liver dysfunction. The appearances are typical of acute rejection of moderate degree. A fairly dense but compact cellular infiltrate occupies the two portal tracts (P), whilst the parenchyma is essentially normal. H & E stain.

**Fig. 9.4** Acute cellular rejection: human liver graft, day 7. A portal tract occupies most of the field and contains a dense cellular infiltrate in which vessels and bile ducts can only be distinguished with difficulty. Note the neutrophil polymorphs which are concentrated at the sites of disrupted bile ducts. The infiltrate is compact and does not spill significantly into the parenchyma. H & E stain.

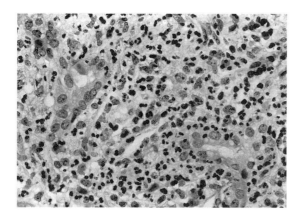

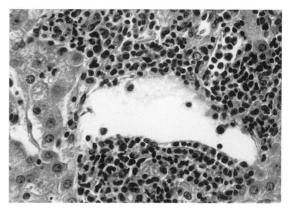

**Fig. 9.5** Acute cellular rejection: human liver graft, day 9. Here the bile ducts are much more easily seen. There is vacuolation and cellular infiltration of the epithelium. Note the prominent neutrophil polymorphs in between the bile ducts, a not infrequent component of acute rejection. No organisms were cultured at any time from this patient. (H & E stain).

**Fig. 9.6** Acute cellular rejection: human liver graft, day 11. Endotheliitis of a large portal venule. Note the adherence of mononuclear cells to the endothelium and, in the lower right part of the vessel wall, infiltration beneath the intima. (H & E stain).

(Hübscher *et al.* 1985), a finding referred to as rejection cholangitis (Ludwig 1988). The infiltrate is often quite compact and well-defined with little interface hepatitis at the limiting plate.

The second feature of the triad (Snover *et al.* 1984a), bile-duct damage, is very variable. The most common finding is vacuolation of biliary epithelium with associated infiltration by lymphocytes and/or neutrophil polymorphs (Figs 9.4 and 9.5). The classic features of apoptosis have recently been described, the number of apoptotic bile-duct cells correlating well with the severity of rejection (Nawaz & Fennell 1994). Occasional cells are in mitosis. The small interlobular ducts and the ducts of Hering are the principal targets of this type of injury, which may lead to the disappearance first of individual nuclei and then subsequently, in severe cases, to loss of ducts altogether (see below).

In both renal (Charpentier *et al.* 1981) and liver grafts (Demetris *et al.* 1985a) T cells have been shown to be the predominant cell in the infiltrate, with helper (CD4+) and cytotoxic (CD8+) T cells present in roughly equivalent numbers in most rejection episodes (Markus *et al.* 1987; Perkins *et al.* 1987; Ibrahim *et al.* 1993), although the cells infiltrating bile-duct epithe-

lium were found to be exclusively CD8+ cytotoxic T cells (McCaughan *et al.* 1989). The infiltrate also includes B cells, macrophages, neutrophils and eosinophils in varying proportions (Adams & Neuberger 1989; Martinez *et al.* 1993; De Groen *et al.* 1994).

The third of the triad (Snover *et al.* 1984a), endotheliitis, is found in both portal (Fig. 9.6) and, less commonly, hepatic venules (Plate 9.2, facing p. 342) although it may be easier to evaluate in the latter because of the intensity of the portal infiltrate. Mononuclear cells adhere to the endothelium but also characteristically infiltrate beneath the endothelium, lifting it from the underlying media. In portal tracts this can result in the vessel being totally obscured. Acute arterial changes are uncommon.

Cholestasis is common and usually takes the form of distension of bile canaliculi in hepatocytes adjacent to hepatic venules, where it may also be associated with some feathery degeneration. It does, however, as a sign, lack both sensitivity and specificity. Williams *et al.* (1985) considered cholestasis to be a manifestation of rejection only when accompanied by mononuclear cells. Cholestasis may have many other causes (Wight 1986) and is an almost invariable feature of liver graft dysfunction, whatever the aetiology. In one series it was found, for example, in over 70% of all biopsies whether or not there was also rejection (Ray *et al.* 1988). Conversely, about one in four of all biopsies which show otherwise typical acute cellular rejection have no cholestasis.

Other changes in uncomplicated rejection are quite unusual. The extensive parenchymal necrosis seen in some rat models (Wight & Portmann 1987) is rare in humans. Occasionally, the infiltrate in the walls of terminal hepatic venules may extend for a short distance into the adjacent parenchyma, producing an appearance which has been called sinusoidal endotheliitis (see Plate 9.2, facing p. 342), and which may be followed by hepatic venular stenosis (Dhillon *et al.* 1994). A similar extension into the parenchyma may also occur at limiting plates. Both forms of extension of the infiltrate into the parenchyma are usually accompanied by canalicular cholestasis of nearby liver cells. Only Sankary *et al.* (1989) regard spillover of inflammation at the limiting plate as a defining feature, which probably accounts for his low incidence of acute rejection. Sometimes the liver cells themselves are swollen with granular clumped bile in their otherwise rarefied cytoplasm, so-called biliary piecemeal necrosis or cellular cholestasis. Kupffer's cells in these areas may contain a little ceroid and bile pigment, and occasionally they may have foamy cytoplasm resembling xanthoma cells. At one time these were regarded as a sign of chronic rejection (Wight 1983) but it has become clear that they correlate only with severe cholestasis, which itself is common in chronic rejection (see below).

*Occurrence of acute rejection.* The true incidence of acute rejection can only be assessed when biopsy is performed frequently. Its incidence seems to vary quite widely in different series but most authors find acute rejection in between 60 and 80% of all patients (de Ville de Goyet *et al.* 1987; Saliba *et al.* 1987; Snover *et al.* 1987; Kemnitz *et al.* 1989; Klintmalm *et al.* 1989; Farges *et al.* 1994; US Multicenter FK506 Liver Study Group 1994).

Because it usually responds so well to treatment, acute rejection as a cause of graft failure is uncommon. Klintmalm *et al.* (1989) attributed graft failure to acute rejection in two of 63 patients, while in the recent US multicentre trial refractory rejection was encountered in 2% of 263 patients treated with FK506 and 12% of 266 treated with cyclosporin (US Multicenter FK506 Liver Study Group 1994).

Most episodes of acute rejection occur in the first few weeks after transplantation, with a peak incidence between day 5 and day 14. In Klintmalm *et al.*'s series (1989) the first episode of rejection occurred within 21 days in no less than 60 of 63 patients who experienced any acute rejection. Occasionally, otherwise typical changes can be seen as early as day 4. Much less commonly, acute rejection may appear for the first time weeks or months after transplantation, when it is frequently related to incomplete or faulty immunosuppression (Mor *et al.* 1992; Yoshida *et al.* 1996).

*Outcome of acute rejection.* Most patients with acute rejection recover both symptomatically and histologically; milder forms may resolve without immunosuppression (Dousset *et al.* 1993). Minor residual portal scarring is also quite common. Increased immunosuppression may cause mononuclear cells to disappear promptly from the portal infiltrate, leaving behind the polymorphonuclear leucocytes, which thus appear more prominent (Snover *et al.* 1984a). The authors who made this observation also stated that in their then small series no liver had fully returned to normal following rejection. This would be contrary to most other experience and may at least in part be a reflection of the fact that only patients who have clinical problems have repeated biopsies. A more recent study by the same group (Nakhleh *et al.* 1990) examined 86 biopsies from 38 patients who had all survived more than a year after transplantation (and up to 4.5 years). They found that one-third of the patients had normal or near normal biopsies, while the remainder all had significant abnormalities. No less than 14 patients had evidence of acute or chronic hepatitis, of unknown cause in most. Interestingly, they also found evidence of acute rejection in four patients, only one of whom had discontinued her medication. Similar findings have been reported from Pittsburgh (Pappo *et al.* 1995).

Various authors have devised grading schemes based on the quantity and/or the quality of acute rejection, and in some cases have been able to relate the grade to outcome. Snover *et al.* (1987), in a detailed study, examined and quantified on a scale of 0–4 a whole range of histological features, but found that only three—arteritis or the simultaneous presence of centrilobular ballooning and areas of liver cell drop-out; confluent necrosis; and paucity of bile-ducts—correlated significantly with outcome. The presence of any one of these features automatically placed the biopsy into the unfavourable grade 3. Grades 1 and 2 were defined on the basis of the traditional triad, biopsies in grade 2 having more than 50% of affected bile-ducts. The weakness of this study, as was acknowledged by the authors, was that the adverse features of grade 3 were not seen in initial biopsies from untreated patients but in all cases developed during attempts at treatment of acute rejection. In reality, all three features represent early changes of chronic rejection (see below). Furthermore, not all authors regard ballooning of centrilobular liver cells as a feature of rejection. Ballooning occurs in a variable number of patients, more than half in one series (Ng *et al.* 1991), and is probably the consequence of ischaemia, which itself may be multifactorial. It may, for example, be related to events around the transplant operation itself (see p. 278).

Other authors have produced their own schemes (Kemnitz *et al.* 1989; McDonald *et al.* 1989; Demetris 1990; Hübscher 1994, 1996; Demetris *et al.* 1995; Gupta *et al.* 1995). The scheme devised by the pathologists participating in the (US) National Institute of Diabetes and Digestive and Kidney Diseases Liver Transplant Database (NIDDK LTD) is relatively simple, with three grades, and has been shown to be both reproducible and to have predictive value for transplant outcome (Demetris *et al.* 1991, 1995). That devised by Gupta *et al.* (1995) has been defined in detail but is as yet untested.

More recently, an international panel of experts in liver transplant pathology met in Banff to define and agree a common nomenclature and set of histopathological criteria for the grading of acute rejection, together with a preferred method of reporting (International Panel 1997). This combines the NIDDK LTD global assessment grades (Demetris *et al.* 1991, 1995) with the European system (Hübscher 1994, 1996),

which forms the basis of a numerical rejection activity index (RAI). The latter is a simple semiquantitative assessment of the three basic criteria defined by Snover *et al.* (1984a), namely portal inflammation, bile-duct inflammation/damage and venous endothelial inflammation, each on a three-point scale. The total RAI score is the sum of the components and thus has a maximum value of 9. The principal difference between the RAI and the scoring system devised by Gupta *et al.* (1995) is the inclusion in the latter scheme of a fourth scored category, namely the number of infiltrating eosinophils.

Immunostaining showed that patients whose portal infiltrates contained predominantly T helper cells responded well to a steroid boost, whereas if the portal infiltrate contained mixed T helper and T cytotoxic suppressor cells only a minority responded (Perkins *et al.* 1989b).

*Differential diagnosis of acute rejection.* Some of the more important differential diagnoses are shown in Table 9.3. In general, the changes in liver transplants are no different from those seen in general pathology (Wight 1994c). However, liver biopsies from transplant patients should always be interpreted with caution and placed in perspective with other data. It is also important to be aware, as already stated, that more than one condition may be present in liver transplant patients. FNAB, because of the attention it necessarily pays to the quality of the infiltrate, can be particularly valuable in the differentiation of viral infection, especially the hepatitis viruses and cytomegalovirus infection (CMV), from rejection (Lautenschlager *et al.* 1994); however, both may be present concurrently (Höckerstedt *et al.* 1989).

Table 9.3 Differential diagnosis of acute rejection.

| |
| --- |
| Reperfusion injury |
| Primary non-function |
| Biliary infection |
| Vascular occlusion |
| Biliary obstruction |
| CMV infection |
| Functional cholestasis |

## Chronic rejection

By analogy with accepted practice in transplantation of other organs (Sibley 1994), chronic rejection is probably the best overall term for the combination of diminished or absent bile-ducts (vanishing bile-duct syndrome) and foam cell endovasculitis of medium and large arteries (Wight 1996). The only problem with the term is the fact that occasional patients develop accelerated disease which may appear within as little as 20 days after transplantation (Ludwig *et al.* 1987); here too, as with acute rejection, Ludwig (1989) argues that terms involving the dimension of time should be reserved for clinical usage and pathologists should only use words based on structural features. He therefore suggests the use of the terms ductopenia and arteriopathy, but this seems unnecessarily cumbersome and pedantic, given established usage.

Chronic rejection is one of the major causes of graft failure beyond the first month after transplantation (Wight & Portmann 1987). The incidence varies from unit to unit but appears to be about 10–20% in those patients who survive beyond the first month (Grond *et al.* 1986; Oguma *et al.* 1989; Freese *et al.* 1991; Deligeorgi-Politi *et al.* 1994) although, interestingly, in most centres it appears to be decreasing in frequency (Pirsch *et al.* 1990). Chronic rejection generally develops insidiously, with progressive cholestasis manifested by a relentless increase in serum bilirubin and alkaline phosphatase. Its course is not influenced by immunosuppression or any other treatment, although the new immunosuppressive drug FK506 was reported to have possibly arrested the progress of chronic rejection in a number of patients in an early trial (Demetris *et al.* 1990a). In one series (Wight 1989) the median time between transplantation and graft loss was 20 weeks but the range was quite wide.

In livers removed at retransplantation or at autopsy the key features are loss of small bile-ducts (Fig. 9.7) and a foam-cell endovasculitis which affects medium and large arteries (Fig. 9.8). The bile-duct loss is fairly uniform throughout the liver and affects mainly the ducts less than 75 μm in diameter (Oguma *et al.* 1989); these are slightly smaller than the ducts affected in primary biliary cirrhosis, which range up to 94 μm

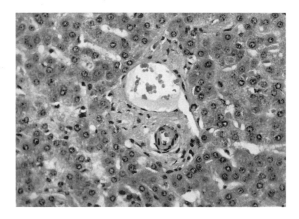

**Fig. 9.7** Chronic rejection (vanishing bile duct syndrome): ABO compatible human liver graft, 6 months after transplantation. Note the complete absence from this small portal tract of a bile duct, whilst the artery can still be clearly seen. Note also the absence of any inflammation. H & E stain.

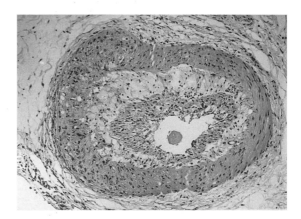

**Fig. 9.8** Chronic rejection: human liver graft, 3 months after transplantation. Note the rather more mature lesion in this main branch of the hepatic artery There is now a subintimal layer of fibromuscular proliferation, separating the foam cells from the medial coat, giving some resemblance to conventional atherosclerosis. H & E stain.

(Nakanuma & Ohta 1979). In fully developed disease portal tracts may have relatively few remaining inflammatory cells and thus have a very bland, almost normal appearance except that the small branches of the hepatic artery are no longer accompanied by a bile-duct of similar size. Limiting plates are often now well defined, and there may or may not be evidence of portal fibrosis. Using histometric analysis Oguma *et al.* (1989) were able to demonstrate that there was also loss of arterioles of the smallest calibre, namely less than 35 μm in diameter. Rarely, larger bile-ducts are totally replaced by foam cells similar to those seen in the arterial lesions (Wight & Portmann 1987) (see below) or are replaced by fibrous scars identical to those seen in primary sclerosing cholangitis. In contrast to most other conditions associated with bile-duct loss, for example primary biliary cirrhosis, there is usually no ductular proliferation (Hübscher 1991).

The arterial lesions, analogous to those called transplant atherosclerosis in heart grafts (Stovin 1984; Billingham 1987), principally affect the first- and second-order branches at the hilum and the medium-sized vessels within the major hepatic septa (Deligeorgi-Politi *et al.* 1994). If these areas are not specifically sampled histologically the lesions may be missed, although sometimes they are easily seen with the naked eye. Not only do the vessels stand out as having thickened walls but they are also bright yellow in colour as a result of the lipid contained within the foam cells, which form the major component of the lesion. Foam cells are found beneath the endothelium and mainly within the intima, and stain positively with macrophage markers. In the larger vessels they may form localized nodules on the wall or they may fill the intima and cause marked narrowing or even total occlusion of the vessel. Only infrequently do the foam cells infiltrate into or beyond the media, when there may also be disruption of the internal elastic lamina. The medium-sized vessels, when involved, are nearly always totally occluded. In about 10% of cases foam cells are also seen in the small vessels (Deligeorgi-Politi *et al.* 1994). Mononuclear inflammatory cells are not usually seen in any number. Because graft failure intervenes quite early more mature lesions are observed only rarely, but when they are it can be seen that the foam cells are gradually replaced by fibromuscular intimal thickening, which comes more and more to resemble conventional atherosclerosis. Very occasionally, similar foam-cell lesions are found in branches of the portal vein or tributaries of the hepatic vein.

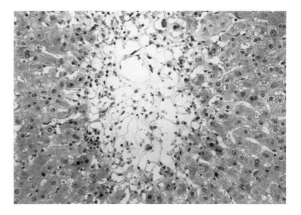

**Fig. 9.9** Chronic rejection: human liver graft, 3 months after transplantation (same case as Plate 9.4). Note the very clearly demarcated zone of liver cell drop-out around the terminal hepatic venule which is a very constant finding in chronic rejection. H & E stain.

Although in most cases both lesions, namely bile-duct loss and foam-cell endovasculitis, are found together, in occasional livers only one or other of the two is seen (Wight 1989; Deligeorgi-Politi *et al.* 1994). This obviously has both pathogenetic (see p. 274) and diagnostic implications.

The other features of established chronic rejection, liver cell loss (Fig. 9.9) and cholestasis (Plate 9.3, facing p. 342), are almost constant but are necessarily less specific. Liver cell loss varies from slight to extensive multilobular collapse, the latter being clearly visible to the naked eye. The less severe loss usually occurs as very sharply demarcated zones of drop-out around terminal hepatic venules, the liver cells being replaced by phagocytes containing ceroid and bile (see Plate 9.3, facing p. 342). The extent of the liver cell loss tends to parallel the degree of arterial occlusion and in practice the more rapid the onset, the more severe the arterial lesions tend to be.

Biochemical cholestasis is virtually invariable and correlates morphologically with severe canalicular cholestasis affecting hepatocytes adjacent to the perivenular drop-out. It is often visible to the naked eye as a yellow–green nutmeg-like appearance. It may be accompanied by feathery degeneration of occasional hepatocytes and sometimes sinusoidal foam cells, as

**Table 9.4** Causes of late graft failure.

Chronic rejection
Recurrent disease
Chronic bacterial infection and sludge
Viral infection (especially hepatitis viruses)
Bile-duct stricture
Vascular occlusion
Drug toxicity

described above (see Plate 9.3, facing p. 342). Eventually there may be centrilobular reticulin condensation and fibrosis and ultimately cirrhosis (Wight & Portmann 1987).

*Diagnosis of chronic rejection.* While it is easy to recognize in a failed graft, chronic rejection is much harder to diagnose on biopsy, yet its early recognition is important to the patient. Because the condition is progressive and irreversible, it is very much in the patient's interest to have a new graft while fit and before liver function has deteriorated too far. Early recognition is, however, difficult and to some extent subjective (Ludwig *et al.* 1987; Demetris 1990), and must be distinguished from other causes of late graft failure (Table 9.4).

As only about 10% of livers with chronic rejection have involvement of small arteries (Deligeorgi-Politi *et al.* 1994), arterial lesions are rarely seen in needle biopsies. When they are, however, diagnosis is confirmed and unequivocal because foam cells in small vessels indicate severe disease. Similarly, when loss of small bile-ducts is total there is no difficulty. Most, but not all, patients who subsequently go on to develop chronic rejection experience initial acute rejection. Serial biopsies may show typical acute rejection cholangitis followed by the gradual development of more chronic changes in bile-duct epithelium. As the inflammatory cells regress, the biliary epithelium becomes more and more uneven. Some nuclei are enlarged while others have apparently disappeared. Bile-ducts become increasingly difficult to identify and instead of about one to two per portal tract, as in the normal liver (Alagille 1979), more and more portal tracts are without ducts.

It has been suggested (Hübscher *et al.* 1991) that a satisfactory definition of chronic rejection would be when more that 50% of portal tracts are without a bile-duct. Special stains such as periodic acid–Schiff after diastase digestion, connective tissue stains and immunostains for cytokeratins (Plate 9.4, facing p. 342) (Harrison *et al.* 1994b) may all assist duct recognition. However, while there is a general belief that ducts cannot regenerate (Sherlock 1987), a recent report casts doubt on this (Hübscher *et al.* 1991). The authors described a series of six patients all of whom were thought to be developing chronic rejection, and whose biopsies met these criteria, yet for a variety of reasons did not receive a new liver. In all cases there was both clinical and biopsy evidence of improvement. While the latter may, of course, represent sampling error, these findings are important and mean that the diagnosis of chronic rejection in such cases (i.e. in the absence of pathognomonic findings such as 100% duct loss or foam-cell arteriopathy) should only be made in the presence of progressive clinical deterioration.

Persistence of centrilobular drop-out is an adverse prognostic factor and greatly increases the possibility that chronic rejection is present (Ludwig *et al.* 1990; Gómez *et al.* 1994).

PATHOGENESIS OF REJECTION

The pathogenenesis of rejection is discussed in detail elsewhere in this book, and thus only those factors relevant to the liver will be considered here.

*Cellular interactions*

Rejection depends on the complex interplay of a variety of cellular interactions involving both cell-associated and soluble mediators (Krams *et al.* 1993). The extravasation and localization of immune cells to the allograft is dependent on recognition and interaction of complementary adhesion molecules expressed on leucocytes and endothelium. Classically, cytotoxic (CD8+) T cells were thought to be the main mediators of graft rejection (Hall & Dorsch 1984), but it is now clear that they also interact with helper (CD4+) cells and macrophages. Helper T cells are probably also the source of the lymphokines that cause recruitment of eosinophils and neutrophils to the site of rejection (see p. 267) (Adams & Neuberger 1989). Allogeneic class II molecules are the main sensitizers of graft rejection and in the liver the dendritic cells, upon which class II antigens are strongly expressed, are found mainly in portal tracts (Demetris *et al.* 1985b). There is good evidence (Gouw *et al.* 1987; Steinhoff *et al.* 1988) that the other rich source of allogeneic class II molecules, on donor Kupffer's cells, is rapidly removed as these cells are replaced in grafts by those of recipient origin. Bile-ducts, liver cells and vascular endothelia of the hepatic artery and portal and hepatic venules are generally class II-negative (Gouw *et al.* 1987).

The liver shows considerable variation of expression of class I antigens between different cell types. Sinusoidal lining cells—endothelium and Kupffer's cells—dendritic cells and bile-duct epithelium normally express antigen (Barbatis *et al.* 1981; Fleming *et al.* 1981; Daar *et al.* 1984; Lautenschlager *et al.* 1984), while hepatocytes do not.

Expression of HLA antigens may be up-regulated in a variety of circumstances. Interferon-α and γ, for example, can induce the appearance of both class I (Pignatelli 1988) and class II antigens (Robbins *et al.* 1988). Interferon-induced HLA display is important in T cell lysis of virus-infected cells, and infection may be one of the triggers causing new expression of HLA antigens in the liver. A number of authors have shown that after transplantation there is increased expression both of class I antigens on bile-duct epithelium and on hepatocytes and of class II antigens on bile-duct epithelium and vascular endothelium but usually not on hepatocytes (Gouw *et al.* 1988b; Steinhoff *et al.* 1988). Although in general there is more antigen expressed during rejection (Nagafuchi *et al.* 1985; So *et al.* 1987), enhancement also occurs in the absence of rejection and in other conditions such as CMV infection and cholangitis (Steinhoff *et al.* 1988). It remains unclear therefore whether the induction of antigens is the cause or the consequence of rejection, although the latter seems the more probable (Wood *et al.* 1988; Snover 1990b). In this respect it is interesting to note that renal allograft rejection in dogs caused increased expression of HLA-DR on the host's own (untransplanted) liver cells (Belitsky *et al.* 1990).

*Bile-duct damage*

The pattern of cellular infiltration in acute liver graft rejection corresponds very much to the sites of HLA antigen expression, with lymphocytes concentrated in the portal tracts (where the dendritic cells are found), in bile-duct epithelium (where class II is newly expressed and where class I is increased) and in vascular endothelium (where class I and II are enhanced). The major exception remains the hepatocytes, where there is dramatic enhancement of class I expression yet parenchymal lymphocytic infiltration and liver cell necrosis are most unusual (So *et al.* 1987). From the foregoing discussion it would seem reasonable to attribute the disappearance of bile-ducts in chronic rejection to this immunological damage, particularly in view of the close similarity with the hepatic lesion in graft vs. host disease (Snover *et al.* 1984b). Furthermore, in a number of cases it is possible to observe a linear progression from acute bile-duct damage in acute rejection through to complete disappearance of bile-ducts in chronic rejection (Wight & Portmann 1987).

Alternative explanations for bile-duct damage have been put forward (Wight & Portmann 1987). Portal tracts and their contained bile-ducts obtain their blood mainly from the hepatic artery and thus any compromise of that supply, for example in the presence of foam-cell endovasculitis, could lead to disappearance of ducts. A histometric study of chronic liver graft rejection (Oguma *et al.* 1989) showed that the severity of arteriolar and bile-duct loss was directly proportional to the severity of the arterial lesions. However, this study also showed that bile-duct loss occurred in the absence of obliterative arterial lesions, and so the authors concluded that both lymphocytotoxicity and ischaemia could be responsible for the lesion. Others have come to a similar conclusion (Wiesner *et al.* 1991).

*Chronic rejection*

The pathogenesis of the atherosclerosis-like lesions of chronic rejection may well be multifactorial (Häyry 1994). Traditionally, the vascular lesions of chronic rejection have been thought to be antibody-mediated

(Demetris *et al.* 1987b; Tilney *et al.* 1991). However, as in atherosclerosis itself (Ross 1993), it is becoming increasingly apparent that the lesions are attributable to the triggering of a whole variety of adhesion molecules and cytokines in the vessel wall (Azuma *et al.* 1994), leading to migration of lymphocytes and macrophages into the vessel wall. These events are perhaps triggered by allogeneic class II molecules on the endothelium (Libby & Tanaka 1994), which might be activated by a whole variety of stimuli (Orosz 1994). These include any cause of tissue damage, such as poor preservation, prior acute rejection, antibody, drugs, cytokines and inflammatory mediators, viral infections and even the lipid status of the recipient (Tullius & Tilney 1995). This great variety of different potential initiators of the process perhaps explains why it is so difficult to identify why particular patients go on to develop chronic rejection while others do not.

Adams *et al.* (1989a) found increased expression of the adhesion molecule ICAM-1 (CD54) in patients with acute rejection and, in particular, greater expression on bile-duct epithelium in those patients who went on to develop chronic rejection than those who responded to increased immunosuppression. Also, ICAM-1 expression is more specific than class II MHC because it is less likely to be expressed in conditions such as cholestasis and, following successful treatment of rejection, the ICAM-1 expression rapidly decreases while class II antigen persists. The role of other adhesion molecules, particularly those on vascular endothelium (Sedmak & Orosz 1991), is being actively explored (Steinhoff *et al.* 1990, 1993; Bacchi *et al.* 1993).

There is good evidence that HLA matching of recipient with donor improves survival of both renal and heart grafts and the improvement is maintained in those patients treated with cyclosporin (Persijn *et al.* 1989), but at the moment the evidence with liver grafts is at best equivocal (Neuberger & Adams 1990). Two studies have shown inferior results for patients in whom HLA-DR matching was good (Donaldson *et al.* 1987; Markus *et al.* 1988). Markus *et al.* (1988) found a higher incidence of primary non-function when there was a good class II match. Donaldson *et al.* (1987) further showed that if there was also a mismatch of class I antigens the risk of chronic rejection was greatly

increased. In addition, high-titre anti-class I antibodies were present in six of 14 patients with chronic rejection and none of those without. Another group found the opposite result (Batts *et al.* 1988), namely that chronic rejection was associated with a class II mismatch, while the Hanover group (Gubernatis *et al.* 1988) found that a class II mismatch was often followed by persistent cholestasis and cholangitis. A recent large study (Donaldson *et al.* 1993) was unable to confirm any link between outcome and class II status. There is thus insufficient evidence at present to know whether or not prospective matching of liver grafts would be beneficial.

Cytomegalovirus infection has been found to be another independent risk factor for chronic rejection in liver grafts (O'Grady *et al.* 1988a; Martelius *et al.* 1997). The better control of CMV infections by prophylactic use of antiviral agents, and the matching of donor organs with the recipient with respect to CMV antibody status, could possibly account for the falling incidence of chronic rejection. It is not clear, however, why a similar effect of viral infection has not been seen in other series (van Hoek *et al.* 1992), or following heart and other organ grafts (Steinhoff 1990; Wallwork 1994). Indeed, at the Mayo Clinic (van Hoek *et al.* 1992) a multivariate analysis showed that the most significant risk factor was immunosuppression using only two (cyclosporin and prednisolone) as opposed to three immunosuppressive drugs (with azathioprine), suggesting that better management of immunosuppression is the key factor (Soin *et al.* 1995). The other significant risk factors in this study were found to be a primary diagnosis of primary sclerosing cholangitis and a positive lymphocytotoxic cross-match.

### Cholestasis

The pathogenesis of the cholestasis seen so regularly in liver transplants is far from clear and may well be multifactorial (Wight 1986; Wight & Portmann 1987), including a variety of non-immunological mechanisms (Forker & Runyon 1978; Hübscher 1991), especially in view of the relative paucity of immunological cells within the parenchyma of rejecting grafts. Drugs may be implicated in some cases. Azathioprine can cause cholestasis and liver cell loss in dogs (Porter 1969) and in humans (Haas *et al.* 1978). Cyclosporin is also known to be hepatotoxic in renal transplant patients (Calne *et al.* 1979; Klintmalm *et al.* 1981), in whom it causes a mild elevation in serum bilirubin but no morphological cholestasis. With the lower doses of both drugs now currently in use it seems unlikely that either drug is a major cause of cholestasis. In some patients the mechanism may be similar to that of the benign postoperative cholestasis (Schmid *et al.* 1965) thought to be caused by bilirubin overload from transfused blood and the resorption of haematomas. Other systemic factors such as shock, haemolysis and bacterial infections (Fahrlander *et al.* 1964) may cause cholestasis without direct hepatic involvement. Increased levels of tumour necrosis factor $\alpha$ (TNF$\alpha$) have been found in patients undergoing renal (Maury & Teppo 1987) and heart (Chollet-Martin *et al.* 1990) allograft rejection. Conversely, antibody to TNF$\alpha$ prolongs cardiac allograft survival in rats with acute rejection (Imagawa *et al.* 1991). The liver is a very rich source of TNF$\alpha$ and it has recently been proposed (Jones *et al.* 1990) that TNF might be an important cause of cholestasis in a variety of acute and chronic liver diseases. Similarly, parenteral nutrition is a well-known cause of cholestasis in the neonatal period (Pallarés *et al.* 1983) and may well be implicated in liver transplant patients. Any or all of these factors are frequently present in an individual transplant patient. Eggink *et al.* (1984) was the first to coin the term functional cholestasis for those cases in which no other obvious cause was found.

### Liver cell drop-out

Hepatocyte ballooning and cell loss (drop-out), mainly affecting zone 3, may be attributable to ischaemia in the perioperative period (Ng *et al.* 1991; Gómez *et al.* 1994) or to the foam-cell endovasculitis of chronic rejection. However, ischaemia cannot readily explain the drop-out sometimes seen in acute rejection. Ludwig *et al.* (1990) suggested that it might be caused by rejection-induced endophlebitis causing outflow blockage, but if this is the case it is surprising that there is not accompanying sinusoidal congestion. Gómez *et al.*, in a

controlled study (Gómez *et al.* 1994), found a significant relationship between drop-out and ischaemia time and the number and early onset of acute rejection episodes. They also showed, as had Ludwig *et al.* (1990), an increased risk of progression to chronic rejection. Alternatively, it might be a consequence of direct hepatotoxicity caused by bile retention (Wight & Portmann 1987). Centrilobular fibrosis is a rare sequel to acute rejection and is probably proportional to the degree of inflammation, although the possibility of azathioprine toxicity as a significant cause (see below) has not been thoroughly explored.

### Technical complications

#### VASCULAR COMPLICATIONS

The liver is inserted into a normal position after recipient hepatectomy, the so-called orthotopic procedure. The operation is itself a most complex procedure with multiple anastomoses of vessels and of the bile-duct. In recent years, because of the shortage of donors in the paediatric age group, increasing use has been made of reduced-size adult livers (Bismuth & Houssin 1984; Broelsch *et al.* 1988; Ryckman *et al.* 1991), usually based upon the left lobe. This same technique (Czerniak *et al.* 1989) has been used to remove the left lobe *in vivo* from living donors and to split the liver from one deceased donor for implantation into two recipients (Broelsch *et al.* 1990).

The patient is often in liver failure or, at least, has compromised liver function and therefore a tendency to haemorrhage and an increased susceptibility to infection. Any one of the anastomoses may break down or become narrowed, or alternatively one of the vascular anastomoses, especially that of the hepatic artery (Sánchez-Bueno *et al.* 1994), may become thrombosed. The incidence of hepatic artery thrombosis is about 1.5% in adults and, because of its small size, 11.8% in children (Esquivel *et al.* 1985). Paradoxically, one of the advantages of the reduced-size adult donor livers (Bismuth & Houssin 1984; Broelsch *et al.* 1988) is that the calibre of the donor arteries is greater than in a child donor's liver and therefore is technically easier to handle. Again, the presence of one pathological state may actually lead to another. Haemorrhagic or bacteraemic shock, for example, may cause hepatic artery or portal vein thrombosis. Similarly, some cases at least may be a manifestation of antibody-mediated rejection (Samuel *et al.* 1989; Yanaga *et al.* 1989) (see p. 264). Measurement of various clotting factors in the blood may predict subsequent thrombosis (Boutiere *et al.* 1994; Himmelreich *et al.* 1994; Jennings *et al.* 1994).

Infarcts may subsequently become infected and result in abscess formation; this may well be the most important pathogenesis of abscesses (Hesselink *et al.* 1987). Hepatic artery occlusion may also be an important cause of breakdown of the biliary anastomosis (Hesselink *et al.* 1987). Perhaps because of the denervated state of the transplanted liver, thromboses of the portal vein, which in the intact liver would give rise to infarcts of Zahn, may also lead to typical ischaemic infarction. Conversely, occlusive thrombosis of the hepatic artery does not always result in infarction. At least two patients with a chronic rejection-like syndrome proved to have underlying hepatic artery thrombosis (Wight & Portmann 1987).

PRIMARY NON-FUNCTION AND
REPERFUSION INJURY

Once the concept of brainstem death was accepted (Conference of Medical Royal Colleges and the Faculties in the United Kingdom 1976) it became possible to excise the liver in one institution and then transport it to the transplant centre for insertion into the recipient. A new perfusate developed at the University of Wisconsin (UW solution), based upon lactobionate, represented a very significant advance because it allowed cold storage of canine livers for up to 48 h (Jamieson *et al.* 1988), far in excess of the previous 8 h maximum. This solution has been universally adopted clinically and has transformed the whole logistics of transplantation. It is now possible to plan operations semielectively—at times convenient for operating-theatre usage, for example—and it has also opened up the potential for planned matching of donor transplantation antigens with those of the recipient, as is now usual with kidney transplants but was not previously

possible, because of lack of time, with the liver (see above).

However, even following the use of the UW solution, the liver may fail to function as expected, a state now generally referred to as preservation injury (Katz *et al.* 1994), which is the most important determinant of early graft function. In its most severe form, the liver may fail to function at all: so-called primary non-function. Clinically, it is manifested by a failure of bile flow, persistent coagulopathy and progressive elevation of enzymes, and it has a very high mortality unless the liver is immediately replaced, although treatment with prostaglandin $E_1$ may have some benefit (Greig *et al.* 1989). Less severe injury, which has been called initial poor function (Ploeg *et al.* 1993; Cillo *et al.* 1994), can resolve spontaneously although full recovery of function may take weeks or months (Demetris 1990). Although uncommon in some series (Ploeg *et al.* 1993; Strasberg *et al.* 1994), it affects up to 23% of livers in other units (Greig *et al.* 1989). Important risk factors in the donor include steatosis, serum sodium concentration, cold preservation of longer than 12 h and donor age greater than 50 years and, in the recipient, retransplantation, poor medical status including renal failure, raised transaminases, low factor V and prolonged prothrombin time (Cillo *et al.* 1994; González *et al.* 1994; Strasberg *et al.* 1994).

Within the liver, sinusoidal lining cells are probably the most susceptible to this kind of damage, but electron microscopy is necessary for full evaluation (McKeown *et al.* 1988; Kakizoe *et al.* 1990; Carles *et al.* 1994a,b). Histologically, the earliest change seen is a diffuse fine vesiculation of hepatocytes, representing fat, associated with sinusoidal neutrophil infiltration and patchy liver cell necrosis (Plate 9.5, facing p. 342) (Tillery *et al.* 1989). The latter is presumably secondary to ischaemia caused by disruption of the microvasculature and varies from extensive zonal necrosis, sometimes periportal (Demetris 1990), to spotty acidophilic necrosis. However, some of the injury may be the consequence of Kupffer's cell and endothelial activation which occurs on revascularization of the graft (Carles *et al.* 1994a,b). There is some evidence that the denervated liver is more susceptible to hypovolaemic injury (Henderson *et al.* 1992); primary non-function has also been described following long-standing hypertension in the donor (Wisecaver *et al.* 1994). Antibody-mediated rejection (see above) may cause a very similar picture (Demetris *et al.* 1992b).

Less severe injury may take the form of diffuse hepatocyte ballooning (Plate 9.6, facing p. 342) in the second or third week after transplantation (Goldstein *et al.* 1991; Ng *et al.* 1991). Occasional acidophil bodies, as isolated findings, are quite commonly seen in biopsies taken during the first week after transplantation and probably represent minor degrees of the same phenomenon. As with any apparent ischaemic necrosis in transplant material, the diagnosis must be made in the appropriate clinical and biochemical context (see above) to avoid overestimating the degree of damage.

Changes associated with reperfusion injury probably take at least some hours to become visible microscopically in sections prepared by routine paraffin processing and thus the biopsy, often taken at the end of the transplant operation (the time zero biopsy), may be deceptively normal. The value of the time zero biopsy lies in the diagnosis of donor disease, for example fatty change (Adam *et al.* 1991), and the provision of a baseline for subsequent developments. In our own material we generally see minor focal neutrophil infiltration of occasional perivenular liver cells, an appearance which closely resembles the 'surgical artefact' described in non-transplant livers (Christoffersen & Poulsen 1970) and itself thought to result from hypoxia, but there is clearly some overlap between this and true preservation injury (Katz *et al.* 1994). A study of time zero biopsies from 38 patients (Abraham & Furth 1996) defined risk factors both for subsequent severe acute rejection, namely hepatocyte swelling, and for primary graft failure, namely apoptotic hepatocytes, centrilobular haemorrhage, hepatocyte swelling and centrilobular necrosis. Confirmation of these results would define a patient subpopulation who should be carefully monitored for signs of graft failure or rejection.

### BILE-DUCT COMPLICATIONS

Complications of the bile-duct anastomosis were once a major cause of graft and patient loss (Starzl *et al.* 1977). Indeed Starzl once referred to the bile-duct as the 'Achilles' heel of liver transplantation' (Starzl *et al.* 1979). With improved technique, the incidence of both bile leak and late duct obstruction has been greatly reduced (Klein *et al.* 1991). End-to-end duct-to-duct anastomosis is now preferred in all major centres, with duct-to-Roux loop being reserved for those cases where there is no duct (e.g. biliary atresia) or where the duct is unsuitable (e.g. primary sclerosing cholangitis).

The bile-ducts within and outside the liver are supplied by branches of the hepatic artery. Anastomotic duct stricture usually occurs more than 2 months after surgery (Lerut *et al.* 1987), and is mainly a technical problem following direct injury to the arterial supply. It has recently been recognized that anatomical aberrations in the supply of the common bile-duct and the main hepatic ducts are unexpectedly frequent (Saxena *et al.* 1995), and may make the ducts especially vulnerable to ischaemic damage, especially with reduced-size livers. However, both anastomotic and non-anastomotic stricture—when strictures may occur throughout the intra- as well as the extrahepatic biliary tree—may follow a variety of different insults to the peribiliary arterial microvasculature (Fisher & Miller 1995). Anything which leads to endothelial injury may be followed by thrombosis; damage incurred during cold preservation (Popescu *et al.* 1994) and reperfusion, warm ischaemia (Sankary *et al.* 1995), ABO incompatibility and immunological damage have all been implicated (Fisher & Miller 1995). In a number of cases duct stricture has proved to be an early manifestation of chronic rejection (see above), the stricturing process being the consequence of foam-cell endovasculitis affecting the blood supply of the donor duct.

Amorphous concretions of biliary sludge filling the biliary tree were a major problem in the King's College Hospital, Cambridge, series at one time (Portmann & Wight 1987). Sludge is almost always associated with obstruction and/or bile leak and associated bacterial cholangitis, and commonly with underlying arterial occlusion (Ludwig *et al.* 1992; Ludwig & Batts 1995). However, it is not always clear whether the latter is the primary event or whether it is vascular occlusion caused by bile injury (Syrakos *et al.* 1979; McMaster *et al.* 1980; Bauer *et al.* 1995).

## Recurrent disease

As with other grafted organs, it had been expected that the original disease might recur in the transplanted liver if it were caused by host and/or environmental factors rather than intrinsic hepatic disorders. In fact, relatively few conditions have been found to recur; those diseases which may do so are shown in Table 9.5 (van Thiel & Gavaler 1987; Hart *et al.* 1990). Viral infections, whether new or recurrent, are all discussed below.

Slapak *et al.* (1997) examined the prevalence of biochemical and histological abnormalities in a series of 116 patients who had lived longer than 5 years since transplantation (mean 8.4 years, range up to 19.5 years). This interesting study showed that 72% of the patients had an abnormal biopsy but, of the one-third with normal biochemistry, only half (19), had biopsy changes, as compared to 65 of the 75 patients (87%) with abnormal biochemistry. About a quarter of the abnormal biopsies had evidence of chronic hepatitis, attributable to viral infection or autoimmune disease in most, but also to possible recurrent primary biliary cirrhosis (PBC) or to poorly treated rejection. Eight other patients had definite changes of recurrence of PBC. A further quarter showed structural abnormalities, which were attributable mainly to vascular complications around the time of transplantation or to azathioprine therapy. Varying degrees of cholangitis were also commonly seen. This study demonstrated an unexpectedly high prevalence of histological abnormalities, even in the face of normal biochemistry, and thus the

authors recommended protocol biopsies at 5 years and thereafter at 2-yearly intervals, to allow for earlier beneficial therapeutic intervention. Broadly similar results were obtained in a similar study in Pittsburgh (Pappo *et al.* 1995).

MALIGNANT DISEASE

Because their ultimate fate was certain, yet their liver function and therefore their ability to stand up to the trauma of transplantation were quite reasonable, patients with hepatic malignancy formed the bulk of the candidates for transplantation in the early series (MacDougall & Williams 1979; Pichlmayr *et al.* 1984). However, it soon became clear that there was a very high risk of recurrence of all types of malignancy (Iwatsuki *et al.* 1985; Portmann *et al.* 1986) and, contrary to the position with other diagnoses, results in patients with malignancy have shown no improvement in the cyclosporin era (Scharschmidt 1984). Most patients develop their recurrence between 6 and 18 months after transplantation. As a consequence fewer patients with malignancy are accepted for transplantation, and those who are are very intensively investigated to try to exclude the presence of extrahepatic spread.

Most patients with malignancy have hepatocellular (HCC) or cholangiocarcinoma (CCA). HCC carries about a 70% risk of recurrence (O'Grady *et al.* 1988b; O'Grady & Williams 1988; Ringe *et al.* 1991), although tumours discovered incidentally in the excised liver may have a very much better prognosis (Starzl *et al.* 1986). There is some debate about whether fibrolamellar carcinoma has a better prognosis than typical HCC (Portmann *et al.* 1986; Starzl *et al.* 1986) although survival is probably only extended in the short term. CCA has a uniformly poor prognosis, with probably as many as 90% of patients dying of recurrence (O'Grady *et al.* 1988b). This applies also to tumours found incidentally, usually in cases of primary sclerosing cholangitis (PSC) in which the tumour extends to the resection margin at the hilum. A second problem with CCA is confirmation of the diagnosis. Because there are no wholly specific features, particularly for peripheral tumours, at least some are probably adeno-

**Table 9.5** Diseases which may recur after liver transplantation.

Malignant tumours
Primary biliary cirrhosis
Autoimmune chronic active hepatitis
Viral hepatitis
   Hepatitis B
   Hepatitis C
   Hepatitis D
Budd–Chiari syndrome
Primary sclerosing cholangitis

carcinomas which have metastasized to the liver from another site. Particular attention should be paid to the colon in patients with PSC, many of whom also have inflammatory bowel disease with a known increased risk of colonic adenocarcinoma (Goss *et al.* 1997). A single-centre study of transplantation for PSC (Goss *et al.* 1997) showed that although 8% of patients had an incidental cholangiocarcinoma (of less than 1 cm diameter) this did not affect patient or graft survival.

Epithelioid haemangioendothelioma has a very variable clinical course and may simultaneously involve organs other than the liver so it is difficult to judge the success of liver transplantation (O'Grady *et al.* 1988b). There are few data on other primary malignant tumours, such as angiosarcoma. Results have been uniformly poor in all our patients in whom metastatic tumours were thought to be confined to the liver (O'Grady *et al.* 1988b). In contrast, some potential cures have been reported from Vienna (Mulbacher & Piza 1987).

### PRIMARY BILIARY CIRRHOSIS

Primary biliary cirrhosis (PBC) is one of the major indications for transplantation of the liver. Neuberger *et al.* (1982) described three patients with PBC who showed changes suggestive of a recurrence of primary disease. In all cases there was evidence of bile-duct damage with basement-membrane breaks, lymphoid aggregates and accumulation of copper-associated protein, but no morphological cholestasis. In one case there was also a poorly formed granuloma in one portal tract. Similar changes were seen in a further four patients (Portmann *et al.* 1986).

This finding has been controversial. Polson *et al.* (1989) found changes compatible with PBC recurrence in nine of 10 patients surviving longer than 1 year (including the seven mentioned above) and IgM levels were elevated in 80%. Others are more sceptical (Demetris *et al.* 1988b; Gouw *et al.* 1994). Analysis of a very large group of 196 patients transplanted for PBC at Pittsburgh (Demetris *et al.* 1988b) did not reveal any instance of recurrent disease. Interestingly, the latter authors did find a slightly higher incidence of chronic rejection in the PBC patients. A more recent analysis of long-surviving Pittsburgh patients presents a contrary view (Pappo *et al.* 1995). Perhaps the best study of PBC recurrence comes from Birmingham (Hübscher *et al.* 1993). This was a blinded study of 172 biopsies from 83 patients who received transplants for PBC from amongst 181 biopsies from 105 control patients who did not have PBC. No changes were found in any of the control patient's biopsies, whereas there were changes strongly suggestive of PBC in 16 biopsies from 13 of the PBC patients, representing 16% of the total. Most of these showed only stage 1 or 2, but one patient (1%) was already cirrhotic. It seems clear that the risk of recurrence of PBC is relatively low and when recurrence does occur there is as yet little evidence that it shortens patient survival.

### AUTOIMMUNE CHRONIC ACTIVE HEPATITIS

Recurrence of this condition is thought to have occurred in a small number of patients in our series (O'Grady & Williams 1988) and at Pittsburgh (Demetris 1990), although it may be difficult to distinguish from viral hepatitis (hepatitis C) on histopathological grounds alone (Bach *et al.* 1992). Furthermore, a number of earlier studies undoubtedly overestimated the prevalence of antibody to hepatitis C (Lok *et al.* 1991), especially in the presence of hyperglobulinaemia. One study (Wright *et al.* 1992a) showed that recurrence was much more likely to occur if an HLA-DR3-negative graft was transplanted into an HLA-DR3-positive recipient.

### BUDD–CHIARI SYNDROME

There is a small but definite risk of recurrent thrombosis in patients transplanted with this condition (Portmann *et al.* 1986). This is perhaps unsurprising because most patients with idiopathic Budd–Chiari syndrome probably have a subclinical haematological disorder which is unaffected by liver transplantation (Levy *et al.* 1985; Valla *et al.* 1985).

### PRIMARY SCLEROSING CHOLANGITIS

Occasional reports suggest that PSC may recur in

about 10% of patients (Lerut *et al.* 1988; Harrison *et al.* 1994a; Goss *et al.* 1997). Interestingly, patient and graft survival was unaffected by recurrence (Goss *et al.* 1997).

## Drug and toxic injury

Drug and/or toxic injury to the allograft liver is difficult to identify with certainty (Demetris 1990). All transplant patients receive a variety of potentially hepatotoxic drugs, but it may be very difficult to distinguish their effects from those of rejection or other factors, such as infection, which may also directly affect the graft. Nevertheless, cyclosporin, azathioprine, corticosteroids, multiple antibiotic therapy and parenteral nutrition have all been implicated.

Cyclosporin is undoubtedly hepatotoxic because it causes abnormalities of liver function tests in up to 50% of renal transplant recipients (Klintmalm *et al.* 1981; Lorber *et al.* 1987). Although dogs are relatively resistant, rats and monkeys both show morphological changes which include ballooning degeneration, cholestasis and fatty change (Ryffel *et al.* 1983; Stone *et al.* 1987). Although suspected of causing cholestasis, no consistent histological pattern of injury has been described in humans. Isometric vacuolation, comparable to that seen in the renal tubule (Thiru 1984), is occasionally seen in hepatocytes in cytological preparations (Lautenschlager *et al.* 1988; Di Tondo *et al.* 1989). The changes correspond to deposits of cyclosporin demonstrated by immunofluorescence and are generally regarded as a manifestation of toxicity, although they may merely be sites of drug storage (Ruben 1987). The dose of cyclosporin currently in use is well below that used in all the above studies.

Azathioprine has been associated with cholestatic hepatitis in renal transplant patients (Sparberg *et al.* 1969). More recently, it has been associated with veno-occlusive disease (Weitz *et al.* 1982) and with nodular regenerative hyperplasia (NRH) (Ihara *et al.* 1982). Sterneck *et al.* (1991) believe that the initial target is the sinusoidal endothelium, damage to which leads to sinusoidal dilatation followed by hepatocyte necrosis. If azathioprine is not withdrawn this may progress first to veno-occlusive disease and then to NRH (Gane *et al.*

1994). Azathioprine was considered to be the main cause of the structural abnormalities found in 17% of 84 patients who had survived for more than 5 years (Slapak *et al.* 1997).

Corticosteroids have been implicated in NRH as well as fatty change (Stromeyer & Ishak 1981), while a number of antibiotics may also cause liver injury (Snover 1990a). Parenteral nutrition can undoubtedly cause severe liver damage, particularly in neonates, and may well be implicated in the cholestasis and ballooning degeneration seen in some transplants (Snover 1990a).

Furthermore, the immunosuppressive drugs may interact with the other medications that the patient is receiving (Mignat 1997).

## Infectious complications

Infections have been a major complication of all transplant programmes (Warren 1984; Wreghitt *et al.* 1987; Kusne *et al.* 1988; Paya *et al.* 1989a; Wade *et al.* 1995), although with improved management of immunosuppression and of the infections themselves, and improved technique over the biliary anastomosis, they probably cause less morbidity and mortality now than 10 years ago. Major infectious complications are more common in patients who were given transplants for chronic hepatitis C (Singh *et al.* 1996b).

Opportunist infections include bacterial, viral, fungal and protozoal infections. The immunosuppressive drugs necessary to prevent and control rejection increase susceptibility to all infections. The increased use of these drugs to treat rejection crises exacerbates the problem. Infections may be acquired from four main sources: namely the donor organ, transfused blood, the environment and the patient him- or herself.

In Pittsburgh (Kusne *et al.* 1988) no less than 83% of patients had one or more infective complications following transplantation and 67% had severe infections. The overall mortality was 26%, and 88% of the deaths in this modern era were cause by infection. The vast majority of infections, in this and other series (Paya *et al.* 1989a), occurred in the first 2 months after transplantation. The histopathologist plays a subsidiary part in the diagnosis of most infections, but he or she may make the first diagnosis of a number of viral infections and, should the patient come to post-mortem, it is most important that all the appropriate samples are taken for microbiological as well as histo-logical examination. Patients subjected to prolonged surgery, for whatever reason (Kusne *et al.* 1988), are particularly at risk of developing severe bacterial or fungal infections.

Gram-positive aerobic bacteria account for most bacterial infections, with bacteraemia, peritonitis and pneumonia the most common manifestations (Wade *et al.* 1995). Liver abscess may be encountered on biopsy and often follows ischaemic necrosis caused by arterial thrombosis.

Fungal infections were particularly common in the early days of transplantation; many patients, by the time they died, had systemic candidiasis. Although now less common, fungal infections were found in 36 of 284 adult patients (13%) in one recent series (Wade *et al.* 1995). Four independent variables predicted fungal infection: low haemoglobin, high bilirubin pre-transplantation, further surgery and prolonged therapy with ciprofloxacin.

Protozoal infections are uncommon, compared to experience with grafts of other organs, although both *Pneumocystis carinii* and *Toxoplasma gondii* are occasionally encountered (Kusne *et al.* 1988; Salt *et al.* 1990). As with CMV infection (see below), tox-oplasmosis is transmitted mainly by the donor organ (Wreghitt 1987).

VIRAL INFECTIONS

The most important of the opportunist viruses are the hepatitis viruses (mainly hepatitis B and C), four members of the herpesvirus group (CMV, herpes simplex virus (HSV), HSV 6 and Epstein–Barr virus (EBV)) and adenovirus (Dussaix 1991).

*Hepatitis viruses*

Liver transplantation remains difficult in end-stage liver disease caused by chronic viral hepatitis because of the high frequency of recurrent infection in the graft (Pons 1995), presumably arising from non-hepatic sources within the host. Furthermore, the rate of progression is in all cases greater than in the general population.

*Hepatitis B and hepatitis D virus infection.* The occur-rence of hepatitis B in liver transplant patients is largely confined to those previously infected, because blood and organ donors are universally screened for hepatitis B. Although the liver is the main site of viral replication, virus has been demonstrated in a number of extrahep-atic sites (Feray *et al.* 1990; Yoffe *et al.* 1990), and only a few virus particles are necessary to establish infection in the new liver. Recurrent disease is extremely common (Angus 1997) and is most likely to occur in HBeAg- or HBV-DNA-positive patients with chronic liver disease (O'Grady *et al.* 1992), but up to 50% of recipients who are HbsAg-negative anti-HbcAg-positive may also resume active replication (Chazouillèresm *et al.* 1994; Wachs *et al.* 1995). Patients transplanted for fulminant disease may fare much better (Todo *et al.* 1991), because the fulminant disease is associated with rapid clearance of the virus (O'Grady & Williams 1988), although recurrence did occur in three patients (Hart *et al.* 1990). Superinfection with hepatitis D (delta virus) in untransplanted patients is associated with progressive disease ending in cirrhosis or liver failure (Purcell *et al.* 1984). It is therefore somewhat surprising that clearance of HBV is more likely to occur in HDV-positive than HDV-negative patients after transplantation (Feray *et al.* 1990), although fulminant hepatic failure does occur (Rizzetto *et al.* 1987). Even when it does recur, HDV does not appear to worsen prognosis (Lake & Wright 1991).

Infection does not recur before 4–8 weeks have elapsed (Hart *et al.* 1990). Recurrent HBV hepatitis may be more aggressive than the original condition (Demetris *et al.* 1986; Rizzetto *et al.* 1987; Benner *et al.* 1992; Wachs *et al.* 1995), with widespread expression of both HBsAg and HBcAg (Demetris *et al.* 1990c). An unusual reaction associated with rapidly progressive disease was noted in six patients in one series (Davies *et al.* 1991), and was termed fibrosing cholestatic hepatitis (FCH). FCH was characterized by slender bands of fibrous tissue radiating from portal tracts into the adjacent parenchyma where they surrounded plates of ductular type epithelium. There was also extensive ground-glass transformation, which correlated with strong diffuse cytoplasmic and membranous staining for HBsAg and mainly nuclear HBcAg and HBeAg. All the patients deteriorated rapidly. Others have described a similar syndrome (Phillips *et al.* 1992; Harrison *et al.* 1993).

Long-term passive immunization with hepatitis B immunoglobulin following transplantation may prevent or delay recurrence (Samuel *et al.* 1991). Recombinant α-interferon failed to prevent recurrence or reduce HBV replication (Rakela *et al.* 1989; Hopf *et al.* 1991). Newer antiviral drugs such as lamivudine may also have a role (Ben Ari *et al.* 1997), although early indications are that drug resistance may develop quite quickly (Grellier & Dusheiko 1997).

*Hepatitis C (non-A, non-B hepatitis).* Since the discovery of antigens associated with hepatitis C (Choo *et al.* 1990), the genome has been defined (Choo *et al.* 1991) and the virus is related both to the flaviviruses and the pestiviruses (Houghton *et al.* 1991). Non-fulminant hepatitis C can both recur and, as a result of blood transfusion (Demetris 1990)—a risk now removed by the screening of transfused blood—or transplantation from a carrier (Pereira *et al.* 1995), arise *de novo* in liver transplant patients. Recurrent infection is virtually universal after transplantation, whether measured serologically or by polymerase chain reaction for hepatitis C RNA (Ferrell *et al.* 1992; König *et al.* 1992; Poterucha *et al.* 1992; Shah *et al.* 1992; Wright *et al.* 1992b; Belli *et al.* 1993; Donataccio *et al.* 1994; Pereira *et al.* 1995). Early indications are that the disease recurs more slowly than hepatitis B, and is generally less likely to cause progressive graft damage (Martin *et al.* 1991; Shiffman *et al.* 1994; Boker *et al.* 1997; Shuhart *et al.* 1997), although a few patients have a more rapidly progressive course (Schluger *et al.* 1996). Patients with episodes of acute rejection have a shorter recurrence-free survival (Sheiner *et al.* 1995; Singh *et al.* 1996a; Shuhart *et al.* 1997), particularly if treated with OKT3 (Rosen *et al.* 1997b). Viruses of genotype 1b recur earlier and are more likely to progress to cirrhosis compared to those with other genotypes (Feray *et al.* 1995; Gordon *et al.* 1997; Shuhart *et al.*

1997). Episodes of CMV viraemia also increase the risk of HCV recurrence (Rosen *et al.* 1997a). Hepatitis G coinfection has no influence on the outcome (Vargas *et al.* 1997).

Histologically, the appearances are similar to those in non-transplant patients (Bach *et al.* 1992; Scheuer *et al.* 1992) and recurrent hepatitis C should be distinguishable from acute rejection (Petrovic *et al.* 1997). Eosinophils and bile-duct damage are important markers of rejection, while portal inflammation with lymphoid aggregates and lobular inflammation are pointers to recurrence of hepatitis C. This can be confirmed by RT-PCR on liver biopsies (Svoboda Newman *et al.* 1997). FNAB may help in this respect, as the quality of the infiltrate differs in the two conditions (Lautenschlager *et al.* 1994).

### Herpesviruses

After primary infection all the herpesviruses probably remain latent in the various tissues of the body for the lifetime of the host. This is a particular problem in the transplant patient in two respects. First, if the recipient has been previously infected, the immunosuppressive drugs may allow reactivation of the virus. Secondly, if the patient has not previously been infected, he or she may acquire a primary infection from the donor organ or from transfused blood while immunocompromised. There is also a third possibility, that the patient may acquire a new 'first' infection (see below).

*Cytomegalovirus hepatitis.* Primary infection is thought to be acquired mainly from the donor graft, although it may also be acquired from transfused blood. Although the exact site of the viral latency is not known it is thought to be within white cells (Winston *et al.* 1980). There is evidence that the disease is more serious when acquired from the donor organ than when blood or blood products are its source, at least in heart transplant patients (Wreghitt 1987), perhaps because of the larger dose of virus acquired from the former. There is also evidence in heart transplant patients that a recipient who is already seropositive is more likely to have clinically manifest CMV infection if he or she receives an organ from a seropositive than from a seronegative patient, suggesting that reinfection may be more important than reactivation in terms of patient illness. Donor CMV seropositivity was also found to be the most important risk factor for subsequent CMV infection in a series of liver transplant patients (Gorensek *et al.* 1990).

For these reasons it is now customary to match donors with recipients. The proportion of patients who are seropositive for CMV rises steadily throughout life. Only about 20% of patients under 10 years are positive, while this figure rises to 67% in those over 50 years (Wreghitt & Hakim 1989). If the recipient is seronegative, as is particularly likely if he or she is a child, he or she is only given an organ from a negative donor, except in cases of emergency.

CMV is the most common cause of viral hepatitis in the allograft (Bronsther *et al.* 1988), but it may also cause systemic disease with involvement of the lungs, gastrointestinal tract—especially as a cause of ulceration and haemorrhage in its upper or lower parts—or CNS. Fifty per cent of our patients had evidence of active CMV infection (Wreghitt *et al.* 1987). Culture methods together with histological examination are jointly better for early diagnosis than serology (Paya *et al.* 1989b). Infection can become manifest at any time between 21 and 56 days after the transplantation but very frequently presents between 21 and 28 days with fever. In the liver CMV infection is similar to that in non-transplant patients, with a lobular focal neutrophilic infiltration around classic cytomegalic inclusions. Diagnosis can be confirmed by immunohistochemical staining or *in situ* hybridization. A recent study comparing the two techniques (Strickler *et al.* 1990) found the former to be superior, and that both techniques correlated better with the demonstration of viral inclusions in infected cells than with the results of culture. PCR may be too sensitive for clinically relevant infection (Brainard *et al.* 1994).

Demetris (1990) suggests that inclusions might be less frequent in the most immunocompetent patients, although it is difficult to correlate this observation with sporadic CMV hepatitis in healthy individuals. It is certainly true that the most immunosuppressed patients often have numerous inclusions in cells of all types, yet negligible evidence of a host response or, indeed, any clinical features specifically referable to CMV. These patients may not even have serum antibody and the CMV, as a marker of immunosuppression, is only one of a number of opportunistic infections found at postmortem. CMV inclusions may also be found quite widely in other tissues in such patients.

CMV infection and acute rejection may coincide in the same patient (Demetris 1990), when each should be treated on its own merits. The possible association of CMV infection with chronic rejection has been referred to above.

Treatment of CMV infection has been transformed with the appearance of the drug ganciclovir (Paya *et al.* 1988), which can also be given prophylactically when it is necessary to place an organ from a positive donor into a seronegative patient.

*Epstein–Barr virus.* Reactivation of Epstein–Barr virus (EBV) occurs in up to 40% of liver transplant patients, but is generally asymptomatic (Roberts *et al.* 1991). Small numbers of EBV-infected cells are commonly found in allograft livers, but there is no evidence that the virus is responsible for the otherwise unexplained hepatitis found is some grafts (Hübscher *et al.* 1994; Slapak *et al.* 1997). True EBV hepatitis is uncommon, but the use of antilymphocyte preparations is a significant risk factor (Langnas *et al.* 1994). EBV may also cause a number of clinical syndromes in liver transplant patients (Demetris 1990), and presentation usually occurs in the first 2 or 3 months (Langnas *et al.* 1994). In some patients it is associated with an infiltrate composed of large atypical mononuclear blast cells and this picture may be difficult to distinguish from acute rejection. Diagnosis is then confirmed by detection of viral antigen on immunostaining (Markin *et al.* 1990) or by *in situ* hybridization (Telenti *et al.* 1991).

EBV infection in immunosuppressed patients may also be associated with lymphoma-like lymphoproliferative disorders (see 'New tumours', below) (Ho *et al.* 1985; Wilkinson *et al.* 1989; Randhawa *et al.* 1990).

*Other herpesviruses.* Both types of herpes simplex virus (HSV) and varicella-zoster virus (VZV) have been identified as a cause of allograft hepatitis (Demetris *et al.* 1987a; Dussaix 1991). Both may be fatal in transplant patients and both can be successfully treated with acyclovir. The pathology of both is similar, with 'geographic' areas of coagulative necrosis of the parenchyma and Cowdry type A intranuclear inclusions visible in viable cells at the edge of the necrotic zones. Serious infections are almost always primary, but nearly 20% of patients may show reactivation of HSV and 10% of VZV (Wreghitt *et al.* 1987). These may be clinically manifest—with cold sores and shingles, respectively—or silent. Human herpes virus 6 (HHV 6) may also be responsible for some cases of unexplained hepatitis (Dussaix 1991).

*Other virus infections.* Adenoviruses are an occasional cause of a severe haemorrhagic clinical illness associated with hepatic necrosis and/or pneumonia, especially in children (Koneru *et al.* 1987; Salt *et al.* 1990; Dussaix 1991; Cames *et al.* 1992). Characteristic smudgy basophilic nuclear inclusions are seen in viable tissue at the margins of the necrosis.

## New tumours

The increased incidence of neoplastic diseases in transplant recipients is well recognized. A large proportion of the reported instances has been made up of lymphoproliferative tumours and non-melanotic cutaneous cancers (Penn 1979, 1983). Penn (1987) noted that, following the introduction of cyclosporin, lymphoproliferative disorders were more common than skin tumours, while previously the reverse had been the case (Penn 1979). Patients with PSC and inflammatory bowel disease already have an increased risk of colorectal neoplasia, which seems to be increased about fourfold after liver transplantation (Loftus *et al.* 1998).

There is good evidence that EBV is responsible for most lymphoproliferative disease in immunosuppressed patients (Cherqui 1991). As well as causing an infectious mononucleosis-like syndrome (see above), the virus is also responsible for widespread lymphoma-like infiltrates as well as true B cell malignant lymphoma. Although the lymphoma-like infiltrates resemble malignant lymphoma, with tumour-like dissemination through many organs, the cells remain phenotypically polyclonal and there is usually no gene rearrangement (Nalesnik *et al.* 1988b). Frequently, this condition is not suspected before autopsy or it may be confused clinically with acute rejection. *In situ* hybridization is the most sensitive method for detection of EBV RNA in liver biopsies (Lones *et al.* 1997).

The risk of lymphoproliferative disease after transplantation ranges between 2 and 20% and is probably greatest when immunosuppression is highest as, for example, following heart–lung transplantation (Armitage *et al.* 1991) or use of antilymphocyte preparations (Morgan & Superina 1994). As with CMV infection, virus acquired from the graft may be more clinically important than reactivation of dormant infections in the host because tumour risk is much higher in patients who are EBV-seronegative at the time of transplantation (Dosch *et al.* 1991). Armes *et al.* (1994), using microsatellite DNA fingerprinting, were able to prove that donor lymphocytes were the source of the lymphoproliferative disease. Reduction of immunosuppression may be followed by remarkable regression of both polyclonal and clonal disease (Nalesnik *et al.* 1988a,b), although the latter is the less likely to respond.

## Graft vs. host disease

Graft vs. host disease (GVHD) occurs in up to 50% of patients after bone marrow transplantation (Thomas *et al.* 1975). It has also been reported after solid organ transplantation (Jamieson *et al.* 1991) and after blood transfusion (Brubaker 1986). It depends upon the introduction into the recipient of immunocompetent cells which are incompatible and therefore capable of mounting a response against the host's own lymphoid cells (Billingham 1966). At the same time the host is incapable of mounting an effective immune response against the graft because of immunosuppression. Because donor immunocompetent cells regularly persist in the donor liver and in the peripheral blood (Schlitt *et al.* 1993a,b), it is perhaps pertinent to question not why GVHD occurs, but why it does not occur more often.

Two types of GVHD are seen after liver transplantation. The more common, but less important, is caused by the production of humoral antibody to red cell antigens following ABO-mismatched grafts (Ramsey *et al.* 1984). This takes the form of haemolytic anaemia which is generally mild and self-limited.

The second type of GVHD is the cellular type, of which the main manifestations are rashes, diarrhoea and liver dysfunction. The last feature is caused by an attack on the cells of the biliary epithelium (Snover *et al.* 1984b; Dilly & Sloane 1985) and is, of course, absent when the liver is the source of the foreign immunocompetent cells. A number of cases have now been reported (Burdick *et al.* 1988; Jamieson *et al.* 1991; Roberts *et al.* 1991). Patients generally present with fever, diarrhoea, skin rashes and pancytopenia in the second month after transplantation. Biopsy of skin or rectum shows distinctive changes, with focal epithelial necrosis associated with infiltration by lymphoid cells (Roberts *et al.* 1991); cells with donor HLA antigens are detectable in the blood and bone marrow (Jamieson *et al.* 1991).

The prognosis of GVHD is very poor (Neumann *et al.* 1994). The condition may well be more common than previously appreciated (Jamieson *et al.* 1991) and awareness may lead to its earlier recognition and the institution of appropriate therapeutic measures, which include increased immunosuppression and antibiotic cover.

## Medical complications

Central nervous system complication of liver transplantation can be life-threatening (Singh *et al.* 1994); central pontine myelinolysis as a result of a sudden change in serum sodium concentration is perhaps the best known.

## Auxiliary liver transplantation

Auxiliary heterotopic transplantation has many theoretical advantages over the orthotopic procedure, particularly if there is a prospect that the liver may recover or if transplantation is being undertaken to replace a missing enzyme as, for example, in primary oxaluria.

However, results have mostly been disappointing, largely because when either the new liver or the old is deprived of portal blood it undergoes atrophy (Starzl *et al.* 1989b). However, workers in Rotterdam appear to have solved many of the technical problems (Terpstra *et al.* 1988; Willemse *et al.* 1992) and so the technique may be more widely applied in future, especially as a means of temporary support during acute hepatic failure (Boudjema *et al.* 1993). A preliminary European study of 36 patients has shown very encouraging early results, with two-thirds of the patients showing complete recovery of the native liver (Chenard Neu *et al.* 1996). It remains to be seen whether the pathological problems will be the same as those encountered in orthotopic grafts.

## References

Abraham, S. & Furth, E.E. (1996) Quantitative evaluation of histological features in 'time-zero' liver allograft biopsies as predictors of rejection or graft failure: receiver-operating characteristic analysis application. *Human Pathology* 27, 1077–1084.

Adam, R., Reynès, M., Johann, M. *et al.* (1991) The outcome of steatotic grafts in liver transplantation. *Transplantation Proceedings* 23, 1538–1540.

Adams, C.M., Danks, D.M. & Campbell, P.E. (1974) Comments upon the classification of infantile polycystic diseases of the liver and kidney, based upon three-dimensional reconstruction of the liver. *Journal of Medical Genetics* 11, 234–243.

Adams, D.H. & Neuberger, J.M. (1989) Patterns of graft rejection following transplantation. *Journal of Hepatology* 10, 113–119.

Adams, D.H., Hübscher, S.G., Shaw, J., Rothlein, R. & Neuberger, J. (1989a) Intercellular adhesion molecule 1 on liver allografts during rejection. *Lancet* 2, 1122–1125.

Adams, D.H., Wang, L. & Neuberger, J.M. (1989b) Serum hyaluronic acid following liver transplantation: evidence of hepatic endothelial damage. *Transplantation Proceedings* 21, 2274.

Alagille, D. (1979) Cholestasis in the first three months of life. In: *Progress in Liver Disease*, Vol. VI (eds H. Popper & F. Schaffner), pp. 471–475. Grune and Stratton, New York.

Angus, P.W. (1997) Review: hepatitis B and liver transplantation. *Journal of Gastroenterology and Hepatology* 12, 217–223.

Armes, J.E., Angus, P., Southey, M.C. *et al.* (1994)

Lymphoproliferative disease of donor origin arising in patients after orthotopic liver transplantation. *Cancer* 74, 2436–2441.

Armitage, J.M., Kormos, R.L., Stuart, R.S. *et al.* (1991) Posttransplant lymphoproliferative disease in thoracic organ transplant patients: ten years of cyclosporine-based immunosuppression. *Journal of Heart and Lung Transplantation* 10, 877–886.

Azuma, H., Heemann, U.W., Tullius, S.G. & Tilney, N. (1994) Cytokines and adhesion molecules in chronic rejection. *Clinical Transplantation* 8, 168–180.

Bacchi, C.E., Marsh, C.L., Perkins, J.D. *et al.* (1993) Expression of vascular cell adhesion molecule (VCAM-1) in liver and pancreas allograft rejection. *American Journal of Pathology* 142, 579–591.

Bach, N., Thung, S.N. & Schaffner, F. (1992) The histological features of chronic hepatitis C and autoimmune chronic hepatitis: a comparative analysis. *Hepatology* 15, 572–577.

Barbatis, C., Wood, J., Morton, J.A. *et al.* (1981) Immunohistochemical analysis of HLA (A, B, C) antigens in liver disease using a monoclonal antibody. *Gut* 22, 985–991.

Batts, K.P., Moore, S.B., Perkins, J.D. *et al.* (1988) Influence of positive lymphocyte crossmatch and HLA mismatching on vanishing bile-duct syndrome in human liver allografts. *Transplantation* 45, 376–379.

Bauer, T., Britton, P., Lomas, D. *et al.* (1995) Liver transplantation for hepatic arteriovenous malformation in hereditary haemorrhagic telangiectasia. *Journal of Hepatology* 22, 586–590.

Belitsky, P., Miller, S.M., Gupta, R., Lee, S. & Ghose, T. (1990) Induction of MHC Class II expression in recipient tissues caused by allograft rejection. *Transplantation* 49, 472–476.

Belli, L.S., Alberti, A., Rondinara, G.F. *et al.* (1993) Recurrent hepatitis C after liver transplantation. *Transplantation Proceedings* 25, 2635–2637.

Ben Ari, Z., Shmueli, D., Mor, E., Shapira, Z. & Tur Kaspa, R. (1997) Beneficial effect of lamivudine in recurrent hepatitis B after liver transplantation. *Transplantation* 63, 393–396.

Benner, K.G., Lee, R.G., Keefe, E.B. *et al.* (1992) Fibrosing cytolytic liver failure secondary to recurrent hepatitis B after liver transplantation. *Gastroenterology* 103, 1308–1312.

Billingham, M.E. (1987) Cardiac transplant atherosclerosis. *Transplantation Proceedings* 19, 19–25.

Billingham, R.E. (1966) The biology of graft-versus-host reactions. *Harvey Lectures* 62, 21–78.

Bird, G., Friend, P., Donaldson, P. *et al.* (1989) Hyperacute rejection in liver transplantation: a case report. *Transplantation Proceedings* 21, 3742–3744.

Bismuth, H. (1994) Consensus conference on indications for liver transplantation. *Hepatology* 20 (Suppl.), S1–S68.

Bismuth, H. & Houssin, D. (1984) Reduced size orthotopic liver graft in hepatic transplantation in children. *Surgery* 95, 367–370.

Bismuth, H., Castaing, D., Ericzon, B.G. *et al.* (1987) Hepatic transplantation in Europe. First report of the European Liver Transplant Registry. *Lancet* 2, 674–676.

Boker, K.H., Dalley, G., Bahr, M.J. *et al.* (1997) Long-term outcome of hepatitis C virus infection after liver transplantation. *Hepatology* 25, 203–210.

Boudjema, K., Jaeck, D., Siméoni, U. *et al.* (1993) Temporary auxiliary liver transplantation for subacute liver failure in a child. *Lancet* 342, 778–779.

Boutiere, B., Arnoux, D., Boffa, M.C. *et al.* (1994) Plasma thrombomodulin in orthotopic liver transplantation. *Transplantation* 58, 1352–1355.

Brainard, J.A., Greenson, J.K., Vesy, C.J. *et al.* (1994) Detection of cytomegalovirus in liver transplant biopsies. A comparison of light microscopy, immunohistochemistry, duplex PCR and nested PCR. *Transplantation* 57, 1753–1757.

Broelsch, C.E., Emond, J.C., Thistlethwaite, J.R. *et al.* (1988) Liver transplantation with reduced size donor organs. *Transplantation* 45, 519–524.

Broelsch, C.E., Emond, J.C., Whitington, P.F. *et al.* (1990) Application of reduced-size liver transplants as split grafts, auxiliary orthotopic grafts, and living related segmental transplants. *Annals of Surgery* 212, 368–375.

Bronsther, O., Makowka, L., Jaffe, R. *et al.* (1988) Occurrence of cytomegalovirus hepatitis in liver transplant patients. *Journal of Medical Virology* 24, 423–434.

Brubaker, D.B. (1986) Transfusion associated graft-versus-host disease. *Human Pathology* 17, 1085–1088.

Brunot, B., Petras, S., Germain, P., Vinee, P. & Constantinesco, A. (1994) Biopsy and quantitative hepatobiliary scintigraphy in the evaluation of liver transplantation. *Journal of Nuclear Medicine* 35, 1321–1327.

Burdick, J.F., Vogelsang, G.B., Smith, W.J. *et al.* (1988) Severe graft-versus-host disease in a liver-transplanted recipient. *New England Journal of Medicine* 318, 689–691.

Calne, R.Y. (1980) Hepatic transplantation. *Springer Seminars in Immunopathology* 3, 385–393.

Calne, R.Y., Rolles, K., White, D.J.G. *et al.* (1979) Cyclosporine A initially as the only immunosuppressant in 34 recipients of cadaveric organs: 32 kidneys, 2 pancreases, and 2 livers. *Lancet* 2, 1033–1036.

Cames, B., Rahier, J., Burtomboy, G. *et al.* (1992) Acute adenovirus hepatitis in liver transplant recipients. *Journal of Pediatrics* 120, 33–37.

Carles, J., Fawaz, R., Hamoudi, N.E. *et al.* (1994a) Preservation of human liver grafts in UW solution.

Ultrastructural evidence for endothelial and Kupffer cell activation during cold ischemia and after ischemia-reperfusion. *Liver* 14, 50–56.

Carles, J., Fawaz, R., Neaud, V. *et al.* (1994b) Ultrastructure of human liver grafts preserved with UW solution. Comparison between patients with low and high postoperative transaminases levels. *Journal of Submicroscopy and Cytological Pathology* 26, 67–73.

Chapman, R.W., Forman, D., Peto, R. & Smallwood, R. (1990) Liver transplantation for acute hepatic failure? *Lancet* 335, 32–35.

Charpentier, B., Lang, P., Martin, B. & Fries, B. (1981) Cells infiltrating rejected human kidney allografts: composition and *in vitro* functional capabilities. *Transplantation Proceedings* 13, 84–89.

Chazouillèresm, I., Mamish, D., Kim, M. *et al.* (1994) 'Occult' hepatitis B virus as a source of infection in liver transplant recipients. *Lancet* 343, 142–146.

Chenard Neu, M.P., Boudjema, K., Bernuau, J. *et al.* (1996) Auxiliary liver transplantation: regeneration of the native liver and outcome in 30 patients with fulminant hepatic failure—a multicenter European study. *Hepatology* 23, 1119–1127.

Cherqui, D. (1991) Lymphoproliferative disorders in organ transplant recipients. In: *Immunological, Metabolic and Infectious Aspects of Liver Transplantation* (eds D.A. Vuitton, C. Balabaud, D. Houssin & D. Dhumeaux), pp. 83–89. John Libby Eurotext, Paris.

Chollet-Martin, S., Depoix, J.P., Hvass, U. *et al.* (1990) Raised plasma levels of tumour necrosis factor in heart allograft rejection. *Transplantation Proceedings* 20, 283–286.

Choo, Q.-L., Weiner, A.J., Overby, L.R., Kuo, G. & Houghton, M. (1990) Hepatitis C virus: the major causative agent of viral non-A, non-B hepatitis. *British Medical Bulletin* 46, 423–441.

Choo, Q.L., Richman, K.H., Han, J.H. *et al.* (1991) Genetic organization and diversity of the hepatitis C virus. *Proceedings of the National Academy of Sciences (USA)* 88, 2451–2455.

Christoffersen, P. & Poulsen, H. (1970) Histological changes in human liver biopsies following extrahepatic biliary obstruction. *Acta Pathologica, Microbiologica et Immunologica Scandinavica* 212, 150–157.

Cillo, U., Tedeschi, U., Carraro, P. *et al.* (1994) Early predictive markers of irreversible graft dysfunction after liver transplantation. *Transplantation Proceedings* 26, 3599–3601.

Clements, D., McMaster, P. & Elias, E. (1988) Indocyanine green clearance in acute rejection after liver transplantation. *Transplantation* 46, 383–385.

Colina, F., Mollejo, M., Moreno, E. *et al.* (1991) Effectiveness of histopathological diagnoses in dysfunction of hepatic transplantation. Review of 146

histopathological studies from 53 transplants. *Archives of Pathology and Laboratory Medicine* 115, 998–1005.

Colletti, L.M., Johnson, K.J., Kunkel, R.G. & Merion, R.M. (1994) Mechanisms of hyperacute rejection in porcine liver transplantation. Antibody-mediated endothelial injury. *Transplantation* 57, 1357–1363.

Conference of Medical Royal Colleges and the Faculties in the United Kingdom (1976) Diagnosis of brain-stem death. *British Medical Journal* 2, 1187–1188.

Cramer, D.V. (1995) Brequinar sodium. *Pediatric Nephrology* 9, S52–S55.

Czerniak, A., Lotan, G., Hiss, Y. *et al.* (1989) The feasibility of *in vivo* resection of the left lobe of the liver and its use for transplantation. *Transplantation* 48, 26–32.

Daar, A.S., Fuggle, S.V., Fabre, J.W., Ting, A. & Morris, P.J. (1984) The detailed distribution of HLA-A, B, C antigens in normal human organs. *Transplantation* 38, 287–292.

Davies, S.E., Portmann, B.C., O'Grady, J.G. *et al.* (1991) Hepatic histological findings after transplantation for chronic hepatitis B virus infection, including a unique pattern of fibrosing cholestatic hepatitis. *Hepatology* 13, 150–157.

De Groen, P.C., Kephart, G.M., Gleich, G.J. & Ludwig, J. (1994) The eosinophil as an effector cell of the immune response during hepatic allograft rejection. *Hepatology* 20, 654–662.

De Ville de Goyet, J., Buts, J.P., Claus, D., Rahier, J. & Otte, J.B. (1987) Monitoring of orthotopic liver transplantation in children by means of serial graft biopsies. *Transplantation Proceedings* 19, 3323–3326.

Deligeorgi-Politi, H., Wight, D.G.D. & Calne, R.Y. (1994) Chronic rejection of liver transplants revisited. *Transplant International* 7, 442–447.

Demetris, A.J. (1990) The pathology of liver transplantation. *Progress in Liver Disease* 9, 687–709.

Demetris, A.J., Lasky, S., van Thiel, D.H., Starzl, T.E. & Dekker, A. (1985a) Pathology of hepatic transplantation. A review of 62 adult allograft recipients immunosuppressed with a cyclosporine/steroid regimen. *American Journal of Pathology* 118, 151–161.

Demetris, A.J., Lasky, S., van Thiel, D.H., Starzl, T.E. & Whiteside, T. (1985b) Induction of DR/IA antigens in human liver allografts. *Transplantation* 40, 504–509.

Demetris, A.J., Jaffe, R., Sheahan, D.G. *et al.* (1986) Recurrent hepatitis B in liver allograft recipients: differentiation between viral hepatitis B and rejection. *American Journal of Pathology* 125, 161–172.

Demetris, A.J., Jaffe, R. & Starzl, T.E. (1987a) A review of adult and pediatric posttransplant liver pathology. *Pathology Annual* 22 (2), 347–386.

Demetris, A.J., Markus, B.H., Burnham, J. *et al.* (1987b) Antibody deposition in liver allografts with chronic rejection. *Transplantation Proceedings* 19, 121–125.

Demetris, A.J., Jaffe, R., Tzakis, A. *et al.* (1988a) Antibody-mediated rejection of human orthotopic liver allografts. A study of liver transplantation across ABO blood group barriers. *American Journal of Pathology* **132**, 489–502.

Demetris, A.J., Markus, B.H., Esquivel, C.O. *et al.* (1988b) Pathologic analysis of liver transplantation for primary biliary cirrhosis. *Hepatology* **8**, 939–947.

Demetris, A.J., Jaffe, R., Tzakis, A. *et al.* (1989) Antibody-mediated rejection of human liver allografts: transplantation across ABO blood group barriers. *Transplantation Proceedings* **21**, 2217–2220.

Demetris, A.J., Fung, J.J., Todo, S. *et al.* (1990a) Pathologic observations in human allograft recipients treated with FK506. *Transplantation Proceedings* **22**, 25–34.

Demetris, A.J., Qian, S.G., Sun, H. & Fung, J.J. (1990b) Liver allograft rejection: an overview of morphological findings. *American Journal of Surgical Pathology* **14**, 49–63.

Demetris, A.J., Todo, S., Van Thiel, D.H. *et al.* (1990c) Evolution of hepatitis B virus liver disease after hepatic replacement. Practical and theoretical considerations. *American Journal of Pathology* **137**, 667–676.

Demetris, A.J., Belle, S.H., Hart, J. *et al.* (1991) Intraobserver and interobserver variation in the histopathological assessment of liver allograft rejection. The Liver Transplantation Database (LTD) Investigators (see comments). *Hepatology* **14**, 751–755.

Demetris, A.J., Murase, N., Nakamura, K. *et al.* (1992a) Immunopathology of antibodies as effectors of orthotopic liver allograft rejection. *Seminars in Liver Disease* **12**, 51–59.

Demetris, A.J., Nakamura, K., Yagihashi, A. *et al.* (1992b) A clinicopathological study of human liver allograft recipients harbouring preformed IgG lymphocytotoxic antibodies. *Hepatology* **3**, 671–681.

Demetris, A.J., Seaberg, E.C., Batts, K.P. *et al.* (1995) Reliability and predictive value of the National Institute of Diabetes and Digestive and Kidney Diseases Liver Transplantation Database nomenclature and grading system for cellular rejection of liver allografts. *Hepatology* **21**, 408–416.

Dhillon, A.P., Burroughs, A.K., Hudson, M. *et al.* (1994) Hepatic venular stenosis after orthotopic liver transplantation. *Hepatology* **19**, 106–111.

Di Tondo, U., Ciardi, A., Pecorella, I. *et al.* (1989) Postoperative liver transplant monitoring with fine-needle aspiration biopsy. *Transplantation Proceedings* **21**, 2311–2312.

Dilly, S.A. & Sloane, J.P. (1985) An immunohistological study of human hepatic graft-versus-host disease. *Clinical and Experimental Immunology* **62**, 545–553.

Donaldson, P.T., Alexander, G.J.M., O'Grady, J. *et al.* (1987) Evidence for an immune response to HLA Class I antigens in the vanishing bile-duct syndrome after liver transplantation. *Lancet* **1**, 945–948.

Donaldson, P., Underhill, J., Doherty, D. *et al.* (1993) Influence of HLA matching on liver allograft survival and rejection: the dualistic effect. *Hepatology* **17**, 1008–1015.

Donataccio, M., Lerut, J., Ciccarelli, O. *et al.* (1994) Hepatitis C viral infection and adult liver transplantation: a difficult clinical problem. *Transplantation Proceedings* **26**, 3588–3590.

Dosch, H.M., Cochrane, D.M., Cook, V.A., Leeder, J.S. & Cheung, R.K. (1991) Exogenous but not endogenous EBV induces lymphomas in beige/nude/xid mice carrying human lymphoid xenografts. *International Immunology* **3**, 731–735.

Dousset, B., Hübscher, S.G., Padbury, R.T. *et al.* (1993) Acute liver allograft rejection—is treatment always necessary? *Transplantation* **55**, 529–534.

Duquesnoy, R.J. (1989) Is there hyperacute rejection of the liver? *Transplantation Proceedings* **21**, 3506–3507.

Dussaix, E. (1991) Incidence and prognosis of viral infections due to herpes viruses (other than cytomegalovirus), adenoviruses and hepatitis C virus in liver transplant recipients. In: *Immunological, Metabolic and Infectious Aspects of Liver Transplantation* (eds D.A. Vuitton, C. Balabaud, D. Houssin & D. Dhumeaux), pp. 77–81. John Libby Eurotext, Paris.

Editorial (1990) Non-randomised controls and assessment of survival in liver transplantation. *Lancet* **335**, 509–510.

Eggink, H.F., Hofstee, N., Gips, C.H., Krom, R.A.F. & Houthoff, H.J. (1984) Histopathology of serial graft biopsies from liver transplant recipients. *American Journal of Pathology* **114**, 18–31.

Emond, J.C., Aran, P.P., Whitington, P., Broelsch, C.E. & Baker, A.L. (1989) Liver transplantation in the management of fulminant hepatic failure. *Gastroenterology* **96**, 1583–1588.

Esquivel, C.O., Jaffe, R., Gordon, R.D. & Starzl, T.E. (1985) Liver rejection and its differentiation from other causes of graft dysfunction. *Seminars in Liver Disease* **5**, 369–373.

Fahrlander, H., Huber, F. & Gloor, F. (1964) Intrahepatic retention of bile in severe bacterial infections. *Gastroenterology* **47**, 590–599.

Farges, O., Ericzon, B.G., Bresson Hadni, S. *et al.* (1994) A randomized trial of OKT3-based versus cyclosporine-based immunoprophylaxis after liver transplantation. Long-term results of a European and Australian multicenter study. *Transplantation* **58**, 891–898.

Feray, C., Zignegno, A.L., Samuel, D. *et al.* (1990) Persistent hepatitis B virus infection of blood mononuclear cells without concomitant liver infection: the liver transplantation model. *Transplantation* **49**, 1155–1158.

Feray, C., Gigou, M., Samuel, D. *et al.* (1995) Influence of the genotypes of hepatitis C virus on the severity of recurrent liver disease after liver transplantation (see comments). *Gastroenterology* **108**, 1088–1096.

Ferrell, L.D., Wright, T.L., Roberts, J., Ascher, N. & Lake, J. (1992) Hepatitis C viral infection in liver transplant recipients. *Hepatology* 16, 865–876.

Fisher, A. & Miller, C.M. (1995) Editorial: Ischemic-type biliary strictures in liver allografts: the Achilles' heel revisited. *Hepatology* 21, 589–591.

Fleming, K.A., McMichael, A., Morton, J.A., Woods, J. & McGee, J.O.D. (1981) Distribution of HLA class I antigens in normal human tissue and in mammary cancer. *Journal of Clinical Pathology* 34, 779–784.

Forker, E.L. & Runyon, B.A. (1978) Canalicular cholestasis. *Gastroenterology* 75, 535–537.

Foster, P.F., Sankary, H.N., Hart, M., Ashmann, M. & Williams, J.W. (1989) Blood and graft eosinophilia as predictors of rejection in human liver transplantation. *Transplantation* 47, 72–74.

Freese, D.K., Snover, D.C., Sharp, H.L. et al. (1991) Chronic rejection after liver transplantation: a study of clinical, histological and immunological features. *Hepatology* 13, 882–891.

Gane, E., Portmann, B., Saxena, R. et al. (1994) Nodular regenerative hyperplasia of the liver graft after liver transplantation. *Hepatology* 20, 88–94.

Goldstein, N.S., Hart, J. & Lewin, K.J. (1991) Diffuse hepatocyte ballooning in liver biopsies from orthotopic liver transplant patients. *Histopathology* 18, 331–338.

Gómez, R., Colina, F., Moreno, E. et al. (1994) Etiopathogenesis and prognosis of centrilobular necrosis in hepatic grafts. *Journal of Hepatology* 21, 441–446.

González, F.X., Rimola, A., Grande, L. et al. (1994) Predictive factors of early postoperative graft function in human liver transplantation. *Hepatology* 20, 565–573.

Gordon, R.D., Fung, J., Markus, B. et al. (1986a) The antibody cross-match in liver transplantation. *Surgery* 100, 705–715.

Gordon, R.D., Iwatsuki, S., Esquivel, C.O., Tzakis, A. & Starzl, T.E. (1986b) Liver transplantation across ABO blood groups. *Surgery* 100, 342–348.

Gordon, F.D., Poterucha, J.J., Germer, J. et al. (1997) Relationship between hepatitis C genotype and severity of recurrent hepatitis C after liver transplantation. *Transplantation* 63, 1419–1423.

Gorensek, M.J., Carey, W.D., Vogt, D. & Goormastic, M. (1990) A multivariate analysis of risk factors for cytomegalovirus infectionin liver transplant recipients. *Gastroenterology* 98, 1326–1332.

Goss, J.A., Shackleton, C.R., Farmer, D.G. et al. (1997) Orthotopic liver transplantation for primary sclerosing cholangitis. A 12-year single center experience. *Annals of Surgery* 225, 472–481.

Gouw, A.S.H., Houthoff, H.J., Huitema, S. et al. (1987) Expression of major histocompatibility complex antigens and replacement of donor cells by recipient ones in human liver grafts. *Transplantation* 43, 291–296.

Gouw, A.S., Snover, D.C., Grond, J. et al. (1988a) Acute rejection in human liver grafts: a comparative histologic study of cases maintained on azathioprine and prednisone versus cyclosporine A and low-dose steroids. *Human Pathology* 19, 1036–1042.

Gouw, A.S.H., Huitema, S., Grond, J. et al. (1988b) MHC antigen expression in human liver grafts: its rôle in rejection. *American Journal of Pathology* 133, 82–94.

Gouw, A.S., Haagsma, E.B., Manns, M. et al. (1994) Is there recurrence of primary biliary cirrhosis after liver transplantation? A clinicopathologic study in long-term survivors. *Journal of Hepatology* 20, 500–507.

Greig, P.D., Woolf, G.M., Sinclair, S.B. et al. (1989) Treatment of primary liver graft non-function with prostaglandin E$_1$. *Transplantation* 48, 447–453.

Grellier, L. & Dusheiko, G.M. (1997) Hepatitis B virus and liver transplantation: concepts in antiviral prophylaxis. *Journal of Viral Hepatitis* 1, 111–116.

Grond, J., Gouw, A.S., Poppema, S., Sloof, M.J.H. & Gips, C.H. (1986) Chronic rejection in liver transplant: a histopathologic analysis of failed grafts and antecedent serial biopsies. *Transplantation Proceedings* 18, 128–135.

Gubernatis, G., Lauchart, W., Jonker, M. et al. (1987) Signs of hyperacute rejection of liver grafts in rhesus monkeys after donor-specific presensitization. *Transplantation Proceedings* 19, 1082–1083.

Gubernatis, G., Kemnitz, J., Tusch, G. & Pichlmayr, R. (1988) HLA compatibility and different features of liver allograft rejection. *Transplant International* 1, 155–160.

Gubernatis, G., Kemnitz, J., Bornscheuer, A., Kuse, E.R. & Pichlmayr, R. (1989) Potential various appearances of hyperacute rejection in human liver transplantation. *Langenbeck's Archives of Surgery (Berlin)* 374, 240–244.

Gugenheim, J., Samuel, D., Fabiani, B. et al. (1989) Rejection of ABO incompatible liver allografts in man. *Transplantation Proceedings* 21, 2223–2224.

Gugenheim, J., Samuel, D., Reynès, M. & Bismuth, H. (1990) Liver transplantation across ABO blood group barriers. *Lancet* 336, 519–523.

Gupta, D.G., Hudson, M., Burroughs, A.K. et al. (1995) Grading of cellular rejection after orthotopic liver transplantation. *Hepatology* 21, 46–57.

Haas, J., Patzold, U. & Stamm, T. (1978) Intrahepatische Cholestase, eine allergische Reaktion bei Azathioprine-Therapie? *Deutsche Medizinische Wochenschrift* 103, 1576–1577.

Hall, B.M. & Dorsch, S.E. (1984) Cells mediating allograft rejection. *Immunological Reviews* 77, 31–59.

Hanto, D.W., Snover, D.C. & Sibley, R.K. (1987) Hyperacute rejection of a human liver allograft in a presensitized recipient. *Clinical Transplantation* 1, 304–310.

Harrison, R.F., Davies, M.H., Goldin, R.D. & Hübscher, S.G. (1993) Recurrent hepatitis B in liver allografts: a distinctive form of rapidly developing cirrhosis. *Histopathology* 23, 21–28.

Harrison, R.F., Davies, M.H., Neuberger, J.M. & Hübscher, S.G. (1994a) Fibrous and obliterative cholangitis in liver allografts: evidence of recurrent primary sclerosing cholangitis? *Hepatology* 20, 356–361.

Harrison, R.F., Patsiaoura, K. & Hübscher, S.G. (1994b) Cytokeratin immunostaining for detection of biliary epithelium: its use in counting bile-ducts in cases of liver allograft rejection. *Journal of Clinical Pathology* 47, 303–308.

Hart, J., Busuttil, R.W. & Lewin, K.J. (1990) Disease recurrence following liver transplantation. *American Journal of Surgical Pathology* 14, 79–91.

Häyry, P. (1994) Chronic allograft rejection: an update. *Clinical Transplantation* 8, 155–159.

Häyry, P. & von Willebrand, E. (1984) Transplant aspiration cytology. *Transplantation* 38, 7–12.

Henderson, J.M., Mackay, G.J., Lumsden, A.B. *et al.* (1992) The effect of liver denervation on hepatic haemodynamics during hypovolaemic shock in swine. *Hepatology* 15, 130–133.

Hesselink, E.J., Slooff, M.J., Schuur, K.H., Bijleveld, C. & Gips, C. (1987) Consequences of hepatic artery pathology after orthotopic liver transplantation. *Transplantation Proceedings* 19, 2476–2477.

Hickman, P.E., Lynch, S.V., Potter, J.M. *et al.* (1994) Gamma glutamyl transferase as a marker of liver transplant rejection. *Transplantation* 57, 1278–1280.

Himmelreich, G., Riewald, M., Rosch, R. *et al.* (1994) Thrombomodulin: a marker for endothelial damage during orthotopic liver transplantation. *American Journal of Hematology* 47, 1–5.

Ho, M., Miller, G., Atchison, R.W. *et al.* (1985) Epstein–Barr virus infections and DNA hybridization studies in post-transplantation lymphoma and lymphoproliferative disease: the role of primary infection. *Journal of Infectionus Diseases* 152, 876–886.

Höckerstedt, K., Lautenschlager, I., Ahonen, J. *et al.* (1989) Differentiation between acute rejection and infection in liver transplant patients. *Transplantation Proceedings* 21, 2317–2318.

Hopf, U., Neuhaus, P., Lobeck, H. *et al.* (1991) Follow-up of recurrent hepatitis B and delta infection in liver allograft recipients after treatment with recombinat interferon-α. *Journal of Hepatology* 13, 339–346.

Houghton, M., Weiner, A., Kuo, G. & Choo, Q.-L. (1991) Molecular biology of the hepatitis C viruses: implications for diagnosis, development and control of viral disease. *Hepatology* 14, 381–388.

Hübscher, S.G. (1991) Histological findings in liver allograft rejection—new insights into the pathogenesis of hepatocellular damage in liver allografts (comment). *Histopathology* 18, 377–383.

Hübscher, S.G. (1994) Pathology of liver allograft rejection. *Transplant Immunology* 2, 118–123.

Hübscher, S.G. (1996) Diagnosis and grading of liver allograft rejection: a European perspective. *Transplantation Proceedings* 28, 504–507.

Hübscher, S.G., Clements, D., Elias, E. & McMaster, P. (1985) Biopsy findings in cases of rejection of liver allograft. *Journal of Clinical Pathology* 38, 1366–1373.

Hübscher, S.G., Buckels, J.A., Elias, E., McMaster, P. & Neuberger, J. (1991) Vanishing bile-duct syndrome following liver transplantation—is it reversible? *Transplantation* 51, 1004–1010.

Hübscher, S.G., Elias, E., Buckels, J.A. *et al.* (1993) Primary biliary cirrhosis. Histological evidence of disease recurrence after liver transplantation. *Journal of Hepatology* 18, 173–184.

Hübscher, S.G., Williams, A., Davison, S.M., Young, L.S. & Niedobitek, G. (1994) Epstein–Barr virus in inflammatory diseases of the liver and liver allografts: an *in situ* hybridization study. *Hepatology* 20, 899–907.

Ibrahim, S., Dawson, D.V., Killenberg, P.G. & Sanfilippo, F. (1993) The pattern and phenotype of T-cell infiltration associated with human liver allograft rejection. *Human Pathology* 12, 1365–1370.

Ihara, H., Ichikawa, Y., Nagano, S., Fukunishi, T. & Shinji, Y. (1982) Peliosis hepatis and nodular regenerative hyperplasia of the liver in renal transplant recipients. *Medical Journal of Osaka University* 33, 13–18.

Imagawa, D.K., Millis, J.M., Seu, P. *et al.* (1991) The role of tumour necrosis factor in allograft rejection. III. Evidence that anti-TNF antibody therapy prolongs allograft survival in rats with acute rejection. *Transplantation* 51, 57–62.

International Panel (1997) Banff schema for grading liver allograft rejection: an international consensus document. *Hepatology* 25, 658–663.

International Working Party (1995) Terminology for hepatic allograft rejection. *Hepatology* 22, 648–654.

Iwatsuki, S., Gordon, R.D., Shaw, B.W. & Starzl, T.E. (1985) Rôle of liver transplantation in cancer therapy. *Annals of Surgery* 202, 401–407.

Jaffe, R. & Yunis, E.J. (1989) Pediatric liver transplantation: diagnostic pathology. *Perspectives in Pediatric Pathology* 13 (44), 44–81.

Jamieson, N.V., Sundberg, R., Lindell, S. *et al.* (1988) Preservation of the canine liver for 24–48 hours using simple cold storage with UW solution. *Transplantation* 46, 517–522.

Jamieson, N.V., Joysey, V., Friend, P.J. *et al.* (1991) Graft-versus-host disease in solid organ transplantation. *Transplant International* 4, 67–71.

Jennings, I., Calne, R.Y. & Baglin, T.P. (1994) Predictive value of von Willebrand factor to ristocetin cofactor ratio and thrombin–antithrombin complex levels for hepatic vessel thrombosis and graft rejection after liver transplantation. *Transplantation* 57, 1046–1051.

Jones, A., Selby, P.J., Viner, C. *et al.* (1990) Tumour necrosis factor, cholestatic jaundice, and chronic liver disease. *Gut* 31, 938–939.

Kakizoe, S., Yanaga, K., Starzl, T.E. & Demetris, A.J. (1990) Evaluation of protocol before transplantation and after reperfusion biopsies from human orthotopic liver allografts: considerations of preservation and early immunological injury. *Hepatology* 11, 932–941.

Kamada, N. & Calne, R.Y. (1979) Orthotopic liver transplantation in the rat. Technique using cuff for portal vein anastomosis and biliary drainage. *Transplantation* 28, 47–50.

Kamada, N., Davies H.F.S. & Roser, B. (1981) Reversal of transplant immunity by liver grafting. *Nature* 292, 840–842.

Katz, E., Mor, E., Schwartz, M.E., Theise, N.T.P. & Miller, C.M. (1994) Preservation injury in clinical liver transplantation: incidence and effect on rejection and survival. *Clinical Transplantation* 8, 492–496.

Kawarasaki, H., Iwanaka, T., Tsuchida, Y. *et al.* (1994) Partial liver transplantation from a living donor: experimental research and clinical experience. *Journal of Pediatric Surgery* 29, 518–522.

Kemnitz, J. & Cohnert, T.R. (1987) Diagnostic criteria for liver allograft rejection. *American Journal of Surgical Pathology* 11, 737–738.

Kemnitz, J., Gubernatis, G., Cohnert, T.R. & Georgii, A. (1989) Histopathologic diagnosis of rejection in liver allografts (letter). *Human Pathology* 20, 1030–1031.

Kirby, R.M., Young, J.A., Hübscher, S.G., Elias, E. & McMaster, P. (1988) The accuracy of aspiration cytology in the diagnosis of rejection following orthotopic liver transplantation. *Transplant International* 1, 119–126.

Kissmeyer-Nielsen, F., Olsen, S., Peterson, V.P. & Fjeldborg, O. (1966) Hyperacute rejection of kidney allografts associated with pre-existing humoural antibodies against donor cells. *Lancet* 2, 662–665.

Kiuchi, T., Kato, H., Kanaya, S. *et al.* (1994) Spontaneous proliferation of peripheral blood lymphocytes as an indicator of intragraft immune activation in liver transplant patients. *Clinical Transplantation* 8, 382–387.

Klein, A.S., Savader, S., Burdick, J.F. *et al.* (1991) Reduction of morbidity and mortality from biliary complications after liver transplantation. *Hepatology* 14, 818–823.

Klintmalm, G.B.G., Iwatsuki, S. & Starzl, T.E. (1981) Cyclosporin A toxicity in 66 renal allograft recipients. *Transplantation* 32, 488–489.

Klintmalm, G.B., Nery, J.R., Husberg, B.S., Gonwa, T.A. & Tillery, G.W. (1989) Rejection in liver transplantation. *Hepatology* 10, 978–985.

Klupp, J., Bechstein, W.O., Platz, K.P. *et al.* (1997) Mycophenolate mofetil added to immunosuppression after

liver transplantation—first results. *Transplant International* 10, 223–228.

Knechtle, S.J., Kolbeck, P., Tsuchimoto, S. *et al.* (1987) Hepatic transplantation into sensitized recipients. Demonstration of hyperacute rejection. *Transplantation* 43, 8–12.

Knechtle, S.J., Yamaguchi, Y., Harland, R.C., Coundouriotis, A. & Bollinger, R.R. (1989) Mediation of rat hepatic allografts by RT-1 antigens. *Transplantation* 48, 723–725.

Koneru, B., Jaffe, R., Esquivel, C.O. *et al.* (1987) Adenovirus infections in pediatric liver transplant recipients. *Journal of the American Medical Association* 258, 489–492.

König, V., Bauditz, J., Lobeck, H. *et al.* (1992) Hepatitis C virus reinfection in allografts after orthotopic liver transplantation. *Hepatology* 16, 1137–1143.

Krams, S.M., Ascher, N.L. & Martinez, O.M. (1993) New immunologic insights into mechanisms of allograft rejection. *Gastroenterology Clinics of North America* 22, 381–400.

Kubota, K., Ericzon, B.G. & Reinholt, F.P. (1991) Comparison of fine-needle aspiration biopsy and histology in human liver transplants. *Transplantation* 51, 1010–1013.

Kusne, S., Dummer, J.S., Singh, N. *et al.* (1988) Infections after liver transplantation. An analysis of 101 consecutive cases. *Medicine (Baltimore)* 67, 132–143.

Lake, J.R. & Wright, T.L. (1991) Editorial: Liver transplantation for patients with hepatitis B: what have we learned from our results? *Hepatology* 13, 796–799.

Langnas, A.N., Markin, R.S., Inagaki, M. *et al.* (1994) Epstein–Barr virus hepatitis after liver transplantation. *American Journal of Gastroenterology* 89, 1066–1070.

Lautenschlager, I., Taskinen, E., Inkinen, K. *et al.* (1984) Distribution of the major histocompatibility complex antigens on different cellular components of human liver. *Cellular Immunology* 85, 191–200.

Lautenschlager, I., von Willebrand, E. & Häyry, P. (1985) Blood eosinophilia, steroids and rejection. *Transplantation* 40, 354–357.

Lautenschlager, I., Höckerstedt, K., Ahonen, J. *et al.* (1988) Fine needle aspiration biopsy in the monitoring of liver allografts. II Applications to human liver allografts. *Transplantation* 46, 47–52.

Lautenschlager, I., Höckerstedt, K. & Häyry, P. (1991) Fine-needle aspiration biopsy in the monitoring of liver grafts. *Transplant International* 4, 54–61.

Lautenschlager, I., Nashan, B., Schlitt, H.J. *et al.* (1994) Different cellular patterns associated with hepatitis C virus reactivation, cytomegalovirus infection, and acute rejection in liver transplant patients monitored with transplant aspiration cytology. *Transplantation* 58, 1339–1345.

Lerut, J., Gordon, R.D., Iwatsuki, S. *et al.* (1987) Biliary tract complications in 393 human liver transplantations. *Transplantation* 43, 47–51.

Lerut, J., Demetris, A.J., Stieber, A.C. *et al.* (1988) Intrahepatic bile-duct strictures after human orthotopic liver transplantation. Recurrence of primary sclerosing cholangitis or unusual presentation of allograft rejection? *Transplant International* 1, 127–130.

Levy, V.G., Ruskone, A., Baillou, C. *et al.* (1985) Polycythaemia and the Budd–Chiari syndrome: study of erythropoietin and bone marrow erythroid progenitors. *Hepatology* 5, 858–861.

Libby, P. & Tanaka, H. (1994) The pathogenesis of coronary arteriosclerosis ('chronic rejection') in transplanted hearts. *Clinical Transplantation* 8, 313–318.

Loftus, E.V., Aguilar, H.I., Sandborn, W.J. *et al.* (1998) Risk of colorectal neoplasia in patients with primary sclerosin cholangitis and ulcerative colitis following orthotopic liver transplantation. *Hepatology* 27, 685–690.

Lok, A.S.F., Ma, O.C.K., Chan, T.-M. *et al.* (1991) Overestimation of the prevalence of antibody to hepatitis C virus in retrospective studies on stored sera. *Hepatology* 14, 756–762.

Lones, M.A., Shintaku, I.P., Weiss, L.M. *et al.* (1997) Posttransplant lymphoproliferative disorder in liver allograft biopsies: a comparison of three methods for the demonstration of Epstein–Barr virus. *Human Pathology* 28, 533–539.

Lorber, M.I., van Buren, C.T., Flescher, S.M., Williams, C. & Kahan, B.D. (1987) Hepatobiliary and pancreatic complications of cyclosporine therapy in 466 renal transplant recipients. *Transplantation* 43, 35–54.

Ludwig, J. (1988) Histopathology of the liver following transplantation. In: *Transplantation of the Liver* (ed. W.C. Maddrey), pp. 191–218. Elsevier, New York.

Ludwig, J. (1989) Classification and terminology of hepatic allograft rejection: whither bound? *Mayo Clinic Proceedings* 64, 676–679.

Ludwig, J. (1994) Terminology of chronic hepatitis, hepatic allograft rejection, and nodular lesions of the liver: summary of recommendations developed by an international working party, supported by the World Congresses of Gastroenterology, Los Angeles, 1994. *American Journal of Gastroenterology* 89, S177–S181.

Ludwig, J. & Batts, K.P. (1995) Transplantation pathology including liver injury in graft versus host disease and in recipients of renal and other allografts. In: *Pathology of the Liver* (eds R.N.M. MacSween, P.P. Anthony, P.J. Scheuer, A.D. Burt & B.C. Portmann), pp. 765–786. Churchill Livingstone, Edinburgh.

Ludwig, J., Wiesner, R.H., Batts, K.P., Perkins, J.D. & Krom, R.A.F. (1987) The acute vanishing bile-duct syndrome (acute irreversible rejection) after orthotopic liver transplantation. *Hepatology* 7, 476–483.

Ludwig, J., Gross, J.B., Perkins, J.D. & Moore, S.B. (1990) Persistent centrilobular necroses in hepatic allografts. *Human Pathology* 21, 656–661.

Ludwig, J., Batts, K.P. & MacCarty, R.L. (1992) Ischemic cholangitis in hepatic allografts. *Mayo Clinic Proceedings* 67, 519–526.

McCaughan, G.W., Davies, S., Waugh, J. *et al.* (1989) Cell surface phenotype of mononuclear cells infiltrating bile-ducts during acute and chronic liver allograft rejection. *Transplantation Proceedings* 21, 2201–2202.

McDiarmid, S.V. (1996) Mycophenolate mofetil in liver transplantation. *Clinical Transplantation* 10, 140–145.

McDonald, J.A., Painter, D.M.R., Gallagher, N.D., Sheil, A.G.R. & McCaughan, G.W. (1989) Human liver allograft rejection: severity, prognosis and response to treatment. *Transplantation Proceedings* 21, 3792–3793.

MacDougall, B.R.D. & Williams, R. (1979) The indications for orthotopic liver transplantation. *Transplantation Proceedings* 11, 247–251.

McKeown, C.M.B., Edwards, V., Phillips, M.J. *et al.* (1988) Sinusoidal lining cell damage: the critical injury in cold preservation of liver allografts in the rat. *Transplantation* 46, 178–191.

McMaster, P., Walton, R.D., Wight, D.G.D., Medd, R.K. & Syrakos, T.P. (1980) The influence of ischaemia on the biliary tract. *British Journal of Surgery* 67, 321–324.

Mañez, R., Kobayashi, M., Takaya, S. *et al.* (1993) Humoral rejection associated with antidonor lymphocytotoxic antibodies following liver transplantation. *Transplantation Proceedings* 25, 888–890.

Manzarbeitia, C., Rustgi, V.K., Jonsson, J. & Oyloe, V.K. (1995) Absolute peripheral blood eosinophilia. An early marker for rejection in clinical liver transplantation. *Transplantation* 59, 1358–1360.

Markin, R.S., Wood, R.P., Shaw, B.J., Brichacek, B. & Purtilo, D.T. (1990) Immunohistologic identification of Epstein–Barr virus-induced hepatitis reactivation after OKT-3 therapy following orthotopic liver transplant. *American Journal of Gastroenterology* 85, 1014–1018.

Markus, B.H., Fung, J.J., Zeevi, A. *et al.* (1987) Analysis of lymphocytes infiltrating human hepatic allografts. *Transplantation Proceedings* 19, 2470–2473.

Markus, B.H., Duquesnoy, R.J., Gordon, R.D. *et al.* (1988) Histocompatibility and liver transplant outcome. Does HLA exert a dualistic effect? *Transplantation* 46, 372–377.

Martelius, T., Krogerus, L., Hockerstedt, K. *et al.* (1997) CMV causes bile-duct destruction and arterial lesions in rat liver allografts. *Transplantation Proceedings* 29, 796–797.

Martin, P., Muñoz, S.J., Di Bisceglie, A.M. *et al.* (1991) Recurrence of hepatitis C virus infection after orthotopic liver transplantation. *Hepatology* 13, 719–721.

Martinez, O.M., Ascher, N.L., Ferrell, L. *et al.* (1993) Evidence for a nonclassical pathway of graft rejection involving interleukin 5 and eosinophils. *Transplantation* 55, 909–918.

Maury, C.P.J. & Teppo, A.M. (1987) Raised serum levels of

cachectin/tumour necrosis factor α. *Journal of Experimental Medicine* **166**, 1132–1137.

Mignat, C. (1997) Clinically significant drug interactions with new immunosuppressive agents. *Drug Safety* **16**, 267–278.

Moore, F.D., Wheeler, H.B. & Demissianos, H.V. (1959) One-stage homotransplantation of the liver following total hepatectomy in dogs. *Transplant Bulletin* **6**, 103–106.

Mor, E., Gonwa, T.A., Husberg, B.S., Goldstein, R.M. & Klintmalm, G.B. (1992) Late-onset acute rejection in orthotopic liver transplantation—associated risk factors and outcome. *Transplantation* **54**, 821–824.

Morgan, G. & Superina, R.A. (1994) Lymphoproliferative disease after pediatric liver transplantation. *Journal of Pediatric Surgery* **29**, 1192–1196.

Mulbacher, F. & Piza, F. (1987) Orthotopic liver transplantation for secondary malignancies of the liver. *Transplantation Proceedings* **19**, 2396–2398.

Munn, S.R., Tominaga, S., Perkins, J.D. *et al.* (1988) Increasing peripheral lymphocyte counts predict rejection in human orthotopic liver allografts. *Transplantation Proceedings* **20**, 674–675.

Murgia, M.G., Jordan, S. & Kahan, B.D. (1996) The side effect profile of sirolimus: a phase I study in quiescent cyclosporine-prednisone-treated renal transplant patients. *Kidney International* **49**, 209–216.

Nagafuchi, Y., Hobbs, K.E.F., Thomas, H.C. & Scheuer, P.J. (1985) Expression of beta-2-microglobulin on hepatocytes after transplantation. *Lancet* **2**, 551–554.

Nakanuma, Y. & Ohta, G. (1979) Histometric and serial section observations of the intrahepatic ducts in primary biliary cirrhosis. *Gastroenterology* **76**, 1326–1332.

Nakhleh, R.E., Schwarzenberg, S.J., Bloomer, J., Payne, W. & Snover, D.C. (1990) The pathology of liver allografts surviving longer than one year. *Hepatology* **11**, 465–470.

Nalesnik, M.A., Jaffe, R., Starzl, T.E. *et al.* (1988a) The pathology of post-transplant lymphoproliferative disorders occurring in the setting of cyclosporine A-prednisone immunosuppression. *American Journal of Pathology* **133**, 173–192.

Nalesnik, M.A., Makowka, L. & Starzl, T.E. (1988b) The diagnosis and treatment of post-transplant lymphoproliferative disorders. *Current Problems in Surgery* **25**, 371–472.

National Institutes of Health (1984) National Institutes of Health Consensus Development Conference statement: liver transplantation – June 20–23, 1983. *Hepatology* **4** (Suppl. 1), S107–110.

Nawaz, S. & Fennell, R.H. (1994) Apoptosis of bile-duct epithelial cells in hepatic allograft rejection. *Histopathology* **25**, 137–142.

Neuberger, J.M. & Adams, D.H. (1990) Is HLA matching important for liver transplantation? *Journal of Hepatology* **11**, 1–4.

Neuberger, J., Portmann, B., MacDougall, B.R.D., Calne, R.Y. & Williams, R. (1982) Recurrence of primary biliary cirrhosis after liver transplantation. *New England Journal of Medicine* **306**, 1–4.

Neumann, U.P., Kaisers, U., Langrehr, J.M. *et al.* (1994) Fatal graft-versus-host-disease: a grave complication after orthotopic liver transplantation. *Transplantation Proceedings* **26**, 3616–3617.

Ng, I.O.L., Burroughs, A.K., Rolles, K., Belli, L.S. & Scheuer, P.J. (1991) Hepatocellular ballooning after liver transplantation: a light and electronmicroscopic study with clinicopathological correlation. *Histopathology* **18**, 323–330.

O'Grady, J. & Williams, R. (1988) Long-term management, complications, and disease recurrence. In: *Transplantation of the Liver Current Topics in Gastroenterology* (ed. W.C. Maddrey), pp. 143–165. Elsevier, New York.

O'Grady, J., Alexander, G.J.M., Sutherland, S. *et al.* (1988a) Cytomegalovirus infection and donor/recipient HLA antigens: interdependent co-factors in pathogenesis of vanishing bile-duct syndrome after liver transplantation. *Lancet* **2**, 302–305.

O'Grady, J., Polson, R.J., Rolles, K., Calne, R.Y. & Williams, R. (1988b) Liver transplantation for malignant disease. Results in 93 consecutive patients. *Annals of Surgery* **207**, 373–379.

O'Grady, J.G., Smith, H.M., Davies, S.M. *et al.* (1992) Hepatitis B virus reinfection after orthotopic liver transplantation. *Journal of Hepatology* **14**, 104–111.

Oguma, S., Belle, S., Starzl, T.E. & Demetris, A.J. (1989) A histometric analysis of chronically rejected human liver allografts: insights into the mechanisms of bile-duct loss: direct immunologic and ischaemic factors. *Hepatology* **9**, 204–209.

Ohzato, H., Monden, M., Yoshizaki, K. *et al.* (1993) Serum interleukin-6 levels as an indicator of acute rejection after liver transplantation in cynomologous monkeys. *Surgery Today* **23**, 521–527.

Olson, L.M., Klintmalm, G.B., Husberg, B.S. & Nery, J. (1988) Physiologic aberrations diagnostic of hepatic graft malfunction: a case report. *Transplantation Proceedings* **20**, 667–668.

Orosz, C.G. (1994) Endothelial activation and chronic allograft rejection. *Clinical Transplantation* **8**, 299–303.

Otte, J.B. (1991) Recent developments in liver transplantation. Lessons from a 5-year experience. *Journal of Hepatology* **12**, 386–393.

Pallarés, R., Sitges-Serra, A., Fuentes, J., Sitges-Creus, A. & Guardia, J. (1983) Cholestasis associated with total parenteral nutrition. *Lancet* **i**, 758–759.

Pappo, O., Ramos, H., Starzl, T.E., Fung, J.J. & Demetris, A.J. (1995) Structural integrity and identification of causes of liver allograft dysfunction occurring more than 5 years after transplantation. *American Journal of Surgical Pathology* **19**, 192–206.

Paya, C.V., Hermans, P.E., Smith, T.F. *et al.* (1988) Efficacy of gancyclovir in liver and kidney transplant recipients with severe cytomegalovirus infection. *Transplantation* **46**, 229–234.

Paya, C.V., Hermans, P.E., Washington, A. *et al.* (1989a) Incidence, distribution, and outcome of episodes of infection in 100 orthotopic liver transplantations. *Mayo Clinic Proceedings* **64**, 555–564.

Paya, C.V., Smith, T.F., Ludwig, J. & Hermans, P.E. (1989b) Rapid shell vial culture and tissue histology compared with serology for the rapid diagnosis of cytomegalovirus infection in liver transplantation. *Mayo Clinic Proceedings* **64**, 670–675.

Penn, I. (1979) Tumour incidence in human allograft recipients. *Transplantation Proceedings* **11**, 1047–1052.

Penn, I. (1983) Lymphomas complicating organ transplants. *Transplantation Proceedings* **15**, 2790–2797.

Penn, I. (1987) Cancers following cyclosporine therapy. *Transplantation* **43**, 32–35.

Pereira, B.J.G., Wright, T.L., Schmid, C.H. & Levey, A.S. (1995) A controlled study of hepatitis C transmission by organ transplantation. *Lancet* **345**, 484–487.

Perkins, J.D., Wiesner, R.H., Banks, P.M. *et al.* (1987) Immunohistologic labeling as an indicator of liver allograft rejection. *Transplantation* **43**, 105–108.

Perkins, J.D., Nelson, D.L., Rakela, J., Grambsch, P.M. & Krom, R.A.F. (1989a) Soluble interleukin-2 receptor level as an indicator of liver allograft rejection. *Transplantation* **47**, 77–81.

Perkins, J.D., Rakela, J., Sterioff, S. *et al.* (1989b) Immunohistologic pattern of the portal T-lymphocyte infiltration in hepatic allograft rejection. *Mayo Clinic Proceedings* **64**, 565–569.

Persijn, G.G., De D'Amaro, J. & Lange, P. (1989) The effect of mismatching and sharing HLA-A, B and DR antigens on kidney graft survival in Eurotransplant 1982–88. In: *Clinical Transplantation* (ed. P. Terasaki), pp. 237–248. UCLA Typing Laboratories, Los Angeles.

Petrovic, L.M., Villamil, F.G., Vierling, J.M., Makowka, L. & Geller, S.A. (1997) Comparison of histopathology in acute allograft rejection and recurrent hepatitis C infection after liver transplantation. *Liver Transplant Surgery* **3**, 398–406.

Phillips, M.J., Cameron, R., Flowers, M.A. *et al.* (1992) Post-transplant recurrent hepatitis B viral liver disease. Viral-burden, steatoviral, and fibroviral hepatitis B. *American Journal of Pathology* **140**, 1295–1308.

Pichlmayr, R., Brölsch, C.H., Wonigeit, K. *et al.* (1984) Experiences with liver transplantation in Hannover. *Hepatology* **4**, 56–60.

Pignatelli, M. (1988) Methods for quantitating HLA gene product expression in the liver during hepatitis B virus infection. *Ricerca in Clinica e in Laboratorio* (Milano) **18**, 233–239.

Pirsch, J.D., Kalayoglu, M., Hafez, G.R. *et al.* (1990) Evidence that the vanishing bile-duct syndrome is vanishing. *Transplantation* **49**, 1015–1018.

Ploeg, R.J., D'Alessandro, A.M., Knechtle, S.J. *et al.* (1993) Risk factors for primary dysfunction after liver transplantation: a multivariate analysis. *Transplantation* **55**, 807–813.

Polson, R.J., Portmann, B., Neuberger, J., Calne, R.Y. & Williams, R. (1989) Evidence for disease recurrence after liver transplantation for primary biliary cirrhosis. Clinical and histologic follow-up studies. *Gastroenterology* **97**, 715–725.

Pons, J.A. (1995) Role of liver transplantation in viral hepatitis. *Journal of Hepatology* **22**, 146–153.

Popescu, I., Sheiner, P., Mor, E. *et al.* (1994) Biliary complications in 400 cases of liver transplantation. *Mount Sinai Journal of Medicine* **61**, 57–62.

Porter, K.A. (1969) Pathology of the orthotopic homograft and heterograft. In: *Experiences in Hepatic Transplantation* (ed. T.E. Starzl), pp. 422–471. W.B. Saunders, Philadelphia.

Portmann, B. & Wight, D.G.D. (1987) Pathology of liver transplantation. In: *Liver Transplantation* (ed. R.Y. Calne), pp. 435–470. Grune and Stratton, London.

Portmann, B., O'Grady, J. & Williams, R. (1986) Disease recurrence following liver transplantation. *Transplantation Proceedings* **18**, 136–141.

Poterucha, J.J., Rakela, J., Lumeng, L. *et al.* (1992) Diagnosis of chronic hepatitis C after liver transplantation by the detection of viral sequences with polymerase chain reaction. *Hepatology* **15**, 42–45.

Purcell, R.H., Rizzetto, M. & Gerin, J.L. (1984) Hepatitis delta infection of the liver. *Seminars in Liver Disease* **4**, 340–346.

Rakela, J., Wooten, R.S., Batts, K.P. *et al.* (1989) Failure of interferon to prevent recurrent hepatitis B infection in hepatic allograft. *Mayo Clinic Proceedings* **64**, 429–432.

Ramsey, G., Nusbacher, J., Starzl, T.E. & Lindsay, G.D. (1984) Isohemagglutinins of graft origin after ABO-unmatched liver transplantation. *New England Journal of Medicine* **311**, 1167–1170.

Randhawa, P.S., Markin, R.S., Starzl, T.E. & Demetris, A.J. (1990) Epstein–Barr virus-associated syndromes in immunosuppressed liver transplant recipients. Clinical profile and recognition on routine allograft biopsy. *American Journal of Surgery and Pathology* **14**, 538–547.

Ray, R.A., Lewin, K.J., Colonna, J., Goldstein, L.I. & Busuttil, R.W. (1988) The rôle of liver biopsy in evaluating acute allograft dysfunction following liver transplantation: a clinical histologic correlation of 34 liver transplants. *Human Pathology* **19**, 835–848.

Riely, C.A. & Vera, S.R. (1990) Liver biopsy in the long-term follow-up of liver transplant patients: still the gold standard. *Gastroenterology* **99**, 1182–1183.

Ringe, B. (1994) Quadrennial review on liver transplantation. *American Journal of Gastroenterology* **89**, S18–26.

Ringe, B., Pichlmayr, R., Wittekind, C. & Tusch, G. (1991) Surgical treatment of hepatocellular carcinoma: experience with liver resection and transplantation in 198 patients. *World Journal of Surgery* **15**, 270–285.

Rizzetto, M., Macagno, S., Chiaberge, E. *et al.* (1987) Liver transplantation in hepatitis delta virus disease. *Lancet* **2**, 469–471.

Robbins, P.A., Maino, V.C., Warner, N.L. & Brodsky, F.M. (1988) Activated T cells and monocytes have characteristic patterns of class II antigen expression. *Journal of Immunology* **141**, 1281–1287.

Roberts, J.P., Ascher, N.L., Lake, J. *et al.* (1991) Graft vs host disease after liver transplantation in humans: a report of four cases. *Hepatology* **14**, 274–281.

Rosen, H.R., Chou, S., Corless, C.L. *et al.* (1997a) Cytomegalovirus viremia: risk factor for allograft cirrhosis after liver transplantation for hepatitis C. *Transplantation* **64**, 721–726.

Rosen, H.R., Shackleton, C.R., Higa, L. *et al.* (1997b) Use of OKT3 is associated with early and severe recurrence of hepatitis C after liver transplantation (see comments). *American Journal of Gastroenterology* **92**, 1453–1457.

Ross, R. (1993) The pathogenesis of atherosclerosis: a perspective for the 1990s. *Nature* **362**, 801–809.

Ruben, Z. (1987) The pathobiologic significance of intracellular drug storage. *Human Pathology* **18**, 1197–1198.

Ryckman, F.C., Flake, A.W., Fisher, R.A. *et al.* (1991) Segmental orthotopic hepatic transplantation as a means to improve patient survival and diminish waiting-list mortality. *Journal of Pediatric Surgery* **26**, 422–427.

Ryffel, B., Donatsch, P., Madorin, M. *et al.* (1983) Toxicological evaluation of cyclosporin A. *Archives of Toxicology* **53**, 107–141.

Saliba, F., Gugenheim, J., Samuel, M. *et al.* (1987) Orthotopic liver transplantation in humans: monitoring by serial graft biopsies. *Transplantation Proceedings* **19**, 2454–2456.

Salt, A., Sutehall, G., Sargaison, M. *et al.* (1990) Viral and *Toxoplasma gondii* infections in children after liver transplantation. *Journal of Clinical Pathology* **43**, 63–67.

Samuel, D., Gillet, D., Castaing, D., Reynès, M. & Bismuth, H. (1989) Portal and arterial thrombosis in liver transplantation: a frequent event in severe rejection. *Transplantation Proceedings* **21**, 2225–2227.

Samuel, D., Bismuth, A., Mathieu, D. *et al.* (1991) Passive immunoprophylaxis after liver transplantation in HBsAg-positive patients. *Lancet* **337**, 813–815.

Sánchez-Bueno, F., Robles, R., Ramírez, P. *et al.* (1994)

Hepatic artery complications after liver transplantation. *Clinical Transplantation* **8**, 399–404.

Sanchez-Urdazpal, L., Batts, K.P., Gores, G.J. *et al.* (1993) Increased bile-duct complications in liver transplantation across the ABO barrier. *Annals of Surgery* **218**, 152–158.

Sankary, H., Foster, P., Hart, M. *et al.* (1989) An analysis of the determinants of hepatic allograft rejection using step-wise logistic regression. *Transplantation* **47**, 74–77.

Sankary, H.N., McChesney, L., Frye, E. *et al.* (1995) A simple modification in operative technique can reduce the incidence of non-anastomotic biliary strictures after orthotopic liver transplant. *Hepatology* **21**, 63–69.

Saxena, R., Toxat, Y., Soin, A.S. *et al.* (1995) Relationship between patterns of hepatobiliary vascular supply and biliary complications in liver transplantation: an anatomical and clinical analysis. *Transplantation Proceedings* **27**, 1199–1200.

Scharschmidt, B.F. (1984) Human liver transplantation: analysis of data on 540 patients from four centres. *Hepatology* **4**, 95S–101S.

Scheuer, P.J., Ashrafzadeh, P., Sherlock, S., Brown, D. & Dusheiko, G.M. (1992) The pathology of hepatitis C. *Hepatology* **15**, 567–571.

Schlitt, H.J. & Nashan, B. (1993) Transplant aspiration cytology of the liver. In: *Acute Rejection of Liver Grafts* (ed. G. Gubernatis), pp. 62–77. R.G. Landes, Austin.

Schlitt, H.J., Nashan, B., Ringe, B. *et al.* (1991) Differentiation of liver graft dysfunction by transplant aspiration cytology. *Transplantation* **51**, 786–793.

Schlitt, H.J., Kanehiro, H., Raddatz, G. *et al.* (1993a) Persistence of donor lymphocytes in liver allograft recipients. *Transplantation* **56**, 1001–1007.

Schlitt, H.J., Raddatz, G., Steinhoff, G., Wonigeit, K. & Pichlmayr, R. (1993b) Passenger lymphocytes in human liver allografts and their potential role after transplantation. *Transplantation* **56**, 951–955.

Schluger, L.K., Sheiner, P.A., Thung, S.N. *et al.* (1996) Severe recurrent cholestatic hepatitis C following orthotopic liver transplantation. *Hepatology* **23**, 971–976.

Schmid, M., Hefti, M.L., Gattiker, R. & Kistler, H.J. (1965) Benign postoperative intrahepatic cholestasis. *New England Journal of Medicine* **272**, 545–550.

Sedmak, D.D. & Orosz, C.G. (1991) The role of vascular endothelial cells in transplantation. *Archives of Pathology and Laboratory Medicine* **115**, 260–265.

Shah, G., Demetris, A.J., Gavaler, J.S. *et al.* (1992) Incidence, prevalence, and clinical course of hepatitis C following liver transplantation. *Gastroenterology* **103**, 323–329.

Sheiner, P.A., Schwartz, M.E., Mor, E. *et al.* (1995) Severe or multiple rejection episodes are associated with early recurrence of hepatitis C after orthotopic liver transplantation. *Hepatology* **21**, 30–34.

Sherlock, S. (1987) The syndrome of disappearing intrahepatic bile-ducts. *Lancet* **2**, 493–496.

Shiffman, M.L., Contos, M.J., Luketic, V.A. *et al.* (1994) Biochemical and histologic evaluation of recurrent hepatitis C following orthotopic liver transplantation. *Transplantation* 57, 526–532.

Shuhart, M.C., Bronner, M.P., Gretch, D.R. *et al.* (1997) Histological and clinical outcome after liver transplantation for hepatitis C. *Hepatology* 26, 1646–1652.

Sibley, R.K. (1994) Morphologic features of chronic rejection in kidney and less commonly transplanted organs. *Clinical Transplantation* 8, 293–298.

Simmons, W.D., Rayhill, S.C. & Sollinger, H.W. (1997) Preliminary risk–benefit assessment of mycophenolate mofetil in transplant rejection. *Drug Safety* 17, 75–92.

Singh, N., Yu, V.L. & Gayowski, T. (1994) Central nervous system lesions in adult liver transplant recipients: clinical review with implications for management. *Medicine (Baltimore)* 73, 110–118.

Singh, N., Gayowski, T., Ndimbie, O.K. *et al.* (1996a) Recurrent hepatitis C virus hepatitis in liver transplant recipients receiving tacrolimus: association with rejection and increased immunosuppression after transplantation. *Surgery* 119, 452–456.

Singh, N., Gayowski, T., Wagener, M.M. & Marino, I.R. (1996b) Increased infections in liver transplant recipients with recurrent hepatitis C virus hepatitis. *Transplantation* 61, 402–406.

Slapak, G.I., Saxena, R., Portmann, B. *et al.* (1997) Graft and systemic disease in long-term survivors of liver transplantation. *Hepatology* 25, 195–202.

Snover, D.C. (1990a) Liver transplantation. In: *The Pathology of Organ Transplantation* (ed. G.E. Sale), pp. 103–132. Butterworths, Boston.

Snover, D.C. (1990b) MHC antigen expression in human liver grafts: its role in rejection. *Hepatology* 11, 704–706.

Snover, D.C. (1993) General aspects of the pathology of rejection of kidney and liver in the early posttransplant period. *Transplantation Proceedings* 25 (4), 2649–2651.

Snover, D.C., Sibley, R.K., Freese, D.K. *et al.* (1984a) Orthotopic liver transplantation: a pathological study of 63 serial liver biopsies from 17 patients with special reference to the diagnostic features and natural history of rejection. *Hepatology* 4, 1212–1222.

Snover, D.C., Weisdorf, S.A., Ramsay, N.K., McGlave, P. & Kersey, J.H. (1984b) Hepatic graft-versus-host disease: a study of the predictive value of liver biopsy in diagnosis. *Hepatology* 4, 123–130.

Snover, D.C., Freese, D.K., Sharp, H.L. *et al.* (1987) Liver allograft rejection. An analysis of the use of biopsy in determining the outcome of rejection. *American Journal of Surgical Pathology* 11, 1–10.

So, S.K.S., Platt, J.L., Ascher, N.L. & Snover, D.C. (1987) Increased expression of Class I major histocompatibility complex antigens on hepatocytes in rejecting human liver allografts. *Transplantation* 43, 79–85.

Soin, A.S., Rasmussen, A., Jamieson, N.V. *et al.* (1995) CsA levels in the early posttransplant period—predictive of chronic rejection in liver transplantation? *Transplantation* 59, 1119–1123.

Sparberg, M., Simon, N. & Del Greco, F. (1969) Intrahepatic cholestasis due to azathioprine. *Gastroenterology* 57, 439–441.

Starzl, T.E. (1969) *Experiences in Hepatic Transplantation.* W.B. Saunders, Philadelphia.

Starzl, T.E., Machioro, T.L., von Kaulla, K. *et al.* (1963) Homotransplantation of the liver in humans. *Surgery, Gynecology and Obstetrics* 117, 659–676.

Starzl, T.E., Machioro, T.L. & Porter, K.A. (1965) Factors determining short- and long-term survival after orthotopic liver homotransplantation in the dog. *Surgery* 58, 131–155.

Starzl, T.E., Putnam, C.W., Hansborough, J.R., Porter, K.A. & Reid, H.A.S. (1977) Biliary complications after liver transplantation: with special reference to the biliary cast syndrome and techniques of secondary duct repair. *Surgery* 81, 212–221.

Starzl, T.E., Koep, L.J., Halgrimson, C.F. *et al.* (1979) Fifteen years of clinical liver transplantation. *Gastroenterology* 115, 815–819.

Starzl, T.E., Iwatsuki, S., Shaw, B.W. *et al.* (1986) Treatment of fibrolamellar hepatoma with partial or total hepatectomy and transplantation of the liver. *Surgery, Gynecology and Obstetrics* 162, 145–148.

Starzl, T.E., Demetris, A.J., Todo, S. *et al.* (1989a) Evidence for hyperacute rejection of human liver grafts: the case of the canary kidneys. *Clinical Transplantation* 3, 37–48.

Starzl, T.E., Demetris, A.J. & van Thiel, D.H. (1989b) Liver transplantation. *New England Journal of Medicine* 321, 1014–1022 and 1092–1099.

Steinhoff, S. (1990) Major histocompatibility complex antigens in human liver transplants. *Journal of Hepatology* 11, 9–15.

Steinhoff, G., Wonigeit, K. & Pichlmayr, R. (1988) Analysis of sequential changes in major histocompatibility complex expression in human liver grafts after transplantation. *Transplantation* 45, 394–401.

Steinhoff, G., Behrend, M. & Wonigeit, K. (1990) Expression of adhesion molecules on lymphocytes/monocytes and hepatocytes in human liver grafts. *Human Immunology* 28, 123–127.

Steinhoff, G., Schrader, B. & Behrend, M. (1993) Endothelial adhesion molecules in human liver grafts: overview on the differential expression of leukocyte ligand molecules. *Transplantation Proceedings* 25, 874–876.

Sterneck, M., Wiesner, R.H., Ascher, N. *et al.* (1991) Azathioprine toxicity after liver transplantation. *Hepatology* 14, 806–810.

Stone, B.G., Udani, M., Sanghvi, A. *et al.* (1987) Cyclosporin A-induced cholestasis. The mechanism in a rat model. *Gastroenterology* 93, 344–351.

Stovin, P.G.I. (1984) The morphology of myocardial rejection and transplant pathology. In: *Transplant Immunology, Clinical and Experimental* (ed. R.Y. Calne), pp. 78–100. Oxford University Press, Oxford.

Strasberg, S.M., Howard, T.K., Molmenti, E.P. & Hertl, M. (1994) Selecting the donor liver: risk factors for poor function after orthotopic liver transplantation. *Hepatology* 20, 829–838.

Strickler, J.G., Manivel, J.C., Copenhaver, C.D. & Kubic, V.L. (1990) Comparison of *in situ* hybridization and immunohistochemistry for the detection of cytomegalovirus and herpes simplex virus. *Human Pathology* 21, 443–448.

Stromeyer, F.W. & Ishak, K.G. (1981) Nodular transformation (nodular 'regenerative' hyperplasia) of the liver. A clinicopathological study of 30 cases. *Human Pathology* 12, 60–71.

Svoboda Newman, S.M., Greenson, J.K., Singleton, T.P., Sun, R. & Frank, T.S. (1997) Detection of hepatitis C by RT-PCR in formalin-fixed paraffin-embedded tissue from liver transplant patients. *Diagnoses in Molecular Pathology* 6, 123–129.

Syrakos, T.P., Wight, D.G.D., McMaster, P., Marni, A. & Alfani, D. (1979) Damage to the biliary tract during preservation. *Transplantation* 28, 166–171.

Tanaka, A., Tanaka, K., Kitai, T. *et al.* (1994a) Living related liver transplantation across ABO blood groups. *Transplantation* 58, 548–553.

Tanaka, K., Uemoto, S., Tokunaga, Y. *et al.* (1994b) Living related liver transplantation in children. *American Journal of Surgery* 168, 41–48.

Telenti, A., Smith, T.F., Ludwig, J. *et al.* (1991) Epstein–Barr virus and persistent graft dysfunction after liver transplantation. *Hepatology* 14, 282–286.

Terasaki, P.I. & Cecka, J.M. (eds) (1995) *Clinical Transplants 1994*. UCLA Tissue Typing Laboratory, Los Angeles.

Terpstra, O.T., Schalm, S.W., Weimar, W. *et al.* (1988) Auxiliary partial liver transplantation for end-stage chronic liver disease. *New England Journal of Medicine* 319, 1507–1511.

Thiru, S. (1984) The morphology of rejection of renal transplants. In: *Transplant Immunology, Clinical and Experimental* (ed. R.Y. Calne), pp. 9–52. Oxford University Press, Oxford.

Thomas, E.D., Storb, R., Clift, R.A. *et al.* (1975) Bone marrow transplantation. *New England Journal of Medicine* 292, 895–902.

Thung, S.N. & Gerber, M.A. (1991) Editorial. Histological features of allograft rejection: do you see what I see? *Hepatology* 14, 949–951.

Tillery, W., Demetris, J., Watkins, D. *et al.* (1989) Pathologic recognition of preservation injury in hepatic allografts with six months follow-up. *Transplantation Proceedings* 21, 1330–1331.

Tilney, N.L., Whitley, W.D., Diamond, J.R., Kupiec-Weglinski, J.W. & Adams, D.H. (1991) Chronic rejection: an undefined conundrum. *Transplantation* 52, 389–398.

Todo, S., Demetrius, A.J., Van Thiel, D.H. *et al.* (1991) Orthotopic liver transplantation for patients with hepatitis B virus-related disease. *Hepatology* 13, 619–626.

Trull, A.K., Facey, S.P., Rees, G.W. *et al.* (1994) Serum alpha-glutathione S-transferase—a sensitive marker of hepatocellular damage associated with acute liver allograft rejection. *Transplantation* 58, 1345–1351.

Tullius, S.G. & Tilney, N.L. (1995) Both alloantigen-dependent and -independent factors influence chronic allograft rejection. *Transplantation* 59, 313–318.

US Multicenter FK506 Liver Study Group. (1994) A comparison of tacrolimus (FK506) and cyclosporine for immunosuppression in liver transplantation. The US Multicenter FK506 Liver Study Group (see comments). *New England Journal of Medicine* 331, 1110–1115.

Valla, D., Casadevall, N., Lacombe, C. *et al.* (1985) Primary myeloproliferative disorder and hepatic vein thrombosis. A prospective study of erythroid colony formation *in vitro* in 20 patients with Budd–Chiari syndrome. *Annals of Internal Medicine* 103, 329–334.

Van Hoek, B., Wiesner, R.H., Krom, R.A.F., Ludwig, J. & Moore, S.B. (1992) Severe ductopenic rejection following liver transplantation: incidence, time of onset, risk factors, treatment and outcome. *Seminars in Liver Disease* 12, 41–50.

Van Thiel, D.H. & Gavaler, J.S. (1987) Recurrent disease in patients with liver transplantation: When does it occur and how can we be sure? *Hepatology* 7, 181–183.

Vargas, H.E., Laskus, T., Radkowski, M. *et al.* (1997) Hepatitis G virus coinfection in hepatitis C virus-infected liver transplant recipients. *Transplantation* 64, 786–788.

Wachs, M.E., Amend, W.J., Ascher, N.L. *et al.* (1995) The risk of transmission of hepatitis B from HBsAg(–), HBcAb(+), HBIgM(–) organ donors. *Transplantation* 59, 230–234.

Wade, J.J., Rolando, N., Hayllar, K. *et al.* (1995) Bacterial and fungal infections after liver transplantation: an analysis of 284 patients. *Hepatology* 21, 1328–1336.

Wallwork, J. (1994) Risk factors for chronic rejection in heart and lungs—why do hearts and lungs rot? *Clinical Transplantation* 8, 341–344.

Warren, R.E. (1984) Bacterial and fungal infections. In: *Transplant Immunology* (ed. R.Y. Calne), pp. 331–363. Oxford University Press, Oxford.

Weitz, H., Gokel, S.M., Loeschke, K., Possinger, K. & Eder, M. (1982) Venoocclusive disease of the liver in patients receiving immunosuppressive therpay. *Virchows Archives A* **395**, 245–256.

Wiesner, R.H., Ludwig, J., van Hoek, B. & Krom, R.A.F. (1991) Current concepts in cell-mediated hepatic allograft rejection leading to ductopenia and liver failure. *Hepatology* **14**, 721–729.

Wight, D.G.D. (1983) Pathology of liver transplantation. In: *Liver Transplantation* (ed. R.Y. Calne), pp. 247–277. Grune and Stratton, London.

Wight, D.G.D. (1984) The morphology of rejection of liver of liver transplants. In: *Transplant Immunology, Clinical and Experimental* (ed. R.Y. Calne), pp. 385–435. Oxford University Press, Oxford.

Wight, D.G.D. (1986) Differential diagnosis of cholestasis in liver allografts. *Transplantation Proceedings* **18**, 152–156.

Wight, D.G.D. (1989) Analysis of the pathological features of 40 cases of chronic liver transplant rejection. *Gut* **30**, A1500–A1501.

Wight, D.G.D. (1994a) Aspects of liver transplant pathology with emphasis on rejection and its mechanisms. *Journal of Clinical Pathology* **47**, 296–299.

Wight, D.G.D. (1994b) Development, anatomy, physiology, patterns ofjury. In: *Liver, Biliary Tract and Exocrine Pancreas*, Vol. 11 (ed. D.G.D. Wight), pp. 1–52. Churchill Livingstone, Edinburgh.

Wight, D.G.D. (1994c) The pathology of liver transplantation. In: *Liver, Biliary Tract and Exocrine Pancreas*, Vol. 11 (ed. D.G.D. Wight), pp. 543–596. Churchill Livingstone, Edinburgh.

Wight, D.G.D. (1996) Chronic liver transplant rejection: definition and diagnosis. *Transplantation Proceedings* **28**, 465–467.

Wight, D.G.D. & Portmann, B. (1987) Pathology of rejection. In: *Liver Transplantation* (ed. R.Y. Calne), pp. 385–435. Grune and Stratton, London.

Wilkinson, A.H., Smith, J.L., Hunsicker, L.G. *et al.* (1989) Increased frequence of posttransplant lymphomas in patients treated with cyclosporine, azathioprine and prednisolone. *Transplantation* **47**, 293–296.

Willemse, P.J.A., Ausema, L., Terpstra, O.T. *et al.* (1992) Graft regeneration and host liver atrophy after auxiliary heterotopic liver transplantation for chronic liver failure. *Hepatology* **15**, 54–57.

Williams, J.W., Peters, T.G., Vera, S. *et al.* (1985) Biopsy directed immunosuppression following hepatic transplantation. *Transplantation* **39**, 589–596.

Williams, J.W., Foster, P.F. & Sankary, H.N. (1992) Role of liver allograft biopsy in patient management. *Seminars in Liver Disease* **12**, 60–72.

Williams, R. & Wendon, J. (1994) Indications for orthotopic liver transplantation in fulminant liver failure. *Hepatology* **20**, 5S–10S.

Williams, R., Smith, M., Shilkin, K.B. *et al.* (1973) Liver transplantation in man: the frequency of rejection, biliary tract complications, and recurrence of malignancy based on an analysis of 26 cases. *Gastroenterology* **64**, 1026–1048.

Winston, D.J., Ho, W.G., Howell, C.L. *et al.* (1980) Cytomegalovirus infections associated with leucocyte transfusions. *Annals of Internal Medicine* **93**, 671–675.

Wisecaver, J.L., Radio, S.J., Shaw, B.W. Jr, Langnas, A.N. & Markin, R.S. (1994) Intrahepatic arteriopathy associated with primary nonfunction of liver allografts. *Human Pathology* **25**, 960–963.

Wood, K.J., Hopley, A., Dallman, M.J. & Morris, P.J. (1988) Lack of correlation between the induction of donor class I and class II major histocompatibility antigens and graft rejection. *Transplantation* **45**, 759–767.

Wreghitt, T.G. (1987) Viral and *Toxoplasma gondii* infections. In: *Liver Transplantation* (ed. R. Calne), pp. 365–383. Grune and Stratton, London.

Wreghitt, T.G. & Hakim, M. (1989) Donor-transmitted disease. In: *Heart and Heart-Lung Transplantation* (ed. J. Wallwork), pp. 341–358. W.B. Saunders, London.

Wright, H.L., Bou Abboud, C.F., Hassanein, T. *et al.* (1992a) Disease recurrence and rejection following liver transplantation for autoimmune chronic active liver disease. *Transplantation* **53**, 136–139.

Wright, T.L., Donegan, E., Hsu, H.H. *et al.* (1992b) Recurrent and acquired hepatitis C viral infection in liver transplant recipients. *Gastroenterology* **103**, 317–322.

Yanaga, K., Makowka, L. & Starzl, T.E. (1989) Is hepatic artery thrombosis after liver transplantation really a surgical complication? *Transplantation Proceedings* **21**, 3511–3513.

Yoffe, B., Burns, D.K., Bhatt, H.S. *et al.* (1990) Extrahepatic B virus DNA sequences in patients with acute hepatitis B infection. *Hepatology* **12**, 187–192.

Yoshida, E.M., Shackleton, C.R., Erb, S.R. *et al.* (1996) Late acute rejection occurring in liver allograft recipients. *Canadian Journal of Gastroenterology* **10**, 376–380.

# Chapter 10/Heart transplantation

NATHANIEL CARY

## Introduction

Orthotopic heart transplantation has become widely established as a treatment for end-stage cardiac failure, mainly resulting from ischaemic heart disease or dilated cardiomyopathy (Schofield 1991). Heterotopic heart transplantation is generally a less satisfactory procedure though may be indicated in cases where a raised pulmonary vascular resistance is a contraindication for orthotopic transplantation. In 1996 the International Society for Heart and Lung Transplantation (ISHLT) registry (Hosenpud *et al.* 1996) shows 34 326 heart transplantations worldwide from 271 centres and 1567 combined heart–lung transplantation from 105 centres. Donor organ availability greatly restricts the number of cardiac transplants that can be performed and consequently the potential pool of patients who would benefit from cardiac transplant greatly exceeds the number of organs that become available. Long-term survival following transplant is principally limited by the development of graft vascular disease (Mullins *et al.* 1992). In the first few months the inability to control the immune system effectively is manifested by deaths caused by rejection and/or oppor-

tunistic infection, though with considerable improvements in immunosuppression regimens and post-transplant management these are becoming much less common.

## Rejection in the heart

The immunopathology of rejection of solid organ grafts is complicated and incompletely understood. The heart is no exception, with humoral as well as cellular mechanisms likely to be involved. The basic immunological phenomena are covered elsewhere. This section will deal with the morphology of rejection in cardiac allografts.

Right ventricular endomyocardial biopsy, as originally described by Caves *et al.* (1973), remains the mainstay in the monitoring of cardiac allograft recipients for the presence of rejection. Grading systems for rejection, of which there are many (Billingham 1989), are mainly focused on lymphocytic infiltrates in the myocardium, in terms of both their intensity and what they are doing, e.g. damaging myocytes. This recognizes the key role of acute cellular rejection as a potential factor which may ultimately result in clinically significant graft malfunction: acute dysrhythmia or heart failure. Some have emphasized the importance of humoral mechanisms, advocating staining for antibodies and complement in biopsies (Hammond *et al.* 1989). However, it must be remembered that many humoral phenomena ultimately lead to cellular infiltration and consequently a proportion of the cellular infiltrate assessed in biopsies may well be the end result of such phenomena. From a practical point of view it is the author's experience that severe cardiac malfunction related to rejection is very unlikely without a significant myocardial cellular infiltrate at some stage (hyperacute rejection excepted). Biopsies may be seen that are 'clear' of infiltrate in the face of poor cardiac function. These tend to be in complex cases, often with repeated rejection episodes, where enhanced immunosuppression has been given recently. Any lymphocytic infiltrate has thus been eliminated, having already done its damage, much of which may not be histologically manifest though functionally important. The finding of complement and immunoglobulin deposits in biopsies from such cases does not make them examples of predominant humoral rejection, as such deposits may equally be seen in 'clear' biopsies from patients who are clinically well. Reports in the literature on the usefulness of such investigations are conflicting (Hammond *et al.* 1989; Bonnaud *et al.* 1995; Lones *et al.* 1995).

In the grading of cardiac rejection it is fortunate that there are very few differential diagnoses to consider as a cause for lymphocytic infiltration of the transplanted heart. The main differential diagnoses to consider are toxoplasma myocarditis, cytomegalovirus (CMV) myocarditis and lymphoproliferative disease. These are all dealt with below. In brief, toxoplasma myocarditis is now very seldom encountered as a result of pyremethamine or co-trimoxazole prophylaxis in mismatches; CMV myocarditis appears to be rare despite the relatively high incidence of CMV infections in this transplant population; and lymphoproliferative disease may be recognized by the clinical setting and the atypical nature of the lymphocytic infiltrate.

At the instigation of the International Society of Heart Transplantation (ISHT), a grading system for cardiac rejection was devised in 1990 (Billingham *et al.*

1990). The purpose of the grading system was to produce a standardized means of conveying the histological features seen in post-transplant endomyocardial biopsies. Therefore there are not only precise definitions of the various grades of rejection but also quite specific requirements for adequacy of the specimen and technical aspects of histological examination, e.g. number of levels examined. This standardization enables comparison of results between different centres and, perhaps more importantly as new immunosuppressive agents are developed, it allows for multicentre drug trials.

The group which met to produce the standardized grading system all came from large centres with long-standing experience of endomyocardial biopsies in post-transplant patients. It was proposed to reconvene in the light of experience of the 1990 grading system and in December 1994 most of the previous group reassembled at Stanford University Medical Center. The aim on this occasion was to modify the grading system where required, while at the same time not to alter it so much as to make a new system incompatible with the 1990 system, which had come into widespread use worldwide. In 1994 the members of the group not only applied their own experience but also that of others around the world, both through personal communication prior to the meeting and through knowledge of the published literature.

The proposed modified version of the grading system for cardiac biopsies is illustrated in Table 10.1, with the 1990 system alongside for comparison. As the 1990 grading system is currently in widespread use the following discussion will incorporate both its histological features and any proposed changes. To date, the modified grading system has not been adopted by the ISHLT. However, whether or not it is ultimately adopted it is the opinion of those who devised it that it represents a sensible progression from the 1990 system which others may wish to adopt in their own centres.

## Adequacy of biopsy sampling

As grading is based on the worst changes present in a biopsy set and cellular rejection is frequently a focal process it is crucial that adequate amounts of tissue are

**Table 10.1** The ISHLT grading of cardiac rejection (1990).

| Old terms | Grades | Notes | Proposed simplification (1994) |
|---|---|---|---|
| No rejection | 0 | Biopsies with very sparse lymphoid infiltrates should be included in this grade | Grade 1 |
| Mild rejection | 1A | Focal perivascular or interstitial infiltrates. The mild intensity and lack of myocyte damage distinguish this from higher grades | |
| | 1B | Diffuse but sparse infiltrate. As with 1A, there must be no myocyte damage | |
| Focal moderate rejection | 2 | One focus only with aggressive infiltration and/or focal myocyte damage. The choice of a single focus as the cut-off from higher grades is arbitrary. In practice, with the amount of tissue usually submitted, one is unlikely to be faced with the problem of biopsy fragments with only two foci | |
| ------------------ | ------ | *Usual treatment threshold* ------------------ | ------------------ |
| Low moderate rejection | 3A | Multifocal aggressive infiltrates and/or myocyte damage. The multiple foci may be present in only one fragment or may be scattered throughout several fragments | Grade 3A |
| | 3B | Diffuse inflammatory process. The intensity of the lymphoid infiltrate varies considerable. It may be little more than 1B, the important feature distinguishing it being the presence of myocyte damage. This damage must be present in least two fragments, but some degree of infiltration is present in most fragments | Grade 3B |
| Severe acute rejection | 4 | A diffuse and polymorphous infiltrate with or without oedema, haemorrhage and vasculitis. The infiltrate is more intense and more widespread than 3B and myocyte damage is conspicuous. There are often neutrophils and/or haemorrhage, though neither is essential for diagnosis of this grade | Grade 4 |

examined to exclude the presence of clinically significant rejection. As a minimum requirement for grading, four biopsy fragments are required. At least 50% of each fragment must be free from fibrosis or biopsy site change. In order to achieve this number of gradable biopsy fragments, it is advisable to take a minimum of six fragments at a biopsy session as ungradable fragments mainly or entirely composed of epicardial tissue are frequently encountered but may be difficult to recognize grossly by the person performing the biopsies. The choice of four fragments of myocardium as a minimum for grading purposes was largely based on the practical experiences of those formulating the grading system. Zerbe and Arena (1988), using autopsy-derived material, showed the potential role of fragment number in establishing an overall rejection grade. However, autopsy-derived material showing

rejection is already self-selected and the pattern of rejection present may not represent that present in the overall heart transplant population at endomyocardial biopsy. In particular, focal areas of rejection—a frequent phenomenon in biopsies—may be relatively unrepresented in autopsy material.

Subsequently, Sharples *et al.* (1992) have demonstrated a statistical basis for choosing four fragments as a minimum to establish the 'true' grade of rejection present in a biopsy set using endomyocardial biopsy material. When less than four assessable fragments are obtained, however, some useful evaluation is usually possible. If all fragments are entirely free of infiltrate then significant underlying rejection is unlikely, though it cannot be entirely excluded. However, in some instances, e.g. when ≥3 fragments show infiltrates indicative of mild rejection (grade 1), there is a significant risk of missing higher-grade rejection and in these cases rebiopsy or empirical treatment may be justified. This dilemma, which is relatively unusual, can be avoided if more than four fragments are obtained as a matter of routine. Clearly clinically significant rejection, i.e. grade 3A or 3B may be manifest in less than four fragments. Although technically a grade cannot be ascribed, the biopsy nevertheless provides the necessary information to justify the giving of enhanced immunosuppression.

## Technical considerations

As a routine it is recommended that biopsies should be fixed in 10% neutral buffered formalin and paraffin-processed. Sections are then cut at a minimum of three levels through the block with a minimum of three sections at each level stained routinely with haematoxylin and eosin. Other fixatives may be used, as may plastic embedding. The key feature is that an adequate area of tissue is examined as this is as relevant from a sampling point of view as the number of fragments obtained. At Papworth this minimal requirement is exceeded significantly. Every endomyocardial biopsy is serial-sectioned to produce 10 slides with a ribbon of five or six sections on each slide. Alternate slides are then stained with haematoxylin and eosin and the remainder are stored. Thus the biopsies are examined at five levels with five or six sections at each level. Special stains, such as trichrome for connective tissue, may be employed but in the 1994 recommendations this was not considered to be mandatory for every biopsy. Additional fragments may be snap-frozen for immunofluorescence or other purposes or processed for electron microscopy, though neither is necessary for routine patient management.

## Grading of rejection

The ISHT grading system (1990) and the proposed revised version are essentially an extension of the original Billingham criteria (Billingham *et al.* 1990). The critical factor is what constitutes moderate rejection. This is not simply the identification of myocyte necrosis. Indeed, immunological attack of myocytes is more likely to be manifest as the less conspicuous process of

apoptosis. To diagnose moderate rejection there needs to be a combination of both intensity of mononuclear cell infiltrate and a tendency of it to encroach on and, by inference, replace myocytes. Evidence of myocyte damage is therefore essentially circumstantial in many instances. Useful histological features in assessing this encroachment are the tendency of the infiltrate to surround myocytes entirely, with indentation and overlapping of their cytoplasm, and a tendency to persist in adjacent sections and in levels through a biopsy set.

The various grades of rejection represent histological entities and it is not clear whether cellular rejection proceeds through several grades and whether diffuse and focal rejection are different processes. Treatment thresholds for the various histological grades of rejection may vary between different centres. However, cases of grade 3 rejection—whether A or B—will generally be automatically treated with enhanced immunosuppression even if diagnosed in an apparently stable clinical situation, e.g. routine follow-up biopsy. Examples of the various grades of rejection are illustrated in Figs 10.1–10.9.

## The 1990 ISHLT grading system and proposed modifications — rejection grades

### Grade 0

This grade is used for biopsies showing no evidence of rejection or its associated damage. In practice, biopsies showing a few small, randomly scattered foci of mononuclear cells should be graded as 0 (Fig. 10.1). Swollen endothelial cell nuclei and nuclei of interstitial cells may give the false impression of a diffuse sparse inflammatory infiltrate. Biopsies showing infiltrates confined to intramyocardial or epicardial fat or scar related to previous biopsy sites should also be graded as 0.

### Grades 1A and 1B

Grades 1A and 1B represent mild focal and diffuse mononuclear cell infiltration, respectively. In grade 1A the infiltrate is sparse, not associated with myocyte

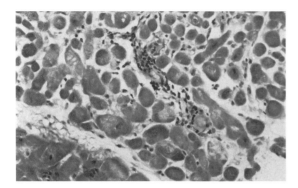

**Fig. 10.1** Grade 0 rejection. Biopsies showing very small collections of mononuclear cells such as that present around a small vessel here should be included in this grade.

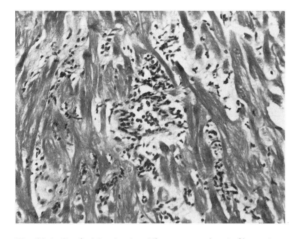

**Fig. 10.2** Grade 1A rejection. The mononuclear infiltrate is centred on a small intramyocardial vessel. Scattered cells are spreading out into the interstitial tissue of the surrounding myocardium. However, there is no tendency for the infiltrate to replace and, by implication, damage myocytes, features which are indicative of moderate rejection.

damage as described above and usually perivascular in distribution (Fig. 10.2). In grade 1B the infiltrate is more diffuse, extending into the interstitium between myocytes but not obviously encroaching on or replacing myocytes (Fig. 10.3). In terms of the total area of myocardial tissue examined in a biopsy set, grade 1B is still a relatively focal process and in a significant proportion the myocardium may show little, if any, infil-

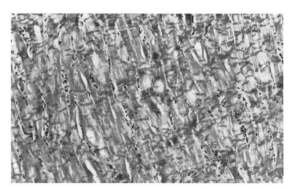

**Fig. 10.3** Grade 1B rejection. Diffuse predominantly interstitial infiltrate which has neither the intensity nor the tendency to replace myocytes as seen in moderate rejection.

trate. Experience has shown that these two different patterns, which essentially represent a continuum, do not appear to have different outcomes (Riseq *et al.* 1994). Apart from higher grades of rejection the main differential diagnoses to consider are inflammatory infiltrates associated with previous biopsy site or peri-transplant injury; the former usually becomes apparent in serial sections and the latter is distinguished by the prominence of myocyte damage compared to the inflammatory infiltrate.

## Grade 2

Grade 2 represents a single focus of moderate rejection amongst the whole biopsy set (Fig. 10.4). This grade has been the most problematic area of the 1990 grading system. Nevertheless, the recognition of the features of grade 2 rejection as an entity was one of the strengths of the 1990 system. Compared to the previous Billingham criteria this clearly distinguished a form of focal moderate rejection which generally did not need enhanced immunosuppression, thus potentially reducing the overall load of immunosuppression.

The 1990 system has been in use at Papworth since its inception and during this period there have been no examples of sudden death following untreated grade 2 rejection, supporting the concept that this degree of moderate rejection is generally clinically insignificant. In establishing grade 2 rejection as an entity the choice

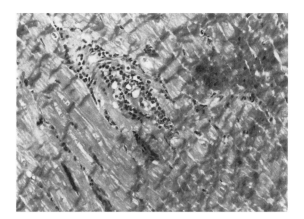

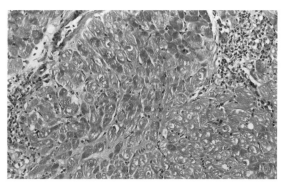

Fig. 10.5 Grade 3A rejection. Multiple foci of moderate rejection were present in this biopsy set. Fortuitously for the purpose of illustration two foci fulfilling the criteria for moderate grade are present in this single field (top right and bottom left).

Fig. 10.4 Grade 2 rejection. Single focus of moderate rejection amongst all the biopsy fragments and serial sections examined. This is a small focus. Nevertheless, in terms of both intensity of mononuclear infiltrate and its tendency to replace myocytes it fulfils the criteria for moderate rejection.

of one focus of moderate rejection in an average biopsy set was an arbitrary one. In practice, though, it is unusual to encounter borderline cases with only two foci and most cases diagnosed as 3A rejection, the next grade up, have several foci. The benign nature of this grade has also been the experience of others (Riseq *et al.* 1994; Winters *et al.* 1995). A recent study suggests that in fact many apparent cases of grade 2 rejection actually represent tangentially sectioned encroaching endocardial infiltrates (Fishbein *et al.* 1994). Clearly, the less sectioning that biopsies are subjected to, the more likely it is that the true endocardial nature of an infiltrate will be missed. However, at Papworth, where endomyocardial biopsies are routinely serial-sectioned, there does appear to be a genuine entity of a single focus of moderate-grade rejection in the deep myocardium, as multiple sections both above and below such foci fail to demonstrate any endocardial connection.

Given that there is now considerable experience of the benign nature of grade 2 rejection, there seems little point from a patient management point of view in continuing to separate off the histological entity of a single focus of myocyte damage associated with myocardial inflammatory infiltrate from grades 1A and 1B or these

different patterns of mild rejection from one another. This was the consensus view at the meeting of pathologists at Stanford University in December 1994.

A new grade 1 rejection is therefore proposed, representing a mild perivascular or interstitial mononuclear cell infiltrate which may be focal or diffuse and may involve any number of the biopsy fragments with up to one focus of myocyte damage associated with infiltrate, i.e. one focus which would otherwise fulfil the criteria of a focus of 'moderate' rejection.

## Grade 3A

This grade is characterized by multiple foci of mononuclear inflammatory cell infiltration, with two or more of the foci associated with myocyte damage as defined on p. 303 (Figs 10.5 and 10.6). The foci may be spread amongst the biopsy fragments or may all be present in one fragment. There may be other foci of mild-grade rejection either in the same fragments or in others.

The presence of widespread intervening uninvolved myocardium helps to distinguish this grade from 3B. Apart from the presence of myocyte damage, the intensity of infiltrate helps to distinguish this from mild-grade rejection. Other differential diagnoses to consider are previous biopsy site and encroaching

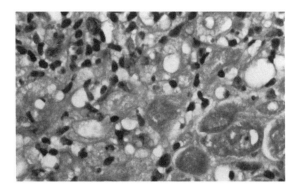

**Fig. 10.6** Grade 3A rejection. High-power view of one of the foci of moderate rejection from the case illustrated in Fig. 10.5. The mononuclear infiltrate is replacing myocyte cytoplasm and myocyte nuclei appear admixed with the infiltrating cells.

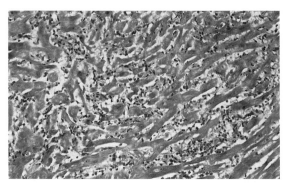

**Fig. 10.7** Grade 3B rejection. Compared to Fig. 10.3 the mononuclear infiltrate is both more intense and is associated with myocyte damage. This latter feature is seen towards the lower right side of the field.

Quilty lesions (see p. 307), both of which usually become apparent on serial sections. Infectious conditions, such as toxoplasmosis and CMV myocarditis, both of which are rare, are distinguished by their specific morphological features and the presence of a mixed inflammatory infiltrate. Eosinophils are often seen amongst the rejection infiltrate. However, their presence is not mandatory for designation of this grade of rejection.

### Grade 3B

There is a diffuse mononuclear inflammatory cell infiltrate involving most of the biopsy fragments, with associated myocyte damage in at least two of the fragments and often in all those showing infiltrate (Fig. 10.7). Eosinophils and neutrophils may be present, though neither are required to diagnose this grade. Some haemorrhage may be seen. The differential diagnosis includes diffuse mild rejection, which is less intense, tends to involve fewer fragments and should not be associated with significant myocyte damage. However, problems can arise in patients already treated with some enhanced immunosuppression, particularly if biopsies are within the first few weeks post-transplant, where there may be superimposed resolving myocyte damage from peritransplant injury.

Thus, although the rejection grades are purely histological, it is important that the pathologist is aware of the clinical circumstances to avoid possible misinterpretation of changes such as these, which may be present in biopsies. Infectious conditions may be confused with this grade but are usually more focal and mainly need to be differentiated from grade 3A.

### Grade 4

This grade is rare (Fig. 10.8). It represents the upper end of the spectrum of the changes seen in grade 3B, being more intense and more widespread in a biopsy set. All biopsy fragments should be involved by the inflammatory process, though it may be more intense in some than others. The infiltrate is polymorphous, with both eosinophils and neutrophils present. Oedema and haemorrhage are frequently, though not invariably, present and small intramyocardial vessels usually show a destructive vasculitis. Partial treatment with enhanced immunosuppression prior to biopsy may modify the infiltrate somewhat, making oedema and haemorrhage more conspicuous. Inflammatory granulation tissue from recent previous biopsy may be confused with this grade but usually becomes obvious in serial sections and is very unlikely to involve all the fragments. Areas of infarction should also be distinguished

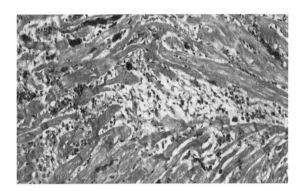

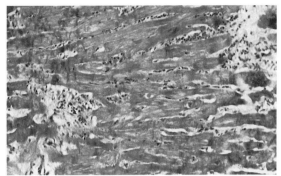

**Fig. 10.8** Grade 4 rejection. There is a diffuse infiltrate which involves all fragments and includes neutrophils. In this field there is severe oedema, most apparent centrally. Haemorrhage, seen as dark areas, is present towards the upper left side of the field. Myocyte damage is widespread. In this field it is best seen towards the lower left side.

**Fig. 10.9** Resolving grade 3A rejection. There are two foci of myocyte loss (bottom left and top right), associated with sparse mononuclear infiltrate. There is no active myocyte damage in terms of a more intense infiltrate replacing viable-looking myocytes. This would be graded as 1A. Some resolution would be implied if the previous grade had been 3A and these biopsies followed treatment with enhanced immunosuppression.

from this grade. Here frank myocyte necrosis is usually much more extensive than the inflammatory infiltrates. Infection is unlikely to produce such diffuse changes.

### Resolving and resolved rejection

As there are no reliable specific features to indicate resolving or resolved rejection, biopsies taken soon after treated rejection are much better dealt with by grading using the usual histological criteria. In this case, resolving rejection is implied by the presence of a grade lower than that seen previously (Fig. 10.9) and resolved rejection is indicated by grade 0.

### Clinical context of the rejection grades

If adequate biopsies show grades 0, 1A, 1B or 2 rejection, then any symptoms or signs referable to the cardiovascular system are highly unlikely to be a result of cellular rejection. Grade 3A rejection frequently causes little in the way of signs or symptoms, though minor enlargement of the cardiac silhouette on chest X-ray or atrial dysrhythmias may be seen. Less frequently, the usual signs and symptoms of heart failure may be seen. However, this grade is often discovered on

routine biopsy in an asymptomatic patient. Grades 3B and 4 are most likely to be associated with features of heart failure, though the former is by no means invariably so.

## Additional features in the biopsy

In grading biopsies, assessment is also made in relation to endocardial lymphoid infiltrates, ischaemic injury, the possibility that changes are caused by infection and the presence of lymphoproliferative disease. Examples of these are illustrated in Figs 10.10–10.14.

### Endocardial infiltrates

In the 1990 ISHLT grading system the presence of endocardial lymphoid infiltrates is recorded and whether they encroach on underlying myocardium (Figs 10.10 and 10.11). The significance of these infiltrates, which may be very florid, as in the Quilty lesions first described by Billingham (Joshi *et al.* 1995), is not clear. Moderate rejection in the deep myocardium is almost always accompanied by a degree of endocardial lymphoid infiltration, suggesting that it is an integral part of the cellular rejection process. On the other

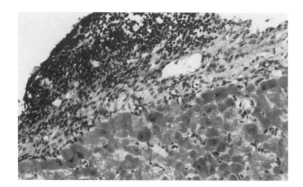

**Fig. 10.10** Small non-encroaching endocardial infiltrates such as that present here are common in post-transplant biopsies.

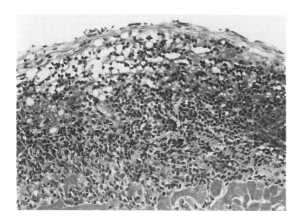

**Fig. 10.11** Encroaching endocardial infiltrate. Towards the lower part of the field the mononuclear infiltrate is replacing myocytes and myocyte nuclei can be seen intimately admixed. These features, which imply myocyte damage, should not be taken to indicate moderate rejection in this context.

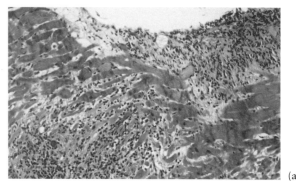

(a)

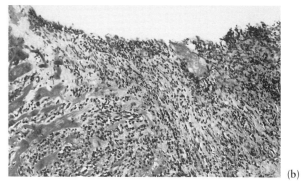

(b)

**Fig. 10.12** (a) In the bottom left side of the field there appears to be a large area of mononuclear infiltrate associated with myocyte damage in deep myocardium and apparently separate from an overlying endocardial infiltrate. (b) Deeper serial sections, however, reveal the true encroaching endocardial nature of this deeper infiltrate, which should not be confused with moderate rejection.

hand, biopsies may be encountered with florid endocardial lymphoid infiltration and underlying myocardial encroachment and damage but with no evidence of infiltration or damage in the deeper myocardium. Experience has shown that this type of lesion can safely be ignored and does not warrant enhancement of immunosuppression. Morphologically these lesions can cause problems as they may on occasion be sectioned tangentially and therefore appear to be foci of moderate rejection in the deep myocardium, which

could lead to an erroneous diagnosis of significant rejection. Cutting of multiple serial sections helps to resolve this problem as such foci will usually be recognized for what they are in deeper or more superficial levels through the biopsy (Fig. 10.12). Nevertheless, some cases graded as showing rejection may actually only have endocardial infiltrates. This possibility particularly applies to occasional cases of what appears to be grade 2 rejection in the 1990 grading system in an otherwise 'clean' biopsy set. This problem has been addressed by Fishbein *et al.* (1994).

The cellular composition of endocardial infiltrates varies. In association with myocardial rejection these infiltrates generally show a similar mixture of cells to that present in the deep myocardium, i.e. lymphocytes of various sizes and maturity together with macrophages and, in some cases, eosinophils. Some of the more florid examples of endocardial lymphoid infiltration seen in the absence of significant myocardial rejection may show conspicuous plasma cells and there may be dilated blood-vessels with high endothelium. Some pleomorphism and atypia of lymphocytes may be seen but when these are marked the possibility of endocardial involvement by lymphoproliferative disease should be considered (see p. 314).

Epstein–Barr virus (EBV) has been implicated in the aetiology of endocardial lymphoid infiltration (Kemmitz & Cohnert 1988). However, the study concerned used the polymerase chain reaction (PCR) to detect EBV genome and it is probable that this highly sensitive method was simply detecting infected 'passenger' B cell clones expanded by cyclosporin A therapy. Subsequent *in situ* hybridization studies have failed to detect EBV genomic sequences in endocardial lymphoid infiltrate (Nakhleh *et al.* 1991). Forbes *et al.* (1990) have suggested that endocardial lymphoid infiltrates in the absence of manifestations of cellular rejection in deep myocardium may be a low-grade form of allograft rejection, possibly reflecting fluctuating cyclosporin A levels.

Long-term studies (Joshi *et al.* 1995) suggest that there is no prognostic difference between cases showing encroaching endocardial infiltrates (Quilty A) and those that do not encroach (Quilty B) and therefore in the proposed 1994 simplified grading system it is suggested that these two forms of endocardial infiltrate do not need to be separated.

## Hyperacute rejection

This is very rarely seen and results in rapid rejection of the cardiac allograft within minutes of reperfusion. Rejection is a result of the presence of preformed complement-fixing antibodies. Histologically there is widespread myocardial haemorrhage and fragmentation, with microvascular thrombosis. Antibody and complement factors are demonstrable within the myocardium. Both the haemorrhagic and thrombotic manifestations are caused by complement activation with associated endothelial cell activation and platelet aggregation. Because of its rarity hyperacute rejection is not incorporated into the ISHLT grading system.

## Ischaemic injury

Early post-transplant evidence of ischaemic injury is frequently seen in biopsies in the form of small foci of myocytolysis, usually subendocardially (Fig. 10.13). As the exact nature of the insult is often not clear, these changes are probably best described under the broad term of peritransplant injury. Catecholamine-related myocyte injury may occur in the donor as a result of endogenous release, e.g. in head injury, subarachnoid haemorrhage or as a result of exogenous administration for donor cardiovascular support. Such injury may also occur post-transplant if catecholamines are administered. Donor organ preservation and reperfusion essentially produce similar histological changes. The myocyte damage is distinguished from rejection-related damage by the relative disproportion of damage compared to the extent of cellular infiltrate, which is usually minimal. However, as lesions resolve, some macrophage infiltration may be seen and the knowledge that biopsies are early post-transplant as well as the tendency of lesions to be subendocardial

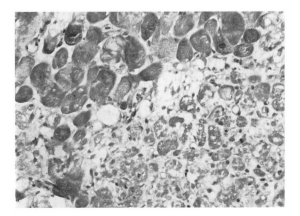

**Fig. 10.13** Peritransplant injury. Pale dead and dying myocytes with little, if any, infiltrate characterize this lesion. In this case the features are particularly florid. Often changes will involve only scattered adjacent myocytes.

generally helps to distinguish this from significant rejection. The changes may persist for some weeks post-transplant and in some instances have a tendency to calcify. Later on, various manifestations of ischaemic injury proceeding to frank infarction may be seen in association with graft vascular occlusive disease.

## Infection

Compared to lung transplants, the possibility that inflammatory infiltrates in the heart are caused by infection is relatively unlikely, particularly with matching and prophylaxis for *Toxoplasma*. Nevertheless, myocarditis as a manifestation of infections, including disseminated *Aspergillus* infection, CMV disease or some other infection, should always be considered and knowledge of the clinical status of the patient allows such possibilities to be addressed. In one patient at Papworth, septic cardiac mural thrombus seen in biopsies associated with a giant-cell reaction was a manifestation of *Nocardia* infection, readily demonstrable in the biopsies by Gram-staining.

## Opportunistic infection

### Toxoplasmosis

*Toxoplasma gondii* is a coccidian parasite which in the non-immunosuppressed is usually associated with asymptomatic infection or, in some cases, a glandular fever-like illness. In the immunosuppressed it may produce more serious and, in some instances, life-threatening infections and these are well recognized in those infected with HIV as well as transplant recipients. In the latter the organism may be acquired from the donor organ and this is particularly a feature of heart transplant recipients compared to recipients of other solid organ grafts, reflecting the fact that cardiac muscle is an important reservoir of infection in antibody-positive donors (Wreghitt *et al.* 1989).

Prior to the introduction of pyremethamine prophylaxis, the incidence of donor-acquired infection in mismatches, i.e. *Toxoplasma gondii* antibody-negative recipients of grafts from antibody-positive donors, has been reported as 57% in heart recipients compared to

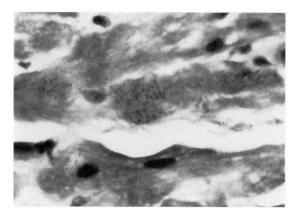

**Fig. 10.14** *Toxoplasma* cyst, donor-acquired *Toxoplasma* infection.

20% in liver and <1% in kidney recipients (Wreghitt *et al.* 1989). Infection in these circumstances is serious and may be fatal. Myocardial involvement is an important feature, with cysts demonstrable in biopsy or autopsy material (Fig. 10.14). Pneumonitis and encephalitis may also be present.

Pyremethamine prophylaxis and, more recently, co-trimoxazole prophylaxis have considerably reduced the incidence of primary donor-acquired toxoplasmosis and, furthermore, those who develop it do so much later with little, if any, morbidity. This has largely obviated the need to exclude *Toxoplasma* infection in post-transplant endomyocardial biopsy specimens. This is fortunate as the *Toxoplasma* cysts tend to be few and far between and may easily be overlooked. In addition, areas of inflammation caused by infection are difficult to differentiate from cellular rejection as they tend to be spatially separate from the cysts, presumably because they only occur when the cysts have ruptured and individual organisms are no longer identifiable as such.

The *Toxoplasma* genome can be detected in biopsy material in cases of active primary *Toxoplasma* infection with a sensitivity equal to or greater than conventional hisopathological analysis (Holliman *et al.* 1992) and this may in the future prove to be the method of choice in establishing a tissue diagnosis of *Toxoplasma* myocarditis on small biopsy material. Heart transplant recipients who were *Toxoplasma gondii* antibody-positive prior to transplant may rarely develop recrudescence of *Toxoplasma* infection (Wreghitt *et al.* 1989). In the Papworth series this was seen in only three of 75 patients and in these the clinical features were generally milder than in primary infection and in no case fatal. *Toxoplasma* cysts were not seen in endomyocardial biopsy material either before or during infection suggesting that myocardial involvement was minimal or absent.

## Cytomegalovirus infection

This virus is a significant cause of morbidity and mortality amongst heart and combined heart–lung transplant recipients. The most serious infections occur in those mismatched for CMV, that is antibody-negative recipients of organs from antibody-positive donors. Furthermore, the primary infection that results from such mismatches is generally more severe than that acquired from other sources, e.g. blood products.

Cytomegalovirus infection usually occurs 4–8 weeks post-transplant and is characterized by multisystem involvement. Fever and leucopenia are frequent manifestations. Pneumonitis is seen in some cases and may be fatal. Myocarditis is uncommon both in the transplant setting and in sporadic cases in apparently healthy individuals. Amongst renal transplant recipients Baandrup and Mortensen (1984) found evidence of CMV myocarditis in terms of the presence of both inflammatory infiltration and associated CMV inclusions in only one out of 16 fatal cases of primary CMV infection. This was in spite of the fact that cardiovascular manifestations were common in this group. Amongst heart transplant recipients evidence of CMV myocarditis has been seen in only one out of 2249 endomyocardial biopsies at Papworth during a 3-year period despite the fact that many more patients were known to be suffering from active CMV infection at the time of biopsy. One potential area for confusion is the possibility of CMV infection causing a myocardial lymphocytic infiltrate in the allograft, which, in the absence of classic inclusions, would be interpreted as rejection. Stovin *et al.* (1989) showed that this was unlikely to be a significant factor, on the basis that there is no evidence of increased cellular infiltration in endomyocardial biopsies taken at the time of active primary CMV infection compared to a control group who did not develop CMV. Even when the CMV genome is specifically sought in the myocardium using *in situ* hybridization and immunohistochemistry in those showing evidence of severe infection elsewhere, myocardial involvement appears to be rare (Bruneval *et al.* 1992). Furthermore, when it occurs it is probably more a manifestation of the systemic nature of CMV infection than an indicator of true cardiac disease, with only occasional infected cells and no significant degree of myocarditis.

## Chronic rejection and graft vascular disease

Several features of the long-term transplanted heart may be manifestations of chronic rejection. Endocardial lymphoid infiltrates have already been discussed. Other chronic changes which should be considered are cardiomegaly, the long-term sequelae of repeated acute rejection episodes and graft vascular disease.

Cardiomegaly is an almost invariable feature of the long-term transplanted heart and appears to develop before clinically significant graft vascular disease (Rowan & Billingham 1990). In combination with the latter it is a potential contributory factor in sudden cardiac death. It does not appear to be related to ischaemic time or immunosuppression regimen. Hypertension, common in post-heart-transplant patients, may contribute to hypertrophy, particularly of the left ventricle.

The long-term effects of acute rejection are difficult to quantify, although both endocardial and interstitial fibrosis is seen in hearts that have been subject to repeated episodes of cellular rejection. Relatively small amounts of fibrosis may stiffen the ventricular muscle and therefore impair function. The frequency of this is undetermined as this form of damage often coexists with graft vascular disease. However, cases are encountered where ventricular function appears impaired in the face of apparently normal or minimally abnormal coronary angiography, although the latter is insensitive for small-vessel occlusive disease.

Graft vascular disease is the principal manifestation of chronic rejection in the transplanted heart and remains the main factor limiting long-term survival. Detailed angiographic criteria exist for diagnosis in life. At Papworth Hospital the angiographic prevalence of graft vascular disease in 193 orthotopic heart transplant recipients studied was 3% and 40% at 1 and 5 years, respectively (Mullins *et al.* 1992). Nitkin *et al.* (1985) have reported a similar angiographic incidence of 40% at 5 years post-transplant.

There are many misconceptions in relation to post-transplant coronary graft vascular disease, at least some of which are related to misconceptions about atherosclerosis. The principal differences compared to native atherosclerosis are first the rate of progression and, secondly, the diffuseness of the disease process throughout the arterial tree, with small epicardial arteries conspicuously involved. The concentric nature of occlusive lesions has been overemphasized as a difference. Concentric lesions are well described in native atherosclerosis, particularly in advanced disease (Davies 1987). The occurrence of native atherosclerosis and preatherosclerosis in the coronary arteries of the donor organ prior to implantation has generally been overlooked. Fragmentation of the elastic lamina is a frequent finding in such early disease, as is intimal thickening. Furthermore, fully developed coronary atherosclerosis is not unusual in the donor population. In a personal study of persons dying of non-cardiovascular causes in the age range 11–38 years and therefore approximately equivalent to the brain-dead donor population, there was widespread evidence of non-stenotic preatherosclerotic and atherosclerotic disease in large epicardial coronary arteries of 27 left anterior descending (LAD) coronary arteries (16 males, 11 females), with only seven entirely free from fatty or fibrous plaques. A further 13 showed fatty plaques only and the remaining seven showed fibrous plaques, i.e. fully developed atherosclerosis in a background of fatty plaques. Overt disease was largely confined to the proximal LAD. However, histological study showed that preatherosclerotic intimal thickening, frequently associated with fragmentation of the internal elastic lamina, was much more widespread. Fully developed fibrous plaques were also seen in the left circumflex right main coronaries.

The recipient will therefore often acquire a degree of coronary artery pathology from the donor and acceleration of these changes may at least in part account for the features of graft vascular disease seen in the larger epicardial coronary arteries. Histologically this essentially resembles conventional atherosclerosis, with necrotic lipid cores, macrophage foam cells and T lymphocytes, although the cellular component in these large-vessel lesions is often more florid than in native atherosclerosis. The rupture of such plaques, with resultant thrombosis, in larger epicardial coronary arteries was a common mode of death in the Papworth series of graft vascular disease (Mullins *et al.* 1992). During the period studied, there were 131 graft failures and 25 of these were caused by graft vascular disease. Thirteen of these had an autopsy and in seven there was acute thrombosis affecting a large epicardial coronary artery. This emphasizes the importance of large-vessel disease, at least from the point of view of mortality. It also demonstrates the similarity to sudden death in conventional coronary atherosclerosis, where plaque rupture and resultant mural thrombosis appear to be the principal mechanism (Davies 1987).

Small-vessel disease appears to be a more specific form of vascular occlusion confined to allografts. Histological analysis of smaller epicardial vessels, i.e. second- and third-order branches, in known cases of graft vascular disease coming to retransplant or autopsy shows a spectrum of changes. Many vessels simply show bland occlusion by proliferated intima, which includes smooth muscle cells (Fig. 10.15). However, some vessels show a greater or lesser infiltration by mononuclear cells (Figs 10.16 and 10.17) and it is generally assumed, though by no means established, that those with bland occlusion have at some state shown a similar infiltrate which has subsided. These infiltrates have been shown to include T cells, with a mixture of both CD4 and CD8+ cells, predominantly in the subendothelial core of the intima (Salomon *et al.* 1991).

## Pathogenesis

### ANTIBODIES

There is an inverse relationship between degree of HLA disparity between recipient and donor and actuarial

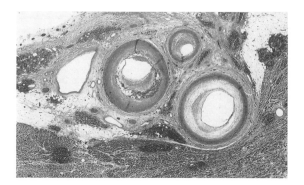

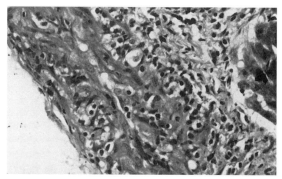

**Fig. 10.15** Intimal proliferation, predominantly concentric and involving second- and third-order epicardial coronary arteries, characterizes graft vascular disease. The proliferation in these three arteries is bland and gives no clue as to pathogenesis.

**Fig. 10.17** True destructive vasculitis with an intense mononuclear infiltrate throughout the wall of this small intramyocardial artery. Such changes may occasionally be seen in endomyocardial biopsies otherwise free of any features of significant rejection. Such changes do not readily fit into the ISHLT grading system. However enhancement of immunosuppression is probably advisable. Such lesions could represent acute cellular rejection of the blood-vessel wall and might be representative of a more generalized process in the coronary arterial tree and possibly related to the pathogenesis of chronic rejection.

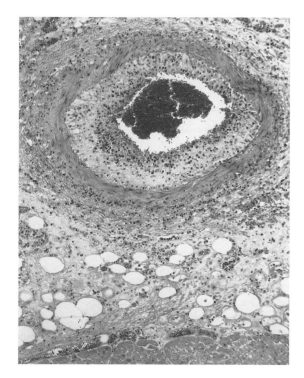

**Fig. 10.16** Concentric intimal proliferation in a small epicardial artery associated with a conspicuous mononuclear infiltrate, particularly towards the endothelial aspect. Vessels of this appearance are only seen occasionally, in this case in a heart retransplanted for graft vascular disease. The appearances provide important clues as to the possible aetiology of chronic rejection.

survival (Opelz 1989). Furthermore, those who produce anti-HLA antibodies have been shown to have a much higher angiographic incidence of graft vascular disease at 2 years than those who do not (Petrossian *et al.* 1989). However, a direct pathogenetic role for anti-HLA antibodies has not been demonstrated in graft vascular disease and associations may simply be epiphenomena.

Hammond has emphasized the importance of 'vascular' (humoral) rejection as a risk factor for subsequent development of graft vascular disease (Hammond *et al.* 1991; Ensley *et al.* 1991). This may, at least in part, be simply a manifestation of sensitization to mouse immunoglobulin as a result of administration of OKT3 therapy (Hammond *et al.* 1992). The possible role of a purely humoral rejection process, both as a cause for primary cardiac dysfunction and as a risk factor in the subsequent development of graft vascular disease, remains unresolved.

CELLULAR MECHANISMS

The finding of T cells in the expanded intima of graft

vascular disease has led to the suggestion that the disease is the result of a chronic delayed-type hypersensitivity reaction, with HLA-DR expression by T cells and adjacent endothelium. This in turn is a consequence of cytokine release, predominantly IFN-γ, by CD8+ lymphocytes recognizing donor MHC class I antigen on donor endothelium. The consequence of this chronic inflammatory process would be a cascade effect, with adjacent cells such as macrophages stimulated to produce growth factors, including platelet-derived growth factor (PDGF), which would promote vasculopathy by smooth muscle proliferation.

OVERVIEW

Rather than graft vascular disease being a manifestation of either cellular or humorally mediated mechanisms, it may in fact be caused by a combination. The cellular mechanism described above, with damage to endothelium and induction of endothelial HLA expression, may in turn lead to release and exposure of endothelial HLA and other antigens, giving rise to an antibody response. The potential role for cellular rejection as an initiator of graft vascular disease is supported by studies showing an association between episodes of cellular rejection and subsequent development of graft vascular disease (Uretsky *et al.* 1987; Narrod *et al.* 1989; Radovancevic *et al.* 1990; Zerbe *et al.* 1992). However, such an association has not been demonstrated in all studies (Hess *et al.* 1983; Gao *et al.* 1989; Hammond *et al.* 1992). This is perhaps not surprising bearing in mind the spectrum of biopsy regimens, rejection episode definitions and treatment protocols worldwide. Furthermore, cellular rejection cannot be the whole answer because the occurrence of graft vascular disease has failed to decline despite significant improvements in immunosuppressive regimens, which have reduced both the severity and the incidence of cellular rejection. This may be a manifestation of the fact that both current and past immunsuppressive protocols have never adequately addressed the control of potential humoral rejection mechanisms.

While the primary damage involved in graft vascular disease has always been assumed to be immunological, other risk factors are undoubtedly important in the development of clinically significant disease. CMV infection has been associated with an increased incidence of graft vascular disease (McDonald *et al.* 1989; Loebe *et al.* 1990; Everett *et al.* 1992). However, this association is likely to be complex in nature because of the association of CMV infection with so many other aspects of heart transplantation. Nevertheless, there are possible direct roles for CMV in the pathogenesis, either through viral cytotoxic damage to the vessel wall or through virally induced up-regulation of HLA expression.

Hyperlipidaemia has also been shown to be an important risk factor (Parameshwar *et al.* 1996) and this is clearly particularly relevant to those receiving transplants for ischaemic heart disease, many of whom have lipid abnormalities prior to transplant. Peritransplant injury around the time of transplant also appears to be a significant risk factor for the development of graft vascular disease (Gaudin *et al.* 1994).

## Lymphoproliferative disease

Lymphoproliferative disease, usually of B cell type and related to Epstein–Barr virus, is a recognized long-term complication of solid organ transplantation (Penn 1990). It is relatively frequent following heart transplantation (Coueteil *et al.* 1990), reflecting necessarily higher levels of cyclosporin immunosuppression than in kidney recipients. Extranodal involvement is common and may on occasion be seen in the transplanted heart, where infiltration tends to be mainly endocardial (Figs 10.18 and 10.19). Such infiltrates are usually readily distinguished from Quilty lesions by the nature of the lymphoid cells, which may form a monomorphic or polymorphic infiltrate (Nalesnic *et al.* 1988). Knowledge of the clinical status of the patient is helpful and histological comparison may be made between nodal and cardiac infiltrates. There is evidence that use of OKT3 in the immunosuppressive regimen makes lymphoproliferative disease more likely to develop (Goldman *et al.* 1992) and the relationship between the development of lymphoproliferative disease and the level of immunosuppression in general is clearly established. As a corollary to this, in some cases infiltrates may regress simply with reduction or

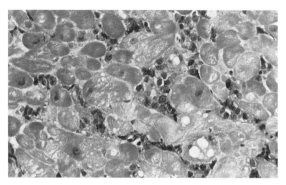

**Fig. 10.19** Post-transplant lymphoproliferative disease. Higher-power view of the myocardial infiltrate illustrated in Fig. 10.18. Compared to the infiltrate of rejection there is considerable atypia and the differential diagnosis is not usually a problem.

## References

Baandrup, U. & Mortensen, S.A. (1984) Histopathological aspects of myocarditis with special reference to mumps, cytomegalovirus infection and the role of endomyocardial biopsy. In: *Viral Heart Disease* (ed. H.D. Bolte), pp. 13–25. Springer-Verlag, New York.

Billingham, M.E. (1989) Dilemma of variety of histopathological grading systems for acute cardiac allograft rejection by endomyocardial biopsy. *Journal of Heart Transplantation* **9**, 272–276.

Billingham, M.E., Cary, N.R.B., Hammond, M.E. *et al.* (1990) A working formulation for the standardization of nomenclature in the diagnosis of heart and lung rejection: Heart Rejection Study Group. *Journal of Heart Transplantation* **9**, 587–593.

Bonnaud, E.V., Lewis, N.P., Masek, M.A. & Billingham, M.E. (1995) Reliability and usefulness of immunofluorescence in heart transplantation. *Journal of Heart and Lung Transplantation* **14**, 163–171.

Bruneval, P., Amrein, C., Guillemain, R. *et al.* (1992) Poor diagnostic value of *in situ* hybridisation and immunohistochemistry in endomyocardial biopsies to detect cytomegalovirus after heart transplantation. *Journal of Heart and Lung Transplantation* **11**, 773–777.

Caves, P.K., Stinson, E.B., Billingham, M.E. & Shumway, N.E. (1973) Percutaneous transvenous endomyocardial biopsy in human heart recipients (experience with a new technique). *Annals of Thoracic Surgery* **16**, 325–336.

Coueteil, J.P., McGoldrick, J.P., Wallwork, J. & English, T.A.H. (1990) Malignant tumours after heart transplantation. *Journal of Heart Transplantation* **9**, 622–626.

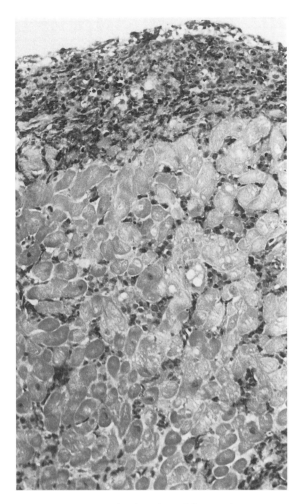

**Fig. 10.18** Post-transplant lymphoproliferative disease involving the endocardium and underlying myocardium.

withdrawal of cyclosporin A and introduction of acyclovir therapy (Nalesnik *et al.* 1992). This is important to bear in mind, as overdiagnosis of what in other circumstances would histologically constitute malignant lymphoma may lead to unnecessary and hazardous cytotoxic chemotherapy and/or radiotherapy. Apart from lymphoproliferative disease, as with other solid organ recipients, cutanuous malignancies are relatively frequently seen in long-term heart transplant recipients (Coueteil *et al.* 1990).

Davies, M.J. (1987) The pathology of ischaemic heart disease. In: *Recent Advances in Histopathology 13* (eds P.P. Anthony & R.N. MacSween). Churchill Livingstone, London.

Ensley, R.D., Hammond, E.H., Renlund, D.G. *et al.* (1991) Clinical manifestations of vascular rejection in cardiac transplantation. *Transplantation Proceedings* 23, 1130–1132.

Everett, J.P., Hershberger, R.E., Norman, D.J. *et al.* (1992) Prolonged cytomegalovirus infection with viremia is associated with development of cardiac allograft vasculopathy. *Journal of Heart and Lung Transplantation* 11, S133–137.

Fishbein, M.C., Bell, G., Lones, M.A. *et al.* (1994) Grade 2 cellular heart rejection: does it exist? *Journal of Heart and Lung Transplantation* 13, 1051–1057.

Forbes, R.D., Rowan, R.A. & Billingham, M.E. (1990) Endocardial infiltrates in human heart transplants: a serial biopsy analysis comparing four immunosuppression protocols. *Human Pathology* 21, 850–855.

Gao, S.Z., Schroeder, J.S., Alderman, E.L. *et al.* (1989) Prevalence of accelerated coronary artery disease in heart transplant survivors: comparison of cyclosporin and azathioprine regiments. *Circulation* 80 (III), 100–105.

Gaudin, P.B., Rayburn, B.K. & Hutchins, G.M. (1994) Peritransplant injury to the myocardium associated with the development of accelerated arteriosclerosis in heart transplant recipients. *American Journal of Surgical Pathology* 18, 338–346.

Goldman, M., Gerard, C., Abramowicz, D. *et al.* (1992) Induction of interleukin-6 and interleukin-10 by the OKT3 monoclonal antibody: possible relevance to post-transplant lymphoproliferative disorders. *Clinical Transplantation* 6, 265–268.

Hammond, E.H., Yowell, R.L., Nunoda, S. *et al.* (1989) Vascular (humoral) rejection in heart transplantation: pathologic observations and clinical implications. *Journal of Heart Transplantation* 8, 430–443.

Hammond, E.H., Ensley, R.D., Yowell, R.L. *et al.* (1991) Vascular rejection of human cardiac allografts and the role of humoral immunity in chronic allograft rejection. *Transplantation Proceedings* 23, 26.

Hammond, E.H., Yowell, R.L. & Price, G.D. *et al.* (1992) Vascular rejection and its relationship to allograft coronary artery disease. *Journal of Heart and Lung Transplantation* 11, S111–119.

Hess, M.L., Hastillo, A., Mohanakumar, T. *et al.* (1983) Accelerated atherosclerosis in cardiac transplantation: role of cytotoxic B-cell antibodies and hyperlipidaemia. *Circulation* 68 (II), 94–101.

Holliman, R., Johnson, J., Savva, D. *et al.* (1992) Diagnosis of toxoplasma infection in cardiac transplant recipients using the polymerase chain reaction. *Journal of Clinical Pathology* 45, 931–932.

Hosenpud, J.D., Novick, R.J., Bennett, L.E. *et al.* (1996) The Registry of the International Society for Heart and Lung Transplantation 1996: Thirteen Official Report—1996. *Journal of Heart and Lung Transplantation* 15, 655–674.

Joshi, A., Masek, M.A., Brown, B.W., Weiss, L.M. & Billingham, M.E. (1995) 'Quilty revisited': a 10 year perspective. *Human Pathology* 26, 547–557.

Kemmitz, J. & Cohnert, T.R. (1988) Lymphoma like lesion in human orthotopic cardiac allografts. *American Journal of Clinical Pathology* 89, 430 (abstract).

Loebe, M., Schüler, S., Zais, O. *et al.* (1990) Role of cytomegalovirus infection in the development of coronary artery disease in the transplanted heart. *Journal of Heart Transplantation* 9, 707.

Lones, M.A., Czer, L.S.C., Trento, A. *et al.* (1995) Clinical-pathology features of humoral rejection in cardiac allografts: a study in 81 consecutive patients. *Journal of Heart and Lung Transplantation* 14, 162–171.

McDonald, K., Rector, T.S., Braunlin, E.A. *et al.* (1989) Association of coronary artery disease in cardiac transplant recipients with cytomegalovirus. *American Journal of Cardiology* 64, 359.

Mullins, P.A., Cary, N.R., Sharples, L. *et al.* (1992) Coronary occlusive disease in late graft failure after cardiac transplantation. *British Heart Journal* 68, 260–265.

Nakhleh, R.E., Copenhaver, C.M., Werdin, K. *et al.* (1991) Lack of evidence for involvement of Epstein–Barr virus in the development of the 'Quilty' lesion of transplanted hearts: an *in situ* hybridisation study. *Journal of Heart and Lung Transplantation* 10, 504–507.

Nalesnic, M., Jaffe, R., Starze, T.E. *et al.* (1988) The pathology of post-transplant lymphoproliferative disorders occurring in the setting of cyclosporine A–prednisolone immunosuppression. *American Journal of Pathology* 133, 173–192.

Nalesnik, M.A., Locker, J., Jaffe, R. *et al.* (1992) Experience with post-transplant lymphoproliferative disorders in solid organ transplant recipients. *Clinical Transplantation* 6, 249–252.

Narrod, J., Kormos, R., Armitage, J. *et al.* (1989) Acute rejection and coronary artery disease in long-term survivors of heart transplantation. *Journal of Heart Transplantation* 8, 418–420.

Nitkin, R.S., Hunt, S.A. & Schroeder, J.S. (1985) Accelerated coronary artery disease risk in heart transplant patients. *Journal of the American College of Cardiology* 6, 243–245.

Opelz, G. (1989) Effects of HLA matching in heart transplantation. *Transplantation Proceedings* 21, 794–796.

Parameshwar, J., Foote, J., Sharples, L. *et al.* (1996) Lipids, lipoprotein (a) and coronary artery disease in patients following cardiac transplant. *Transplant International* 9, 481–485.

Penn, I. (1990) Cancers complicating organ transplantation. *New England Journal of Medicine* **323**, 1767–1769.

Petrossian, G.A., Nichols, A.B., Marboe, C.C. *et al.* (1989) Relation between survival and development of coronary artery disease and anti-HLA antibodies after cardiac transplant. *Circulation* **80** (III), 122–125.

Radovancevic, B., Poindexter, S., Birovljev, S. *et al.* (1990) Risk factors for development of accelerated coronary artery disease in cardiac transplant recipients. *European Journal of Cardiothoracic Surgery* **4**, 309–312.

Riseq, M.N., Masek, M.A. & Billingham, M.E. (1994) Acute rejection: significance of elapsed time post-transplant. *Journal of Heart and Lung Transplantation* **13**, 862–868.

Rowan, R.A. & Billingham, M.E. (1990) Pathologic changes in the long-term transplanted heart: a morphometic study of myocardial hypertrophy, vascularity and fibrosis. *Human Pathology* **21**, 767–772.

Salomon, R.N., Hughes, C.C.W., Schoen, F.J. *et al.* (1991) Human coronary transplantation-associated arteriosclerosis: evidence of a chronic immune reaction to activated graft endothelial cells. *American Journal of Pathology* **138**, 791–798.

Schofield, P.M. (1991) Indications for cardiac transplantation. *British Heart Journal* **65**, 55–56.

Sharples, L.D., Cary, N.R.B., Large, S.R. & Wallwork, J. (1992) Error rates with which endomyocardial biopsies are graded for rejection following cardiac transplantation. *American Journal of Cardiology* **70**, 527–530.

Stovin, P.G.I., Wreghitt, T.G., English, T.A.H. & Wallwork, J. (1989) Lack of association between cytomegalovirus infection of the heart and rejection-like inflammation. *Journal of Clinical Pathology* **42**, 81–83.

Uretsky, B.F., Murali, S., Reddy, P.S. *et al.* (1987) Development of coronary artery disease in cardiac transplant patients receiving immunosuppressive therapy with cyclosporine and prednisolone. *Circulation* **76**, 827–834.

Winters, G., Loh, E. & Schoen, F. (1995) Natural history of focal moderate cardiac allograft rejection: is treatment warranted? *Circulation* **91**, 1975–1980.

Wreghitt, T.G., Hakin, M., Gray, J.J. *et al.* (1989) Toxoplasmosis in heart and lung transplant recipients. *Journal of Clinical Pathology* **42**, 194–199.

Zerbe, T.R. & Arena, V. (1988) Diagnostic reliability of endomyocardial biopsy for assessment of cardiac allograft rejection. *Human Pathology* **19**, 1307.

Zerbe, T., Uretsky, B., Kormos, R. *et al.* (1992) Graft atherosclerosis: effects of cellular rejection and human lymphocyte antigen. *Journal of Heart and Lung Transplantation* **11**, S104–110.

# Chapter 11/Lung transplantation

SUSAN STEWART

## Introduction

Lung transplantation is now an accepted surgical treatment for both end-stage pulmonary vascular and pulmonary parenchymal diseases (Reitz et al. 1982; Griffith et al. 1987; Penketh et al. 1987; Dark & Corris 1989; Smyth et al. 1991a; Hosenpud et al. 1997). It can be performed in combination with the heart, as single or double lung grafts and, rarely, as lobar transplantation.

The International Society for Heart and Lung Transplantation (ISHLT) maintains a register of procedures (Hosenpud et al. 1997). By the end of 1996, 2186 heart–lung transplantations, 3939 single lung and 2543 double lung transplantations had been reported. The number of lung transplants grew until 1993 compared with heart–lung transplantation, which peaked as a result of the limited numbers of donor organs.

Combined heart–lung transplantation was initially developed for patients with pulmonary hypertension and right heart failure, mainly Eisenmenger's syndrome and primary pulmonary hypertension (Reitz et al. 1982). It was then offered to patients with advanced parenchymal disease and right heart failure (Smyth et al. 1991a). The ISHLT registry report shows that combined heart–lung transplantation is most often performed for primary pulmonary hypertension, Eisenmenger's complex and cystic fibrosis (Hosenpud et al. 1997). Not all end-stage pulmonary conditions are associated with cardiac failure and under these circumstances single or double lung transplantation can be performed. As these procedures increase, in response to donor organ shortage the number of combined heart–lung grafts is decreasing and there is inevitably rising donor age for both groups.

Single and double lung transplantation is now performed more frequently for patients with pulmonary parenchymal disease. Double lung transplantation is favoured for cystic fibrosis and bronchiectasis, as both infected lungs are replaced. Single lung transplantation is reserved for those parenchymal conditions without suppuration or infection that would pose a threat to the new graft, particularly under immunosuppression (Dark & Corris 1989). Single lung grafting is therefore indicated in emphysema, including α-1-antitrypsin deficiency, idiopathic pulmonary fibrosis, sarcoidosis and, more rarely, retransplantation (Hosenpud et al. 1997). However, there are limitations associated with single lung replacement for bilateral disease and native lungs can cause problems of infection, compression and pneumothorax. More controversially, single lung transplants have been performed for pulmonary hypertension (Higenbottam 1992). Where this is a result of congenital heart disease it may be possible to combine this with operative repair of the defect. There is considerable haemodynamic improvement after single lung transplantation for pulmonary hypertension.

The choice of procedure is also influenced by donor availability. The greater use of single and double lung transplants compared to combined heart–lung transplantation releases greater numbers of hearts for cardiac transplantation. Patients retaining their own heart are not at risk of developing cardiac rejection or accelerated coronary occlusive disease. It is, however, possible to use the explanted heart of a heart–lung recipient for a cardiac recipient, thus increasing donor supply. This is known as the domino procedure (Kells *et al*. 1992).

There have been considerable improvements in outcome of lung transplants (Hosenpud *et al*. 1997). Heart–lung transplant survival rates are 60% at 1 year and less than 20% at 11 years. Double lung transplantation has a patient half time of 4.5 years and single lung transplantation of 3.7 years, indicating no significant difference in actuarial survival. Survival is greater for patients with pulmonary parenchymal disease than for those undergoing transplantation for pulmonary vascular disease. The most common causes of death in both heart–lung and lung transplantation are infection and chronic rejection (Bando *et al*. 1995; Hosenpud *et al*. 1997). There is also a high incidence of non-specific graft failure, which relates both to donor selection and to methods of organ preservation. It is likely that lung transplantation has been maintained at a level limited by donor organ availability (Egan *et al*. 1992; Hosenpud *et al*. 1997) and the long-term survival will be influenced by the quality of organs grafted.

The postoperative complications of lung transplantation are monitored and assessed by transbronchial biopsy of the graft (Higenbottam *et al*. 1988a,b; Starnes *et al*. 1989a,b; Guilinger *et al*. 1995; Kesten *et al*. 1996). The early investigation, diagnosis and prompt treatment of the main complications, i.e. rejec-

tion and infection, have contributed to improved graft survival (Hutter *et al*. 1988; Scott *et al*. 1990; Guilinger *et al*. 1995). The pathological changes are similar in all types of lung transplants (Keenan *et al*. 1991a). There is a higher incidence of ischaemic complications of the airways in double (up to 40%) and single lung transplants (15%) compared with combined heart–lung blocks (less than 10%) (Cooper *et al*. 1989; Courand & Nashef 1995). The combined grafts have a tracheal anastomosis which is more vascular and also bronchial–coronary collateral vessels, which may further reduce local airway ischaemia. Ischaemic airways are susceptible to infection, particularly by *Aspergillus*, and also to dehiscence with mediastinitis. Fibrosis or narrowing and bronchomalacia may require long-term stenting of the airways (Yousem *et al*. 1990c; Frost *et al*. 1993).

The pathology of lung transplantation centres mainly on rejection, both acute and chronic, and opportunistic infection (Stewart *et al*. 1988; Stewart 1992; Berry & Yousem 1995; Stewart & Cary 1996). In addition, the lung is susceptible to common pathogens, lymphoproliferative disease and recurrence of primary disease. The morphological appearances of these conditions will be considered in this chapter.

## Donor lung injury and preservation

A significant number of lung transplant recipients suffer early mortality as a result of primary graft failure (Zenati *et al*. 1990b; Hosenpud *et al*. 1997). This is related partly to preservation injury and partly to factors inherent in the donor lung. Preservation of the lung lags behind that of other organs in many ways and the procedure is still limited to 4–6 hours' ischaemic time. Methods of preservation have included topical cooling, flush perfusion with Euro-Collins solution or cold blood and cooling with cardiopulmonary bypass (Locke *et al*. 1988). More recently, autoperfusion of the ventilated heart–lung block has been performed.

Damage may occur to the lung at the time of reperfusion and may be mediated by neutrophils and platelets. The generation of oxygen free radicals is important in the pathogenesis of reperfusion damage. It is likely that those early deaths showing the pathological changes of adult respiratory distress syndrome represent ischaemic or reperfusion damage to the grafted lung. It is difficult, however, to exclude other causes particularly if there has been early infection or excessive operative bleeding. Interleukin 6 (IL-6) has been used as a marker of preservation injury in clinical lung transplantation (Pham *et al.* 1992; Yoshida *et al.* 1993). Interleukin 6 is a cytokine produced by alveolar macrophages and other pulmonary cellular constituents in response to injury and infection. The serum IL-6 level in the immediate postoperative period (4 h) has been shown to be a useful marker of preservation injury and a level of more than 1000 pg/mL is associated with a poor outcome (Pham *et al.* 1992). In this study, preservation injury was assessed by the need for prolonged intubation, the arteriolar:alveolar oxygen tension ratio, the presence of diffuse alveolar damage on the first lung biopsy and the 30-day graft survival rate. Infection was excluded by examination of the sputum, bronchoalveolar fluid and lung biopsy specimens. In the future it will be of great benefit to find a marker, possibly a cytokine that is predictive of graft function, before implantation. However, the pressure on donor organs is such that less than optimal organs have to be considered.

The availability of suitable pulmonary donors will probably limit the growth of lung transplantation (Egan *et al.* 1992; Hosenpud *et al.* 1997). By definition, the donors will have suffered brain death and artificial ventilation. The harvested lungs are therefore very likely to be infected or have suffered aspiration. A pathological study of unused donor lungs confirmed these and other abnormalities and targeted areas for improvement in the care of the donor, possibly thereby increasing the supply of organs (Stewart *et al.* 1993). The unused donor lungs examined comprised both unsuitable lungs and unplaced lungs. The latter included unused partners of single transplants where a suitable recipient was not available for the second lung.

The donors were assessed perioperatively by accepted clinical, radiological, physiological and microbiological criteria. These included age, smoking history, chest radiograph, arterial blood gases and evidence of aspiration or sepsis. Six pairs of lungs were available for pathological study after the heart alone

was donated for transplantation. A further four lungs remained after one partner was used for single lung recipients. Histological abnormalities were demonstrated in all the lungs examined even if the macroscopic appearance was normal. The most common abnormality was purulent bronchitis and/or bronchiolitis. This was present in 13 lungs (81%) and had progressed to bronchopneumonia in eight of these (50%). Interstitial emphysema and subpleural blebs were probably related to barotrauma caused by high ventilatory pressures. These were seen in one pair of unused lungs and an unused single lung. A surprising finding was the high incidence of thrombo-emboli in the young donors. These were present in eight lungs (50%) and were usually accompanied by evidence of early organization confirming their origin prior to donor harvesting. Fat or bone marrow emboli were seen in a further four lungs (25%), which may have been pre- or perioperative. One donor was thought preoperatively to have fat embolism and showed features of diffuse alveolar damage. An unused single lung also showed diffuse alveolar damage in association with a severe bronchopneumonia and the donor had suffered long-bone fractures. Airway abnormalities included goblet-cell hyperplasia and/or respiratory bronchiolitis with pigment accumulation strongly suggestive of smoking. These changes were seen in 44% of lungs but a clinical history of smoking was obtained in only three donors. Neither common nor opportunistic organisms were demonstrated in histological material from the lungs. The pathological findings are summarized in Table 11.1. The clinical decision to reject some pairs of lungs as unsuitable and use only the heart from a donor is vindicated in this study. These donors have the highest incidence of bronchopneumonia and thrombo-emboli.

The pathological abnormalities in those lungs considered suitable but not placed imply that many transplanted lungs also have these abnormalities. The postoperative management of lung transplant cases should therefore take into account the very high likelihood of infectious bronchitis and bronchiolitis (Zenati *et al.* 1990a). Intubation and ventilation eliminate the upper airway protective mechanisms, predisposing the lung to infection and aspiration. The successful trans-

**Table 11.1** Pathology of unused donor lungs.

| Donor no. | Acute bronchiolitis | Bronchopneumonia | Interstitial emphysema | Emboli | Haemorrhage | Goblet cell hyperplasia respiratory bronchiolitis | Diffuse alveolar damage |
|---|---|---|---|---|---|---|---|
| 1* | + | | | | | | |
| 2* | | + | | F | | + | |
| 3* | + | | | | + | + | |
| 4 | + | | + | BM | + | + | |
| 5 | + | + | + | FT | | | |
| 6 | + | + | | | + | | |
| 7 | + | | | T | | + | |
| 8 | + | + | | T | | | With aspiration |
| 9 | | + | + | T | | + | |
| 10 | + | + | | | | | + |
| 11 | + | | | | | | |
| 12 | + | + | | | | | |
| 13 | + | | | T | + | | |
| 14 | + | + | | BM | | | |
| 15 | + | + | | T | | | |
| 16 | + | + | | T | + | | |
| 17 | + | + | | | | | |
| 18* | + | + | | T | | | |
| 19* | + | | | T | + | | |
| 20 | + | + | | | | | |
| 21 | + | + | | T | + | | |
| 22 | + | + | | T | | + | |

BM, bone marrow; F, fat; T, thrombo-embolus.
* Lungs considered suitable but not placed.

plantation of single lungs where the unused partner has shown this type of pathological abnormality suggests, though, that this does not preclude use of the organ. This study also indicates that some histological features in early postoperative transbronchial biopsies may be donor-related. In particular, the perivascular and peribronchiolar cellular infiltrates that accompany many common infections may be impossible to distinguish from early rejection.

## Morphology of acute lung rejection

### Experimental models

The histopathological appearances of acute lung rejection have now been extensively studied in both experimental and clinical material. The experimental studies have shown similar features in rats, dogs and primates (Casteneda *et al.* 1972; Veith *et al.* 1973; Prop *et al.* 1985a,b). Transplantation between inbred strains of rat has allowed greater immunogenetic standardization.

Prop *et al.* (1985a,b) described the histological features of rejection in the rat under standardized immunogenetic conditions. The initial *latent* phase is followed by a *vascular* phase in which rejection is accompanied by prominent perivascular and peribronchial mononuclear cell infiltrates. These cuff the vessels and bronchioles intensely and are composed predominantly of lymphocytes. Macrophages and plasma cells are also seen with progression of the rejection process. These infiltrates extend into the interstitium, with cellular accumulation within alveolar walls and spaces. This is described as the *alveolar* phase and, in the absence of immunosuppression, leads to acute inflammatory cell infiltration, necrosis and haemorrhage in the final *destructive* stage. The rat has prominent bronchus-associated lymphoid tissue (BALT), which makes the airway changes difficult to extrapolate to other species, including humans. In rats the mucosa-associated lymphoid tissue is thought to facilitate infiltration of the graft by recipient lymphocytes, thus providing a strong stimulus for a local immune response (Prop *et al*. 1985a). The presence of lymphoid material in grafted human lungs may similarly explain the high incidence of rejection compared with other solid organ grafts.

## Vessels in acute rejection

The descriptions of acute rejection in human lung transplantation relate to patients on immunosuppressive therapy (Yousem *et al*. 1985; Stewart *et al*. 1988; Clelland *et al*. 1990; Yousem *et al*. 1990a; Stewart 1992; Yousem *et al*. 1996). This is generally a combination of cyclosporin, azathioprine and steroid therapy, augmented as necessary (Hutter *et al*. 1988). Antithymocyte globulin and OKT3 are also used in some centres, together with FK506 and mycophenolate.

Acute rejection of the lung is most common in the first 3–6 months after transplantation although the precise incidence is not known. Clinical features include breathlessness, cough and pyrexia and these may be accompanied by an abnormal radiograph with new or changing infiltrates (Millet *et al*. 1989). Pulmonary function tests may deteriorate but patients can be completely asymptomatic. The radiographic changes are more common and more specific within 1 month of transplantation. Perihilar and lower zone shadowing may be present, with pleural effusions (Judson & Sahn 1996; Judson *et al*. 1997). However, after the first month the radiograph is only abnormal in a few rejection episodes (Millet *et al*. 1989). Routine surveillance biopsies show an alarmingly high rate of rejection in the absence of any of the above features (Trulock *et al*. 1992; Sibley *et al*. 1993).

The histopathology of acute lung rejection has been studied mainly in transbronchial biopsy material

(Stewart *et al*. 1988; Yousem *et al*. 1990a, 1996; Stewart 1992; Clelland *et al*. 1993). Open biopsy and autopsy material is often complicated by other pathological processes, particularly infection. The following description is based largely on biopsy material in which other pathology, in particular infection, has been excluded. The earliest change is mononuclear cell infiltration around small vessels (Fig. 11.1). The infiltrates are usually within and around the adventitia, cuffing both venules and arterioles. Infiltrates comprise mainly small lymphocytes of mature appearance but admixed with some larger lymphocytes (Stewart *et al*. 1988). The infiltrate in the early stages is up to two to three cells thick and may be associated with very mild perivascular oedema. These minimal infiltrates require high-power magnification for their identification. With increasing severity the infiltrates become more easily visible at scanning magnification (Yousem *et al*. 1990a, 1996). The cellularity increases as does the proportion of large transformed-looking lymphocytes (Fig. 11.2). Macrophages and plasma cells are seen at this mild grade and there may be endotheliitis. The cellular infiltrate within the intima is composed of similar cells and may be associated with hyperplasia of the overlying endothelial cells. It is not usually of sufficient magnitude to encroach on the vascular lumen. The media of the vessels is not infiltrated

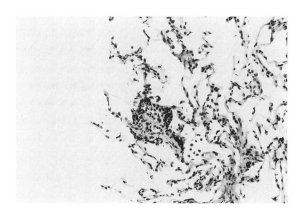

**Fig. 11.1** Minimal acute lung rejection showing a single perivascular infiltrate of mononuclear cells, small and mature in appearance. Adjacent parenchyma is unremarkable. Grade A1 rejection. Medium power: transbronchial biopsy; H & E stain.

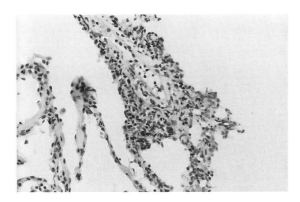

**Fig. 11.2** Mild acute lung rejection with larger infiltrate composed of small and large lymphocytes and showing endotheliitis. Adjacent parenchyma is normal. Similar infiltrates were present in other biopsy fragments. Grade A2 rejection. Medium power: transbronchial biopsy; H & E stain.

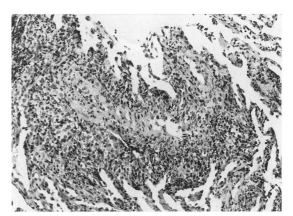

**Fig. 11.3** Moderate acute lung rejection with extension of perivascular infiltrates into adjoining interstitium and alveoli, which also contain inflammatory cells. Endotheliitis is conspicuous and mononuclear infiltrate contains polymorphs and eosinophils. Uninvolved parenchyma at the periphery of the field confirms that this is a discrete process. Grade A3 rejection. Medium power: transbronchial biopsy; H & E stain.

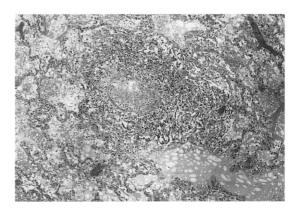

**Fig. 11.4** Severe acute lung rejection showing extension of perivascular cellular infiltrates into interstitium with confluence and prominent alveolar involvement. Alveoli show cellular infiltration, haemorrhage, hyaline membranes and epithelial hyperplasia. Grade A4 rejection. Medium power: autopsy lung; H & E stain.

in acute rejection. Endotheliitis is seen in both venous and arteriolar vessels (see Fig. 11.2). Advancing rejection is associated with extension of the perivascular infiltrates from the perivascular adventitia into the interstitium (Fig. 11.3). The alveolar septa become expanded with mononuclear cells and at this moderate stage polymorphs and eosinophils may be seen but not usually in great numbers. The alveolar epithelial cells undergo hyperplastic changes and mononuclear inflammatory cells accumulate in the adjacent alveolar spaces including alveolar macrophages. Moderate acute rejection is a patchy pathological process but rejection becomes more confluent in its most severe grade, with haemorrhage, necrosis and hyaline membrane formation (Fig. 11.4). Pulmonary rejection of this severity is not commonly seen in clinical material as a result of the use of immunosuppression but may occur in patients particularly prone to rejection or where immunosuppression has been reduced because of severe infection or lymphoproliferative disease. Cystic fibrosis recipients with absorption problems may also suffer severe acute rejection.

## Airways in acute rejection

The vascular features of rejection are mirrored in the small airways. The earliest change is peribronchiolar cuffing by mononuclear cells, most of which are small, round and mature. With advancing rejection the infiltrate extends into the mucosa, with lymphocytic infiltration of the epithelium (Fig. 11.5). This epithelium

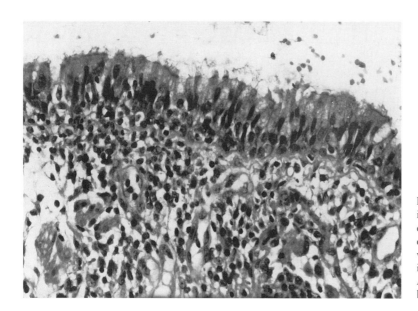

**Fig. 11.5** Mononuclear cell infiltration of bronchial respiratory epithelium and submucosa without epithelial damage or ulceration. This was not accompanied by perivascular infiltrates. Lymphocytic bronchiolitis A0 B2. High power: transbronchial biopsy; H & E stain.

remains intact in low-grade rejection but undergoes degeneration and finally necrosis as rejection becomes more severe (Stewart *et al.* 1988; Yousem *et al.* 1990a, 1996). The airways then show polymorph infiltration of the ulcerated mucosa. Similar extension from the peribronchiolar adventitial tissue into the interstitium is seen.

Both perivascular and peribronchiolar infiltrates can occur independently but most commonly occur together. It is important to have adequate sampling of both transbronchial lung parenchyma and small airways and mucosa in assessing acute rejection. In open biopsy and autopsy material it is possible to see similar adventitial infiltrates around larger vessels and bronchi (Tazelaar & Yousem 1988). The epithelium of larger airways may undergo squamous metaplasia as a result of repeated episodes of acute rejection (Higenbottam & Stewart 1989; Yousem *et al.* 1990c). The epithelium may also show individual cell necrosis associated with Leu 7-positive (CD57) intraepithelial lymphocytes (Hruban *et al.* 1988a). Acute rejection therefore appears to affect all the airway distal to the tracheal or bronchial anastomosis and predisposes to the development of obliterative bronchiolitis and bron-

chitis as a manifestation of chronic rejection of the lung (Hruban & Hutchins 1990). Rejection of the airways involves both a direct immunological attack on the epithelium and the effect of perivascular infiltration of vessels supplying the airway wall.

Studies on stable lung transplant recipients have demonstrated a significant increase in CD8-positive lymphocytes and HLA-DR positivity, with a probable increase in macrophages in endobronchial mucosa (Snell *et al.* 1997). This indicates that there is ongoing inflammation in healthy lung transplant recipients despite triple immunosuppression and this may contribute to the development of obliterative bronchiolitis.

## Morphology of chronic rejection

### Obliterative bronchiolitis

The success of lung transplantation is limited by a progressive fibrosing condition of the airways (Burke *et al.* 1984; Yousem *et al.* 1985; Scott *et al.* 1990; Stewart 1992; Levine & Bryant 1995; Reichenspurner *et al.* 1996). This process is identical to obliterative bronchiolitis of other non-transplant aetiologies (Epler &

Colby 1983) but is thought to be a manifestation of chronic lung rejection (Tazelaar *et al.* 1987; Yousem *et al.* 1990a). It is accompanied by a progressive decline in pulmonary function, with clinical deterioration which is not reversed by augmented immunosuppression (Scott *et al.* 1990; Paradis *et al.* 1993). Chronic vascular changes similar to chronic rejection in other solid organ transplants usually accompany this condition but the obliterative bronchiolitis (OB) dominates the clinical picture rather than the vascular pathology. The patient may suffer from cough, copious sputum, breathlessness and recurrent infections. There may be radiological abnormalities, including bronchiectasis and lower lobe shadowing, and these can be confirmed on computerized tomography (Burke *et al.* 1984; Tazelaar & Yousem 1988). The irreversible decline of pulmonary function can be monitored and is an essential part of the clinical diagnosis.

In 1993 a working formulation for the standardization of nomenclature and clinical staging of chronic dysfunction in lung allografts was proposed by the ISHLT (Cooper *et al.* 1993). The progressive airways disease for which no other cause is identified is referred to as the bronchiolitis obliterans syndrome (BOS). Stage 0 (no OB) is defined by an $FEV_1$ of 80% or greater than baseline; stage 1 (mild OB) by an $FEV_1$ of 66–80% of baseline; stage 2 (moderate OB) by an $FEV_1$ of 51–65% of baseline; and stage 3 (severe OB) by an $FEV_1$ less than 50% of baseline. Each stage is subcategorized as 'a' or 'b' for histological evidence of OB or not, respectively. Subsequently, a drop in FEF of 25–75% has been found to be an earlier and more sensitive indicator of OB (Maurer 1994). Nathan *et al.* (1995) described three clinical subgroups of OB consisting of:
1 rapid onset and relentless progressive course;
2 initial rapid decline but subsequent stabilization of lung function; and
3 insidious onset and course.
Neither steroids nor antilymphocytic treatment is beneficial in most cases of OB, any initial remission inevitably leading to relapse with death caused by respiratory failure and/or infection.

Histologically, the fibrosis involves membranous and respiratory bronchioles in an eccentric or concentric fashion, reducing the bronchiolar lumen (Fig. 11.6). In

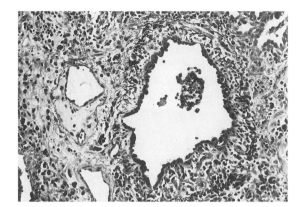

**Fig. 11.6** Chronic lung rejection involving a small bronchiole and accompanying vessel. The bronchiole shows inflammatory cells and fibrosis to the elastica, reducing the lumen, which is lined by hyperplastic cuboidal cells. The vessel shows marked intimal sclerosis with few mononuclear cells. Grade Ca, D. Medium power: open lung biopsy; trichrome stain.

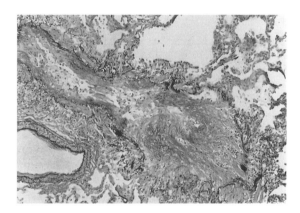

**Fig. 11.7** Obliterative bronchiolitis with a tiny residual bronchiolar lumen. The bronchiolar elastica is fragmented where the fibrosis has extended into the muscular wall. Few inflammatory cells remain at this stage. The accompanying arteriole shows mild medial hypertrophy only. Grade Cb. Low power: open lung biopsy; elastic van Gieson stain.

the early stages the lumen is reduced but finally the bronchiole may be totally obliterated and only recognized by connective tissue stains demonstrating its proximity to an accompanying arteriole (Fig. 11.7). In the early phases the fibrosis is accompanied by a cellular infiltrate (Yousem *et al.* 1990a, 1996). This can involve the full thickness of the bronchiolar wall with dense periadventitial cellular infiltrates of predominantly mononuclear cells. The essential diagnostic feature, however, is fibrosis within the lumen leading to eventual obliteration. This distinguishes obliterative bronchiolitis from lymphocytic bronchiolitis, in which there is mononuclear cell infiltration but no scarring.

In obliterative bronchiolitis the bronchiolar epithelium may simply be infiltrated by lymphocytes or may show degenerative changes and necrosis with ulceration. Polymorphs are seen but if present in large numbers should suggest superimposed infection. Granulation tissue appears in association with the epithelial damage and may grow into the lumen in a polypoid fashion prior to eccentric or concentric scarring. The cellular infiltrate and fibrosis can destroy the smooth muscle and extend the scarring into the interstitium. This is periadventitial only and must be distinguished from the intra-alveolar granulation tissue of organizing pneumonia (Abernathy *et al.* 1991; Milne *et al.* 1994; Stewart & Cary 1996). Obliterative bronchiolitis may exist with features of acute rejection elsewhere in the lung and with lymphocytic bronchiolitis. It may also be accompanied by chronic vascular rejection (Yousem *et al.* 1989a, 1990a). Obliterative bronchiolitis may be seen on biopsy material when the patient is apparently well (Sibley *et al.* 1993). It is initially a patchy process and the patient may not be symptomatic until a significant proportion of bronchioles have been compromised.

It is essential to distinguish the clinical and pathological diagnosis of obliterative bronchiolitis in lung transplant recipients until more precise correlation is known. In practice most patients with progressive loss of function in the second year or later following transplantation are confirmed to have established obliterative bronchiolitis at autopsy or, rarely, at retransplantation (Sharples *et al.* 1996). Biopsy evidence of subtotal active inflammatory obliterative bronchiolitis often prompts augmented immunosuppression in the hope of slowing its progression or possibly even reversing the process (Glanville *et al.* 1987; Levine & Bryant 1995; Sundaresan *et al.* 1995). Inac-

tive total obliteration is clearly irreversible. The early subtotal phases can be easily overlooked if connective tissue stains are not performed on all biopsy material (Higenbottam *et al.* 1988a; Yousem *et al.* 1990a, 1996). The diagnosis should always be sought when foamy macrophages are prominent in distal airspaces resulting from obstruction, with further serial sections and connective tissue stains of biopsy material if necessary.

Obliterative bronchiolitis is the result of bronchiolar damage from numerous causes in the non-transplant population (Epler & Colby 1983). These include toxic fumes, connective tissue disorders and other immunological disorders, such as graft vs. host disease and drug effects (Wyatt *et al.* 1984). There are also infectious causes including respiratory syncytial virus, adenovirus and mycoplasma (Veecroft 1971). In the context of lung transplantation the most likely causes are rejection and/or infection. The weight of evidence is now in favour of rejection as the main cause (Burke *et al.* 1987; Scott *et al.* 1991; Yousem *et al.* 1991). Obliterative bronchiolitis is associated with severe and frequent acute rejection episodes. The severity of acute rejection can be assessed according to a grading system which also takes into account the presence or absence of rejection involving small airways (Yousem *et al.* 1990a, 1996). However, frequent high-grade acute rejection does not inevitably lead to the development of obliterative bronchiolitis and in some studies a clinical diagnosis of acute rejection would appear to be a better predictor (Scott *et al.* 1991). The presence of airways involvement in histologically proven acute rejection correlates with the development of histological obliterative bronchiolitis (Yousem *et al.* 1991; Ohori *et al.* 1994). It appears that intense and persistent immune damage to bronchioles is associated with epithelial loss and later airway fibrosis. Not all institutions follow the same protocols for performing biopsies on transplant patients and clinical diagnoses of rejection are not always confirmed histologically (Higenbottam *et al.* 1988a,b). It is therefore necessary to distinguish between clinical and histological relationships in the development of obliterative bronchiolitis and its response, if any, to new immunosuppressive regimes.

It has been demonstrated that the respiratory epithelium within the graft is an immune target. It expresses class II antigens and some studies have linked the increased expression of these antigens to the development of obliterative bronchiolitis (Romaniuk *et al.* 1987; Glanville *et al.* 1989; Yousem *et al.* 1990b). However, the induction of class II antigens on bronchial and bronchiolar epithelium is not specific to rejection and may be associated with infection, particularly by viruses or *Pneumocystis* (Hruban *et al.* 1989). As well as inducing class II antigens an infectious episode may also non-specifically up-regulate lymphocyte alloreactivity (Zeevi *et al.* 1985). The degree of histocompatibility mismatch has been shown to relate to the extent of bronchiolar damage in animal studies (Romaniuk *et al.* 1987). Harjula *et al.* (1987) reported that their longest surviving lung transplant patient who did not develop obliterative bronchiolitis had the closest HLA match compared with other recipients in their programme. Lung allografts show both histological and functional correlation of obstructive airways disease with positive primed lymphocyte tests performed on bronchoalveolar lavage (Zeevi *et al.* 1985). All these features confirm the importance of acute rejection in the development of obliterative bronchiolitis. Clinically there can be a beneficial effect of augmenting immunosuppression to slow the progression of this fibrosing condition in its early stages (Glanville *et al.* 1987) but relapse appears inevitable (Levine & Bryant 1995), with OB accounting for most long-term deaths (Hosenpud *et al.* 1997).

Infection must be considered as a contributory cause of obliterative bronchiolitis in lung transplant patients. These patients have a greatly increased susceptibility to infection by both common pathogens and opportunistic organisms (Brooks *et al.* 1985; Dummer *et al.* 1986; Maurer *et al.* 1992). Infection can result in chronic persistent epithelial injury with inadequate healing and this may result in mucosal granulation tissue and eventually total obliteration.

Amongst the infectious agents known to cause obliterative bronchiolitis, respiratory syncytial virus, adenovirus, mycoplasma and chlamydia are all known to occur in lung transplant recipients (Veecroft 1971). Cytomegalovirus (CMV) has also been suggested as a cause of obliterative bronchiolitis in graft recipients. It

has been described as producing this pathological change in non-immunosuppressed hosts as a direct effect of viral infection (Katzenstein & Askin 1990a). However, CMV infection has not been identified as a risk factor for the development of obliterative bronchiolitis in all transplant centres (Duncan *et al.* 1991; Keenan *et al.* 1991b; Smyth *et al.* 1991; Sharples *et al.* 1996). There was evidence of a higher incidence of obliterative bronchiolitis in seropositive recipients and mismatched recipients and this association was greater in well-documented CMV pneumonitis (Keenan *et al.* 1991b).

There are several mechanisms by which CMV could increase the risk of developing chronic rejection. There may be a direct viral cytopathic effect on the graft in CMV pneumonitis. Viral inclusions are seen in alveolar epithelial cells, alveolar macrophages and endothelial cells (Stewart *et al.* 1988). However, the bronchiolar epithelium does not usually show viral inclusions or severe inflammatory changes. Cross-reactive antibodies may be formed during CMV infection. Alternatively, the virus may release cytokines or induce cytokines from other inflammatory cells, leading to an increased expression of class II antigens on alveolar epithelial and endothelial cells (Sissons & Borysiewicz 1989; Humbert *et al.* 1992). Such increased expression of class II antigens on bronchial epithelium has been described in obliterative bronchiolitis in human lung transplant patients (Yousem *et al.* 1990b). In all organ grafts the relationship between CMV infection and rejection is complex. The acute lung damage associated with active CMV pneumonitis seems to be related to direct viral cytopathic damage and activation of both macrophages and cytotoxic cells within the lungs. Damage to small airways may occur through any of these mediators even in a predominantly interstitial viral infection (Craigen & Grundy 1996).

Obliterative bronchiolitis does not occur in experimental autografts, which suggests that non-immunological factors, such as ligation of the bronchial circulation, interruption of lymphatics and denervation, are not significant factors in its development (Al-Dossari *et al.* 1995). The most significant effect of denervation and loss of cough reflex is the retention of secretions and an increased risk of pulmonary infections, which may contribute to the development of obliterative bronchiolitis but do not seem to be primary causes. The final common pathology, regardless of specific aetiology, is inflammatory damage to the small airways in the grafted lung.

Obliterative bronchiolitis in lung allograft recipients caused by chronic rejection should be distinguished from bronchiolitis obliterans organizing pneumonia (Abernathy *et al.* 1991). This is seen in transplant recipients as a form of organizing pneumonia and shows granulation tissue in the distal airspaces, often cellular and polypoid. The process may be more patchily distributed than the rejection-related obliterative bronchiolitis, which does not extend distally. This pattern resembles bronchiolitis obliterans organizing pneumonia in non-immunosuppressed patients, which is often associated with chronic interstitial pneumonitis. Bronchiolitis obliterans organizing pneumonia in transplant patients may be postinfectious, as a result of aspiration or drugs (Camus *et al.* 1989). Histological evidence of foreign material, vegetable matter and giant cells usually helps to make the diagnosis of aspiration.

## Large airway pathology

The proximal cartilage-containing airways also show changes in chronic rejection (Hruban & Hutchins 1990; Yousem *et al.* 1990c). Bronchitis and bronchiectasis are common findings. The bronchi are cylindrically dilated with viscid secretions (Tazelaar & Yousem 1988). Acute and chronic inflammatory cell infiltration of the airways occurs with squamous metaplasia and submucosal scarring, including loss of submucosal glands. Smooth muscle may be replaced by fibrous tissue in these larger airways in a similar pattern to that in distal obliterative bronchiolitis. This is probably an important factor in the development of bronchiectasis. The segmental and small subsegmental bronchi can show obliteration with scarring and fulfil the criteria for obliterative bronchitis. This large-airway dilatation, together with air-trapping, is a useful feature of obliterative bronchiolitis at high-resolution computed tomography scanning.

## Chronic vascular rejection

Chronic vascular rejection occurs in pulmonary grafts with a similar morphological appearance to that in other solid organ grafts (Yousem *et al.* 1989a, 1990a). At the present time the pulmonary deterioration in long-term survivors is dominated by the fibrosis of small airways and the vascular abnormalities do not appear to be of clinical relevance. However, if the incidence of obliterative bronchiolitis is reduced and its onset delayed, the vascular abnormalities may have greater clinical implications in the future.

The morphological appearances are those of fibrointimal cellular proliferation involving pulmonary vessels of all sizes (Figs 11.6 and 11.8). On the arterial side all vessels, from the large elastic to smaller muscular arteries and pulmonary arterioles, are involved. The process is initially patchily distributed but becomes more diffuse in advanced cases. The cellularity varies from vessel to vessel and within segments of individual vessels. The main cellular constituents are lymphocytes, both small and large, with macrophages and plasma cells. Neutrophils are not a common feature. The cellular infiltrates can involve the full thickness of the wall with an active endotheliitis. This is similar to the endotheliitis which is seen in acute rejection and represents the active component. In contrast to acute rejection, however, the infiltrates of chronic vasculopathy are more often transmural and are associated with fibrosis and significant narrowing of the lumen (Fig. 11.8). This form of vasculopathy is associated with fibrosis in all layers of the vessel wall (Tazelaar & Yousem 1988). The vascular elastica can be focally destroyed or reduplicated and in many vessels elastic tissue stains demonstrate a combination of these two processes. Thrombosis within the lumen is not a common feature. The venous circulation shows less cellular fibrosis, with hyaline sclerosis involving all sizes of veins. The sclerosis is dense and acellular and does not resemble the looser fibrotic occlusion seen, for example, in veno-occlusive disease. However, this latter pattern can be found in rare cases.

It is also possible to find foamy lipid-laden macrophages within both the arterial and the venous

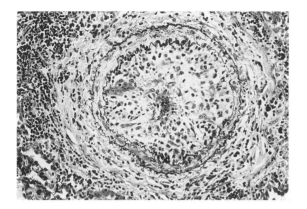

**Fig. 11.8** Chronic vascular rejection of the lung with prominent fibrointimal proliferation occluding the lumen. The elastica is focally disrupted and duplicated. There is periadventitial inflammation indicating transmural infiltration. Grade D. Medium power: open lung biopsy; elastic van Gieson stain.

lesions. The pulmonary capillaries can also show fibrosis and narrowing of the lumen. It is important to distinguish these features from thrombosis and thrombo-embolism, in which there is definite evidence of intraluminal organization of thrombus with recanalization. In patients transplanted for thrombo-embolic pulmonary hypertension, these features may coexist with the distinctive features of allograft vasculopathy. In addition to the features of fibro-occlusive vascular disease, some cases show mild to moderate medial hypertrophy and arterialization of pulmonary arterioles and veins of the type seen in pulmonary hypertension. It is uncertain whether this is a manifestation of chronic vascular rejection. Some patients have right heart catheterization and correlation of the pathological features of the pulmonary vascular bed can be made with the recorded pressures. This is not the case for most patients and pulmonary hypertension does not seem to be a clinical problem as yet in lung transplant recipients.

Yousem *et al.* (1989a) studied the features of pulmonary arteriosclerosis in patients who survived more than 3 months and graded the pulmonary vascular lesions. Grade 1 lesions consisted of mild (less than one-third of diameter) diffuse intimal hyperplasia, Grade 2 lesions reduced the lumen to half of the original diameter and Grade 3 lesions showed complete occlusion. Patients who died with evidence of obliterative bronchiolitis showed Grade 3 pulmonary vascular occlusive disease. A group of five patients without evidence of obliterative bronchiolitis showed only one case of significant arterial disease. Evidence of small recent and organizing thrombo-emboli were seen in two patients dying with obliterative bronchiolitis, one of whom showed Grade 3 changes. Venous sclerosis was also more pronounced in the obliterative bronchiolitis group. All four patients with obliterative bronchiolitis and one non-obliterative bronchiolitis case showed endovasculitis with infiltration of the fibrotic plaques by inflammatory cells. There was no evidence of necrotizing vasculitis. The morphological appearances suggested that the occlusive process began on the luminal aspect of the internal elastic lamina, which later became fragmented. The muscular wall then became attenuated. Advanced vascular occlusive disease can be associated with lipid-rich macrophages and cholesterol clefts resembling an atheromatous plaque.

Pulmonary occlusive disease shares similar risk factors to obliterative bronchiolitis (Scott *et al.* 1990). It is associated with frequent and high-grade acute rejection and in some centres also with CMV infection. In combined grafts there is some correlation between pulmonary and coronary occlusive disease (Stewart & Cary 1991). Indeed some patients with combined grafts die as a result of severe coronary occlusive disease causing extensive myocardial infarction. This occurs in patients with evidence of obliterative bronchiolitis but may be as an isolated manifestation of chronic rejection (Yousem *et al.* 1985; Stewart & Cary 1991; Hosenpud *et al.* 1997). The appearances of the coronary occlusive disease are similar to those in isolated cardiac transplants. The effects of preservation injury and donor vascular pathology on the development of pulmonary occlusive disease are not yet known. The study of unused donor lungs (Stewart *et al.* 1993) showed a high incidence of vascular abnormalities in donors, mainly of an embolic nature. These changes, together with ischaemic damage as a result of preservation and reperfusion, may render the vessels abnormal and more susceptible to the effects of rejection and/or viral infection.

## Grading of lung rejection

In July 1990 the International Society of Heart and Lung Transplantation sponsored a meeting to devise a grading system for rejection in the lung (Yousem *et al.* 1990a). This was to be a histological grading system not dependent on the clinical state of the patient but with meticulous exclusion of infection both in histological, cytological and accompanying microbiological samples (Martin *et al.* 1987). The essential features of the grading system are shown in Table 11.2.

The 1995 modification of the ISHLT scheme (Yousem *et al.* 1996) will be described for each grade, the principles of the earlier scheme being important to the understanding of pulmonary rejection (Table 11.3). Grade A is the acute rejection grade and is based on the frequency, nature and extent of perivascular mononuclear cell infiltration of the lung parenchyma, as

Table 11.2 Working formulation for classification and grading of pulmonary rejection (Lung Rejection Study Group, Yousem *et al.* 1990a).

| Grade | Notes |
| --- | --- |
| **Grade A: Acute rejection** | |
| 1 (Minimal) acute rejection | Scattered infrequent perivascular infiltrates, not obvious at low power; approx. 2–3 cells in perivascular adventitia; may be eosinophils |
| 2 (Mild) acute rejection | Frequent perivascular infiltrates seen at low magnification; lymphocytes, plasmacytoid cells, macrophages, eosinophils; subendothelial infiltration; endothelialitis; no infiltration of alveolar septa or spaces; lymphocytic bronchiolitis (Grade A2a) |
| 3 (Moderate) acute rejection | Dense perivascular infiltrates extending into perivascular and peribronchiolar (a) alveolar septa and spaces; endothelialitis common; eosinophils and neutrophils |
| 4 (Severe) acute rejection | Diffuse perivascular, peribronchiolar, interstitial and airspace infiltrates; alveolar epithelial cell damage; haemorrhage; hyaline membranes, necrosis, infarction; necrotizing vasculitis |
| *Additional suffixes* | |
| a  With evidence of bronchiolar inflammation | |
| b  Without evidence of bronchiolar inflammation | |
| c  With large airway inflammation | |
| d  No bronchioles present | |
| **Grade B: Active airway damage without fibrous scarring** | |
| B1  Lymphocytic bronchitis | No perivascular infiltrates, i.e. no A grade |
| B2  Lymphocytic bronchiolitis | Important to assess in relation to obliterative bronchiolitis |
| **Grade C: Chronic airway damage** | Differs from B by having fibrosis |
| C1  Bronchiolitis obliterans: subtotal | |
| C2  Bronchiolitis obliterans: total | |
|    a  Active | |
|    b  Inactive | |
| **Grade D: Chronic vascular rejection** | Fibrointimal thickening of arteries and veins. Correlation with pulmonary and coronary occlusive disease (in HLT) |
| **Grade E: Vasculitis** | Disproportionate to other inflammation. Necrosis of vessel wall |

**Table 11.3** Revised working formulation for classification and grading of lung allograft rejection (Yousem *et al.* 1996).

Grade A: acute rejection
  Grade 0 None
  Grade 1 Minimal
  Grade 2 Mild   } with/without Grade B
  Grade 3 Moderate
  Grade 4 Severe

Grade B*: airway inflammation
Lymphocytic bronchitis/bronchiolitis

Grade C: chronic airway rejection
Bronchiolitis obliterans
  a Active
  b Inactive

Grade D: chronic vascular rejection
Accelerated graft vascular sclerosis

* Pathologist may choose to grade B lesions, B0–4, none–severe.

assessed semiqualitatively and semiquantitatively. There are four grades of acute rejection with additional suffixes to denote the presence or absence of airways inflammation if these are present in the submitted material. Grade A1 (minimal) acute rejection shows infrequent perivascular infiltrates not obvious at low power and generally only two to three cells thick in the perivascular adventitia. Grade A2 (mild) acute rejection shows more frequent perivascular infiltrates easily visible at low magnification and comprises larger lymphocytes with plasma cells, macrophages and eosinophils. Endotheliitis is common in this grade but there is no infiltration of alveolar septa or spaces. Accompanying airways inflammation is frequently present, i.e. Grade A2a. The next grade, A3 (moderate) acute rejection, is defined by perivascular infiltrates extending into the perivascular and peribronchiolar alveolar septa and spaces. This has to be distinguished from the expansion of the adventitia in Grade A2, in which true interstitial extension is not seen. Endotheliitis is more common in Grade A3, as is the presence of eosinophils and neutrophils. Grade A4 (severe) acute rejection shows progression from A3 with confluence of the interstitial and airspace infiltrates, often involving all the pulmonary tissue in biopsy material. There is

more conspicuous alveolar epithelial cell damage with haemorrhage, hyaline membranes, necrosis and, ultimately, infarction. There may also be necrotizing vasculitis of small vessels but this is extremely uncommon. The separate recording of airways inflammation allowed prospective correlation of the development of obliterative bronchiolitis with the presence of acute rejection involving bronchioles and bronchi. Correlation has varied with different centres (Yousem *et al.* 1996) and has been compounded by difficulties in distinguishing infection-related airway inflammation.

When there is no evidence of perivascular infiltration an A grade cannot be assigned. In this circumstance, if there is active airways inflammation without scarring Grade B is denoted. In the 1990 classification this was divided into lymphocytic bronchitis (B1) and lymphocyte bronchiolitis (B2). This is another category which is important to assess in relation to the development of obliterative bronchiolitis as it may represent the progenitor lesion. In practice it is much less common than Grade A rejection. With adequate sampling of biopsy material perivascular infiltrates are usually found. The 1995 ISHLT working formulation modification retains the A grades 0–4 as the defining features of acute rejection based on perivascular infiltrates. However, suffixes to denote airways changes have been replaced by the category of lymphocytic bronchitis/bronchiolitis, which can be graded B0–4 according to severity. Ungradable biopsies with few airways, tangential cutting or concomitant infection are indicated by BX. The original B category of 1990 is therefore denoted AO, B and the distinction between bronchiolitis and bronchitis is no longer required.

Obliterative bronchiolitis is denoted by Grade C and was divided into a subtotal (C1) and total (C2) form in 1990. The revised formulation appreciates the difficulty of making this distinction in transbronchial biopsies and a single category of C is suggested. Within each category the process is further classified as to the presence (a) or absence (b) of an active inflammatory component. The distinction from Grade B is made by the presence of fibrosis. The most common Grade C found on biopsy material was C1a. This may be because patients with established total, inactive bronchiolitis are less often biopsied after the firm diagnosis of chronic airways rejection had been made (Yousem *et al.* 1989a).

Chronic vascular rejection is designated Grade D and includes the fibrointimal thickening of both arteries and veins. The cellular and acellular hyaline types are not separated on this classification. There may be a correlation with obliterative bronchiolitis and also with coronary occlusive disease in combined grafts (Billingham 1995). Grade D remains unchanged in the revised formulation.

Finally, Grade E referred to the presence of vasculitis which was disproportionate to other inflammation present in the lung material and required the presence of vessel wall necrosis. This change was seen more often in open biopsy material than transbronchial biopsies and may have represented severe acute rejection affecting larger vessels than those present in small biopsy material. This category was abolished in the revised working formulation.

The working formulation for the grading of lung rejection made several recommendations for its application (Yousem *et al.* 1990a, 1996). A minimum of five parenchymal samples is required from the transplanted lung and these should be examined at a minimum of three levels. In practice, many centres use serial sections for more thorough sampling. The biopsies are stained with haematoxylin and eosin, connective tissue stains to demonstrate elastica and fibrosis and silver stains for *Pneumocystis* and fungi. Immunohistochemical or *in situ* hybridization techniques can be applied but are not mandatory. These may be useful to exclude infection, particularly viral, and also for the demonstration of cytokines.

The classifications have been designed to allow communication of results between centres by the standardization of rejection grading. They also aim to incorporate the grading systems that may be in use in individual centres and to allow for easy assessment of new immunosuppression protocols. In practice they have been relatively straightforward to use, the main difficulty being the high incidence of infections in these patients, which can preclude grading of rejection because of the histological overlap of these two processes. When biopsies are taken for both clinical reasons and routine surveillance, specimens are sent for culture and serology, including biopsy material, lavage and sputum. If infection has been suspected, blood cultures and throat swabs may have also been submitted. It is important to review all this material for evidence of infection before assigning a confident rejection grade to biopsy material. This means that biopsy grading for compilation of a database should be a retrospective activity. In practice the diagnosis and grading of rejection for immediate patient management can be performed but the additional caveat 'exclude infection' may be needed.

The main histological features suggestive of concomitant bacterial infection are purulent inflammation in the airways, abundant polymorphs within bronchioles or bronchiolar epithelium and excessive numbers of polymorphs in the lung parenchyma, either diffusely distributed or forming microabscesses (Fig. 11.9). The patient can then be treated both for rejection and infection with augmented immunosuppression and appropriate antimicrobial therapy. A repeat biopsy may be necessary to diagnose the episode correctly and to confirm that the illness has cleared. Biopsies apparently showing rejection only histologically may be associated with positive cultures or serology, emphasizing the need for retrospective review (Wreghitt *et al.* 1990). Other histological features strongly suggestive of infection are necrosis, granulomas and eosinophilia (Stewart & Cary 1996). In a study of 100 consecutive transbronchial biopsies from 43 lung transplant recipients, 54 biopsies were confidently graded as showing rejection only and 14 had evidence of infection on culture or serology (Hunt *et al.* 1992). These biopsies did not show an excess of airways inflammation (suffix a or c on old formulation, B on revised formulation). In a further 22 transbronchial biopsies not graded for rejection as they showed features strongly suggestive of infection histologically, the infection was confirmed by the appropriate culture or serology in 20 instances. The two cases with histological features of infection which were not confirmed showed non-specific pneumonitis and changes suggestive of a viral pneumonitis, respectively. This study showed that 54% of transbronchial biopsies could be retrospectively assigned a final rejection grade having excluded infection and also demonstrated the usefulness of transbronchial biopsy in the

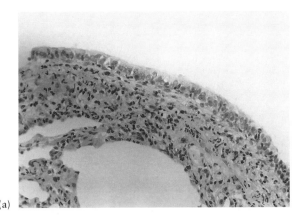

(a)

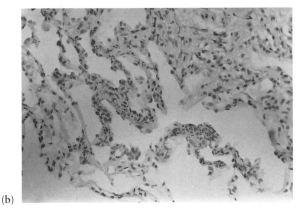

(b)

**Fig. 11.9** Histological features suggestive of concomitant infection are common in (a) the airways and (b) the parenchyma. Collections of polymorphs or more diffusely distributed polymorphs should always raise the possibility or infection. In this case CMV inclusions were seen in areas of inflammation in other biopsy fragments. (a) Medium power, (b) low power: transbronchial biopsy; H & E stain.

diagnosis of pulmonary infections. There is high specificity of the histological appearances of infection in this biopsy material.

## Infections of the transplanted lungs

Lung transplant recipients are particularly prone to infectious complications by both common and opportunistic pathogens (Brooks *et al.* 1985; Dummer *et al.* 1986; Gryzan *et al.* 1988; Maurer *et al.* 1992). This is related to the fact that the immunosuppressed graft is itself in constant exposure to pathogens in the environment. The incidence of infections seems to be greatest after periods of augmented immunosuppression and also when obliterative bronchiolitis has become established. Bacterial superinfections are also common after viral infections (Duncan *et al.* 1991). The diagnosis of bacterial bronchitis, bronchiolitis or pneumonia does not usually require transbronchial material and is generally made by examination and culture of sputum. Gram-negative bacterial infections constitute the largest group of infections in lung transplants but are associated with less mortality than viral and fungal infections (Dummer *et al.* 1986; Maurer *et al.* 1992; Snell *et al.* 1993). The latter two are less common but are more likely to be fatal.

The incidence and nature of infections are broadly similar in combined heart, double and single lung grafts but a diseased native lung can act as a reservoir of infection in an immunosuppressed single lung recipient. The higher risk of ischaemia in the airway in double and single grafts predisposes particularly to infection by *Aspergillus* and this fungus appears to be of greater significance in these patients. Also airway narrowing and stents associated with the double and single lung procedures predispose to distal infection by common as well as opportunistic pathogens.

## Cytomegalovirus

Cytomegalovirus is an important opportunistic viral pathogen of lung allografts, causing significant morbidity and mortality (Burke *et al.* 1986; Hutter *et al.* 1989; Duncan *et al.* 1991; Smyth *et al.* 1991). The virus probably has a role in modulating rejection through immune mechanisms in addition to its direct cytopathic effect (Craigen & Grundy 1996). The prevalence of CMV pulmonary infections has been reported to exceed 75% amongst lung transplant recipients who survive at least 2 weeks after transplantation (Duncan *et al.* 1991). CMV infection can be transmitted via the donor organs or blood, so-called primary infection, or may be caused by reactivation of the virus in a seropositive recipient.

Initially no attempt was made to match donor and

recipient for CMV status but the high mortality associated with primary CMV pneumonitis in the seronegative recipient led to the introduction of a matching policy in most institutions (Hutter *et al.* 1989; Smyth *et al.* 1991). Matching was done on the basis of serological status and reduced the incidence of primary CMV considerably, before instigation of prophylactic regimes of ganciclovir. Reactivation of CMV infection has now assumed greater importance. Prior exposure to CMV is indicated by CMV seropositivity. CMV infection is defined as the identification of the virus by culture or in histological material in a seropositive patient and this must be distinguished from CMV disease, in which the virus is not only identified but causes an inflammatory process (Smyth *et al.* 1991b). Any patient seropositive for CMV may show occasional viral inclusions in tissue samples while under the effects of immunosuppression. In transbronchial biopsy material these infected cells are occasionally seen without any associated inflammatory reaction.

In contrast, CMV pneumonitis is the manifestation of CMV disease in the lung. The histopathological appearances are typical of viral alveolitis. There are alveolar cell hyperplasia, cuboidal metaplasia and epithelial necrosis in severe cases, with hyaline membrane formation (Stewart *et al.* 1988). The interstitium contains an inflammatory cell infiltrate which is a mixture of polymorphs, lymphocytes and macrophages. The polymorphs may be diffusely or focally distributed throughout the alveolar walls and may form microabscesses within these septa (Fig. 11.10). The alveolar spaces contain macrophages and some acute inflammatory cells together with fibrin and haemorrhage. The inflammation tends not to be perivascular in this form of diffuse viral alveolitis. In contrast to rejection, the vessels show marked perivascular oedema with loose collections of cells external to the adventitia. These infiltrates are again rich in polymorphs, further aiding distinction. The hallmark of CMV pneumonitis is the presence of diagnostic inclusions against these background changes. CMV-infected cells contain intranuclear inclusions described as 'owl's eyes' (see Fig. 11.10). The inclusions are variably haematoxyphilic with a perinuclear halo, they are solitary and occur in cells with a single nucleus. In addition, there are intracyto-

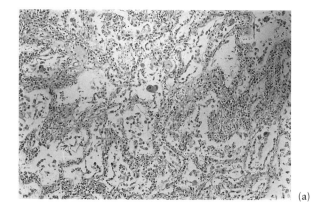

(a)

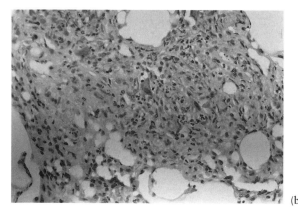

(b)

**Fig. 11.10** (a) Cytomegalovirus disease in grafted lung. CMV pneumonitis at autopsy with well-developed owl's eye inclusions, prominent enlargement of infected cells and interstitial inflammatory reaction. (b) Partially treated CMV pneumonitis with degenerate inclusions, minor cytomegaly and prominent polymorph infiltration of alveolar walls. Patient had been taking ganciclovir prophylaxis and treatment. (a) Low power: autopsy lung, (b) high power: transbronchial biopsy; H & E stain.

plasmic granules which are intensely eosinophilic and can be easily missed if they are out of the plane section of the intranuclear inclusion. They should not be confused with toxoplasma trophozoites. Some biopsies show all the features of alveolitis without the diagnostic inclusions and it is usually possible to suggest the correct diagnosis in a seropositive patient, particularly after augmented immunosuppression, on the basis of these findings (Myerson *et al.* 1984; Stewart *et al.*

1988). Immunohistochemical staining and *in situ* hybridization methods can be useful in these circumstances to confirm the presence of CMV in the lung tissue but have not been shown to have a significant role when diagnostic inclusions are visible on haematoxylin and eosin sections (Niedobitek *et al.* 1988; Weiss *et al.* 1990; Theise *et al.* 1991). These special staining methods increase sensitivity of detection but the important differentiation of infection from pneumonitis is not helped.

There are several difficulties in the diagnosis of CMV pneumonitis in lung transplant patients. First, the patient may have been receiving antiviral therapy either with ganciclovir or acyclovir. Both these drugs have an effect on CMV viral replication which affects the appearance of the inclusions (see Fig. 11.10). The viral inclusions may appear more eosinophilic and degenerate and may be difficult to recognize as viral inclusions in general or CMV in particular (Stewart 1992). The modified inclusions may also be confused with those of other viruses, most commonly herpes simplex virus (HSV). The latter has a different histological appearance, which will be discussed later, but may coexist with CMV in some patients (Smyth *et al.* 1990). Secondly, some biopsies show features of both viral alveolitis and rejection (Higenbottam *et al.* 1988a; Sibley *et al.* 1993). It is not possible to grade rejection according to the working formulation when viral infection is present (Yousem *et al.* 1990a, 1996). It may appear that the two processes are concomitant and a clinician may be advised under these circumstances to treat both. CMV pneumonitis has been associated with perivascular infiltrates in non-transplant patients (Tazelaar 1991) but these tend to be more loosely cellular with oedema compared with the infiltrates associated with acute rejection. Although it may be possible to suggest a diagnosis of CMV pneumonitis with rejection, CMV infection and rejection can be very difficult to differentiate. In some patients it may be necessary to treat and rebiopsy in order to classify the illness correctly. Finally, antiviral prophylaxis and treatment produce a more localized patchy viral pneumonitis, which can only be appreciated by adequate sampling, meticulous screening and a high index of suspicion when a focal neutrophil alveolitis is present.

Primary CMV pneumonitis was almost uniformly fatal until the introduction of ganciclovir (Hutter *et al.* 1989; Smyth *et al.* 1991). It rarely occurs now, as a result of either matching policies between donor and recipient or use of prophylaxis protocols. Fatal CMV pneumonitis involves CMV dissemination to many extrathoracic sites. Non-fatal CMV pneumonitis is a risk factor for the development of obliterative bronchiolitis in some series (Duncan *et al.* 1991, 1992; Ettinger *et al.* 1993) but not others (Keenan *et al.* 1991b; Sharples *et al.* 1996). It is associated with an increase of respiratory superinfections by bacteria and decreased survival. Patients particularly at risk are those who have biopsy-proven CMV pneumonitis. They may develop fungal pneumonias independently of obliterative bronchiolitis. Ganciclovir prophylaxis is now routinely used and this is decreasing the incidence of CMV infections with a corresponding reduction in respiratory superinfections. It is hoped that long-term patient survival will also improve. Ganciclovir treatment of CMV pneumonitis has not been shown to prevent the development of chronic rejection but it may be that prophylaxis will have a beneficial effect on these long-term complications (Keenan *et al.* 1991b). It may also decrease the unexpectedly high incidence of CMV pneumonia found in surveillance biopsies (Trulock *et al.* 1992).

## Herpes simplex infection

Herpes simplex infection (HSV) occurs in lung transplant recipients, usually in seropositive patients (Smyth *et al.* 1990). Its incidence has been significantly reduced by the use of prophylactic acyclovir following transplantation and also during any periods of augmented immunosuppression. It is less common than CMV infection and may be associated with the characteristic mucocutaneous lesions. These lesions are not present in all patients with herpes simplex infection of the graft and the diagnosis of unsuspected HSV pneumonia can be difficult.

The virus causes ulcerating tracheobronchitis, bronchiolitis and necrotizing bronchopneumonia, in contrast to the alveolitis or interstitial pattern of CMV (Smyth *et al.* 1990; Stewart 1992). Necrosis is a prominent feature, with abundant polymorph debris, and this again is useful in distinguishing it from CMV pneumonitis (Fig. 11.11). In biopsy material there may be evidence of viral inclusions in the small airways or in endobronchial biopsy samples (Fig. 11.11). The inclusions are less easy to find than those of CMV. Infected cells are typically bronchoepithelial, squamous metaplastic and alveolar epithelial cells. The HSV inclusions exist in two forms. One shows

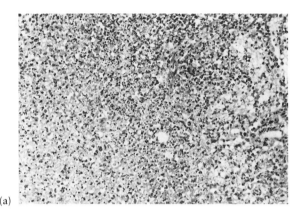

(a)

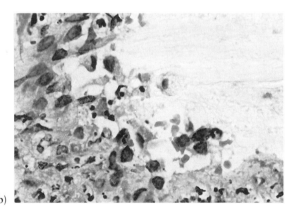

(b)

**Fig. 11.11** (a) Herpes simplex pneumonia in the grafted lung. Necrosis is much more prominent than in CMV pneumonitis and there is no evidence of cytomegaly. The inflammatory process is distributed in a bronchopneumonic pattern. This patient died of unsuspected HSV pneumonia in his second post-transplant year. (b) HSV inclusions in bronchial epithelium. Autopsy lung; H & E stain.

eosinophilic, ground-glass change in infected nuclei with a thin peripheral rim of condensed chromatin. The second form is a Cowdry A type inclusion with a round eosinophilic central body and a clear halo. Multinucleation may be seen but it is not as common as in herpes simplex outside the respiratory tract. Herpes simplex does not produce cytoplasmic inclusions or evidence of cytomegaly. Immunohistochemical staining of biopsy material can be useful in demonstrating the herpetic inclusions but thorough examination of accompanying bronchial aspirate often yields greater numbers of infected cells from the airways with diagnostic inclusions. An intensely purulent aspirate with eosinophilic and pyknotic debris should always prompt a search for HSV in lung transplant patients. Necrotizing bronchopneumonia and tracheobronchitis are associated with intubation and ventilation and have also been seen in patients without obvious risk factors of herpes infection (Geradts *et al.* 1990). In the context of transplantation similar predisposing factors include airway ischaemia, lymphatic interruption and the effects of repeated infections (Katzenstein & Askin 1990b).

Herpes simplex infection can be fatal in transplant patients and may show dissemination to other organs including lymph nodes, oesophagus, liver and brain (Smyth *et al.* 1990). The diagnosis should always be considered when a lung recipient presents with features suggestive of encephalitis. The allograft can be heavily infected in the absence of mucocutaneous lesions to suggest the diagnosis and also acyclovir can clear mucocutaneous HSV without affecting the graft. At autopsy inclusions are more difficult to find because of autolysis. They may be present in viable cells in the residual intact mucosa of the tracheobronchial tree or in the underlying glands. In fatal cases the herpetic pneumonia can advance to diffuse alveolar damage with marked necrosis and identification of the virus may then be extremely difficult.

### *Aspergillus*

*Aspergillus* is a ubiquitous fungus which has emerged as a significant opportunistic pathogen in lung transplant patients. In the non-immunosuppressed host it can produce a range of pathological manifestations ranging from colonization of cavities to hypersensitivity pneumonitis (Pennington 1980). In the immunosuppressed patients other than pulmonary transplants, aspergillosis is a significant problem in those receiving high-dose steroids and many organs may be involved in addition to the lung (Boon *et al.* 1991).

Cerebral aspergillosis has been described particularly in liver transplant recipients. Disseminated *Aspergillus* infection is often diagnosed only at necropsy and this is the experience in some lung transplant patients. However, the regular monitoring of the lung transplant population by sputum culture, lavage and transbronchial biopsies usually leads to identification of the fungus in life. There are many pathological manifestations of *Aspergillus* infection in lung grafts (Table 11.4) and the simple isolation of *Aspergillus* must be interpreted in the light of any other clinicopathological findings (Stewart 1992).

It is helpful to consider *Aspergillus* infection as causing saprophytic, minimally invasive and frankly invasive disease. The large airways are frequent sites of saprophytic colonization, particularly when bronchiectatic as a result of repeated infections and the development of obliterative bronchiolitis (Higenbottam *et al.* 1988a). In this circumstance *Aspergillus* may be cultured from sputum or identified in bronchial aspirates. Aggressive use of antifungal agents with their own serious side effects may not be indicated in patients suffering from this manifestation alone.

Another variant of non-invasive large-airway disease is obstructive tracheobronchial aspergillosis (OTBA) (Kramer *et al.* 1991). In this condition masses of fungal hyphae physically occlude the major airways but show no invasion of the tracheal or bronchial walls. This can be recognized at bronchoscopy by thick greyish yellow occlusive material, which may be lavaged as a therapeutic procedure. Total eradication may require appropriate antifungal therapy.

*Aspergillus* can also cause bronchocentric granulomatous mycosis in lung transplant patients (Tazelaar *et al.* 1989). This is best regarded as a form of minimally invasive disease as the fungal hyphae are not confined to the airway lumen. In this condition there is giant-cell granulomatous inflammatory reaction in the airways. The mucosa can be completely replaced by granulomatous tissue, which may involve all layers of the bronchial or bronchiolar wall eventually (Fig. 11.12). It may be associated with bronchiectasis in larger airways. This type of *Aspergillus* infection is often accompanied by a distal eosinophilic pneumonia. The fungal hyphae are often fragmented and confined to the areas of granulomatous inflammation, not being present in the areas of eosinophilic pneumonia. The granulomatous inflammation may be associated with very small fungal fragments, which require numerous sections and meticulous screening of silver-stained sections for their detection. The granulomas may show necrosis and other organisms, particularly acid-fast bacilli, should be excluded. In severe cases bronchioles

Table 11.4 Histopathological classification of *Aspergillus* disease in transplanted lungs.

|  | Non-invasive | Minimally invasive | Invasive |
|---|---|---|---|
| **Large airways** | Saprophytic colonization | Bronchocentric granulomatous mycosis | Pseudomembranous tracheobronchitis |
|  | Obstructive tracheobronchial aspergillosis |  | Invasion of ischaemic tracheobronchial wall<br>*Aspergillus* bronchitis |
| **Small airways** | Saprophytic colonization | Bronchocentric granulomatous mycosis | *Aspergillus* bronchiolitis |
| **Parenchyma** | Colonization of cavity | Colonization of cavity; focal invasion of wall | Suppurative pneumonia with or without cavitation and abscess formation |

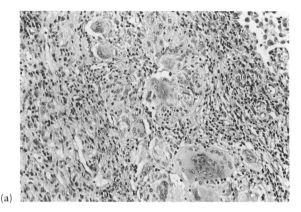

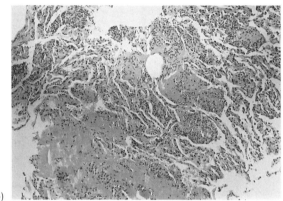

(a)

(b)

**Fig. 11.12** Two manifestations of *Aspergillus* infection in the grafted lung. (a) Bronchocentric granulomatous mycosis with multinucleated giant cells, macrophages and lymphocytes lining a bronchiole and replacing its mucosa. Eosinophilic pneumonia was seen in surrounding parenchyma. Small fungal hyphal fragments were present in a few giant cells in the Grocott methenamine silver stain (not shown). (b) Suppurative pneumonia with prominent intra-alveolar polymorphs and fibrin. Fungal fragments were more frequent than in (a) and were present in large numbers in the accompanying bronchial aspirate. (a) Medium power: resected lung lobe, (b) low power: transbronchial biopsy; H & E stain.

may be totally destroyed by this necrotizing granulomatous process and the bronchocentric nature may only be evident on connective tissue stains. The fungal hyphae do not invade widely into the lung parenchyma, hence its designation of a minimally invasive

form, but, in the setting of immunosuppression, the potential for further invasion is great. This is emphasized by the eventual dissemination in two patients reported by Tazelaar *et al.* (1989). In a patient with severe right upper lobe bronchiectasis a lobectomy performed at our institution revealed extensive bronchocentric granulomatous mycosis and eosinophilic pneumonia in the intervening parenchyma. Resection and antifungal treatment have led to apparent eradication of the *Aspergillus* in this case. Histological examination of lung tissue is critical for the diagnosis of bronchocentric granulomatous *Aspergillus* disease.

Invasive *Aspergillus* infection can involve the airways primarily or the lung parenchyma. It can also exist in a bronchopneumonic form with widespread pulmonary involvement. In the airways *Aspergillus* is seen early after transplantation when there is ischaemia of the anastomosis or distal bronchus. The airway becomes ulcerated with pseudomembrane formation in which fungal hyphae can be demonstrated (Hines *et al.* 1991). Ischaemic cartilage is particularly prone to invasion and this is a potentially lethal complication of airways ischaemia in single and double lung transplant patients (Shumway *et al.* 1993). The less well-vascularized bronchial anastomosis compared with the tracheal anastomosis of combined heart–lung grafts is responsible for the increased risk. Dehiscence of the airway may occur and the fungus may also invade the adjacent pulmonary artery, leading to fatal haemoptysis. Access to the bloodstream allows dissemination of fungus and even aggressive antifungal treatment is not generally successful.

In single lung transplants this invasive *Aspergillus* of the airways is confined to the grafted side, emphasizing the importance of local defence factors. Invasion of the native lung occurs later as a result of blood-borne dissemination. Fungal infection in the ischaemic airway can lead to an early suppurative *Aspergillus* pneumonia in the distal lung tissue, with parenchymal necrosis. *Aspergillus* bronchopneumonia, with *Aspergillus* bronchitis and suppuration is usually seen in the setting of widespread *Aspergillus* infection (Fig. 11.12). Prolonged immunosuppression and obliterative bronchiolitis may predispose to this form of infection. A widely disseminated pulmonary *Aspergillus* infection has also been seen in a patient fulfilling some criteria of graft vs. host disease with persistent chimerism and depletion of lymphoid tissue, but this is an unusual association.

Invasive parenchymal disease may also arise on the basis of colonization of a parenchymal cavity with subsequent tissue extension. Such cavities may be caused by areas of infarction or even previous biopsy sites. *Aspergillus* pneumonia may cavitate *de novo* and this may be difficult to distinguish from a pre-existing cavity. The very different pathological manifestations of *Aspergillus* infection require the careful assessment of patients in whom *Aspergillus* has been identified in sputum, lavage or biopsy material. Antifungal therapy has toxic side effects and the total dose is usually limited. The incidence of *Aspergillus* infection is high, with over a third of lung transplant patients showing histological or cytological evidence either on biopsy material or at autopsy. The incidence may increase further with the increasing use of single and double lung grafts and with increasing numbers of long-term survivors developing obliterative bronchiolitis. Judicious use of immunosuppression in patients with established obliterative bronchiolitis reduces the incidence of *Aspergillus* infection.

## *Pneumocystis carinii*

*Pneumocystis carinii* is an important opportunistic pathogen in lung transplant patients (Gryzan *et al.* 1988). It is important to recognize for two reasons. First, it is readily treatable and, secondly, of all the opportunistic infections it is the closest mimic of rejection (Yousem *et al.* 1990a; Tazelaar 1991). The histopathological features of *Pneumocystis* in a grafted lung differ from those described in other groups of immunosuppressed patients and AIDS patients. In these latter patients *Pneumocystis* is readily identified in abundant intra-alveolar foamy exudate, which is associated with a variable amount of interstitial inflammation (Weber *et al.* 1977). There is conspicuous alveolar cell hyperplasia. Atypical manifestations are also well described and are increasingly recognized in the AIDS population (Travis *et al.* 1990).

Lung transplant recipients, in contrast, show a granulomatous response as the most common reaction to

*Pneumocystis* (Higenbottam *et al.* 1988a; Stewart 1992). There is marked interstitial inflammation with perivascular mononuclear cell infiltrates (Fig. 11.13). Plasma cells are usually very conspicuous and there is often accompanying intra-alveolar organization of exudate. Well-formed giant-cell and epithelioid granulomas may be present but more often there is a diffuse granulomatous inflammation with ill-defined granulomas and scattered giant cells. Serial sections are useful in demonstrating small amounts of foamy exudate in association with these granulomatous areas but this is not always identified. Methenamine silver staining is necessary to demonstrate the organisms, which occur in the centre of the granulomatous areas. The organisms are sparse in number. The features of conspicuous plasma cells and intra-alveolar organization should always raise the possibility of *Pneumocystis* in transbronchial biopsies. It is a mandatory requirement of the working formulation (original and revised) that silver stains for *Pneumocystis* should be screened in all biopsy material from transplant patients in order to exclude this infection (Yousem *et al.* 1990a, 1996). Only then can a diagnosis of rejection be made. The

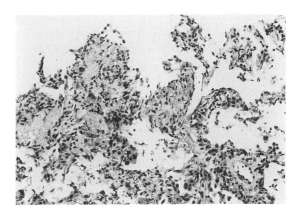

**Fig. 11.13** *Pneumocystis carinii* pneumonia in a grafted lung showing foamy intra-alveolar exudate, intra-alveolar organization and perivascular infiltration. Alveolar cell hyperplasia is prominent and should prompt a search for CMV (not present in this case). Other areas of the biopsy showed epithelioid granulomas with scanty foamy exudate. Medium power: transbronchial biopsy; H & E stain.

**Table 11.5** Histological features of *Pneumocystis carinii* pneumonia in 22 transbronchial biopsies from lung and heart transplant recipients.

|  | Lung transplants* | Heart transplants |
| --- | --- | --- |
| Total number in group | 10 | 12 |
| Granulomas/granulomatous | 8 | 6 |
| Intra-alveolar foam | 4 | 9 |
| Organisms |  |  |
| Scanty | 3 | 0 |
| Intermediate | 6 | 7 |
| Numerous | 1 | 5 |

* Eight biopsies from six heart–lung transplant patients and two biopsies from a single lung transplant patient: one transplant, one own lung.

small numbers of organisms means that transbronchial biopsies are usually required for the diagnosis. Occasionally organisms are identified in lavage material but reliance on these specimens would seriously underdiagnose the condition. The reason for the atypical histological pattern is not clear. *Pneumocystis* may elicit an atypical reaction when it occurs in a graft which is itself susceptible to immunological attack. The immunosuppressive therapy may also be a factor and it is noted that granulomatous *Pneumocystis carinii* pneumonia is seen in heart transplant recipients on similar drug regimes though not in the same high proportion of patients (Table 11.5).

## Mycobacterial infections

Mycobacterial infections occur in lung transplants but are uncommon compared with other opportunistic infections in the UK. Infection by both typical and atypical mycobacteria are described (Schulman *et al.* 1997) and the main risk factor for these infections appears to be obliterative bronchiolitis (Trulock *et al.* 1989) although donor transmission has been described (Ridgeway *et al.* 1996). The relatively low incidence of mycobacterial infections means that stains for acid-fast bacilli are not mandatory when examining transbronchial biopsy material. They should be performed, however, whenever there is granulomatous inflamma-

tion with well- or ill-defined granulomas. The presence of necrosis is a helpful feature but this may occur in other infections, including those caused by fungus. It is also useful to be aware of the primary diagnosis requiring transplantation. Patients transplanted for pulmonary sarcoidosis may experience recurrence in the graft with non-caseating granulomas. The most likely cause of granulomas in immunosuppressed patients is infection and this must be excluded before a diagnosis of recurrent primary disease can be entertained.

## Toxoplasmosis

Toxoplasmosis can occur as primary (donor-transmitted) and recrudescent infection (Wreghitt *et al.* 1989). In cardiac transplants the *Toxoplasma* cysts and trophozoites can be demonstrated in biopsy material but the organisms have not been seen on lung biopsy material. The diagnosis is therefore made by serology. Infection may follow increased immunosuppression and its incidence is decreased by the use of prophylaxis in the early weeks following transplantation in seropositive and mismatched patients. It is important on biopsy material not to confuse the intracytoplasmic inclusions of CMV infection with *Toxoplasma* trophozoites.

## Epstein–Barr virus

Epstein–Barr virus (EBV) causes pulmonary infection and is associated with lymphoproliferative disease in the grafted lung. The diagnosis of acute EBV pneumonitis in lung transplants is extremely difficult as the histological appearances overlap considerably with those of acute pulmonary rejection (Yousem *et al.* 1990a). In non-immunosuppressed patients EBV pneumonitis has been described as showing interstitial infiltration with atypia and necrosis (Veal *et al.* 1990).

## Non-infectious differential diagnosis of acute rejection

The histological appearances of rejection are characteristic but entirely non-specific (Stewart *et al.* 1988; Yousem *et al.* 1990a, 1996). The most important differential diagnoses are those of common and opportunistic infections. BALT is not usually prominent in human lungs. In the first few weeks and months after transplantation it may become exuberant and be confused with lymphocytic bronchitis or bronchiolitis. It can be distinguished by the follicular and parafollicular architecture and the prominent vascularity, including high endothelial venules. The overlying epithelium contains infiltrating lymphocytes, fulfilling the criterion for a lymphoepithelium. Hyperplasia of the BALT following transplantation is probably related to antigen stimulation. The development of BALT has been described in human fetal and infant lung (Gould & Isaacson 1993). It was well developed in almost half of the fetal lungs in cases of stillbirth with intrauterine pneumonia but in only 10% of fetuses without infection. This strongly suggests that its appearance is dependent on antigenic stimulation. Animal studies in the rat have suggested that the BALT is the site of an *in vivo* mixed lymphocyte reaction critical to the rejection of the grafted lung (Prop *et al.* 1985a). Following transplantation the BALT may become depleted and this may be another factor in the increased susceptibility to infections in this group of patients (Hruban *et al.* 1988b).

Recurrence of the primary disease has to be considered in the differential diagnosis of rejection (Stewart & Cary 1991). The aetiology of many of the parenchymal conditions necessitating transplantation is not clear and the likelihood of recurrence in the graft is therefore not known (Stewart *et al.* 1995). Sarcoidosis appears to recur as early as 3–4 months after transplantation but this inevitably remains a diagnosis of exclusion of other causes of granulomas, particularly infectious organisms. Langerhans' cell histiocytosis may recur in the graft but many of its features could be difficult to detect in small biopsies involving many pathological processes. Similarly the features of cryptogenic fibrosing alveolitis or desquamative interstitial pneumonia recurring in the graft would be extremely difficult to differentiate with certainty. The end-stage lung of chronic rejection does not show honeycomb or microcystic change and true recurrence of cryptogenic fibrosis in the graft may be expected to have dissimilar macroscopic and microscopic appearances. Chronic

rejection does not cause this pattern of architectural disruption.

Many patients have numerous transbronchial biopsies performed as part of the postoperative management and many centres exceed the minimum recommendation of five samples of parenchyma. Previous biopsy sites may therefore be encountered in fresh biopsy material and the presence of fibrosis and inflammation should not be confused with rejection. Lung recipients take a variety of medications in addition to their immunosuppressive drugs. It is always possible that a drug effect may be present in biopsy material but, resulting from lack of specificity, its definitive diagnosis is extremely difficult (Camus *et al.* 1989). The effects of drug toxicity, such as that caused by azathioprine, are hard to distinguish from viral infections, which are very common in transplant recipients.

## Post-transplant lymphoproliferative disease in the lung

Heart–lung and lung transplantation appear to be associated with an increased risk of post-transplant lymphoproliferative disorders (LPD) (Yousem *et al.* 1989b; Nalesnik *et al.* 1992). The approximate frequencies are 1% of kidney allograft patients, 2.7% of liver, 3.3% of heart and 3.8% of combined heart–lung or lung recipients. This may be related to the level of immunosuppression used in heart and lung transplants. The pathology of post-transplant lymphoproliferative disease is dealt with in a subsequent chapter but features particularly relevant to lung transplant recipients are described here.

In many other solid organ grafts post-transplant lymphoproliferative disease tends to involve extranodal sites but may also involve the allograft itself. In the lung there is an apparent predilection for involvement of the transplanted organ (Randhawa *et al.* 1989). In an early series of cases, Yousem *et al.* (1989b) reported 60% of LPD in heart–lung transplant recipients presenting primarily in the lung itself. They had an incidence of ~10% in heart–lung transplantation survivors. The lymphoid proliferations are commonly of B cell origin and are frequently preceded by infection with EBV (Nalesnik *et al.* 1988; Swerdlow 1992). The condition can be considered as another manifestation of opportunistic infection, as there are well-documented series of tumour regressing after a reduction of immunosuppression. Within the lung LPD comprises a range of disorders, from non-clonal hyperplasia to monoclonal or oligoclonal tumours (Hanto 1992).

The disease in the lung may be associated with non-specific clinical symptoms and signs or may be found incidentally on chest X-ray or computed tomography. It commonly occurs as multiple nodules of varying sizes. These can be biopsied successfully by the transbronchial biopsy technique under fluoroscopic control or fine needle aspiration biopsy and often a generous bronchial biopsy can be helpful (Egan *et al.* 1995).

Alternative methods of diagnosis include open lung biopsy and some cases are discovered at autopsy.

The disease process is best described from open biopsy and autopsy material, where the architecture of the nodules is apparent. There is consolidation of the pulmonary parenchyma into nodular areas with ill-defined margins. The cellular infiltrate often extends from these margins along perivascular and lymphatic and peribronchiolar routes as well as extending into interlobular septa. The consolidation is caused by sheet-like infiltration of lymphoid cells (Fig. 11.14). These is a mixture of large and small lymphoid cells but either can predominate. Some have cleaved, others non-cleaved nuclei and there may be immunoblasts

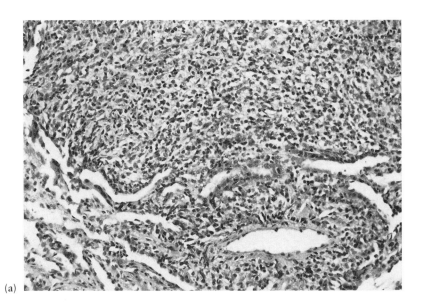

(a)

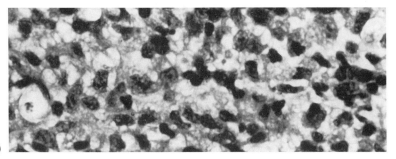

(b)

**Fig. 11.14** (a) Lymphoproliferative disease in the transplanted lung showing sheet-like infiltration from a perivascular distribution of variably sized lymphoid cells. These are atypical and pleomorphic (b) compared to the infiltrate of acute rejection. This patient died of disseminated disease. Transbronchial biopsy; H & E stain.

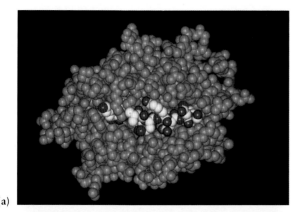

(a)

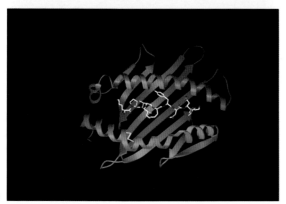

(b)

**Plate 2.1** Computer simulation of a viral peptide presented by an MHC class I molecule: (a) shows a space-filling representation; (b) shows a ribbon diagram of the same complex.

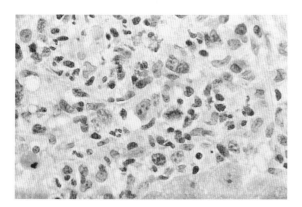

**Plate 9.1** Acute cellular rejection: human liver graft, day 6. High power view of the portal cellular infiltrate which includes many blast cells with large open nuclei with several nucleoli and a number of mitotic figures, and many eosinophils. H & E stain.

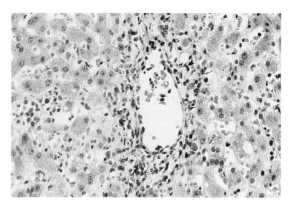

**Plate 9.2** Acute cellular rejection, high grade: human liver graft, day 6. Endotheliitis of a terminal hepatic venule. Note also the extension of the infiltrate into the adjacent sinusoids—'sinusoidal endotheliitis'. H & E stain.

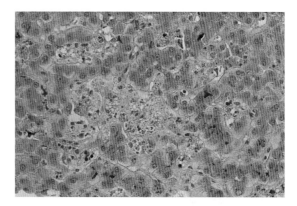

**Plate 9.3** Chronic rejection: human liver graft, 8 months after transplantation. Note the profound canalicular cholestasis in hepatocytes. In addition, many of the sinusoidal Kupffer cells have taken up bile pigment and/or have a foamy cytoplasm. H & E stain.

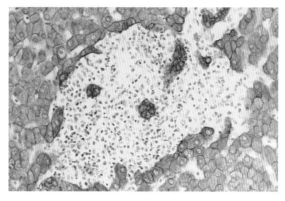

**Plate 9.4** Actue rejection: use of an immunostain for cytokeratins to demonstrate bile-duct epithelium. In this case there has been no loss and the small bile-ducts are intact and normal, despite being surrounded by a dense cellular infiltrate. Haematoxylin, anticytokeratin stain.

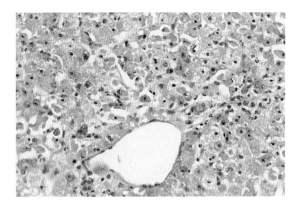

**Plate 9.5** Primary non-function: human liver graft. The liver never showed any evidence of synthetic function and had to be replaced on day 5. Note the very irregular non-zonal pattern of acidophilic necrosis with, in a number of places around this terminal venule, alternating necrotic and viable hepatocytes. H &E stain.

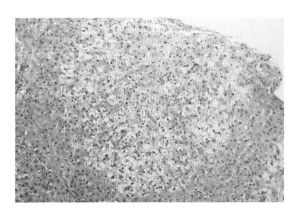

**Plate 9.6** Hepatocyte ballooning: human liver graft, day 8. Note the well-defined area of hepatocyte ballooning in acinar zones 2 and 3, which was attributable to initial poor function. Complete recovery occurred in time. H & E stain.

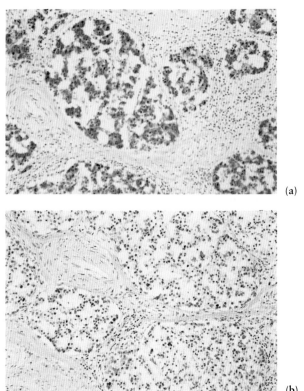

(a)

(b)

**Plate 12.1** Post-mortem sections of fully functioning segmental duct occluded pancreas graft 9.5 years post-transplantation. Sections stained brown for (a) human insulin, and (b) human glucagon by immunohistochemical staining procedure (magnification ×200).

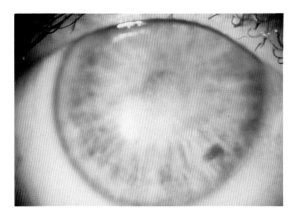

**Plate 13.1** Corneal scarring secondary to herpes simplex keratitis.

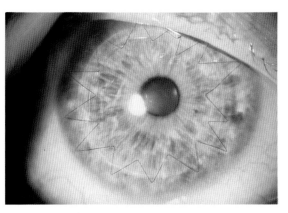

**Plate 13.2** Successful penetrating keratoplasty.

with large nuclei and multiple nucleoli (Nalesnik *et al.* 1988). Cytoplasm may be abundant. Occasionally, Reed–Sternberg-like cells can be identified. Mitotic activity is nearly always present and the lesions very commonly show areas of coagulative necrosis. Plasma cells and plasmacytoid cells are variable but can be a striking component which is readily identifiable on fine needle aspiration material. Infiltration of vascular walls of both arterioles and veins involves the full thickness and includes fibrinoid necrosis. Nodules close to the pleura often show invasion through the pleural elastica. Diagnosis on transbronchial biopsy is more difficult but LPD should always be considered when coagulative necrosis, with sheets of rather monotonous ghost cells, is present. Sheet-like proliferations of viable lymphoid cells may also occur and their diffuse nature should alert pathologists to the correct diagnosis.

The main differential diagnosis is acute rejection (Rosendale & Yousem 1995; Yousem *et al.* 1996), which does not show extensive sheet-like infiltration or the pleomorphism and mitoses. Also acute rejection is not associated with coagulative necrosis or transmural infiltration. Fibrinoid necrosis is seen in larger vessels than those usually sampled on transbronchial biopsies in very advanced rejection grades only. Despite the great variation in clonality (Hanto 1992; Swerdlow 1992) the histopathological pattern can be uniform in this disease and it should always be suspected when unusual lymphoid infiltrates are present in biopsy material. The nodular form of LPD confined to the lungs may regress on a combination of acyclovir treatment and reduction of immunosuppression. Lymphoproliferative disease can, however, be fatal, behaving as a malignant lymphoma and necessitating aggressive chemotherapy. The findings at autopsy are typical of disseminated malignant lymphoma. Extranodal disease is common, including involvement of the central nervous system. Initial presentation in the small bowel has been seen in several of the Papworth cases.

Phenotypic, genotypic and EBV studies show a range of abnormalities in common with LPD in other transplant groups (Hanto 1992). Complete characterization of the LPD requires studies of this nature, as classification on the basis of morphology alone is difficult (Swerdlow 1992). There are two principal classifications. Frizerra *et al.* (1981) describe polymorphic B cell hyperplasia, polymorphic B cell lymphoma and atypical polymorphic B cell hyperplasia. Their classification attaches importance to atypical immunoblasts and necrosis as well as plasmacytic differentiation. An alternative classification on histological grounds is that of Nalesnik *et al.* (1988), which recognizes polymorphic, monomorphic and minimally polymorphic categories. This classification concentrates on the proportions of small and large lymphocytes, cleaved and non-cleaved, plasmacytoid cells, plasma cells and immunoblasts. Necrosis and atypical immunoblasts are not essential criteria. It is not only difficult to distinguish with certainty benign from malignant proliferations on these histological features but it is also difficult to classify these processes using conventional lymphoma classification schemes. Genotypic studies suggest that many LPD cases represent polyclonal or oligoclonal disease subsequently evolving into a monoclonal proliferation in a subset of cases.

In lung transplant recipients the presence of nodules on radiographic, computed tomography or tissue samples should raise the possibility of lymphoproliferative disease. Other causes of similar nodules include opportunistic pneumonias, mainly *Aspergillus* and herpes simplex pneumonias, and bronchiolitis obliterans organizing pneumonia. Recent biopsy sites can produce haemorrhagic subpleural nodules, which are occasionally detected at autopsy and should not be confused with a neoplastic or infectious process.

## Cytological aspects of lung transplantation

Bronchoalveolar lavage (BAL) is a non-invasive technique which can be used to assess the inflammatory and immune responses of the lung. It has been applied to both experimental and clinical lung transplantation. The assumption is made that the cells obtained at lavage are representative of those within the lung parenchyma and studies looking at both biopsies and synchronous lavages have confirmed this to a large extent (Clelland *et al.* 1993). The differential cell count, however, may not be valid if the airways are inflamed with purulent or retained secretions. In the clinical setting lavage has had a major role with the analysis of cell populations and functional testing of lymphocytes (Paradis *et al.* 1985; Griffith *et al.* 1987; Gryzan *et al.* 1988). Analysis of cells recovered by lavage has shown that most donor lymphocytes within the graft are replaced by the recipient cells within the first 6 weeks. Macrophages and lymphocytes of donor HLA may persist as late as 32 weeks after transplantation and this may be reflected in the lower incidence of rejection after this period. Zeevi *et al.* (1985) showed that during rejection episodes cells obtained by lavage were cytolytic to donor spleen cells and showed spontaneous proliferation and interleukin 2 responsiveness. However, high levels of cell-mediated lympholysis were also seen during infection and rejection could not be distinguished from infection by the cellular profile alone.

Clelland *et al.* (1993) studied concurrent transbronchial lung biopsies and bronchoalveolar lavages in 48 heart–lung transplant recipients. Paired samples were available on 135 occasions and total lavage cell counts were increased slightly during episodes of illness, whether caused by infection or rejection. High lymphocyte counts greater than 15% were supportive of a diagnosis of rejection but were only found in 23% of rejection episodes. Neutrophils were increased in both rejection and infection but cell counts returned to normal after treatment. There was no evidence that bronchoalveolar cell counts or profiles were diagnostic for lung rejection and there was no correlation with the histological grade of rejection on the corresponding biopsy. The use of immunocytochemistry to determine lymphocyte phenotypes did not provide additional discrimination. CD3 and CD8 cells were increased in both acute and chronic rejection, with considerable overlap between these and infected patients. CD8 cells always predominated but these are the most common cells in both normal and diseased respiratory epithelium anyway (Fournier *et al.* 1989). Reinsmoen *et al.* (1992) demonstrated that BAL cells cultured from patients undergoing acute rejection showed a predominance of CD4, consistent with class II-directed reactivity. In contrast, cultured BAL cells from patients with obliterative bronchiolitis demonstrated a CD8 predominant phenotype, consistent with class I-directed reactivity. The percentage BAL lymphocytosis during rejection has been studied prospectively. De Hoyos *et al.* (1993) found that the percentage lymphocytosis was significantly greater in Grade 2–3 rejection than in Grade 1 or Grade 0 rejection. There was, however, no significant difference between Grade 0 and 1. They found that a 20% BAL lymphocytosis had a sensitivity of 40% and specificity of 96%. For 15% lymphocytosis, sensitivity improved to 59% but specificity declined to 86%, similar to the results obtained by Clelland *et al.* (1993).

The main role of lavage cytology is in the diagnosis of opportunistic infections, as discussed in other sections of this chapter and as described in non-transplant patients (Martin *et al.* 1987).

## Conclusions

The morphological appearances of lung transplants are many and varied. The principal pathologies are those of rejection, both acute and chronic, and infection by herpes viruses, *Pneumocystis* and *Aspergillus*. Lymphoproliferative disease may occur primarily in the graft. The differentiation of these various disorders can be extremely difficult and can be further confused by the possible recurrence of primary disease in the graft. In common with other groups of transplant patients there is often more than one diagnosis in the grafted organ and the biopsy material submitted for the evaluation of postoperative complications should always be examined with this possibility in mind. It is likely that transbronchial biopsy material will remain a gold standard for the diagnosis of complications in this group of patients for some time to come (Trulock *et al.* 1992; De Hoyos *et al.* 1993; Sibley *et al.* 1993; Guilinger *et al.* 1995; Boehler *et al.* 1996; Yousem *et al.* 1996). Clinical and radiological assessment combined with pulmonary function testing is less specific. The future will bring developments in the diagnosis of rejection in tissue samples and its differentiation from other similar processes by identifying specific subsets of effector cells. Cytological monitoring of the graft through the examination of the bronchoalveolar lavage fluid will also continue to grow in importance (Clelland *et al.* 1993). At present it has largely research applications in the phenotyping and alloreactivity of the cellular constituents. The measurements of cytokines may yield more useful and specific profiles with an impact on therapy. This is an exciting area where molecular techniques will have a significant role in the diagnosis of immunological complications of grafting.

# References

Abernathy, E.C., Hruban, R.H., Baumgartner, W.A., Reitz, B.A. & Hutchins, G.M. (1991) The two forms of bronchiolitis obliterans in heart–lung transplant recipients. *Human Pathology* 22, 1102–1110.

Al-Dossari, G.A., Jessurun, J., Bolman, R.M. *et al.* (1995) Pathogenesis of obliterative bronchiolitis. *Transplantation* 59, 143–145.

Bando, K., Paradis, I.L., Komatsu, K. *et al.* (1995) Analysis of time-dependent risks for infection, rejection and death after pulmonary transplantation. *Journal of Thoracic and Cardiovascular Surgery* 109, 49–59.

Berry, G.J. & Yousem, S.A. (1995) Lung transplantation In: *Diagnostic Immunopathology* (eds R.B. Colvin, A.K. Bhan & R.T. McCluskey), pp. 397–411. Raven Press, New York.

Billingham, M.E. (1995) Pathology of graft vascular disease after heart and heart–lung transplantation and its relationship to obliterative bronchiolitis. *Transplantation Proceedings* 27, 2013–2016.

Boehler, A., Vogt, P., Zollinger, A., Weder, W. & Speich, R. (1996) Prospective study of the value of transbronchial lung biopsy after lung transplantation. *European Respiratory Journal* 9, 658–662.

Boon, A.P., O'Brien, D. & Adams, D.H. (1991) 10 year review of invasive aspergillosis detected at necropsy. *Journal of Clinical Pathology* 44, 452–254.

Brooks, R.G., Hofflin, J.M., Jamieson, S.W., Stinson, E.B. & Remington, J.S. (1985) Infectious complications in heart–lung recipients. *American Journal of Medicine* 79, 412–422.

Burke, C.M., Theodore, J., Dawkins, K.D. *et al.* (1984) Posttransplant obliterative bronchiolitis and other late lung sequelae in human heart–lung transplantation. *Chest* 86, 824–829.

Burke, C.M., Glanville, A.R., Macoviak, J.A. *et al.* (1986) The spectrum of cytomegalovirus infection in human heart–lung transplantation. *Journal of Heart Transplantation* 5, 267–272.

Burke, C.M., Glanville, A.R., Theodore, J. & Robin, E.D. (1987) Lung immunogenicity, rejection and obliterative bronchiolitis. *Chest* 92, 547–549.

Camus, P., Lombard, J.-N., Perrichon, M. *et al.* (1989)

Bronchiolitis obliterans organising pneumonia in patients taking acebutalol or amiodarone. *Thorax* 44, 711–715.

Casteneda, A.R., Arnor, O., Schmidt-Habelbaum, P., Moller, J.H. & Zamora, R. (1972) Cardiopulmonary autotransplantation in primates. *Journal of Cardiovascular Surgery* 37, 523–531.

Clelland, C.A., Higenbottam, T.W., Stewart, S., Scott, J.P. & Wallwork, J. (1990) The histological changes in transbronchial biopsy after treatment of acute lung rejection in heart–lung recipients. *Journal of Pathology* 161, 105–112.

Clelland, C.A., Higenbottam, T.W., Stewart, S. *et al.* (1993) Bronchoalveolar lavage and transbronchial lung biopsy during acute rejection and infection in heart–lung transplant patients. *American Review of Respiratory Disease* 147, 1386–1392.

Cooper, J.D., Patterson, G.A., Grossman, R. & Maurer, J. (1989) Double lung transplant for advanced chronic obstructive lung disease. *American Review of Respiratory Disease* 139, 303–307.

Cooper, J.D., Billingham, M.E., Egan, T. *et al.* (1993) A working formulation for the standardization of nomenclature and for clinical staging of chronic dysfunction in lung allografts. *Journal of Heart and Lung Transplantation* 12, 713–716.

Courand, L. & Nashef, S.A.M. (1995) Airway complications. In: *Lung Transplantation—Current Topics in General Thoracic Surgery* (ed. G.A. Patterson), pp. 483–496. Elsevier Science, Amsterdam.

Craigen, J.L. & Grundy, J.E. (1996) Cytomegalovirus induced up-regulation of LFA-3 (CD58) and ICAM-1 (CD54) is a direct viral effect that is not prevented by ganciclovir or foscarnet treatment. *Transplantation* 62, 1102–1108.

Dark, J. & Corris, P.A. (1989) The current state of lung transplantation. *Thorax* 44, 689–692.

De Hoyos, A., Chamberlain, D., Schwartzman, R. *et al.* (1993) Prospective assessment of a standardised pathologic grading system for acute rejection in lung transplantation. *Chest* 103, 1813–1818.

Dummer, S.J., Montero, C.G., Griffith, B.P. *et al.* (1986) Infections in heart–lung transplant recipients. *Transplantation* 41, 725–729.

Duncan, A.J., Dummer, J.S., Paradis, I.L. *et al.* (1991) Cytomegalovirus infection and survival in lung transplant recipients. *Journal of Heart and Lung Transplantation* 10, 638–646.

Duncan, S.R., Paradis, I.L., Yousem, S.A. *et al.* (1992) Sequelae of cytomegalovirus pulmonary infections in lung allograft recipients. *American Review of Respiratory Disease* 146, 1419–1425.

Egan, J.J., Hasleton, P.S., Yonan, N. *et al.* (1995) Necrotic, ulcerative bronchitis, the presenting feature of lymphoproliferative disease following heart–lung transplantation. *Thorax* **50**, 205–207.

Egan, T.M., Boychuk, J.E., Rosato, K. & Cooper, J.D. (1992) Whence the lungs? A study to assess suitability of donor lungs for transplantation. *Transplantation* **53**, 420–422.

Epler, G.R. & Colby, T.V. (1983) The spectrum of bronchiolitis obliterans. *Chest* **83**, 161–162.

Ettinger, N.A., Bailey, T.C., Trulock, E.P. *et al.* (1993) Cytomegalovirus infection and pneumonitis: impact after isolated lung transplantation. *American Review of Respiratory Disease* **147**, 1017–1023.

Fournier, M., Lebargy, F., Ladurie, F.L.R., Lenormand, E. & Pariente, R. (1989) Intraepithelial T-lymphocyte subsets in the airways of normal subjects and of patients with chronic bronchitis. *American Review of Respiratory Disease* **140**, 737–742.

Frizerra, G., Hanto, D.W., Gajl-Peczalska, K.J. *et al.* (1981) Polymorphic diffuse B-cell hyperplasia and lymphomas in renal transplant recipients. *Cancer Research* **41**, 4262–4279.

Frost, A.E., Keller, C.A. & Cagle, P.T. (1993) Severe ischaemic injury to the proximal airway following lung transplantation. Immediate and long-term effects on bronchial cartilage. *Chest* **103**, 1899–1901.

Geradts, J., Warnock, M. & Yen, B. (1990) Use of the polymerase chain reaction in the diagnosis of unsuspected herpes simplex viral pneumonia: report of a case. *Human Pathology* **21**, 118–121.

Glanville, A.R., Baldwin, J.C., Burke, C.M., Theodore, J. & Robin, E.D. (1987) Obliterative bronchiolitis after heart–lung transplantation: apparent arrest by augmented immunosuppression. *Annals of Internal Medicine* **107**, 300–304.

Glanville, A.R., Tazelaar, H.D., Theodore, J. *et al.* (1989) The distribution of MHC class I and class II antigens on bronchial epithelium. *American Review of Respiratory Disease* **139**, 330–334.

Gould, S.J & Isaacson, P.G. (1993) Bronchus-associated lymphoid tissue (BALT) in human fetal and infant lung. *Journal of Pathology* **169**, 229–234.

Griffith, B.P., Hardesty, R.L., Trento, A. *et al.* (1987) Heart–lung transplantation: lessons learned and future hopes. *Annals of Thoracic Surgery* **43**, 6–16.

Gryzan, S., Paradis, I.L., Zeevi, A. *et al.* (1988) Unexpectedly high incidence of *Pneumocystis carinii* infection after heart–lung transplantation: implications for lung defence and allograft survival. *American Review of Respiratory Disease* **137**, 1268–1274.

Guilinger, R.A., Paradis, I.L., Dauber, J.H. *et al.* (1995) The importance of bronchoscopy with transbronchial biopsy and bronchoalveolar lavage in the management of lung transplant recipients. *American Journal of Respiratory and Critical Care Medicine* **152**, 2037–2043.

Hanto, D.W. (1992) Polyclonal and monoclonal post

transplant lymphoproliferative disease (LPD). *Clinical Transplantation* **6**, 227–234.

Harjula, A.J.L., Baldwin, J.C., Glanville, A.R. *et al.* (1987) Human leukocyte antigen compatibility in heart–lung transplantation. *Journal of Heart Transplantation* **6**, 162–166.

Higenbottam, T.W. (1992) Single lung transplantation and pulmonary hypertension. *British Heart Journal* **62**, 121.

Higenbottam, T.W. & Stewart, S. (1989) Transbronchial lung biopsy in the diagnosis of rejection of the transplanted lung. In: *Heart and Lung Transplantation* (ed. J. Wallwork), pp. 523–532. W.B. Saunders, Philadelphia.

Higenbottam, T.W., Stewart, S., Penketh, A.R.L. & Wallwork, J.L. (1988a) Transbronchial lung biopsy for the diagnosis of rejection in heart–lung transplant patients. *Transplantation* **46**, 532–539.

Higenbottam, T.W., Stewart, S. & Wallwork, J. (1988b) Transbronchial lung biopsy to diagnose lung rejection and infection of heart–lung transplants. *Transplantation Proceedings* **20**, 767–769.

Hines, D.W., Hauber, M.H., Yaremko, L. *et al.* (1991) Pseudomembranous tracheobronchitis caused by aspergillus. *American Review of Respiratory Disease* **143**, 1408–1411.

Hosenpud, J.D., Bennett, L.E., Keck, B.M., Fiol, B. & Novick, R.J. (1997) The Registry of the International Society for Heart and Lung Transplantation, Fourteenth Official Report. *Journal of Heart and Lung Transplantation* **16**, 691–712.

Hruban, R.H. & Hutchins, G.M. (1990) The pathology of lung transplantation. In: *Heart–Lung Transplantation* (eds W.A. Baumgartner, S.C. Achuff & B.A. Reitz), pp. 372–389. W.B. Saunders, Philadelphia.

Hruban, R.H., Beschorner, W.E., Baumgartner, W.A. *et al.* (1988a) Diagnosis of lung allograft rejection by bronchial intraepithelial Leu-7 positive T-lymphocytes. *Journal of Thoracic and Cardiovascular Surgery* **96**, 939–946.

Hruban, R.H., Beschorner, W.E., Baumgartner, W.A. *et al.* (1988b) Depletion of bronchus-associated lymphoid tissue with lung allograft rejection. *American Journal of Pathology* **132**, 6.

Hruban, R.H., Beschorner, W.E., Baumgartner, W.A. *et al.* (1989) Evidence that the expression of class II MHC antigens is not diagnostic of lung allograft rejection. *Transplantation* **48**, 529–530.

Humbert, M., Devergne, O., Cerrina, J. *et al.* (1992) Activation of macrophages and cytotoxic cells during cytomegalovirus pneumonia complicating lung transplants. *American Review of Respiratory Disease* **145**, 1178–1184.

Hunt, J.B., Stewart, S., Cary, N. *et al.* (1992) Evaluation of the International Society for Heart Transplantation grading of pulmonary rejection in 100 consecutive biopsies. *Transplant International* **5**, S249–S251.

Hutter, J.A., Despins, P., Higenbottam, T.W., Stewart, S. & Wallwork, J.L. (1988) Heart–lung transplantation: better use of resources. *American Journal of Medicine* 85, 4–11.

Hutter, J.A., Scott, J.P., Wreghitt, T., Higenbottam, T. & Wallwork, J. (1989) The importance of cytomegalovirus in heart–lung transplant recipients. *Chest* 95, 627–631.

Judson, M.A. & Sahn, S.A. (1996) Pleural space and the organ transplantation. *American Journal of Respiratory and Critical Care Medicine* 153, 1153–1165.

Judson, M.A., Handy, J.R. & Sahn, S.A. (1997) Pleural effusion from acute lung rejection. *Chest* 111, 1128–1130.

Katzenstein, A.L. & Askin, F.B. (1990a) *Surgical Pathology of Non-neoplastic Lung Disease*, pp. 323–328. W.B. Saunders. Philadelphia.

Katzenstein, A.L. & Askin, F.B. (1990b) *Surgical Pathology of Non-neoplastic Lung Disease*, pp. 326–333. W.B. Saunders. Philadelphia.

Keenan, R.J., Bruzzone, P., Paradis, I.L. *et al.* (1991a) Similarity of pulmonary rejection patterns among heart–lung and double lung transplant recipients. *Transplantation* 51, 176–180.

Keenan, R.J., Lega, M.E., Dummer, S. *et al.* (1991b) Cytomegalovirus serologic status and postoperative infection correlated with risk of developing chronic rejection after pulmonary transplantation. *Transplantation* 51, 433–438.

Kells, C.M., Marshall, S. & Kramer, M. (1992) Cardiac function after domino-donor heart transplantation. *American Journal of Cardiology* 69, 113–116.

Kesten, S., Chamberlain, D. & Maurer, J. (1996) Yield of surveillance transbronchial biopsies performed beyond two years after lung transplantation. *Journal of Heart and Lung Transplantation* 15, 384–408.

Kramer, M.R., Denning, D.W., Marshall, S.E. *et al.* (1991) Ulcerative tracheobronchitis after lung transplantation: a new form of invasive aspergillosis. *American Review of Respiratory Disease* 144, 552–556.

Levine, S.M. & Bryant, C.L. (1995) Bronchiolitis obliterans in lung transplant recipients. *Chest* 107, 894–896.

Locke, T.J., Hooper, T.L., Flecknell, P.A. & McGregor, C.G.A. (1988) Preservation of the lung. Comparison of topical cooling and cold crystalloid pulmonary perfusion. *Journal of Thoracic and Cardiovascular Surgery* 96, 789–795.

Martin, W.F., Smith, T.F., Bruntinel, W.M., Cockerill, F.R. & Douglas, W.M. (1987) Role of bronchoalveolar lavage in the assessment of opportunistic pulmonary infections: utility and complications. *Mayo Clinic Proceedings* 62, 549–557.

Maurer, J.R. (1994) Lung transplantation bronchiolitis obliterans. In: *Diseases of the Bronchioles* (ed. Gary R. Epler), pp. 275–289. Raven Press, New York.

Maurer, J.R., Tullis, E., Grossman, R.F. *et al.* (1992)

Infectious complications following isolated lung transplantation. *Chest* 101, 1056–1059.

Millet, B., Higenbottam, T.W., Flower, C.D.R., Stewart, S. & Wallwork, J. (1989) The radiographic appearances of infection and acute infection of the lung after heart–lung transplantation. *American Review of Respiratory Disease* 140, 62–67.

Milne, D.S., Gascoigne, A.D., Ashcroft, T. *et al.* (1994) Organizing pneumonia following pulmonary transplantation and the development of obliterative bronchiolitis. *Transplantation* 57, 1757–1762.

Myerson, D., Hackman, R.C., Nelson, J.A., Ward, D.C. & McDougall, J.K. (1984) Widespread presence of histologically occult cytomegalovirus. *Human Pathology* 15, 430–439.

Nalesnik, M.A., Jaffe, R., Starzl, T.E. *et al.* (1988) The pathology of post-transplant lymphoproliferative disorders occurring in the setting of cyclosporin A prednisolone immunosuppression. *American Journal of Pathology* 133, 173–192.

Nalesnik, M.A., Locker, J., Jaffe, R. *et al.* (1992) Experience with posttransplant lymphoproliferative disorders in solid organ transplant recipients. *Clinical Transplantation* 6, 249–252.

Nathan, S.D., Ross, D.J., Belman, M.J. *et al.* (1995) Bronchiolitis obliterans in single-lung transplant recipients. *Chest* 107, 967–972.

Niedobitek, G., Finn, T., Herbst, H. *et al.* (1988) Detection of cytomegalovirus by in-situ hybridisation and histochemistry using a monoclonal antibody CCH2: a comparison of methods. *Journal of Clinical Pathology* 41, 1005–1009.

Ohori, N.P., Iacono, A.T., Grgurich, W.F. & Yousem, S.A. (1994) Significance of acute bronchiolitis/bronchiolitis in the lung transplant recipient. *American Journal of Surgical Pathology* 18 (12), 1192–1204.

Paradis, I.L., Marrari, M., Zeevi, A. *et al.* (1985) HLA phenotype of lung lavage cells following heart–lung transplantation. *Journal of Heart Transplantation* 4, 422–425.

Paradis, I.L., Yousem, S.A. & Griffith, B. (1993) Airway obstruction and bronchiolitis obliterans after lung transplantation. *Clinics in Chest Medicine* 14, 751–763.

Penketh, A.R.L., Higenbottam, T.W.H., Hakim, M. & Wallwork, J. (1987) Heart and lung transplantation in patients with end-stage lung disease. *British Medical Journal* 295, 311–314.

Pennington, J.E. (1980) Aspergillus lung disease. *Medical Clinics of North America* 64, 475–491.

Pham, S.M., Yoshida, Y., Aeba, R. *et al.* (1992) Interleukin-6, a marker of preservation injury in clinical lung transplantation. *Journal of Heart and Lung Transplantation* 11, 1017–1024.

Prop, J., Nieuwenhuis, P. & Wildevuur, C.R.H. (1985a) Lung

allograft rejection in the rat. I. Accelerated rejection caused by graft lymphocytes. *Transplantation* **40**, 25–30.

Prop, J., Wildevuur, C.R.H. & Nieuwenhuis, P. (1985b) Lung allograft rejection in the rat III. Corresponding morphological rejection phases in various rat strain combinations. *Transplantation* **40**, 132–137.

Randhawa, P.S., Yousem, S.A., Paradis, I.L. *et al.* (1989) The clinical spectrum, pathology and clonal analysis of Epstein–Barr virus associated lymphoproliferative disorders in heart–lung transplant recipients. *American Journal of Clinical Pathology* **92**, 177–185.

Reichenspurner, M., Girgis, R.E., Robbins, R.C. *et al.* (1996) Stanford experience with obliterative bronchiolitis after lung and heart–lung transplantation. *Annals of Thoracic Surgery* **62**, 1467–1472.

Reinsmoen, N.L., Bolman, R.M., Savik, K., Butters, K. & Hertz, M. (1992) Differentiation of class I and class II directed donor specific alloreactivity in bronchoalveolar lavage lymphocytes from lung transplant recipients. *Transplantation* **53**, 181–189.

Reitz, B.A., Wallwork, J., Hunt, S.A. *et al.* (1982) Heart–lung transplantation: successful therapy for patients with pulmonary vascular disease. *New England Journal of Medicine* **306**, 557–564.

Ridgeway, A.L., Warner, G.S., Phillips, P. *et al.* (1996) Transmission of *Mycobacterium tuberculosis* to recipients of single lung transplants from the same donor. *American Journal of Respiratory and Critical Care Medicine* **153**, 1166–1168.

Romaniuk, A., Prop, J., Peterson, A.H., Wildevuur, C.R.H. & Nieuwenhuis, P. (1987) Expression of class II major histocompatability complex antigens by bronchial epithelium in rat lung allografts. *Transplantation* **44**, 209–214.

Rosendale, B. & Yousem, S.A. (1995) Discrimination of Epstein–Barr virus-related posttransplant lymphoproliferations from acute rejection in lung allograft recipients. *Archives of Pathology and Laboratory Medicine* **119**, 418–423.

Schulman, L.L., Scully, B., McGregor, C.C. & Austin, J.H.M. (1997) Pulmonary tuberculosis after lung transplantation. *Chest* **111**, 1459–1462.

Scott, J.P., Higenbottam, T.W., Clelland, C.A. *et al.* (1990) Natural history of chronic rejection in heart–lung transplant recipients. *Journal of Heart Transplantation* **9**, 510–515.

Scott, J.P., Higenbottam, T.W., Sharples, L. *et al.* (1991) Risk factors of obliterative bronchiolitis in heart–lung transplant recipients. *Transplantation* **51**, 813–817.

Sharples, L.D., Tamm, M., McNeil, K. *et al.* (1996) Development of bronchiolitis obliterans syndrome in recipients of heart–lung transplantation: early risk factors. *Transplantation* **61**, 560–566.

Shumway, S.J., Hertz, M.I., Maynard, R., Kshetty, V.R. & Bolman, I.I.I. (1993) Airway complications after lung and heart–lung transplantation. *Transplantation Proceedings* **25**, 1165–1166.

Sibley, R.K., Berry, G.J., Tazelaar, H.D. *et al.* (1993) The role of transbronchial biopsies in the management of lung transplant recipients. *Journal of Heart and Lung Transplantation* **12**, 308–324.

Sissons, J.G.P. & Borysiewicz, L.K. (1989) Human Cytomegalovirus infection. *Thorax* **44**, 241–246.

Smyth, R.L., Higenbottam, T.W., Scott, J.P. *et al.* (1990) Herpes simplex virus infection in heart–lung transplant recipients. *Transplantation* **49**, 735–739.

Smyth, R.L., Higenbottam, T.W., Scott, J. & Wallwork, J. (1991a) The current state of lung transplantation for cystic fibrosis. *Thorax* **46**, 213–216.

Smyth, R.L., Scott, J.P., Borysiewicz, L.K. *et al.* (1991b) Cytomegalovirus infection in heart–lung transplant recipients: risk factors, clinical associations and response to treatment. *Journal of Infectious Diseases* **164**, 1045–1050.

Snell, G.I., de Hoyos, A., Krajden, M., Winton, T. & Maurer, J.R. (1993) *Pseudomonas cepacia* in lung transplant recipients with cystic fibrosis. *Chest* **103**, 466–471.

Snell, G.I., Ward, C., Wilson, J.W. *et al.* (1997) Immunopathological changes in the airways of stable lung transplant recipients. *Thorax* **52**, 322–328.

Starnes, V.A., Theodore, J., Oyer, P.E. *et al.* (1989a) Evaluation of heart–lung transplant recipients with prospective, serial transbronchial biopsies and pulmonary function studies. *Journal of Thoracic and Cardiovascular Surgery* **98**, 683–690.

Starnes, V.A., Theodore, J., Oyer, P.E. *et al.* (1989b) Pulmonary infiltrates after heart–lung transplantation: evaluation by serial transbronchial biopsies. *Journal of Thoracic and Cardiovascular Surgery* **98**, 945–950.

Stewart, S. (1992) Pathology of lung transplantation. *Seminars in Diagnostic Pathology* **9**, 210–219.

Stewart, S. & Cary, N. (1991) The pathology of heart and lung transplantation: an update. *Journal of Clinical Pathology* **44**, 803–811.

Stewart, S. & Cary, N.R.B. (1996) The pathology of heart and lung transplantation. *Current Diagnostic Pathology* **3**, 69–79.

Stewart, S., Higenbottam, T.W., Hutter, J.A. *et al.* (1988) Histopathology of transbronchial biopsies in heart–lung transplantation. *Transplantation Proceedings* **20**, 764–766.

Stewart, S., Ciulli, F., Wells, F. & Wallwork, J. (1993) Pathology of unused donor lungs. *Transplantation Proceedings* **25**, 1167–1168.

Stewart, S., McNeil, K., Nashef, S.A.M. *et al.* (1995) Audit of referral and explant diagnoses in lung transplantation: a pathologic study of lungs removed for parenchymal disease. *Journal of Heart and Lung Transplantation* 14, 1173–1186.

Sundaresan, S., Trulock, E.P., Mohanakumar, T., Cooper, J.D., Patterson, G.A. & The Washington University Lung Transplant Group (1995) Prevalence and outcome of bronchiolitis obliterans syndrome after lung transplantation. *Annals of Thoracic Surgery* 60, 1341–1347.

Swerdlow, S. (1992) Post-transplant lymphoproliferative disorders: a morphologic, phenotypic and genotypic spectrum of disease. *Histopathology* 20, 373–385.

Tazelaar, H.D. (1991) Perivascular inflammation in pulmonary infections: implications for the diagnosis of lung rejection. *Journal of Heart and Lung Transplantation* 10, 437–441.

Tazelaar, H.D. & Yousem, S.A. (1988) The pathology of combined heart–lung transplantation. An autopsy study. *Human Pathology* 19, 1403–1416.

Tazelaar, H.D., Prop, J., Nieuwenhuis, P., Billingham, M.E. & Wildevuur, C.R.H. (1987) Obliterative bronchiolitis in the transplanted rat lung. *Transplantation Proceedings* 19, 1052.

Tazelaar, H.D., Baird, A.M., Mill, M. *et al.* (1989) Bronchocentric mycosis occurring in transplant recipients. *Chest* 96, 92–95.

Theise, N.D., Haber, M.M. & Grimes, M.M. (1991) Detection of *Cytomegalovirus* in lung allografts. Comparison of histologic and immunohistochemical findings. *American Journal of Clinical Pathology* 96, 762–766.

Travis, W.D., Pittaluga, S., Lipschik, G.Y. *et al.* (1990) Atypical pathologic manifestations of *Pneumocystis carinii* pneumonia in the acquired immune deficiency syndrome. *American Journal of Surgical Pathology* 14, 615–625.

Trulock, E.P., Bolman, R.M. & Genton, R. (1989) Pulmonary disease caused by mycobacterium chelonae in a heart–lung transplant recipient with obliterative bronchiolitis. *American Review of Respiratory Disease* 140, 802–805.

Trulock, E.P., Ettinger, N.A., Brunt, E.M. *et al.* (1992) The role of transbronchial lung biopsy in the treatment of lung transplant recipients. *Chest* 102, 1049–1054.

Veal, C.F., Carr, M.B. & Briggs, D.D. (1990) Diffuse pneumonia and acute respiratory failure due to infectious mononucleosis in a middle aged adult. *American Review of Respiratory Disease* 141, 502–504.

Veecroft, D.M.O. (1971) Bronchiolitis obliterans, bronchiectasis and other sequelae of adenovirus type 21 infection in young children. *Journal of Clinical Pathology* 24, 72–82.

Veith, F.J., Koerner, S.K., Siegelman, S.S. *et al.* (1973) Diagnosis and reversal of rejection in experimental and clinical lung allografts. *Annals of Thoracic Surgery* 16, 172–183.

Weber, W.R., Askin, F.B. & Dehner, L.P. (1977) Lung biopsy in *Pneumocystis carinii* pneumonia. A histopathological study of typical and atypical features. *American Journal of Clinical Pathology* 67, 11–19.

Weiss, L.M., Movahed, L.A., Berry, G.J. & Billingham, M.E. (1990) In situ hybridisation studies for viral nucleic acids in heart and lung allograft biopsies. *American Journal of Clinical Pathology* 93, 675–679.

Wreghitt, T.G., Hakim, M., Gray, J.J. *et al.* (1989) Toxoplasmosis in heart and lung transplant recipients. The Papworth Hospital Series. *Journal of Clinical Pathology* 42, 194–199.

Wreghitt, T.G., Smyth, R.L., Scott, J.P. *et al.* (1990) Value of culture of biopsy material in diagnosis of viral infections in heart–lung transplant recipients. *Transplantation Proceedings* 22, 1809–1810.

Wyatt, S.E., Nunn, P., Hows, J.M. *et al.* (1984) Airways obstruction associated with graft versus host disease after bone marrow transplantation. *Thorax* 39, 887–894.

Yoshida, Y., Iwaki, Y., Pham, S. *et al.* (1993) Benefits of post-transplantation monitoring of interleukin 6 in lung transplantation. *Annals of Thoracic Surgery* 55, 89–93.

Yousem, S.A., Burke, C.M. & Billingham, M.E. (1985) Pathologic pulmonary alterations in long-term human heart–lung transplantation. *Human Pathology* 16, 911–923.

Yousem, S.A., Paradis, I.L., Dauber, J.H. *et al.* (1989a) Pulmonary arteriosclerosis in long-term human heart–lung transplant recipients. *Transplantation* 47, 564–569.

Yousem, S.A., Randhawa, P., Locker, J. *et al.* (1989b) Post transplant lymphoproliferative disorders in heart lung transplant recipients: primary presentation in the allograft. *Human Pathology* 20, 361–369.

Yousem, S.A., Berry, G.J., Brunt, E.M. *et al.* (1990a) A working formulation for the standardisation of nomenclature in the diagnosis of heart and lung rejection: lung rejection study group. *Journal of Heart Transplantation* 9, 593–601.

Yousem, S.A., Curley, J.M., Dauber, J.A. *et al.* (1990b) HLA class II antigen expression in human heart–lung allografts. *Transplantation* 49, 991–995.

Yousem, S.A., Paradis, I.L., Dauber, J.A. *et al.* (1990c) Large airway inflammation in heart–lung recipients—its significance and prognostic implications. *Transplantation* 49, 654.

Yousem, S.A., Dauber, J.A., Keenan, R. *et al.* (1991) Does histologic acute rejection in lung allografts predict the development of bronchiolitis obliterans? *Transplantation* 52, 306–309.

Yousem, S.A., Berry, G.J., Cagle, P.T. *et al.* (1996) A revision of the 1990 working formulation for the classification of lung allograft rejection. *Journal of Heart and Lung Transplantation* 15, 1–15.

Zeevi, A., Fung, J.J., Paradis, I.L. *et al.* (1985) Lymphocytes of bronchoalveolar lavages from heart–lung transplant recipients. *Journal of Heart Transplantation* **4**, 417–421.

Zenati, M., Dowling, R.D., Dummer, S. *et al.* (1990a) Influence of the donor lung on development of early infections in lung transplant recipients. *Journal of Heart Transplantation* **9**, 502–509.

Zenati, M., Yousem, S.A., Dowling, R.D., Stein, K.L. & Griffith, B.P. (1990b) Primary graft failure following pulmonary transplantation. *Transplantation* **50**, 165–167.

# Chapter 12/Pancreas and islet transplantation

I. GABRIELLE M. BRONS

## Introduction

With the discovery of the blood glucose-lowering hormone, insulin, by Banting and Best (1922), hopes were raised that a cure for diabetes mellitus (DM) had been found. Exogenous insulin therapy effectively abolished early mortality and extended the lifespan of insulin-dependent diabetic patients. However, it was soon realized that DM was really a multifactorial disease and over a period of time could result in diabetic micro- and macroangiopathy affecting, amongst others, specific cells of the kidney, heart, nervous tissue and the highly sensitive retinal cells. These secondary complications, rarely seen before, affect about 50% of all patients within 5–20 years after the onset of the disease. So far no clear evidence of the mechanism for the development of life-threatening secondary complications has been demonstrated despite extensive research throughout the twentieth century.

However, it has been confirmed that perfect metabolic control delays the onset of secondary complications and slows down the progression of diabetic retinopathy, nephropathy and neuropathic lesions (DCCT 1993). However, it is difficult for the patient to achieve tight glucose control over a prolonged period with multiple exogenous insulin injections or devices such as insulin pumps with continuous subcutaneous insulin infusions (CSII) or intensive intermittent subcutaneous (ISII) insulin injections. It is tedious for the patient, requires effective patient education, discipline and compliance over many years for these measures to result in long-term euglycaemia. Frequent self-monitoring of blood glucose levels throughout the day and multiple clinic visits are the norm. These measures also carry a high risk of potentially lethal hypoglycaemic episodes and other side effects, such as ketoacidosis.

Although important developments in insulin therapy have improved the quality of life of the diabetic patient, they are still 25 times more prone to blindness, 17 times more likely to acquire renal disease resulting in renal failure, five times more afflicted with neuropathic alterations resulting in gangrene and amputations and run the risk of heart disease twice as often as non-diabetic individuals. The cumulative incidence of nephropathy was calculated at 45% after 40 years of diabetes. Of patients referred for dialysis or renal transplantation

20–30% have end-stage renal disease caused by diabetic microangiopathy.

No common indicator has been found to predict at an early stage which patient may be more susceptible to the effects of rapidly changing high and low glucose levels and thus more liable to develop macro- and/or microangiopathy. However, there are protocols to identify individuals at risk of acquiring DM and for identifying subjects where DM is already in progress, though at a subclinical level, by testing for islet cell autoantibodies (ICA), insulin autoantibodies (IAA) and a range of metabolic glucose tolerance tests. With identification of patients at high risk of developing diabetes it is possible to set up trials for the prevention of further progression of this disease.

Moreover, large trials have been undertaken to test new immunosuppressive agents for their ability to arrest or even reverse the autoimmune process of type 1 DM and inhibit the selective destruction of insulin-secreting islet cells in newly diagnosed patients, especially young children, before clinical diabetes becomes manifest (Dupre *et al.* 1988). Despite early promising results (Stiller *et al.* 1984) this immunotherapy, using the powerful agent cyclosporin A (CyA), did not seem to be able, upon cessation of treatment, to prevent or reverse the progression of DM. Also, nephrotoxicity was seen in some patients relative to dosage and duration of this treatment.

Strategies for preventing type 1 DM have been suggested by Verge and Eisenbarth (1996), resulting in several large clinical trials to test whether the onset of disease can be prevented by administration of low-dose exogenous insulin therapy or the use of nicotinamide.

Transplantation of pancreatic tissue with normal β cells, programmed to release insulin on demand to maintain euglycaemic glucose levels within a very narrow range, would provide physiological glucose control and remove the threat of ketoacidosis or potentially lethal hypoglycaemic episodes. In DM it is only the insulin-producing tissue which is failing and thus pancreatic islet tissue in the form of isolated islets as a free graft or a segmental or whole organ pancreas graft as a vascular graft can be used. Both these concepts have developed concurrently since the mid-1960s as a potential form of therapy for DM.

Extensive experimental research in the large-animal model was mainly concerned with the development and improvement of surgical techniques and assessment of new preservation solutions. It has contributed enormously to the clinical applicability and success of vascular pancreas grafting, which is now recognized as a true alternative therapy for DM.

Experimental islet transplantation has been successful in the small-animal model for many years and to a lesser extent in the larger-animal model. Using animal models with autoimmune diabetes has made a significant contribution not only towards the immunological and metabolic implications of transplanting insulin-secreting tissue, but also towards our understanding of the aetiology of diabetic disease. However, the transformation to clinical islet transplantation has only recently been made in a very limited number of selected patients in a few centres worldwide and with only a few patients achieving consistent insulin independence for prolonged periods.

## Vascularized pancreas transplantation

The first human segmental pancreas transplant was performed by Kelly *et al.* in 1966 at the University of Minnesota. Since then pancreatic transplant cases have been reported to the International Pancreas Transplant Registry (IPTR) and analysed by Dr Sutherland, University of Minnesota, USA. A series of 13 segmental pancreas transplants were performed between the end of 1966 and 1973. Only one of these transplants functioned for more than 1 year, but this was proof that a segmental pancreas graft could produce the insulin needed to support the patient's requirements at least for a limited timespan. By 1977 information on 57 transplants was collected. The 1-year graft survival was only 3% with a 1-year patient survival of 40% (Sutherland 1980). This early experience was not encouraging because most grafts failed as a result of inadequate immunosuppression or technical problems, such as thrombosis and leakage of exocrine fluid resulting in fistulae and infections.

Dubernard *et al.* (1978) overcame the complications of exocrine leakage seen in the earlier studies by occluding the ductal system with neoprene, a synthetic rubber, which results in necrosis of the exocrine tissue without damaging the endocrine system. This new technique, together with the discovery of the immuno-suppressive properties of CyA by Borel *et al.* (1976) and its clinical application as a steroid-sparing yet powerful immunosuppressant by Calne *et al.* (1978, 1979), has been instrumental in advancing pancreas transplantation. Improvement of graft survival increased pancreas transplant activity dramatically. To date over 10 000 cases from over 150 institutions worldwide have been reported to the IPTR (Sutherland *et al.* 1998).

## Indication and timing

Many diabetic patients lead a satisfactory life on exogenous insulin injections with little disturbance of their daily routine. If, however, macro- and/or microangiopathic alterations occur and their quality of life is deteriorating, replacement therapy should be considered.

Renal grafting is the treatment of choice for renal failure in DM; 1-year graft survival results are nearly as good as in non-diabetic patients with end-stage renal failure of different aetiology (Cedea & Terasaki 1991). However, the development of diabetic nephropathy in renal grafts 2–4 years after transplantation was of great concern (Mauer *et al.* 1983, 1989; Hariharan *et al.* 1996), but there is now ample evidence that an additional pancreas graft can protect the newly trans-planted kidney from recurrent disease (Bohman *et al.* 1985; Bilous *et al.* 1989). Thus, simultaneous pancreas and kidney (SPK) from the same donor or pancreas after a previously transplanted kidney (PAK) is indi-cated in insulin-dependent diabetic patients with end-stage renal failure.

Indications for solitary pancreas grafts (pancreas transplant alone, PTA) (Sutherland 1991), however, are still hotly debated. Here the side effects of immuno-suppression have to be set off against simply achieving insulin independence and improvement of quality of life if it is accepted that the effect of pancreas transplan-tation on arresting or even reversing the progression of nephropathy, retinopathy and neuropathy have so far been minimal. Current criteria for a solitary pancreas graft include insulin-dependent diabetes with first signs of diabetic nephropathy with a creatinine clearance above 70 ml/min, proven neuropathy and/or progressive retinopathy, labile diabetes and unaware-ness of hypoglycaemia. As a general rule, candidates should be selected on the basis that their predicted secondary complications are potentially more dan-gerous than the combined risk of chronic immuno-suppressive treatment and operative intervention (Tattersal 1989).

One-year graft survival results have improved con-siderably in this category over the last few years from 37% to 61% and over 70% if a pancreas from a 0–1 HLA A, B and DR antigen-matched donor is trans-planted (Sutherland 1991). With the improvement of graft survival the indications for this procedure should be continuously redefined, especially if one can wait for a good HLA-matched donor organ and if the risks of immunosuppressive treatment can be reduced or if donor-specific tolerance can be induced by simple strategies. However, it is important to realize that pan-creas transplantation is not a life-saving operation but certainly an improvement in the quality of life (AIDSPIT Conference Report 1991; Bartlett *et al.* 1996) and should therefore be carried out in carefully selected patients to achieve maximum benefit. Never-theless, the risks should be weighed against the possi-bility of halting or even preventing the secondary complications which are now the major cause of diabetic mortality and morbidity.

## Living related pancreas donation

The rationale for the use of living related pancreas donation is the shortage of cadaver donors and the likely reduction of rejection occurring with HLA histo-compatible organs and thus the reduced need for immunosuppression. Living related grafts are techni-cally more difficult and therefore have resulted in a higher failure rate, but this is offset by a lower inci-dence of graft rejection compared to cadaveric donor grafts. The most extensive experiences with grafts from related donors have been reported by Sutherland *et al.* (1984, 1989a,b) and provide an opportunity to study the effect of hemipancreatectomy on glucose metabolism in the non-diabetic donating patient (Kendall *et al.* 1989). Preliminary results showed metabolic changes in over one-third of otherwise healthy patients. In three donors non-insulin-dependent diabetes mellitus (NIDDM) developed. Later they reported on the metabolic consequences of hemipancreatectomy in 28 healthy living related donors. Although these donors had normal fasting blood glucose and insulin levels and normal 24 h glucose profiles, there were abnormalities in insulin secretion and deterioration in glucose tolerance in seven of 28 patients studied 1 year after hemipancreatectomy (Kendall *et al.* 1990). No further decline in glucose tolerance was shown 2–7 years after hemipancreatectomy. Whether clinical insulin-dependent DM will develop later in some of the donors is not yet clear and further long-term studies are called for. As a result of this study much stricter criteria for the selection of living related donors have been instituted.

These results are not surprising, considering the 50% reduction in pancreatic tissue with an even higher reduction in islet cell mass, as it is generally agreed that islets and β cells are more numerous in the tail than the head or body. The reduction in insulin storage capacity, resulting in the loss of first-phase insulin secretion and the time required to resynthesize insulin, may result in abnormal glucose tolerance during stimulation but normal levels during fasting. The metabolic effects of the resection of various amounts of pancreatic tissue have been studied in dogs and were reported by Sun *et al.* (1974), who found significant metabolic changes when more than 50% of the pancreas was removed. Metabolic studies in two non-diabetic patients after resection of over 50% of pancreatic tissue (Whipple's operation) for adenocarcinoma showed normal fasting glucose levels but similarly impaired glucose tolerance (Brons *et al.* 1987).

## Segmental versus whole pancreas grafting

On the basis of the aforementioned study concerning hemipancreatectomy, it would seem to be logical to transplant whole cadaveric pancreas rather than a segmental graft in order to provide sufficient insulin-secreting cells for synthesis and storage and as a func-

tional reserve in case of graft injury as a result of prolonged ischaemia, preservation damage or rejection. In terms of metabolic control, differences were seen in a study by La-Rocca *et al.* (1987), Caldara *et al.* (1991) and Christiansen *et al.* (1996). Responses to glucose stimulation were more adequate with whole-organ than with segmental grafts. Even so, segmental grafts sustained normal glucose metabolism over a long period of time, as evidenced by several reports on the long-term function of segmental grafts (Brons *et al.* 1991; Holdas *et al.* 1991; Landgraf *et al.* 1991; Robertson *et al.* 1991; Secchi *et al.* 1991).

## Surgical techniques

The development of surgical techniques for pancreas transplantation has gone through many stages with several techniques being rediscovered over the years. Three main duct management techniques have emerged: duct injection (DI), as advocated by Dubernard *et al.* (1978); intestinal drainage (ID), further developed by the Stockholm group (Groth *et al.* 1982, 1989); and bladder drainage (BD), reintroduced by Cook *et al.* (1983) and Sollinger *et al.* (1987) and modified by Corry *et al.* (1986). These techniques use non-physiological systemic endocrine drainage leading to potential peripheral hyperinsulinaemia. Calne (1984) developed a surgical technique with physiological insulin delivery, the paratopic technique, with portal endocrine drainage and diversion of the exocrine secretion into the stomach (Calne 1984; Calne & Brons 1985; Brons & Calne 1991).

In this institution (Department of Surgery, University of Cambridge, England) >46 pancreas transplants have been performed using these four different surgical techniques. The earliest was in 1979 with a segmental duct-injected graft. This patient had long-term pancreatic function, being insulin-independent for 9.5 years when she died suddenly from a myocardial infarction. Post-mortem revealed the pancreatic graft had shrunk to the size of a thumbnail, consisting entirely of well-vascularized pancreatic islets surrounded by fibrous tissue (Plate 12.1, facing p. 342), demonstrating for the first time that a vascularized islet graft could function satisfactorily in the long term. In the paratopic group several patients are insulin-independent and have ongoing long-term function of both their segmental pancreas and simultaneous kidney grafts for >15, >13.5 and >12 years and one patient who received a bladder-drained pancreas graft has had a functioning graft for >8.5 years.

## Graft survival results

Worldwide, SPK transplant outcome for 1-year patient survival was 94%, with 90% for kidney and 83% for pancreas graft survival (Sutherland *et al.* in press). For 5-year graft survival the outcome was 81%, 70% and 62%, respectively (Fig. 12.1) (Sutherland & Gruessner 1995a). In the USA, 15% of transplants are carried out as solitary grafts of either PAK or PTA. Survival of the pancreatic graft was significantly higher ($P<0.001$) in the SPK group than the PAK or PTA category, with 1-year graft survival of 68% vs. 45% and 37%, respectively. Patient survival was higher in the PAK and PTA groups, with 94% and 91% compared with 88% in the SPK recipient category (Sutherland & Gruessner 1995b). This, of course, is not surprising as this group includes patients with more severe secondary complications.

When comparing SPK pancreas graft survival rates with the PAK or PTA rates, the better outcome is probably influenced by the immunosuppressive effect of uraemia (Lawrence 1965) and the use of a simultaneously transplanted kidney as a marker for rejection episodes. With serum creatinine being a very sensitive marker, early treatment of an immune response directed initially towards the renal graft could prevent the progression of the rejection process towards the pancreas, whereas in the PAK and PTA groups the undetected destruction of islets may already be too far advanced to be reversible by antirejection treatment. However, the change in immunosuppressive therapy from triple therapy to tacrolimus (FK506) and mycophenolate mofetil (MMF) in the PTA group has increased the 1-year graft survival to >68% (Sutherland *et al.* 1998) without any apparent detrimental effect on the islet cell function.

## Diagnosis of rejection

Rejection involves the combined forces of cellular and humoral host products responding to the invading foreign antigen. The detection of rejection is well defined in organ grafts other than pancreas by bio-

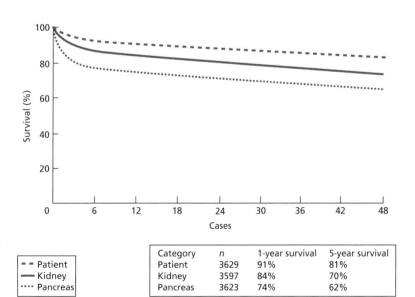

**Fig. 12.1** One- and 5-year world transplant outcome in cadaveric simultaneous pancreas and kidney grafted patients during the period 1 October 1987 to 30 April 1994. From data presented at the 5th Congress of the International Pancreas and Islet Transplant Association (IPITA), Miami Beach, Florida, USA, 1995.

| Category | *n* | 1-year survival | 5-year survival |
|----------|------|-----------------|-----------------|
| Patient  | 3629 | 91%             | 81%             |
| Kidney   | 3597 | 84%             | 70%             |
| Pancreas | 3623 | 74%             | 62%             |

chemical markers and histological assessment of biopsy material. However, the early diagnosis of pancreatic rejection remains a problem. It is very difficult to detect rejection at an early stage by monitoring plasma glucose levels. A rise in fasting blood glucose is almost always a late manifestation of ongoing rejection. It normally only occurs after over 80% of islet tissue has been destroyed by undetected rejection and rescue treatment may already be too late.

Simultaneously transplanted kidneys are being used as markers of immunological activity, though in several instances ongoing rejection did not always occur in both organs and one graft may be lost while the other continues to function. Nevertheless, results from combined kidney and pancreas grafting are better than pancreas grafts alone. This suggests that the kidney graft and thus serum creatinine measurements or renal biopsy may act as indirect diagnostic tools for assessment of rejection in the pancreas.

With the bladder drainage technique it is possible to monitor rejection, based on the observation that rejection first attacks the exocrine portion of the pancreas and thus a decrease in the enzyme content and pancreatic juice output precedes hyperglycaemia by several days (Prieto *et al.* 1987; Tyden *et al.* 1987b). Urinary amylase concentrations will vary considerably and therefore amylase content is calculated from 24 h urine collections, having established a baseline for each patient. A decrease of more than 40% is suggestive but not diagnostic of rejection and careful observation of other signs of rejection have to be taken into account to avoid overtreatment with antirejection therapy.

Fasting and postprandial serum c-peptide measurements can give a more accurate estimate of insulin secretion if renal function is normal. As c-peptide is metabolized by the kidneys, high levels of c-peptide may accumulate during the first few days after a kidney and pancreas graft until kidney function is normalized. On the other hand, false high levels may be seen with nephrotoxic levels of immunosuppressive agents such as CyA. However, routine monitoring may be helpful in recipients of a single pancreas graft (PAK, PTA) when it is not possible to monitor amylase content and output of the excreted pancreatic juice.

Many other pancreas-specific markers for diagnosis of rejection have been developed, such as serum anodal trypsinogen (Marks *et al.* 1990; Perkal *et al.* 1992), pancreatic-specific protein measurements (Kernstad *et al.* 1989), pancreatic juice neopterin excretion (Margreiter *et al.* 1983; Tilg *et al.* 1992) and pancreatic juice cytology (Tyden *et al.* 1987c). The transcytoscopic biopsy of bladder-drained grafts (Perkins *et al.* 1990), cytoscopic transduodenal biopsy under ultrasound guidance (Stratta *et al.* 1995) or the percutaneous biopsy technique described by Allen *et al.* (1990), may be less difficult and dangerous than fine needle (Egidi *et al.* 1995) or open biopsies and provide a good assessment of graft rejection.

Pancreatic tissue obtained by biopsy, pancreatectomy or autopsy from 100 pancreas grafts were immunohistologically and histopathologically examined and reported by Sibley and Sutherland (1987). This series represents the largest experience of histological findings correlated with clinical observations. The authors showed that although rejection accounted for many episodes of post-transplant hyperglycaemia and graft loss there were other causes as well. These included preservation injury, pancreatitis, isletitis and recurrence of disease. The histological diagnosis of acute pancreatic graft rejection features infiltrates of transformed lymphocytes within the exocrine pancreas with vascular lesions consisting of endotheliitis and/or fibrinoid necrosis and an increase in the intensity of Ia antigen expression by duct–ductular epithelium and acinar tissue. Most infiltrating mononuclear cells were CD8+ T cells. The islets appear to be normal without infiltrates and with normal or near normal numbers of β cells despite hyperglycaemia. It has been suggested that interleukin 1 release during the rejection process could have a toxic effect on insulin secretion (Mandrup-Poulsen *et al.* 1986) resulting in hyperglycaemia.

## Immunosuppression

Pancreas transplant centres have developed their own immunosuppressive regimes in the quest for improved graft survival on one hand and a reduction of their potentially dangerous side effects on the other. Increasing numbers of reports, reviewed by Jindal (1994), have shown the development of post-transplant diabetes mellitus (PTDM) in recipients of immunosuppressive drugs.

Although steroid treatment is highly diabetogenic, it is still used in combination with other immunosuppressive agents and as a first-line agent in rejection episodes. Cyclosporin A, developed by Borel *et al.* (1976) and introduced into the clinic by Calne *et al.* (1979), was hailed initially as the drug of choice for pancreas transplant patients because of its steroid-sparing effect, but soon Gunnarsson *et al.* (1983) reported the diabetogenic action of CyA. The nephrotoxic effect, especially in cases with renal injury as a result of ischaemic preservation damage, and diabetogenic effect of CyA (Tyden *et al.* 1987a; Cantarovitch *et al.* 1988) are controlled by the reduction of CyA dosage with addition of azathioprine or prednisolone to compensate for the potential risk of underimmunosuppression.

Azathioprine, developed by Calne (1960) and first used clinically in 1963, has maintained its place as a non-diabetogenic immunosuppressant within the protocols applied to transplantation.

The antirejection agent FK506 (tacrolimus) has been used in vascular pancreas transplantation but has since been shown to decrease glucose-induced insulin release from rodent and human islets *in vitro* (Tze *et al.* 1990) and to be diabetogenic in animals (Calne *et al.* 1987) and resulted in a dose-dependent 20% incidence of new-onset diabetes in kidney transplant patients (Scantlebury *et al.* 1991). FK506 has been shown to result in PTDM in liver transplanted patients (Tabasco-Minguilan *et al.* 1993). However, several centres have reported the advantageous use of tacrolimus for induction and maintenance and rescue therapy, achieving pancreatic graft survival rates of over 80% for all categories of recipients (Gruessner *et al.* 1996).

Many centres are using quadruple induction therapy where either antilymphocyte globulin (ALG), antithymocyte globulin (ATG) or OKT3 is given during the first 10 days. A comparison between ATG and OKT3 therapy as prophylactic treatment in SPK cases was made by Le Francois *et al.* (1990) and showed no statistically significant differences, though kidney rejection episodes were more frequent and occurred earlier in the OKT3 group. Similar trials were conducted by Melzer *et al.* (1990), where patient and graft survival were similar but OKT3 induction therapy was associated with fewer rejection episodes and less morbidity. International Pancreas Transplant Registry results for 1986–90 showed significantly higher graft survival rates with the use of anti-T cell agents and no significant difference between OKT3 and ALG: OKT3 71% ($n=$319) vs. ALG 63% ($n=1025$) vs. neither 59% ($n=711$) (OKT3 and ALG vs. neither $P<0.001$) (IPTR 1994).

The diabetogenicity of new agents, including rapamycin, RS-61443, Leflunomide, brequinar and 15-deoxyspergualin (DSG), has not been well defined so far and more data are required at the molecular level. Other forms of immunosuppressive strategies under development include the reduction of immunogenicity by graft pretreatment with specific monoclonal antibodies, as studied clinically in renal grafting (Brewer *et al.* 1989). This has been investigated in rat (Lloyd *et al.* 1989) and dog pancreas allografting (Miyoshi *et al.* 1992) and dog islet grafting (Brons *et al.* 1991, 1992, 1994) resulting in moderate prolongation, but it has so far not been tried in the clinical setting.

The future of pancreas transplantation will clearly benefit from the development of new non-diabetogenic agents or different regimens of current general immunosuppression producing fewer side effects. Tolerance-inducing therapies with reduction in maintenance immunosuppression may become available, resulting in rapid expansion of pancreas transplant units worldwide instead of the few centres currently offering this service.

## HLA typing

The role of tissue typing for HLA-A, B and DR antigens for donor–recipient matching has been analysed by the Minnesota group, using the typing data submitted to the IPTR as well as data from their own single centre study. Functional survival rates were significantly higher for cadaveric grafts with no mismatch for DR, compared to grafts with one or two DR antigen mismatches (Squifflet *et al.* 1988; So *et al.* 1990). However, the effect of DR matching seems to be less strong in the current IPTR analysis of 1986–90 (Sutherland 1991), with 1-year functional graft survival rates in technically successful SPK cases with 2, 1, and 0 DR matched grafts being 87% (*n*=41), 82% (*n*=459) and 80% (*n*=698), respectively. Although pancreas graft survival varies according to recipient category and duct management technique, every comparison within the various groups showed graft survival rates to be progressively higher from DR mismatch to DR match, but not statistically significant. The SPK bladder-drainage subgroup matched for 2, 1 and 0 DR showed a 1-year graft survival of 77%, 72% and 73%, respectively. Data from SPK transplants reported from a single institution (Madison, Wisconsin, USA) with DR-match data in 166 cases collected between 1985 and 1991 showed, however, a significant difference in pancreas and kidney graft survival between 2 DR and 1 DR mismatch. This difference was maintained over 4 years of observation (Sasaki *et al.* 1991). These different sets of results need further clarification with respect to patient numbers in single institutions vs. large cohorts of patients collected and analysed by the IPTR. Thus, final conclusions about the effect of HLA DR matching on the outcome of pancreas grafts and thereby on the use of prospective DR matching have to await further long-term analysis and, as the differences seemed to be small, most centres do not advocate prospective HLA matching for SPK transplants. However, in PTA grafting it is worthwhile to wait for a well matched organ (Sutherland *et al.* 1991).

### Recurrence of disease

Recurrence of autoimmune diabetes has been documented in recipients of cadaveric grafts. There were eight cases of documented isletitis with selective loss of β cells, defined as recurrence of disease, in the Minnesota series (Sibley & Sutherland 1987; Sutherland *et al.* 1989b). This isletitis was seen in several grafts of HLA-identical recipients, three without any immunosuppressive treatment (identical twin donors), others on low-dose CyA alone or on much reduced immuno-

suppression. In order to prevent this process all patients from identical siblings or twins receive low-dose immunosuppression and no further recurrence of disease has been seen.

The authors suggested that the selective destruction of β cells in the three identical grafts represented an anamnestic cytotoxic T-lymphocyte-mediated autoimmune response, whereas the isletitis in the non-identical recipients represented a rejection phenomenon caused by class I and class II alloantigen disparity. It was possible to obtain pancreatic tissue from one such patient undergoing isletitis and recurrent diabetes without any evidence of rejection 8 years after a pancreas and kidney transplant from a class I and class II HLA-matched normal sibling (Santamaria *et al.* 1992). Immunohistopathological analysis of the pancreas revealed selective loss of β cells and the presence of peri- and intraislet leucocyte infiltrates, which were predominantly CD8+ lymphocytes. Cells from this tissue have been expanded in tissue culture by anti-CD3 monoclonal antibody. This strategy may allow further characterization of the putative autoreactive T lymphocytes mediating type 1 diabetes.

As type 1 diabetes is an autoimmune disease and may be MHC-restricted, it is not surprising that recurrence of diabetes may occur in closely matched patients; matching at the DR locus of donor–recipient HLA antigens could thus result in a higher incidence of recurrence of disease. On the other hand, Tyden *et al.* (1996) reported recently on recurrent disease in two mismatched patients. Drachenberg *et al.* (1996) examined biopsy material obtained from 55 patients with whole cadaveric pancreas allografts. Isolated islet insulitis as a histological indication of selective cell-mediated cytotoxicity against β cells, usually associated with type 1 DM, was not observed between 6 and 52 months post-transplant in this patient group. In contrast, Stegall *et al.* (1996) reported evidence of recurrent autoimmunity in a human allogeneic islet transplant with preferential loss of insulin-staining cells.

Conventional immunosuppression, as currently used, seems to prevent recurrent disease in cadaveric grafts. However, low-level autoimmune destruction of islet tissue could be the underlying cause in many instances of isolated late graft failure without any signs of rejection in simultaneously transplanted kidney or liver grafts where patients were maintained on low-dose immunosuppressive therapy over several years. Moreover, recurrence may become a problem when newly developed immunosuppressive strategies, such as tolerance induction or immunomodulation of grafts, resulting in a drastic reduction in immunosuppression, are employed.

## Metabolic function

After successful pancreatic transplantation, patients become insulin-independent and fasting and postprandial blood glucose levels usually normalize within 24 h. Glycosylated haemoglobin A1 (HbA1) levels fall within a short time and satisfactory pancreatic function is shown by normal or near normal levels of HbA1 in the long term. Twenty-four-hour glucose profiles have been shown to be virtually normal in most patients. Diurnal patterns of free fatty acids, 3-hydroxybutyrate and alanine were found to be normal, with blood lactate and glycerol slightly higher after combined renal and pancreatic grafting in comparison with kidney transplanted non-diabetic patients (Ostman *et al.* 1989). Results of oral and intravenous glucose tolerance tests have been shown to vary from patient to patient without regard to the transplant technique, but over 70% of patients have a normal response while 20–30% have impaired glucose tolerance and a small proportion of patients have a diabetic response despite a functioning graft and normal fasting glucose levels (Bolinder *et al.* 1991; Landgraf *et al.* 1991; Robertson *et al.* 1991). Reasons for impaired glucose control include reduced islet cell mass as a result of the use of segmental grafts, preservation injury or rejection episodes or immunosuppressive treatment with diabetogenic drugs, such as CyA, FK506 and steroids, or impaired renal function.

Whether denervation impairs glucose tolerance and reduces the incretin effect, which is produced by the enteroinsular axis, has been investigated in patients with paratopic pancreas transplant and physiological insulin delivery. The enteroinsular axis was preserved in these patients despite denervation (Clark *et al.*

1989). Insulin levels during glucose stimulation have been found to be elevated in many pancreas and kidney transplanted patients in comparison with levels seen in healthy volunteers or non-diabetic kidney transplanted patients on similar immunosuppressive treatment. This was seen in spite of virtually normal glucose control and irrespective of the transplant technique. Insulin resistance, common in diabetic patients (De Fronzo *et al.* 1982) but also seen during immunosuppressive therapy, or the persistence of lower insulin sensitivity, as seen in uraemic patients pretransplant, may be responsible for this stimulatory hyperinsulinaemia. Another explanation may be the development of NIDDM in some patients, where resistance to insulin-stimulated glucose uptake results in a compensatory response of the β cells to release more insulin and thus stimulatory hyperinsulinaemia (Reaven 1988).

The failure of the pancreas after satisfactory long-term glucose control, where no rejection in simultaneously transplanted organs was evident or other factors such as diabetogenic immunosuppressive therapy or pancreatitis were excluded, has been a puzzle to many transplant surgeons (see above). An explanation could be severe exhaustion of insulin production. With reduced insulin storage capacity as a result of acute or chronic rejection processes, fewer insulin-secreting cells are present to fulfil the insulin requirements needed because the regeneration potential of endocrine cells is below 1% in the adult pancreas. The exhaustion or ageing phenomenon of insulin-secreting cells is a very slow process and difficult to diagnose. Kinetic measurements of the precursor, pro-insulin, may give some indication of decreasing intracellular insulin transport and storage potential, evident by progressive differences in the pro-insulin : insulin ratio.

However, normal metabolic control was maintained during a successful pregnancy 3 years after combined renal and segmental paratopic pancreas grafting. In spite of the reduced islet cell mass (segmental graft) β cells seemed to have sufficient functional reserve to cope with the additional physiological stress of pregnancy. This patient had another successful pregnancy 8 years post-transplant, again without any distress to the pancreatic graft. Other successful cases showing good metabolic control during pregnancy have been reported from different centres (Calne *et al.* 1988; Tyden *et al.* 1989; Moudry-Munns *et al.* 1996).

### Effect on secondary complications

With the increase in graft survival rates in pancreas transplantation the potentially beneficial effect of successful long-term normoglycaemia on secondary complications of diabetes has been studied in several centres. A review of observations from a single institution was reported by Sutherland (1992a). Ample evidence on the prevention of recurrence of diabetic nephropathy in the transplanted kidney is available (Bohman *et al.* 1985, 1987; Bilous *et al.* 1989). However, reversal or arrest of diabetic lesions in pre-uraemic patients transplanted with a pancreas only has been disappointing (Groth *et al.* 1991). The expected stabilization of renal function by prolonged normoglycaemia was actually reversed and renal function deteriorated further during the first year post-transplantation. This effect was ascribed to the nephrotoxic effect of CyA; however, a similar deterioration of diabetic complications occurred in patients with advanced proliferative retinopathy during the first 2 years after pancreas grafting despite good glucose control (Ramsay *et al.* 1988). This was also seen in diabetic patients with intensive conventional therapy (ICT) and CSII, where retinopathy deteriorated initially despite better glucose control (KROC Collaborative Study Group 1988; Rosenlund *et al.* 1988). However, advanced retinopathy appears to be stabilized or at least slowed down in recipients with long-term functioning pancreas grafts (Ulbig *et al.* 1987; Scheider *et al.* 1991) reassessed after several years. This trend was also seen in patients with neuropathic alterations (Van der Vliet *et al.* 1988; Kennedy *et al.* 1990) but whether these improvements are entirely a result of the correction of diabetes or uraemia was difficult to distinguish because most long-term follow-up cases come from the combined kidney–pancreas transplant group and uraemic and diabetic neuropathic complications can be rather similar in their clinical appearance (Solders *et al.* 1987, 1991). A positive effect of pancreas grafting on skin microcirculation was shown by Abendroth *et al.* (1990). An increased basal blood flow in skin microcirculation but impaired reactivity of the microvascular bed was documented by Jorneskog *et al.* (1991).

### Conclusions

Results of pancreas transplantation have continued to improve, especially in the combined pancreas and kidney graft category with bladder drainage. Results in this group are approaching those of other solid organs, but results of solitary pancreas grafting in non-uraemic or pre-uraemic diabetic patients have been slow to follow. Vascular pancreas transplantation is currently the only treatment that can truly provide endocrine replacement therapy over a prolonged period. It is important, however, to realize that pancreas transplantation is not an immediate life-saving operation, but should be considered as a procedure to improve quality of life and many studies have been published to this effect. Ideally, pancreas grafting should be applied at an earlier stage in the disease process before secondary complications become established and thus irreversible.

## Islet transplantation

Transplantation of isolated islets as a free graft can be a safer and more simple procedure than vascular pancreas grafting. However, the potential risk of lifelong immunosuppressive treatment to prevent rejection of the free graft needs to be reduced considerably before this procedure can be offered as a low-risk therapeutic alternative treatment to the young diabetic patient, who would most profit from an islet graft before the onset of complications.

The concept of isolated islets as a free graft is not a new one but was made possible by Moskalewsky (1965) with the discovery of the separation of islets by digestion of the pancreas with the powerful enzyme, collagenase. Amelioration of diabetes was subsequently achieved by successful islet transplantation in the rodent model by Ballinger and Lacy (1972). Since then considerable effort has been invested in further developing islet isolation techniques as well as immunosuppressive therapies and antirejection schemes; excellent review articles are available (Gray & Morris 1987; Hering *et al.* 1988; Ricordi *et al.* 1992; Warnock *et al.* 1992).

## Clinical islet transplantation

Despite years of intensive experimental research and many attempts at clinical islet transplantation, amelioration of diabetes in these patients has been elusive. However, advances in the isolation and purification methods of human pancreatic islets together with improved antirejection therapy have allowed clinical trials of islet transplantation, which have been collected and documented by the international Islet Transplant Registry (ITR) based at the University of Giessen in Germany and the North American Islet Transplant Interchange (NITI), Philadelphia, PA, USA. Between 1974 and 1990 (90) and during the last 7 years (286) a total of 376 cases of adult islet allografts in patients with type 1 DM were reported and analysed by the ITR.

The first patient to stop exogenous insulin therapy 15 days after islet grafting was reported from St Louis in 1989 (Scharp *et al.* 1991). This was the first essential step towards establishing that islet transplants can function and can result in insulin independence in type 1 diabetic patients on immunosuppressive therapy. Although the islet tissue had been immunomodulated pregrafting by 7 days of *in vitro* tissue culture in order to reduce its immunogenicity and immunosuppressive therapy similar to that used in vascular organ grafting had been given, graft function ceased after 25 days because of rejection. A comprehensive review of the first experiences of adult human islet transplants has been published by Warnock and Rajotte (1992).

The definition of successful islet function is insulin independence. It is common practice with islet grafting to reduce exogenous insulin dosage very slowly in many stages to allow for engraftment and adjustment to the needs of the patient. Thus, a considerable reduction of exogenous insulin requirements shows that there is function of the grafted tissue with persistence of basal c-peptide production over 1 ng/ml. However, c-peptide measurements, their interpretation and the sensitivity of the assay need careful assessment with respect to renal function and immunosuppressive treatment.

Analysis of 200 well-documented cases performed during 1990–97 revealed a 1-year patient survival of 96% with a graft survival of 35% in type 1 diabetic recipients (Fig. 12.2). Islet grafts were performed either simultaneously with a kidney from the same donor (SIK) or after a functioning kidney graft (IAK); islets were from multiple donors, either freshly prepared or cryopreserved. Four common characteristics observed in 60 of 200 recipients showed a successful influence on the graft outcome:

1 islet isolation procedure < 8 h;
2 > 6000 islet equivalents (number of islets if all had a diameter of 150 mm) per kg body weight;
3 implantation into liver via portal vein; and
4 induction of immunosuppression by anti-T cell agents ALG or ATG but not OKT3.

Seventeen of these 60 selected recipients were insulin-independent at 1-year follow-up and had significantly higher basal c-peptide levels at 1 month and at 1 year. All other parameters were not statistically different, which seems to suggest that other factors difficult to record, such as the degree of islet implantation, susceptibility of islets towards adverse effects of immunosuppressive drugs and/or exhaustion of insulin production by β cells (see above), may also determine the outcome. Tables 12.1 and 12.2 summarize insulin-independent cases from 1978 to 1997 (*n*=36). Metabolic glucose control follow-up in some of the longer-term graft survival patients has been described excellently by Luzi *et al.* (1996).

It seems to be easier to achieve insulin independence in non-diabetic patients with an additional liver graft, as seen in the Pittsburgh cases, where long-term insulin independence was seen in patients receiving islet grafts in combination with a liver graft following upper abdominal exenteration for extensive tumours (*n*=11). This is in contrast to diabetic patients with kidney–islet allografts (*n*=11) performed at the same institution (Tzakis *et al.* 1990; Ricordi *et al.* 1992). Whether these results are a result of diabetes being a multifactorial disease and thus more difficult to control or whether a liver graft protects the islets from the same donor from rejection has not been clearly established. Such protec-

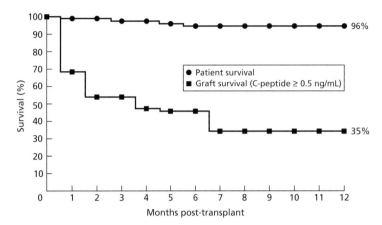

Fig. 12.2 Cumulative 1-year patient and graft survival in 200 pre-transplant c-peptide-negative type 1 diabetic recipients (1990–97). Data from the International Islet Transplant Registry Newsletter No. 8, presented at the 7th World Congress of the IPITA, Sydney, Australia, August 1999.

tion has been shown in patients grafted with a liver and kidney from the same donor. Kidney graft rejection episodes were reduced compared to kidney-alone transplants under similar immunosuppressive treatment (Rasmussen *et al.* 1995).

The experience of intraportal autotransplantation of islets after total pancreatectomy for benign disease is even more interesting. In total, 222 cases of adult islet autografts from 1974 to December 1998 have been reported to the ITR with the largest series of >50 cases performed in Minnesota (Wahoff *et al.* 1995; ITR 1996). After intraportal islet grafting 50% of well-documented cases showed insulin independence. In 15 of 21 patients, who had received more than 300 000 islets, 71% were insulin-independent >1 year post-transplant with the longest follow-up of >7 years of insulin independence after total pancreatectomy. In this situation immunosuppressive drugs are not employed, thus avoiding any diabetogenic stress on the islets. This clearly shows that free islet grafts can survive within the liver parenchyma even when the purity of these isolated islets is low and contaminated with digestive enzyme containing exocrine tissue or ductal remnants (Gores & Sutherland 1993; Gores *et al.* 1993). Moreover, it has recently been confirmed that islet stem cells are recruited from ductal precursors (Bouwens *et al.* 1997); thus the success rate of islet

autografts may be determined by the low purity of these grafts. Also, the remnant pancreas, in patients who have not undergone a total pancreatectomy, contributes to the overall insulin production. Figure 12.3 shows insulin independence comparing different recipient categories.

## Advances in islet separation

What have been the advances in islet transplantation which made clinical trials a possibility? The developments in islet transplantation up to 1987 were extensively and excellently described by Gray and Morris (1987). Since then islet isolation, purification and preservation methods have been improved further. The semiautomated digestion technique described by Ricordi *et al.* (1989) allows the immediate removal of separated islets from the action of collagenase. Collagenase contains many factors and proteases that are vital for the release of islets from the surrounding tissue but they can also be damaging and toxic to the function of the islets and need to be removed as soon as possible (Johnson *et al.* 1996).

Purification of islets from the digested gland is generally achieved by density-gradient methods (Tze *et al.* 1976; Lake *et al.* 1989; Ricordi *et al.* 1989), with either ficoll dissolved in hypo-osmolar preservation solu-

**Table 12.1** Summary of insulin-independent cases ($n = 36$) through 31 December 1997. Type I diabetic recipients of adult islet allografts. Data from the International Islet Transplant Registry Newsletter No. 8, presented at the 7th World Congress of the IPITA, Sydney, Australia, August 1999.

| Case no. | Institution | Year of transplant | Previous pancreas/ islet transplant | Pre-transplant c-peptide (ng/mL) | No. of donors (fresh/cryo) | | IEQ/kg | Purity (%) | Period of insulin independence (days post-transplant) | Last update |
|---|---|---|---|---|---|---|---|---|---|---|
| 1 | Zurich | 1978 | – | B 0.00 | 1 | – | 3846* | 5 | 245–550 | |
| 2 | Paris† | 1988 | – | S 0.03 | 1 | – | 2143* | 80 | 206–1470 | |
| 3 | St. Louis | 1989 | P 83 | S 0.06 | 2 | – | 12661 | 95 | 10–25 | |
| 4 | St. Louis | 1990 | I 89 | S 0.18 | 1 | +2 | 14735 | 98 | 33–341 | |
| 5 | St. Louis | 1993 | I 89, I 90 | S 0.42 | 2 | +6 | 22055 | 92 | 92–948 | Mar. 96 |
| 6 | St. Louis | 1993 | – | S 0.08 | 3 | +2 | 26494 | 87 | 274–355 | |
| 7 | Edmonton | 1990 | – | S 0.00 | 1 | +4 | 9692 | 70 | 70–821 | |
| 8 | Edmonton | 1992 | – | S 0.00 | 1 | +5 | 9866 | 58 | 155–166 + 837 – 992 | |
| 9 | Milan | 1990 | – | S 0.00 | 1 | – | 10773 | 95 | 120–330 | |
| 10 | Milan | 1990 | P 88 | B 0.15 | 2 | – | 8610 | 78 | 122–1178 | |
| 11 | Milan | 1991 | P 87 | B 0.00 | 1 | +2 | 16859 | 80 | 210–360 + 480 – 635 | |
| 12 | Milan | 1992 | – | B 0.00 | 2 | – | 11567 | 80 | 150–1537 | |
| 13 | Milan‡ | 1994 | P 91, P 92 | B 0.15 | 1 | +2 | 28995 | 55 | 41–65 + 92 – 133 | |
| 14 | Milan‡ | 1995 | P 85 | B 0.00 | 1 | – | 9600 | 50 | 56–121 | |
| 15 | Miami | 1990 | – | S 0.03 | 3 | – | 18700 | 55 | 42–78 | |
| 16 | Miami | 1990 | – | S 0.03 | 3 | – | 18884 | 50 | 87–125 | |
| 17 | Miami | 1995 | – | B 0.03 | 1 | – | 15691 | 85 | 49–69 | |
| 18 | Minneapolis | 1992 | – | S 0.00 | 1 | – | 7882 | 5 | 326–1241 | |
| 19 | Minneapolis | 1992 | – | S 0.39 | 1 | – | 13319 | 5 | 123–321 | |
| 20 | Minneapolis | 1995 | P 92 | NA | 1 | – | 9004 | 5 | 43–340 | |
| 21 | Giessen | 1992 | – | S 0.10 | 1 | – | 6156 | 92 | 401–1150 | |
| 22 | Giessen | 1995 | – | S 0.00 | 1 | – | 7246 | 95 | 13–25 | |
| 23 | Giessen | 1995 | – | B 0.08 | 1 | – | 12031 | 90 | 312–844 | |
| 24 | Giessen | 1995 | – | B 0.05 | 1 | – | 8251 | 90 | 371–769 | |
| 25 | Giessen | 1995 | – | B 0.00 | 1 | – | 6376 | 85 | 382–650 | |
| 26 | Giessen | 1996 | – | B 0.00 | 1 | – | 5475 | 87 | 230–965 | |
| 27 | Giessen | 1996 | – | B 0.00 | 1 | – | 7777 | 90 | 547–724 | |
| 28 | Giessen | 1996 | – | S 0.29 | 1 | – | 5472 | 85 | 388–1188 | Aug. 99 |
| 29 | Giessen | 1997 | – | B 0.10 | 1 | – | 6548 | 85 | 382–696 | |
| 30 | Giessen | 1997 | – | S 0.05 | 1 | – | 7896 | 90 | 249–646 | Mar. 98 |
| 31 | Pittsburgh | 1994 | – | S 0.00 | 1 | – | 8137 | 80 | 118–850 | Aug. 99 |
| 32 | Brussels | 1995 | – | S 0.00 | 6 | – | 4400 | 70 | 218–745 | Aug. 97 |
| 33 | Brussels | 1996 | – | S 0.00 | 8 | – | 2600 | 59 | 194–365 | May. 97 |
| 34 | Odense/Milan§ | 1995 | – | S 0.00 | 2 | – | 9360 | 80 | 85–522 | |
| 35 | Geneva | 1996 | – | B 0.19 | 2 | – | 8800 | 28 | 61–1139 | Aug. 99 |
| 36 | Los Angeles VA | 1996 | – | NA | 1 | +3 | NA | NA | 231–262 | |

B, basal; I islet; IEQ, islet equivalents (150 μm islets per kg body weight of recipient); P, pancreas; NA, not available; S, stimulated.
* Islets/kg.
† Cholangiocarcinoma.
‡ Previous transplants and follow-up in Nantes; haemochromatosis and type 1 diabetes.
§ Islet Transplant/Islet Isolation Institution.

tions, euroficoll (Olac *et al.* 1991) or iso-osmotic bovine serum albumin (BSA) density gradients (Lake *et al.* 1989).

These improvements in islet isolation made large-scale purification of islets possible, but are still not ade-

quate to produce sufficient viable purified islet tissue from one organ, compared to the number of islets available in, for example, a successful vascularized segmental pancreas graft.

Cryopreservation protocols have been improved

**Table 12.2** Summary of insulin-independent cases ($n = 36$) through 31 December 1997. Type I diabetic recipients of adult islet allografts. Data from the International Islet Transplant Registry Newsletter No. 8, presented at the 7th World Congress of the IPITA, Sydney, Australia, August 1999.

| Case no. | Institution | Year of transplant | Site of transplant | Recipient category | No. of shared HLA-Ag | | Immunosuppression | | |
|---|---|---|---|---|---|---|---|---|---|
| | | | | | AB | DR | Induction | | Maintenance |
| 1 | Zurich | 1978 | Spleen | SIK | 1 | 0 | ALG | +S+A+CPM | S+A |
| 2 | Paris | 1988 | Epiploic flap | SIL | 1 | 1 | ALG | +S+C+A | S+C+A |
| 3 | St. Louis | 1989 | Liver | IAK | 3/1 | 2/1 | ALG | +S(SD)+C+A | C+A |
| 4 | St. Louis | 1990 | Liver | IAK | 1/2/2 | 1/1/0 | ALG | +S+A | S+A |
| 5 | St. Louis | 1993 | Liver | SIK | 1/0/0/0/0/1/0/0 | 1/0/1/0/1/0/1 | OKT3 | +S+C+A | S+C+A |
| 6 | St. Louis | 1993 | Liver | SIK | 1/1/3/1/1 | 1/1/1/2/1 | ATG | +S+C+A | S+C+A |
| 7 | Edmonton | 1990 | Liver | SIK | 3/1/0/1/0 | 0/0/0/0/0 | ALG | +S+C+A | S+C+A |
| 8 | Edmonton | 1992 | Liver | SIK | 3/1/0/0/1/0 | 1/1/1/0/0/1 | ALG | +S+C+A | S+C+A |
| 9 | Milan | 1990 | Liver | IAK | 1 | 0 | ALG | +S+C+A | S+C+A |
| 10 | Milan | 1990 | Liver | IAK | 1/2 | 1/0 | ALG | +S+C+A | S+C+A |
| 11 | Milan | 1991 | Liver | SIK | NA | NA | ALG | +S+C+A | S+C+A |
| 12 | Milan | 1992 | Liver | IAK | NA | NA | ALG | +S+C+A | S+C+A |
| 13 | Milan | 1994 | Liver | IAK | 0/1/2 | NA | ATG | +S+C+A | C+A |
| 14 | Milan | 1995 | Liver | IAK | 0 | NA | ATG | +S+C+A | S+C+A |
| 15 | Miami | 1990 | Liver | IAK | 0/2/0 | 1/1/0 | OKT3 | +S+C+A | S+C+A |
| 16 | Miami | 1990 | Liver | IAK | 0/0/0 | 0/1/0 | OKT3 | +S+C+A | S+C+A |
| 17 | Miami | 1995 | Liver | SIK | 0 | 0 | ATG | +S+T+MMF | S+T+MMF |
| 18 | Minneapolis | 1992 | Liver | SIK | 1 | 1 | ALG | +S+C+A+D | S+C+A |
| 19 | Minneapolis | 1992 | Liver | SIK | 2 | 0 | ALG | +S+C+A+D | S+C+A |
| 20 | Minneapolis | 1995 | Liver | IFPP | 2 | 1 | None | +S+C+MMF | S+C+MMF |
| 21 | Giessen | 1992 | Liver | IAK | 2 | 1 | ATG | +S+C | S+C |
| 22 | Giessen | 1995 | Liver | ITA | 1 | 0 | Anti-CD4 | +S(SD)+C | – |
| 23 | Giessen | 1995 | Liver | SIK | 1 | 1 | ATG | +S+C+A | S+C+A |
| 24 | Giessen | 1995 | Liver | SIK | 2 | 1 | ATG | +S+C+A | S+C+A |
| 25 | Giessen | 1995 | Liver | IAK | 2/0 | 1/0 | ALG | +S+C+A | S+C+A |
| 26 | Giessen | 1996 | Liver | IAK | 1 | 0 | ALG | +S+C+A | S+C+A |
| 27 | Giessen | 1996 | Liver | SIK | 0 | 1 | ATG | +S+C+A | S+C+A |
| 28 | Giessen | 1996 | Liver | SIK | 1 | 1 | ATG | +S+C+MMF | S+C+MMF |
| 29 | Giessen | 1997 | Liver | IAK | 1 | 0 | ALG | +S+C+A | S+C+A |
| 30 | Giessen | 1997 | Liver | SIK | 2 | 0 | ATG | +S+C+A | S+C+MMF |
| 31 | Pittsburgh | 1994 | Liver | SIK | 3 | 2 | None | +S+T | S+C+A |
| 32 | Brussels | 1995 | Liver | IAK | 0/0/1/0/1/1 | 0/1/1/0/1/1 | None | +S+C+A | C+A |
| 33 | Brussels | 1996 | Liver | IAK | 0/0/0/0/1/0/1/0 | 0/1/1/0/1/1/1/0 | None | +S+C+A | S+C+A |
| 34 | Odense/Milan* | 1995 | Liver | SIK | 2/NA | 1/NA | ATG | +C | C+MMF |
| 35 | Geneva | 1996 | Liver | IAK | 1/2 | 1/0 | ATG | +S+C+A | S+C+A |
| 36 | Los Angeles VA | 1996 | Liver | SIL | NA | NA | None | +S+T+MMF | S+C+MMF |

A, azathioprine; ALG, antilymphocyte globulin; ATG, antithymocyte globulin; C, cyclosporin A; CPM, cyclophosphamide; D, deoxyspergualin; IAK, islet after kidney; IFPP, islets from previous pancreas (i.e. isolated from a previously removed vascularized pancreas graft); ITA, islet transplant alone; MMF, mycophenolate mofetil; NA, not available; S, steroids; SD, single dose; SIK, simultaneous islet kidney; SIL, simultaneous islet liver; T, tacrolimus.
* Islet Transplant/Islet Isolation Institution.

(Rajotte *et al.* 1990) making it possible to store tissue-typed human islets in tissue banks for later use. Tissue culture after the isolation and purification as well as before and after the preservation process may have a beneficial effect on initiating repair processes and removing dying cells. Although the recovery of viable islet cells is reduced after cryopreservation, this technique has overcome the problem of inadequate islet yields from a single donor by adding cryopreserved islet tissue from multiple donors to increase the islet

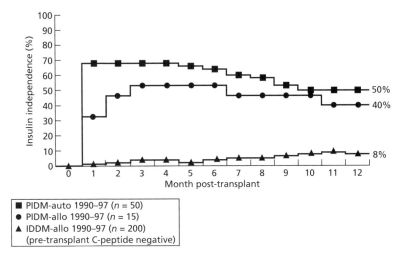

**Fig. 12.3** One-year insulin independence following islet transplantation in different recipient groups. allo, allograft; auto, autograft; IDDM, insulin-dependent diabetes mellitus; PIDM, pancreatomy-induced diabetes mellitus.

quantity beyond the critical mass that is required to reverse diabetes.

It has been established that a critical number of islets, >5000 islets/kg body weight, is necessary to reverse diabetes in autografts in large animals (Warnock *et al.* 1990). This number has to be more than doubled for allotransplantation to be successful. Allostimulated inflammatory reactions are not the only reason to account for these differences. The vulnerability of relatively small amounts of purified or semipurified islet tissue to non-specific macrophage-mediated inflammatory processes attacking the grafted tissue was demonstrated by Gores *et al.* (1993). Islet grafts, unprotected by their usual stromal elements, are usually dispersed by intraportal infusion into the liver, where there is a high content of phagocytosing macrophages and Kupffer cells. The damage induced by non-specific macrophage-mediated cytokine release on the insulin-secreting tissue can be immediate and may result in primary non-function. Although the idea that low purity of islet preparations is detrimental to the hormone-secreting function and contamination with exocrine tissue can damage the grafted islets and the surrounding tissue has been put forward as an important factor in primary non-function, experiences with unpurified autografted islets have shown contrasting results (see above). Moreover, the recently reported

allograft cases from Minneapolis (Gores *et al.* 1993) were undertaken with unpurified islets and a new immunosuppressive drug, 15-deoxyspergualin (DSG), to inhibit the non-specific action of macrophages during the first days of engraftment.

## Immunosuppression

Attempts at improving immunosuppressive regimes for free islet grafts have to take into account non-specific inflammatory processes, reduce the risk of primary non-function and minimize the risk of islet cell loss caused by early rejection episodes. Moreover, they should also have no adverse effects on the production and secretion of insulin and should not interfere with the neovascularization and engrafting process of the islets.

The induction of donor-specific tolerance towards histoincompatible tissue is a prime but as yet unfulfilled objective in the clinic. The development of monoclonal antibodies directed against specific cells of the immune system has made it possible to deplete cells or inhibit their function selectively without affecting the islet cells and insulin secretion. In murine and rodent animal models long-term unresponsiveness and even donor-specific tolerance can be achieved in strongly MHC-mismatched strain combinations by severe manipulation of the host immune system using Mab therapies or by intrathymic inoculation with donor antigen as cells or peptides. Transfer of these therapies into higher animal models have been mostly unsuccessful, with chronic rejection, toxicity or infections common in these models. Prolonged graft survival without chronic immunosuppression was achieved in only a few selected cases.

## Clinical protocols

Advances in the clinical situation have included the induction of immunosuppression with polyclonal ALG, ATG or DSG followed by triple therapy with low-dose CyA, prednisolone and azathioprine (AZA), as used in vascular pancreas grafting. Although some drugs impair graft function they are still the only immunosuppressive agents available in the clinic to combat graft rejection. Both CyA and FK506 have been shown to reduce insulin production and inhibit insulin secretion (see above; Ricordi *et al.* 1991; Tabasco-Minguilan *et al.* 1993). Cyclosporin A also reduces neovascularization of the islets and steroid treatment is well known to induce insulin resistance.

The detection of rejection episodes and their reversal by immunosuppressive agents is even more disappointing. Usually bolus doses of steroids are given for 3 days or a course of ALG/OKT3 in cases of steroid unresponsiveness. There is very little functional reserve in islets during rejection episodes which is directly related to the barely optimal numbers of islets grafted. Moreover, the adverse effects of immunosuppressive drugs on the biosynthesis and secretion of insulin may drive the remaining cells into exhaustion. Most centres are very careful in reducing exogenous insulin therapy after grafting and certainly higher insulin doses need to be given during rejection episodes. This underlines the importance of grafting sufficient numbers of viable and intact islets, first to overcome drug dosage-related islet toxicity and provide enough insulin-storage capacity and, secondly, to overcome rejection episodes. On the other hand, increasing the islet yield by using unpurified or semipurified or multiple islet donors also increases the antigenicity of the transplant tissue considerably.

## Experimental protocols

The antigenicity of tissues varies according to their level of expression of MHC antigens, class I and class II, on the surface of their respective cells. In the pancreas the endocrine cells do not usually express MHC class II and express only weakly class I antigens. However, distributed within the islet matrix are passenger leucocytes and capillary endothelial cells which express strong class II antigens on their surface. These passenger leucocytes, lymphocytes, macrophages and dendritic cells—of which the dendritic cell is the most powerful—together with endothelial cells, are effective inducers of graft rejection by direct presentation of donor allogeneic MHC antigens to the host's T lymphocytes, providing the second signal for T cell activation (Lafferty & Cunningham 1975; Gill *et al.* 1996). This direct allorecognition represents initial T cell priming to alloantigen on donor antigen-presenting cells (APC) in recipient lymphoid organs and is the first line of defence against the foreign tissue. The indirect T cell recognition of donor peptides presented by APC of recipient origin provides help for cytotoxic T cell activation and production of donor-directed antibodies by B cells (Lechler & Batchelor 1982).

As MHC class II antigens are a major target for the allogeneic immune response, the modification of antigenicity by eliminating these APC or inhibiting their action would help diminish potentially dangerous immunosuppressive treatment needed to achieve graft acceptance. Moreover, a reduction of diabetogenic immunosuppressive agents may be beneficial to the insulin-producing function of the transplanted islet tissue during the engraftment period and revascularization process. *In vitro* islet immunomodulation before grafting is therefore an attractive strategy and islet cells are probably the most suitable tissue for this kind of immune alteration.

This passenger leucocyte concept was first demonstrated by Steinmuller (1967) (for review see Steinmuller 1980). Since then many pretreatment protocols have been developed and tested (for review see Gray & Morris 1987). In small animals these procedures resulted in successful prolongation of graft survival and long-term unresponsiveness. In rodents endothelium does not express class II antigen (Hart & Fabre 1981), hence the protocols altering the immunogenicity of rodent islets were almost invariably successful. In the large-animal model and in humans endothelium does express class II antigens (Fabre 1982; Fuggle *et al.* 1983) and thus may present problems. Also, expression of class II antigens is up-regulated after allotransplantation, thus potent immunomodulatory manipulation would be necessary in higher animals and humans.

In large-animal experiments perfusion of the pancreas with anti-MHC class II monoclonal antibodies before isolation of islets (Lloyd *et al.* 1989) showed only moderate prolongation of graft function, as did islet modulation without recipient immunosuppression in dogs using synergistic autologous complement-fixing monoclonal antibodies directed against the leucocyte common antigen (LCA CD45) present on white blood cells (Brons *et al.* 1994).

In humans immunomodulation of whole-organ donor kidney grafts before transplantation by *ex vivo* perfusion with a mixture of two synergistically acting anti-LCA Mabs showed reduced rejection episodes in renal transplants (Brewer *et al.* 1989). Uptake, effective distribution and Mab concentration, with assessment of total depletion or inhibition of target cells distributed within the whole organ, are not only difficult to investigate just before transplantation but also difficult to achieve.

In rodents donor immunomodulation, together with recipient Mab therapy, directed against specific lymphocyte subsets CD4 and CD8, has resulted in tolerance (Benjamine & Waldmann 1986; Cobbold *et al.* 1992). This type of Mab-induced tolerance induction has been investigated in the pre-clinical large-animal model using dog islet allografts. Islet immunomodulation, together with selective immunosuppressive therapy, including anti-Thy 1, CD4 and CD8 Mabs given from −2 to +10 days post-transplantation plus AZA, to suppress any recipient immune response directed against the rat antibody, has resulted in prolonged islet cell function with normal glucose control and maintenance of body weight (Brons *et al.* 1994). Further studies of the tolerogenic potential of this protocol using different treatment regimes and immunosuppressive therapies have improved islet graft function and survival considerably (Brons *et al.* 1995).

## Intrathymic tolerance induction

Posselt *et al.* (1990) reported the induction of tolerance towards islet tissue by intrathymic inoculation of donor islet cells under cover of transient immunosuppression. Residence of allogeneic islets in the thymus induced unresponsiveness to extrathymically placed donor strain islets 200 days after intrathymic implantation, but third-party islets were rejected normally. This confirmed the donor-specific nature of tolerance induced by the intrathymic inoculation technique (Barker *et al.* 1991). These first studies were later successfully extended to the BB rat (Posselt *et al.* 1991) and to islet xenografts (Mayo *et al.* 1994).

Posselt *et al.* utilized islet tissue harbouring APC to achieve this tolerance; but when these islets were immunomodulated by prolonged tissue culture, thus eliminating antigen-presenting cells, extrathymic donor-type islet grafts were rejected in the normal fashion (Campos *et al.* 1994).

Intrathymic inoculation with donor-type soluble peptides has been successful in producing unresponsiveness to rat organ grafts (Oluwole & Jin 1993; Chowdhury *et al.* 1996).

Oluwole *et al.* (1994) examined the cellular components of splenic intrathymic preparations. They demonstrated that highly purified B cells, macrophages or dendritic cells failed to prevent acute rejection of heart grafts, but highly purified T cells led to indefinite graft survival. Purified dendritic cells isolated from the spleen and contaminated with some splenic B cells were used for intrathymic inoculation under cover of intraperitoneal ALS (Chaib *et al.* 1993). These cells failed to induce prolongation of subsequently transplanted islets infused into the liver. These studies suggest that intrathymic MHC class I T cell antigen may also be necessary to induce donor-specific unresponsiveness by the intrathymic inoculation route. These results are in contrast to Goss *et al.* (1992), who showed that resting T cells failed to induce tolerance. However, class I antigen-expressing cells are contained in all inoculation preparations, such as islet cells, renal glomeruli, bone marrow, splenocytes and liver non-parenchymal cells (NPC).

The generation of suppressor cells by the intrathymic inoculation route has been tested by Goss *et al.* (1992) and Oluwole *et al.* (1995). These authors reported that adoptive transfer of splenocytes obtained from tolerant cardiac allograft recipients into naïve syngeneic rats did not prolong the survival of donor-type heart grafts, suggesting that suppressor mechanisms are unlikely.

The thymus is a privileged transplant site. It was thought that it was protected from immune surveillance by the blood–thymus barrier (Agus *et al.* 1991) and thus the inoculated cells may not be destroyed within the thymic microenvironment. Moreover, the blood–thymus barrier protects the thymic cortex from blood-borne macromolecules and thus developing thymocytes seem not to be affected by injections of anti-lymphocyte serum (ALS); only medullary lymphocytes are exposed to bloodborne substances, such as ALS and Mabs (Monaco *et al.* 1966; Raviola & Karuovski 1972). However, new research suggests that the immune privileged thymus may contain special cell surface factors to combat immune surveillance (see below).

The use of temporary non-specific but powerful immunosuppression with ALS to deplete the peripheral T cell pool of the host is necessary for the successful achievement of graft survival, thus removing cells capable of acutely destroying extrathymically placed allografts. It may also make room for the repopulation of secondary peripheral lymphoid tissues by emigrated, newly educated T cells from the microchimeric thymus.

The mechanism underlying the development of the intrathymic donor-specific tolerance induction is still under intense investigation (Naji 1996). There is very little information on intrathymic tolerance induction in large animals and humans. Knechtle *et al.* (1997) evaluated in an MHC-mismatched monkey renal allograft model a novel, highly potent, anti-T cell agent, FN18-CRM9, which is composed of an anti-rhesus monkey CD3 Mab and a binding site mutant diphtheria toxin, CRM9. Tolerance, proven by donor-specific skin grafts, developed in several animals, whether donor

lymphocytes or just saline was injected intrathymically. The immunosuppressive agent, given in three consecutive doses starting on day −7 before the renal graft, depleted peripheral as well as lymph node T cells dramatically, with peripheral T cell recovery to baseline levels within 3–4 weeks.

In an attempt to use the thymus as a privileged site Levy *et al.* (1996) showed intrathymic islet allograft survival in dogs under CyA therapy and limited prolongation after withdrawal of the treatment. However, extrathymic grafts were not performed to prove tolerance induction.

Brons and colleagues evaluated short-term anti-CD4 + CD8 Mab therapy (day −5 to +7) plus low-dose AZA in the MHC-mismatched beagle to mongrel islet allograft model. Intrathymic islet inoculation and concurrent extrathymic grafting of the majority of the islet cell mass demonstrated islet graft function and survival for over 50 days in several animals. The extrathymic graft functioned in one animal for over 2.9 years, even after intravenous infusion of viable donor lymphocytes on day +470, demonstrating the establishment of donor-specific unresponsiveness.

From these results it seems that the timing between satisfactory depletion of the mature T cell pool and the intra- and extrathymic placement of the allogeneic graft is of vital importance for the establishment of tolerance. To be of clinical relevance this interval needs to be within a very short time limit for organs other than islet grafts; using cryopreserved islets, tissue typed and held in tissue banks, islet transplants could be performed at any time after successful intrathymic inoculation.

## Immune privileged transplant site

An interesting study by Selawry *et al.* (1985) showed the survival of mismatched islets transplanted into the testis of spontaneously diabetic rats. Even when composite islet and Sertoli cells were grafted under the renal capsule the allografts were protected from rejection and survived indefinitely (Selawry & Cameron 1993). The testis has been known to be one of the immune privileged transplant sites. Immune privileged sites are defined as regions where the immune system seems to be incapable of mounting an immune response (Barker & Billingham 1977) and it is suggested that this is because the response could irreversibly damage sensitive tissues at this site (Griffith *et al.* 1995).

It now becomes clear that the mechanism of this tolerance-inducing privileged site may be mediated by the discovery of the cell death factor and its receptor (Nagata & Golstein 1995), which regulate programmed cell death, apoptosis (Raff 1992). The protection of these tissues seems to be regulated by the control of the immune response mediated by interaction of Fas or CD95 receptor with its ligand Fas-L or CD95 L, resulting in death of the target cell within hours. Fas-L is expressed on a variety of lymphoid and non-lymphoid tissues and was recently detected also on cells at immune privileged sites, such as the brain, eyes, testis, ovary and adrenal glands (Bellgrau *et al.* 1995; Griffith *et al.* 1995; Brunner *et al.* 1996). Induction of apoptosis is thus providing protection from invading immune cells and immune damage of sensitive cells within the vicinity. In general terms, interaction of Fas-L and Fas are thought to play a major part in homoeostasis and coexpression may contribute to physiological cell turnover and regulation of cell numbers (French & Tschopp 1996).

Developments in genetic engineering allowed the expression of Fas-L by transfected myoblasts. When transplanted as a composite graft with allogeneic islet cells, the islet graft was protected from rejection by provision of the Fas-L death signal to invading alloactivated Fas-positive immune cells. This manipulation of the local environment resulted in normoglycaemia for over 80 days in diabetic mice; however, loss of Fas-L expression correlated with islet rejection, indicating that continued expression of Fas-L within the islet graft transplant site is necessary for immune protection (Lau *et al.* 1996).

This immune protection was recently confirmed in the rat model in the absence of systemic immunosuppression by transplantation of syngeneic, naturally Fas-L-expressing Sertoli cells, aggregated together with allogeneic islet tissue. The composite graft survived indefinitely. These results are interesting as no gene protocol was necessary (Korbutt *et al.* 1997). Added

to this, Selawry *et al.* (1996) studied the preservation and functionality of cryopreserved islets cocultured with Sertoli cells. It improved significantly the islet yield, viability and glucose responsiveness of adult cryopreserved islets.

Clearly, this new and stimulating approach to islet transplantation needs to be tested in the large-animal model. Should it prove to be a feasible strategy using both male and female syngeneic Fas-L-expressing cells, application in the clinical situation may become a possibility in the near future. Whether this approach will also hold true for xenogeneic islet tissue needs to be explored so that islet grafting could be freed from problems of islet cell yield, purity and viability.

## Xenografting

The most suitable and readily available xenograft donor species is the pig, because of its breeding characteristics, comparable organ size and consistency and physiological similarity to humans. Porcine insulin has been used for many decades as exogenous insulin replacement therapy in diabetic patients. Thus isolated and purified pig islets may promise to function well, despite a lower insulin secretion rate upon glucose stimulation compared with human islets (Crowther *et al.* 1989).

However, in discordant species combination, such as pig to human, preformed natural antibodies, present in varying degrees, are highly reactive against donor tissue. Binding of xenoreactive natural antibodies to vascular donor endothelial cells activates these and other surrounding cells and factors and initiates a cascade of complement activation, ending in hyperacute rejection (HAR) and destruction of the foreign tissue.

The antigen against which these human antibodies are directed has been identified as the terminal carbohydrate disaccharide gal$\alpha$ (1–3) gal (Galili *et al.* 1984). This epitope is expressed on cells of non-primate mammals, prosimians and New World monkeys but is absent in Old World monkeys, apes and humans (Galili *et al.* 1988). The preformed antibody against this epitope, anti-gal, is continuously synthesized in humans in large amounts by as many as 1% of circulating B cells (Sandrin & McKenzie 1994; Sandrin *et al.* 1994).

The target epitope is expressed on many cell types of the pig and is seen at a high density on vascular endothelial cells in all types of tissues and organs. In contrast to, for example, liver or kidney parenchymal cells, pancreatic endocrine as well as exocrine cells are devoid of this epitope and only the capillary endothelial cells and the lining of the pancreatic ducts express the galα (1–3) gal epitope (McKenzie *et al.* 1995a,b). Purified islets have lost most of the endothelial lining of the vascular tree within the islet during the isolation procedure and thus the prime source of binding sites for xenoreactive natural antibodies is absent. Moreover, the revascularization process takes place from the host side by ingrowth of vessels using the existing channels and thus the endothelial lining of the vessel will be of recipient type. However, in most purified islet preparations some impurities remain, such as ductal cells, a few exocrine cell clumps of similar size to the islet tissue and thus not removed by the purification process, and single cells of many different cell types, all of which could be target cells for antibody binding. There are also passenger leucocytes residing within the islet. These cells are distributed within the cluster of hormone-producing islet cells and may act as target cells for natural antibody binding once the revascularization process has started and blood-borne substances have access to these targets.

In the case of fetal pig islet xenografts given to immunosuppressed patients, evidence has shown that some of the tissue survived for a prolonged period and that these cells could escape from the destructive onslaught by natural antibodies (Groth *et al.* 1994; Satake *et al.* 1994) although analysis of antibodies with anti-gal activity demonstrated a marked increase in titre and affinity post-transplantation (Galili *et al.* 1995). Graft function in terms of reduced insulin requirements was not seen, but c-peptide could be measured occasionally in the urine in some patients.

There is also evidence that fetal pig islets survived for some time in primates immunosuppressed with CyA, azathioprine and steroids, a regimen that does not prevent HAR (Mandel *et al.* 1995). Transplantation of islet tissue from normal pigs and pigs transgenic for human regulators of complement (White 1996) into non-immunosuppressed cynomolgus monkeys has shown viable graft tissue with minimal infiltration by day 3, but by day 7 these grafts were rejected (Mandel *et al.* 1997). In contrast, immediate (within hours after transplantation) destruction of purified rabbit islets transplanted under the kidney capsule occurred in non-immunosuppressed cynomolgus monkeys with influx of neutrophils, macrophages and eosinophils, but a few islets situated near the kidney capsule survived until they were finally destroyed by day 4 (Hamelmann *et al.* 1994). Again, non-specific macrophage damage through generation of nitric oxide, reactive oxygen intermediates and cytokine release is one of the first defence mechanisms of the host. Most islet grafts are infused into the liver, where they are immediately targeted by a very hostile environment of macrophages and Kupffer cells. These cells are also able to recruit other cells, including cytotoxic T cells and natural killer (NK) cells, potentiating the destructive reaction. However, prolonged tissue culture before implantation seems to prevent HAR of islet xenografts in the same animal model (Gray *et al.* 1995). Pretransplant tissue culture is advisable because it may help in the repair process of islets after the damaging isolation procedure, removing dying and dead cells and debris, thus limiting early non-specific signals for damage clearance.

Thus, it seems from these reports that HAR may not be a problem in islet xenotransplantation but in higher animals immunosuppression, using high doses of a cocktail of potentially dangerous chemical agents, seems to be needed to suppress the ensuing xenogeneic graft rejection.

## Immunoisolation of islets

Immunoprotection of islets could be achieved by semipermeable membranes which are permeable for glucose and nutrients in one direction and passage of insulin in the other direction but are impermeable to immune cells and large-molecule immunoglobulins. These membranes also need to be inert and biocompatible so as not to induce a foreign-body reaction from the recipient, resulting in fibrous overgrowth of the membrane. As the membrane inhibits the process of neovascularization the diffusion potential of the membrane needs to be fast and the distance between the membrane and the islet tissue needs to be small.

There are several approaches to immunoprotection of islet tissue from the onslaught of rejection. Various diffusion chambers, intravascular devices and macro- and microencapsulated islets have been designed and assessed by *in vitro* assays and in small-animal models. A few have been used in large animals, mainly dogs.

Problems associated with diffusion chambers or encapsulation procedures, such as biocompatibility, resulting in fibrosis, adhesion to the implant site and breakage of the chamber and thus sensitization of the host to the implanted tissue, are not yet solved, although these chambers can provide restoration of euglycaemia without the use of immunosuppressive agents (Weber *et al*. 1990; Lanza *et al*. 1995; Lanza & Chick 1997).

Intravascular devices require vascular surgery. Islets protected by a semipermeable membrane within the double lumen of a vascular prothesis are connected to the circulation of the recipient. Promising results from a large-animal model using allogeneic and xenogeneic islets were reported by Maki *et al*. (1996), achieving normoglycaemia for over 8 months in one particular case. However, patency of the vascular device presented difficulties; also larger amounts of islet tissue needed for a human-sized body mass were difficult to accommodate within one device.

Many substances and materials have been investigated for their biocompatibility and diffusion rate for the encapsulation of islets. Moreover, the host response to low-molecular-weight antigens released by the implanted islets diffusing through the membrane may result in non-specific inflammatory immune destruction, cytokine crossover and induction of nitric oxide production. Although immunoisolation of islets has shown some success in ameliorating diabetes in animal models, many questions about the host immune reaction need to be answered and long-term viability and metabolic glucose control need to be assessed.

Alginate poly-L-lycine-coated islets have successfully been used to reverse diabetes in rodents, dogs and, in one case, have resulted in prolonged function in a diabetic patient on a regimen of immunosuppressive drugs (Soon-Shiong *et al*. 1994). However, the longevity of encapsulated islets is questionable (De Vos *et al*. 1996) and rarely have they survived and functioned for more than 6 months in large-animal models, with the exception of porcine islets encapsulated in alginate-polylysine and transplanted intraperitoneally into spontaneously diabetic cynolmogus monkeys (Sun *et al*. 1996), which survived in two cases with partial glucose control for over 2 years. This is the first report on discordant pig xenografted islets without immunosuppression in a small primate animal. More studies using larger animals comparable to humans need to be carried out before any of these procedures could become a viable proposition for the young diabetic patient.

## Conclusions

Islet transplantation has shown some success in ameliorating diabetes in type 1 diabetic patients. Moreover, islet autografts and islet allografts in non-diabetic patients seem to achieve a higher rate of functional survival. Whether this is a reflection on some factors of insulin-dependent diabetes not yet discovered or whether it may be a failure of developing techniques for the detection of early graft rejection and/or safer immunosuppressive therapies is questionable. It is a constant surprise that whole organ or segmental pancreas transplantation seems to function so well, yet the simple procedure of injecting a small amount of endocrine tissue seems to result in such a destructive rejection reaction that similar antirejection therapies to those used in whole organ grafting are not able to overcome it consistently. This seems to suggest that allo- or even xenogeneic islet tissue should be transplanted using immunoisolation procedures or as a composite graft, enveloped by a mass of host-type cells aggregated with islet tissue, to overcome the first line of the host's defence by non-specific immune damage. In this respect, the new idea of composite grafts containing Fas-L-positive cells seems to provide mechanisms of hiding and protecting functional islet tissue from destruction and recurrence of the diabetic disease without the need of chronic and potentially dangerous immunosuppressive therapy.

# References

Abendroth, D., Landgraf, R., Illner, W.D. & Land, W. (1990) Beneficial effect of pancreatic transplantation in insulin dependent diabetes mellitus patients. *Transplantation Proceedings* **22**, 696–697.

Agus, D.B., Surh, C.D. & Sprent, J. (1991) Re-entry of T cells to the adult thymus is restricted to activated T cells. *Journal of Experimental Medicine* **173**, 1039–1046.

AIDSPIT Conference Report (1991) AIDSPIT Conference report. *Diabetologia* **34** (Suppl. 1).

Allen, R.D.M., Wilson, T.G., Grierson, J.M. *et al.* (1990) Percutaneous pancreas transplant fine needle aspiration and needle core biopsies are useful and safe. *Transplantation Proceedings* **22**, 663–664.

Ballinger, W.F. & Lacy, P.E. (1972) Transplantation of intact pancreatic islets in rats. *Surgery* **72**, 175.

Banting, F.G. & Best, C.H. (1922) The internal secretion of the pancreas. *Journal of Laboratory and Clinical Medicine* **7**, 251–266.

Barker, C.F. & Billingham, R.E. (1977) Immunologically privileged sites. *Advances in Immunology* **25**, 1–25.

Barker, C.F., Markmann, J.F., Posselt, A.M. & Naji, A. (1991) Studies of privileged sites and islet transplantation. *Transplantation Proceedings* **23**, 2138–2142.

Bartlett, S.T., Dela Torre, A., Johnson, L.B., Kuo, P.C. & Schweitzer, E.J. (1996) Long-term pancreatic function: potential benefits. *Transplantation Proceedings* **28**, 2128–2130.

Bellgrau, D., Gold, D., Selawry, H. *et al.* (1995) A role for CD95 ligand in preventing graft rejection. *Nature* **377**, 630–632.

Benjamine, R.J. & Waldmann, H. (1986) Induction of tolerance by monoclonal antibody therapy. *Nature* **320**, 449.

Bilous, R.W., Mauer, S.M., Sutherland, D.E.R. *et al.* (1989) The effects of pancreas transplantation on the glomerular stucture of renal allografts in patients with insulin dependent diabetes. *New England Journal of Medicine* **321**, 80–85.

Bohman, S.O., Tyden, G. & Wilczek, H. (1985) Prevention of kidney graft diabetic nephropathy by pancreas transplantation in man. *Diabetes* **34**, 306–308.

Bohman, S.O., Wilzek, H., Tyden, G. *et al.* (1987) Recurrent diabetic nephropathy in renal allografts placed in diabetic patients and protective effect of simultaneous pancreatic transplantation. *Transplantation Proceedings* **19**, 2290–2293.

Bolinder, J., Tyden, G., Tibell, A. & Groth, C.G. (1991) Long-term metabolic control after pancreatic transplantation with enteric exocrine diversion. *Diabetologia* **34**, 76–80.

Borel, J.F., Ruegger, A. & Stahelin, H. (1976) Cyclosporin A: a new anti-lymphocytic agent. *Experimentia* **32**, 777.

Bouwens, L., Lu, W.G. & de-Krijger, R. (1997) Proliferation and differentiation in the human fetal endocrine pancreas. *Diabetologia* **40**, 398–404.

Brewer, Y., Taube, D., Parlmer, A. *et al.* (1989) Effect of graft perfusion with two CD45 monoclonal antibodies on incidence of kidney allograft rejection. *Lancet* **1**, 935–937.

Brons, I.G.M. & Calne, R.Y. (1991) Pancreas transplantation at Cambridge, more than 10 years of experience in the cyclosporin era. *Transplantation Proceedings* **23**, 2215–2216.

Brons, I.G.M., Calne, R.Y., Rolles, K. *et al.* (1987) Glucose control after segmental pancreas with simultaneous kidney transplantation. *Transplantation Proceedings* **19**, 2288–2289.

Brons, I.G.M., Tavora, P.F., Cobbold, S.P. *et al.* (1991) Synergistic monoclonal antibodies for *in vitro* immunomodulation of dog islets. *Transplantation Proceedings* **24**, 1032–1033.

Brons, I.G.M., Champenay, R., Cobbold, S.P. *et al.* (1992) Immunomodulation of dog islets using a cocktail of monoclonal antibodies. *Transplant International* **5**, 484–486.

Brons, I.G.M., Davies, H.ff.S., Makisalo, H. *et al.* (1994) Transplantation of immunomodulated islets. *Transplantation Proceedings* **26** (2), 754.

Brons, I.G.M., Davies, H.ff.S., Watson, C.J., Cobbold, S.P., Waldmann, M. & Calne, R.Y. (1995) Substantial peripheral T-cell depletion before grafting is beneficial in islet transplantation. *Transplantation Proceedings* **27**, 3181.

Brunner, T., Yoo, N.J., Griffith, T.S., Ferguson, T.A. & Green, D.R. (1996) Regulation of CD95 ligand expression: a key element in immune regulation? *Behring Institute Mitteilungen* **97**, 161–174.

Caldara, R., Martin, X., Secchi, A. *et al.* (1991) Metabolic control after kidney and pancreas transplantation: whole series results and effects of segmental duct obstruction versus whole pancreas with bladder diversion technique. *Diabetologia* **34** (Suppl. 1), S51–S53.

Calne, R.Y. (1960) The rejection of renal homografts. Inhibition in dogs by 6 mercaptopurine. *Lancet* **1**, 417–418.

Calne, R.Y. (1984) Paratopic segmental pancreas grafting: a technique with portal venous drainage. *Lancet* **i**, 595–597.

Calne, R.Y. & Brons, I.G.M. (1985) Observations on paratopic segmental pancreas grafting with splenic venous drainage. *Transplantation Proceedings* **17**, 340–341.

Calne, R.Y., White, D.J.G., Thiru, S. & Evans, D.B. (1978) Cyclosporin A in patients receiving renal allografts from cadaveric donors. *Lancet* **ii**, 323.

Calne, R.Y., Rolles, K., White, D.J.G. *et al.* (1979) Cyclosporin A initially as the only immunosuppressant in 34 recipients of cadaveric organs: 32 kidneys, 2 pancreata and 2 livers. *Lancet* **ii**, 1033–1036.

Calne, R.Y., Collier, D.StJ. & Thiru, S. (1987) Observations about FK506 in primates. *Transplantation Proceedings* **19**, 63.

Calne, R.Y., Brons, I.G.M., Williams, P.F. *et al.* (1988) Successful pregnancy after paratopic segmental pancreas and kidney transplantation. *British Medical Journal* **296**, 1709.

Campos, L., Posselt, A.M., Deli, B.C. *et al.* (1994) The failure of intrathymic transplantation of nonimmunogenic islet allografts to promote induction of donor-specific unresponsiveness. *Transplantation* **57**, 950–953.

Cantarovitch, D., Murat, A., Hourmant, M., Bardet, S. & Soulillou, J.P. (1988) Is cyclosporine toxic for human pancreas? *Transplantation Proceedings* **20**, 449–452.

Cedea, J.M. & Terasaki, P.I. (1991) The UNOS Scientific Renal Transplant Registry, 1991. In: *Clinical Transplants 1991* (eds P. Terasaki & J.M. Cedea), UCLA Tissue Typing Laboratory, Los Angeles, California.

Chaib, E., Brons, I.G.M., Papalois, A. & Calne, R.Y. (1993) Does intra-thymic injection of allo antigen-presenting cells before islet allo-transplantation prolong graft survival? *Transplant International* **7**, 423–425.

Chowdhury, N.C., Murphy, B., Sayed, M.H. *et al.* (1996) Acquired systemic tolerance to rat cardiac allografts induced by intrathymic inoculation of synthetic polymorphic MHC class I allopeptides. *Transplantation* **62**, 1878–1882.

Christiansen, E., Tibell, A., Volung, A. *et al.* (1996) Pancreatic endocrine function in recipients of segmental and whole pancreas transplantation. *Journal of Endocrinological Metabolism* **81**, 3972–3979.

Clark, J.D.A., Wheatley, T., Brons, I.G.M., Bloom, S.R. & Calne, R.Y. (1989) Studies of the entero–insular axis following pancreas transplantation in man: neural or hormonal control. *Diabetic Medicine* **6**, 813–817.

Cobbold, S.P., Qin, S., Leong, L.Y.W., Martin, G. & Waldmann, H. (1992) Reprogramming the immune system for peripheral tolerance with CD4 and CD8 monoclonal antibodies. *Immunological Reviews* **129**, 165–201.

Cook, K., Sollinger, H.W., Warner, T., Kamps, D. & Belzer, F.O. (1983) Pancreticocystostomy: an alternative method for exocrine drainage of segmental pancreatic allografts. *Transplantation* **35**, 634–636.

Corry, R.J., Nghiem, D.D. & Schulak, J.A. (1986) Surgical treatment of diabetic nephropathy with simultaneous pancreatic duodenal and renal transplantation. *Surgery, Gynecology and Obstetrics* **162**, 547–555.

Crowther, N.J., Gotfredsen, C.F., Moody, A.J. & Green, I.C. (1989) Porcine islet isolation, cellular composition and secretory response. *Hormonal Metabolism Research* **21**, 590–595.

DCCT Research Group (1993) The effect of intensive treatment of diabetes on the development and progression of long-term complications in insulin-dependent diabetes mellitus. *New England Journal of Medicine* **329**, 977.

De Fronzo, R.A., Hender, R. & Simonson, D. (1982) Insulin resistance is a prominent feature of insulin dependent diabetes. *Diabetes* **31**, 795–801.

De Vos, P., De Haan, B., Pater, J. & Van Schilfgaarde, R. (1996) Association between capsule diameter, adequacy of encapsulation and survival of microencapsulated of rat islet allografts. *Transplantation* **62**, 893–899.

Drachenberg, C.B., Papadimitriou, J.C., Weir, M.R. *et al.* (1996) Histological findings in islets of whole pancreas allografts. Lack of evidence for recurrent cell-mediated diabetes mellitus. *Transplantation* **62**, 1770–1773.

Dubernard, J.M., Traeger, J., Neyra, P. *et al.* (1978) A new method of preparation of segmental pancreatic grafts for transplantation and trials in dogs and in man. *Surgery* **84**, 633–639.

Dupre, J., Stiller, C.R., Gent, M. *et al.* (1988) Effects of immunosuppression with CyA in insulin dependent diabetes mellitus of recent onset. The Canadian Open study of 44 months. *Transplantation Proceedings* **20**, 184–192.

Egidi, M.F., Shapiro, R., Khanna, A., Fung, J.J. & Corry, R.J. (1995) Fine-needle aspiration biopsy in pancreatic transplantation. *Transplantation Proceedings* **27**, 3055–3056.

Fabre, J. (1982) The rat kidney allograft model: was it all too good to be true? *Transplantation* **34**, 223.

French, L.E. & Tschopp, J. (1996) Constitutive Fas ligand expression in several non-lymphoid mouse tissues: implications for immune protection and cell turnover. *Behring Institute Mitteilungen* **97**, 156–160.

Fuggle, S.V., Errasti, P., Daar, A.S. *et al.* (1983) Localisation of MHC (HLA-ABC and DR) antigens in 46 kidneys. Differences in HLA-DR staining of tubules between kidneys. *Transplantation* **35**, 385.

Galili, U., Rachminiwitz, E.A., Peleg, A. & Flechner, I. (1984) A unique natural human IgG antibody with anti agalactosyl specificity. *Journal of Experimental Medicine* **160**, 1519.

Galili, U., Shohet, S.B., Kobrin, E., Stults, C.L.M. & Macher, B.A. (1988) Man, apes and old world monkeys differ from other mammals in the expression of agalactosyl epitopes on nucleated cells. *Journal of Biological Chemistry* **263**, 17755–17762.

Galili, U., Tibell, A., Samuelsson, B., Rydberg, L. & Groth, C.G. (1995) Increased anti Gal activity in diabetic patients transplanted with fetal porcine islet cell clusters. *Transplantation* **59**, 1549–1556.

Gill, R.G., Coulombe, M. & Lafferty, K.J. (1996) Pancreatic islet allograft immunity and tolerance: the two signal hypothesis revisited. *Immunological Reviews* **149**, 75–96.

Gores, P.F. & Sutherland, D.E.R. (1993) Pancreatic islet

transplantation: is purification necessary? *American Journal of Surgery* **166**, 538–542.

Gores, P.F., Najarian, J.S., Stephanian, E. *et al.* (1993) Insulin independence in type I diabetes after transplantation of unpurified islets from single donor with 15-deoxyspergualin. *Lancet* **341** (8836), 19–21.

Goss, J.A., Nakafusa, Y. & Flye, M.W. (1992) MHC Class II presenting cells are necessary for the induction of intrathymic tolerance. *Annals of Surgery* **217**, 492–501.

Gray, D.W. & Morris, P.J. (1987) Developments in isolated pancreatic islet transplantation. *Transplantation* **43**, 321–331.

Gray, D.W., Song, Z., Glover, L., Welsh, K.I. & Morris, P.J. (1995) Tissue culture prevents hyperacute rejection of islet xenografts. *Xenotransplantation* **2**, 157–158.

Griffith, T.S., Brunner, T., Fletcher, S.W., Green, D.R. & Ferguson, T.A. (1995) Fas (CD95) Fas ligand induced apoptosis as a mechanism of immune privilege. *Science* **270**, 1189–1192.

Groth, C.G., Lungren, G. & Colliste, H. (1982) Successful outcome on segmental human pancreatic transplantation with enteric exocrine diversion after modifications in technique. *Lancet* **1**, 522–524.

Groth, C.G., Tyden, G. & Ostman, J. (1989) Fifteen years' experience with pancreas transplantation with pancreatico-enterostomy. *Diabetes* **38** (Suppl. 1), 13–15.

Groth, C.G., Tyden, G. & Tibell, A. (1991) Why is the pancreas special? *Transplantation Proceedings* **23**, 2183–2185.

Gruessner, R.W.G., Burke, G.W., Stratta, R. *et al.* (1996) A multicenter analysis of the first experience with FK506 for induction and rescue therapy after pancreas transplantation. *Transplantation* **61**, 261–273.

Gunnarsson, R., Klintmalm, G., Umdgren, G. *et al.* (1983) Deterioration in glucose metabolism in pancreatic transplant recipients given CyA. *Lancet* **2**, 571–572.

Hamelmann, W., Gray, D.W., Cairns, T.D. *et al.* (1994) Immediate destruction of xenogeneic islets in a primate model. *Transplantation* **58**, 1109–1114.

Hariharan, S., Smith, R.D., Viero, R. & First, M.R. (1996) Diabetic nephropathy after renal transplantation. *Transplantation* **62**, 632–635.

Hart, D.N.J. & Fabre, J.W. (1981) Major histocompatibility complex antigens in rat kidney, ureter and bladder: localisation with monoclonal antibodies and demonstration of Ia-positive dendritic cells. *Transplantation* **31**, 318.

Hering, B.J., Bretzel, R.G. & Federlin, K. (1988) Current status of clinical islet transplantation. *Hormone and Metabolic Research* **20**, 537.

Holdas, H., Brekke, I.B., Hartmann, A. *et al.* (1991) Long-term metabolic control in recipients of combined pancreas and kidney transplants. *Diabetologia* **34** (Suppl. 1), S68–S71.

International Islet Transplant Registry (ITR) Newsletter, No. 1 (1991) (ed. K. Federlin *et al.*). Department of Medicine, Justus Liebig University of Giessen, Giessen, Germany.

International Islet Transplant Registry (ITR) Newsletter, No. 6, Vol. 5, No. 1. (1995) (ed. B.J. Hering *et al.*). Department of Medicine, Justus Liebig University of Giessen, Giessen, Germany.

International Islet Transplant Registry (ITR) Newsletter, No. 7, Vol. 6, No. 1. (1996) (ed. B.J. Hering *et al.*). Third Medical Department, Justus Liebig University of Giessen, Giessen, Germany.

International Pancreas Transplant Registry (ITR) Newsletter, Vol. 7, No. 1. (1994) (ed. D.A. McKeehen). Department of Surgery, University of Minnesota, Minneapolis, USA.

Jindal, R.M. (1994) Posttransplant diabetes mellitus: a review. *Transplantation* **58**, 1289–1298.

Johnson, P.R., White, S.A. & London, N.J. (1996) Collagenase and human islet isolation. *Cell Transplantation* **5**, 437–452.

Jorneskog, G., Tyden, G., Bolinder, J. & Fagnell, B. (1991) Skin microvascular reactivity in fingers of diabetic patients after combined kidney and pancreas transplantation. *Diabetologia* **34**, 135–137.

Kelly, W.D., Lillehei, R.C., Merkel, F.K., Idezuki, Y. & Goetz, F.C. (1966) Allotransplantation of the pancreas and duodenum along with the kidney in diabetic nephropathy. *Surgery* **61**, 827–837.

Kendall, D.M., Sutherland, D.E.R., Goetz, F.C. & Najarian, J.S. (1989) Metabolic effect of hemipancreatectomy in donors. *Diabetes* **38** (Suppl. 1), 101–103.

Kendall, D.M., Sutherland, D.E.R., Najarian, J.S., Goetz, F.C. & Robertson, P.P. (1990) Effects of hemipancreatectomy on insulin secretion and glucose tolerance in healthy humans. *New England Journal of Medicine* **322**, 898–903.

Kennedy, W.R., Navarro, X., Goetz, F.C. *et al.* (1990) Effects of pancreatic transplantation on diabetic neuropathy. *New England Journal of Medicine* **322**, 1031–1037.

Kernstad, R., Tyden, G., Brattstrom, C. *et al.* (1989) Pancreas-specific protein new serum marker for graft rejection in pancreas transplant recipients. *Diabetes* **38** (Suppl. 1), 55–56.

Knechtle, S.J., Vargo, D., Fechner, J. *et al.* (1997) FN18-CRM9 immunotoxin promotes tolerance in primate renal allografts. *Transplantation* **63**, 1–6.

Korbutt, G.S., Elliott, J.F. & Rajotte, R.V. (1997) Co-transplantation of allogeneic islets with allogeneic testicular cell aggregates allows long-term graft survival without systemic immunosuppression. *Diabetes* **46**, 317–322.

KROC Collaborative Study Group (1988) Diabetic retinopathy after two years of intensified insulin treatment: follow-up of the KROC Collaborative Study. *Journal of the American Medical Association* **260**, 37–41.

La-Rocca, E., Traeger, J., Cantarowitch, D. *et al.* (1987) Segmental or whole pancreatic graft? Further comparison of metabolic control between segmental pancreatic grafts and whole pancreas grafts in the long term. *Transplantation Proceedings* 19, 3872–3873.

Lafferty, K.J. & Cunningham, A.J. (1975) A new analysis of allogeneic interactions. *Australian Journal of Experimental Biological and Medical Science* 53, 27–42.

Lake, S.P., Bassett, P.D. & Larkins, A. (1989) Large scale purification of human islets utilising discontinuous albumin gradient on IBM 2991 cell separator. *Diabetes* 38, 143.

Landgraf, R., Nusser, J., Riedl, R.L. *et al.* (1991) Metabolic and hormonal studies of type 1 (insulin dependent) diabetic patients after successful pancreas and kidney transplantation. *Diabetologia* 34, 61–67.

Lanza, R.P. & Chick, W.L. (1997) Immunoisolation: at a turning point. *Review of Immunology Today* 18, 135–139.

Lanza, R.P., Kuhtreiber, W.M., Ecker, D., Staruk, J.E. & Chick, W.L. (1995) Xenotransplantation of porcine and bovine islets without immunosuppression using uncoated alginate microspheres. *Transplantation* 59, 1377–1384.

Lau, H.T., Yu, M., Fontana, A. & Stoeckert, C.J. Jr (1996) Prevention of islet allograft rejection with engineered myoblasts expressing FasL in mice. *Science* 273, 109–112.

Lawrence, H.S. (1965) Uraemia: nature's immunosuppressive device. *Annals of Internal Medicine* 2, 166–168.

Le Francois, N., Raffaele, P., Martinenghi, S. *et al.* (1990) Prophylactic polyclonal versus monoclonal antibodies in kidney and pancreas transplantation. *Transplantation Proceedings* 22, 632–633.

Lechler, R.I. & Batchelor, J.R. (1982) Immunogenicity of retransplanted rat kidney allografts: route I and route II. *Journal of Experimental Medicine* 156, 1835–1841.

Levy, M.M., Ketchum, R.J., Perloff, J.R. *et al.* (1996) A model for successful engraftment of intrathymic islet allografts in dogs: the role for delayed native pancreatectomy and short term islet culture. Presentation at the XVIth International Congress of the Transplantation Society 1996. Abstract.

Lloyd, D.M., Cother, S.J., Letai, A.G., Stuart, F.P. & Thistlethwaite, J.R. (1989) Pancreas graft immunogeneicity and pretreatment with anti class II monoclonal antibodies. *Diabetes* 38 (Suppl. 1), 104–108.

Luzi, L., Hering, B.J., Socci, C. & Raptis, G. (1996) Metabolic effects of successful intraportal islet transplantation in insulin-dependent diabetes mellitus. *Journal of Clinical Investigation* 97, 2611–2618.

McKenzie, I.F.C., Koulmanda, M., Mandel, T.E., Xing, P.X. & Sandrin, M.S. (1995a) Pig to human xenotransplantation: the expression of gal a (1,3) gal epitopes on pig islet cells. *Xenotransplantation* 2, 1–7.

McKenzie, I.F.C., Koulmanda, M., Sandrin, M.S. & Mandel, T.E. (1995b) Fetal pig islet xenografts in NOD/Lt mice: the

effect of peritransplant anti CD4 monoclonal antibody and graft immunomodification on graft survival, and lack of gal α (1,3) gal expression on endocrine cells. *Xenotransplantation* 2, 295.

Maki, T., Otsu, I. & O'Neill, J.J. (1996) Treatment of diabetes by xenogeneic islets without immunosuppression: use of a vascularised bioartificial pancreas. *Diabetes* 45, 342–347.

Mandel, T.E., Koulmanda, M., Kovarik, J. *et al.* (1995) Transplantation of organ cultured fetal pig pancreas in non-obese diabetic (NOD) mice and primates. *Xenotransplantation* 2, 128–132.

Mandel, T.E., Koulmanda, M., Cozzi, E. *et al.* (1997) Transplantation of normal and DAF-transgenic fetal pig pancreas into cynomolgus monkeys. *Transplantation Proceedings* 29, 940.

Mandrup-Poulsen, T., Bendtzen, K., Nerup, J. *et al.* (1986) Affinity purified human interleukin 1 is cytotoxic to isolated islets of Langerhans. *Diabetologia* 29, 63–67.

Margreiter, R., Fuchs, D., Hansen, A. *et al.* (1983) Neopterin as a new biochemical marker for diagnosis of allograft rejection. *Transplantation* 36, 650–653.

Marks, W.H., Borgstrom, A., Sollinger, H. & Marks, C. (1990) Serum immunoreactive anodal trypsinogen and urinary amylase as biochemical markers for rejection of clinical whole-organ pancreas allografts having exocrine drainage into the urinary bladder. *Transplantation* 49, 112–115.

Mauer, M., Steffes, M., Connett, J. *et al.* (1983) The development of lesions in the glomerular basement membrane and mesangium after transplantation of normal kidneys into diabetic patients. *Diabetes* 32, 948–952.

Mauer, S.M., Goetz, F.C., McHugh, L.E. *et al.* (1989) Long-term study of normal kidneys transplanted into patients with type I diabetes. *Diabetes* 38, 516–523.

Mayo, G.L., Posselt, A.M., Campos, L. *et al.* (1994) Induction of donor-specific tolerance by intrathymic cellular transplantation. In: *Rejection and Tolerance* (eds J.L. Touraine *et al.*). Kluwer Academic Publishers, Netherlands.

Melzer, J.S., D'Allessandro, A.M., Kalayolu, M. *et al.* (1990) The use of OKT3 in combined pancreas–kidney allotransplantaiton. *Transplantation Proceedings* 22, 634–635.

Miyoshi, K., Sakagami, K. & Orita, K. (1992) *Ex vivo* perfusion of canine pancreaticoduodenal allografts using Class II specific monoclonal antibody delays the onset of acute rejection. *Transplant International* 5 (Suppl. 1), 516–520.

Monaco, A.P., Wood, M.L., Gray, J.G. & Russel, P.S. (1966) Studies on heterologous anti-lymphocyte serum in mice. II: effects on the immune system. *Journal of Immunology* 96, 229.

Moskalewsky, S. (1965) Isolation and culture of the islets of

Langerhans of the guinea pig. *General and Comparative Endocrinology* 5, 342.

Moudry-Munns, K.C., Barrou, B. & Sutherland, D.E. (1996) Pregnancy after pancreas transplantation: report from the International Pancreas Transplant Registry. *Transplantation Proceedings* 28, 3639.

Nagata, S. & Golstein, P. (1995) The Fas death factor. *Science* 267, 1449–1456.

Naji, A. (1996) Induction of tolerance by intrathymic inoculation of alloantigen. *Current Opinion in Immunology* 8, 704–709.

Olac, B.J., Swanson, G.S., McLear, M.A. *et al.* (1991) Islet purification using Euroficoll gradients. *Transplantation Proceedings* 23, 774.

Oluwole, S.F. & Jin, M. (1993) Induction of donor specific tolerance in rat cardiac allograft by intrathymic inoculation of allogeneic soluble peptides. *Transplantation* 56, 1523.

Oluwole, S.F., Chowdhury, N.C. & Jin, M.X. (1994) The relative contribution of intrathymic inoculation of donor leukocyte subpopulations in the induction of specific tolerance. *Cellular Immunology* 153, 163–170.

Oluwole, S.F., Jin, M.X., Chowdhury, N.C. *et al.* (1995) Induction of peripheral tolerance by intrathymic inoculation of soluble alloantigens: evidence for the role of host antigen-presenting cells and suppressor cell mechanism. *Cellular Immunology* 162, 33–41.

Ostman, J., Bolinder, J., Gunnarsson, R. *et al.* (1989) Effect of pancreas transplantation on metabolic and hormonal profiles in IDDM patients. *Diabetes* 38 (Suppl. 1), 88–93.

Perkal, M., Marks, C.G., Lorber, M.I. & Marks, W.H. (1992) A three year experience with serum anodal trypsinogen as a biochemical marker for rejection in pancreatic allografts. *Transplantation* 53, 415–419.

Perkins, J.D., Munn, S.R., Marsh, C.L. *et al.* (1990) Safety and efficacy of cystoscopically directed biopsy in pancreas transplantation. *Transplantation Proceedings* 22, 665–666.

Posselt, A.M., Barker, C.F., Tomaszewski, J.E. *et al.* (1990) Induction of donor-specific unresponsiveness by intrathymic islet transplantation. *Science* 249, 1293–1295.

Posselt, A.M., Naji, A., Roark, J.H., Markmann, J.F. & Barker, C.F. (1991) Intrathymic transplantation in the spontaneously diabetic BB rat. *Annals of Surgery* 214, 363–373.

Prieto, M., Sutherland, D.E.R., Fernandez Cruz L., Heil, J. & Najarian, J.S. (1987) Experimental and clinical experience with urine amylase monitoring for early diagnosis of rejection in pancreas transplantation. *Transplantation* 43, 73–79.

Raff, M.C. (1992) Social controls on cell survival and cell death. *Nature* 356, 397–400.

Rajotte, R.V., Evans, M.G., Warnock, G.L. & Kneteman,

N.M. (1990) Islet cryopreservation. *Hormonal Metabolism Research Supplement* 25, 72–81.

Ramsay, R.C., Goetz, F.C., Sutherland, D.E.R. *et al.* (1988) Progression of diabetic retinopathy after pancreas transplantation for insulin-dependent diabetes mellitus. *New England Journal of Medicine* 318, 208–214.

Rasmussen, A., Davies H.ff.S., Jamieson, N.V. *et al.* (1995) Combined transplantation of liver and kidney from the same donor protects the kidney from rejection and improves kidney graft survival. *Transplantation* 59, 919–921.

Raviola, E. & Karuovski, M. (1972) Evidence for a blood–thymus barrier using electron opaque tracers. *Journal of Experimental Medicine* 136, 466–498.

Reaven, G.M. (1988) Role of insulin resistance in human disease. *Diabetes* 37, 1595–1607.

Ricordi, C., Lacy, P.E. & Scharp, D.W. (1989) Automated islet isolation from human pancreas. *Diabetes* 38, 140–142.

Ricordi, C., Zeng, Y., Alejandro, R. *et al.* (1991) In vivo effect of FK506 on human pancreatic islets. *Transplantation* 52, 519–522.

Ricordi, C., Tzakis, A.G., Carroll, P.B. *et al.* (1992) Human islet isolation and allotransplantation in 22 consecutive cases. *Transplantation* 53, 407–414.

Robertson, R.P., Diem, P. & Sutherland, D.E.R. (1991) Time related cross-sectional and prospective follow-up of pancreatic endocrine function after pancreas allograft transplantation in type 1 diabetic patients. *Diabetologia* 34 (Suppl. 1), S57–S61.

Rosenlund, E.F., Haakens, K., Brinchmann, H.O., Dahl, J.K. & Hanssen, K.F. (1988) Transient proliferative diabetic retinopathy during intensified insulin treatment. *American Journal of Ophthalmology* 105, 618–625.

Sandrin, M.S. & McKenzie, I.F.C. (1994) Gal α (1,3) gal, the major xenoantigens recognised in pigs by human natural antibodies. *Immunological Reviews* 141, 169–189.

Sandrin, M.S., Vaughan, H.A. & McKenzie, I.F.C. (1994) Identification of gal α (1,3) gal as the major epitope for pig to human vascularised xenografts. *Transplantation Reviews* 8, 134–149.

Santamaria, P., Nakhleh, R.E., Sutherland, D.E.R. & Barbosa, J.J. (1992) Characterization of T lymphocytes infiltrating human pancreas allograft affected by isletitis and recurrent disease. *Diabetes* 41, 53–61.

Sasaki, T., Pirsch, J.D., Alessandro, A.M. *et al.* (1991) Simultaneous pancreas–kidney transplantation at University of Wisconsin–Madison Hospital. In: *Clinical Transplants 1991* (ed. P. Terasaki). UCLA Tissue Typing Laboratory, Los Angeles, California.

Satake, M., Korsgren, O., Ridderstad, A. *et al.* (1994) Immunological characteristics of islet cell xenotransplantation in humans and rodents. *Immunological Reviews* 141, 191–211.

Scantlebury, V., Shapiro, R., Fung, J. *et al.* (1991) New onset of diabetes in FK506 vs. cyclosporin-treated kidney transplant recipients. *Transplantation Proceedings* 23, 3169–3170.

Scharp, D.W., Lacy, P.E., Santiago, J.V. *et al.* (1991) Results of our first nine intraportal islet allografts in type 1 insulin dependent diabetic patients. *Transplantation* 51, 76–85.

Scheider, A., Meyer-Schwickerath, E., Nasser, J., Land, W. & Landgraf, R. (1991) Diabetic retinopathy and pancreas transplantation: a 3 year follow-up. *Diabetologia* 34, 95–99.

Secchi, A., Dubernard, J.M., Larocca, E. *et al.* (1991) Endocrinometabolic effects of whole versus segmental pancreas allotransplantation in diabetic patients: a two-year follow-up. *Transplantation* 51, 625–629.

Selawry, H.P. & Cameron, D.F. (1993) Sertoli cell-enriched fractions in successful islet cell transplantation. *Cell Transplantation* 2, 123.

Selawry, H.P., Fojaco, R. & Whittington, K. (1985) Intratesticular islet allografts in the spontaneously diabetic BB/W rat. *Diabetes* 34, 1019–1024.

Selawry, H.P., Wang, X. & Alloush, L. (1996) Sertoli cell-induced effects on functional and structural characteristics of isolated neonatal porcine islets. *Cell Transplantation* 5, 517–524.

Sibley, R.K. & Sutherland, D.E.R. (1987) Pancreas transplantation: an immunohistologic and histopathologic examination of 100 grafts. *American Journal of Pathology* 128, 151–170.

So, S.K.S., Minford, E.J., Moudry-Munn, K., Gillingham, K. & Sutherland, D.E.R. (1990) DR matching improves cadaveric pancreas transplant results. *Transplantation Proceedings* 22, 687–688.

Solders, G., Gunnarsson, R., Persson, A. *et al.* (1987) Effect of combined pancreatic and renal transplantation on diabetic neuropathy: a two-year follow-up study. *Lancet* 2, 1232–1235.

Solders, G., Tyden, G., Persson, A. & Groth, C.G. (1991) Improvements in diabetic neuropathy 4 years after successful pancreatic and renal transplantation. *Diabetologia* 34, 125–127.

Sollinger, H.W., Sratta, R.J., Kalayoglu, M., Pirsch, J.D. & Belzer, F.O. (1987) Pancreas transplantation with pancreaticocystostomy and quadruple immunosuppression. *Surgery* 102, 674–679.

Soon-Shiong, P., Heintz, R.E., Merideth, N. *et al.* (1994) Insulin independence in a type 1 diabetic patient after encapsulated islet transplantation. *Lancet* 343, 950–951.

Squifflet, J.P., Moudry-Munn, K. & Sutherland, D.E.R. (1988) Is HLA matching relevant in pancreas transplantation? *Transplant International* 1, 26–29.

Stegall, M., Lafferty, K.J., Kam, I. & Gill, R.G. (1996) Evidence of recurrent autoimmunity in human allogeneic islet transplantation. *Transplantation* 61, 1272–1274.

Steinmuller, D. (1967) Immunisation with skin isografts taken from tolerant mice. *Science* 158, 127–129.

Steinmuller, D. (1980) Passenger leukocytes and immunogenicity of skin allografts. *Journal of Investigative Dermatology* 75, 107–115.

Stiller, C.R., Dupre, J., Gent, M. *et al.* (1984) Effects of CyA immunosuppression in insulin-dependent diabetes mellitus of recent onset. *Science* 223, 1362–1367.

Stratta, R.J., Taylor, R.J., Grune, M.T. *et al.* (1995) Experience with protocol biopsies after solitary pancreas transplantation. *Transplantation* 60, 1431–1437.

Sun, A.M., Coddling, J.A. & Haist, R.E. (1974) A study of glucose tolerance and insulin response in partially depancreatectomised dogs. *Diabetes* 23, 424–432.

Sun, Yl., Ma, X., Zhou, D., Vacek, I. & Sun, A.M. (1996) Normalization of diabetes mellitus in spontaneously diabetic cynomologus monkeys by xenografts of microencapsulated porcine islets without immunosuppression. *Journal of Clinical Investigation* 98, 1417–1422.

Sutherland, D.E.R. (1980) International human pancreas and islet transplant registry. *Transplantation Proceedings* 12, 2229–2236.

Sutherland, D.E.R. (1991) Report from the International Pancreas Transplant Registry. *Diabetologia* 34 (Suppl. 1), S28–S39.

Sutherland, D.E.R. (1992a) Effect of pancreas transplants on secondary complications of diabetes: review of observations at a single institution. *Transplantation Proceedings* 24, 859–860.

Sutherland, D.E.R. (1992b) Pancreas transplantation: state of the art. *Transplantation Proceedings* 24, 762–766.

Sutherland, D.E.R. & Gruessner, A.C. (1995a) Long-term function (>5 years) of pancreas grafts from the International Pancreas Transplant Registry database. *Transplantation Proceedings* 27, 2977–2980.

Sutherland, D.E.R. & Gruessner, A.C. (1995b) Pancreas transplantation in the United States as reported to the United Network for Organ Sharing (UNOS) and analysed by the International Pancreas Transplant Registry. *Clinical Transplantation* 49–67.

Sutherland, D.E.R., Goetz, F.C. & Najarian, J.S. (1984) Pancreas transplants from related donors. *Transplantation* 38, 625–633.

Sutherland, D.E.R., Dunn, D.L., Goetz, F.C. *et al.* (1989a) A 10 year experience with 290 pancreas transplants at a single institution. *American Surgery* 210, 274–288.

Sutherland, D.E.R., Goetz, F.C. & Sibley, R.K. (1989b) Recurrence of disease in pancreas transplants. *Diabetes* 38 (Suppl. 1), 85–87.

Sutherland, D.E.R., Gruessner, R., Gillingham, K. *et al.* (1991) A single institution's experience with solitary pancreas transplantation: a multivariant analysis of factors leading to improved outcome. In: *Clinical Transplants 1995* (ed. P.I. Terasaki), p. 67. UCLA Tissue Typing Laboratory, Los Angeles, California.

Sutherland, D.E.R., Gruessner, R.W., Gores, P.F. *et al.* (1995) Pancreas transplantation: an update. *Diabetes Metabolism Reviews* 11, 337–363.

Sutherland, D.E.R., Cecka, M. & Gruessner, A.C. (in press) Report from the International Pancreas Transplant Registry (IPTR), 1998. *Transplantation Proceedings*, in press.

Tabasco-Minguilan, J., Mieles, L., Carroll, P. *et al.* (1993) Insulin requirements after liver transplantation and FK-506 immunosuppression. *Transplantation* 56, 862–867.

Tattersal, R. (1989) Is pancreas transplantation for insulin dependent diabetics worthwhile? *New England Journal of Medicine* 321, 112–114.

Tilg, H., Konigsrainer, A., Krausler, R. *et al.* (1992) Urinary and pancreatic juice neopterin excretion after combined pancreas–kidney transplantation. *Transplantation* 53, 804–808.

Tyden, G., Brattstrom, G., Gunnarsson, R. *et al.* (1987a) Metabolic control 2 months to 4.5 years after pancreas transplantation with special reference to the role of cyclosporin A. *Transplantation Proceedings* 19, 2294–2296.

Tyden, G., Brattstrom, C., Haggmark, A. & Groth, C.G. (1987b) Studies on the exocrine secretion of segmental pancreatic grafts in humans. *Surgery, Gynecology and Obstetrics* 164, 404–408.

Tyden, G., Reinholt, F., Brattstrom, D. *et al.* (1987c) Diagnosis of rejection in recipients of pancreatic grafts with enteric exocrine diversion by monitoring pancreatic juice cytology and amylase excretion. *Transplantation Proceedings* 19, 3892–3894.

Tyden, G., Brattstrom, C., Bjorkman, U. *et al.* (1989) Pregnancy after combined pancreas–kidney transplantation. *Diabetes* 38 (Suppl. 1), 43–45.

Tyden, G., Finn, P.R., Sundkvist, G. & Bolinder, J. (1996) Recurrence of autoimmune diabetes mellitus in recipients of cadaveric pancreatic grafts. *New England Journal of Medicine* 335, 860–863.

Tzakis, A.G., Ricordi, C., Alejandro, R. *et al.* (1990) Pancreatic islet transplantation after upper abdominal exenteration and liver replacement. *Lancet* 336, 402–405.

Tze, W.J., Wong, F.C. & Tingle, A.J. (1976) The use of Hypaque Ficoll in the isolation of pancreatic islets in rats. *Transplantation* 22, 201.

Tze, W.J., Tai, J. & Cheung, S. (1990) *In vitro* effects of FK506 on human and rat islets. *Transplantation* 49 (6), 1172–1174.

Ulbig, M., Kampik, A., Landgraf, R. & Land, W. (1987) The influence of combined pancreatic and renal transplantation on advanced diabetic retinopathy. *Transplantation Proceedings* 19, 3554–3556.

Van der Vliet, J.A., Navarro, X., Kennedy, W.R. *et al.* (1988) The effect of pancreas transplantation on diabetic polyneuropathy. *Transplantation* 45, 368–370.

Verge, C.F. & Eisenbarth, G.S. (1996) Strategies for preventing type 1 diabetes mellitus. *West Journal of Medicine* 164, 249–255.

Wahoff, D.C., Papalois, B.E., Najarrian, J.S. *et al.* (1995) Autologous islet transplantation to prevent diabetes after pancreatic resection. *Annals of Surgery* 222, 562–575 (discussion 575–579).

Warnock, G.L. & Rajotte, R.V. (1992) Human pancreatic islet transplantation. *Transplantation Review* 6, 195–208.

Warnock, G.L., Dabbs, K.D., Evans, M.G. *et al.* (1990) Critical mass of islets that function after implantation in a large mammalian. *Hormone and Metabolic Research Supplement* 25, 156–161.

Warnock, G.L., Kneteman, N.M., Ryan, E.A. *et al.* (1992) Long-term follow-up after transplantation of insulin producing pancreatic islets into patients with type I diabetes mellitus. *Diabetologia* 35, 89.

Weber, C.J., Zabinski, S., Koschitzky, T. *et al.* (1990) The role of CD4+ T helper cells in the destruction of microencapsulated islet xenografts in NOD mice. *Transplantation* 49, 396–404.

White, D.J.G. (1996) hDAF transgenic pig organs: are they concordant for human transplantation? *Xeno* 4, 50–54.

# Chapter 13/Corneal transplantation

SUSAN M. NICHOLLS, JEREMY P. DIAMOND,
BENJAMIN A. BRADLEY & DAVID L. EASTY

## Introduction

Corneal transplantation has been the mainstay of treatment for serious corneal disease for over a century. The operation was proposed by Franz Reisinger in the early 19th century (Reisinger 1824) and was first attempted in humans as a xenograft from pig by Richard Sharp Kissam in 1838 (Kissam 1844). Kissam had been inspired by the experience of S.S.L. Bigger, an Irishman imprisoned in North Africa, who had performed a successful corneal allograft on a blind gazelle. The first human allograft is credited to S. Sellerbeck in 1878, who transplanted the cornea of a 2.5-year-old donor eye removed for glioma to a man blinded with ophthalmic gonorrhoea. The cornea remained clear for 20 days before clouding over (Sellerbeck 1878). The first successful full-thickness corneal transplant is attributed to Eduard Zirm. He transplanted a cornea from an 11-year-old boy, whose eye was removed because of an iron splinter, to Alois Glogar, who had blinded himself with lime when whitewashing his chicken hutch (Zirm 1906).

## Structure of the cornea

The cornea constitutes a transparent avascular tissue devoid of lymphatic drainage and possessing a unique blood–aqueous barrier (Fig. 13.1). It is a continuation of the white sclera, the two blending at the corneoscleral limbus, and has five distinct layers: epithelium and

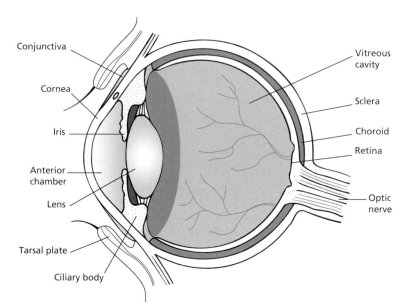

Conjunctiva

Cornea

Iris

Anterior
chamber

Lens

Tarsal plate

Ciliary body

Vitreous
cavity

Sclera

Choroid

Retina

Optic
nerve

**Fig. 13.1**  Schematic drawing of a transverse section of the eye.

its basement membrane, stroma, Bowman's layer, Descemet's membrane and endothelium.

EPITHELIUM

The epithelium is stratified, five to six cells thick and lacks the keratin found in skin epithelium (Fig. 13.2). A single layer of tall germinal cells abut the basement membrane, opposing a mid-layer, two or three cells thick, of polyhedral 'wing' cells, which in turn meet an outermost layer of flat cells. These outer cells are joined via tight junctions, an important factor in limiting drug penetration. They also exhibit microvilli and microplicae, to which adheres a thin layer of hydrophilic mucus. The mucus, secreted by conjunctival goblet cells, supports the aqueous tear film, which is itself protected from evaporation by an oily layer. This triple layer of tears is the main refractive surface of the eye. Langerhans' cells (LC) are present, as in skin, but are restricted almost entirely to the limbus, this being an ill-defined transition zone between cornea and sclera.

Loss or damage to the epithelium may affect the tear film, resulting in reduction of visual acuity. A discontinuity in the epithelium also increases the potential for pathogenic bacteria to gain access to the deeper layers of the cornea, from where infection may invade intraocular structures. Damaged epithelial cells are normally replaced rapidly by mitosis of stem cells at the limbus, which are also a source of replacement cells for the conjunctival epithelium.

The cornea receives sensory innervation via terminal branches of the ophthalmic division of the trigeminal (fifth) cranial nerve. These form a net in the anterior stroma below the Bowman's zone and send branches into the epithelium. Free nerve endings induce considerable pain following epithelial loss in eyes with intact innervation.

STROMA AND BOWMAN'S LAYER

The stroma constitutes 90% of the corneal thickness. The thin Bowman's layer, immediately below the epithelium, is an acellular lamella of randomly organized collagen bundles in continuity with the remaining stroma. The remaining stroma is composed of regular lamellae of collagen fibres which extend uninterrupted across the width of the cornea. Each lamella consists of parallel fibres embedded in a ground substance composed of mucoprotein and glycoprotein and each fibre is separated from its neighbours by its own

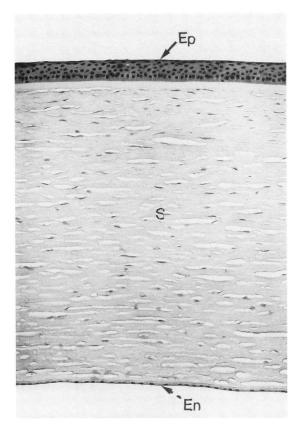

**Fig. 13.2** Photomicrograph of a transverse section of the cornea. En, endothelium; Ep, epithelium; S, stroma. H & E stain, ×26. (Courtesy Dr M. Berry.)

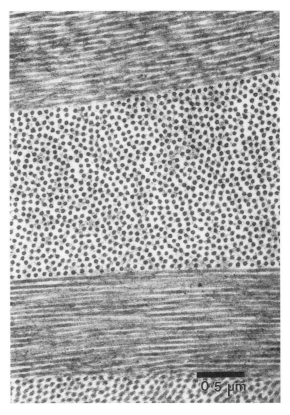

**Fig. 13.3** Transmission electromicrograph of a transverse section of corneal stroma demonstrating the arrangement of collagen fibres. (Courtesy Dr R. Young.)

width, ~200 nm or half the wavelength of blue light (Fig. 13.3). Keratocytes are fibroblast-like cells scattered infrequently throughout the stroma that lay down collagen. Dendritic accessory cells are present, mainly at the periphery, as with epithelium. Keratocytes are relatively inactive and their extracellular matrix is normally turned over very slowly in comparison with sclera and dermis (Dohlman & Boström 1955), presumably because of the special requirement for transparency. However, after corneal injury, migration and mitosis of keratocytes rapidly increase (Maumenee & Kornblueth 1949), with new collagen being produced and keratocytes lost at the centre being

replaced from the periphery in approximately 3 weeks (Dunnington & Smelser 1958).

### DESCEMET'S MEMBRANE

Descemet's membrane is the homogeneous basement membrane laid down by endothelial cells and may undergo repair after surgery or other trauma.

### ENDOTHELIUM

The endothelium is a monolayer of hexagonal cells with large central nuclei and multiple intracellular organelles. They are attached anteriorly to their basement membrane and exposed to the aqueous humour of the anterior chamber (Fig. 13.4a). They are bound at their apex by tight junctions, forming a permeability barrier, and play a crucial part in maintaining corneal transparency.

Unlike epithelial and stromal cells, endothelial cells do not replicate significantly in adults and there is a gradual loss with age, accommodated by sliding of adjacent cells, with consequent increase in overall cell size. In normal individuals, 6000 endothelial cells per mm² present at birth have been observed to decrease to 2700 at 10 years of age and 2500 in adulthood (Hiles *et al.* 1979; Bahn *et al.* 1986). The natural decrease is exacerbated by surgery, such as cataract extraction and

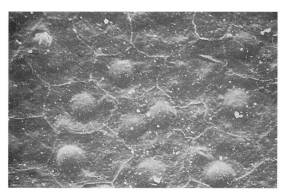

(a)

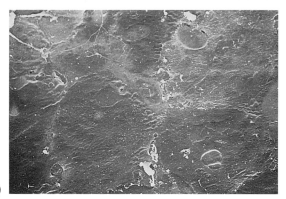

(b)

Fig. 13.4 Scanning electron micrographs of corneal endothelium. (a) Normal endothelium demonstrating cell margins and nuclei. (b) Endothelium from a patient with secondary endothelial dystrophy. Note the decreased number of nuclei. (Courtesy Mr B. Amer.)

transplantation, resulting in further enlargement of cells (Fig. 13.4b). It is this lack of replacement of endothelial cells by mitosis that ultimately leads to corneal graft failure and blindness after alloimmune attack (see p. 392). By contrast, in some mammals, including the rabbit and rat, the endothelium can replicate *in vivo*, leading to repair of this layer and the eventual resolution of rejection.

Blood-vessels arborize at the limbus, where they extend less than 1 mm into the clear cornea. The central cornea receives metabolic support from these vessels and via diffusion from the aqueous humour and overlying tear film.

## Embryology

While the epithelium is ectodermal, keratocytes and endothelium are mesenchymal cells derived from the neural crest. These cells migrate inwards from the periphery of the optic cup between the surface ectoderm and the lens to form the stroma (homologous to the dermis of the skin), endothelium and iris. The presence of the lens with its outer layer of cells is essential for their ordered migration and the formation of the anterior chamber (Beebe & Coats 1998). The endothelium has no homology with vascular endothelium.

## Functions of the cornea

An understanding of the functions of the cornea is valuable when considering indications for and outcome of corneal transplantation. The functions of the cornea include transmission of light, refraction of light and maintenance of the structural integrity of the eye. Successful corneal transplantation demands that each of these functions is reproduced by the transplanted tissue.

## Transmission of light

There is no fundamental biochemical difference between the structure of the transparent cornea and the opaque sclera. Corneal transparency arises from an absence of blood-vessels and pigment and from the regular arrangement of evenly sized collagen fibrils orientated in a lattice and separated by less than the wavelength of visible light, scattered light being eliminated by destructive interference (Maurice 1957). Lipid deposition, scar tissue and oedema fluid compromise the regular arrangement of fibrils with consequent loss of corneal transparency.

The cornea is maintained in a relatively dehydrated state by the epithelium and endothelium acting as permeability barriers and the endothelium pumping ions from the stroma into the anterior chamber with subsequent movement of water down a concentration gradient. The mechanism is not well understood, but if the endothelium is removed or exposed to ouabain, which blocks sodium–potassium ATPase, the cornea swells to three times normal thickness and the resulting oedema causes loss of corneal transparency. Active transport of sodium, bicarbonate and probably of chloride ions occurs. Endothelial cell loss becomes of pathological importance if cell density falls below ~400–700 cells per mm$^2$ (Klyce & Beuerman 1988). Below this threshold the loss of equilibrium between water influx and efflux leads to stromal oedema. Fluid also collects below the relatively impermeable epithelium, where it forms cysts. These may break, resulting in epithelial defects. The corneal fluid balance may also be disturbed if the intraocular pressure (IOP) rises. An increase in IOP shifts the equilibrium in favour of fluid influx, inducing corneal oedema.

## Refraction of light

The quality of image falling upon the retina depends largely upon the optics of the cornea with its normal refractive power of approximately +40 dioptres (two-thirds of the total refractive power of the eye). Many normal corneas include a small cylindrical lens element, resulting in astigmatism. Corneal disease and corneal transplantation (see p. 388) may compromise visual acuity as a result of inducing large cylindrical errors upon the anterior corneal surface.

Loss of corneal transparency results in reduced light transmission but not necessarily in impaired light refraction. However, many lesions, e.g. corneal scarring, also cause increased light scattering, while others, e.g. surface epithelial irregularity or loss, adversely affect the refraction of light without necessarily reducing its transmission.

## Maintenance of structural integrity of the eye

The cornea provides anatomical continuity with the anterior segment of the eye. Any lesion which compromises anatomical integrity rapidly results in derangement of intraocular anatomy, contributing to loss of vision. Secondary infection is common and may result in loss of the eye.

## Ocular pharmacology

The cornea is exposed to the external environment, thereby facilitating topical administration of pharmacological agents. By contrast, it is relatively isolated from the systemic circulation by a blood–aqueous barrier similar to the blood–brain barrier, which tends to exclude drugs administered systemically.

Drugs can be applied in the form of drops, viscous solutions or ointments. Increasing the viscosity of the vehicle prolongs exposure of the eye to the drug. Drugs in routine use to treat or prevent corneal graft rejection attain therapeutic concentration within the cornea and anterior chamber following local administration, thereby minimizing the side effects inherent in systemic drug administration. Topically administered medications eventually leave the conjunctival sac, eluted with the flow of tears via the nasolacrimal duct into the nose, and may thus result in systemic side effects following absorption via the nasal or gastrointestinal mucosa.

The tight junctions of the corneal epithelium allow passage of fat-soluble compounds while restricting those that are water-soluble. Subsequent transfer across the corneal stroma is potentiated by water solubility, while penetration of the endothelium is again dependent upon the hydrophobic nature of the compound. Thus, biphasic drugs are most able to enter the cornea and anterior chamber. Corneal inflammation, trauma or surgery may diminish these barriers and increase drug penetration.

Systemically administered drugs may be excluded from the intraocular tissues. Only highly lipid-soluble compounds pass through the tight junctions present in the ciliary body. This barrier to drug transfer is lowered in the presence of local inflammation and corneal vascularization. Many drugs are actively transported out of the eye by the ciliary epithelium.

## Keratoplasty

Corneal transplantation may involve full-thickness (penetrating keratoplasty) or partial-thickness (lamellar) grafts.

### Penetrating keratoplasty

This requires removal of all layers of the host cornea with subsequent transplantation of a full-thickness donor cornea. This surgical approach is indicated where the host disease process involves the entire stromal thickness and/or the endothelium. Full-thickness corneal grafts accounted for 96% of transplants performed using tissue supplied via the United Kingdom Transplant Support Service Authority (UKTSSA) (1996) during 1991–94.

### Lamellar keratoplasty

Where the host corneal disease involves the anterior structures (epithelium or anterior stroma) the deeper structures (posterior stroma and endothelium) may be normal. In such circumstances the host cornea is cleaved deep to the lesion and a donor disc of similar thickness is grafted into the defect. In this case the host endothelium is retained. Donor tissue preparation can involve freezing corneal tissue with liquid nitrogen to facilitate machine cutting with a cryolathe. Lamellar transplants are less prone to rejection than are full-thickness grafts (Richard *et al.* 1977).

### Endothelial cell transplantation

Several endothelial disorders that currently necessitate corneal transplantation would benefit from replacement of this layer alone. This might reduce the antigenic load on the recipient and subsequent risk of rejection. Two experimental techniques of endothelial transplantation have been mooted: a gelatine membrane method (Maurice *et al.* 1977) and seeding of cultured cells directly on to the denuded Descemet's membrane (Gospodarowicz *et al.* 1979). Studies using human tissue have been carried out using extended incubation times for culture of infant human endothelial cells (Insler & Lopez 1991). Human endothelial cells transplanted into African green monkeys became stable much more quickly than controls and subsequently were shown to present a healthy endothelial cell monolayer. Although impracticable at the present time, these experiments indicate that therapeutic transplantation may be attainable with endothelial cells alone. Research to reconstruct the entire cornea by tissue engineering is in progress, but in its early stages (Hicks *et al.* 1997).

### Indications for keratoplasty

Keratoplasty has four prime indications:
1 *Visual* to improve vision reduced by corneal disease;
2 *Therapeutic* to effect the removal of infected, damaged or painful corneal tissue;
3 *Tectonic* to establish corneal integrity following tissue perforation or thinning; and
4 *Cosmetic* to improve the appearance of a cosmetically unacceptable cornea.

Most keratoplasties are performed to improve vision. The indications for surgery and their relative frequency are listed in Table 13.1. The common indications for keratoplasty are briefly described below.
1 *Keratoconus.* A degenerative condition affecting younger patients in which the cornea adopts a conical shape. Vision is reduced as a consequence of distorted light refraction.
2 *Endothelial failure.* Loss of the corneal endothelium causes corneal oedema. Primary failure is of idiopathic origin, while secondary failure usually arises as a consequence of surgical trauma. The most common surgical cause of corneal damage is cataract extraction. An aphakic eye is devoid of a lens, hence aphakic endothelial failure. If the patient received a prosthetic lens implant the failure becomes pseudophakic.
3 *Herpes simplex keratitis* (Plate 13.1, facing p. 342).

Table 13.1 Indications for keratoplasty in the UKTSSA Corneal Transplant Follow-up Study (modified from Vail *et al.* 1993, with permission).

| Diagnosis | Total | (%) |
|---|---|---|
| Keratoconus | 634 | (19.9) |
| Primary endothelial failure | 407 | (12.8) |
|   363 Füchs' dystrophy | | |
|   44 Congenital or juvenile | | |
| Secondary endothelial failure | 804 | (25.3) |
|   481 Pseudophakic | | |
|   221 Aphakic | | |
|   102 Other | | |
| Herpes simplex keratitis | 338 | (10.6) |
|   288 Chronic | | |
|   50 Acute | | |
| Other inflammation | 495 | (15.5) |
|   355 Chronic | | |
|   112 Acute | | |
|   28 Unspecified | | |
| Stromal dystrophy | 151 | (4.7) |
|   62 Lattice | | |
|   43 Granular | | |
|   37 Macular | | |
|   9 Unspecified | | |
| Trauma | 148 | (4.6) |
|   102 Mechanical | | |
|   28 Chemical (alkaline) | | |
|   18 Chemical (other) | | |
| Other diagnoses | 207 | (6.5) |
|   63 Congenital malformation | | |
|   31 Epithelial degeneration | | |
|   14 Contact lens-related | | |
|   6 Unspecified endothelial failure | | |
|   35 Miscellaneous | | |
|   58 Aetiology uncertain | | |
| TOTAL | 3184 | (100) |

This arises as a consequence of herpes simplex virus (HSV) reactivation in the trigeminal ganglion and egress along the fifth cranial nerve. Although a self-limiting condition, repeated infection leads to permanent corneal scarring.

4 *Corneal dystrophy.* This is a disparate group of conditions of largely unknown aetiology, often hereditary, leading to progressive deposition of opaque material within the layers of the cornea. Anterior corneal dystrophies may be treated by lamellar keratoplasty, while deeper disease requires full-thickness grafts.

### Technique for penetrating keratoplasty

For a full discussion of surgical technique the reader is referred to a textbook on surgical ophthalmology (Figueiredo & Easty 1999). For example, the donor tissue, a 'button' usually between 6.5 and 8.5 mm in diameter, is cut using a trephine. The recipient cornea is then cut using a trephine 0.25–0.5 mm smaller than the donor tissue to ensure a watertight fit. The donor tissue is sutured into place using either a continuous zigzag or individual sutures, leaving a recipient rim or bed of 1.5–2.5 mm in diameter. At the end of the procedure the anterior chamber is inflated with balanced salt solution. Leaks are identified and sealed with extra sutures if necessary (Plate 13.2, facing p. 342).

### Donor corneal tissue and eye banking

Transplant surgeons have a common need for good-quality donor tissue, HLA-matched if necessary and available when required. Corneal surgeons have less difficulty than other surgeons in procuring suitable tissue because cadaver corneas remain viable for donation up to 24 h after circulatory death if the body is refrigerated. However, most tissue obtained (80%) is typed neither for ABO antigens nor for HLA.

There are a variety of storage techniques for donor corneal tissue.

*Refrigeration.* Donor eyes were originally stored in moist chambers at 4°C for 48 h (Filatov 1937). Within this period, however, the endothelial cells begin to demonstrate evidence of collapse with granular change appearing on the cell membrane.

*McCarey–Kaufman medium.* Tissue culture medium containing 5% dextran is now used to store corneoscleral discs (the entire cornea removed with a rim of sclera) for up to 4 days at 4°C (McCarey & Kaufman 1974). Addition of chondroitin sulphate (as in K-sol) has been shown to extend storage time up to 14 days (Kaufman *et al.* 1985). However, the more prolonged the preoperative storage time, the greater the postoperative loss of endothelial cells.

*Organ culture*. Corneoscleral discs can be stored in organ culture medium at 34–37°C for up to 30 days (Doughman *et al.* 1976; Pels & Schuchard 1983). In 1983 the Corneal Transplant Service (CTS) was inaugurated under the auspices of the United Kingdom Transplant Service (UKTS) in Bristol. In 1986 the University of Bristol Department of Ophthalmology established an eye bank in collaboration with the CTS to exploit organ-culture techniques. Three years later a similar bank was set up in Manchester. By 1996 these eye banks supplied a total of 2460 organ-cultured corneas for transplantation, the remainder being supplied locally after short-term storage (Fig. 13.5).

Organ-cultured corneas lose endothelial cells exponentially after transplantation with a half-life of 41 months (Redmond *et al.* 1992). This endothelial cell loss is comparable to that seen for corneas stored using the McCarey–Kaufman technique (Bourne 1983).

Extended tissue storage has several advantages: it enables surgery to be planned electively, it facilitates emergency penetrating keratoplasty — usually performed for therapeutic or tectonic reasons (repair of anatomical defects) — and it allows a full search for HLA-matched recipients.

The Corneal Transplant Act 1986 enabled corneas to be collected by non-medically qualified personnel within the UK; thus donor eyes are now retrieved by suitably trained eye bank technicians, nurses or morticians, reducing pressure on corneal transplant surgeons and increasing collection rates. Corneal donors may be any age. Donors suffering from HIV, hepatitis B and C and Creutzfeldt–Jakob disease are excluded (Allan & Tuft 1998).

## Graft failure

The term graft failure indicates the permanent loss of tissue transparency, caused by corneal oedema, scarring or stromal deposition of opaque material, e.g. lipid or calcium. Oedema arises secondarily to endothelial cell loss as a consequence of immunological rejection or trauma. Scarring and deposition may be the result of infection, trauma or recurrence of the primary disease process. The visual outcome is an important measure of the success of a corneal graft and this is usually measured in terms of Snellen visual acuity, normal acuity being 6/6 while 6/60 is the legal definition of blindness (a person standing at 6 m can see a letter that a person with normal acuity could see at 60 m).

### Risk factors influencing graft outcome

The results of corneal transplantation may be influenced for better or for worse by a wide variety of visual factors that have their impact on the preoperative, operative and postoperative epochs (Table 13.2).

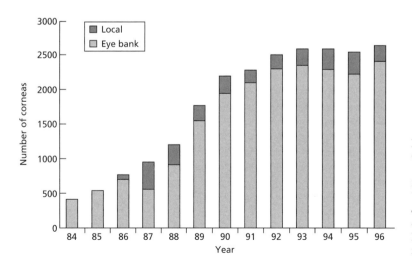

Fig. 13.5 Number of corneal transplants notified to UKTSS between 1984 (when the Corneal Transplant Study was initiated) and 1996. Eye banks supplying organ-cultured corneas were opened at the University of Bristol and Manchester Royal Eye Hospital in 1986 and 1989, respectively.

**Table 13.2** Examples of risk factors influencing outcome of transplants.

(a) *Preoperative*
Quality of donor tissue
Vascularization
Inflammation: previous or concurrent
Breakdown of blood–aqueous barrier
Recipient age
Histoincompatibility
Previous ocular surgery
Previous corneal transplantation

(b) *Operative*
Endothelial cell loss
Suture material
Poor accuracy and tension of sutures
Lack of watertight interface
Operative haemorrhage
Excessive tissue manipulation
Complications involving iris and vitreous
Additional concurrent procedures (e.g. cataract extraction, intraocular lens implant)

(c) *Postoperative*
Loss of anterior chamber depth
Poor control of intraocular pressure
Inflammation
Vascularization
Premature suture removal
Postoperative astigmatism: improved by selective suture removal

## PREOPERATIVE FACTORS

Risk of failure is increased when surgery is performed on vascularized corneas and in the presence of infection or inflammation, because these factors promote immunological rejection. Certain preoperative diagnostic categories carry risk of recurrence of the original disease, e.g. herpes simplex keratitis and the corneal dystrophies. Other host factors relevant to outcome (Table 13.2a) will be discussed further below.

## OPERATIVE FACTORS

There is an abundance of operative complications that may lead to poor graft survival (Table 13.2b). The key to success is the avoidance of undue manipulative damage to the donor endothelium, thereby maintaining the highest possible cell count postoperatively. This is assisted today by a viscoelastic material, sodium hyaluronate, that helps maintain a deep anterior chamber during the surgical procedure. If the iris closes off the drainage angle of the chamber as a result of adhesion formation, often between the iris and the graft interface, elevation of IOP results and may lead to permanent loss of vision caused by endothelial cell death. Care is taken to avoid these adhesions by maintaining the chamber during and immediately after surgery by ensuring that the graft–host junction is watertight. Sutures should distribute tension evenly to the graft, thereby maintaining its spherical refractive power and minimizing induced astigmatism. A crucial improvement in success rates occurred with the introduction of monofilament nylon suture material (10–11/0) in the mid-1960s, following earlier use of antigenic 8/0 silk, which had been responsible for encouraging vascular ingrowth and frequent rejection episodes.

## PRIMARY GRAFT FAILURE

This is defined as irreversible graft oedema arising in the immediate postoperative period. It should not be confused with primary endothelial failure, which is a preoperative indication for transplantation. Oedema results if endothelial cell numbers are reduced to the point where the endothelial pump mechanism fails to control influx of water. The failure becomes irreversible when cell numbers are so diminished that sliding and enlargement of the remaining cells cannot restore the layer. Primary graft failure usually arises as a result of damage to the donor endothelium consequent upon inadequate donor selection, tissue preservation or surgical trauma (Wilson & Kaufman 1990).

## POSTOPERATIVE FACTORS

In the immediate postoperative period, early graft failure may result from loss of the anterior chamber with subsequent elevation of IOP (Table 13.2c). The inflammatory response excited by the operative procedure may be suppressed effectively with topical corticosteroid. Short-term systemic therapy may be beneficial in some cases. Suture ends or knots on the corneal surface may become foci for rapid ingrowth of superficial blood-vessels, which can be avoided by burying suture knots in corneal stroma. It is more difficult to prevent vessel invasion where corneal vascularization existed prior to graft surgery.

Donor corneal endothelial cell density declines following transplantation. Redmond *et al.* (1992) demonstrated a fall from a preoperative mean count of 2334 cells/mm$^2$ to a mean of 2158 cells/mm$^2$ (8% reduction) in 2 months. Four years after transplantation the cell loss was 46%. The mode of initial cell loss may be influenced by the mode of preservation. Corneas that suffered a rejection episode had a greater cell loss. Fifty per cent of the corneas that failed in the Corneal Transplant Follow-up Study (CTFS) failed as a consequence of donor endothelial failure (Vail *et al.* 1996). The CTFS was launched by the United Kingdom Transplant Service in 1987 to identify indications and donor and histocompatibility factors pertaining to the outcome of corneal transplantation. Data were collected on patients at the time of transplantation and at 3 and 12 months after transplantation, using detailed questionnaires. Figure 13.6 illustrates the age range and sex of patients in the major diagnostic categories. Multifactorial analysis was performed on the data to identify factors influencing graft outcome as reflected in graft rejection (Table 13.3a) and visual acuity (VA) (Table 13.3b). In the analysis the importance of each level of each factor is expressed as a ratio relative to a chosen baseline level (relative risk) and expressed as the mean plus 95% confidence interval.

## Corrected visual acuity

Distributions of preoperative and 3- and 12-month postoperative visual acuity in functioning grafts performed for visual reasons (i.e. not cosmetic or therapeutic) showed improvement at each stage. Whereas 15% of grafts had a preoperative visual acuity of 6/24 or better, 58% and 70% had reached this level by 3 and 12 months (Fig. 13.7a). Multiple factors, both immunological and non-immunological, influence postgraft visual acuity (Vail *et al.* 1994, 1997).

## Astigmatism

Astigmatism is correctable by cylindrical lenses. The power of the cylinder and therefore the degree of astigmatism is measured in dioptres (a dioptre being the power of a lens that refracts light from infinity to a point 1 m from the lens) and expressed as dioptres cylinder (DC). Distribution of preoperative and 3 and 12 month postoperative DC in functioning grafts shows that, whereas 77% had less than 4 DC of astigmatism preoperatively, 51% and 57% had less than 4 DC at 3 and 12 months postoperatively (Fig. 13.7b). 4 DC is an acceptable visual standard for near vision with appropriate spectacle correction.

Astigmatism may be induced by irregular stresses arising from asymmetrical suture tension. It can be minimized by utilizing good surgical technique in conjunction with optical devices designed to give the surgeon feedback on corneal topography. Once established, astigmatism may be neutralized using rigid contact lenses. If these are not tolerated, refractive surgical techniques may be applied (Binder 1985; Limberg *et al.* 1989).

## High intraocular pressure

Elevation of IOP has an adverse influence on graft survival when occurring either prior to or following graft surgery. Arentsen and Laibson (1982) attributed 2% of graft failures to uncontrolled IOP; elevated IOP is associated with reduced endothelial cell density (Bigar 1982). Williams *et al.* (1997) reported that raised IOP was a significant risk factor for graft failure ($P > 0.0001$). In the CTFS, preoperative glaucoma (i.e. optic nerve damage, associated with raised IOP) was a significant risk factor for acute rejection (Table 13.3a and Vail *et al.* 1997).

## Recurrence of original disease

In a few cases the donor cornea may become opaque following recurrence of the primary disease. In the CTFS this only accounted for 7.5% of graft failures (Vail *et al.* 1996). The corneal dystrophies, including

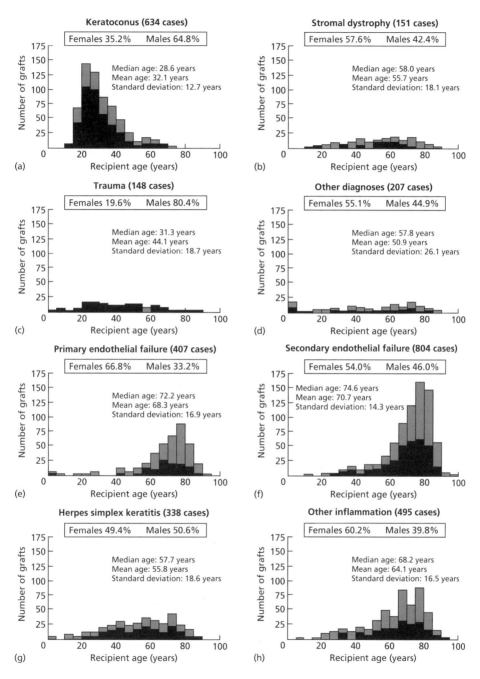

**Fig. 13.6** Age distribution and sex ratio in the main diagnostic groups evaluated in the Corneal Transplant Follow-up Study (CTFS) (from Vail *et al.* 1993, with permission).

**Table 13.3** Factors influencing (a) time to first rejection and (b) visual acuity 12 months after corneal transplantation. Risk is significant at the 5% level (a) or 1% level (b) if the confidence interval lies outside the baseline for the factor (i.e. 1 in (a) and 0 in (b)). Below the baseline denotes decreased risk, above denotes increased risk. (From Vail *et al.* 1997, with permission.)

**(a)**

| Factor | Relative risk (95% confidence interval) |
|---|---|
| Recipient age (years) | |
| 0–9 | 4.32 (1.43, 13.01) |
| 10–19 | 2.60 (0.99, 6.85) |
| 20–29 | 2.40 (1.16, 5.00) |
| 30–39 | 1.93 (0.97, 3.87) |
| 40–49 | 1.55 (0.78, 3.08) |
| 50–59 | 1.43 (0.76, 2.71) |
| 60–69 | 1.32 (0.75, 2.34) |
| 70–79 | 1.19 (0.70, 2.04) |
| 80+ | 1.00 |
| Previous grafts in operated eye | |
| None | 1.00 |
| One | 1.39 (0.92, 2.11) |
| Two | 2.66 (1.56, 4.54) |
| More | 2.75 (1.34, 5.65) |
| Diagnosis of original disease | |
| Keratoconus | 1.00 |
| Primary endothelial failure | 1.48 (0.68, 3.24) |
| Secondary endothelial failure | 2.35 (1.17, 4.69) |
| Herpes simplex keratitis | 1.99 (0.99, 3.98) |
| Other inflammation | 2.43 (1.21, 4.86) |
| Stromal dystrophy | 0.98 (0.30, 3.20) |
| Trauma | 1.94 (0.88, 4.30) |
| Others | 2.28 (1.09, 4.76) |
| Glaucoma | |
| No | 1.00 |
| Yes | 1.52 (1.05, 2.21) |
| Graft size | |
| Donor + recipient | |
| ≤14.5 mm | 1.00 |
| ≤15.5 mm | 1.43 (0.99, 2.06) |
| >15.5 mm | 1.58 (1.08, 2.31) |
| Donor − recipient | |
| =0 mm | 1.00 |
| ≤0.25 mm | 0.90 (0.59, 1.37) |
| >0.25 mm | 1.19 (0.86, 1.66) |

**(b)**

| Factor | Coefficient (99% confidence interval) 12 months post-transplant |
|---|---|
| Recipient age (years) | |
| 0–9 | −0.46 (−1.50, 0.58) |
| 10–19 | 0.48 (0.05, 0.93) |
| 20–29 | 0.32 (−0.02, 0.66) |
| 30–39 | 0.43 (0.11, 0.76) |
| 40–49 | 0.38 (0.06, 0.70) |
| 50–59 | 0.37 (0.07, 0.67) |
| 60–69 | 0.28 (0.03, 0.52) |
| 70–79 | 0.20 (−0.02, 0.43) |
| 80+ | 0.00 |
| Previous grafts | |
| None | 0.00 |
| One | −0.21 (−0.43, 0.01) |
| Two | −0.50 (−0.93, −0.07) |
| More | −0.49 (−1.00, 0.02) |
| Diagnosis | |
| Keratoconus | 0.00 |
| Primary EF | −0.09 (−0.41, 0.23) |
| Secondary EF | −0.63 (−0.95, −0.31) |
| HSK | −0.37 (−0.68, −0.07) |
| Other inflammation | −0.43 (−0.74, −0.13) |
| Stromal dystrophy | 0.03 (−0.34, 0.41) |
| Trauma | −0.89 (−1.28, −0.50) |
| Others | −0.92 (−1.27, −0.58) |
| Glaucoma | |
| No | 0.00 |
| Yes | −0.63 (−0.85, −0.41) |
| Preoperative VA | |
| <6/60 | 0.00 |
| <6/24 | 0.41 (0.24, 0.58) |
| ≥6/24 | 0.47 (0.27, 0.67) |
| Unrecorded | 0.08 (−0.63, 0.79) |
| Graft size | |
| Sum | |
| ≤14.5 mm | 0.00 |
| ≤15.5 mm | 0.08 (−0.08, 0.24) |
| >15.5 mm | 0.19 (0.01, 0.37) |
| Difference | |
| =0 mm | 0.00 |
| ≤0.25 mm | 0.16 (−0.03, 0.34) |
| >0.25 mm | 0.11 (−0.05, 0.27) |
| Vitreous surgery | |
| No | 0.00 |
| Yes | −0.07 (−0.30, 0.15) |

EF, endothelial failure; HSK, herpes simplex keratitis; VA, visual acuity.

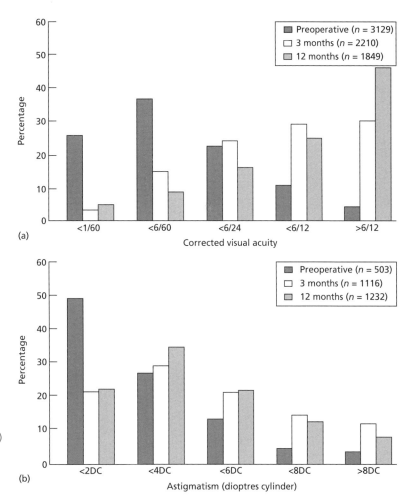

**Fig. 13.7** Distribution of corrected (a) visual acuity and (b) astigmatism before transplantation and 3 and 12 months after transplantation. (From Vail *et al.* 1997, with permission.)

Reis–Bücklers, lattice, macular and granular dystrophy, are recognized to recur in transplanted tissue (Wilson & Kaufman 1990).

Where herpes simplex keratitis is the indication for surgery, viral infection may reactivate in 15% of patients during the first year following surgery (Cobo *et al.* 1980; Coster 1982). Recrudescent herpes simplex keratitis usually causes a superficial keratitis at the graft–host interface and it may sometimes be difficult to differentiate this from immunological rejection. The sequelae of recrudescent herpes simplex keratitis include scarring, vascularization and genuine immunological rejection (Foster & Duncan 1981), often requir-

ing repeat penetrating keratoplasty. Herpes simplex keratitis was the indication for surgery in 10.6% of all corneal grafts in the UK (Vail *et al.* 1993 and Table 13.1).

### Infection or trauma

Donor corneal tissue may develop subepithelial scarring as a consequence of operative trauma or infection. Infections may arise following keratoplasty as a consequence of corticosteroid use, suture breakage or contact lens wear. Bacterial and fungal infection may originate from the host—particularly where the graft is performed for therapeutic reasons—from contaminated donor tissue or from the environment. However, contamination via the donor occurs much less with cultured corneas, the incidence of endophthalmitis being ~20-fold less in the UK than that reported by Aiello *et al.* (1993) in the USA for non-cultured cornea (0.04% as opposed to 0.8%). Avascular scars may directly reduce visual acuity while vascularized scars carry additional elevated risk of rejection. Infection *per se* accounted for 12% of graft failures in the CTFS (Vail *et al.* 1994).

## Immunology of graft rejection

When the first successful human corneal transplant was performed early this century, it was at a time when immunological rejection was not a recognized phenomenon. Other organ grafts did not survive until suppression of the immune response with drugs became part of the clinical postoperative treatment. Hence the cornea was viewed at an early stage as immunologically privileged.

Maumenee (1951), experimenting with rabbits, definitively demonstrated immunological rejection as a cause of corneal graft failure by showing that opacification was induced by donor-specific sensitization. However, earlier animal studies (e.g. Greene & Lund 1944; Medawar 1948), in which foreign tissue transplanted to the anterior chamber was protected from rejection, supported the idea of privilege. Several explanations for corneal privilege were suggested. Medawar (1948) hypothesized that the total antigenic load was insufficient to excite a host immunological response and/or that the mobile host epithelium gradually replaced that of the donor. Duke-Elder (1956) suggested that the donor stromal cells were physically separated from host antibodies by a barrier of scar tissue at the edge of the graft. Woodruff (1952) attributed the immunological privilege to the lack of lymphatic drainage common to the eye and to other such privileged sites, so that donor antigens were not 'seen' by the host immune system. Raju & Grogan (1971) undermined these concepts when they demonstrated that tissue grafted to the anterior chamber resulted in accelerated rejection of a second graft derived from the same donor transplanted to another site on the recipient animal. Subsequent work has shown that antigen injected directly into the anterior chamber is not sequestered within the eye but escapes via venous drainage channels to initiate an aberrant systemic response in which delayed-type hypersensitivity (DTH) is suppressed (Niederkorn & Streilein 1983), termed anterior chamber-associated immune deviation (ACAID; see p. 406).

Many of these findings encouraged the misconception, particularly among transplantation scientists, that corneal graft rejection is an insignificant problem. For this reason and perhaps because loss of vision is not itself life-threatening, early research into corneal graft rejection was apportioned low priority. Despite this, clinicians have continued to recognize rejection as an important cause of graft failure.

Corneal transplants interface with host tissue at four sites.

**1** The junction between donor and host corneal epithelium and stroma. The division between host and donor stromal cells is initially sited at the graft margin. Postoperative inflammation encourages movement of host dendritic cells into donor tissue (Ross *et al.* 1991a; Figueiredo *et al.* 1993).

**2** The anterior surface of the donor Bowman's zone, where donor epithelial cells may eventually be replaced by those of the host.

**3** The junction between host and donor endothelium. This interface is plastic as donor endothelial cells have been shown to migrate into host tissue and vice versa (Imaizumi 1990).

**4** The contact between graft endothelium and aqueous humour. The host may be exposed to donor antigen carried with the aqueous humour via the trabecular drainage apparatus into the systemic circulation (Sonoda & Streilein 1992).

Any of these sites may be involved in modulating the immunological interaction between graft and host.

### Clinical rejection

Immunological rejection (Fig. 13.8) is the most common single cause of graft failure, accounting for approximately one-third of cases. Signs of rejection include corneal epithelial and stromal oedema, endothelial folding, keratic precipitates (lymphocyte aggregates) on the endothelium and anterior chamber cells and flare. They are associated with reduction in vision, discomfort, redness and mild photophobia, which must be promptly treated if irreversible graft failure is to be avoided. Past reports of the incidence of rejection episodes in 'low-risk' cases range from 2% to 35% (Khodadoust 1973; Polack 1973; Chandler & Kaufman 1974; Donshik *et al.* 1979). Episodes can occur as early as 2 weeks or as long as 15 years or more after transplantation (Maumenee 1973). However, rejection reactions are most likely to occur within the first year (Fine & Stein 1973; Collaborative Corneal Transplantation Studies (CCTS) Research Group 1992; Pleyer *et al.* 1992; Vail *et al.* 1997). In the most recent US study (CCTS Research Group 1992) two-thirds of high-risk individuals experienced mild graft reactions by 3 years after transplantation, involving cell infiltration of any layer or an increase in corneal thickness in the absence of cell infiltration. In the UK CTFS study, rejection episodes occurred in 14% of first grafts by 12 months and accounted for 34% of graft failures (Vail *et al.* 1994). Of 6011 grafts documented by the Australian Corneal Graft Registry for up to 10 years, 16% of grafts experienced at least one rejection episode. After 8–9 years, the probability of graft survival was only 28% if one or more rejection episodes had occurred, compared with 74% if there had been no rejection (Williams *et al.* 1997).

## Risk factors for human rejection and graft failure

Human corneal graft outcome is very often analysed with reference to failure rather than to immunological rejection, which is only one cause of failure. This should be borne in mind when data pertaining to rejection are sought. A rejection episode may frequently be reversed by increasing dosage of topical corticosteroids and/or initiating systemic treatment, sometimes combined with other systemic immunosuppressive drugs. Early recognition of rejection by the patient and clinician is essential but does not always occur. Vascularization, a history of inflammation in the grafted eye, recipient age, previous failed ipsilateral graft, diagnosis, raised IOP, graft size, HLA matching, removal of sutures and blood transfusion have all been implicated in graft rejection and failure.

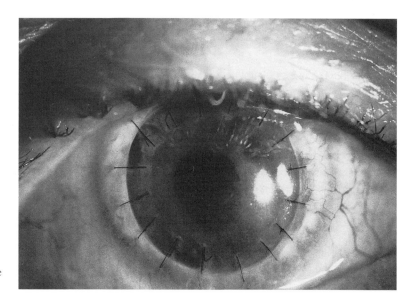

**Fig. 13.8** Early stage of rejection of a human corneal transplant showing corneal opacity (right hand side) in the vicinity of host blood vessels.

## Vascularization

Corneal vascularization, including lymphatic vessel ingress, may occur in inflammatory corneal disease, ranging from a single vascular arcade to complete circumferential vessel invasion involving four quadrants. Vessels may be superficial, derived from the conjunctival plexus or deep within the stroma. The Australian Corneal Graft Registry indicated that recipient vascularization of four quadrants has a significant detrimental effect on graft survival, no distinction being made between deep and superficial vascularization (Williams *et al.* 1997). Vessel penetration of the graft itself was highly predictive of failure, probability of survival being 36% after 8–9 years as opposed to 64% if there had been no postgraft vascularization. Interestingly, in the CTFS, deep vascularization was a significant risk factor for graft failure but not for rejection (Vail *et al.* 1997).

## Previous graft

A previous graft increases the risk of rejection of a subsequent graft in the same eye. The reasons for this may include increased numbers of antigen-presenting cells in the recipient bed and sensitization to foreign antigens on the previous graft. Kirkness *et al.* (1990) reported in a single-centre study that the 5-year survival in 99 regrafts was 49% and that visual acuity reached 6/12 or better in only 18% of patients. Allograft rejection was responsible for failure in most patients. Rapuano *et al.* (1990) reviewed data on 150 repeat grafts, 52% of which were performed because of endothelial failure, and found that 26% of these had failed in a minimum follow-up period of 6 months. Allograft rejection was the cause of failure in 32% of cases. The CTFS revealed a significant increment in the relative risk of graft failure, time to first rejection (Table 13.3a) and visual acuity below 6/24 (Table 13.3b) after two or more failed grafts (Vail *et al.* 1997), while Williams *et al.* (1997) found a significantly increased risk of failure after more than one graft.

## Age and diagnosis

Risk of rejection (Vail *et al.* 1997) and failure (Vail *et al.* 1997; Williams *et al.* 1997) are increased in younger age groups and lowest in the oldest recipients. This is consistent with widespread observations of dwindling T cell immunity with age. In the CTFS, certain diagnoses were associated with increased risk of rejection, including secondary endothelial failure and 'other inflammation' (Vail *et al.* 1997).

## Blood transfusion and/or pregnancy

The impact of a few blood transfusions prior to transplantation is regarded as favourable to kidney transplants but numerous transfusions are associated with a detrimental outcome resulting from sensitization. Very little experimental work has been performed in corneal transplantation and no definitive clinical studies have been carried out. A single donor-specific blood transfusion shortly before rabbit corneal transplantation had a detrimental effect on graft survival (Liu *et al.* 1989), but certain rat strain combinations, termed high responders, showed a significant benefit from such transfusions (Ayliffe *et al.* 1992a). In humans both random transfusion and pregnancy were associated with poorer graft survival in unifactorial analyses but this effect failed to reach significance as an independent variable on multifactorial analyses (Williams *et al.* 1997). The clinical benefits, if any, of prior blood transfusion must await further research.

## HLA mismatch

Allograft rejection involving the endothelium provides a decisive clinical end-point for determining the role of HLA matching in the outcome of corneal transplantation. Although a number of single-centre studies have investigated the importance of HLA matching, there remains some uncertainty regarding its importance and there is still no conclusive investigation that supports a beneficial effect of matching, even in high-risk cases. Some early univariate studies of transplants with variable degrees of matching showed some correlation between graft failure and HLA-A and B mismatching (Batchelor *et al.* 1976), while other studies did not confirm this (Fine & Payne 1974; Stark 1980). Some more recent studies report that matching at the HLA-A and B loci reduces the risk of failure (Volker-Dieben *et al.* 1982, 1984) and rejection reactions (Boisjoly *et al.* 1986, 1990; Sanfilippo *et al.* 1986). Boisjoly *et al.* (1990) found a strong association between failure caused by immunological reactions and HLA-A or B incompatibility in low-risk recipients, defined as unvascularized recipients of a small corneal graft. Conflicting results have emerged from HLA-DR matching (Völker-Dieben *et al.* 1987; Baggesen *et al.* 1991, 1996; CCTS Research Group 1992; Vail *et al.* 1997).

More recent multicentre studies have used increasingly sophisticated statistical analysis to address these uncertainties. The CCTS Research Group in the USA (1992) evaluated the effect of donor–recipient histocompatibility matching and cross-matching in high-risk patients. This randomized and double-blind prospective assessment showed that neither HLA-A or B or HLA-DR matching substantially reduced the likelihood of graft rejection or failure. In addition, a negative donor–recipient cross-match provided no benefit over a positive cross-match. Contrary to previous observations (Batchelor *et al.* 1976) ABO blood group matching seemed to reduce the risk of graft failure, this being 30% in the incompatible group and 40% in the compatible group. One explanation for the lack of significance for HLA arising from such a study was the use of a comprehensive immunosuppressive regime, which may have masked differences in rejection responses. Indeed, it is concluded that high-dose postoperative steroid therapy, good compliance and close follow-up are the keys to successful corneal transplantation in the high-risk recipient. Nevertheless, topical steroid medication is known to present a number of unwanted effects, which include cataract, glaucoma and herpes simplex recurrence, that are common enough to indicate the need for a clear answer to the question of histocompatibility matching in corneal transplantation.

A different approach was taken in the UK by the CTFS (Vail *et al.* 1997). High-risk patients were registered with the UKTS and suitable donor matches identified. Donors and recipients were matched using the same criteria as for renal transplants, i.e. minimizing the number of mismatches first at HLA-DR, then at HLA-B and finally at HLA-A. Data collected at 12 months showed that HLA-A and B matching was beneficial but that, contrary to expectations, zero mismatches for HLA-DR, irrespective of the level of mismatch for HLA-A or B, seemed to be associated with a higher risk of rejection when compared to one or two mismatches for HLA-DR (Fig. 13.9). Further scrutiny of these data may reveal whether or not this apparent detrimental effect of DR matching is a surrogate for other risk factors or whether it has an independent biological basis.

In contrast, Baggesen *et al.* (1996) used DNA-based technology to obtain more accurate assessment of HLA-DR matching and concluded that 'precise HLA-DRB1 genotype matching significantly improves the outcome'. Unfortunately, such a conclusion for the HLA-DRB1-matched and mismatched groups contained an imbalance in the proportion of recipients who had previously failed transplants. In the matched group, there were only 29% and in the mismatched groups 53%, an imbalance that could account for the observed survival decrement attributed to mismatching. Gore *et al.* (1995) concluded from a systematic review of published evidence that, whereas minimizing the number of HLA class I mismatches significantly reduces the risk of rejection, HLA-DR mismatching was associated with less rejection. This supported the finding of the CTFS study that HLA-DR mismatching was beneficial (Vail *et al.* 1997).

In summary, we feel that the weight of evidence suggests a limited clinical benefit from HLA-A and B matching. The role of HLA-DR remains *sub judice*. Further studies are underway using molecular rather than serological typing techniques.

## Human graft outcome

Multifactorial analysis of factors affecting time to first rejection in the final analysis of the CTFS database showed that recipient age, graft number, glaucoma,

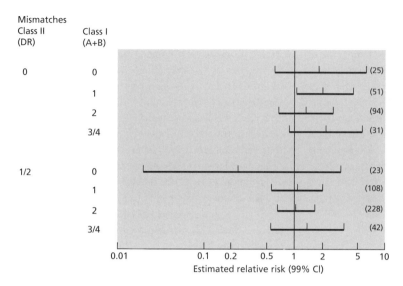

**Mismatches**

Class II (DR)     Class I (A+B)

Fig. 13.9 Influence of HLA mismatching on rejection-free graft survival, adjusted for other factors. The vertical bar represents the estimated risk of rejection of grafts where the donor was untyped. If the 99% CI bar bisects the baseline the relative risk does not deviate from 1.00 at the 1% level of significance. Numbers in brackets are the numbers of patients. (From Vail *et al.* 1997, with permission.)

secondary endothelial failure and inflammation all constituted significant risk factors (Vail *et al.* 1997) (Table 13.3a). As each diagnostic scenario consists of a different constellation of risk factors, corneal transplant outcome is reviewed for each of these disease groups.

### Keratoconus

High success rates of corneal transplantation for keratoconus have been regularly reported since Castroviejo's first description (1949). Transparency was achieved in 78–85% of patients in the 1950s, improving to 90–100% from 1960 onwards. Paglen *et al.* (1982) and Payne (1982) reported success rates of 90 and 92%, respectively, in a series of 300 patients. Where multiple surgeons—including those in training—performed transplants, the success rates were reduced to 78% (Tullo 1982).

Failure of penetrating keratoplasty in keratoconus because of immunological rejection is rare because the graft bed is not inflamed or vascularized. The percentage of keratoconus patients experiencing reversible rejection episodes has been reported to be as high as 37% by Chandler and Kaufman (1974), but is gener-

ally around a level of 7–18% (Moore & Aronson 1978; Donshik *et al.* 1979; Troutman & Gaster 1980; Alldredge & Krachmer 1981; Paglen *et al.* 1982). Graft failure caused by rejection has been reported to vary between 0 and 9.4% (Malbran & Fernandez-Meijide 1982, 0%; Paglen *et al.* 1982, 2.4%; Troutman & Gaster 1980, 2.4%; Chandler & Kaufman 1974, 9.4%).

### Stromal dystrophies

These are a variety of hereditary conditions that present with progressive opacities in the corneal stroma. They are not associated with corneal vascularization and therefore carry a prognosis for graft survival similar to that for keratoconus.

### Endothelial failure

Failure of the metabolic function of the endothelium leads to corneal oedema and subsequent reduction in vision. Füchs' endothelial dystrophy involves a slow progressive loss of endothelial function in later life. Bullous keratopathy (subepithelial oedema) arises as a complication of intraocular surgery and may lead to secondary endothelial failure. In this disease the marginal population of recipient endothelial cells is reduced, thereby limiting the potential for movement of host endothelial cells to repopulate the donor tissue. It is a painful condition because surface epithelial bullae rupture, exposing subepithelial free nerve endings. Furthermore, other factors related to previous surgery may compromise visual function after transplantation. The eye may be inflamed or anatomically deranged, for example by rupture of the capsular diaphragm between the anterior and posterior segments, with the presence of vitreous gel within the anterior chamber.

## Inflammatory keratitis

In the past, graft survival in cases of HSV disease has been poor (Ficker *et al.* 1988) because of the background of previous ocular inflammation, which increases the risk of rejection. There is also risk of recurrence of HSV disease in the donor tissue. The introduction of second-generation antiviral drugs such as acyclovir (Zovirax) appears to be improving the long-term survival of these grafts because of their low toxicity and superior penetration into the corneal stroma.

Other inflammatory conditions present prior to or at the time of transplantation demonstrate reduced graft survival and visual function. These conditions include corneal scarring from previous inflammatory disease, e.g. interstitial keratitis, or resolved infective keratitis.

## Animal models of rejection

The earliest experimental work involved clinical and histological studies in the rabbit. Orthotopic full-thickness corneal allografts (Maumenee 1951; Nelken *et al.* 1961) and interlamellar allografts (i.e. grafts into pockets made in the stromal layer) (Basu & Ormsby 1956) and xenografts (Choyce 1952) were performed. Corneal allograft rejection was encouraged by grafts of donor-specific skin. The importance of the local ocular environment for corneal privilege was established by the extended survival of other tissues, such as skin

(Medawar 1948) and tumours (Greene & Lund 1944), when transplanted to the anterior chamber of the eye, or of skin transplanted to the corneal stroma (Billingham & Boswell 1953). This was further substantiated by transplantion of corneas to extraocular vascularized sites, e.g. the skin, where they were rapidly rejected (Billingham & Boswell 1953).

Inbred strains of rodent, as they became available, were increasingly used. Early experiments involved either interlamellar models in rats (Lang *et al.* 1975; Gronemeyer *et al.* 1978) or heterotopic subcutaneous transplantation in mice (Chandler *et al.* 1982; Streilein *et al.* 1982) and in rats (Treseler & Sanfilippo 1985; Treseler *et al.* 1985). This gave an insight into the role played by the MHC and different effector processes in rejection.

In 1985 Williams and Coster published a method for performing full-thickness penetrating keratoplasty in the rat, largely obviating the need for heterotopic grafts and giving new impetus to experimental studies on matching and the involvement of leucocyte subsets, cytokines and other immunologically active molecules in the rejection response. More recently, the technical difficulties of penetrating grafts in mice have been overcome (She *et al.* 1990; Sonoda & Streilein 1992).

However, although rodents have many advantages, a drawback shared with rabbits is that the recipient endothelium can proliferate and will migrate inwards to replace donor cells (Tuft *et al.* 1986), thereby often partially or completely restoring corneal clarity (Williams & Coster 1985; Nicholls *et al.* 1991), in some cases within 10 days after rejection. Therefore animals must be monitored frequently to distinguish instances of rejection followed by rapid recovery from the genuine absence of rejection. Other investigators have favoured the use of larger animals, such as sheep (Williams *et al.* 1999) and the cat (Bahn *et al.* 1982; Meyer 1986; Cohen *et al.* 1990), in which the endothelium does not proliferate (Van Horn *et al.* 1977) and in which cell loss, migration and repair characteristics are similar to those of humans. Moreover, the kinetics of rejection and perhaps responses to drugs are also more akin to those of humans, making them more suitable for evaluating potential agents to reverse established rejection.

## Rejection of individual cell layers

In the absence of blood-vessels, the targets of rejection are the graft parenchymal cells (i.e. epithelium, stromal fibroblasts (keratocytes) and endothelium). Rejection of the endothelium receives the most clinical attention because of the supreme importance of a healthy endothelium to corneal function and because in humans it cannot regenerate. However, epithelial (Khodadoust & Silverstein 1969a; Kanai & Polack 1971a) and stromal (Khodadoust & Silverstein 1969a; Khodadoust 1973) rejection are also recognized in humans and animals and can occur concurrently with or independently of endothelial rejection. Khodadoust and Silverstein (1969b), by transplanting the three layers of the cornea separately in rabbits, showed that each layer had the dual potential to sensitize the recipient and act as a target for rejection.

### ENDOTHELIUM

The hallmark of endothelial rejection is the appearance of leucocytes in the form of keratic precipitates on the posterior surface of the donor endothelium. Precipitates occur either as an opaque linear deposit, a rejection line ('Khodadoust line'; Fig. 13.10), beginning to one side and advancing across the graft over a few days, or as an increasing number of scattered punctate foci. A line of advancing cells leaves dead endothelial cells in its wake, above which the stroma becomes oedematous. If the precipitates are scattered rather than linear, oedematous foci occur, which gradually coalesce if untreated (Polack 1973). A possible explanation for these two different manifestations of rejection—linear or diffuse—lies in the origin of the destructive cells. Those in scattered punctate precipitates may have come via the anterior chamber from the iris or ciliary body. The rejection line, on the other hand, in both humans (Khodadoust 1973) and rabbit (Silverstein & Khodadoust 1973) generally appears adjacent to stromal blood-vessels and these authors propose that the cells in this case have come directly from the stroma. They may penetrate through a gap or a thin area of Descemet's membrane at the

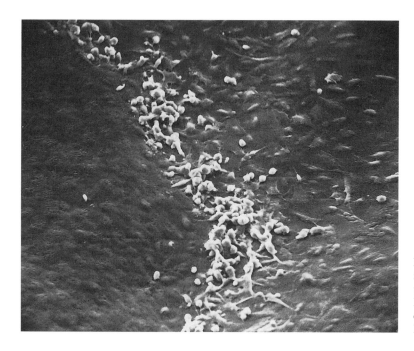

**Fig. 13.10** Scanning electron micrograph of rabbit endothelium undergoing rejection, demonstrating a line of adherent leucocytes. Damaged endothelial cells lie to the right of the line (×200). (Courtesy Dr F. Polack.)

graft–host junction (Polack 1962). However, the origin of the cells is not proven. In humans and in rabbits (Inomata *et al.* 1970; Polack & Kanai 1972), an opaque retrocorneal membrane containing fibroblast-like cells often develops after endothelial destruction. These may be stromal keratocytes that have grown through the wound. However, ultrastructural studies of membranes associated both with rejection and with other corneal pathologies in humans and rabbits suggests that they are actually metaplastic endothelial cells (Kanai *et al.* 1972; Michels *et al.* 1972; Maumenee 1973). A retrocorneal membrane has also been reported in rats (Williams & Coster 1985; Callanan *et al.* 1989).

EPITHELIUM

Epithelial rejection is seen as a 'rejection line' of infiltrating cells in humans (Polack 1973), rabbits (Khodadoust & Silverstein 1969a) and rats (Figueiredo *et al.* 1993). The line represents a zone of leucocytes and donor epithelial cell destruction, which stains with the vital dye fluorescein. It moves over the graft surface if left untreated (Wilson & Kaufman 1990). In rabbits a line has been observed as long as 6 months after transplantation (Khodadoust & Silverstein 1969b), indicating that unrejected donor epithelium can persist for at least this period. Electron microscope observation of rabbit epithelium undergoing rejection showed cytoplamic disorganization, vacuolation and rupture of plasma membranes (Kanai & Polack 1971a). Lymphocytes were found within the epithelium and in some areas the basal layer was fragmented and invaded by macrophages. Similar changes occur in the epithelium of the rat (Figueiredo 1996), with T cells (both CD4+ and CD8+) being the predominant infiltrating cell type.

Clinically, epithelial rejection is of little importance and may often not be recognized because epithelial cells, if lost, are rapidly replaced by those of the host. Indeed, in the past preoperative removal of donor epithelium has been advocated (Khodadoust 1973; Tuberville *et al.* 1983) to reduce the antigenic load and minimize rejection, but this benefit has not been confirmed (Sundmacher 1985; Stulting *et al.* 1988) and the

practice has been largely abandoned as it may lead to stromal damage (Dohlman 1973) followed by corneal infection.

STROMA

Here, a discrete rejection line does not occur and stromal rejection is defined as increasing diffuse opacity, spreading from invading blood-vessels. In humans it often appears as 'localized subepithelial haze' (Krachmer & Alldredge 1978) restricted to the donor cornea, although full-thickness stromal haze may sometimes occur (Stark 1980). Stromal infiltration without accompanying signs of epithelial and/or endothelial rejection is relatively rare (14% of rejection episodes, Alldredge & Krachmer 1981; 1%, Pleyer *et al.* 1992), but the extent to which 'stromal' rejection involves destruction of the scattered keratocytes is not clear. Physical damage to the epithelial layer alone can induce apoptosis of underlying keratocytes (Mohan *et al.* 1997). Definition of stromal cell rejection is further complicated by the fact that mild infiltration of the stroma is difficult to distinguish clinically from the oedema caused by loss of endothelial cells.

In rabbits monitored for at least a year after transplantation, donor stromal keratocytes were not replaced by those of the host unless the cornea was rejected (Hanna & Irwin 1962; Polack & Smelser 1962). By electron microscopy, Kanai and Polack (1971b) found keratocyte damage during the early stages of rejection especially below areas of epithelial rejection. In the absence of endothelial rejection, if keratocytes are destroyed, it is likely that they are replaced from the host without permanent damage to the stromal architecture.

Cell infiltration into the stroma is more pronounced in animal models than in humans, particularly when no immunosuppressive therapy is given. It is the predominant clinical sign of rejection in small rodents, the endothelium generally becoming obscured by the opaque stroma (Fig. 13.11). Vessels gradually migrate into the graft, often to the centre in allografts, while in isografts these rarely progress beyond the vicinity of sutures.

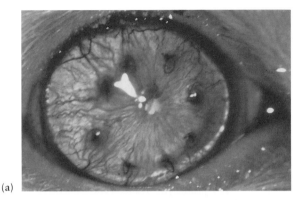

(a)

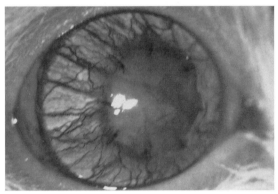

(b)

**Fig. 13.11** (a) Clear corneal allograft (DA to LEW). (b) Rejected allograft (DA to LEW) 12 days after transplantation showing opaque donor cornea and vessels extending to the centre of the graft. The bright spots are reflection artefacts.

## Antigenicity of the cornea

Undoubtedly the antigenic load of the cornea in terms of number of cells is relatively low, because the cellular component of the stroma is small (see Fig. 13.2). In particular, it has no vascular endothelium, a prime target for rejection in other organ grafts, and few class II+ antigen-presenting cells. It has been found that smaller grafts fare better in animals (Khodadoust & Silverstein 1972; Katami 1991) and some human studies (Völker-Dieben *et al.* 1987; Hoffmann & Pahlitzsch 1989). In addition to their low antigenic load this may be because they are further from limbal blood-vessels. In the CTFS the time to first rejection was correlated with larger graft size (Vail *et al.* 1997).

However, in one human study lower rejection rates were found in grafts larger than 8 mm and very small grafts (<7 mm) fared badly (Sanfilippo & Foulks 1989). Williams *et al.* (1997) also found that the smallest grafts had a decreased chance of survival, although the effect of graft size was excluded in multivariate analysis.

## MHC expression

MHC class I antigens are present on all three layers of normal corneas, in both rats (e.g. Treseler & Sanfilippo 1986; Figueiredo 1996) and humans (e.g. Treseler *et al.* 1984), but expression is strongest on the epithelium and weakest on the endothelium. Some studies failed to detect class I on normal adult human endothelium (Whitsett & Stulting 1984; Pepose *et al.* 1985b; Williams *et al.* 1985a). Such low or absent expression may help to protect the endothelium from CD8-mediated cytolysis, although there is evidence of its up-regulation or induction on rejected corneas (Pepose *et al.* 1985b).

Class II antigens are normally only seen on passenger cells, but Pepose *et al.* (1985b) found that they were induced on basal epithelium, stroma and endothelium during rejection in humans. However, Williams *et al.* (1985a) did not find class II expression, on either healthy or diseased human keratocytes or epithelium, antigen being present only on passenger cells and invading vascular endothelium. In the rat, patchy class II expression was found on donor epithelium (Figueiredo *et al.* 1993 and Fig. 13.12) and endothelium undergoing rejection (Figueiredo *et al.* 1998), which may be induced by IFN-γ (Young *et al.* 1985; Abu El-Asrar *et al.* 1989; Brandt *et al.* 1990; Foets *et al.* 1991). The role of this induced class II and whether or not it exacerbates rejection are unclear.

## Vascularization

Animal experiments have confirmed that vascularization abrogates the privilege of tissue in the ocular environment. In rats (Gebhardt 1981; Williams & Coster 1985), rabbits (Williams *et al.* 1986) and mice (Sano *et al.* 1995) prevascularization of the recipient bed pro-

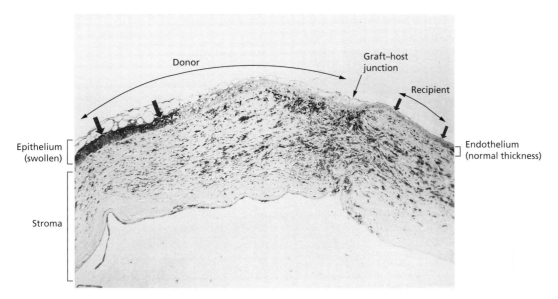

**Fig. 13.12** MHC class II-expressing cells in an allografted rat cornea (LEW to PVG) 13 days after transplantation and 2 days after the onset of clinical rejection. The micrograph spans the graft–host junction. The recipient epithelium on the right appears normal (small arrows), but the oedematous and vacuolated donor epithelium expresses MHC class II (large arrows). Immunoperoxidase staining with light haematoxylin counterstain, original magnification×76.

motes rejection. Lymphatic vessels, present in the conjunctiva, accompany invading blood-vessels (Faure *et al.* 1970) and Indian ink injected into a rabbit cornea is transported to the preauricular and cervical lymph nodes (Smolin & Hyndiuk 1971) and in mice to the cervical lymph nodes (Easty *et al.* 1997). In rodents, secondary *in vitro* T cell proliferation responses have been demonstrated in the ipsilateral draining lymph nodes within 2 weeks of transplantation. However, they were not found at this stage in contralateral lymph nodes or spleen (Easty *et al.* 1997). Thus, it appears that sensitization occurs via the lymphatics, blood-vessels being important for the efferent response and for augmenting the afferent response by increasing the number of local antigen-presenting cells. These are features that the cornea shares with skin (Barker & Billingham 1968), although a second possible route of priming to corneal graft antigens is from the endothelium via the anterior chamber to the systemic circulation (Niederkorn & Streilein 1983).

## Direct vs. indirect antigen presentation

The strongest stimulus to early alloactivation of T cells after vascularized organ transplantation are the class II+ antigen-presenting cells in the graft (Lechler & Batchelor 1982), which present antigen directly to host T cells. Such cells are very sparse or absent in the central corneal epithelium of mice, hamsters, guinea-pigs and rats (Streilein *et al.* 1979; Bergstresser *et al.* 1980; Figueiredo *et al.* 1992) and sparse (7/mm$^2$ of cross-section) in the central cornea, including the stroma, of humans (Williams *et al.* 1985a) and in the stroma (2/mm$^2$) of rats (Treseler & Sanfilippo 1986; F. Figueiredo *et al.*, unpublished). The relative lack of these cells is associated with low or absent systemic Th1-type DTH responses in both heterotopic (Peeler & Niederkorn 1986) and orthotopic corneal transplantation models (Callanan *et al.* 1988), although cytotoxic T lymphocyte (CTL) responses are still generated. Rat donor buttons taken from the periphery of the cornea, where there are more class II+ cells, are rejected more rapidly and frequently than those of equivalent size from the centre (Katami *et al.* 1991). Grafts are also more readily rejected if the number of LC in the donor cornea is artificially increased before transplantation (Rubsamen *et al.* 1984; Callanan *et al.* 1988; He & Niederkorn 1996), when they elicit strong DTH responses (Callanan *et al.* 1988). Peeler *et al.* (1988) found that if H-Y was the sole disparity, only LC-enriched grafts were able to stimulate rejection. However, an LC-enriched graft disparate for class II alone was not rejected unless the animal had been preimmunized, although it could sensitize the host, as demonstrated by the rejection of a second corneal graft in the contralateral eye (Ross *et al.* 1991c).

Whether or not the relatively few LC transplanted in a fully allogeneic donor cornea have a significant immunological effect is still not clear. The potency of LC is considerable; as few as 10 injected subcutaneously into mice can stimulate a systemic CTL response, compared with a minimum of $10^4$ class II-negative keratinocytes (McKinney & Streilein 1989). Gebhardt (1990) found that $2 \times 10^7$ allogeneic class II-positive spleen cells injected into normal rat corneas failed to elicit detectable immunity in spleen or blood lymphocytes. However, the crucial draining lymph node cells were not tested.

Because of the possibility that the few antigen-presenting cells present are important, depletion of these cells before transplantation by a variety of methods has been tested in animal models. These include culture in hyperbaric oxygen (Chandler *et al.* 1982; Ray-Keil & Chandler 1985; Coster & Williams 1989; He & Niederkorn 1996) and UV-B irradiation (Ray-Keil & Chandler 1986; Dana *et al.* 1990; Niederkorn *et al.* 1990; Katami 1991; He & Niederkorn 1996). The latter, particularly, has some potential to prolong survival. For example, in mice, neither systemic DTH nor CTL responses were detected after heterotopic or orthotopic transplantation of a UV-irradiated cornea in which the number of LC had been artificially increased (Niederkorn *et al.* 1990; He & Niederkorn 1996) and, after heterotopic transplantation, animals were found to be tolerant to DTH and CTL induction after receiving a second non-irradiated LC-rich graft (Niederkorn *et al.* 1990). Although *in*

*vitro* studies indicate that low doses of UVB (100 mJ/cm$^2$) do not cause irreversible morphological damage to human corneas (Borderie *et al.* 1995), the danger of critical damage to parenchymal cells, particularly the endothelium, has meant that these procedures have not been tested in clinical practice.

The relatively large interface between graft and host tissue offers recipient antigen-presenting cells relatively rapid access to the graft in comparison with a vascularized organ graft. This can occur, even in the absence of corneal blood-vessels, by direct migration of antigen-presenting cells across recipient epithelium and stroma. Such migration can be induced experimentally by the same stimuli that induce vessel ingress, i.e. infection (Lewkowicz-Moss *et al.* 1987), chemical (Rubsamen *et al.* 1984) and mechanical trauma (McLeish *et al.* 1989), including transplantation (Ross *et al.* 1991a), and is initiated by secretion of cytokines and/or chemokines by epithelial cells, e.g. interleukin 1 (Niederkorn *et al.* 1989). Langerhans' cell infiltration begins within hours of transplantation and is increased in allografts if rejection ensues (Figueiredo *et al.* 1992). There is a parallel migration of dendritic cells into the stroma, augmented from ingrowing blood-vessels. Infiltrating cells may enhance the immune response, once initiated, by migrating back out of the cornea to the lymph nodes or by remaining in the cornea and presenting antigen *in situ* to host T cells. In humans, poor graft survival has been strongly linked to recipient leucocytes in the graft bed (Williams *et al.* 1986, 1989; Philipp & Gottinger 1990). Williams *et al.* (1987a) have also shown that accessory cells extracted from vascularized inflamed rat corneas can present an artificial antigen (dinitrophenyl-ovalbumin) to T cells *in vitro*.

The easy access of recipient antigen-presenting cells to the graft accounts for the rapid indirect alloactivation of T cells (Sonoda *et al.* 1995; Nicholls *et al.* 1997) and graft rejection between 7 and 14 days in many rat strain combinations, which is within a comparable time-frame to normal reponses to pathogens. This contrasts with renal and heart grafts, in which indirect presentation is thought to account for delayed chronic rejection (e.g. Sherwood *et al.* 1986; Benichou *et al.* 1992; Parker *et al.* 1992). Indirectly and directly activated T cells will recognize different spectra of antigenic epitopes, the former being biased towards non-MHC rather than MHC class II. This may account for the relative importance of non-MHC mismatches in experimental corneal graft rejection (Katami 1991; Nicholls *et al.* 1991; Sano *et al.* 1996) (see below) and the difficulty in detecting a beneficial effect of class II matching in human high-risk cases (Bradley *et al.* 1995; Nicholls 1996).

## Conjunctiva-associated lymphoid tissue

In addition to the number and distribution of professional antigen-presenting cells and the extent of corneal neovascularization, other poorly understood local ocular factors may contribute to rejection, especially in a previously inflamed eye. In common with other mucosal surfaces, the conjunctiva possesses conjunctiva-associated lymphatic tissue (CALT). Mitosis has been observed in the lymphocytes in CALT and the epithelial cells overlying this tissue have elongated microvilli and may thus be specialized to pick up antigen from the ocular surface (Chandler & Gillette 1983). T cells in human conjunctiva express a β-integrin that is expressed on T cells at other mucosal sites (Dua *et al.* 1994). The area can become packed with lymphocytes during rejection, especially in pre-sensitized individuals (Polack 1966) and a clear follicular structure has been seen in rabbits receiving xenografts (Polack & Gonzales 1968). Chandler and Gillette (1983) proposed that sensitized T cells locate to CALT, while B cells are retained in the lacrimal glands and secrete IgA into the tears. However, if this distinction exists it is certainly not absolute, as B cells can be found in CALT and T cells in the lacrimal gland (Wieczorek *et al.* 1988). Moreover, a strong response in CALT is not always identifiable by histology after transplantation (Figueiredo 1996) and the extent to which rejection is influenced by local T cell activation remains to be determined. There is also evidence of species differences in the structure and immunological activity of the conjunctiva (Setzer *et al.* 1987).

## Effect of matching

In rat models there is a wide strain-dependent variation in survival of corneal grafts (Katami 1991), whether matched or not. Thus, with an isolated class I mismatch, survival in naïve hosts was 18% (RT1ᵒ to RT1ᵃ; Ross *et al.* 1991b), 58% (RT1ᵃ to RT1ᶜ; Katami *et al.* 1989) or 100% (RT1ᵃ to RT1ᵘ; S.M. Nicholls, unpublished). However, an isolated class II incompatibility did not provoke rejection (Katami *et al.* 1990; Ross *et al.* 1991c), even in corneas artificially enriched with LC, unless the recipient was preimmunized (Ross *et al.* 1991c). The authors' explanation for this was that class II expression occurred on parenchymal cells only transiently after transplantation and in naïve, but not in sensitized animals, subsided before effector cells capable of recognizing class II reached the graft. In mice, Sonoda and Streilein (1992) also found class I to be more potent, but a class II disparity elicited rejection in some naïve individuals. In general, the evidence from animals indicates that it is more important to match for class I than class II, at least in unsensitized individuals, as might be expected in a tissue deficient in class II+ antigen-presenting cells.

The H-Y antigen is expressed on corneal grafts and can be a rejection target (Ray-Kiel & Chandler 1985; Peeler *et al.* 1988; He *et al.* 1991a). Other, as yet unidentified, non-MHC genes are also involved. Katami (1991) first recorded that grafts between two donor–recipient strain combinations of identical MHC mismatch (RT1ᶜ to RT1ᵘ), but with different background disparities, exhibited very different median survival, i.e. 13 days (PVG to AO) and >100 days (AUG to WAG). More recently, the use of congenic rats in three different strain combinations has confirmed that non-MHC disparity makes a substantial but variable, strain-dependent contribution to rejection (Table 13.4). In this respect corneas resemble skin. Matching tends to have an overall beneficial effect, but does not necessarily improve survival, as shown in the PVG to DA combination. Furthermore, reciprocal grafts between two strains do not have the same outcome.

The hybrid strain combination shown in Table 13.4 was used to mimic more closely the unknown variability of the human population. Because the backcross (DA × LEW) $F_1$ × LEW recipients possesed a random selection of DA genes, the precise non-MHC disparity between donor and recipient was unknown. However, MHC typing of recipients (either RT1ᵃ/ˡ or RT1ˡ/ˡ) as in humans, enabled matching or mismatching with the

**Table 13.4** Relative effect of MHC and non-MHC mismatches on rejection in the rat.

| Donor | Recipient | Mismatch | Number rejected* | Day of rejection Median | Day of rejection Range | Reference |
|---|---|---|---|---|---|---|
| DA | PVG | MHC (RT1a) + non-MHC | 25/29 | 21 | 13–>100 | Katami *et al.* (1991) |
| DA | PVG.RT1a | Non-MHC | 11/22 | 95 | 33–>100 | |
| PVG | DA | MHC (RT1c) + non-MHC | 10/10 | 12 | 9–14 | Nicholls *et al.* (1997) |
| PVG.RT1a | DA | Non-MHC | 15/15 | 12 | 10–14 | |
| DA | (DA × LEW) F₁ × LEW | MHC (RT1a) + non-MHC† | 37/37 | 11 | 7–17 | Nicholls *et al.* (1991, |
| DA | (DA × LEW) F₁ × LEW | Non-MHC† | 35/40 | 17 | 7–>100 | 1995) |

* Within 100 days.
† Partial mismatch at a variable number of non-MHC loci — see text for details.

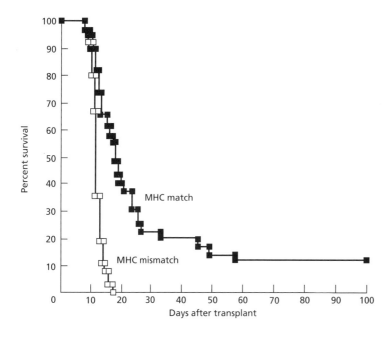

**Fig. 13.13** Survival of 77 corneal grafts in the rat, approximately half of which were MHC-matched. Matching significantly prolonged survival (*P*=0.00002), but 87% of matched grafts were ultimately rejected. (From Nicholls *et al.* 1995, with permission.)

donor (RT1a/a). The resulting high incidence of rejection of MHC-matched grafts (87%; see Fig. 13.15), compared with an average non-MHC disparity of only 50%, showed that there were several independently segregating non-MHC genes involved. The survival of individual grafts in this group is presumably related to the precise number of mismatched loci. In mice, Streilein and coworkers have found a strong non-MHC effect in the C57BL to BALB/c mouse combination. In

this case, such antigens were more potent than those of the MHC alone (H-2k to H-2d), both in terms of clinical rejection (Sonoda & Streilein 1992; Sano *et al.* 1996) and donor-specific cell-mediated reponses (Joo *et al.* 1995; Sonoda *et al.* 1995; Sano *et al.* 1996).

In combination, the above factors may account for the disappointing overall clinical effect of MHC matching. In humans, a significant beneficial effect of matching may be achievable only in a subgroup in which there are few other mismatches. A future course of action in humans might be to type and, if necessary, to match for non-MHC antigens. If the non-MHC effect in transplantion is due to a limited number of immunodominant loci (Simpson 1998), this might not be insuperably difficult. Non-MHC gene products, in addition to acting as targets for rejection, may also play a role in modulating the immune response, e.g. via cytokine polymorphisms (Hutchinson *et al.* 1998).

## Effector mechanisms of rejection

These are still not fully elucidated, although rejection appears to be predominantly cell-mediated (Polack 1966) and Th-1-like, at least in unsensitized individuals. Early functional studies of immunity after heterotopic corneal transplantation provided evidence of CTL-mediated effector mechanisms (Peeler *et al.* 1985; Treseler *et al.* 1985), while systemic DTH responses were not detected unless donor corneas were enriched with LC. Experiments in which thymectomized irradiated mice were reconstituted with T-cell subsets further implicated CTL in rejection (Matoba *et al.* 1986). In humans, reports of differential rejection of penetrating and patch lamellar grafts from different donors placed in the same eye also support a specific CTL effector mechanism (Rozenman *et al.* 1985). Rejection is associated with the development of primed donor class I-reactive CTL in the blood of humans (Roelen *et al.* 1995). However, from other experiments, CD8+ cells seem to be less important than CD4+ cells. He *et al.* (1991b) in mice and Ayliffe *et al.* (1992b) in rats found that only depletion of the CD4+ subset prolonged graft survival, while rejection in perforin knock-out or CD8 knock-out mice is not delayed (Hegde & Niederkorn 1999). A DTH-type response is implicated from the work of Gebhardt (1988). He found that only a combination of specific CD4+ cells and class II+ cells were able to cause pathological damage when injected into the stroma of rats. An important role for macrophages is confirmed by evidence that depletion of these cells prolongs graft survival (Van der Veen *et al.* 1994).

Histological examination of human rejection is hampered by a lack of useful tissue, because biopsies are inadvisable and there is a better prognosis for regrafts if they are performed well after the acute inflammatory response has died down. Early electron microscope studies of acute endothelial rejection in humans identified lymphocytes and macrophages. Immunohistological examination of corneal sections shows a mixed infiltrate in humans at the time of regraft (Pepose *et al.* 1985a) and during acute rejection in rabbits and in rats (Otsuka *et al.* 1990; Holland *et al.* 1991, 1994; Figueiredo 1996). Up to 20% of infiltrating T cells in rats are CD25 (IL-2R)+ (Fig. 13.14) and a large number of infiltrating cells express class II (Otsuka *et al.* 1990; Holland *et al.* 1994; Fig. 13.12). There appears to be differential migration of T cells—compared with macrophages and neutrophils—into the epithelium (Fig. 13.15), which are concentrated in clinically defined rejection lines similar to those seen in humans. Although natural-killer-like cells can adhere to and kill corneal endothelial cells *in vitro* (Opremcak *et al.* 1985), few natural killer cells were found in rejected human grafts (Pepose *et al.* 1985a) or on rat endothelium undergoing rejection (S.M. Nicholls, unpublished data). Few infiltrating plasma cells (Kanai & Polack 1971b) or B cells are found in humans (Pepose *et al.* 1985a) or rats (Figueiredo 1996) and a positive cross-match does not prejudice graft survival (CCTS Research Group 1992). However, the development of anti-HLA antibodies after keratoplasty is associated with increased risk and this effector mechanism may be more important in individuals that have previously rejected a graft and in xenograft rejection (Polack & Gonzales 1968; Ross *et al.* 1993; Larkin *et al.* 1995).

Because of the difficulty of viewing the thin endothelial cell layer in cross-section, there has been very little detailed immunohistological study of this layer, despite its supreme importance. Figueiredo *et al.* (1998), by careful removal of the endothelium from rats as a sheet, showed rejection-associated morphological changes typical of other species, including a distinct rejection line. At the ultrastructural level, Takano and Williams (1995) identified CD4+, CD8+, CD25+, class II+ cells and macrophages adhering to the endothelium. CD4+ cells predominated over CD8+ cells. Using a different CD4-reactive monoclonal antibody, Nicholls *et al.* (1996) found a much lower ratio of CD4+ to CD8+

Epithelium [

Stroma

Endothelium [

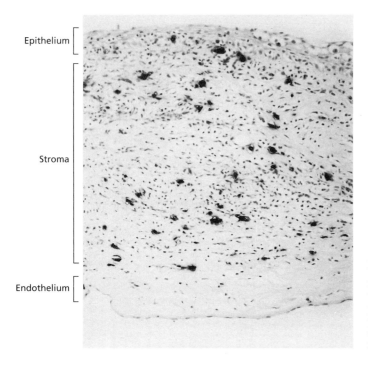

**Fig. 13.14** Cells expressing the interleukin-2 receptor in a rat corneal allograft (LEW to PVG) 13 days after transplantation and 1 day after the onset of clinical rejection. Immunoperoxidase staining with light haematoxylin counterstain, original magnification ×176.

T cells on endothelial sheets (1:15), rising only in the later stages of rejection. This contrasted with a ratio of 1:1, in the epithelium, stroma (Figueiredo 1996) and anterior chamber at the same time point. A possible explanation for the absence of CD4+ cells is that they are more susceptible than CD8+ cells to apoptosis induced by Fas ligand, known to be expressed on the endothelium (Griffith *et al.* 1995) and to be a component of corneal privilege (see below). As most cells adhering to the endothelium were either macrophages or CD8+ T cells, it is likely that rejection was effected by either or both of these cell types. The predominant cytokines expressed in grafts at the time of rejection appear to be TNFα (Torres *et al.* 1996; Larkin *et al.* 1997; Pleyer *et al.* 1997) and the Th-1 cytokines IFN-γ (Torres *et al.* 1996; Larkin *et al.* 1997) and IL-2 (Torres *et al.* 1996).

### Anterior chamber-associated immune deviation

Skin and tumour allografts are partially protected from immune destruction if placed in the anterior chamber

of the eye. Protection is greater with lower levels of antigenic disparity but is abrogated by vascularization. The immune response to viral antigens injected into the anterior chamber is also suppressed (Whittum *et al.* 1983). The phenomenon is characterized not by a lack of immune recognition but by specific suppression of DTH, while antibody (Niederkorn & Streilein 1982) and CTL (Niederkorn & Streilein 1983) responses remain intact. Streilein and coworkers have called this anterior chamber-associated immune deviation (ACAID). Antigen apparently escapes from the anterior chamber via the systemic circulation to the spleen, where antigen-specific suppressor cells are generated (Niederkorn & Streilein 1983). The phenomenon is associated with a predominantly Th-2 pattern of cytokine secretion in the spleen, i.e. a lack if IL-2 and IFN-γ (but also of IL-4) and high levels of IL-10 (Li *et al.* 1996). In addition, CD45− cells of the iris and ciliary body are able to secrete TGFβ (Wilbanks *et al.* 1992), which inhibits T cell proliferation (Cousins *et al.* 1991) and induces a Th-2-type cytokine secretion pattern in T cells (Takeuchi *et al.* 1997; Taylor *et al.*

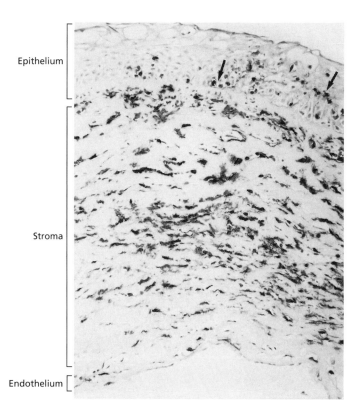

Epithelium

Stroma

Endothelium

**Fig. 13.15** Section of a rat corneal allograft (LEW to PVG) 13 days after transplantation and 2 days after the onset of clinical rejection. Peripheral donor cornea showing numerous CD8+ T cells in the stroma and epithelium (arrows). Immunoperoxidase staining with light haematoxylin counterstain, original magnification×159.

1997). Streilein and Wegmann (1987) proposed that this suppression of DTH is a unique adaptation to protect the visual axis from cell-mediated damage by intraocular pathogens or autoimmune reactions to antigens such as retinal S antigen. Sonoda and Streilein (1993) first reported that acceptance of corneal grafts in mice was associated with such suppression of DTH reactivity and the induction of specific suppressor cells in the spleen. A further aspect of ACAID is the more recent finding that corneal endothelial cells express Fas ligand and can induce apoptosis of leucocytes (Griffith *et al.* 1995). This has been confirmed in mutant mice lacking Fas ligand or Fas itself, which suffer more acute allograft rejection (Stuart *et al.* 1997).

There is no direct evidence that human corneal transplants are protected by this mechanism, although Fas-L-mediated apoptotic cell death appears to contribute to the local immune regulation of ocular inflammatory disease (Dick *et al.* 1999). Presentation of corneal graft

antigens in animals clearly occurs efficiently via the limbus and the conjunctival lymphatic supply and this elicits immunity with a cell infiltrate and cytokine profile characteristic of a Th-1 response. Moreover, corneal infection with HSV provokes normal DTH responses, indicating that antigen within the epithelium and stroma does not induce deviant immunity. Although some corneal graft antigens may escape via the anterior chamber, activation of T cells via the draining lymph nodes is clearly sufficient to override ACAID-inducing signals that may tend to suppress the response. The situation is further complicated in rats and rabbits by the proven ability of endothelial cells to proliferate. Thus it is not clear whether the recovery from rejection that is seen in these species is a result of replacement of all donor cells by those of the recipient or whether some donor cells remain, perhaps protected by active suppressive mechanisms generated via release of antigen into the anterior chamber during rejection.

However, in humans the balance between possible ACAID-inducing signals and other factors governing immunity and privilege is likely to be different from that in rodents and it is unknown whether the phenomenon has any effect in protecting human corneal grafts.

## Xenotransplantation

The cornea is susceptible to antibody-mediated xenograft rejection (Ross *et al.* 1994; Larkin & Williams 1995), but this is delayed in comparison with solid organ grafts. Corneas from guinea pigs transplanted to discordant rats remained clear for up to a week without immunosuppression (Ross *et al.* 1993). This was probably due to the lack of target blood vessels and the blood–ocular barrier delaying the arrival of immunoglobulin in the eye. Immunoglobulin from naïve as well as transplanted rats adhered to cells in sections of guinea pig cornea, indicating that natural antibodies were involved. In the cell infiltrates, the proportion of neutrophils relative to mononuclear cells and T cells was increased in comparison with allografts (Ross *et al.* 1994).

The lack of hyperacute rejection and the fact that allosensitization does not accelerate rejection of a xenograft (Ross *et al.* 1993) show some promise for the success of corneal xenotransplantation. However, because of the critical importance of the curvature and thickness of the cornea for proper apposition and visual function after transplantation, the size of the donor eye is of critical importance. The most likely candidate, the pig, has a cornea almost twice the human thickness, so that either young animals or minipig strains would be required.

## Immunosuppression

### CORTICOSTEROIDS

Since their introduction many years ago, topically applied steroids have remained the most useful immunosuppressants in corneal transplantation, despite the success of more recently developed drugs, notably cyclosporin. Steroids are easily absorbed through the cornea, having a direct immunosuppressive and lympholytic (apoptotic) effect. Gillette *et al.* (1982) have demonstrated depletion of corneal LC in mice by both topical and systemic corticosteroid. They are also potent inhibitors of angiogenesis, thereby helping to maintain the cornea's architectural privilege.

### CYCLOSPORIN A

Cyclosporin administered systemically to both rabbits (Shepherd *et al.* 1980; Bell *et al.* 1982) and rats (Nishi *et al.* 1990; Nicholls *et al.* 1995) for limited periods of time (up to 28 days from the day of transplantation) delays graft rejection. Rejection ensues after cessation of treatment. Systemic treatments are relatively less effective in corneal transplantation because of the lack of a direct blood supply to the cornea. Thus systemically administered drug is not detected in ocular structures of rabbits unless there is significant intraocular inflammation (i.e. vascularization) (BenEzra & Maftzir 1990a).

The topical use of cyclosporin A (CsA) in humans has been hampered by its poor solubility and the difficulty of finding an efficient vehicle that does not itself cause inflammation. Although in animals the drug is absorbed into the stroma after topical treatment, it does not penetrate well to the anterior chamber when dissolved in oil (BenEzra & Maftzir 1990b). Moreover, a drug such as CsA that acts on the afferent arm of the immune response is likely to have limited effectiveness when only administered locally. Nevertheless, rabbit studies indicate that rejection is delayed by local administration in drops (Foets *et al.* 1985; Williams *et al.* 1985b; Newton *et al.* 1988) or in collagen shields (a form of contact lens from which the drug is slowly released) (Mahlberg *et al.* 1991). When used alone in rabbits it is less effective than topical steroid (Williams *et al.* 1985b) but in rats, when combined with topical steroid, it is more effective than steroid alone (Williams *et al.* 1987b).

## Immunosuppression in humans

Immunosuppression is used both in prophylaxis against rejection and in treatment of established rejection. The agent(s) employed to prevent rejection, their strength, frequency and duration of use depend upon the perceived risk. In general, low-risk grafts receive topical steroid preparations alone while higher-risk cases may receive additional systemic steroids with or without further systemic immunosuppresive agents (Rinne & Stulting 1992).

For prophylaxis, low-risk cases receive topical corticosteroid drops, e.g. dexamethasone four times daily, reducing over a period of up to 12 months, while high-risk cases may receive topical corticosteroids every 30 min. Prophylactic systemic steroids are used in doses of 20–30 mg, either daily or alternate daily. A placebo-controlled double-blind trial to test the effect of topical cyclosporin on the prevention of rejection in 'high-risk' graft recipients was begun in 1991 in the UK. The trial was not completed because early results did not suggest that topical cyclosporin was of value. However, the trial patients had received high doses of topical steroids in addition to cyclosporin, which may have obscured a beneficial effect.

Systemic CsA was used prophylactically by Miller *et al.* (1988) to prevent rejection of high-risk corneal grafts in humans, while Hill (1989) used systemic CsA in combination with topical and systemic steroids and concluded that this combination therapy was superior to steroid alone. Cyclosporin is given in a dose of 4.0–4.5 mg/kg body weight and adjusted to give therapeutic serum levels of 250–400 μg/L. At the Bristol Eye Hospital, systemic cyclosporin is usually employed as short-term immunosuppressant for high-risk patients to cover the post-transplantation period during which the risk of rejection is greatest. Long-term use is rarely justified after corneal transplantation as the risk of drug-related side effects may exceed the problems associated with graft failure.

Because the cornea is exposed and relatively permeable and rejection symptoms may be rapidly recognized by an alert patient, aggressive immunosuppressive therapy can often be delivered directly to the graft before a critical reduction in endothelial cell density has been reached. Smiddy *et al.* (1986) showed that earlier presentation of the patient for treatment significantly improved the prognosis. To treat rejection episodes topical steroid is supplemented with systemic cyclosporin or systemic steroids. Hill *et al.* (1991) report successful treatment of established rejection using a single 500 mg dose of intravenous methylprednisolone.

Azathioprine has been advocated in penetrating keratoplasty (Barraquer 1985; Coster 1989) and may be used as a steroid-sparing agent at a dose of 1–2 mg/kg/day but, as with cyclosporin, the toxic side effects demand that patients have their haemopoetic, hepatic and renal function monitored closely.

Kobayashi *et al.* (1989) demonstrated that tacrolimus (Prograf) will prevent allograft rejection in rabbits and Nishi *et al.* (1990, 1993) found that it is effective at 1/10 of the concentration of cyclosporin. It may be useful as an alternative to cyclosporin in human corneal transplantation but it is likely to have similar drawbacks to cyclosporin because of its poor solubility.

## The future of immunosuppression

### MONOCLONAL ANTIBODIES

Some success in preventing or delaying rejection has been achieved with systemically injected anti-CD4+ antibody in rodents (He *et al.* 1991b; Ayliffe *et al.* 1992b), with locally injected anti-T cell antibodies in humans (Ippoliti & Fronterrè 1987) and antimyeloid antibodies in rabbits (Williams *et al.* 1992). Intraperitoneal, but not subconjunctival injection of CTLA4-Ig daily for 1 week after transplantation gave modest delay in rejection of mouse corneal grafts (Hoffmann *et al.* 1997). Antibodies to adhesion molecules, given systemically, have also achieved limited success in inhibiting rejection in rodents (Muramatsu *et al.* 1993; He *et al.* 1994; Hori *et al.* 1997). In general, injection of antibodies into the anterior chamber, with the attendant risks of inflammation, infection and damage to the endothelium, are not currently justified for the level of benefit provided. Systemically injected antibody is likely to be less effective for corneas than for other organs because of the regional, rather than systemic, nature of the initial immune response and because of the blood–ocular barrier. Moreover, the success of some antibodies, e.g. anti-CD4, may rely on continuous release of antigens from the graft into the systemic circulation (Hamano *et al.* 1996), which, because of this barrier and because of the relatively small size of the graft, would not occur efficiently after transplantation of cornea.

GENE TRANSFER

Because of its accessiblity, the cornea is a good model to test the possibility of transfecting genes coding for immunomodulatory proteins into transplanted tissue. Constructs can be injected into the anterior chamber, transferred via tissue culture before transplantation or applied topically. Experimental work has so far achieved expression for limited periods of time (2–4 weeks) using adenovirus vectors, which seem preferentially to infect endothelial cells. Thus, the reporter β-galactosidase gene has been introduced into such cells by injection into the anterior chamber of mice (Budenz *et al.* 1995) or by exposing rat or rabbit (Fehervari *et al.* 1997) or human (Oral *et al.* 1997) corneas to constructs in tissue culture. Potentially therapeutic proteins have also been transferred, including the stress protein haem oxygenase-1 (Abrahams *et al.* 1995) and functionally active CTLA4-Ig fusion protein (Oral *et al.* 1997). It may be possible to transfect with genes that are only switched on under inflammatory conditions, e.g. in the presence of TNFα (Arancibia-Carcamo *et al.* 1998). A different approach has been adopted by Shewring *et al.* (1997). They have targeted β-galactosidase to cultured rabbit, pig and human corneas using synthetic or natural peptides comprising a polylysine segment for DNA-binding and an integrin-binding fragment for cell attachment and internalization. They demonstrated efficient transfer (to 30% of endothelial cells), indicating the promise of this approach, which avoids the potential adverse effects of virus transfer.

INDUCTION OF DONOR-SPECIFIC TOLERANCE

As indicated above, the special characteristics of the cornea mean that suppressive regimens found appropriate for other organs will not necessarily be successful for corneas. However, protocols that target T cells activated by indirect presentation pathways are particularly appropriate. One such treatment exploits the capacity of donor antigen administered via mucosal sites—the gut and respiratory tract—to induce specific unresponsiveness. It was first shown to be effective in preventing or alleviating disease in experimental models of allergy and autoimmunity and has now also been successful in mouse corneal transplantation, via oral administration of whole freshly isolated or cultured corneal cells, immortalized by human papilloma virus (He *et al.* 1996). The tolerizing effect was significantly enhanced by conjugating the cells to the B subunit of cholera toxin, a potent adjuvant (Ma *et al.* 1997). Success has also been achieved using crude donor cell extracts via the nasal route (Filipec *et al.* 1998). Tolerizing agents might in theory be whole cells or cell extracts, purified proteins or immunogenic peptides derived from these proteins, each of which has potential advantages. The necessary recipient pretreatment would be greatly facilitated in human corneal transplantation because donor corneas can be stored for up to a month in tissue culture before use, allowing time for tolerance to develop. In humans, tolerizing donor cells might be blood leucocytes, keratinocytes or cells cultured from the donor conjunctiva. However, there are attendant risks of disease transmission, which would not arise with the use of artificially manufactured donor-specific proteins or peptides. These could be stored for long periods and a potential graft recipient could be tissue-typed and pretreated with an appropriate mixture of such molecules. However, realistically, only a limited number of potential tolerizing epitopes could be used and success would depend on the induction of strong bystander suppression. Although this has proved possible in other models, its potential has yet to be tested in corneal transplantation.

## Acknowledgements

The authors would like to thank Dr Francisco Figueiredo for reviewing the manuscript and Mrs Gill Bennerson and Mr Cliff Jeal for photography.

# References

Abrahams, N.G., Da Silva, J.-L., Lavrovsky, Y. *et al.* (1995) Adenovirus-mediated heme oxygenase-1 gene transfer into rabbit ocular tissues. *Investigative Ophthalmology and Visual Science* 36, 2202–2210.

Abu El-Asrar, A.M., van den Oord, J.J., Billiau, A. *et al.* (1989) Recombinant interferon-gamma induces HLA-DR expression on human corneal epithelial cells and endothelial cells *in vitro*: a preliminary report. *British Journal of Ophthalmology* 73, 587–590.

Aiello, L.P., Javitt, J.C. & Canner, J.K. (1993) National outcomes of penetrating keratoplasty: risks of endophthalmitis and retinal detachment. *Archives of Ophthalmology* 111, 509–513.

Allan, B. & Tuft, S. (1998) Transmissson of Creutzfeldt-Jakob disease in corneal grafts: observing the exclusion criteria for donated grafts should ensure the risk is small. *British Medical Journal* 315, 1553–1554.

Alldredge, O.C. & Krachmer, J.H. (1981) Clinical types of corneal transplant rejection: their manifestations, frequency, preoperative correlates, and treatment. *Archives of Ophthalmology* 99, 599–604.

Arancibia-Carcamo, C.V., Oral, H.B., Haskard, D.O., Larkin, D.F.P. & George, A.J.T. (1998) Lipoadenofection-mediated gene delivery to the corneal endothelium: prospects for modulating graft rejection. *Transplantation* 65, 62–67.

Arentsen, J.J. & Laibson, P.R. (1982) Surgical management of pseudophakic corneal oedema: complications and visual results following penetrating keratoplasty. *Ophthalmic Surgery* 13, 371–373.

Ayliffe, W., McCleod, D. & Hutchinson, I.V. (1992a) The effect of blood transfusions on rat corneal graft survival. *Investigative Ophthalmology and Visual Science* 33, 1974–1978.

Ayliffe, W., Alam, Y., Bell, E.B. *et al.* (1992b) Prolongation of rat corneal graft survival by treatment with anti-CD4 monoclonal antibody. *British Journal of Ophthalmology* 76, 602–606.

Baggesen, K., Ehlers, N. & Lamm, L.U. (1991) HLA-DR/RFLP compatible corneal grafts. *Acta Ophthalmologica* 69, 229–233.

Baggesen, K., Lamm, L.U. & Ehlers, N. (1996) Significant effect of high-resolution HLA-DRB1 matching in high risk corneal transplantation. *Transplantation* 62, 1273–1277.

Bahn, C.F., Meyer, R.F., MacCallum, D.K. *et al.* (1982) Penetrating keratoplasty in the cat: a clinically applicable model. *Ophthalmology* 89, 687–699.

Bahn, C.F., Glassman, R.M., MacCallum, D.K. *et al.* (1986) Postnatal development of corneal endothelium.

*Investigative Ophthalmology and Visual Science* 27, 44–51.

Barker, C.F. & Billingham, R.E. (1968) The role of afferent lymphatics in the rejection of skin homografts. *Journal of Experimental Medicine* 128, 197–221.

Barraquer, J. (1985) Immunosuppressive agents in penetrating keratoplasty. *American Journal of Ophthalmology* 100, 61–64.

Basu, P.K. & Ormsby, H.L. (1956) Interlamellar frozen-stored corneal homografts in rabbits. *American Journal of Ophthalmology* 42, 71–75.

Batchelor, J.R., Casey, T.A., Gibbs, D.C. *et al.* (1976) HLA matching and corneal grafting. *Lancet* 1, 551–554.

Beebe, D.C. & Coats, J.M. (1998) The lens controls the early development of the cornea. *Investigative Ophthalmology and Visual Science* 39 (Suppl.), 223.

Bell, T.A.G., Easty, D.L. & McCullagh, K.G. (1982) A placebo-controlled blind trial of cyclosporin-A in prevention of corneal graft rejection in rabbits. *British Journal of Ophthalmology* 66, 303–308.

BenEzra, D. & Maftzir, G. (1990a) Ocular penetration of cyclosporin A. I. The rabbit eye. *Investigative Ophthalmology and Visual Science* 31, 1362–1366.

BenEzra, D. & Maftzir, G. (1990b) Ocular penetration of cyclosporine A in the rat eye. *Archives of Ophthalmology* 108, 584–587.

Benichou, G., Takizawa, P.A., Olson, C.A. *et al.* (1992) Donor major histicompatibility complex (MHC) peptides are presented by recipient MHC molecules during graft rejection. *Journal of Experimental Medicine* 175, 305–308.

Bergstresser. P.R., Fletcher, C.R. & Streilein, J.W. (1980) Surface densities of Langerhans cells in relation to rodent epidermal sites with special immunologic properties. *Journal of Investigative Dermatology* 74, 77–80.

Bigar, F. (1982) Specular microscopy of the endothelium. *Developmental Ophthalmology* 6, 1–9.

Billingham, R.E. & Boswell, T. (1953) Studies on the problem of corneal homografts. *Proceedings of the Royal Society of London (B)* 141, 392–406.

Binder, P.S. (1985) Selective suture removal can reduce postkeratoplasty astigmatism. *Ophthalmology* 92, 1412–1416.

Boisjoly, H.M., Raynald, R., Dube, I. *et al.* (1986) HLA-A, B and DR matching in corneal transplantation. *Ophthalmology* 93, 1290–1297.

Boisjoly, H.M., Raynald, R., Bernard, P.M. *et al.* (1990) Association between corneal allograft reactions and HLA compatibility. *Ophthalmology* 97, 1689–1698.

Borderie, V.M., Kantelip, B.M. & Delbosc, B.Y. (1995) Ultrastructure of UVB-irradiated and organ-cultured donor corneas. *Transplantation Proceedings* 27, 1652–1653.

Bourne, W.M. (1983) Chronic endothelial cell loss in transplanted corneas. *Cornea* **2**, 289–294.

Bradley, B.A., Vail, A., Gore, S.M. *et al.* (1995) Negative effect of HLA-DR matching on corneal transplantation. *Transplantation Proceedings* **27**, 1392–1393.

Brandt, C.R., Knupfer, P.B., Boush, G.A. *et al.* (1990) *In vivo* induction of Ia expression in murine cornea after intravitreal injection of interferon-γ. *Investigative Ophthalmology and Visual Science* **31**, 2248–2253.

Budenz, D.L., Bennett, J., Alonso, L. & Maguire, A. (1995) *In vivo* gene transfer into murine endothelial and trabecular meshwork cells. *Investigative Ophthalmology and Visual Science* **36**, 2211–2215.

Callanan, D., Peeler, J. & Niederkorn, J.Y. (1988) Characteristics of rejection of orthotopic corneal allografts in the rat. *Transplantation* **45**, 437–443.

Callanan, D.G., Luckenbach, M.W., Fischer, B.J. *et al.* (1989) Histopathology of rejected orthotopic corneal grafts in the rat. *Investigative Ophthalmology and Visual Science* **30**, 413–424.

Castroviejo, R. (1949) Keratoplasty in the treatment of keratoconus. *Archives of Ophthalmology* **42**, 776–800.

Chandler, J.W. & Gillette, T.E. (1983) Immunological defense mechanisms of the ocular surface. *Ophthalmlogy* **90**, 585–591.

Chandler J.W., Kaufman, H.E. (1974) Graft reactions after keratoplasty for keratoconus. *American Journal of Ophthalomology* **77**, 543–547.

Chandler, J.W., Ray-Keil, L. & Gillette, T.E. (1982) Experimental corneal allograft rejection: description of murine model and a new hypothesis of immunopathogenesis. *Current Eye Research* **2**, 387–397.

Choyce, D.P. (1952) Successful transplantation of human and cat corneal tissue into rabbit corneae. *British Journal of Ophthalmology* **36**, 537–542.

Cobo, L.M., Coster, D.J., Rice, N.S.C. & Jones, B.R. (1980) Prognosis and management of corneal transplantation for herpetic keratitis. *Archives of Ophthalmology* **98**, 1755–1759.

Cohen, K.L., Tripoli, N.K., Cervantes, G. & Smith, D. (1990) Cat endothelial morphology after corneal transplant. *Current Eye Research* **9**, 445–450.

Collaborative Corneal Transplantation Studies (CCTS) Research Group (1992) The Collaborative Corneal Transplantation Studies (CTTS). Effectiveness of histocompatibility matching in high-risk corneal transplantation. *Archives of Ophthalmology* **110**, 1392–1403.

Coster, D.J. (1982) Management of herpes keratitis. *Transactions of the Ophthalmological Society of New Zealand* **34**, 48–55.

Coster, D.J. (1989) Mechanisms of corneal graft failure: the erosion of privilege. *Eye* **2**, 251–262.

Coster, D.J. & Williams, K.A. (1989) Surgical manoeuvres to reduce the impact of corneal allograft rejection. *Developmental Ophthalmology* **18**, 156–164.

Cousins, S.W., Mc Cabe, M.M., Danielpour, D. & Streilein, J.W. (1991) Identification of transforming growth factor-beta as an immunosuppressive factor in aqueous humour. *Investigative Opthalmology and Visual Science* **32**, 2201–2211.

Dana, M.R., Olkowski, S.T., Ahmadian, H. *et al.* (1990) Low-dose ultraviolet-B irradiation of donor corneal endothelium and graft survival. *Investigative Ophthalmology and Visual Science* **31**, 2261–2268.

Dick, A.D., Siepmann, K., Dees, C. *et al.* (1999) Fas-Fas ligand-mediated apoptosis within aqueous during idiopathic acute anterior uveitis. *Investigative Ophthalmology and Visual Science* **40**, 2258–2267.

Dohlman, C.H. (1973) Pathophysiology of graft failure. In: *Corneal Graft Failure: Ciba Foundation Symposium 15* (eds R. Porter & J. Knight), pp. 25–41. Elsevier, Amsterdam.

Dohlman, Ch. & Boström, H. (1955) Uptake of sulfate by mucopolysaccharides in the rat cornea and sclera. *Acta Ophthalmologica* **33**, 455–467.

Donshik, P.C., Cavanagh, H.D., Boruchoff, S.A. & Dohlman, C.H. (1979) Effect of bilateral and unilateral grafts on the incidence of rejections in keratoconus. *American Journal of Ophthalmology* **87**, 823–826.

Doughman, D.J., Harris, J.E. & Schmitt, M.K. (1976) Penetrating keratoplasty using 37 C organ cultured cornea. *Transactions of the American Academy of Ophthalmology and Otolaryngology* **81**, 778–793.

Dua, H.S., Gomes, J.A.P., Jindal, V.K. & Appa, S.N. (1994) Mucosa specific lymphocytes in the human conjunctiva, corneoscleral limbus and lacrimal gland. *Current Eye Research* **13**, 87–93.

Duke-Elder, S. (1956) The problems of homoplastic grafting as applied to the cornea. *Journal of Royal College of Surgeons (Edinburgh)* **1**, 187–212.

Dunnington J.H. & Smelser, G.K. (1958) Incorporation of S[35] in healing wounds in normal and devitalized corneas. *Archives of Ophthalmology* **60**, 116–129.

Easty, D.L., Lau, C.H., Nicholls, S.M. & Williams, N.A. (1997) Differential mixed lymphocyte reaction kinetics in the draining lymph nodes in a murine corneal intralamellar transplantation model. *Investigative Ophthalmology and Visual Science* **38** (Suppl.), S8.

Faure, J.P., Kozak, Y., Graf, B. & Pouliquen, Y. (1970) Lymphatiques dans la cornée vascularisée avec cours de rejet d'héterogreffes expérimentales. *Archives of Ophthalmology (Paris)* **30**, 575–588.

Fehervari, Z., Rayner, S.A., Oral, H.B. *et al.* (1997) Gene transfer to ex-vivo stored corneas. *Cornea* **16**, 459–464.

Ficker, L.A., Kirkness, C.M., Rice N.S.C. & Steele A.D.McG. (1988) Longterm prognosis for corneal grafting in herpes simplex keratitis. *Eye* **2**, 400–408.

Figueiredo, F. (1996) *Immunopathology of corneal graft rejection in a rat model*. PhD thesis, University of Bristol.

Figueiredo, F., Nicholls, S.M., Easty, D.L. & Shimeld, C. (1992) Langerhans cell infiltration of the cornea after orthotopic corneal transplantation in rats. *Investigative Ophthalmology and Visual Science* 33 (Suppl.), 983.

Figueiredo, F., Nicholls, S.M., Easty, D.L. & Shimeld, C. (1993) Cells infiltrating the corneal epithelium after penetrating keratoplasty in rats. *Investigative Ophthalmology and Visual Science* 34 (Suppl.), 1101.

Figueiredo, F., Pendergrast, D., Zhang, L. *et al.* (1998) An improved method for examining the corneal endothelium during graft rejection in the rat. *Experimental Eye Research* 67, 625–630.

Filatov, V.P. (1937) Transplantation of the cornea from preserved cadavers' eyes. *Lancet* 1, 1395–1397.

Filipec, M., Kuffova, L., Krulova, M. *et al.* (1998) Mucosal tolerance as a strategy for preventing rejection of corneal graft. *Ophthalmic Research* 30 (Suppl. 1), 109.

Fine, M. & Payne, R. (1974) Histocompatibility typing and corneal transplantation. *Transactions of the American Academy of Ophthalmology and Otolaryngology* 78, 445–456.

Fine, M. & Stein, M. (1973) The role of corneal vascularization in human corneal graft reactions. In: *Corneal Graft Failure: Ciba Foundation Symposium 15* (eds R. Porter & J. Knight), pp. 193–208. Elsevier, Amsterdam.

Foets, B., Missotten, L., Vanderveeren, P. & Goossens, W. (1985) Prolonged survival of allogeneic corneal grafts in rabbits treated with topically applied cyclosporin A: systemic absorption and local immunosuppressive effect. *British Journal of Ophthalmology* 69, 600–603.

Foets, B.J.J., Van den Oord, J.J., Billiau, A. *et al.* (1991) Heterogeneous induction of major histocompatibility complex class II antigens on corneal endothelium by interferon-γ. *Investigative Ophthalmology and Visual Science* 32, 341–345.

Foster, C.S. & Duncan, J. (1981) Penetrating keratoplasty for herpes simplex keratitis. *American Journal of Ophthalmology* 92, 336–343.

Gebhardt, B.M. (1981) Factors affecting corneal allograft rejection in inbred rats. *Transplantation Proceedings* 13, 1091–1093.

Gebhardt, B.M. (1988) Cell-mediated immunity in the cornea. *Transplantation* 46, 273–280.

Gebhardt, B.M. (1990) The role of class II antigen-expressing cells in corneal allograft immunity. *Investigative Ophthalmology and Visual Science* 31, 2254–2260.

Gillette, T.E., Chandler, J.W. & Greiner, J.V. (1982) Langerhans cells of the ocular surface. *Ophthalmology* 89, 700–710.

Gore, S.M., Vail, A., Bradley, B.A. *et al.* (1995) HLA-DR matching in corneal transplantation: systematic review of published evidence, *Transplantation* 69, 1033–1039.

Gospodarowicz, D., Greenburg, G. & Alvarodo, J. (1979) Transplantation of cultured bovine endothelial cells to species with non-regenerative endothelium. The cat as an experimental model. *Archives of Ophthalmology* 97, 2163–2169.

Greene, H.S.N. & Lund, P.K. (1944) The heterologous transplantation of human cancers. *Cancer Research* 4, 352–363.

Griffith, T.S., Brunner, T., Fletcher, S.M. *et al.* (1995) Fas ligand-induced apoptosis as a mechanism of immune privilege. *Science* 270, 1189–1192.

Gronemeyer, U., Pülhorn, G. & Müller-Ruchholtz, W. (1978) Allogeneic corneal grafting in inbred strains of rats. *Graefes Archive for Clinical and Experimental Ophthalmology* 208, 247–262.

Hamano, K., Rawsthorne, M.A., Bushell, A.R., Morris, P.J. & Wood, K.J. (1996) Evidence that the continued presence of the organ graft and not peripheral microchimerism is essential for maintenance of tolerance to alloantigens *in vivo* in anti-CD4-treated recipients. *Transplantation* 62, 856–860.

Hanna, C. & Irwin, E.S. (1962) Fate of cells in the corneal graft. *Archives of Ophthalmology* 68, 810–817.

He, Y.-G. & Niederkorn, J.Y. (1996) Depletion of donor-derived Langerhans cells promotes corneal allograft survival. *Cornea* 15, 82–89.

He, Y.-G., Ross, J., Callanan, D. & Niederkorn, J.Y. (1991a) Acceptance of H-Y-disparate corneal grafts despite concomitant immunization of the recipient. *Transplantation* 51, 1258–1262.

He, Y.-G., Ross, J. & Niederkorn, J.Y. (1991b) Promotion of murine heterotopic corneal graft survival by systemic administration of anti-CD4 monoclonal antibody. *Investigative Ophthalmology and Visual Science* 32, 2723–2728.

He, Y., Mellon, J., Apte, R. & Niederkorn, J.Y. (1994) Effect of LFA-1 and ICAM-1 antibody treatment on murine corneal allograft survival. *Investigative Ophthalmology and Visual Science* 35, 3218–3225.

He, Y.-G., Mellon, J. & Niederkorn, J.Y. (1996) The effect of oral immunization on corneal allograft survival. *Transplantation* 61, 920–926.

Hegde, S. & Niederkorn, J.Y. (1999) Cytotoxic T lymphocytes are not essential for corneal graft rejection. *Investigative Ophthalmology and Visual Science* 40 (Suppl.), 250.

Hicks, C.R., Fitton, J.H., Chirila, T.V. *et al.* (1997) Keratoprosthesis: advancing towards a true artificial cornea. *Surveys in Ophthalmology* 42, 175–189.

Hiles, D.A., Biglan, A.W. & Fetherolf, E.C. (1979) Central corneal endothelial counts in children. *Journal of the American Intraocular Implant Society* 5, 292–300.

Hill, J.C. (1989) The use of cyclosporin in high risk keratoplasty. *American Journal of Opthalmology* **107**, 506–510.

Hill, J.C., Maske, R. & Watson, P.G. (1991) The use of a single pulse oftravenous methylprednisolone in the treatment of corneal graft rejection. A preliminary report. *Eye* **5**, 420–424.

Hoffmann, F. & Pahlitzsch, T. (1989) Predisposing factors in corneal graft rejection. *Cornea* **8**, 215–219.

Hoffmann, F., Zhang, E.-P., Pohl, T. *et al.* (1997) Inhibition of corneal allograft reaction by CTLA4-Ig. *Graefes Archive for Clinical and Experimental Ophthalmology* **235**, 535–540.

Holland, E.J., Chan, C.-C., Wetzig, R.P. *et al.* (1991) Clinical and immunohistologic studies of corneal rejection in the rat penetrating keratoplasty model. *Cornea* **10**, 374–380.

Holland, E.J., Olsen, T.W., Chan, C.-C. *et al.* (1994) Kinetics of corneal transplant rejection in the rat penetrating keratoplasty model. *Cornea* **13**, 317–323.

Hori, J., Isobe, M., Yamagami, S. *et al.* (1997) Specific immunosuppression of corneal allograft rejection by combination of anti-LVA-4 and anti-LFA-1 monoclonal antibodies in mice. *Experimental Eye Research* **65**, 89–98.

Hutchinson, I.V., Turner, D.M., Sankaran, D. *et al.* (1998) Influence of cytokine genotypes on allograft rejection. *Transplantation Proceedings* **30**, 862–863.

Imaizumi, T. (1990) Movement of corneal endothelium after penetrating keratoplasty. Observation of sex chromatin as a cell marker. *Acta Societatis Ophthalmologica Japan* **94**, 928–936.

Inomata, H., Smelser, G.K. & Polack, F.M. (1970) Fine structure of regenerating endothelium and Descemet's membrane in normal and rejecting corneal grafts. *American Journal of Ophthalmology* **70**, 48–64.

Insler, M.S. & Lopez, J.H. (1991) Extended incubation times improve corneal endothelial cell transplantation success. *Investigative Ophthalmology and Visual Science* **32**, 1828–1836.

Ippoliti, G. & Fronterrè, A. (1987) Use of locally injected anti-T monoclonal antibodies in the treatment of acute corneal graft rejection. *Transplantation Proceedings* **19**, 2579–2580.

Joo, C.-K., Pepose, J.S. & Stuart, P.M. (1995) T-cell mediated responses in a murine model of orthotopic corneal transplantation. *Investigative Ophthalmology and Visual Science* **36**, 1530–1540.

Kanai, A. & Polack, F.M. (1971a) Ultramicroscopic alterations in corneal epithelium in corneal grafts. *American Journal of Ophthalmology* **72**, 119–126.

Kanai, A. & Polack, F.M. (1971b) Ultramicroscopic changes in the corneal graft stroma during early rejection. *Investigative Ophthalmology* **10**, 415–423.

Kanai, A., Mustakallio, A.H. & Kaufman, H.E. (1972) Electron microscopic studies of corneal endothelium: the abnormal endothelium associated with retrocorneal membrane. *Annals of Ophthalmology* **4**, 564–576.

Katami, M. (1991) Corneal transplantation—immunologically privileged status. *Eye* **5**, 528–548.

Katami, M., White, D.J.G. & Watson, P.G. (1989) An analysis of corneal graft rejection in the rat. *Transplantation Proceedings* **21**, 3147–3149.

Katami, M., Lim, S.M.L., Kamada, N. *et al.* (1990) A pure class II MHC disparity does not induce rejection of cornea or heart grafts in the rat. *Transplantation Proceedings* **22**, 2200–2201.

Katami, M., Graudenz, M.S., White, D.J.G. & Watson, P.G. (1991) The role of antigen-presenting cells in rat corneal graft rejection. *Transplantation Proceedings* **23**, 93–95.

Kaufman, H.E., Varnell, E.D., Kaufman, S. *et al.* (1985) K-sol corneal preservation. *American Journal of Ophthalmology* **100**, 299–304.

Khodadoust, A.A. (1973) The allograft rejection reaction: the leading cause of late faillure of clinical corneal grafts. In: *Corneal Graft Failure: Ciba Foundation Symposium 15* (eds R. Porter & J. Knight), pp. 151–167. Elsevier, Amsterdam.

Khodadoust A.A., Silverstein, A.M. (1969a) The survival and rejection of epithelium in experimental corneal transplants. *Investigative Ophthalmology* **8**, 169–179.

Khodadoust, A.A. & Silverstein, A.M. (1969b) Transplantation and rejection of individual cell layers of the cornea. *Investigative Ophthalmology* **8**, 180–195.

Khodadoust, A.A. & Silverstein, A.M. (1972) Studies on the nature of the privilege enjoyed by corneal allografts. *Investigative Ophthalmology* **11**, 137–148.

Kirkness, C.M., Ezra, E., Rice, N.S.C. & Steele, A.D.McG. (1990) The success and survival of repeat corneal grafts. *Eye* **4**, 58–64.

Kissam, R.S. (1844) Ceratoplastice in man. *New York Journal of Medicine* **2**, 281–283.

Klyce, S.D. & Beuerman, R.W. (1988) Structure and function of the cornea. In: *The Cornea* (eds H.E. Kaufman, B.A. Barron, M.B. McDonald & S.R. Waltman), pp. 3–54. Churchill Livingstone, New York.

Kobyashi, C., Kanai, A., Nakajimi, A. & Okumura, K. (1989) Suppression of corneal graft rejection in rabbits by a new immunosuppressive agent, FK-506. *Transplantation Proceedings* **21**, 3156–3158.

Krachmer, J.H. & Alldredge, O.C. (1978) Subepithelial infiltrates. A probable sign of corneal transplant rejection. *Archives of Ophthalmology* **96**, 2234–2237.

Lang, R.F., Riekhof, F.T. & Steinmuller, D. (1975) Interlamellar corneal grafts in rats. Effect of histocompatibility. *Archives of Ophthalmology* **93**, 349–353.

Larkin D.F.P. & Williams, K.A. (1995) The host response to corneal xenotransplantation. *Eye* **9**, 254–260.

Larkin, D.F.P., Takano, T., Standfield, S.D. & Williams, K.A.

(1995) Experimental orthotopic corneal xenotransplantation in the rat: mechanisms of graft rejection. *Transplantation* **60**, 491–497.

Larkin, D.F.P., Calder, V.L. & Lightman, S.L. (1997) Identification and characterization of cells infiltrating the graft and aqueous humour in rat corneal allograft rejection. *Clinical and Experimental Immunology* **107**, 381–391.

Lechler, R.I. & Batchelor, J.R. (1982) Restoration of immunogenicity to passenger cell-depleted kidney allografts by the addition of donor strain dendritic cells. *Journal of Experimental Medicine* **155**, 31–41.

Lewkowicz-Moss, S.J., Shimeld, C., Lipworth, K. *et al.* (1987) Quantitative studies on Langerhans cells in mouse corneal epithelium following infection with herpes simplex virus. *Experimental Eye Research* **45**, 127–140.

Li, X.-Y., D'Orazio, T. & Niederkorn, J.Y. (1996) Role of Th1 and Th2 cells in anterior chamber-associated immune deviation. *Immunology* **98**, 34–40.

Limberg, M.B., Dingeldein, S.A., Green, M.T. *et al.* (1989) Corneal compression sutures for the reduction of astigmatism after penetrating keratoplasty. *American Journal of Ophthalmology* **108**, 36–42.

Liu, E.Y., Raizman, M.B., Rosner, B. *et al.* (1989) Effects of blood transfusion and cyclosporin on rabbit corneal graft survival. *Current Eye Research* **8**, 523–531.

Ma, D., Mellon, J. & Niederkorn, J.Y. (1997) Oral immunisation as a strategy for enhancing corneal allograft survival. *British Journal of Ophthalmology* **81**, 778–784.

McCarey, B.E. & Kaufman, H.E. (1974) Improved corneal storage. *Investigative Ophthalmology and Visual Science* **13**, 165–173.

McKinney, E.C. & Streilein, J.W. (1989) On the extraordinary capacity of allogeneic epidermal Langerhans cells to prime cytotoxic T cells *in vivo*. *Journal of Immunology* **143**, 1560–1564.

McLeish, W., Rubsamen, P., Atherton, S.A. & Streilein, J.W. (1989) Immunobiology of Langerhans cells on the ocular surface. II. Role of central corneal Langerhans cells in stromal keratitis following experimental HSV-1 infection in mice. *Regional Immunology* **2**, 236–243.

Mahlberg, K., Uusitalo, R.J., Gebhardt, B. & Kaufman, H.E. (1991) Prevention of experimental corneal allograft rejection in rabbits using cyclosporin-collagen shields. *Graefes Archive for Clinical and Experimental Ophthalmology* **229**, 69–74.

Malbran, E.S. & Fernandez-Meijide, R.E. (1982) Bilateral versus unilateral penetrating graft in keratoconus. *Ophthalmology* **89**, 38–43.

Matoba, A.Y., Peeler, J.S. & Niederkorn, J.Y. (1986) T cell subsets in the immune rejection of heterotopic corneal allografts. *Investigative Ophthalmology and Visual Science* **27**, 1244–1254.

Maumenee, A.E. (1951) The influence of donor-recipient sensitization on corneal grafts. *Ophthalmology* **34**, 142–152.

Maumenee, A.E. (1973) Clinical patterns of corneal graft failure. In: *Corneal Graft Failure: Ciba Foundation Symposium 15* (eds R. Porter & J. Knight), pp. 5–23. Elsevier, Amsterdam.

Maumenee, A.E. & Kornblueth, W. (1949) Regeneration of the corneal stromal cells. II. Review of literature and histologic study. *American Journal of Ophthalmology* **32**, 1051–1064.

Maurice, D.M. (1957) The structure and transparency of the cornea. *Journal of Physiology* **136**, 263–286.

Maurice, D.M., McCulley, J.P. & Perlman, M. (1977) Donor endothelium from tissue culture. *Investigative Ophthalmology and Visual Science* **16** (Suppl.), 103.

Medawar, P.B. (1948) Immunity to homologous grafted skin. III. The fate of skin homografts transplanted to the brain, to subcutaneous tissue, and to the anterior chamber of the eye. *British Journal of Pathology* **29**, 58–69.

Meyer, R.F. (1986) Corneal allograft rejection in bilateral penetrating keratoplasty: clinical and laboratory studies. *Transactions of the American Ophthalmological Society* **84**, 664–742.

Michels, R.G., Kenyon, K.R. & Maumenee, A.E. (1972) Retrocorneal fibrous membrane. *Investigative Ophthalmology* **11**, 822–831.

Miller, K., Huber, C., Neiderwieser, D. *et al.* (1988) Succesful engraftment of high-risk corneal allografts with short-term immunosuppresson with cyclosporin. *Transplantation* **45**, 651–653.

Mohan, R.R., Liang, Q., Kim, W.-J. *et al.* (1997) Apoptisis in the cornea: further characterization of Fas/Fas ligand system. *Experimental Eye Research* **65**, 575–589.

Moore, T.E. & Aronson, S.B. (1978) Results of penetrating keratoplasty in keratoconus. *Advances in Ophthalmology* **37**, 106–111.

Muramatsu, R., Kumakura, S., Shimizu, N. *et al.* (1993) Monoclonal antibodies to ICAM-1 and LFA-1 prolong corneal allograft survival in a rat penetrating keratoplasty model. *Investigative Ophthalmology and Visual Science* **34** (Suppl.), 1101.

Nelken, E., Nelken, D., Michaelson, I.C. & Gurevitch, J. (1961) Late clouding of experimental corneal grafts. *Archives of Ophthalmology* **65**, 584–590.

Newton, C., Gebhardt, B.M. & Kaufman, H.E. (1988) Topically applied cyclosporin in azone prolongs corneal allograft survival. *Investigative Ophthalmology and Visual Science* **29**, 208–215.

Nicholls, S.M. (1996) Non-HLA antigens and HLA-DR matching in corneal transplantation. *British Journal of Ophthalmology* **80**, 780–782.

Nicholls, S.M., Bradley, B.A. & Easty, D.L. (1991) Effect of mismatches for major histocompatibility complex and minor antigens on corneal graft rejection. *Investigative Ophthalmology and Visual Science* **32**, 2729–2734.

Nicholls, S.M., Bradley, B.A. & Easty, D.L. (1995) Non-MHC antigens and their relative resistance to immunosuppression after corneal transplantation. *Eye* **9**, 208–214.

Nicholls, S.M., Figueiredo, F.C. & Easty, D.L. (1996) Infiltration of leukocytes and MHC and ICAM-1 expression on the rat corneal endothelium during graft rejection. *Investigative Ophthalmology and Visual Science* **37** (Suppl.), 1113.

Nicholls, S.M., Williams, N.A., Bradley, B.A. & Easty, D.L. (1997) Characterisation of antigenic determinants in corneal transplantation. *Ophthalmology* **92** (Suppl.), 48.

Niederkorn, J.Y. & Streilein, J.W. (1982) Analysis of antibody production induced by allogeneic tumor cells inoculated into the anterior chamber of the eye. *Transplantation* **33**, 573–577.

Niederkorn, J.Y. & Streilein, J.W. (1983) Alloantigens placed into the anterior chamber of the eye induce specific suppression of delayed-type hypersensitivity but normal cytotoxic T lymphocyte and helper T lymphocyte responses. *Journal of Immunology* **131**, 2670–2674.

Niederkorn, J.Y., Peeler, J.S. & Mellon, J. (1989) Phagocytosis of particulate antigens by corneal epithelial cells stimulates interleukin-1 secretion and migration of Langerhans cells into the central cornea. *Regional Immunology* **2**, 83–90.

Niederkorn, J.Y., Callanan, D. & Ross, J.R. (1990) Prevention of the induction of allospecific cytotoxic T lymphocyte and delayed-type hypersensitivity responses by ultraviolet irradiation of corneal allografts. *Transplantation* **50**, 281–286.

Nishi, M., Matsubara, M., Sugawara, I. *et al.* (1990) An immunohistochemical study of rejection process in a rat penetrating keratoplasty model. In: *Ocular Immunology Today* (eds M. Usui, S. Ohno & K. Aoki), pp. 99–102. Elsevier, Amsterdam.

Nishi, M., Herbort, C.P., Matsubara, M. *et al.* (1993) Effects of the immunosuppressant FK506 on a penetrating keratoplasty model in the rat. *Investigative Ophthalmology and Visual Science* **34**, 2477–2486.

Opremcak, E.M., Whisler, R.L. & Dangel, M.E. (1985) Natural killer cells against human corneal endothelium. *American Journal of Ophthalmology* **99**, 524–529.

Oral, H.B., Larkin, D.F.P., Fehervari, Z. *et al.* (1997) *Ex vivo* adenovirus-mediated gene transfer and immunomodulatory protein production in human cornea. *Gene Therapy* **4**, 639–647.

Otsuka, H., Muramatsu, R. & Usui, M. (1990) Immunohistochemical study of corneal allograft rejection in inbred rats. In: *Ocular Immunology Today* (eds M. Usui, S. Ohno & K. Aoki), pp. 147–151. Elsevier, Amsterdam.

Paglen, P.G., Fine, M., Abbot, R.L. & Webster, R.G. (1982) The prognosis for keratoplasty in keratoconus. *Ophthalmology* **89**, 651–654.

Parker, K.E., Dalchau, R., Fowler, V.J. *et al.* (1992) Stimulation of CD4+ T lymphocytes by allogeneic MHC peptides presented on autologous antigen-presenting cells. Evidence of the indirect pathway of allorecognition in some strain combinations. *Transplantation* **53**, 918–924.

Payne, J.W. (1982) Primary penetrating keratoplasty for keratoconus: a long-term followup. *Cornea* **1**, 21–28.

Peeler, J.S. & Niederkorn, J.Y. (1986) Antigen presentation by Langerhans cells *in vivo*: donor-derived Ia+ Langerhans cells are required for induction of delayed-type hypersensitivity but not for cytotoxic T lymphocyte responses to alloantigens. *Journal of Immunology* **138**, 4362–4371.

Peeler, J., Niederkorn, J. & Matoba, A. (1985) Corneal allografts induce cytotoxic T cell but not delayed hypersensitivity responses in mice. *Investigative Ophthalmology and Visual Science* **26**, 1516–1523.

Peeler, J.S., Callanan, D.G., Luckenbach, M.W. & Niederkorn, J.Y. (1988) Presentation of the H-Y antigen on Langerhans' cell-negative corneal grafts downregulates the cytotoxic T cell response and converts responder strain mice into phenotypic nonresponders. *Journal of Experimental Medicine* **168**, 1749–1766.

Pels, E. & Schuchard, Y. (1983) Organ-culture preservation of human corneas. *Documenta Ophthalmologica* **56**, 147–153.

Pepose J.S., Nestor M.S., Gardner J.M. *et al.* (1985a) Composition of cellular infiltrates in rejected human corneal allografts. *Graefes Archive for Clinical and Experimental Ophthalmology* **222**, 128–133.

Pepose, J.S., Gardner, K.M., Nestor, M.S. *et al.* (1985b) Detection of HLA class I and II antigens in rejected human corneal allografts. *Ophthalmology* **92**, 1480–1484.

Philipp, W. & Gottinger, W. (1990) Incidence and function of Langerhans cells in various corneal diseases. *Fortschritte der Ophthalmologie* **87**, 124–127.

Pleyer, U., Steuhl, K.P., Weidle, E.G. *et al.* (1992) Corneal graft rejection: incidence manifestation, and interaction of clinical subtypes. *Transplantation Proceedings* **4**, 2034–2037.

Pleyer, U., Milani, J.K., Ruckert, D. *et al.* (1997) Determinations of serum tumor necrosis factor alpha in corneal allografts. *Ocular Immunology and Inflammation* **5**, 149–155.

Polack, F.M. (1962) Histopathological and histochemical alterations in the early stages of corneal graft rejection. *Journal of Experimental Medicine* **116**, 709–717.

Polack, F.M. (1966) The pathologic anatomy of corneal graft rejection. *Surveys in Ophthalmology* **11**, 391–404.

Polack, F.M. (1973) Corneal graft rejection: clinico-pathological correlation. In: *Corneal Graft Failure: Ciba*

*Foundation Symposium* 15 (eds R. Porter & J. Knight), pp. 127–150. Elsevier, Amsterdam.

Polack, F.M. & Gonzales, C.E. (1968) The response of the lymphoid tissue to corneal heterografts. *Archives of Ophthalmology* **80**, 321–324.

Polack, F.M. & Kanai, A. (1972) Electron microscopic studies of graft endothelium in corneal graft rejection. *American Journal of Ophthalmology* **73**, 711–717.

Polack, F.M. & Smelser, G.K. (1962) The persistence of isotopically labeled cells in corneal grafts. *Proceedings of the Society for Experimental Biology and Medicine* **110**, 60–61.

Raju, S. & Grogan, J.B. (1971) Immunology of the anterior chamber of the eye. *Transplantation Proceedings* **3**, 605–608.

Rapuano, C.J., Cohen, E.J., Brady, S.E. *et al.* (1990) Indications for and outcomes of repeat penetrating keratoplasty. *American Journal of Ophthalmology* **109**, 689–695.

Ray-Keil, L. & Chandler, J.W. (1985) Rejection of murine heterotopic corneal transplants. *Transplantation* **39**, 473–477.

Ray-Keil, L. & Chandler, J.W. (1986) Reduction in the incidence of rejection of heterotopic murine corneal transplants by pretreatment with ultraviolet radiation. *Transplantation* **42**, 403–406.

Redmond, R.M., Armitage, W.J., Whittle, J., Moss, S.J. & Easty, D.L. (1992) Long-term survival of endothelium following transplantation of corneas stored by organ culture. *British Journal of Ophthalmology* **76**, 479–481.

Reisinger, F. (1824) Die Keratoplastik: ein Versuch zur Erweiterung der Augenheilkunde. *Bayerische Annalen Chirogische Augenheilkunde* **1**, 207.

Richard, J.M., Paton, D. & Gasset, A.R. (1977) A comparison of penetrating and lamellar keratoplasty in the surgical management of keratoconus. *American Journal of Ophthalmology* **86**, 807.

Rinne, J.R. & Stulting, R.D. (1992) Current practices in the prevention and treatment of corneal graft rejection. *Cornea* **11**, 326–328.

Roelen, D.L., Van Beelen, E., Van Bree, S.P.M.J. *et al.* (1995) The presence of activated donor class I-reactive T lymphocytes is associated with rejection of corneal grafts. *Transplantation* **59**, 1039–1042.

Ross, J., He, Y.-G., Pidherney, M., Mellon, J. & Niederkorn, J.Y. (1991a) The differential effect of donor versus host Langerhans cells in the rejection of MHC-matched corneal allografts. *Transplantation* **52**, 857–861.

Ross, J., He, Y.-G. & Niederkorn, J.Y. (1991b) Class I disparate corneal grafts enjoy afferent but not efferent blockade of the immune response. *Current Eye Research* **10**, 889–892.

Ross, J., Callanan, D., Kunz, H. & Niederkorn, J. (1991c) Evidence that the fate of class II-disparate corneal grafts is determined by the timing of class II expression. *Transplantation* **51**, 532–536.

Ross, J.R., Howell, D.N. & Sanfilippo, F.P. (1993) Characteristics of corneal xenograft rejection in a discordant species combination. *Investigative Ophthalmology and Visual Science* **34**, 2469–2476.

Ross, J.R., Sanfilippo, F.P. & Howell, D.N. (1994) Histopathologic features of rejecting orthotopic corneal xenografts. *Current Eye Research* **13**, 725–730.

Rozenman, J., Arentsen, J.J. & Laibson, P.R. (1985) Corneal transplant allograft reactions in unilateral, double corneal transplants. *Cornea* **4**, 25–29.

Rubsamen, P.E., McCulley, J., Bergstresser, P.B. & Streilein, J.W. (1984) On the Ia immunogenicity of mouse corneal allografts infiltrated with Langerhans cells. *Investigative Ophthalmology and Visual Science* **25**, 513–518.

Sanfilippo, F. & Foulks, G.N. (1989) The role of histocompatibility in human corneal transplantation. *Transplantation Proceedings* **21**, 3127–3129.

Sanfilippo, F., MacQueen, J.M., Vaughn, W.K. & Foulks, G.N. (1986) Reduced graft rejection with good HLA-A and B matching in high-risk corneal transplantation. *New England Journal of Medicine* **315**, 29–35.

Sano, Y., Ksander, B.R. & Streilein, J.W. (1995) Fate of corneal allografts in eyes that cannot support anterior chamber-associated immune deviation induction. *Investigative Ophthalmology and Visual Science* **36**, 2176–2185.

Sano, Y., Ksander, B.R. & Streilein, J.W. (1996) Minor H, rather than MHC, alloantigens offer the greater barrier to successful orthotopic corneal transplantation in mice. *Transplant Immunology* **4**, 53–56.

Sellerbeck, S. (1878) Über Keratoplastik. *Graefes Archive for Clinical and Experimental Ophthalmology* XXIV **4**, 1–46.

Setzer, P.Y., Nichols, B.A. & Dawson, C.R. (1987) Unusual structure of rat conjunctival epithelium. *Investigative Ophthalmology and Visual Science* **27**, 531–537.

She, S.-C., Steahly, L.P. & Moticka, E.J. (1990) A method for performing full thickness, orthotopic, penetrating keratoplasty in the mouse. *Ophthalmic Surgery* **21**, 781–785.

Shepherd, W.F.I., Coster, D.J., Chin Fook, T. *et al.* (1980) Effect of cyclosporin A on the survival of corneal grafts in rabbits. *British Journal of Ophthalmology* **64**, 148–153.

Sherwood, R.A., Brent, L. & Rayfield, L.S. (1986) Presentation of alloantigens by host cells. *European Journal of Immunology* **16**, 569–574.

Shewring, L., Collins, L., Lightman, S.L. *et al.* (1997) A non-viral vector system for efficient gene transfer to corneal endothelial cells via membrane integrins. *Transplantation* **64**, 763–769.

Silverstein, A.M. & Khodadoust, A.A. (1973) Transplantation immunobiology of the cornea. In: *Corneal Graft Failure: Ciba Foundation Symposium 15* (eds R. Porter & J. Knight), pp. 105–125. Elsevier, Amsterdam.

Simpson, E. (1998) Minor transplantation antigens. Animal models for human host-versus-graft, graft-versus-host, and graft-versus-leukemia reactions. *Transplantation* **65**, 611–616.

Smiddy, W.E., Stark, W.J., Young, E. *et al.* (1986) Clinical and immunological results of corneal allograft rejection. *Ophthalmic Surgery* **17**, 644–649.

Smolin, G. & Hyndiuk, R.A. (1971) Lymphatic drainage from vascularized rabbit cornea. *American Journal of Ophthalmology* **72**, 147–151.

Sonoda, Y. & Streilein, J.W. (1992) Orthotopic corneal transplantation in mice—evidence that the immunogenetic rules of rejection do not apply. *Transplantation* **54**, 694–704.

Sonoda, Y. & Streilein, J.W. (1993) Impaired cell-mediated immunity in mice bearing healthy orthotopic corneal allografts. *Journal of Immunology* **150**, 1727–1734.

Sonoda, Y., Sano, Y., Ksander, B. & Streilein, J.W. (1995) Characterisation of cell-mediated immune responses elicited by orthotopic corneal allografts in mice. *Investigative Ophthalmology and Visual Science* **36**, 427–434.

Stark, W.J. (1980) Transplantation immunology of penetrating keratoplasty. *Transactions of the American Ophthalmological Society* **78**, 1079–1117.

Streilein, J.W. & Wegmann, T.G. (1987) Immunologic privilege in the eye and the fetus. *Immunology Today* **8**, 362–366.

Streilein, J.W., Toews, G.B. & Bergstresser, P.R. (1979) Corneal allografts fail to express Ia antigens. *Nature* **282**, 326–327.

Streilein, J.W., McCulley, J. & Niederkorn, J.Y. (1982) Heterotopic corneal grafting in mice: a new approach to the study of corneal alloimmunity. *Investigative Ophthalmology and Visual Science* **23**, 489–500.

Stuart, P.M., Griffith, T.S., Usui, N. *et al.* (1997) CD95 ligand (FasL) -induced apoptosis is necessary for corneal allograft survival. *Journal of Clinical Investigations* **99**, 396–402.

Stulting, R.D., Waring, G.O., Bridges, W.Z. & Cavanagh, H.D. (1988) Effect of donor epithelium on corneal transplant survival. *Ophthalmology* **95**, 803–812.

Sundmacher, R. (1985) The role of donor epithelium in perforating keratoplasty. *Developmental Ophthalmology* **11**, 61–67.

Takano, T. & Williams, K.A. (1995) Mechanism of corneal endothelial destruction in rejecting rat corneal allografts and xenografts: a role for CD4+ cells. *Transplantation Proceedings* **27**, 260–261.

Takeuchi, M., Kosiewicz, M.M., Alard, P. & Streilein, J.W. (1997) On the mechanism by which transforming growth factor-beta2 alters antigen presenting abilities of macrophages on T cell activation. *European Journal of Immunology* **27**, 1648–1656.

Taylor, A.W., Alard, P., Yee, D.G. & Streilein, J.W. (1997) Aqueous humor induces transforming growth factor-beta (TGF-beta) -producing regulatory T cells. *Current Eye Research* **16**, 900–908.

Torres, P.F., De Vos, A.F., Van der Gaag, R., Martins, B. & Kijlstra, A. (1996) Cytokine mRNA expression during experimental corneal allograft rejection. *Experimental Eye Research* **63**, 453–461.

Treseler, P.A. & Sanfilippo, F. (1985) Humoral immunity to heterotopic corneal allografts in the rat. *Transplantation* **39**, 193–195.

Treseler, P.A. & Sanfilippo, F. (1986) The expression of major histocompatibility complex and leukocyte antigens by cells in the rat cornea. *Transplantation* **41**, 248–252.

Treseler, P.A., Foulks, G.N. & Sanfilippo, F. (1984) The expression of HLA antigens by cells of the human cornea. *American Journal of Ophthalmology* **98**, 763–772.

Treseler, P.A., Treseler, C.B., Foulks, G.N. & Sanfilippo, F. (1985) Cellular immunity to heterotopic corneal allografts in the rat. *Transplantation* **39**, 196–201.

Troutman, R.C. & Gaster, R.N. (1980) Surgical advances and results of keratoconus. *American Journal of Ophthalmology* **90**, 131–136.

Tuberville, A.W., Foster, C.S. & Wood, T.O. (1983) The effect of donor cornea epithelium removal on the incidence of allograft rejection reactions. *Ophthalmology* **90**, 1351–1356.

Tuft, S.J., Williams, K.A. & Coster, D.J. (1986) Endothelial repair in the rat cornea. *Investigative Ophthalmology and Visual Science* **27**, 1199–1204.

Tullo, A.B. (1982) Corneal transplantation in Bristol, 1970–80. *Bristol Medico-Chirurgical Journal* **97**, 17–20.

United Kingdom Transplant Support Service Authority (1996) *Corneal Transplant Audit, 1991–94*, p. 20. UKTSSA.

Vail, A., Gore, S.M., Bradley, B.A. *et al.* (1993) Corneal transplantation in the United Kingdom and Republic of Ireland. *British Journal of Ophthalmology* **77**, 650–656.

Vail, A., Gore, S.M., Bradley, B.A. *et al.* (1994) Corneal graft survival and visual outcome: a multi-center study. *Ophthalmology* **101**, 120–127.

Vail, A., Gore, S.M., Bradley, B.A. *et al.* (1996) Clinical and surgical factors influencing corneal graft survival, visual acuity and astigmatism. *Ophthalmology* **103**, 41–49.

Vail, A., Gore, S.M., Bradley, B.A. *et al.* (1997) Conclusions of the corneal transplant follow up study. *British Journal of Ophthalmology* **81**, 631–636.

Van der Veen, G., Broersma, L., Dijkstra, C.D. *et al.* (1994) Prevention of corneal allograft rejection in rats treated with subconjunctival injection of dichloromethylene diphosphonate. *Investigative Ophthalmology and Visual Science* 35, 3505–3515.

Van Horn, D.L., Sendele, D.D., Seideman, S. & Buco, P.J. (1977) Regenerative capacity of the corneal endothelium in rabbit and cat. *Investigative Ophthalmology and Visual Science* 16, 597–613.

Völker-Dieben, H.J., Kok-van Alphen, C.C., Lansbergen, Q. & Persijn, G.G. (1982) The effect of prospective HLA-A and B matching on corneal graft survival. *Acta Ophthalmologica* 60, 203–213.

Völker-Dieben, H.J., Kok-van Alphen, C.C., D'Amaro, J. & de-Lange, P. (1984) The effect of prospective HLA-A and -B matching in 288 penetrating keratoplasties for herpes simplex keratitis. *Acta Ophthalmologica* 62, 513–523.

Völker-Dieben, H.J., D'Amaro, J.D. & Kok-van Alphen, C.C. (1987) Hierarchy of prognostic factors for corneal allograft survival. *Australian and New Zealand Journal of Ophthalmology* 15, 11–18.

Whitsett, C.F. & Stulting, R.D. (1984) The distribution of HLA antigens on human corneal tissue. *Investigative Ophthalmology and Visual Science* 25, 519–524.

Whittum, J.A., Niederkorn, J.A., McCulley, J.P. & Streilein, J.W. (1983) Intracameral inoculation of herpes simplex virus Type 1 induces anterior chamber-associated immune deviation. *Current Eye Research* 2, 691–697.

Wieczorek, R., Jakobiec, F.A., Sacks, E.H. & Knowles, D.M. (1988) The immunoarchitecture of the normal human lacrimal gland. Relevancy for understanding pathologic conditions. *Ophthalmology* 95, 100–109.

Wilbanks, G.A., Mammolent, M. & Streilein, J.W. (1992) Studies on the induction of anterior chamber-associated immune deviation (ACAID) III. Induction of ACAID depends on intraocular transforming growth factor beta. *European Journal of Immunology* 22, 165–173.

Williams, K.A. & Coster, D.J. (1985) Penetrating corneal transplantation in the inbred rat: a new model. *Investigative Ophthalmology and Visual Science* 26, 23–30.

Williams, K.A., Ash, J.K. & Coster, D.J. (1985a) Histocompatibility antigen and passenger cell content of normal and diseased human cornea. *Transplantation* 39, 265–269.

Williams, K.A., Grutzmacher, R.D., Roussel, T.J. & Coster, D.J. (1985b) A comparison of the effects of topical cyclosporine and topical steroid on rabbit corneal allograft rejection. *Transplantation* 39, 242–244.

Williams, K.A., Mann, T.S., Lewis, M. & Coster, D.J. (1986) The role of resident accessory cells in corneal allograft rejection in the rabbit. *Transplantation* 42, 667–671.

Williams, K.A., Ash, J.K., Mann, T.S. & Coster, D.J. (1987a) Antigen-presenting capabilities of cells infiltrating inflamed corneas. *Transplantation Proceedings* 19, 225.

Williams, K.A., Erickson, S.A. & Coster, D.J. (1987b) Topical steroid, cyclosporin A, and the outcome of rat corneal allografts. *British Journal of Ophthalmology* 71, 239–242.

Williams, K.A., White, M.A., Ash, J.K. & Coster, D.J. (1989) Leukocytes in the graft bed associated with corneal graft failure. Analysis by immunohistology and actuarial graft survival. *Ophthalmology* 96, 38–44.

Williams, K.A., Standfield, S.D., Wing, S.J. *et al.* (1992) Patterns of corneal graft rejection in the rabbit and reversal of rejection with monoclonal antibodies. *Transplantation* 54, 38–43.

Williams, K.A., Muehlberg, S.M., Lewis, R.F., Giles, L.C. & Coster, D.J. (eds on behalf of all contributors) (1997) *The Australian Corneal Graft Registry: 1996 Report.* Mercury Press, Adelaide, Australia.

Williams, K.A., Standfield, S.D., Mills R.A.D. *et al.* (1999) A new model of orthotopic penetrating corneal transplantation in the sheep: graft survival, phenotypes of graft-infiltrating cells and local cytokine production. *Australian and New Zealand Journal of Ophthalmology* 27, 127–135.

Wilson, S.E. & Kaufman, H.E. (1990) Graft failure after penetrating keratoplasty. *Surveys in Ophthalmology* 34, 325–336.

Woodruff, M.E.A. (1952) The transplantation of homologous tissue and its surgical applications. *Annals of the Royal College of Surgeons (England)* 11, 173–194.

Young, E., Stark, W.J. & Prendergast, R.A. (1985) Immunology of corneal allograft rejection: HLA-DR antigens on human corneal cells. *Investigative Ophthalmology and Visual Science* 26, 571–574.

Zirm, E. (1906) Eine erfolgreiche totale Keratoplastik. *Graefes Archive for Clinical and Experimental Ophthalmology* 64, 580–593.

# Chapter 14/Skin transplantation

MARGARET A. STANLEY

## Introduction

The skin is the largest organ of the body; in the average human it exceeds 2 m² in area but in most sites is no more than 2 mm thick. This organ, a sheet-like covering of the whole body, forms a physical barrier with the external environment which, none the less, is exquisitely adapted to the body contours and flexibly adjusts to every movement. The skin barrier prevents fluid loss and desiccation and protects against injury, whether chemical, traumatic or microbial. The skin vasculature and the sweating system are central to thermoregulation and the extensive neuroreceptor network represents a unique sensing system transducing environmental information to the interior of the organism.

Skin transplantation is a special challenge because it involves the problem of organ morphogenesis irrespective of the immunological issues which must be addressed with allografts.

## Skin structure and organization

Skin is a complex organ consisting of two layers: an outer epidermis and an inner dermis. The epidermis varies little in thickness, 75–150 μm, over the whole body except on the palms and soles where it can reach 0.6 mm; it forms a continuous sheet ending at mucocutaneous junctions and is perforated only by the pores of

secretory and excretory glands and the follicles from which hairs emerge. The epidermis is a stratified squamous epithelium consisting mainly of keratinocytes —cells characterized by a keratin polypeptide intermediate filament network. The keratinocytes are arranged in an ordered spatial array with proliferation restricted to the basal layer, cells leaving this layer commit themselves to a differentiation programme which terminates in the production of anucleate squamae or corneocytes, which form a tough protective barrier to the outside. Other minor cell populations of the epidermis include melanocytes, Merkel cells and the antigen-presenting cell of the skin, the Langerhans' cell.

The dermis is a complex tissue supporting extensive vascular and nerve networks and enclosing specialized glandular structures for excretion and secretion and the appendages of nail and hair. It varies considerably in thickness, ranging from 1 mm on the scalp to 4 mm on the back and is divided into an upper papillary and lower 'deep' or reticular dermis, the dominant cell in both being the dermal fibroblast, whose synthetic products, collagens, glycosaminoglycans and glycoproteins, provide the dominant structural elements.

The papillary dermis is highly vascular and cellular with a loosely distributed collagen and elastin network compared to the relatively avascular, acellular, densely collagenous and elastic reticular dermis. Both the dermis and epidermis are infiltrated daily by populations of lymphocytes and phagocytes, all contributing to a dynamic, highly regulated and organized cellular society. The dermo-epidermal junction or basement membrane zone (BMZ) consists of matrix components synthesized by the overlying basal keratinocytes. This is traversed by filamentous structures or anchoring fibrils, composed of collagen type VII, forming macromolecular attachments with the dermal collagens and the epidermal hemidesmosomes, anchoring together dermis and epidermis.

The keratinocytes of the epidermis form a self-renewing population, with basal cells forming the proliferative compartment from which cells migrate upward, differentiating as they progress to be exfoliated or desquamated from the surface and replaced by new cells from below. Such a self-renewing population by definition contains a subset of cells with stem cell properties and there is a keratinocyte lineage extending from primitive stem cell to differentiated anucleate squamae.

In hair-bearing skin in rodents, cells with stem cell properties are found in two sites: in the interfollicular epidermis in the centre of the epidermal proliferative unit or EPU (Morris *et al.* 1985); and the bulge zone of the hair follicle (Miller *et al.* 1993). The stem cells found in the hair follicle are pluripotential, capable of regenerating not only the hair follicle but also sebaceous glands and epidermis. In human hair follicles, cells with the properties of stem cells can be identified in a region outside the bulb at the mid-point of the follicle below the site of insertion of the arrector pili muscle; this point of insertion corresponds with the bulge region, when this can be identified, in human hair follicles (Rochat *et al.* 1994). There is no experimental evidence that these stem cells in human hair follicles are pluripotential. Full-thickness wounds on skin do not result in the regeneration of the organ but instead the process is one of repair, with re-epithelialization of the overlying epidermis and scar formation in the dermis. Partial regeneration of large wounds is achieved by autografting split-thickness skin but in these situations no regeneration of the skin adnexae, hair follicles and sweat glands occurs, illustrating the importance of the anatomical location of the pluripotential stem cells.

## Skin grafts

Skin replacement by transplantation is a life-saving procedure for patients who have suffered extensive skin loss. Burn wounds illustrate the problems of skin grafting in these situations. In most burn centres the accepted treatment for deep partial (second-degree) (see Fig. 14.1) and full-thickness (third-degree) burns is immediate surgical excision and wound coverage with a split-skin autograft. Early wound coverage is important as this reduces fluid loss and sepsis, promotes wound healing and reduces scarring and contracture. The best skin autograft is one from an adjacent undamaged area which matches the defective region in colour, texture and thickness. Unfortunately this is rarely available and skin for grafting is taken from the available and accessible areas.

In patients with extensive skin loss there is a limited availability of donor sites from which skin for autografts can be excised and this fact directly relates to the high mortality rate in extensively burned patients. Various strategies, such as meshing (Tanner *et al.* 1964) or dicing (Nanchahal 1989), are used to increase the area of the donor graft and to minimize the effect of limited donor sites and expansion ratios of up to 1:9 and 1:20, respectively, can be achieved by these techniques. Unexpanded grafts are used preferentially on exposed areas, such as hands and feet, because these grafts give a better cosmetic effect than meshed grafts, which appear to promote the development of contractures and enhanced scarring. Meshed grafts cover larger areas and permit drainage of blood and exudate but grafts expanded by more than 1:4 must be overlaid with biological or synthetic dressings to stabilize the mesh and prevent fluid loss and microbial contamination.

Other strategies (some of which will be considered in detail later) include covering the wound initially with short-term biological dressings, such as cadaveric skin allograft or porcine skin xenograft, or synthetic dressings, such as Biobrane. However, temporary substitutes for wound cover must eventually be replaced by autograft as healed donor sites become available for repeat harvesting. Delays in grafting do result in increased scarring with consequent loss of function and disfigure-

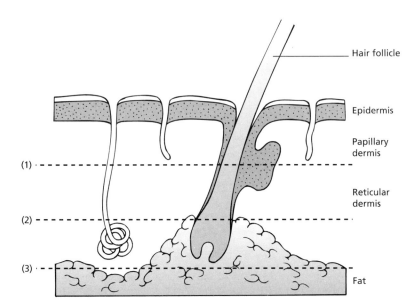

Fig. 14.1 Classification of burn wounds. 1, Superficial partial-thickness burn leaving the skin adnexae intact; 2, deep partial-thickness burn leaving only the deep portion of the hair follicle intact, involving the reticular dermis and breaching the dermis–fat interface; 3, full-thickness burn involving all structures.

ment. The reality is that the size and depth of the wound increases mortality and the survivors of extensive burn injuries who have limited donor sites have long-term functional and cosmetic sequelae which limit the resumption of normal life. All this is well recognized and has fuelled the search for alternatives to the split-skin autograft for long-term wound coverage.

## Cultured autologous keratinocyte grafts

One approach to the problem of limited donor sites for skin coverage would be to culture skin *in vitro* and to graft this on to freshly excised wounds. The technologies to produce skin as a complete organ (epidermis and dermis) *in vitro* do not exist at present but those to generate cultured epidermis in the form of sheets of cultured keratinocytes do.

The serial cultivation of human epidermal keratinocytes was described in seminal experiments in 1975 (Rheinwald & Green 1975). Prior to this work primary cultures of keratinocytes, either from explants or from single-cell suspensions of enzyme-disaggregated tissue, had been relatively easy to pro-

duce but serial cultivation, and hence amplification of these cells had proved elusive. In the Rheinwald and Green technique an enzyme-disaggregated single-cell suspension of epidermis is produced and a cell aliquot inoculated on to a lawn of lethally irradiated mouse fibroblast cells, usually 3T3 cells (Todaro & Green 1963). These cells are then cultured in conventional growth medium consisting of Dulbecco's modification of Eagle's medium supplemented with fetal bovine serum and hydrocortisone. Keratinocyte colony formation in this culture methodology is enhanced substantially by agents which activate adenyl cyclase, particularly cholera toxin (Green 1978), and keratinocyte motility and proliferation is increased by epidermal growth factor (Rheinwald & Green 1977). Insulin, transferrin and tri-iodothyronine stimulate cell growth and promote the *in vitro* longevity of keratinocytes. The most satisfactory medium for epidermal keratinocytes in the feeder support technique is a mixture of Dulbecco's medium and Ham's F12 with the supplements listed above.

The fibroblast feeder layer is of central importance in permitting growth at clonal density and the serial cultivation of keratinocytes. The irradiated fibroblasts both provide matrix proteins and growth factors and induce the overlying keratinocytes to generate these. They may also act as a regulatory barrier degrading or sequestering inhibitory factors and possibly regulating $Ca^{2+}$ gradients. Keratinocytes grown using this technique have an *in vitro* life ranging from 60 to 200 population doublings (four to eight subcultivations) depending upon the age of the donor. In practical terms this means that a 1–2 cm$^2$ biopsy can be expanded by up to 10 000 times in a 30-day period. In these cultures the keratinocytes form confluent sheets from which the 3T3 feeder cells have been expelled as a consequence of expansion and fusion of colonies. However, prior to their use as grafts any remaining 3T3 cells are removed by treatment with EDTA or other chelating agents and growth factors and serum removed by extensive washing. There remains the theoretical possibility of an immune response to residual serum or foreign proteins transferred with the autologous keratinocytes but this does not appear to be a problem in practice. Culture systems which do not require feeder support are available (Boyce & Ham 1983) but have not always permitted the required cell number amplification (Marks & Dykes 1983).

Sheets of autologous cultured keratinocytes were first used successfully for grafting burns patients by O'Connor *et al.* (1981). Several other groups subsequently reported success using cultured autologous keratinocyte (CKG) on burned patients and this technique has been widely used, with many hundreds of patients having received such grafts. CKG have also been used to cover leg and decubitus ulcers (Hefton *et al.* 1986; Leigh & Purkis 1986), defects resulting from the excision of giant naevi (Gallico *et al.* 1989), individuals with epidermolysis bullosa (Carter *et al.* 1987) and toxic epidermal necrolysis (Birchall *et al.* 1987).

The results obtained with CKG have been variable (Meuli & Raghunath 1997). Spontaneous blistering and breakdown of grafts, which then required split-skin grafting, have been reported in several studies, particularly in burns patients (Woodley *et al.* 1988; Paddle Ledinek *et al.* 1997). These defects were prominent in areas of dermal loss (Kumagai *et al.* 1988; Woodley *et al.* 1988). Such instability of the grafted epithelium may be related to abnormal reformation of

the BMZ and anchoring filaments (Desai *et al.* 1991). Studies on CKG grafted on to fascia revealed the presence of most of the normal components of dermis by day 10 post-grafting although there was a marked reduction or complete absence of anchoring filaments up to 7 months post-grafting (Birchall *et al.* 1987) and a paucity of elastic tissue.

The most extensive study on skin regeneration post-CK grafting has been a 5-year follow-up study of 23 paediatric patients with full-thickness burns (Nanchahal & Ward 1992). All CKG in this study were applied to beds of muscle fascia which had been prepared for up to 3 weeks with cadaver allograft or xenograft or the synthetic dressing, Biobrane. A complete dermo-epidermal junction formed within 3–4 weeks post-grafting although full maturation of anchoring fibrils required more than a year. Epidermal rete ridges regenerated within 6 weeks to 1 year post-grafting. Initially the subepidermal connective tissue formed a normal scar but remodelled subsequently to resemble a true dermis within 4–5 years. This contrasted with meshed graft controls, which showed no rete ridge regeneration or connective tissue remodelling.

The degree of contracture has also been variable, as compared to split-skin grafts. In some studies CK grafting has been reported to lead to the same degree of contracture as split-skin grafting (O'Connor *et al.* 1981; Compton *et al.* 1989; Teepe *et al.* 1990b) although no quantitative data on contraction were given in these studies. However, Gallico *et al.* (1989), in a study in which CK were used to graft after excision of giant hairy naevi in eight children, reported 30% contracture in one patient as compared to 95% for split-skin grafts. Others have observed contracture rates of 50% for CKG (Clugston *et al.* 1991).

A major problem with CKG has been the extreme variability of graft 'take'. Encouraging reports, often on small series of patients, gave clinical estimations of take as high as 80% for CKG on burn wounds (Gallico *et al.* 1984; Munster *et al.* 1990). However, other studies, principally from Europe, have reported levels of take varying from 2 to 50%. The crucial factor in all these problems is the nature of the wound bed and the absence of a dermal component (Hunyadi *et al.* 1988).

Studies in the mouse (McKenzie & Fusenig 1983), showed quite clearly that epidermal sheets transplanted without dermis seldom re-formed an organized epidermal structure. Furthermore, they showed that epidermis transplanted in combination with non-dermal connective tissues such as muscle fascia and tendon exhibited poor survival and any epidermis which did survive showed poor organization and maturation.

Comparable observations were made (Blight *et al.* 1991) in a careful clinical study detailing the results of applying CKG to full-thickness burn wounds on 89 sites in 26 patients. The overall estimate of take varied from 0 to 98% with a mean of 15% and graft take was directly related to the constitution of the wound bed. When CKG were applied to freshly excised areas the average graft take was low, of the order of 8%; this is in direct contrast to split-skin grafts, where such wound beds result in good graft take. Granulation tissue was also found to be a poor wound bed for CKG with an average take of 10% and this, in contrast to other studies (Teepe *et al.* 1988; De Luca *et al.* 1989), was not related to bacterial colonization of the wound bed. Bacterial colonization in any wound bed correlated with poor CKG take, an observation confirmed in other reports (Teepe *et al.* 1990b; Barillo *et al.* 1992; Odessey 1992). CKG was most successful when the wound bed had been pretreated with allogeneic split-skin graft as a biological wound dressing, resulting in successful CKG take of 43%. Many other studies confirm this observation and there is no doubt that, when biological dressings, such as allogeneic dermis in the form of fresh or cryopreserved cadaver skin or porcine skin xenograft, are used prior to grafting with CK sheets, success in terms of take and long-term wound coverage is very much enhanced.

Temporary wound coverage with allograft or xenograft combined with expanded split-skin mesh grafts have been used widely to achieve burn wound coverage (Yang *et al.* 1979; Alexander *et al.* 1981; Herndon & Rutan 1992; Kreis *et al.* 1992; Hussmann *et al.* 1994). For reasons discussed later rejection of this foreign tissue is variable but under optimal conditions the allo- or xenograft persists for long enough to permit outgrowth and coverage from the meshed autograft.

Cuono *et al.* (1986) were the first to report successful combination of dermal allograft and autologous CKG. In this study the allograft skin, consisting of epidermis and dermis, was grafted immediately on to excised burn wounds, where it functioned as a true graft and not merely as a biological dressing. The autograft was then abraded, leaving a dermal base which supported the engraftment of the keratinocyte cultures and integration of keratinocyte and dermis into a successful permanent replacement. Light and ultrastructural microscopic studies of these grafts showed that reconstitution of the dermo-epidermal junction commenced at 7 weeks and was complete by 13 weeks (Langdon *et al.* 1988), observations comparable to others (Compton *et al.* 1989).

Clinical studies imply that a dermis is essential for proper epidermal regeneration but experimental systems are essential if the role of the dermis and the mechanisms involved are to be understood. Animal models for studying the significance of dermis for grafting cultured keratinocytes on to full-thickness wounds have been developed in the pig (Kangesu *et al.* 1993; Navsaria *et al.* 1994) and in rodents (Leary *et al.* 1992). Both models use a transplantation technique which allows the isolation of the graft from the host skin by a silicone transplantation chamber, a methodology first described by Worst *et al.* (1974). In brief, full-thickness wounds are made on the dorsal flanks of animals and a skin pocket formed in which the wound bed may be manipulated. The transplantation chamber has a circular flanged base, which is inserted under the skin flaps of the wound edge; the graft is placed in the centre of the chamber and is effectively isolated from the host skin by the physical barrier of the chamber flanges.

Using this system in the porcine model the effect of the wound bed on the take of CKG and the subsequent maturation of the grafted keratinocytes have been carefully detailed (Kangesu *et al.* 1993). In this study keratodermal grafts were prepared in a two-step protocol in which de-epidermized dermis was initially grafted to form a dermal bed, which was overlaid 7 days later with cultured keratinocyte sheets. The fate of these grafts was compared to CKG on granulating wound beds. Graft take of CK on a dermal bed was a mean of 47% compared to 4% on granulating beds. The keratodermal grafts were fragile but durable and histologically the epidermis which re-formed resembled normal skin with rete ridges, normal stratification and cornification. The epidermis which re-formed after CKG on granulating wounds was histologically immature with no rete ridges although ultrastructural studies indicated that the basement membrane zone and basal keratinocytes were the same in both grafts. A crucial element of epidermal stability is the anchoring complex of fibrils and hemidesmosomes of the BMZ. In the porcine model epidermis re-formed after CK grafting on granulating beds showed normal numbers of anchoring fibrils and hemidesmosomes but the length of these elements did not reach the normal size during the period of study. Furthermore, collagen appeared slowly in the granulating wound bed and the epidermis could be easily avulsed from it with the plane of cleavage being at the junction of the basement membrane and the granulation tissue. In keratodermal grafts, neovascularization followed by innervation occurred rapidly and was almost complete 6 weeks post-grafting (Gu *et al.* 1995). This early angiogenesis probably plays a crucial part in the survival of the cultured keratinocyte sheets in the keratodermal grafts.

Further information on the importance of the dermis has come from the work of Leary *et al.* (1992), who examined the role of dermal factors in the maintenance of epidermal stem cells. These studies showed that in the mouse, epidermis grafted in the absence of dermis lost the capacity for self-renewal measured as the ability of the grafted epidermis to grow as proliferative keratinocyte colonies *in vitro*. These experimental observations were supported by clinical studies in which biopsies from cultured keratinocytes grafted on to excised wounds on leg ulcers failed to grow in culture whereas full-thickness skin adjacent to the grafts formed progressively growing keratinocyte colonies in culture. This suggested that keratinocyte stem cells were dependent upon dermal factors for the maintenance of the self-renewal phenotype in a manner analogous to haemopoietic stem cells, which are dependent upon a heterologous cell, the stromal cell, for growth factors and matrix signals (Spooncer *et al.* 1985). This hypothesis has been supported by the observation that keratinocytes grafted on to wound

beds seeded with dermal papilla cells retain self-renewal capacity (D.M. Anderson and M.A. Stanley, unpublished data).

The fate of the allogeneic dermis in the combined keratodermal grafts is not entirely clear. The dermal component of the cadaver allograft is not, or is rarely rejected and this may be attributed to several factors. Major burn injuries are associated with immunosuppression (Deitch 1990) but also the dermal component of a skin allograft is less immunogenic than the epidermis, an observation made in the seminal studies of Medawar (1944, 1945). The take and persistence of allogeneic dermis is enhanced by cryopreservation in glycerol or lyophilization (Hettich *et al.* 1994), procedures which usually result in loss of viable epidermal and dermal cells (Basile 1982) and which decrease the immunogenicity of the graft (Hettich *et al.* 1994; Wu *et al.* 1995). Effectively grafting cryopreserved or lyophilized allogeneic skin is grafting a connective tissue skeleton or scaffold which can be recolonized by host cells. Histological observations both in clinical (Cuono *et al.* 1987; Hickerson *et al.* 1994) and experimental (Hettich *et al.* 1994) studies support this notion because it can be shown that the allodermis is engrafted and does persist. Overall the evidence is that the persistence of the allodermis and abrogation of rejection is a result of the loss of viable endothelial cells and immunocytes.

There are striking similarities between these observations on the role of the dermis for epidermal morphogenesis and the initiation and promotion of bone/bone marrow regeneration by the implantation of demineralized bone matrix (Reddi 1994). The demineralized matrix initiates a regulated cascade of events as a consequence of the release from the matrix of sequestered bone morphogenetic proteins (BMPs) by proteases derived from inflammatory cells. The bone matrix, in addition to being the source of BMPs, forms an architecturally correct skeleton into which mesenchymal stem cells migrating from host connective tissue at the periphery of the graft can reassemble in the appropriate niches and undergo a normal differentiation programme. It seems highly probable that the de-epidermized dermis fulfils a similar function in the keratodermal grafts.

## Skin equivalents

Synthetic alternatives to cadaveric allograft have been developed. A two-layered artificial skin comprising a layer of collagen and chondroitin-6-sulphate overlaid with a sheet of silastic was used by Burke *et al.* (1981). In an initial study 10 patients with extensive third-degree burns were grafted with this material; the silastic layer was removed after a few days and the denuded surface covered with thin (0.15 mm) split-skin grafts. Problems encountered in this technology have included premature separation of the silastic, haematoma formation under the skin and infection (Matsuda *et al.* 1991). In a multicentre randomized trial (Heimbach *et al.* 1988) of 106 patients there was a median take rate of 80% compared to 95% for control sites conventionally grafted with split-skin and/or meshed grafts. Scarring was reduced compared to control grafts and it was considered that the cosmetic appearance was superior compared to meshed autograft. Histological follow-up on patients so treated showed that the dermal component was gradually remodelled over a 4-week period with an apparent reticular and papillary dermis although no rete ridges were present (Stern *et al.* 1990).

A number of strategies to combine a synthetic dermal equivalent with epidermal cells have been devised. In initial studies cultured keratinocytes were overlaid on to the dermal equivalent but the surface failed to support cell growth (Yannas 1984), possibly caused by the cytotoxic effect of glutaraldehyde used for cross-linking the collagen–glycosaminoglycan (CG) membrane (Hey *et al.* 1990). Using the guinea-pig, Yannas *et al.* (1982) showed that seeding CG equivalents with autologous dermal and epidermal cells induced partial regeneration of the dermis. The effectiveness of these seeded CG equivalents in retarding wound contraction and inducing regeneration were shown to be critically dependent upon pore diameter and the resistance to proteolytic degradation of the collagen (Yannas *et al.* 1989). The morphologic events in these grafts were carefully documented (Murphy *et al.* 1990). The synthetic matrix was rapidly invaded by leucocytes and then dermal fibroblasts, which remained in a random orientation. Directed angiogene-

sis occurred early, with the formation of discrete epidermal plexuses by day 14–17. The synthetic matrix disappeared by day 17 but clearly had resulted in effective dermal regeneration because at 1 year post-grafting the graft sites resembled normal dermis. The overlying epidermis was similar to skin.

An alternative strategy for the provision of a dermal component incorporates fibroblasts either into a synthetic dressing material, such as Biobrane (Hansbrough *et al.* 1994), or into a gel of acid-extracted collagen, which then is allowed to contract. These dermal equivalents can then be overlaid with a suspension of keratinocytes to form a 'living skin equivalent' (Bell *et al.* 1991). When the contracted collagen fibroblast gel–keratinocyte sandwich is raised to the air–liquid interface in culture the keratinocytes stratify and exhibit many of the features of epidermal differentiation, such as the expression of differentiation-specific keratins (Kopan *et al.* 1987). The dermo-epidermal junction in these cultures has some features of the *in vivo* structure (Tinois *et al.* 1987) but full epidermal differentiation and reconstitution of the BMZ requires *in vivo* signals (Bosca *et al.* 1988).

The value of cultured autologous skin equivalents of this type as permanent wound dressings has been examined in several studies and they have shown good short-term results for the coverage of both acute surgical wounds (Eaglstein *et al.* 1995) and venous ulcers (Sabolinski *et al.* 1996). However, experimental studies (Medalie *et al.* 1997) suggest that the composition of the dermal analogue is critical for the provision of the appropriate microenvironment permissive for true epidermal differentiation and function and that acellular dermis is superior in this property to collagen impregnated with fibroblasts.

## Allografts

The obvious alternative to split-skin autografts and the problem of limited availability of donor sites is skin allografts. However, the rejection of full-thickness skin allografts by immunocompetent individuals is such a consistent and reproducible phenomenon that it has, since the seminal work of Medawar (Gibson & Medawar 1943), been a central model for the study of immunologically mediated tissue destruction *in vivo*; for review see Rosenberg and Singer (1992). The only accurately documented permanent coverage with skin allografts in humans has been in identical siblings (Converse & Duchet 1947; Stranc 1966; Caruso *et al.* 1996).

However, allograft skin is used as a biological dressing in the management of severely burned patients. Thus widely meshed (>1:6) split skin is interleaved with allograft either by overlaying (Alexander *et al.* 1981; Sawada 1985; Phipps & Clarke 1991; Kreis *et al.* 1992) or insertion of allograft into holes cut in autograft sheets (Yang *et al.* 1979). Except for one isolated case report (Takiuchi *et al.* 1982) allografts do not survive in the long term (Korn *et al.* 1978), rejection always occurring before 3 months and often within the first 3 weeks. Attempts to modify this outcome with general immunosuppression have been made (Burke *et al.* 1974, 1975) but encountered serious problems with sepsis as a result of immunodeficiency.

Experimental studies in animal models showed that skin allograft survival was prolonged by cyclosporin (Borel & Meszaros 1980; Black *et al.* 1988; Hewitt *et al.* 1988). In patients cyclosporin was effective in preventing rejection during the period of administration (Frame *et al.* 1989; Sakabu *et al.* 1990). However, the actual fate of the allograft in many of these studies is not entirely clear. In 1989 Frame *et al.* treated three patients with cyclosporin after allografting. The allografts survived during drug treatment but were rejected in two cases after cessation of therapy. In the third case a meshed allo-autograft sandwich technique was used and, although there was no visible evidence of rejection, it is probable that the allograft was replaced by a creeping substitution with autologous cells. It is likely that the same process occurred in the first reported case (Achauer *et al.* 1986) of long-term allograft survival after a 4-month course of cyclosporin in an adolescent with massive burns as a meshed allograft overlay on widely meshed autograft was used.

## Cultured keratinocyte allografts

One of the major perceived disadvantages of cultured keratinocyte autografts is the 3–4-week delay between taking the biopsy and the provision of large enough sheets of cultured epithelium for grafting. Cultured keratinocyte allografts would overcome this problem and raise the alluring prospect of banks of frozen skin readily available for transplantation. A consideration of how alloantigen is recognized in the skin suggests that cultured keratinocyte allografts could survive without rejection.

The passenger leucocyte concept of Snell (1957) as the basis for alloantigen recognition and presentation has been supported by several experimental models (Lafferty *et al.* 1976, 1983; Faustmann *et al.* 1984) which demonstrate the pivotal role of donor antigen-presenting cells (APCs) in the initiation of graft rejection. The dendritic cells system of APCs is the initiator and modulator of the immune response; for review see Banchereau and Steinman (1998). In the skin the Langerhans' cell (LC) is the dendritic cell and the immunogenicity of skin allografts correlates directly with the density of LCs which they contain. Thus mice tail skin, which has the lowest LC density, is weakly immunogenic when compared to flank or ear skin, which have 5–10 times the LCs (Bergstresser *et al.* 1980; Chen & Silvers 1982).

Functionally, however, LCs are complex because the efficiency with which they process and present antigen and activate naïve T cells depends upon their location and differentiation. *In vitro*, freshly isolated LCs can effectively process and present antigen but are ineffective at activating allospecific T cells; after 3–4 days in culture LCs are potent activators of naïve allospecific T cells but lose their capacity to process antigen (Banchereau & Steinman 1998). This maturation programme is a necessary aspect of *in vivo* function. Naïve LCs in the epidermis encounter antigen, which is then processed and displayed in association with major histocompatibility complex (MHC) class I or II glycoproteins on the cell surface; LCs then migrate to the lymph node and mature in response to a cocktail of cytokine signals. In the lymph node the MHC antigen complex displayed at the LC plasma membrane is presented to any T cell reactive to the original antigen. In skin allograft responses, the evidence is that host T cells are activated by donor LCs which migrate from the graft to the draining lymph node. Thus, if the afferent lymphatics

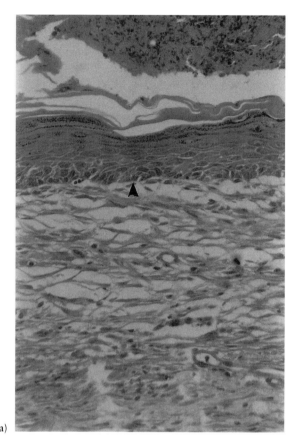

(a)

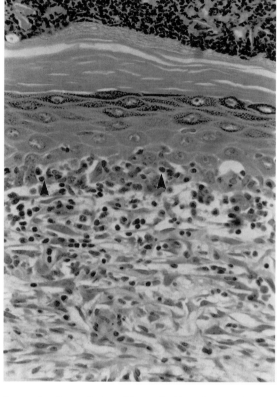

(b)

**Fig. 14.2** Cultured SJL keratinocyte allografts on CBA/CaH recipients. (a) Day 8 post-grafting. The epidermis (arrow) is healthy and keratinizing but a small number of lymphocytes infiltrate the graft bed. (b) Day 14 post-grafting. There is a mononuclear cell infiltrate in the basal epidermal layers (arrows) and vacuolation of the grafted keratinocytes. (c) Day 21 post-grafting. There is a dense mononuclear cell infiltration of the graft bed and epidermal detachment, with the necrosis of all grafted tissue except keratin. H & E stain, ×320.

are severed, graft rejection is either abrogated (Barker & Billingham 1968) or delayed (Tilney & Gowans 1970).

In elegant studies using skin grafts *in vivo* and organ culture *in vitro* (Larsen *et al.* 1990a) LCs were observed to migrate from the epidermis into the dermal lymphatics and out of the graft. Only LCs which migrated from the graft could activate naïve allospecific T cells. The reciprocal migration of dendritic cells from the circulation into the graft could not be shown (Larsen *et al.* 1990b).

Langerhans cells are non-adherent *in vitro* and are eliminated from primary keratinocyte cultures within 7 days as a consequence of medium changing (Morhenn *et al.* 1982; Hammond *et al.* 1987). Cultured keratinocytes do not constitutively express MHC class II glycoproteins or the costimulatory molecules CD80 and CD86 (Nickoloff & Turka 1994) and fail to stimulate autologous lymphocytes in mixed lymphocyte reactions. Sheets of cultured keratinocytes are therefore devoid of donor APCs, are MHC II-negative and could, in theory, be transplanted to incompatible recipients.

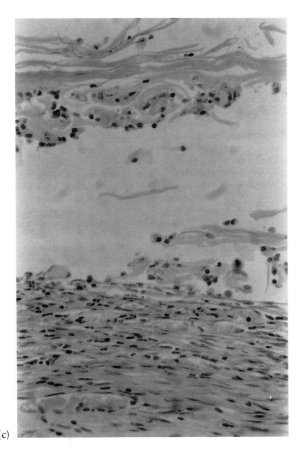

(c)

**Fig. 14.2** *Continued.*

Studies in the mouse using a transplantation technique which prevented wound healing by contraction or host re-epithelialization showed prolonged survival of cultured epidermal keratinocytes grafted on to immunocompetent, MHC incompatible hosts (Worst *et al.* 1980; Hammond *et al.* 1987; Ramrakha *et al.* 1989; Demidem *et al.* 1990). This effect of culture also extended to grafts which were MHC-compatible but differed at minor loci (Ramrakha *et al.* 1989). These non-rejected grafts were repopulated by host APCs within 7–14 days after grafting. Reconstitution of cultured grafts at the time of transplantation with dendritic cells compatible with the graft resulted in graft rejection (Ramrakha *et al.* 1989; Yeoman *et al.* 1989b). Cultured keratinocytes are unable to induce allospe-

cific responses of naïve T cells in MLR but primed T cells from mice presensitized by full-thickness skin grafting or i.p. injection of allo-spleen cells showed weak but significant proliferative responses to allo-cultured keratinocytes and cultured keratinocytes were lysed by alloreactive cytotoxic T cells (Yeoman *et al.* 1989b; Kawai *et al.* 1993). Furthermore, grafted cultured keratinocytes are recognized but are not rejected by CD8+ T cells *in vivo* (Tinois *et al.* 1989), implying that allograft survival is a result of the absence of APC/CD4+ T helper cell interactions necessary to activate functionally poised CD8+ cytotoxic T cells.

However, in marked contrast to the prolonged survival of LC-free CKG in the mouse, such grafts are rejected acutely in the rat (Fabre & Cullen 1989; Yeoman *et al.* 1990) and the pig (Carver *et al.* 1991). In humans cultured keratinocyte allografts do not survive, although little histological evidence of acute rejection has been provided (Aubock *et al.* 1988). This suggests that the observed abrogation of rejection may reflect an atypical post-grafting immune response in the mouse. Interestingly in one mouse strain, the SJL H-2s mouse, this abrogation of rejection is not seen. The SJL mouse is particularly susceptible to autoimmune disease and has been used extensively in such studies.

In a series of experiments (N. Lees, H. Yeoman and M.A. Stanley, unpublished data) SJL cultured keratinocytes were grafted as single-cell suspensions at 2× $10^6$/graft on to the flanks of CBA/CaH (H-2k) recipients using the transplantation chamber technique (Hammond *et al.* 1987). All donor and recipient animals were 6–8-week-old females. An essentially normal epidermis was re-formed at 8 days postgrafting (Fig. 14.2) but subsequently mononuclear cells invaded the graft bed and the grafted epidermal cells underwent necrosis and all grafts were rejected within 21 days (Fig. 14.3). The acute rejection of APC-free keratinocyte allografts seen in the rat and pig models and in humans could have been related to the fact that in all these situations the keratinocytes can be induced during inflammation to express MHC class II molecules. In view of the apparently absolute requirement for CD4+ T cells for allograft rejection in the rat (Mason & Simmonds 1988) this would imply that MHC class II induction could enable transplanted rat keratinocytes to function as alloantigen-presenting cells. However, allografted SJL keratinocytes remain class II-negative, at least by immunostaining, prior to and during rejection, nor can they be induced to express MHC class II *in vitro* after treatment with γ-interferon (IFN-γ), an observation entirely analogous to findings in other mouse strains (Yeoman *et al.* 1989a).

Keratinocytes do not constitutively express MHC class II but can be induced to do so *in vitro*, at least in the case of the human and rat, by cytokines such as IFN-γ and TNFα or *in vivo* during immune-mediated inflammatory responses such as contact hypersensitivity or graft vs. host disease. Mouse keratinocytes cannot be induced to express MHC class II *in vitro* by such cytokine treatment (Yeoman *et al.* 1989a). There are conflicting reports concerning the induction of MHC class II expression *in vivo* in the mouse. Class II expression on uncultured Balb/c keratinocytes undergoing rejection in the chamber transplantation model cannot be shown by immunostaining (Fig. 14.4). However, class II expression on keratinocytes in graft vs. host disease in the mouse was shown by immunostaining (Breathnach & Katz 1987) and by Western blotting in cultured keratinocyte allografts (Cairns *et al.* 1994). Human epidermal keratinocytes induced to express MHC class II by IFN-γ are able to act as accessory cells for T cells following superantigen stimulation but, crucially, do not stimulate allogeneic responses (Nickoloff *et al.* 1993). This keratinocyte costimulatory activity specifically induces a Th-2 cytokine profile with the secretion of IL-2 and IL-4 but no IFN-γ. In the presence of recombinant IL-12, however, keratinocyte-supported T cell cultures generate IFN-γ to levels comparable to those seen when professional APCs are used as accessory cells. Keratinocytes express B7-3, thought to be a member of the B-7 family and a putative ligand for CD28/CTLA-4 (Nickoloff *et al.* 1994). However, blocking this interaction with anti-B7-3 (BB1) antibodies does not prevent class II+ keratinocyte costimulation of superantigen-activated T cells (Goodman *et al.* 1994). Keratinocytes do not express B7-1 or B7-2 and, because alloreactivity *in vivo* is apparently dependent upon CD28/CTLA-4 interaction with these molecules (Zheng *et al.* 1997), the failure of class II+ ker-

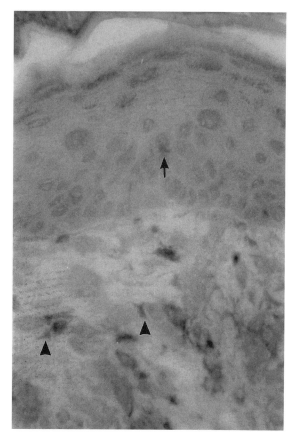

**Fig. 14.3** Immunostaining of cultured SJL keratinocyte allograft on CBA/CaH recipient at day 8 post-grafting. Cryostat section was stained with a 1 : 100 dilution of the monoclonal antibody P7/7 (Serotec) which recognizes mouse I-A. Antibody binding was detected using antimouse biotinylated second antibody and horseradish peroxidase complexes (Vectastain ABC kit, Vector Laboratories). There is no expression of MHC class II molecules on the graft keratinocytes but class II-positive cells of dendritic morphology can be seen sparsely in the graft (arrow) and at a high density in the graft bed.

atinocytes to stimulate allogeneic T cells has been attributed to the absence of B7-1/2. However, even when keratinocytes are transfected with B7-1 (Nickoloff & Turka 1994) or CD28 engagement on the T cell is provided by stimulatory antibody (Nickoloff *et al.* 1993), allogeneic T cells do not proliferate, implying

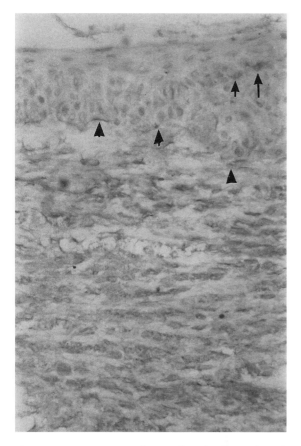

**Fig. 14.4** Immunostaining of an uncultured Balb/c epidermal allograft on CBA/CaH recipient at day 14 post-grafting. Cryostat section was stained with a 1:100 dilution of the monoclonal antibody M5/114 (Serotec) which recognizes I-A$^{b,d,q}$ and I-E$^{k,d}$. Antibody binding was detected by an antimouse biotinylated second antibody and horseradish peroxidase complexes (Vectastain ABC kit, Vector laboratories). The epidermis is undergoing rejection but has not yet undergone destruction. There is no expression by the graft keratinocytes of MHC class II, although dendritic cells (arrow) and mononuclear cells in the graft bed show positive staining. The dermo-epidermal junction is indicated (arrow heads).

that additional signalling pathways must be activated for these responses.

Cultured keratinocyte allografts have been used clinically to treat burn wounds and chronic ulcers. The initial reports (Hefton *et al.* 1983; Thivolet *et al.* 1986)

indicated that these grafts were not rejected and suggested that they served as permanent wound coverage. However, in these studies the evidence for allograft persistence was tenuous because blood group typing was used as the allograft marker.

In more rigorous studies subsequently sex-mismatched grafts were probed with Y-chromosome-specific DNA probes and it became clear that cultured allogeneic keratinocyte grafts did not survive permanently but were replaced by ingrowth of host keratinocytes from the graft edge (Brain *et al.* 1989; Burt *et al.* 1989; van der Merwe *et al.* 1990). Despite their rapid replacement cultured keratinocyte allografts have a beneficial effect on wound healing and act as true biological dressings when applied to chronic ulcers (Phillips & Gilchrest 1989; Phillips *et al.* 1990; Teepe *et al.* 1990a). The mechanisms by which this enhancement of wound healing is effected is again not clear but keratinocytes can express a wide range of cytokines and growth factors, especially in inflammatory situations. Cultured keratinocytes have the wound keratinocyte phenotype and it is likely that the regulated expression and secretion of proinflammatory cytokines and growth factors are of major importance in this situation.

There is very little clinical or histological evidence for acute rejection of cultured keratinocyte allografts on ulcers or burn wounds. Aubock *et al.* (1988) used cultured allografts to partially cover tangentially excised third-degree burns and split-thickness donor sites. These grafts were rejected after 14 days, about 4–5 days longer than that reported for split-thickness allografts. Histologically, rejection was accompanied by a mononuclear cell infiltrate and vacuolation and necrosis of the grafted epithelium. In other studies, however, in which the fate of the allograft was followed by the expression of HLA antigens on the graft (Gielen *et al.* 1987), no histological evidence of rejection could be found. The donor keratinocytes were steadily replaced by host cells with complete coverage by host cells within 6 months of grafting.

The mechanisms by which human keratinocyte allografts are replaced are obscure but overall seem to be distinct from the classical acute rejection seen in the rat models. There is evidence from the mouse that cultured keratinocyte allografts can prime for alloantigen recognition (Cairns *et al.* 1994). This observation has not been confirmed in other studies, which, however, used a different transplantation protocol (Hammond *et al.* 1987). Furthermore, evidence from the murine system (Cairns *et al.* 1993) suggests that, despite evidence of priming from *in vitro* assays, sensitization does not occur *in vivo*.

One should be cautious in the interpretation of the data on the rejection or otherwise of cultured keratinocyte allografts. The keratinocyte is not a passive bystander in immunological responses in the skin and can be induced to express immunologically relevant molecules such as MHC class II, ICAM-1 and LFA-1, to secrete proinflammatory cytokines and up-regulate their receptors after exposure to cytokines such as IFN-γ, IL-1 and TNFα. APC-free keratinocyte allografts represent a situation in which the immunological balance may be pushed toward, as Nickoloff and Turka (1994) phrase it, 'the epithelial sphere of influence'.

In cultured keratinocyte allografts the environment is dominated by keratinocytes in the initial response and when professional APCs enter the epithelium they encounter T cells stimulated to differentiate under conditions driven by the keratinocyte. The T cell differentiation pathway in this situation will depend critically on the cytokine mix in the local environment. The epithelial-driven T cell responses are most likely to be of the Th-2 type, which could be functionally equivalent to T cell anergy if the readout is graft rejection, but this scenario could alter in the presence of IFN-γ and IL-12, a molecule of critical importance in graft rejection (Piccotti *et al.* 1998). Furthermore, the rate of recruitment and differentiation of LCs themselves into cultured keratinocyte grafts may be critically influenced by the hyperproliferative wound phenotype of the keratinocytes in the graft and the intensity of the inflammatory response in the graft bed. These will dictate the cytokine milieu and adhesion molecule expression, both of which are crucial for dendritic cell recruitment and maturation (Banchereau & Steinman 1998). The fate of cultured keratinocyte allografts may therefore be influenced by the degree of inflammation, the size of the allograft, the nature of the graft bed and,

in the experimental models, the species and transplantation technique employed.

## Conclusions

Skin transplantation in which the outcome is the complete regeneration of a morphologically normal organ remains both an experimental and a clinical challenge. None the less, significant advances have been made in understanding the biology of skin morphogenesis and development and skin substitutes, both synthetic and cultured, are in the clinic. Our understanding of the role of the skin in immune responses and the modulation of these responses has advanced significantly although the prospect of skin allotransplantation remains tenuous.

## References

Achauer, B.M., Hewitt, C.W., Black, K.S. *et al.* (1986) Long-term skin allograft survival after short-term cyclosporin treatment in a patient with massive burns. *Lancet* i, 14–15.

Alexander, J.W., MacMillan, B.G., Law, E. & Kittur, D.S. (1981) Treatment of severe burns with widely meshed skin autograft and meshed skin allograft overlay. *Journal of Trauma* 21, 433–438.

Aubock, J., Irschick, E., Romani, N. *et al.* (1988) Rejection, after a slightly prolonged survival time, of Langerhans cell-free allogeneic cultured epidermis used for wound coverage in humans. *Transplantation* 45, 730–732.

Banchereau, J. & Steinman, R.M. (1998) Dendritic cells and the control of immunity. *Nature* 392, 245–252.

Barillo, D.J., Nangle, M.E. & Farrell, K. (1992) Preliminary experience with cultured epidermal autograft in a community hospital burn unit. *Journal of Burn Care and Rehabilitation* 13, 158–165.

Barker, C.F. & Billingham, R.E. (1968) The role of afferent lymphatics in the rejection of skin homografts. *Journal of Experimental Medicine* 128, 197–220.

Basile, A.R.D. (1982) A comparative study of glycerinised and lyophilised porcine skin in dressings for third degree burns. *Plastic and Reconstructive Surgery* 69, 969–972.

Bell, E., Rosenberg, M., Kemp, P. *et al.* (1991) Recipes for reconstituting skin. *Journal of Biomechanical Engineering* 113, 113–119.

Bergstresser, P.R., Fletcher, C.R. & Streilin, J.W. (1980) Surface densities of Langerhans cells in relation to rodent epidermal sites with special immunogenic properties. *Journal of Investigative Dermatology* 74, 77–80.

Birchall, N., Langdon, R., Cuono, C. & McGuire, J. (1987)

Toxic epidermal necrolysis: an approach to management using cryopreserved allograft skin. *Journal of the American Academy of Dermatology* 16, 368–372.

Black, K.S., Hewit, C.W., Smelser, S. *et al.* (1988) Cyclosporine and skin allografts for the treatment of thermal injury. *Transplantation* 45, 13–16.

Blight, A., Mountford, E.M., Cheshire, I.M., Clancy, J.M.P. & Levick, P.L. (1991) Treatment of full skin thickness burn injury using cultured epithelial grafts. *Burns* 17, 495–498.

Borel, J.F. & Meszaros, J. (1980) Skin transplantation in mice and dogs. Effect of cyclosporin A and dihydrocyclosporin. *Transplantation* 29, 161–162.

Bosca, A.R., Tinois, E., Faure, M. *et al.* (1988) Epithelial differentiation of human skin equivalents after grafting onto nude mice. *Journal of Investigative Dermatology* 91, 136.

Boyce, S.T. & Ham, R.G. (1983) Calcium regulated differentiation of normal human epidermal keratinocytes in chemically defined clonal culture and serum free serial culture. *Journal of Investigative Dermatology* 81(1), 33s–40s.

Brain, A., Purkis, P., Coates, P. *et al.* (1989) Survival of cultured allogeneic keratinocytes transplanted to deep dermal bed assessed with probe specific for Y chromosome. *British Medical Journal* 298, 917–919.

Breathnach, S.M. & Katz, S.I. (1987) Immunopathology of cutaneous graft-versus-host disease. *American Journal of Dermatopathology* 9, 343–348.

Burke, J.F., May, J.W., Albright, N., Quinby, W.C. & Russell, P.S. (1974) Temporary skin transplantation and immunosuppression for extensive burns. *New England Journal of Medicine* 290, 269–271.

Burke, J.F., Quinby, W.C., Bondoc, C.C. *et al.* (1975) Immunosuppression and temporary skin transplantation in the treatment of massive third degree burns. *Annals of Surgery* 182, 183–197.

Burke, J.F., Yannas, I.V., Quinby, W.C., Bondoc, C.C. & Jung, W.K. (1981) Successful use of a physiological acceptable artifical skin in the treatment of extensive burn injury. *Annals of Surgery* 194, 413–428.

Burt, A.M., Pallett, C.D., Sloane, J.P. *et al.* (1989) Survival of cultured allografts in patients with burns assessed with probe specific for Y chromosome. *British Medical Journal* 298, 915.

Cairns, B.A., DeSerres, S., Kilpatrick, K., Frelinger, J.A. & Meyer, A.A. (1993) Cultured keratinocyte allografts fail to induce sensitization in vivo. *Surgery* 114, 416–422.

Cairns, B.A., DeSerres, S., Matsui, M., Frelinger, J.A. & Meyer, A.A. (1994) Cultured mouse keratinocyte allografts prime for accelerated second set rejection and enhance cytotoxic lymphocyte response. *Transplantation* 58, 67–72.

Carter, D.M., Lin, A.N., Varghese, M.C. *et al.* (1987) Treatment of junctional epidermolysis bullosa with

apidermal autografts. *Journal of the American Academy of Dermatology* 17, 246–250.

Caruso, D.M., Gregory, M.W. & Schiller, W.R. (1996) The use of skin from a monozygotic twin combined with cultured epithelial autografts as coverage for a large surface area burn: a case report and review of the literature. *Journal of Burn Care and Rehabilitation* 17, 432–434.

Carver, N., Navsaria, H.A., Green, C.J. & Leigh, I.M. (1991) Acute rejection of cultured keratinocyte allografts in nonimmunosuppressed pigs. *Transplantation* 52, 918–921.

Chen, H.-D. & Silvers, W.K. (1982) Influence of Langerhans cells on the survival of H-Y incompatible skin grafts in rodents. *Journal of Investigative Dermatology* 81, 20–23.

Clugston, P.A., Snelling, C.F.T., MacDonald, I.B. *et al.* (1991) Cultured epithelial allografts: three years of clinical experience with eighteen patients. *Journal of Burn Care and Rehabilitation* 12, 533–539.

Compton, C.C., Gill, J.M., Bradford, D.A. *et al.* (1989) Skin regenerated from cultured epithelial autografts on full thickness burn wounds from 6 days to 5 years after grafting. A light, electron microscopic and immunohistochemical study. *Laboratory Investigation* 60, 600–612.

Converse, J.M. & Duchet, G. (1947) Successful homologous skin grafting in a war burn using an identical twin as a donor. *Plastic and Reconstructive Surgery* 2, 342–344.

Cuono, C., Langdon, R. & McGuire, J. (1986) Use of cultured epidermal autografts and dermal allografts as skin replacement after burn injury. *Lancet* i, 1123–1124.

Cuono, C.B., Langdon, R., Birchall, N., Barttelbort, S. & McGuire, J. (1987) Composite autologous-allogeneic skin replacement: development and clinical application. *Plastic and Reconstructive Surgery* 80, 626–635.

De Luca, M., Albanese, E., Bondanza, S. *et al.* (1989) Multicentre experience in the treatment of burns with autologous and allogenic cultured epithelium, fresh or preserved in a frozen state. *Burns* 15, 303–309.

Deitch, E.A. (1990) Management of burns. *New England Journal of Medicine* 323, 1249–1253.

Demidem, A., Chiller, J.M. & Kanagawa, O. (1990) Dissociation of antigenicity and immunogenicity of neonatal epidermal allografts in the mouse. *Transplantation* 49, 966.

Desai, M.H., Mlakar, J.M., McCauley, R.L. *et al.* (1991) Lack of long term durability of cultured keratinocyte burn wound coverage: a case report. *Journal of Burn Care and Rehabilitation* 12, 540–545.

Eaglstein, W.H., Iriondo, M. & Laszlo, K. (1995) A composite skin substitute (graftskin) for surgical wounds. A clinical experience. *Dermatological-Surgery* 21, 839–843.

Fabre, J.W. & Cullen, P.R. (1989) Rejection of cultured keratinocyte allografts in the rat. *Transplantation* 48, 306.

Faustmann, D.L., Steinman. R.M., Gebel, H.M. *et al.* (1984) Prevention of rejection of murine islet allografts by pre-treatment with anti-dendritic cell antibody. *Proceedings of the National Academy of Sciences of the USA* 81, 3864–3868.

Frame, J.D., Sanders, R., Goodacre, T.E.E. & Morgan, B.D.G. (1989) The fate of meshed allograft skin in burned patients using cyclosporin immunosuppression. *British Journal of Plastic Surgery* 42, 27–34.

Gallico, G.G., O'Connor, N.E., Compton, C.C., Kehinde, O. & Green, H. (1984) Permanent coverage of large burn wounds with autologous cultured human epithelium. *New England Journal of Medicine* 311, 448–451.

Gallico, G.G., O'Connor, N.E., Compton, C.C., Remensnyder, J.P., Kehinde, O. & Green, H. (1989) Cultured epithelial autografts for giant congenital nevi. *Plastic and Reconstructive Surgery* 84, 1–9.

Gibson, T. & Medawar, P.B. (1943) The fate of skin homografts in man. *Journal of Anatomy* 77, 299–316.

Gielen, V., Faure, M., Mauduit, G. & Thivolet, J. (1987) Progressive replacement of cultured epithelial allografts by recipient cells as evidenced by HLA class I antigens expression. *Dermatologica* 175, 166–170.

Goodman, R.E., Nestle, F., Naidu, Y.M. *et al.* (1994) Keratinocyte derived T cell costimulation induces preferential production of IL 2 and IL 4 but not IFN gamma. *Journal of Immunology* 152, 5189–5198.

Green, H. (1978) Cyclic AMP in relation to the epidermal cell: a new view. *Cell* 15, 801–811.

Gu, X.H., Terenghi, G., Kangesu, T. *et al.* (1995) Regeneration pattern of blood vessels and nerves in cultured keratinocyte grafts assessed by confocal laser scanning microscopy. *British Journal of Dermatology* 132, 376–383.

Hammond, E.J., Ng, R.L., Stanley, M.A. & Munro, A.J. (1987) Prolonged survival of cultured keratinocyte allografts in the nonimmunosuppressed mouse. *Transplantation* 44, 106–112.

Hansbrough, J.F., Morgan, J., Greenleaf, G. *et al.* (1994) Evaluation of Graftskin composite grafts on full-thickness wounds on athymic mice. *Journal of Burn Care and Rehabilitation* 15, 346–353.

Hefton, J.M., Madden, M.R., Finkelstein, J. & Shires, G.T. (1983) Grafting of burn patients with allografts of cultured epidermal cells. *Lancet* ii, 428–430.

Hefton, J.M., Caldwell, D., Biozes, D.G., Balin, A.K. & Carter, D.M. (1986) Grafting of skin ulcers with cultured autologous epidermal cells. *Journal of the American Academy of Dermatology* 14, 399–405.

Heimbach, D., Luterman, A., Burke, J. *et al.* (1988) Artificial dermis for major burns. A multicentre randomized clinical trial. *Annals of Surgery* 208, 313–320.

Herndon, D.N. & Rutan, R.L. (1992) Comparison of cultured epidermal autograft and massive excision with serial autografting plus homograft overlay. *Journal of Burn Care and Rehabilitation* 13, 154–157.

Hettich, R., Ghofrani, A. & Hafemann, B. (1994) The immunogenicity of glycerol-preserved donor skin. *Burns* 20, S71–S76.

Hewitt, C.W., Black, K.S., Aguinaldo, M.A., Achauer, B.M. & Howard, E.B. (1988) Cyclosporine and skin allografts for the treatment of thermal injury. *Transplantation* 45, 8–12.

Hey, K.B., Jutley, J.K., Cunliffe, W.J. & Wood, E.J. (1990) Growth factors modulate collagen production and collagenase action by skin fibroblasts in a dermal equivalent model system. *Biochemical Society Transactions* 18, 899–900.

Hickerson, W.L., Compton, C., Fletchall, S. & Smith, L.R. (1994) Cultured epidemal autografts and allodermis combination for permanent would coverage. *Burns* 20, S52–S56.

Hunyadi, J., Farkas, F., Bertenyi, C., Olah, J. & Dobozy, A. (1988) Keratinocyte grafting: a new means of transplantation for full-thickness wounds. *Journal of Dermatologic Surgery and Oncology* 14, 75–78.

Hussmann, J., Russell, R.C., Kucan, J.O. *et al.* (1994) Use of glycerolized human allografts as temporary (and permanent) cover in adults and children. *Burns* 20, S61–S66.

Kangesu, T., Navsaria, H.A., Manek, S. *et al.* (1993) Kerato-dermal grafts: the importance of dermis for the in vivo growth of cultured keratinocytes. *British Journal of Plastic Surgery* 46, 401–409.

Kawai, K., Ikarashi, Y., Tomiyama, K., Matsumoto, Y. & Fujiwara, M. (1993) Rejection of cultured keratinocyte allografts in presensitized mice. *Transplantation* 56, 265–269.

Kopan, R., Traska, G. & Fuchs, E. (1987) Retinoids as important regulators of terminal differentiation: examining keratin expression in individual epidermal cells at various stages of keratinization. *Journal of Cell Biology* 105, 427–439.

Korn, G.A., Gaulden, M.E., Baxter, C.R. & Herndon, J.H. (1978) Use of the Y-body for identification of skin source on a successfully grafted burn patient. *Journal of Investigative Dermatology* 70, 285–287.

Kreis, R.W., Hoekstra, M.J., Mackie, D.P., Vloemans, A.F. & Hermans, R.P. (1992) Historical appraisal of the use of skin allografts in the treatment of extensive full skin thickness burns at the Red Cross Hospital Burns Centre, Beverwijk, the Netherlands. *Burns* 18 (Suppl. 2), S19–S22.

Kumagai, M., Nishina, H., Tanabe, H. *et al.* (1988) Clinical application of autologous cultured epithelia for the treatment of burn wounds and burn wound scars. *Plastic and Reconstructive Surgery* 82, 99–108.

Lafferty, K.J., Bootes, A., Dart, G. & Talmage, G.W. (1976)

Effect of organ culture on the survival of thyroid allografts in mice. *Transplantation* 22, 138–149.

Lafferty. K.J., Prowse, S.J. & Simeonovic, C.J. (1983) Immunobiology of tissue transplantation: a return to the passenger leucocyte concept. *Annual Review of Immunology* 1, 143–173.

Langdon, R.C., Cuono, C.B., Birchall, N. *et al.* (1988) Reconstruction and structure and cell functions in human skin grafts derived from cryopreserved allogeneic dermis and autologous cultured keratinocytes. *Journal of Investigative Dermatology* 91, 478–485.

Larsen, C.P., Steinman, R.M., Witmer-Pack, M. *et al.* (1990a) Migration and maturation of Langerhans cells in skin transplants and epithelia. *Journal of Experimental Medicine* 172, 1483–1493.

Larsen, C.P., Barker, H., Morris, P.J. & Austyn, M. (1990b) Failure of mature dendritic cells of the host to migrate from the blood into skin or cardiac allografts. *Transplantation* 50, 294–301.

Leary, T., Jones, P.L., Appleby, M.W. *et al.* (1992) Epidermal keratinocyte self renewal is dependent upon dermal integrity. *Journal of Investigative Dermatology* 99, 422–430.

Leigh, I.M. & Purkis, P.E. (1986) Culture grafted leg ulcers. *Clinical and Experimental Dermatology* 11, 650–652.

McKenzie, I.C. & Fusenig, N.E. (1983) Regeneration of organised epithelial structure. *Journal of Investigative Dermatology* 81, 189s–194s.

Marks, R. & Dykes, P.J. (1983) Cultured epidermal cells and burns. *Lancet* ii, 678–679.

Mason, D.W. & Simmonds, S.J. (1988) The autonomy of CD8+ T cells in vivo and in vitro. *Immunology* 65, 249–252.

Matsuda, K., Susuki, S., Isshiki, N. *et al.* (1991) A bilayer 'artificial skin' capable of sustained release of an antibiotic. *British Journal of Plastic Surgery* 44, 142.

Medalie, D.A., Eming, S.A., Collins, M.E. *et al.* (1997) Differences in dermal analogs influence subsequent pigmentation, epidermal differentiation, basement membrane, and rete ridge formation of transplanted composite skin grafts. *Transplantation* 64, 454–465.

Medawar, P.B. (1944) The behaviour and fate of skin autografts and skin homografts in rabbits. *Journal of Anatomy* 78, 176–199.

Medawar, P.B. (1945) A second study of the behaviour and fate of skin homografts in rabbits. *Journal of Anatomy* 79, 157–199.

Meuli, M. & Raghunath, M. (1997) Burns (Part 2). Tops and flops using cultured epithelial autografts in children. *Pediatric Surgery International* 12, 471–477.

Miller, S.J., Sun, T.-T. & Lavker, R.M. (1993) Hair follicles, stem cells and skin cancer. *Journal of Investigative Dermatology* 100, 289s–94s.

Morhenn, V.B., Benike, C.J., Cox, A.J., Charron, D.J. & Engleman, E.G. (1982) Cultured human epidermal cells do not synthesize HLA-DR. *Journal of Investigative Dermatology* 78, 32–37.

Morris, R.J., Fischer, S.M. & Slaga, T.J. (1985) Evidence that the centrally and peripherally located cells in the murine epidermal proliferative unit are two distinct populations. *Journal of Investigative Dermatology* 84, 277–281.

Munster, A.M., Weiner, S.H. & Spence, R.J. (1990) Cultured epidermis for the coverage of massive burn wounds: a single centre experience. *Annals of Surgery* 211, 676–679.

Murphy, G.F., Orgill, D.P. & Yannas, I.V. (1990) Partial dermal regeneration is induced by biodegradable collagen–glycosaminoglycan grafts. *Laboratory Investigation* 63, 305–313.

Nanchahal, J. (1989) Stretching skin to the limit: a novel technique for split skin graft expansion. *British Journal of Plastic Surgery* 42, 88–91.

Nanchahal, J. & Ward, C.M. (1992) New grafts for old? A review of alternatives to autologous skin. *British Journal of Plastic Surgery* 45, 354–363.

Navsaria, H.A., Kangesu, T., Manek, S., Green, C.J. & Leigh, I.M. (1994) An animal model to study the significance of dermis for grafting cultured keratinocytes on full thickness wounds. *Burns* 20, S57–S60.

Nickoloff, B.J. & Turka, L.A. (1994) Immunological function of non-professional antigen-presenting cells: new insights from studies of T cell interactions with keratinocytes. *Immunology Today* 15, 464–469.

Nickoloff, B.J., Mitra, R.S., Green, J. *et al.* (1993) Accessory cell function of keratinocytes for superantigen. *Journal of Immunology* 150, 2148–2159.

Nickoloff, B.J., Nestle, F.O., Zheng, X.G. & Turka, L.A. (1994) T lymphocytes in skin lesions of psoriasis and mycosis fungoides express B7-1: a ligand for CD28. *Blood* 83, 2580–2586.

O'Connor, N.E., Mulliken, J.B., Banks-Schlegel, S., Kehinde, O. & Green, H. (1981) Grafting of burns with cultured epithelium from cultured autologous epidermal cells. *Lancet* i, 75–78.

Odessey, R. (1992) Addendum: multicenter experience with cultured epidermal autograft for treatment of burns. *Journal of Burn Care and Rehabilitation* 13, 174–180.

Paddle Ledinek, J.E., Cruickshank, D.G. & Masterton, J.P. (1997) Skin replacement by cultured keratinocyte grafts: an Australian experience. *Burns* 23, 204–211.

Phillips, T.J. & Gilchrest, B.A. (1989) Cultured allogenic keratinocyte grafts in the management of wound healing: prognostic factors. *Journal of Dermatologic Surgery and Oncology* 15, 1169–1176.

Phillips, T.J., Bhawan, J., Leigh, I.M., Baum, H.J. & Gilchrest, B.A. (1990) Cultured epidermal autografts and allografts: a study of differentiation and allograft survival.

*Journal of the American Academy of Dermatology* **23**, 189–198.

Phipps, A.R. & Clarke, J.A. (1991) The use of intermingled autograft and parental allograft skin in the treatment of major burns in children. *British Journal of Plastic Surgery* **44**, 608–611.

Piccotti, J.R., Li, K., Chan, S.Y. *et al.* (1998) Alloantigen-reactive Th1 development in IL-12-deficient mice. *Journal of Immunology* **160**, 1132–1138.

Ramrakha, P.S., Sharp, R.J., Yeoman, H. & Stanley, M.A. (1989) The influence of MHC compatible and MHC incompatible antigen presenting cells on the survival of MHC compatible cultured murine keratinocyte allografts. *Transplantation* **48**, 676–680.

Reddi, A.H. (1994) Bone and cartilage differentiation. *Current Opinion in Genetics and Development* **4**, 737–744.

Rheinwald, J.G. & Green, H. (1975) Serial cultivation of strains of human epidermal keratinocytes: the formation of keratinising colonies from single cells. *Cell* **6**, 331–344.

Rheinwald, J.G. & Green, H. (1977) Epidermal growth factor and the multiplication of cultured human keratinocytes. *Nature* **265**, 421–424.

Rochat, A., Kobayashi, K. & Barrandon, Y. (1994) Location of stem cells of human hair follicles by clonal analysis. *Cell* **25**, 1063–1073.

Rosenberg, A.S. & Singer, A. (1992) Cellular basis of skin allograft rejection: an in vivo model of immune-mediated tissue destruction. *Annual Review of Immunology* **10**, 333–358.

Sabolinski, M.L., Avarez, O., Auletta, M., Mulder, G. & Parenteau, N.L. (1996) Cultured skin as a 'smart material' for healing wounds: experience in venous ulcers. *Biomaterials* **17**, 311–320.

Sakabu, S.A., Hansborough, J.F., Cooper, M.L. & Greenleaf, G. (1990) Cyclosporine A for prolonging allograft survival in patients with massive burns. *Journal of Burn Care and Rehabilitation* **11**, 410–418.

Sawada, Y. (1985) Survival of an extensively burned child following use of fragments of autograft skin overlain with meshed allograft skin. *Burns* **11**, 429.

Snell, G.D. (1957) The homograft reaction. *Annual Review of Microbiology* **11**, 439–458.

Spooncer, E., Lord, B.I. & Dexter, T.M. (1985) Defective ability to self renew in vitro of highly purified haemopoietic cells. *Nature* **316**, 62–64.

Stern, R., McPherson, M. & Longaker, M.T. (1990) Histologic study of artificial skin used in the treatment of full thickness thermal injury. *Journal of Burn Care and Rehabilitation* **11**, 7–13.

Stranc, M.F. (1966) Skin homograft survival in a severely burned triplet: study of triplet zygotic type. *Plastic and Reconstructive Surgery* **37**, 280–290.

Takiuchi, L., Higuchi, D., Sei, Y. & Nakajima, T. (1982) Histological identification of prolonged survival of a skin allograft on an extensively burned patient. *Burns* **8**, 164–167.

Tanner, J.C., Vandeput, J. & Olley, J.F. (1964) The mesh skin graft. *Plastic and Reconstructive Surgery* **34**, 287–292.

Teepe, R.G.C., Ponec, M., Kempenaar, J.A., Mauwe, B. & Scheffer, E. (1988) Clinical, histological and ultrastructural aspects of cultured epithelium. In: *Proceedings of Symposium on Cultured Epithelium; 28 March 1987; Leiden: University of Leiden*, pp. 36–44.

Teepe, R.G., Koebrugge, E.J., Ponec, M. & Vermeer, B.J. (1990a) Fresh versus cryopreserved cultured allografts for the treatment of chronic skin ulcers. *British Journal of Dermatology* **122**, 81–89.

Teepe, R.G.C., Kreis, R.W., Koebrugge, E.J. *et al.* (1990b) The use of cultured autologous epidermis in the treatment of extensive burn wounds. *Journal of Trauma* **30**, 269–275.

Thivolet, J., Faure, M., Demidem, A. & Mauduit, G. (1986) Cultured human epidermal allografts are not rejected for a long period. *Archives of Dermatological Research* **278**, 252–254.

Tilney, N.L. & Gowans, J.L. (1970) The sensitisation of rats by allografts transplanted to a lymphatic pedicle. *Journal of Experimental Medicine* **133**, 951–962.

Tinois, E., Faure, M., Kanitakis, J. *et al.* (1987) Growth of human dermal epithelia on human dermal equivalent. *Epithelia* **1**, 141–149.

Tinois, E., Cobbold, S., Faure, M., Yeoman, H. & Stanley, M. (1989) Cultured keratinocyte grafts are recognized, but not rejected by CD8+ T cells in vivo. *European Journal of Immunology* **19**, 1031–1035.

Todaro, J.G. & Green, H. (1963) Quantitative studies of the growth of mouse embryo cells in culture and their development into established cell lines. *Journal of Cell Biology* **17**, 199–213.

Van der Merwe, A.E., Mattheyse, F.J., Bedford, M., van Helden, P.D. & Rossouw, D.J. (1990) Allografted keratinocytes used to accelerate the treatment of burn wounds are replaced by recipient cells. *Burns* **16**, 193–197.

Woodley, D.T., Peterson, H.D., Herzog, S.R. *et al.* (1988) Burn wounds resurfaced by cultured epidermal autografts show abnormal reconstitution of anchoring fibrils. *Journal of the American Medical Association* **259**, 2566–2571.

Worst, P.K.M., Valentine, E.A. & Fusenig, N.E. (1974) Formation of epidermis after reimplantation of pure primary epidermal cell cultures from perinatal mouse skin. *Journal of the National Cancer Institute* **53**, 1061–1064.

Worst, P., Boukamp, P., Schirrmaker, V. & Fusenig, N.E. (1980) Prolonged survival of allografted mouse epidermal cells: lack of Ia antigen in mouse epidermal cells. *Immunobiology* **156**, 303–310.

Wu, J., Barisoni, D. & Armato, U. (1995) An investigation into the mechanisms by which human dermis does not significantly contribute to the rejection of allo-skin grafts. *Burns* **21**, 11–16.

Yang, C.-C., Shih, T.-S., Chu, T.-A. *et al.* (1979) The intermingled transplantation of auto- and homografts in severe burns. *Burns* 6, 141–145.

Yannas, I.V. (1984) What criteria should be used for designing artificial skin replacements and how well do current grafting materials meet these criteria? *Journal of Trauma* 24, S29–S31.

Yannas, I.V., Burke, J.F., Orgill, D.P. & Skrabut, E.M. (1982) Wound tissue can utilise a polymeric template to synthesise a functional extension of skin. *Science* 215, 174–176.

Yannas, I.V., Lee, E., Orgill, D.P., Skrabut, E.M. & Murphy, G.F. (1989) Synthesis and characterization of a model extracellular matrix that induces partial regeneration of mammalian skin. *Proceedings of the National Academy of Sciences of the USA* 86, 933–937.

Yeoman, H., Anderton, J.G. & Stanley, M.A. (1989a) Ia expression is not induced on murine epidermal keratinocytes by interferon gamma alone or in combination with tumour necrosis factor alpha. *Immunology* 66, 100–105.

Yeoman, H., Ramrakha, P.S., Sharp, R.J. & Stanley, M.A. (1989b) The role of antigen presenting cells in the survival of murine cultured keratinocyte allografts. *Transplantation Proceedings* 21, 263.

Yeoman, H., Munro, A.J. & Stanley, M.A. (1990) Rejection of MHC incompatible, Langerhans cell free epidermal keratinocyte allografts in the rat. *Regional Immunology* 3, 75–81.

Zheng, X.X., Sayegh, M.H., Zheng, X.G. *et al.* (1997) The role of donor and recipient B7-1 (CD80) in allograft rejection. *Journal of Immunology* 159, 1170–1173.

# Chapter 15/Graft versus host disease: its control and prospects for allogeneic bone marrow transplantation

HERMAN WALDMANN, STEPHEN COBBOLD & GEOFFREY HALE

## Introduction

Bone marrow provides a convenient source of pluripotential stem cells that can be transplanted so as to replace a defective haemopoietic system with a healthy one. In theory, bone marrow transplantation (BMT) can be used to restore genetically defective elements of the blood system in, for example, immunodeficiencies, osteopetrosis, neutrophil and macrophage dysfunction, and diseases of red cells (thalassaemia and sickle cell anaemia), although in practice some diseases lend themselves to successful BMT more than others. More commonly BMT is used to rescue haemopoiesis after supralethal therapy of leukaemia and in certain acquired disease states, such as aplastic anaemia. There is increasing interest in its application in autoimmune diseases, and in the use of marrow transplants to help induce tolerance in recipients to their donor organ grafts if the transplant-related problems could be controlled. There already exists a large body of work that overviews the history and current practice in the field (Atkinson 1994; Forman *et al.* 1994). The aim of this chapter is to introduce the reader to the complex immunological problems that are currently limiting the success of bone marrow transplantation.

## Procurement of stem cells

Although 'invasive' and carrying a small but significant risk to the marrow donor, pelvic marrow has for a long time provided the most convenient and reliable source of stem cells. The recent advances in using growth factors to mobilize marrow stem cells into the peripheral blood may mean that blood will eventually become the most acceptable stem-cell source (Russell & Hunter 1994; To *et al.* 1994; Andrew *et al.* 1995; Bensinger *et al.* 1995; Russell *et al.* 1995; Schmitz *et al.* 1995; Shpall *et al.* 1995). As cord blood also contains many stem cells, it too has been advocated as a source of stem cells for transplantation (Gluckman 1995). However, the need for pools of donors and a number of other logistical and ethical issues have precluded its routine use.

## Preparation of the recipient

Bone marrow transplant recipients need to be 'conditioned' to ensure graft take while simultaneously eliminating any undesirable haemopoietic elements. This is normally achieved through the administration of marrow-destructive irradiation and/or cytotoxic drugs accomplishing three purposes (see Fig. 15.1):

1 achieving as effective a kill of leukaemic cells as possible;

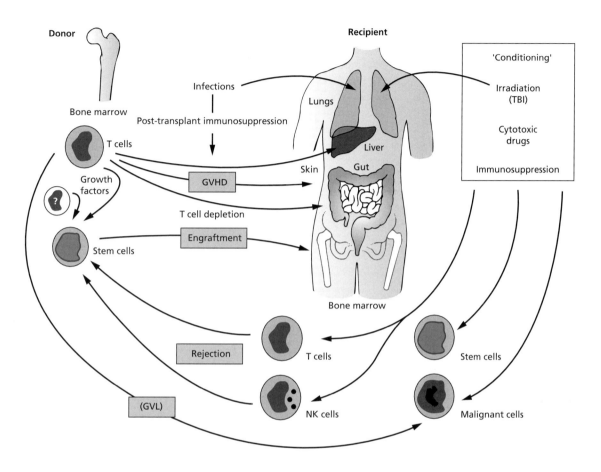

**Fig. 15.1** The problems of BMT. Transfusion of alloreactive host T cells can lead to complex interactions: GVHD, GVL effect and marrow rejection. (Redrawn with permission from Waldmann *et al.* (1994) courtesy of Current Biology Ltd.)

2 creating adequate 'space' for stem cells to engraft and, finally;

3 eliminating many of the host T cells that might have otherwise rejected the graft.

The concept of 'space' is ill-defined and reflects the experience that optimal donor haemopoiesis requires elimination of recipient haemopoiesis. The creation of 'space' can best be thought of as, in some way, reducing competition for critical stromal support niches.

## Immunological constraints

Marrow transplantation between genetically non-identical individuals is, at present, constrained by two major immunological responses. These are graft rejection and graft vs. host disease (GVHD). So serious a problem is GVHD that until recently BMT has largely been limited to HLA-matched siblings, differing only in minor transplantation antigens. Without further immunosupppression all graft recipients would suffer from acute GVHD. This form of GVHD, which usually occurs within 100 days post-transplant, is characterized by a distinctive syndrome comprising dermatitis, hepatitis and enteritis. The severity of the disease is defined by a grading scheme (0–IV) where 0–I represents mild disease, II moderate and III–IV severe and/or life-threatening. Even with optimal immunosuppression, for example the combination of methotrexate and cyclosporin, there still remains a significant degree of morbidity and mortality from acute GVHD. In the longer term—beyond 100 days from transplantation—a different form of GVHD can emerge (chronic) and limit the functional status of patients with so-called successful grafts. Chronic GVHD is considered a more pleiotropic disease process than acute GVHD and is often associated with autoimmune phenomena and relative immunodeficiency. A fuller account of the histopathological assessment and the clinical grading of GVHD is given in a fine article by Sullivan (1994).

Experimental work in animal models shows that both forms of GVHD can be caused by both CD4 and CD8 T cells, and can be prevented by removal of T cells from the inoculum (Cobbold *et al.* 1986a,b; Berger *et al.* 1994). In humans the same is true (Reisner *et al.* 1981; Waldmann *et al.* 1984), the offending T cells being those that spill into and contaminate the marrow inoculum during the bleeding that inevitably occurs during the marrow harvesting procedure. As pluripotential stem cells are rare and T cells common, it is impossible to guarantee a sufficient marrow cell dose for engraftment without transferring many alloreactive T cells. In practice, an inoculum of $3 \times 10^8$ marrow cells/kg for an adult recipient will result in transfer of somewhere in the order of $10^9$ T cells. It seems likely that there is an aspect of T cell quality that determines GVHD risk. T cells with prior experience of cross-reacting environmental antigens may be more likely to effect GVHD than naïve T cells. This may be one explaination of why cord blood T cells are, dose for dose, less potent than T cells from immunologically mature donors.

## T cell purging to prevent GVHD

The removal of T cells is able to reduce the incidence of GVHD. This can be achieved to varying degrees by a number of techniques applicable to the single-cell leucocyte suspension of the marrow harvest: for example,

E-rosetting, monoclonal antibodies and elutriation. Not only can efficient removal of T cells prevent GVHD—both acute and chronic—but it can also obviate the need for any drug-based immunosuppression (Friedrich *et al.* 1984; Noga *et al.* 1986; Reisner *et al.* 1981, 1986b; Hale & Waldmann 1994, 1996; Hale *et al.* 1994; Jacobs *et al.* 1994; Hamblin *et al.* 1996). However, a price is paid for control of GVHD by T cell purging. First, a significant proportion of patients actually reject their marrow graft, suggesting that they have residual immunocompetent T cells remaining after conditioning (Waldmann *et al.* 1984; Reisner *et al.* 1986a; Hale & Waldmann 1994, 1996). Secondly, in certain categories of leukaemia, the incidence of leukaemic relapse increases compared to those patients given T-cell-sufficient grafts (Friedrich *et al.* 1984; Noga *et al.* 1986; Hale *et al.* 1994; Jacobs *et al.* 1994; van Rhee *et al.* 1994; Mackinnon *et al.* 1995; Hale & Waldmann 1996; Hamblin *et al.* 1996). This is particularly the case in chronic myeloid leukaemia.

The conclusion of the numerous studies involving T cell depletion is that allogeneic BMT with T-cell-sufficient marrow is contributing two further therapeutic gains beyond the mere reconstitution of stem cells. First, graft vs. host reactions seem to be able to suppress the capacity of the host to reject the marrow. Secondly, there must be a component(s) of graft vs. host reactivity which has an antileukaemic effect—the so-called graft vs. leukaemia (GVL) effect—operating by mechanisms that are not yet fully understood (Weiden *et al.* 1979; van Rhee *et al.* 1994; Mackinnon *et al.* 1995; Mavroudis & Barrett 1996).

## Overcoming marrow rejection

Rodent models have confirmed that irradiation used for conditioning may still spare some host T cells capable of rejecting marrow grafts (Cobbold *et al.* 1986a,b; Lapidot *et al.* 1988; Mavroudis & Barrett 1996). Whereas T-cell-deficient grafts were rejected by the irradiated host, they were not rejected by irradiated recipients that had been pretreated with anti-CD4 and CD8 antibodies to ablate residual T cells. Primate studies also revealed that many radiation-resistant alloreactive T cells could be found in the spleens of conditioned recipients, probably contributing to the residual resistance to marrow engraftment (Reisner *et al.* 1986a). The predictions of these studies are that, if one is to prevent GVHD by T cell purging, then one also needs strategies to overcome this residual rejection potential. The following are approaches that are currently being investigated. None are mutually exclusive.

1 Combining conventional drug immunosuppresssion of the recipient with T cell depletion of the host. This might be an attractive option for genetically unrelated transplants to enhance their success rates, but is unattractive for HLA-matched sibling transplants as it obviates one of the main benefits of T cell depletion— removal of drug immunosuppression.

2 Additional irradiation selectively directed to lymphoid tissue or total lymphoid irradiation (TLI). This has been shown to help engraftment but requires specialized facilities that may be impracticable in many centres.

3 Direct elimination of host T cells by use of depleting antilymphocyte antibodies. The only study of this type has been performed with CAMPATH-1G, a rat monoclonal antibody that is competent to debulk lymphocytes *in vivo*. Pretreatment of the host with CAMPATH-1G reduces the rate of graft rejection, although the speed of engraftment—time to achieve defined numbers of neutrophils and platelets—may be delayed (Waldmann *et al.* 1984; Hale & Waldmann 1994; Hale *et al.* 1994).

4 Stronger host conditioning and increasing the stem cell dose, for example stem cell mobilization into donor peripheral blood lymphocytes (PBL), are also remarkably able to overwhelm residual rejection capacity, and these observations raise significant hopes for transplantation across stronger genetic barriers (Aversa *et al.* 1994, 1996). In some way, increasing the dose of haemopoietic elements inactivates residual alloreactive T cells. If one could understand the mechanism underlying this, then the veto of rejection capacity might be separately achieved in advance of the stem-cell-containing infusion.

## Problems likely to follow T cell purging of donor and host

A summary of the major problems that can be expected from T cell purging of donor and recipient are the following.

1 Loss of GVL activity. If we knew more of the GVL mechanisms then it might, in time, be possible to restore a GVL effect as a defined therapeutic product in the absence of T cells. This still remains a possibility.

2 Impaired immunity until residual T cells expand or T cells develop anew. There is concern whether the thymus of adult recipients is able to reconstitute adequately the T cell system (see Small 1996 for a review). Additional short-term antimicrobial prophylaxis may be required to guarantee the full benefit of T cell purging until sufficient immune competence is regenerated within the recipient.

It can be seen that the triad of therapeutic goals—the control of GVHD, the benefits of GVL and the facilitation of engraftment—cannot in practice be easily divorced from each other (Waldmann *et al.* 1994). This interdependence has led many exponents of BMT to try and juggle their approaches to each of the problems, for example to add back small numbers of T cells to preserve GVL while still avoiding GVHD, so as to gain in each area.

This approach seems doomed, as (a) it may return matters back to the *status quo*; (b) it does not easily lend itself to dissemination beyond the specialist centres; and (c) it offers no long-term future to BMT outside the HLA-matched sibling combinations. The future must lie in gaining benefit in each of the three areas of GVHD, leukaemia kill and engraftment, with specific modalities targeted to each requirement.

## Future goals

Therapies will need improvement on the following fronts.

1 Enhancing the kill or growth control of leukaemia cells prior to transplant, as well as new methods to monitor early relapse (for review on molecular methods

see Lin & Cross 1995) following BMT. This may enable earlier and more effective intervention designed to kill leukaemic cells selectively.

2 Advancing antibody-based antilymphocyte therapies, by trying to balance the degree of lymphocyte depletion with low-impact use of short-term blockading antibodies to interfere with lymphocyte function. This might ensure that sufficient T cells remain within the system, so diminishing the need for a competent thymus to regenerate new T cells. This would also ensure that immunological memory from previous donor and recipient vaccination would be sustained and, in addition, that sufficient T cells were left on board to participate in antimicrobial responses. For example, blockading antibodies to CD4, CD8, CD40L or CTLA4-Ig could be offered in the short term to mask alloreactivity, giving natural peripheral tolerance mechanisms a chance to ensure mutual tolerance of antihost or antidonor alloreactive T cells. Once blockading antibody is withdrawn, the residual T cells should be able to participate normally in host immunity. The finding that these blocking agents have some benefit on this front in rodent graft vs. host and host vs. graft reactions (Qin *et al.* 1989; Waldmann *et al.* 1994) suggests that they may prove synergistic with the current depletion-based protocols in humans.

3 Enhance the stem cell dose of the inoculum (Aversa *et al.* 1994, 1996). The increasing sophistication of techniques to mobilize stem cells into the blood may facilitate this process (Russell & Hunter 1994; To *et al.* 1994; Andrew *et al.* 1995; Bensinger *et al.* 1995; Russell *et al.* 1995; Schmitz *et al.* 1995; Shpall *et al.* 1995). There has been much interest in purification of stem cells based on their expression of surface markers such as CD34. Commercial kits are available but are not yet refined enough to ensure adequate T cell removal from the enriched stem cell preparations. Even if they were, the enriched stem cell preparations would risk rejection by residual host T cells, and would not remove the need for better antilymphocyte therapies or for preserving donor T cells for reconstitution at a later time.

These ideas are summarized diagrammatically in Fig. 15.2.

## Unrelated donor transplants

The rapid progress of unrelated marrow transplants in recent years has largely resulted from the growing activities of national registries and substantial international communication to ensure adequate donor pools to find potential matches (Marks *et al.* 1993; Anasetti *et al.* 1995; Sierra & Anasetti 1995; Spencer *et al.* 1995b; Oakhill *et al.* 1996). The fact that small differences in MHC class I and II alleles can result in GVHD and marrow rejection, and that large differences can result in severe GVHD, has meant that the use of unrelated donor transplants requires improved tissue-typing methods for matching host and donor. DNA-typing methods for HLA class II alleles are continuously improving, and this permits the registries to follow outcome against the extent of match by the new procedures. The application of similar techniques for class I matching may also lead to more efficient detection of donor–recipient combinations (for review of typing methods see Chapter 3 and Charron 1996). However, it should be clear that improved matching procedures will necessitate a larger pool of donors. The finer the distinctions that can be made become, the harder it becomes to find a 'match'. As a result the potential for improvement will eventually become limited.

Perhaps the most important issue, however, is whether one can, in addition, predict good or bad matches by some *in vitro* tests of T lymphocyte function. Limiting dilution systems have proved of some value in helping the selection, being based on measures of frequencies of cytotoxic and helper precursors (Sharabi & Sachs 1989; Theobald *et al.* 1993; Schwarer *et al.* 1994; Spencer *et al.* 1995a; Theobald 1995). This information might in turn be used to determine the need for T cell depletion and the precise conditioning protocol.

The use of antibodies to control GVHD and graft rejection has been investigated in the UK with CAMPATH-1 antibodies, leading to the view that control of these immunological complications can result in better survival and quality of life in this group (Hale & Waldmann 1996; Marks *et al.* 1993; Spencer *et al.* 1995b; Oakhill *et al.* 1996). Surprisingly, relapse of chronic myeloid leukaemia does not seem as signifi-

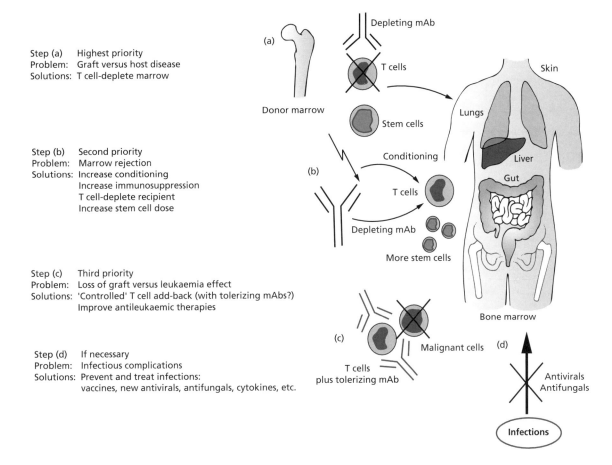

Step (a)    Highest priority
Problem:    Graft versus host disease
Solutions:  T cell-deplete marrow

Step (b)    Second priority
Problem:    Marrow rejection
Solutions:  Increase conditioning
            Increase immunosuppression
            T cell-deplete recipient
            Increase stem cell dose

Step (c)    Third priority
Problem:    Loss of graft versus leukaemia effect
Solutions:  'Controlled' T cell add-back (with tolerizing mAbs?)
            Improve antileukaemic therapies

Step (d)    If necessary
Problem:    Infectious complications
Solutions:  Prevent and treat infections:
            vaccines, new antivirals, antifungals, cytokines, etc.

**Fig. 15.2** The future of BMT reseach. Problems to be solved, in order of descending priority: (a) GVHD; (b) marrow rejection; (c) loss of GVL effect; (d) infectious complications. (Redrawn with permission from Waldmann *et al.* (1994) courtesy of Current Biology Ltd.)

cant a problem as in the HLA-matched groups, and where it arises there is evidence that control can be achieved through reinfusion of donor T cells at the onset of relapse (van Rhee *et al.* 1994).

## Allogeneic bone marrow transplant for the induction of immunological tolerance in transplantation

Ever since Medawar was able to infuse donor marrow

to induce tolerance in the neonate there has been the expectation that marrow transplantation could be used to induce immunological tolerance to organ grafts (Qin *et al.* 1989, 1993; Leong *et al.* 1992). Behind this hope lies the assumption that sufficient donor chimerism may ensure deletion of antidonor T cells in the thymus and their inactivation in the periphery (Leong *et al.* 1992). The reader must realize from the above account that it has proven difficult to achieve engraftment of T-cell-purged marrow mismatched only for minor transplantation antigens. To achieve high-level chimerism of MHC, incompatible or even xenogeneic marrow would probably require such aggressive conditioning that the morbidity and/or mortality risk would be too high for a routine procedure.

However, there is now an increased realization

that immunological tolerance need not arise from clonal deletion but can be enabled through the selective expansion of regulatory T cells that prevent host vs. graft and graft vs. host reactions. The degree and quality of chimerism that might be required for this may well be within the scope of low-impact therapies applicable to patients. This is a strong reason to understand more about the biology of these dominant regulatory mechanisms and 'infectious' tolerance (Qin *et al.* 1993), so that their clinical equivalents could be sought in the future.

# References

Anasetti, C., Etzioni, R., Petersdorf, E.W., Martin, P.J. & Hansen, J.A. (1995) Marrow transplantation from unrelated volunteer donors. *Annual Review of Medicine* **46**, 169–179.

Andrew, P., Haynes, M.D. & Russell, N.H. (1995) Blood stem cell allografting. *Current Opinion in Hematology* **2**, 431–435.

Atkinson K. (ed.) (1994) *Clinical Bone Marrow Transplantation.* Cambridge University Press, Cambridge.

Aversa, F., Tabilio, A., Terenzi, A. *et al.* (1994) Successful engraftment of T cell depleted haploidentical 'three loci' incompatible transplantation in leukemia patients by addition of recombinant granulocyte colony-stimulating factor-mobilised peripheral blood progenitor cells to marrow inoculum. *Blood* **84**, 3948–3955.

Aversa, F., Terenzi, A., Tabilio, A. *et al.* (1996) Addition of PBPCs to the marrow inoculum allows engraftment of mismatched T cell-depleted transplants for acute leukemia. *Bone Marrow Transplantation* **17** (Suppl. 2), S58–S61.

Bensinger, W.I., Weaver, C.H., Appelbaum, F. *et al.* (1995) Transplantation of allogeneic peripheral blood stem cells mobilised by recombinant human granulocyte colony-stimulating factor. *Blood* **85**, 1655–1658.

Berger, M., Wettstein, P.I. & Korngold, R. (1994) T cell subsets involved in lethal grafts versus host disease directed to immunodominant minor histocompatibility antigens. *Transplantation* **47**, 1095–2102.

Charron, D.J. (1996) HLA matching in unrelated donor bone marrow transplantation. *Current Opinion in Hematology* **3**, 416–422.

Cobbold, S.P., Martin, G., Qin, S. & Waldmann, H. (1986a) Monoclonal antibodies to promote marrow engraftment and tissue graft tolerance. *Nature* **323**, 164–166.

Cobbold, S., Martin, G. & Waldmann, H. (1986b) Monoclonal antibodies for the prevention of graft-versus-host disease and marrow graft rejection. The depletion of T cell subsets *in vitro* and *in vivo*. *Transplantation* **42**, 239–247.

Forman S., Blume, K. & Thomas, E.D. (eds) (1994) *Bone Marrow Transplantation.* Blackwell Scientific Publications, Oxford.

Friedrich, W., Goldmann, S.F., Vetter, U. *et al.* (1984) Immunoreconstitution in severe combined immunodeficiency after transplantation of HLA-haploidentical T cell-depleted bone marrow. *Lancet* **1** (8380), 761–764.

Gluckman, E. (1995) Umbilical cord blood biology and transplantation. *Current Opinion in Hematology* **2**, 413–416.

Hale, G. & Waldmann, H. (1994) CAMPATH-1 monoclonal antibodies in bone marrow transplantation *Journal of Hematotherapy* **3**, 15–31.

Hale, G. & Waldmann, H. (1996) Recent results using CAMPATH-1 antibodies to control GVHD and graft rejection. *Bone Marrow Transplantation* **17**(3), 305–308.

Hale, G., Waldmann, H. for CAMPATH users (1994) Control of graft versus host disease and graft rejection by T cell depletion of donor and recipient with CAMPATH-antibodies: results of matched sibling transplants for malignant diseases. *Bone Marrow Transplantation* **13**, 597–611.

Hamblin, M., Marsh, J.C., Lawler, M. *et al.* (1996) Campath-1G *in vivo* confers a low incidence of graft-versus-host disease associated with a high incidence of mixed chimaerism after bone marrow transplantation for severe aplastic anaemia using HLA-identical sibling donors. *Bone Marrow Transplanation* **17**, 819–824.

Jacobs, P., Wood, L., Fullard, L., Waldmann, H. & Hale, G. (1994) T cell depletion by exposure to Campath-1G *in vitro* prevents graft-versus-host disease. *Bone Marrow Transplanation* **13**, 763–769.

Lapidot, T., Singer, T.S., Salomon, O. *et al.* (1988) Booster irradiation to the spleen following total body irradiation. A new immunosuppressive approach for allogeneic bone marrow transplantation. *Journal of Immunology* **141**, 2619–2624.

Leong, L.Y.W., Qin, S., Cobbold, S.P. & Waldmann, H. (1992) Classical transplantation tolerance in the adult: the interaction between myeloablation and immunosuppression. *European Journal of Immunology* **22**, 2825–2830.

Lin, F. & Cross, N.C.P. (1995) Molecular methods for monitoring malignant disease after bone marrow. *Current Opinion in Hematology* **2** (6), 460–467.

Mackinnon, S., Papadopoulos, E.P., Carabasi, M.H. *et al.* (1995) Adoptive immunotherapy evaluating escalating doses of donor leukocytes for relapse of chronic myeloid leukaemia following bone marrow transplantation: separation of graft versus leukaemia from graft versus host disease. *Blood* **86**, 1261–1268.

Marks, D.I., Cullis, J.O., Ward, K.N. *et al.* (1993) Allogeneic bone marrow transplantation for chronic myeloid leukemia using sibling and volunteer unrelated donors. *Annals of Internal Medicine* **119**, 207–214.

Mavroudis, D. & Barrett, J. (1996) The graft-versus-leukemia. *Current Opinion in Hematology* **3**, 423–429.

Noga, S.J., Donnenberg, A.D., Schwartz, C.L. *et al.* (1986) Development of a simplified counterflow centrifugation elutriation procedure for depletion of lymphocytes from human bone marrow. *Transplantation* **41**, 220–229.

Oakhill, A., Pamphilon, D.H., Potter, M.N. *et al.* (1996) Unrelated donor bone marrow transplantation for children with relapsed acute lymphoblastic leukaemia in second complete remission. *British Journal of Haematology* **94**, 574–578.

Qin, S.X., Cobbold, S.P., Benjamin, R. & Waldmann, H. (1989) Induction of classical transplantation tolerance in the adult. *Journal of Experimental Medicine* **169**, 779–794.

Qin, S., Cobbold, S.P., Pope, H. *et al.* (1993) Infectious transplantation tolerance. *Science* **259**, 974–977.

Reisner, Y., Kapoor, N., Kirkpatrick, D. *et al.* (1981) Transplantation for acute leukaemia with HLA-A and B non-identical parental marrow cell fractionated with soybean agglutinin and sheep red cells. *Lancet* **2**, 327–3116.

Reisner, Y., Ben Bassat, I., Douer, D. *et al.* (1986a) Demonstration of clonable alloreactive host T cells in a primate model for bone marrow transplantation. *Proceedings of the National Academy of Sciences (USA)* **83**, 4012–4015.

Reisner, Y., Friedrich, W. & Fabian, I. (1986b) A shorter procedure for preparation E-rosette-depleted bone marrow for transplantation. *Transplantation* **42**, 312–315.

Russell, J.A., Luider, J., Weaver, M. *et al.* (1995) Collection of progenitor cells for allogeneic transplantation from peripheral blood of normal donors. *Bone Marrow Transplantation* **15**, 111–115.

Russell, N.H. & Hunter, A.E. (1994) Peripheral blood stem cells for allogeneic transplantation. *Bone Marrow Transplantation* **13**, 353–355.

Schmitz, N., Dreger, P., Suttorp, M. *et al.* 1995) Primary transplantation of allogeneic peripheral blood progenitor cells mobilised by filgrastim (granulocyte colony-stimulating factor). *Blood* **85**, 1666–1672.

Schwarer, A.P., Zheng, J.Y., Deacock, S. *et al.* (1994) Comparison of helper and cytotoxic anti-recipient T cell frequencies in unrelated bone marrow transplantations. *Transplantation* **58**, 1198–1203.

Sharabi, Y. & Sachs, D.H. (1989) Mixed chimerism and permanent specific transplantation tolerance induced by a non-lethal preparative regimen. *Journal of Experimental Medicine* **169**, 493–502.

Shpall, E.J., Gee, A., Cagnoni, P.J. *et al.* (1995) Stem cell isolation. *Current Opinion in Hematology* **2**, 452–459.

Sierra, J.M.D. & Anasetti, C. (1995) Marrow transplantation from unrelated donors. *Current Opinion in Hematology* **2**, 444–451.

Small, T.N. (1996) Immunologic reconstitution following stem cell transplantation (1996). *Current Opinion in Hematology* **3**, 461–465.

Spencer, A., Brookes, P.A., Kaminiski, E. *et al.* (1995a) Cytotoxic T lymphocyte precursor frequency analyses in bone marrow transplantation with volunteer unrelated donors. Value in donor selection. *Transplantation* **59**, 1302–1308.

Spencer, A., Szydlo, R.M., Brookes, P.A. *et al.* (1995b) Bone marrow transplantation for chronic myeloid leukemia with volunteer unrelated donors using *ex vivo* or *in vivo* T cell depletion: major prognostic impact of HLA class I identity between donor and recipient. *Blood* **86**, 3590–3597.

Sullivan, K. (1994) Graft versus host disease In: *Bone Marrow Transplantation* (eds S. Forman, K. Blume & E.D. Thomas), pp. 339–362. Blackwell Scientific Publications, Oxford.

Theobald, M. (1995) Predicting graft-versus-host disease. *Current Opinion in Immunology* **7**, 649–655.

Theobald, M., Bunjes, D., Nierle, T., Arnold, R. & Hempel, H. (1993) Measurements of recipient specific alloreactivity: is GVHD predictable *Bone Marrow Transplantation* **12** (Suppl. 3), 518–523.

To, L.B., Haylock, D.N., Dowse, T. *et al.* (1994) A comparative study of the phenotype and proliferative capacity of peripheral blood (PB) CD34+ cells mobilised by four different protocols and those of steady-phase PB and bone marrow CD34+ cells. *Blood* **84**, 2930–2939.

Van Rhee, F., Lin, F., Cullis, J.O. *et al.* (1994) Relapse of chronic myeloid leukemia after allogeneic bone marrow transplant: the case for giving donor leukocyte transfusions before the onset of hematologic relapse. *Blood* **83**, 3377–3383.

Waldmann, H., Polliak, A., Hale, G. *et al.* (1984) Elimination of graft versus host disease by in-vitro depletion of alloreactive lymphocytes using monoclonal rat anti-human lymphocyte antibody (CAMPATH-1). *Lancet* **2**, 483–486.

Waldmann, H., Cobbold, S.P. & Hale, G. (1994) What can be done to prevent grafts versus host diseases? *Current Opinion in Immunology* **6**, 777–783.

Weiden, P.L., Flournoy, N., Thomas, E.D. *et al.* (1979) Anti-leukaemic effect of graft versus hosts disease in human recipients of allogeneic marrow grafts. *New England Journal of Medicine* **300**, 1068–1073.

# Chapter 16/Viral infections

## TIM WREGHITT & JIM GRAY

## Introduction

Humans with an impaired immune system are generally more susceptible to virus infections than those who are immunocompetent. Patients with T cell deficiencies, either acquired or iatrogenic, are more liable to experience infections with viruses (notably the herpesviruses), as well as intracellular bacteria, fungi and some protozoa (Hermans & Wilson 1980). Agammaglobulinaemia or B cell deficiency is more likely to predispose to infection with Gram-positive bacteria but not viral or fungal infections (Hermans & Wilson 1980), with the exception of infection with some enteroviruses (Bardelas *et al.* 1977).

In transplant recipients the use of immunosuppressive agents such as cyclosporin A, which inhibits the synthesis of interleukin 2 by T cells (Bach & Strom 1985), and OKT3 (O'Connell *et al.* 1989), a murine monoclonal antibody directed against the CD3 molecule known to be associated with the T cell receptor for antigen recognition, induce a T cell deficiency. OKT3 has no effect on B lymphocytes and cyclosporin A has only a limited effect. Azathioprine and steroids inhibit cell division and cytokine generation by all elements of the immune system. Immunosuppression is often greatest immediately after transplant and during episodes of acute rejection.

T cells play a major part in the defence against virus infections and therefore profound T cell deficiency increases the risk of infection by most viruses. Selective T cell suppression, such as that achieved with immunosuppressive drugs, is associated with a selective predisposition to infection by certain viruses, such as herpesviruses. Endogenous viruses such as the herpesviruses, hepatitis B virus, adenovirus, human immunodeficiency virus, hepatitis C virus and papovaviruses, which produce latent or persistent infections, are more commonly associated with symptomatic infection in transplant recipients than exogenous viruses.

## Herpesviruses

### Cytomegalovirus

Cytomegalovirus (CMV) is the most important virus in transplant recipients, particularly in the first few months after transplantation. In adult heart, heart–lung, liver and kidney transplant recipients in Cambridge, who received broadly similar basic immunosuppressive regimes (cyclosporin A, prednisolone and azathioprine), 34–50% CMV antibody-negative patients had primary CMV infection and 51–80% CMV antibody-positive recipients experienced

CMV reactivation or reinfection after transplant (Wreghitt 1991; Sutherland *et al.* 1992).

The host cell-mediated immune response is essential for recovery from CMV infection. Transplant patients may experience fatal CMV infections despite the presence of circulating antibody. In transplant recipients CMV infection may have several clinical presentations. Infection may be asymptomatic and mild illness may be associated with fever, atypical lymphocytosis, leucopenia, thrombocytopenia and elevated serum transaminase activity. Severe infection may be characterized by interstitial pneumonitis, hepatitis, haemorrhagic gastroenteritis, encephalitis, myocarditis and chorioretinitis (Merigan 1981). Severe CMV infection may also have an immunosuppressive effect on the host. CMV is not responsible for acute organ rejection in heart recipients (Stovin *et al.* 1989) but there is some evidence of a role in chronic organ rejection in kidney, heart and liver recipients (O'Grady *et al.* 1988; Pouteil-Noble *et al.* 1993; Decoene *et al.* 1996; Koskinen *et al.* 1996; Toyoda *et al.* 1997). Toyoda *et al.* (1997) showed that CMV infection was associated with an enhanced humoral immune response to endothelial cell antigens in heart and kidney recipients, which may be a risk factor for vascular rejection, chronic rejection and decreased graft survival. However, Nadasdy *et al.* (1994) showed that obliterative transplant arteriopathy in renal transplant patients was not associated with CMV infection.

Yilmaz *et al.* (1996) showed that, in the rat model, CMV infection enhanced chronic kidney allograft rejection in association with increased interstitial inflammation and vascular endothelial and tubular endothelial ICAM-1 expression.

Decoene *et al.* (1996) showed that there was no correlation with CMV and total rejection episodes in heart transplant recipients with CMV-positive donors. CMV infection has been associated with the development of accelerated heart allograft arteriosclerosis and vascular wall inflammation, an abnormality linked with chronic rejection (Koskinen *et al.* 1994, 1996).

CMV infection has been associated with vanishing bile-duct syndrome, associated with rejection in liver transplant recipients (O'Grady *et al.* 1988). A suppressor T response and reduction in numbers of helper T cells have been observed in transplant patients with CMV infection (O'Toole *et al.* 1986). The immunosuppressive effect exerted by CMV predisposes transplant patients to serious infections with other opportunistic pathogens (Rand *et al.* 1978).

Among patients receiving solid organs the severity of CMV disease will vary according to the organ transplanted, the route by which infection was acquired and on other coexistent opportunistic infections (Wreghitt *et al.* 1986c). Heart–lung and lung transplant recipients experience the most severe CMV disease. The severity is far greater in the CMV antibody-negative group who receive organs from CMV antibody-positive donors (CMV mismatched). Those who also develop primary CMV infection but receive organs from CMV antibody-negative donors are more likely to have acquired infection from blood and in these patients CMV disease is generally much less severe. This is also seen in kidney and liver transplant patients, with those receiving organs from CMV antibody-positive donors having more severe primary CMV infection or CMV reactivation or reinfection than those acquiring organs from CMV antibody-negative donors. By contrast, CMV antibody-positive heart–lung and lung transplant recipients are highly likely to experience CMV reactivation or reinfection after transplantation and the incidence and severity of disease is unaffected by the CMV antibody status of the organ donor (Smyth *et al.* 1991b).

As severe CMV disease is more likely to arise in CMV-mismatched patients the introduction of a CMV matching policy and provision of antiviral prophylaxis in heart–lung, liver and kidney transplant recipients has greatly reduced deaths from primary CMV infection in Cambridge.

Although most children who receive transplants are CMV antibody-negative they are less likely than a CMV antibody-negative adult to acquire CMV infection from the donated organ as most of their donor organs come from young donors, who are less likely to be CMV antibody-positive. The use of reduced-size adult organs (i.e. livers) will increase the risk of CMV infection. In a study of 40 children who received liver transplants in Cambridge, 29 (73%) were CMV antibody-negative pretransplant but only 5 (19%) of these acquired primary CMV (Salt *et al.* 1990).

It is a common misconception that transplant patients are unable to mount a good antibody response to virus infections. In fact, for certain antibodies the reverse is true. Immunocompetent individuals with primary CMV infection have detectable amounts of CMV-specific IgM for 3–6 months, which compares with 1–2 years in solid organ transplant recipients (Wreghitt *et al*. 1986a).

Antibody detection is an important means by which CMV infections are identified. However, not all of those individuals with CMV infection will have CMV disease, which requires the presence of organ damage attributable to CMV together with identification of CMV in the organ (Smyth *et al*. 1991a).

There are many methods for detecting CMV antibody. In the UK the most common method used to be the complement fixation test (CFT) (Bradstreet & Taylor 1962). However, this test is prone to false-positive reactions, particularly in patients awaiting transplantation (Wreghitt & Smith 1989) and CMV IgG enzyme-linked immunosorbent assays (ELISAs) are now usually employed for donor and recipient assessment and for detecting CMV IgG antibody rises (Chandler *et al*. 1990). We regard the competitive ELISA, which is both specific and sensitive, as the ideal means of testing recipients and donors before transplantation (Wreghitt *et al*. 1986b) although some excellent indirect ELISAs have been produced for this purpose. All sensitive tests will be capable of detecting antibody passively acquired by patients from the transfusion of blood and blood products, a fact which must be borne in mind when assessing a patient's antibody status.

In Cambridge we have found the latex agglutination test (CMV scan, Becton Dickinson) to be reliable for determining the CMV antibody status of the donor and recipient prior to transplantation and for detecting CMV antibody rises concurrent with CMV infection (Gray *et al*. 1987). Figure 16.1 shows a typical antibody response in a solid organ transplant recipient with primary CMV infection while Fig. 16.2 shows the corresponding response to CMV reactivation or reinfection.

The availability of antiviral drugs such as ganciclovir (Cymevene) for the treatment of severe CMV disease has made a rapid diagnosis of CMV infection imperative. The detection of CMV-specific IgM, particularly at high concentrations, is the most useful serological method of diagnosing acute primary CMV infection (Wreghitt *et al*. 1986a) because this antibody is produced early.

However, serology has now been largely superseded by the rapid CMV antigen detection tests shell viral assay (Stagno *et al*. 1980), DEAFF test (Griffiths *et al*. 1984), antigenaemia (van der Bij *et al*. 1988) and the polymerase chain reaction (PCR) test, which give more rapid results (Hsia *et al*. 1989; Olive *et al*. 1989; Zipeto *et al*. 1992). The shell viral and DEAFF tests employ monoclonal antibodies directed against CMV immediate early and early antigens, produced early in cell culture infection. While these tests are rapid, they are not always as sensitive as conventional virus culture (Griffiths *et al*. 1984).

In a study carried out in Cambridge with bronchoalveolar lavage and lung biopsy specimens collected

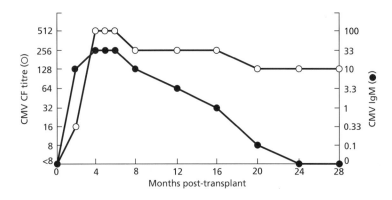

Fig. 16.1 Typical antibody response in a solid organ transplant recipient with primary CMV infection.

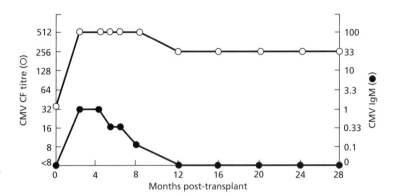

**Fig. 16.2** Typical antibody response in a solid organ transplant recipient with CMV reactivation/reinfection.

from heart and heart–lung transplant recipients, we grew CMV from 8.7% of specimens, while only 5.6% specimens were positive in the DEAFF test. Therefore a positive result may be useful but a negative result is less reliable. Many different PCR tests have been developed; they have varying sensitivies and specificities. The more sensitive PCRs are used for detecting CMV infection and are more sensitive than culture, DEAFF test and antigenaemia tests. The most sensitive PCRs, however, cannot distinguish between latent and replicating CMV (Delgado *et al.* 1992; Kanji *et al.* 1996). Less sensitive PCRs have been developed as a means of diagnosing current or impending disease. Being more sensitive, PCR is capable of detecting infection or disease earlier than culture or DEAFF tests (Gerna *et al.* 1991; Hebart *et al.* 1996). If available, histological examination of biopsy material is a useful means by which CMV disease can be identified (Smyth *et al.* 1991a).

Another useful but expensive means of identifying active CMV infection is by the detection of CMV antigen in peripheral blood leucocytes. This technique has been perfected by Dutch workers (van der Bij *et al.* 1988) and involves the preparation of leucocytes from blood, which are then stained with monoclonal antibodies directed against CMV matrix protein pp65. In their hands the technique is specific and more sensitive than commercial virus culture. The main disadvantage of this technique is that the leucocyte preparations have to be made within 4h of taking the blood sample. However, this test is rapid and has been shown to iden-

tify those patients who require antiviral treatment (van den Berg *et al.* 1991). The level of CMV antigenaemia has been shown to be related to and predictive for the severity of CMV disease (The *et al.* 1990). Quantitative PCRs have also been devised to diagnose current or impending CMV disease with a genome copy number per millilitre being used as the threshold for disease prediction. The detection of late mRNA is more indicative of virus replication in patients treated with antivirals (Gaeta *et al.* 1997).

CMV infection and disease in transplant patients are costly both financially and in terms of patients' quality of life. McCarthy *et al.* (1993) studied the cost impact of CMV disease in renal transplant recipients. Patients developing CMV disease spent 59 days in hospital in the first year after transplant compared with 22 days in control patients without evidence of CMV disease ($P=0.001$). The cost of transplantation was 2.5 times greater in patients with CMV disease compared to controls ($P=0.001$). It is against this setting that the benefit of prophylactic antiviral regimes for reducing CMV infection and disease must be judged.

Several antiviral drugs are now available for the treatment of CMV disease and some have been shown to be useful prophylactically. Several studies have been performed to evaluate the usefulness of prophylactic ganciclovir (Cymevene) and aciclovir (Zovirax) in reducing the impact of CMV disease in transplant patients. Balfour *et al.* (1989) reported that in a randomized placebo-controlled trial, oral aciclovir (3200 mg/day for 12 weeks) reduced the rate of CMV infection and disease in kidney transplant recipients. In the first year after transplant, 7.5% patients receiving aciclovir had symptomatic CMV disease, compared with 29% receiving placebo. The beneficial effect was greatest in CMV-mismatched patients. In a small study using historical controls, Mollison *et al.* (1993) showed that 63% liver transplant patients receiving prophylactic oral aciclovir (3200 mg/day for 12 weeks) developed CMV infection, 16% had CMV viraemia and 5% had CMV disease compared with 100%, 75% and 25%, respectively, for patients receiving no prophylaxis. In a non-randomized clinical trial in CMV-mismatched liver transplant recipients Stratta *et al.* (1991) concluded that prophylactic intravenous immunoglobulin (0.5 g/kg/week for 6 weeks) and intravenous aciclovir (5 mg/kg t.d.s. for 3 months) reduced the incidence of CMV disease from 71 to 24% compared with historical controls. Carefully performed studies in kidney transplant recipients have shown significant but not complete protection against CMV disease with the administration of repeated doses of CMV hyperimmune globulin over a 3-month period (Fassbinder *et al.* 1985; Snydman *et al.* 1987, 1988). Several hyperimmune globulin preparations of varying potency have been used in clinical trials and it is therefore difficult to compare these studies.

As ganciclovir is the drug of choice for treating CMV infections, it should also be the most useful means of providing prophylaxis against CMV disease. Although the drug was well tolerated in solid organ transplant recipients, its main disadvantage was that it had to be administered intravenously. Several studies have shown that a 2-week prophylactic course of ganciclovir is ineffective in preventing CMV disease in heart transplant recipients. Merigan *et al.* (1992), in a randomized double-blind placebo-controlled study employing 5 mg/kg ganciclovir every 12 h from postoperative day 1 to 14, then a daily dose of 6 mg/kg each day for 5 days a week for a further 2 weeks, showed that this regimen was ineffective in preventing CMV disease in CMV-mismatched patients, those at greatest risk of severe or fatal CMV disease. However, ganciclovir did have a significantly beneficial effect in reducing CMV illness in CMV antibody-positive patients. Forty-six per cent of patients on placebo had sympto-

matic CMV illness compared with 9% patients given ganciclovir prophylaxis (*P* < 0.001). It is generally believed that this protocol did not continue the ganciclovir for long enough for it to be effective in CMV-mismatched patients.

Winston *et al.* (1995) compared intravenous ganciclovir (6 mg/kg/day from day 1 to 100 after transplant) with aciclovir (10 mg/kg t.d.s. IV until discharge, then 800 mg q.d.s. orally until day 100 after transplant) as prophylaxis against CMV disease in liver transplant patients. CMV infection occurred in 38% patients given aciclovir and 5% patients on ganciclovir (*P* < 0.0001). Symptomatic CMV disease occurred in 10% patients on aciclovir but in only 0.8% patients receiving ganciclovir (*P* = 0.002). Ganciclovir reduced the incidence of CMV infection in both CMV-positive (*P* = 0.001) and CMV-negative (*P* = 0.06) patients.

In a recently published placebo-controlled study of oral ganciclovir prophylaxis (1 g t.d.s. for 14 weeks) for preventing CMV disease in liver transplant recipients, oral ganciclovir was found to be of significant benefit in reducing the impact of CMV infection and disease in these patients (Gane *et al.* 1997). The incidence of CMV disease (ganciclovir 4.8%, placebo 18.9%, *P* < 0.001) was significantly reduced with oral ganciclovir prophylaxis compared with placebo. CMV disease in the highest-risk group (CMV-positive donor, negative recipients) occurred in 44% patients in the placebo group but in only 14.8% of the patients receiving oral ganciclovir prophylaxis (*P* = 0.02). Despite the availability of anti-CMV drugs and improved methods for the rapid identification of CMV infection, the impact of CMV disease in some centres is considerable. Maybe with an increased use of a CMV matching policy in more transplant centres and the availability of more active antiviral agents or better formulations of existing anti-CMV drugs for prophylaxis and treatment, the impact of CMV disease in transplant patients will be reduced.

## Herpes simplex virus

Herpes simplex virus (HSV) infections are seen most frequently in transplant recipients in the first few weeks after transplantation, when immunosuppression is most severe. They are also found more frequently following enhanced immunosuppressive antirejection therapy. Infection is almost always a result of reactivation of endogenous virus and primary HSV infection is seldom found in transplant recipients. After primary HSV infection, which frequently occurs in childhood or is acquired sexually in later life, the virus remains latent in basal root ganglia in a non-infectious state and may reactivate as a result of a number of stimuli, including T cell immunosuppression.

The humoral response does not play a major part in preventing reactivation of latent virus. Reactivation often takes place in the presence of circulating neutralizing antibody and defects of the humoral immune system do not interfere with the host's ability to control infection with this virus. Reactivation in transplant recipients, at a time when they are receiving high doses of immunosuppressive therapy, particularly in the first weeks after transplantation, is probably a result of the suppression of protective T cells.

Many immunocompromised patients experience symptomatic HSV infection (i.e. mucositis and pharyngitis) in the absence of detectable vesicular herpes simplex-like lesions (Baglin *et al.* 1989) and not all patients with culture-proven herpes simplex lesions mount an antibody response (Salt *et al.* 1990). Therefore it is important, when determining the incidence and impact of HSV infection in transplant recipients, to attempt to culture the virus. HSV can be detected in vesicle fluid by electron microscopy and culture and antigen-detection ELISAs. For patients with HSV encephalitis, PCR of cerebrospinal fluid, which detects HSV DNA, is the method of choice. HSV serology in the diagnosis of infection is rarely useful.

In Cambridge, heart–lung transplant recipients have experienced more severe reactivated HSV infection than heart, liver or kidney recipients. In the absence of aciclovir prophylaxis, we have detected HSV pneumonia (diagnosed by histological examination of transbronchial biopsy and virus culture) in 10% heart–lung transplant recipients, which was fatal in one patient (Smyth *et al.* 1990). Subsequently, a policy of establishing the HSV antibody status of heart–lung and lung recipients and giving HSV antibody-positive patients

prophylactic oral aciclovir (200 mg q.d.s.) for 6 weeks has dramatically reduced the incidence and severity of HSV disease in these patients.

Aciclovir is the drug of choice for treating HSV infections in transplant recipients. Aciclovir-resistant strains of HSV may emerge during treatment of profoundly immunosuppressed patients (Gray *et al.* 1989). Two virus-specific enzymes, thymidine kinase and DNA polymerase, are involved in the antiviral effect of aciclovir against HSV. Most aciclovir-resistant strains isolated from immunosuppressed patients have deficient thymidine kinase activity and therefore will be susceptible to other antiherpes drugs, such as foscarnet and vidarabine, with an alternative mode of action.

As most HSV infections arising in immunosuppressed patients are a result of reactivation of latent virus and resistant strains are selected during treatment, the latent virus will be susceptible to aciclovir and subsequent reactivations should be amenable to treatment with aciclovir. However, it is possible that aciclovir-resistant mutants may be found in these patients, although as yet there is little evidence that these are frequently encountered. In order to reduce the impact of HSV infection in transplant recipients at risk of severe infection, a policy of aciclovir prophylaxis should be adopted. Reactivation of HSV can be prevented or ameliorated with prophylactic doses of aciclovir (200 mg b.d.) started at the time of transplant. We believe the most efficient protocol is based on the serological identification of those patients with previous experience of HSV infection (i.e. HSV antibody-positive before transplant) and restricting aciclovir prophylaxis to this group of patients. The complement fixation test is not sensitive enough for this purpose, and ELISA is probably the test of choice. Some patients will require prolonged aciclovir prophylaxis and, particularly when receiving enhanced immunosuppression, some may need a higher dose to prevent HSV disease.

## Epstein–Barr virus

Epstein–Barr virus (EBV) is a ubiquitous virus, with 90% of adults having experienced infection by 35 years of age (Crawford & Edwards 1987). Infection in immunocompetent patients is usually mild or asymptomatic, but symptomatic EBV infection is associated with glandular fever and characterized by a lymphocytosis and atypical mononuclear cells in peripheral blood.

In adult transplant recipients most infections are caused by reactivation of latent virus, although a few EBV antibody-negative patients will experience primary infection after transplantation. In children, where a higher proportion are EBV antibody-negative before transplant, primary infection will be more common (Salt *et al.* 1990).

In a study of 362 heart and heart–lung recipients transplanted at Papworth Hospital, Cambridge, age range between 12 and 62 years (mean 37 years), 338 (93.3%) were EBV antibody-positive before transplant. A total of 62 (18.3%) EBV antibody-positive patients had evidence of reactivation after transplant. Ninety-two per cent of EBV antibody-negative recipients had serological evidence of primary EBV infection, with the other 8% patients remaining EBV antibody-negative. All the patients who experienced primary EBV infection received organs from EBV antibody-positive donors whereas the patients who remained EBV antibody-negative were transplanted with organs from EBV antibody-negative donors. It therefore seems likely that, like CMV, EBV may be transmitted with the donor organ.

Most primary infections arose within 8 months of transplant although one patient experienced infection 4 years after transplant. Reactivation of EBV infection occurred between 2 months and 5 years, with most occurring 1–2 years after transplant (Fig. 16.3).

Many of the symptoms associated with EBV infection in transplant recipients are non-specific, although post-transplantation lymphoproliferative disorder is a well-recognized, frequently fatal complication of immunosuppression (Nalesnik *et al.* 1988; Leblond *et al.* 1995). Nalesnik *et al.* (1988) reported an incidence of 1% in kidney, 2.2% in liver, 1.8% in heart and 4.6% in heart–lung transplant recipients and Strazzabosco *et al.* (1997) reported an incidence of 3% in orthotopic liver transplant recipients. Post-transplant lymphoproliferative diseases may be benign or malignant with polyclonal or monoclonal, polymorphic or monomorphic lymphocyte proliferation, most commonly of B cell origin (Gray *et al.* 1995). In

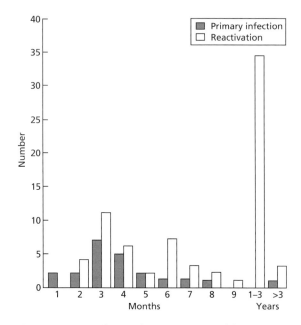

**Fig. 16.3** Timing of EBV infections in Papworth heart and heart–lung transplant recipients.

Papworth, Cambridge, 15 of 600 (2.5%) heart and heart–lung transplant recipients developed lymphoproliferative disease after transplantation. Ten of these had serological evidence of recent EBV reactivation in the months preceding the development of lymphoproliferative disease. Although lymphoproliferative disease may be associated with EBV infection, it may also be a result of the enhanced immunosuppression in this group of patients which would in turn encourage the reactivation of latent EBV. The reported incidence of lymphoproliferative disease in USA organ transplants is higher than in the UK because patients in the USA generally receive more intense immunosuppression.

EBV, in contrast to HSV and varicella-zoster virus (VZV), which establish latency in long-lived neuronal cells, probably persists in the oropharyngeal cells. These short-lived cells are constantly being replaced and therefore the virus must replicate at a low level. It has been postulated that under the influence of immunosuppressive therapy, especially treatment with OKT3 or other anti-CD3 monoclonal antibodies (Swinnen *et al.* 1990; Morgan and Superina 1994), B lymphocytes infected with EBV are liberated from the control of one or more types of T lymphocytes, allowing unlimited proliferation. *In vitro* studies have shown that transplant patients receiving cyclosporin A do not have memory T cells capable of causing regression of autologous EBV-infected B cell cultures (Crawford *et al.* 1981).

It is therefore important to monitor patients for EBV infection and the development of lymphomas after transplant, as reducing the doses of immunosuppressive drugs and treating patients with high-dose aciclovir (1 g t.d.s. orally) and antilymphoma chemotherapy can reverse these potentially fatal tumours (Starzl *et al.* 1984; Benkerrou *et al.* 1993). Bone marrow transplant recipients have donor organ tumours that do not respond to decreases in immunosuppression. Adoptive immunotherapy with donor lymphocytes is the treatment of choice (Lucas *et al.* 1997).

Serology is the most readily available means of detecting EBV infection in transplant patients. However, it is likely that reliance on this method alone provides an underestimate of EBV infection, particularly reactivation. At the time of onset of clinical symptoms in primary EBV infection, IgM and IgG antibodies to virus capsid antigen (VCA) can be detected in the serum as can antibodies to EBV early antigen (EA). Antibodies to EBV nuclear antigen (EBNA) are not detectable in the serum for several weeks or months. We have noted that false-negative EBNA results are common in transplant patients, making this test unreliable for diagnosing recent infection. EBV reactivation infections may be detected by a rise in EBV VCA antibody titre. The avidity of IgG during the acute phase of primary viral infections is low and increases with the maturation of the immune response (Webster 1968). This property of antibodies can be used to determine whether a rise in titre of IgG antibody to EBV VCA is a response to a primary infection or a reactivation of a postinfection (Gray & Wreghitt 1989; Gray 1995).

## Varicella-zoster virus

Primary varicella-zoster virus (VZV) infection (chickenpox) is predominantly seen in children and zoster or shingles, which is a result of VZV reactivation, is found more often in older age groups. After primary infection VZV persists in the sensory ganglia. When the host's cell-mediated immunity is impaired or suppressed the virus may replicate in a sensory ganglion and subsequently be transported down the sensory nerve and released in the area of skin (dermatome) served by that sensory nerve, characteristically producing vesicles.

Primary VZV infection is potentially fatal in transplant recipients. The lack of a competent host cell-mediated response, through immunosuppression, can result in visceral dissemination of virus with intravascular coagulation and cerebral haemorrhage (Bradley *et al.* 1987). Patients who are successfully treated with aciclovir may perish with opportunistic infections (e.g. aspergillosis). In a study in Cambridge, five of 610 adult kidney transplant patients experienced chickenpox between 35 days and 9 years after transplant. Four patients were treated with aciclovir although three, who subsequently died, were given suboptimal doses. In total, four of the five patients died as a result of chickenpox (Bradley *et al.* 1987).

As ~95% UK adults have experienced VZV infection before transplant (Tedder *et al.* 1981) most VZV infections seen after transplant are a result of reactivation of latent virus. Transplant patients are 10 times more likely to experience zoster than non-transplant patients of a similar age (Warrell *et al.* 1980). Zoster is seen most frequently in patients in the first few months after transplantation but it may occur later. Some transplant patients with zoster have extensive vesicles in several dermatomes. Others may have only one or two vesicles but as these usually contain high titres of VZV, they may give rise to nosocomial infections (Wreghitt *et al.* 1992). A prospective study of nosocomial VZV infections in hospital showed a higher incidence of zoster than chickenpox and that zoster is a more likely source of cross-infection than chickenpox (Wreghitt *et al.* 1996).

Aciclovir should be administered promptly during the incubation period to susceptible patients (those with no detectable VZV antibody by a sensitive test, for example ELISA) in contact with VZV (Balfour & Groth 1981). The use of zoster-immune globulin (ZIG), administered prophylactically, should also be considered in high-risk patients (those who are severely immunosuppressed).

Transplant patients presenting after the onset of chickenpox should be given intravenous aciclovir immediately, using the recommended dose of 10 mg/kg t.d.s. and should also be given ZIG (Balfour *et al.* 1983). Prompt treatment may be vital in preventing fatal infection. Patients with zoster should be treated with intravenous aciclovir if symptoms are severe. Mild cases should be treated with famciclovir or valaciclovir, but intravenous aciclovir should always be used if symptoms worsen significantly.

In patients with chickenpox or zoster-like vesicles a provisional diagnosis can be made by collecting a sample of vesicle fluid and demonstrating herpesvirus-like particles in the electron microscope. This is a very rapid technique which can be done within minutes of specimen collection. Because this technique cannot differentiate between the morphologically identical viruses HSV and VZV, the definitive diagnosis of VZV infection requires either virus isolation (which may take up to 6 weeks), the detection of VZV DNA or the demonstration of a significant rise in VZV antibody titre. However, as HSV produces a cytopathic effect in cell culture within a few days of inoculation, the failure to isolate a virus within a few days from a vesicle fluid which contains herpesviruses by electron microscopy suggests that it contains VZV.

In the UK, the complement fixation test and ELISAs are used for the serological diagnosis of most VZV infections. Serum collected within 4 days after the onset of varicella is unlikely to contain complement-fixing or ELISA-detected antibody, whereas high-titre antibody may already be present at this time in sera collected from patients with zoster. A convalescent serum sample collected 10 days after the onset of chickenpox can be used to demonstrate an increase in antibody titre and the presence of VZV-specific IgM. Antibody titre will decline a few months after infection and may become undetectable. Therefore, the complement fixation test is unsuitable for determining the immune status of patients.

Indirect immunofluorescence, with VZV-infected human embryonic lung fibroblasts (Schmidt *et al.* 1965), can be used to determine the immune status of high-risk patients although this test does lack sensitivity. Wreghitt *et al.* (1984) showed that competitive radioimmunoassay and enzyme-linked immunosorbent assay had similar sensitivity and specificity and were 10 times more sensitive than indirect immunofluorescence and 20 times more sensitive than complement fixation for detecting antibody to VZV. There are now several commercially available ELISAs for detecting VZV antibody, which are useful for diagnosing cases of chickenpox and zoster and are sensitive enough to be used to determine the immune status of patients exposed to VZV.

## Human herpesvirus type 6

Human herpesvirus type 6 (HHV-6), a newly recognized human herpesvirus, was first isolated from the blood of six patients with lymphoproliferative disorders, some of whom also had AIDS (Salahuddin *et al.* 1986).

Most HHV-6 infections in transplant recipients will be associated with a reactivation of latent virus although a few individuals who remain seronegative may experience primary HHV-6 infection. Ward *et al.* (1989) described a primary HHV-6 infection in a liver transplant recipient. Virus was isolated from peripheral blood lymphocytes 23 days after transplant and the patient developed pyrexia and grand mal fits, with a liver biopsy and liver function tests revealing evidence of a slow-resolving hepatitis.

Appleton *et al.* (1995) have suggested a role for HHV-6 in graft vs. host disease (GVHD). HHV-6 was detected more frequently in skin or rectal biopsies in allogeneic recipients with severe GVHD than those patients with moderate or mild GVHD.

The frequency of primary and secondary HHV-6 infections and their impact in transplant recipients are as yet unclear. Okuno *et al.* (1990) reported that HHV-6 infection may play a part in rejection after renal transplantation and Carrigan *et al.* (1991) reported interstitial pneumonitis associated with HHV-6 infection after bone marrow transplantation.

Serological studies with HHV-6-infected J-JHAN cells (Tedder *et al.* 1987) used in an indirect immunofluorescence assay indicated that HHV-6 infection is widespread in human populations, with most infections arising in early childhood (Briggs *et al.* 1988). It is the aetiological agent of exanthem subitum, a common benign disease which occurs almost exclusively in infants and young children. Therefore, in common with the other herpesviruses, HHV-6 is ubiquitous. It is thought to establish latency in monocytes after primary infection. DNA homology studies between HHV-6 and CMV show some homology, suggesting a relationship between these viruses, although this relationship has still to be defined (Efstathiou *et al.* 1988).

Irving *et al.* (1990) and Morris *et al.* (1988) described dual antibody rises to CMV and HHV-6 in organ transplant recipients. Ward *et al.* (1991, 1993) demonstrated similar dual antibody rises in recipients experiencing primary CMV infection and showed by absorption studies and later by determining the avidity of the CMV and HHV-6 IgG antibodies that these were not cross-reacting antibodies. These studies indicate that a primary CMV infection may trigger the reactivation of latent HHV-6.

The mechanism for the reactivation of HHV-6 during a primary CMV infection is not clear but it is possible that CMV may trigger the reactivation of HHV-6 by infecting monocytes containing latent HHV-6. The role of HHV-6 infection and the spectrum of diseases caused by this virus in organ transplant recipients have yet to be fully established.

## Human herpesvirus type 8

Human herpesvirus type 8 (HHV-8) or Kaposi's sarcoma-associated herpesvirus (KSHV) has been implicated in various epidemiological forms of Kaposi's sarcoma (KS), including AIDS-associated, classic and endemic types (Chang *et al.* 1994; Engelbrecht *et al.* 1997).

The risk of developing KS in non-HIV-infected immunosuppressed hosts is significantly higher compared to immunologically normal individuals. Alkan *et al.* (1997) retrospectively evaluated 28 organ transplant patients with KS for the presence of the KSHV genome by PCR and detected KSHV DNA in 27 of 28 patients.

## Hepatitis viruses

There are several hepatitis viruses. All may be acquired by transplant patients, some in the course of normal living and some as a result of transplantation (Table 16.1). Hepatitis A virus (HAV) is transmited principally by the faecal–oral route, usually through contam-

Table 16.1 Hepatitis viruses.

| Hepatitis | Virus | Transmission | Disease resulting in transplant | Recurrence after transplant | Donor transmission | Long-term survival |
|-----------|-------|--------------|----------------------------------|------------------------------|---------------------|---------------------|
| A | Picorna | Faecal/oral | Yes* | Yes† | No | Not affected |
| B | Hepadna | Parenteral | Yes | Yes‡ | Yes | Increased morbidity and mortality |
| C | Flavivirus/pestivirus | Parenteral | Yes | Yes | Yes | Increased morbidity and mortality |
| D | Viroid/virusoid | Parenteral | Yes | Yes‡ | Yes | Increased morbidity and mortality |
| E | Calicivirus | Faecal/oral | NA§ | NA | NA | NA |
| G | Flavivirus | Parenteral | No | Yes | Yes | Not affected |

NA, not applicable.
\* Fulminant HAV infection.
† Recurrent HAV infection does not seem to jeopardize long-term survival even when HAV-related antigens are detected in the grafted liver.
‡ Recurrence frequent after transplantation for cirrhosis but uncommon after transplantation for fulminant hepatitis.
§ Disease endemic in developing countries. No reported transplants.

inated water, but may also be contracted from food, notably bivalve mollusc seafood contaminated with sewage. Some patients with fulminant HAV infection will undergo liver transplantation, but transplantation *per se* does not carry any particular risk of severe HAV infection.

Hepatitis B virus (HBV) is transmitted parenterally, either by contaminated blood or blood products, or sexually. Patients with end-stage liver disease (i.e. cirrhosis) may undergo liver transplantation and HBV may be acquired by transplant recipients from the donated organ or from blood or blood products, although blood and organ donors are screened for evidence of HBV infection to minimize the risk of transmission. HBV is discussed in more detail later in this chapter.

Hepatitis C virus (HCV) is the principal non-A, non-B (NANB) hepatitis virus (Choo *et al.* 1990), which is also transmitted parenterally through contaminated blood or blood products and may be acquired from the donor organ. Blood and organ donors are now also screened for HCV to minimize transmission. Patients with chronic HCV infection may undergo liver transplantation. A more detailed account of HCV is given in a later section.

Hepatitis D virus (HDV) is an incomplete virus that depends on HBV to replicate. HDV infection may be acquired at the same time as HBV or as a superinfection.

Hepatitis E virus (HEV) and hepatitis G virus (HGV) have recently been identified. HEV is transmitted by the faecal–oral route. No cases of infection acquired in the UK have been recorded. HGV is transmitted parenterally. Transplantation does not carry an increased risk of infection with HEV.

## Hepatitis B virus

Hepatitis B virus (HBV) may give rise to either clinically apparent or asymptomatic infection. In at least 90% of adult cases patients experience acute hepatitis, with the production of hepatitis B surface antigen (HBsAg) and the subsequent appearance of antibody directed against core (anti-HBc) and surface (anti-HBs) antigens. Approximately 10% of cases are asympto-

matic, with HBsAg detectable for only a few weeks or months. Approximately 5% of infected individuals, who do not mount an anti-HBs response, experience asymptomatic chronic infection with persistent HBsAg and anti-HBc and may be the source of transfusion-associated HBV infection. Some chronic HBsAg carriers also carry 'e' antigen (HBeAg) and HBV DNA in their sera, are prone to chronic active hepatitis and are highly infectious. Chronic carriage of HBsAg is associated with a high risk of developing primary hepatocellular carcinoma in later life (Beasley *et al.* 1981).

Conventional thinking is that HBV-associated hepatitis is immunopathic, caused by CD8-positive cytotoxic T lymphocytes recognizing antigens on the surface of virus-infected hepatocytes. The clearance of HBsAg from the bloodstream probably represents a suppression of the viral genome and not the eradication of infected cells. This suppression is probably achieved through immune surveillance as T lymphocyte abnormalities are associated with chronic antigenaemia (Desaules *et al.* 1976).

In the days before HBV-infected patients could be identified, infection was widespread in haemodialysis and transplant centres throughout the world. The chance discovery of Australia antigen (Blumberg *et al.* 1965), now referred to as HBsAg, led to the development of diagnostic tests. In the UK surveillance of HBV infection began in 1970 (Public Health Laboratory Service Survey 1974). Despite the fact that the incidence of HBV-related clinical hepatitis cases in dialysis units in the UK trebled between 1968 and 1970, they were virtually eliminated by 1973 as a result of screening and the segregation of known HBsAg-positive patients. These policies are still in force today.

In the UK all organ and tissue donors are screened for evidence of active HBV infection by testing for HBsAg. There have been reports of HBsAg-negative anti-HBc-positive donors transmitting infection to transplant recipients who acquire HBV infection at the time of transplant and who then suffer chronic antigenaemia because of the immunosuppressive therapy administered to prevent rejection (Turner *et al.* 1997). This highly infectious chronic carrier state (frequently HBeAg- and HBV DNA-positive) poses an infection risk not only to other patients but also to members of staff who may be exposed to blood from the infected patient. Patients with acute (fulminant) or chronic HBV infection may be potential candidates for liver transplantation. However, the high rate of HBV recurrence after transplantation is responsible for increased morbidity and mortality in this group (Demetris *et al.* 1986; O'Grady *et al.* 1992). Short-term (<6 months) or long-term (>6 months) monoclonal or polyclonal anti-HBs immunoglobulin (1g) prophylaxis has been used to prevent HBV infecting the graft organ (Lauchart *et al.* 1987; Samuel *et al.* 1991).

In a study of liver transplant recipients in Europe (Samuel *et al.* 1991), the rate of HBV recurrence was reduced significantly in patients who received anti-HBs Ig for more than 6 months after transplantation compared with those treated for less than 6 months or given no anti-HBs prophylaxis. However, infection of the graft is more likely if the patient has a high viral load pretransplant (Samuel *et al.* 1991).

HBV employs reverse transcription for its replication. Because this lacks proof-reading ability, it gives rise to mutations in the HBV genome (Summers & Measons 1982). Some of these mutants will be selected by the presence of prophylactically acquired high-titre anti-HBs in liver transplant recipients (Hawkins *et al.* 1996). These are known as escape mutants. This phonemenon is more pronounced when patients receive prophylactic monoclonal anti-HBs because the change in antigenic structure required to avoid neutralization involves the alteration of a single epitope. Carman *et al.* (1996) showed that prophylactic anti-HBs imposes a selection pressure on the S gene, and the resulting mutants result in reinfection.

In an attempt to reduce the HBV DNA viral load in patients before liver transplant and thus reduce the risk of graft infection, patients have been treated with antiviral agents such as lamivudine, but with only limited success to date.

The availability of HBV vaccines has meant that most staff working in dialysis or transplant units can be successfully immunized against HBV although 15% of staff in the Cambridge units failed to produce an adequate immune response after a course of three injections. Dialysis and transplant patients respond poorly to HBV vaccines and in some studies only 55% have

produced an adequate immune response (Bruguera *et al.* 1987). However, there is evidence that dialysis patients who produce a poor response or no response to HBV vaccine may still be protected against HBV infection (Roll *et al.* 1995). It is therefore important that patients are given HBV vaccine as soon as they have been identified as requiring haemodialysis treatment.

Transplant and dialysis patients with HBV infection should be segregated from other patients and should be cared for only by staff with proven immunity to HBV.

## Hepatitis C virus

Hepatitis C virus (HCV) is a small positive-stranded RNA virus and comparative sequence analysis suggests that it is a flavivirus (Choo *et al.* 1989). HCV is responsible for most cases of post-transfusion NANB hepatitis worldwide. Infection is clinically mild and often asymptomatic but more than 50% of patients eventually experience chronic hepatitis and some go on to develop cirrhosis (Realdi *et al.* 1982). Fluctuating amounts of serum transaminases are characteristically found in patients infected with HCV, but the amounts do not correlate with the severity of HCV disease. It has yet to be determined whether HCV is directly cytopathic, like hepatitis A virus, or causes pathological changes in the liver through the destruction of infected cells by the host immune response, like hepatitis B virus.

Organ transplant recipients may acquire primary HCV infection after the administration of infected blood or blood products during transplantation or having received an organ from an HCV antibody-positive donor. However, this is an unlikely event following the introduction of HCV screening in blood and organ donors in 1991. In the UK ~0.2% blood donors are confirmed HCV antibody-positive. The precise relationship between the presence of HCV antibody and infectivity is not known. Garson *et al.* (1990) reported that only one out of six (17%) HCV antibody-positive blood donations transmitted HCV to the recipient, but there is a good correlation between infectivity and the presence of HCV RNA (Garson *et al.* 1990).

The first report of HCV transmission from organ donors to transplant recipients was made in 1990 by Otero *et al*. Forty-five consecutive kidney donors were tested for HCV antibody in a first-generation ELISA and two (4%) were positive. The four kidneys from these two donors were given to three HCV antibody-negative and one HCV antibody-positive recipients. The patient who was HCV antibody-positive before transplantation remained so afterwards and did not develop hepatitis postoperatively. Two of the three HCV antibody-negative recipients of HCV antibody-positive organs did not develop HCV antibody, did not have raised liver enzymes postoperatively and had no evidence of hepatitis. The other patient seroconverted to HCV 7 months after transplantation. He developed persistently raised liver enzymes 5 months later.

There have been several subsequent reports of donor-acquired HCV infection in transplant recipients (Pereira *et al*. 1991, 1992; Pouteil-Noble *et al*. 1992). Pereira *et al*. (1991) found 13 (1.8%) of 716 USA organ donors HCV antibody-positive in a first-generation ELISA. Nineteen kidneys, six hearts and four livers from these donors were given to 29 recipients. Fourteen (48%) recipients developed NANBH after transplantation, which in 92% of cases was shown to be caused by HCV. However, because many of these patients were HCV antibody-positive before transplantation, it is difficult to determine how many acquired the infection from the donated organs. Pouteil-Noble *et al*. (1992) reported that 3% of French organ donors were HCV antibody-positive. Of four HCV antibody-negative patients who received kidneys from HCV antibody-positive donors, two (50%) seroconverted and three (75%) developed liver disease. The problem with these three studies is that they used first-generation assays to screen donors and test recipients after transplantation. Better tests, such as third-generation ELISAs, recombinant immunoblot assays, Western blot assays and RT-PCR, are now available.

Pereira *et al*. (1992) employed second-generation HCV antibody assays and RT-PCR to detect HCV RNA to investigate the transmission of HCV from organ donors to recipients. All 13 HCV antibody-negative recipients who were given organs from HCV RNA-positive donors acquired HCV infection. However, they did not provide evidence of the amount of liver disease in these patients. In the UK we have shown that 100% HCV antibody-negative recipients have acquired HCV infection from HCV antibody-positive donors of hearts, livers and kidneys (Wreghitt *et al*. 1994). These findings are shown in Table 16.2.

In the UK it is estimated that serum samples from ~1% of organ donors will be reactive in second-generation HCV antibody ELISAs (Wreghitt *et al*. 1994). Approximately 0.7% will react in immunoblot assays. Not all assays are suitable for routine testing of organ donors for evidence of HCV infection, principally because of time constraints. Very few donor-testing clinical virology laboratories could provide a service 24 h a day, 7 days a week to test organ donors for evidence of HCV-infection by RT-PCR or immunoblot assays. Therefore, at the present time, ELISAs are most likely to be employed.

HCV antibody is not produced by most HCV-infected organ recipients. Pereira *et al*. (1992) showed that while 100% of patients who acquired HCV from the donor organ had detectable HCV RNA by RT-PCR after transplantation, only 63% developed HCV antibody detectable in second-generation ELISAs. Others have noted similar findings (Poterucha *et al*. 1992).

We are, at the present time, uncertain as to what proportion of transplant patients who acquire HCV from the donor organ will develop liver disease, and over what time-scale. The studies on donor-acquired HCV in transplant patients reported so far have all had a relatively short follow-up period. Approximately 85% of non-transplanted patients with HCV infection have evidence of chronic infection with persistent RNA in their serum (Di Bisceglie 1998). In our own study, we have shown that 47% patients with organ donor-acquired HCV infection had biochemical or histological evidence of liver dysfunction after a follow-up of 4–72 months. This must be an underestimate because all patients were not closely monitored. However, one kidney recipient died of fulminant NANBH 56 months after transplantation.

There is, at present, debate about whether organs from HCV antibody-positive donors should be used

**Table 16.2** Outcome of donor-transmitted HCV infection in solid organ transplant recipients.

| Donor | Recipients | HCV infection diagnosed by | | Period of follow-up (months) | Symptoms |
|---|---|---|---|---|---|
| | | HCV antibody | HCV RNA (PCR) | | |
| A | Heart | + | + | 68 | None |
| | Kidney | − | + | 59 | Abnormal LFTs, hepatitis (died from other causes) |
| | Kidney | + | Not tested | 56 | Hepatitis 5 months after transplant. Died from HCV-related disease |
| B | Heart | + | + | 25 | None |
| | Liver | Non-specific result | + | 12 | Abnormal LFTs. Died from recurrence of hepatocelluar carcinoma |
| | Kidney | − | + | 21 | None |
| | Kidney | + | + | 19 | None |
| C | Heart | − | + | 78 | None |
| | Liver | + | + | 70 | None |
| | Kidney | − | + | 70 | None |
| | Kidney | − | + | 37 | None (died from other causes) |
| D | Heart | − | + | 29 | Acute hepatitis 8 months after transplant |
| | Liver | + | + | 32 | Acute hepatitis 20 months after transplant |
| | Kidney | − | + | 32 | Abnormal LFTs 5 months after transplant |
| | Kidney | − | + | 32 | Abnormal LFTs 5 months after transplant |

LFT, liver function test.

for transplantation. We know that 100% of HCV anti-body-negative patients will acquire infection by this route if they are given HCV-positive organs. We also know that a substantial proportion will develop HCV-related liver disease after transplantation. So far HCV-infected patients have been followed up for only a short period. We must expect that a significant proportion of patients with organ-donor-acquired HCV infection will eventually go on to life-threatening end-stage liver disease and at a faster rate than non-transplanted patients. We would not consider using HIV-positive organs and there is probably a fairly similar long-term morbidity and mortality in recipients of HCV-positive organs.

It has been suggested that organs from HCV anti-body-positive donors could be used for HCV-positive recipients (Pirsch & Belzer 1992). As there are more than one genotype of HCV (Farci *et al.* 1991) and we have insufficient information available at the present time to enable us to be sure that we are not knowingly

infecting a transplant recipient with a potentially fatal infection, this is probably unwise. However, in patients with end-stage liver or heart failure who would otherwise be denied a transplant, some may feel that there is nothing to lose. By excluding the use of HCV antibody-positive organs we would probably reduce the donor pool by ~1%. In our UK study we have been unable to identify risk factors in our HCV antibody-positive donors which would enable us to screen them out by taking a history from relatives. We need more information on the long-term consequences of using HCV-positive donors by following up carefully those patients who have been unwittingly infected. In the meantime we should reject organs from HCV antibody-positive donors.

In Cambridge we have found 15 of 100 (15%) patients being assessed for liver transplantation HCV antibody-positive (Gray *et al.* 1990). Six of these 15 patients had liver disease not normally associated with HCV infection. Their serum samples probably gave false-positive reaction involving non-specific antibodies cross-reacting with the recombinant HCV antigen used in the earlier available immunoassays. When these tests were repeated in the presence of 8 M urea, which dissociates weak-binding or low-avidity antibodies from the antigen, five of six patients with liver disease not normally associated with HCV infection had weak-binding or low-avidity antibody whereas only one of nine patients with cryptogenic cirrhosis had low-avidity antibodies. These non-specific low-avidity antibodies have also been demonstrated in patients with rheumatoid arthritis (Goeser *et al.* 1990) and therefore may indicate autoimmune disease rather than a past HCV infectiion. Currently available HCV ELISAs are more reliable in accurately assessing patients' HCV status.

Almost all patients who are transplanted because of end-stage chronic HCV liver disease infect their new grafts and have an accelerated course of disease. Antiviral treatment is of limited benefit. In non-immunosuppressed patients, IFN-α combined with ribavirin has been shown to be of greater benefit than either drug alone (Reichard *et al.* 1998).

## Hepatitis G virus

Hepatitis G virus (HGV) is a flavivirus related to HCV which is transmitted by the parenteral route but so far has not been associated with human disease (Muerhoff *et al.* 1995; Kao *et al.* 1996; Kuroki *et al.* 1996; Linnen *et al.* 1996). HGV RNA has been found in 0.8% blood donors with normal alanine aminotransferase (ALT) and in 3.9% blood donors with elevated ALT levels (Dawson *et al.* 1996). Persistent infection has been reported in a significant proportion of patients (Dawson *et al.* 1996; Linnen *et al.* 1996) but evidence of HGV-related liver disease in these patients is lacking. HGV-infected dialysis and transplant patients with hepatitis have been shown to also be infected with HCV. HGV and HCV coinfection is found frequently in patients who have been multiply transfused.

Fabrizi *et al.* (1997) reported that 37.5% of HGV RNA-positive patients showed raised serum aminotransferase levels. Dussol *et al.* (1997) reported that, although HGV infection is highly prevalent in kidney transplant recipients, acute and chronic hepatitis were not more prevalent in the HGV-positive patients than in the HGV-negative patients.

## Human immunodeficiency virus

Human immunodeficiency virus (HIV), like HBV, may be transmitted to transplant patients through the donor organ(s), blood or blood products. In 1985 the World Health Organization produced recommendations for screening blood for the presence of HIV, by means of HIV antibody tests (World Health Organization 1985) and in 1991 the UK Department of Health issued similar guidelines for organ donors (Acheson 1990).

Some of the early HIV antibody screening tests were unreliable and frequently associated with non-specific reactions. The early literature should therefore be interpreted with caution. The HIV antibody tests in current use are reliable and sensitive and most are capable of detecting antibodies to both HIV strains: HIV 1 and HIV 2. Despite this, there are no published reports of HIV-2-infected transplant patients but it is probably only a matter of time before this arises. HIV infection may also be diagnosed by culturing the virus or by RNA detection by RT-PCR, but these tests are less widely available.

It is current practice to screen blood from blood and organ donors and transplant recipients for HIV antibody before transplantation and to exclude from donation those persons with identifiable risk factors (e.g. intravenous drug use). Blood and organs from HIV antibody-positive donors must not be given to patients. Several groups have looked at the effect of transplantation on the long-term survival of HIV antibody-positive recipients and the advisability of transplanting and thereby giving further immunosuppression to known HIV antibody-positive patients has been questioned. Several reports have shown a shorter AIDS-free time in patients who were HIV antibody-positive before transplantation compared to those who were not transplanted (Rubin *et al.* 1987; Tzakis *et al.* 1990; Erice *et al.* 1991; Lang & Niaudet 1991), although Dummer *et al.* (1989) did not confirm these findings.

Rubin *et al.* (1987) showed that in HIV antibody-positive renal transplant recipients, 50% had an accelerated onset of HIV-associated disease with early death from opportunistic infections. HIV-infected patients had a much lower survival rate when compared with non-infected recipients. Lang and Niaudet (1991), in a retrospective study of French HIV antibody-positive renal transplant recipients, showed that 70% of patients who remained on immunosuppressive therapy with a retained kidney graft died within 5 years from AIDS or HIV-related disease. By contrast, the mean survival time of patients who had rejected their kidney and reverted to dialysis was approximately twice that of those who had retained their kidney. It is therefore likely that dialysis is the best treatment for HIV antibody-positive patients with chronic renal failure.

Tzakis *et al.* (1990) reviewed 25 patients transplanted between 1981 and 1988 and followed for a mean of 2.75 years (range 0.7–6.6 years). Eleven patients were infected before transplant and 14 were infected perioperatively. Of 10 paediatric patients only one died with AIDS in the study period, which compared with five of 15 adults who died with AIDS. When compared to a control group of HIV antibody-positive haemophiliac and transfusion-acquired patients, the HIV antibody-positive transplant recipients had a more rapid progression to AIDS. Ragni *et al.* (1990) reported on the progress of four HIV antibody-positive liver and one heart transplant patients. The four who survived after transplant developed AIDS, 3, 14, 24 and 41 months later, and three died.

Several factors affect the outcome in HIV antibody-positive transplant recipients. Patients infected with HIV many years before transplantation do less well than those infected a few years before grafting (Ragni *et al.* 1990). The outcome for HIV antibody-positive patients who receive a liver or multiple organs has been reported to be worse than that of patients receiving a heart and much worse than those receiving a kidney transplant (Tzakis *et al.* 1990).

It has been reported in several studies (Rubin *et al.* 1987; Dummer *et al.* 1989; Tzakis *et al.* 1990; Lang & Niaudet 1991) that episodes of rejection resulted in a poorer prognosis for HIV antibody-positive transplant recipients. Rejection of an organ results in stimula-

tion of T cells, particularly CD4-positive lymphocytes, which play a central part in the initiation of allograft rejection. Thus there is an increase in the number of cells which could be infected by HIV. These cells are also in the 'activated' state and it has been shown that HIV replication is limited until cellular activation develops, at which time transcription occurs, with the eventual production of mature virions associated with cell death, lymphocyte depletion and disease advancement (Klatzmann & Gluckman 1986). Variation in the immunosuppressive therapy received by different groups of patients seems to be a very important factor in influencing HIV disease progression. Patients who receive antithymocyte globulin, OKT3 or multiple antirejection agents have the worst outcome (Dummer *et al.* 1989). Two reports have shown that the age of the HIV antibody-positive transplant recipient is inversely related to survival (Rubin *et al.* 1987; Tzakis *et al.* 1990).

In Cambridge, we have only identified one HIV antibody-positive transplant patient who received a liver transplant in 1982 (Jacobson *et al.* 1991). As routine screening for HIV antibody was not introduced until 1985 this patient's pretransplant serum was only found to be HIV antibody-positive retrospectively. He had been given cyclosporin A as the sole immunosuppressive treatment and had only one rejection episode treated with prednisolone early after transplantation. He had no AIDS or HIV-related symptoms 9 years after transplantation. Karpas *et al.* (1992) have shown that the immunosuppressive drugs cyclosporin A and FK506 may inhibit replication of cells infected with HIV.

We have reviewed HIV infections in transplant patients (Jacobson & Wreghitt 1992). The length of time infected with the virus, type and number of organs transplanted, intensity of the initial immunosuppressive therapy, number and severity of rejection episodes, number and severity of other viral infections and age of the patient are all factors which appeared to influence the outcome in HIV antibody-positive organ recipients. Poli *et al.* (1989) reviewed eight transplant patients who had acquired HIV infection postoperatively between 1982 and 1985. These patients were reviewed in 1988 and three had died: one with AIDS and another with Kaposi's sarcoma 5 and 2 years, respectively, after transplant. The third patient died without AIDS. Three other patients were asymptomatic, one had AIDS-related complex and another had persistent lymphadenopathy.

There is an ethical dilemma, particularly in heart and liver transplant recipients, for whom no alternative treatments are available, of whether or not to transplant a known HIV antibody-positive patient. In making this decision, the benefit to the patient, the risk to staff and the denial of scarce organs to other patients who would most probably have a better prognosis should be considered. Combination anti-HIV therapy regimes may improve long-term survival in transplant recipients.

## Adenovirus

Adenovirus infections are an important cause of morbidity and mortality in organ recipients. Infection is common in children but rare in adults. Adenoviruses have been associated with interstitial pneumonia and acute haemorrhagic cystitis in kidney transplant recipients and fulminant infection has been reported in liver, kidney and bone marrow recipients (Zahradnik *et al.* 1980; Wreghitt *et al.* 1989). Infection is not usually acquired from the donor organ, although it may be transmitted with heart–lung or lung grafts. Infection may arise at any time after transplantation. Koneru *et al.* (1987) described adenovirus infection in 22 of 262 (8.4%) paediatric liver transplant recipients, of which 60% were caused by adenovirus types 1 and 2 and associated with mild symptoms. By contrast, all five patients who were infected with adenovirus type 5 had severe fulminant hepatitis, all following treatment for rejection; two patients died. Adenovirus type 7 was isolated from one child with mild symptoms. By contrast, one child developed fatal interstitial pneumonia in Cambridge as a result of adenovirus type 7 infection (Salt *et al.* 1990). In our series, eight of 43 (19%) developed adenovirus infection. Apart from the patient who died, four other patients had symptoms which were characterized by transient fever, coryza, pharyngitis and conjunctivitis (Salt *et al.* 1990).

Adenovirus infection after transplant is usually diagnosed by means of serological tests which employ group-specific antigens. This has resulted in limited data on the adenovirus types associated with infection in these patients although where virus culture has been performed adenovirus types 5, 7, 11, 34 and 35 have been frequently isolated (Shields *et al.* 1985). Intermediate adenovirus types such as adenovirus 11/35 have been isolated from transplant patients.

Adenoviruses have been shown to persist in human tissue at extremely low levels in immunocompetent individuals. Virus may persistently infect about one in 100 million cells of the adenoids or tonsils. The effects of immunosuppression on the virus–host interaction are persistent and the importance of primary and reactivated infections if latency is established needs further investigation.

## Orthomyxo- and paramyxoviruses

Orthomyxo- and paramyxoviruses cause clinically important infections in organ transplant recipients. Patients often develop lower respiratory tract involvement and sometimes respiratory failure, which is often fatal. There is a higher risk of severe disease in bone marrow transplant recipients compared with solid organ transplant recipients (Sable & Hayden 1995).

Wendt *et al.* (1995) reported paramyxovirus infections in 21% of lung transplant recipients and that age was the strongest predictor of infection, with a higher incidence in patients under 18 years old. Lower respiratory tract infection with respiratory syncytial virus or paramyxovirus could be fatal or result in a permanent reduction in pulmonary function.

Apalsch *et al.* (1995) reported that in paediatric organ transplant recipients parainfluenza and influenza infections were important causes of morbidity and mortality. Eight out of 42 patients with influenza or parainfluenza virus infection died; five had parainfluenza and three had influenza virus infection. Factors associated with poor outcome included age, with increased morbidity and mortality in those less than 6 months old, augmentation of immunosuppression and the onset of disease within 1 month of transplantation.

## Papovaviruses

The suppression of cell-mediated immune surveillance with immunosuppressive drugs results in ~90% of organ recipients developing cutaneous warts within 5 years after transplant (Leigh & Glover 1995). Although external anogenital lesions are more rare than cutaneous lesions in organ transplant recipients, their association with dysplastic changes and malignant transformation make regular surveillance necessary (Euvrard *et al.* 1997). A history of warts and the presence of human papillomavirus (HPV) DNA sequences in biopsies of normal areas of epithelium in these patients suggests a reactivation of persistent virus rather than a primary infection after transplantation. It is thought that HPVs, associated with cutaneous warts, may persist in squamous epithelium in the absence of recognizable lesions (McCance & Gardner 1987).

Most infections with polyomaviruses are unapparent. Progressive multifocal leucoencephalopathy, which is associated with polyomavirus infection, is a rare complication of infection after transplantation. In bone marrow transplant recipients transient post-transplant hepatitis (O'Reilly *et al.* 1981) and intestitial pneumonia (Sandler *et al.* 1997) have been associated with polyomavirus infection. Both primary and secondary infections with the human polyomaviruses BK and JC are common after transplantation (Gardner *et al.* 1984). More than 90% of the population in the UK will have experienced infection with BK virus by the age of 5 years. Therefore most infections after transplant are a result of reactivation of latent virus. Both primary infection and reactivation of endogenous virus are seen with JC virus, as only 50% of the population have experienced infection with this virus by the time they reach adulthood. Although many polyomavirus infections occur 4–8 weeks after transplant, infections after 12 or more months have been reported.

## Conclusions

There are many viruses which are associated with morbidity in transplant recipients. The severity of infection is generally associated with the intensity of the immunosuppressive therapy given. The increasing availability of more and better antiviral agents and their use prophylactically and pre-emptively is providing a means to prevent infection or limit the severity of some viral infections, notably the herpesviruses.

## References

Acheson, D. (1990) *HIV Infection, Tissue Banks and Organ Donation.* Department of Health, London; CMO **92**, 2.

Alkan, S., Karcher, D.S., Ortiz, A. *et al.* (1997) Human herpesvirus-8 Karposi's sarcoma-associated herpesvirus in organ transplant patients with immunosuppression. *British Journal of Haematology* **96**, 412–414.

Apalsch, A.M., Green, M., Ledesma-Medina, J., Nour, B. & Wald, E.R. (1995) Parainfluenza and influenza virus infections in pediatric organ transplant recipients. *Clinical Infectious Diseases* **20**, 394–399.

Appleton, A.L., Sviland, L., Peiris, J.S. *et al.* (1995) Human herpes virus-6 infection in marrow graft recipients: role in pathogenesis of graft-versus-host disease. *Bone Marrow Transplantation* **16**, 777–782.

Bach, J.F. & Strom, T. (1985) *The Mode of Action of Immunosuppressive Agents.* Elsevier, Amsterdam.

Baglin, T.P., Gray, J.J., Marcus, R.E. & Wreghitt, T.G. (1989) Antibiotic-resistant fever associated with herpes simplex virus infection in neutropenic patients with haematological malignancy. *Journal of Clinical Pathology* **42**, 1255–1258.

Balfour, H.H. & Groth, K.E. (1981) Zoster immune plasma prophylaxis of varicella: a follow up report. *Journal of Pediatrics* **94**, 743–746.

Balfour, H.H. Jr, McMonigal, K.A. & Bean, B. (1983) Aciclovir therapy of varicella zoster virus infections in immunocompromised patients. *Antimicrobial Agents and Chemotherapy* **12** (Suppl. B), 169–179.

Balfour, H.H. Jr, Chace, B.A., Stapleton, J.T., Simmons, R.L. & Fryd, D.S. (1989) A randomized, placebo-controlled trial of oral acyclovir for the prevention of cytomegalovirus disease in recipients of renal allografts. *New England Journal of Medicine* **320**, 1381–1387.

Bardelas, J.A., Winkelstein, J.A., Seto, D.S.Y., Tsai, T. & Rogol, A.D. (1977) Fatal ECHO 24 infection in a patient with hypogammaglobulinemia. Relationship to dermatomyositis–like syndrome. *Journal of Pediatrics* **90**, 396–399.

Beasley, R.P., Hwang, L.Y., Lin, C.C. & Chien, C.S. (1981) Hepatocellular carcinoma and hepatitis B virus. *Lancet* ii, 1129–1133.

Benkerrou, M., Durandy, A. & Fischer, A. (1993) Therapy for transplant-related lymphoproliferative diseases. *Hematology Oncology Clinics of North America* **7**, 467–475.

Blumberg, B.S., Alter, H.J. & Visnich, S. (1965) A 'new' antigen in leukaemia sera. *Journal of the American Medical Association* **191**, 541–546.

Bradley, J.R., Wreghitt, T.G. & Evans, D.B. (1987) Chickenpox in adult renal transplant recipients. *Nephrology, Dialysis, Transplantation* **1**, 242–245.

Bradstreet, C.M.P. & Taylor, C.E.D. (1962) Technique of complement fixation test applicable to the diagnosis of virus diseases. *Monthly Bulletin of the Ministry of Health and Public Health Laboratory Service* **21**, 96–104.

Briggs, M., Fox, J. & Tedder, R.S. (1988) Age prevalence of antibody to human herpesvirus 6. *Lancet* **i**, 1058–1059.

Bruguera, M., Cremades, M., Mayor, A., Sanchez Tapias, J.M. & Rodes, J. (1987) Immunogenicity of a recombinant hepatitis B vaccine in haemodialysis patients. *Postgraduate Medical Journal* **63** (Suppl.2), 155–158.

Carman, W.F., Trautwein, C., van Deursen, F.J. *et al.* (1996) Hepatitis B virus envelope variation after transplantation with and without hepatitis B immunoglobulin prophylaxis. *Hepatology* **24**, 489–493.

Carrigan, D.R., Drobyski, W.R., Russler, S.K. *et al.* (1991) Interstitial pneumonitis associated with human herpesvirus-6 infection after marrow transplantation. *Lancet* **338**, 147–149.

Chandler, C., Meurisse, E.V. & Wreghitt, T.G. (1990) Herpesviruses. In: *ELISA, in the Clinical Microbiology Laboratory* (eds T.G. Wreghitt & P. Morgan-Capner), pp. 62–86. Public Health Laboratory Service, London.

Chang, Y., Cesarman, E., Pessin, M.S. *et al.* (1994) Identification of herpesvirus-like DNA sequences in AIDS-associated Kaposi's sarcoma. *Science* **266**, 1865–1869.

Choo, Q.-L., Kuo, G., Weiner, A.J. *et al.* (1989) Isolation of a cDNA clone derived from a blood-borne non-A, non-B viral hepatitis genome. *Science* **244**, 359–362.

Choo, Q.-L., Weiner, A.J., Overby, L.R., Kuo, G. & Houghton, M. (1990) Hepatitis C virus: the major causative agent of viral non-A, non-B hepatitis. *British Medical Bulletin* **46**, 423–441.

Crawford, D.H. &. Edwards, J.M.B. (1987) Epstein–Barr virus. In: *Principles and Practice of Clinical Virology* (eds A.J. Zuckerman, J.E. Banatvala & J.R. Pattison), pp. 111–133. John Wiley & Sons, Chichester.

Crawford, D.H., Edwards, J.M.B., Sweny, P., Hoffbrand, A.V. & Janossy, G. (1981) Studies on longterm T cell mediated immunity to Epstein–Barr virus in immunosuppressed renal allograft recipients. *International Journal of Cancer* **28**, 705–709.

Dawson, G.J., Schlauder, G.G., Pilot-Matias, T.J. *et al.* (1996) Prevalence studies of GB virus-C infection using reverse transcriptase-polymerase chain reaction. *Journal of Medical Virology* **50**, 97–103.

Decoene, C., Pol, A., Dewilde, A. *et al.* (1996) Relationship between CMV and graft rejection after heart transplantation. *Transplant International* **9** (Suppl. 1), S241–S242.

Delgado, R., Lumbreras, C., Alba, C. *et al.* (1992) Low predictive value of polymerase chain reaction for diagnosis of cytomegalovirus disease in liver transplant recipients. *Journal of Clinical Microbiology* **30**, 1876–1878.

Demetris, A.J., Jaffe, R., Sheahan, D.G. *et al.* (1986) Recurrent hepatitis B in liver allograft reagents. Differentiation between viral hepatitis B and rejection. *American Journal of Pathology* **125**, 161–172.

Desaules, M., Frei, P.C., Libanska, J. & Wuilleret, B. (1976) Lack of leucocyte migration inhibition by hepatitis B antigen and normal non-specific immunoreactivity in asymptomatic carriers. *Journal of Infectious Diseases* **134**, 505.

Di Bisceglie, A.M. (1998) Hepatis C. *Lancet* **351**, 351–355.

Dummer, J.S., Erb, S., Breinig, M.K. *et al.* (1989) Infection with human immunodeficiency virus in the Pittsburgh transplant population. *Transplantation* **47**, 134–140.

Dussol, B., Charrel, R., De-Lamballerie, X. *et al.* (1997) Prevalence of hepatitis G virus infection in kidney transplant recipients. *Transplantation* **64**, 537–539.

Efstathiou, S., Gompels, U.A., Craxton, M.A., Honess, R.W. & Ward, K.N. (1988) DNA homology between a novel human herpesvirus (HHV-6) and human cytomegalovirus. *Lancet* **i**, 63–64.

Engelbrecht, S., Treurnicht, F.K., Schneider, J.W. *et al.* (1997) Detection of human herpes virus 8 DNA and sequence polymorphism in classical, epidemic, and iatrogenic Kaposi's sarcoma in South Africa. *Journal of Medical Virology* **52**, 168–172.

Erice, A., Rhame, F.S., Heussner, R.C., Dunn, D.L. & Balfour, H.H. (1991) Human immunodeficiency virus infection with solid organ transplants: report of five cases and review. *Reviews of Infectious Diseases* **13**, 537–541.

Euvrard, S., Kanitakis, J., Chardonnet, Y. *et al.* (1997) External anogental lesions in organ transplant recipients. A clinicopathologic and virologic assessment. *Archives of Dermatology* **133**, 175–178.

Fabrizi, F., Lunghi, G., Bacchini, G. *et al.* (1997) Hepatitis G virus infection in chronic dialysis patients and kidney transplant recipients. *Nephrology, Dialysis, Transplantation* **12**, 1645–1651.

Farci, P., Alter, H.J., Wong, D. *et al.* (1991) A long term study of hepatitis C virus replication in non-A, non-B hepatitis. *New England Journal of Medicine* **325**, 98–104.

Fassbinder, W., Scheuermann, E.H., Bechstein, P.B. & Schoeppe, W. (1985) Cytomegalovirus infections after renal transplantation: effect of prophylactic hyperimmune globulin. *Proceedings of the European Dialysis and Transplant Association*. **22**, 630–634.

Gaeta, A., Nazzari, C., Augeletti, S. *et al.* (1997) Monitoring for cytomegalovirus infection in organ transplant recipients: analysis of pp65 antigen, DNA and late mRNA in peripheral blood leukocytes. *Journal of Medical Virology* **53**, 189–195.

Gane, E., Saliba, F., Valdecasas, G.J.C. *et al.* (1997) Randomised trial of efficacy and safety of oral ganciclovir in the prevention of CMV disease in liver transplant recipients. *Lancet* **350**, 1729–1733.

Gardner, S.D., MacKenzie, E.F.D., Smith, C. & Porter, A.A. (1984) Prospective study of the human polyomaviruses BK and JC and cytomegalovirus in renal transplant recipients. *Journal of Clinical Pathology* **37**, 578–586.

Garson, J.A., Tedder, R.S., Briggs, M. *et al.* (1990) Detection of hepatitis C viral sequences in blood donations by 'nested' polymerase chain reaction and prediction of infectivity. *Lancet* **335**, 1419–1422.

Gerna, G., Zipeto, D., Parea, M. *et al.* (1991) Monitoring of human CMV infections and ganciclovir treatment in heart transplant recipients by determination of viraemia, antigenaemia and DNAemia. *Journal of Infectious Diseases* **164**, 488–498.

Goeser, T., Blazek, M., Gmelin, K., Kommerell, B. & Theilmann, L. (1990) Washing with 8mol/1 urea to correct false-positive anti-HCV results. *Lancet* **ii**, 878.

Gray, J.J. (1995) Avidity of EBV VCA-specific IgG antibodies; Distinction between recent primary infection, post infection and reactivation. *Journal of Virological Methods* **52**, 95–104.

Gray, J.J. & Wreghitt, T.G. (1989) Immunoglobulin G avidity in Epstein–Barr virus infections in organ transplant recipients. *Serodiagnosis and Immunotherapy in Infectious Disease* **3**, 389–393.

Gray, J.J., Alvey, B.A., Smith, D.J. & Wreghitt, T.G. (1987) Evaluation of a commercial latex agglutination test for detecting antibodies to cytomegalovirus in organ donors and transplant recipients. *Journal of Virological Methods* **16**, 13–19.

Gray, J.J., Wreghitt, T.G. & Baglin, T.P. (1989) Susceptibility to acyclovir of herpes simplex virus: emergence of resistance in patients with lymphoid and myeloid neoplasia. *Journal of Infection* **19**, 31–40.

Gray, J.J., Wreghitt, T.G., Friend, P.J. *et al.* (1990) Differentiation between specific and non-specific hepatitis C antibodies in chronic liver disease. *Lancet* **335**, 609–610.

Gray, J.J., Wreghitt, T.G., Pavel, P. *et al.* (1995) Epstein–Barr virus infection in heart and heart–lung transplant recipients: incidence and clinical impact. *Journal of Heart and Lung Transplantation* **14**, 640–646.

Griffiths, P.D., Panjwani, D.D., Stirk, P.R. *et al.* (1984) Rapid diagnosis of cytomegalovirus infection in immunocompromised patients by detection of early antigen fluorescent foci. *Lancet* **ii**, 1242–1245.

Hawkins, A.E., Gilson, R.J.C., Gilbert, N. *et al.* (1996) Hepatitis B virus surface mutations associated with infection after liver transplantation. *Journal of Hepatology* **24**, 8–14.

Hebart, H., Muller, C., Loffler, J., Jahn, G. & Einsele, H. (1996) Monitoring of CMV infection: a comparison of PCR from whole blood, plasma—PCR, pp 56 antigenaemia and virus culture in patients after bone marrow transplantation. *Bone Marrow Transplantation* **17**, 861–868.

Hermans, P.E. & Wilson, W.R. (1980) Immunoglobulin deficiency—pathogenisis and type of infection. In: *Infections in the Immunocompromised Host: Pathogenesis, Prevention and Therapy* (ed. J. Verokoefer), pp. 5–21. Elsevier, Amsterdam.

Hsia, K., Spector, D.H., Lawne, J. & Spector, S. (1989) Enzymatic amplification of human cytomegalovirus sequences by polymerase chain reaction. *Journal of Clinical Microbiology* **27**, 1802–1809.

Irving, W.L., Mala Ratnamohan, V., Hueston, L.C., Chapman, J.R. & Cunningham, A.L. (1990) Dual antibody rises to cytomegalovirus and human herpesvirus type 6: frequency of occurrence in CMV infections and evidence for genuine reactivity to both viruses. *Journal of Infectious Diseases* **161**, 910–916.

Jacobson, S.K. & Wreghitt, T.G. (1992) HIV infection in transplant patients. *Reviews of Medical Virology* **2**, 221–224.

Jacobson, S.K., Calne, R.Y. & Wreghitt, T.G. (1991) Outcome of HIV infection in a transplant patient on Cyclosporin. *Lancet* **337**, 794.

Kanji, S.S., Sharara, A.I., Clavien, P.A. & Hamilton, J.D. (1996) Cytomegalovirus infection following liver transplantation: review of the literature. *Clinical Infectious Diseases* **22**, 537–549.

Kao, J.-H., Chen, P.-J. & Chen, D.-S. (1996) GBV-C in the aetiology of fulminant hepatitis. *Lancet* **347**, 120.

Karpas, A., Lowell, M., Jacobson, S.K. & Hill, F. (1992) Inhibition of human immunodeficiency virus and growth of infected T cells by the immunosuppressive drugs cyclosporin A and FK 506. *Proceedings of the National Academy of Sciences (USA)* **89**, 8351–8355.

Klatzmann, D. & Gluckman, J.C. (1986) HIV infection: facts and hypotheses. *Immunology Today* **7**, 291–296.

Koneru, B., Jaffe, R., Esquivel, C.O. *et al.* (1987) Adenovirus infections in paediatric liver transplant recipients. *Journal of the American Medical Association* **258**, 489–492.

Koskinen, P., Lemstrom, K., Bruggeman, C., Lautenschlager, J. & Hayry, P. (1994) Acute CMV infection induces a subendothelial inflammation in the allograft vascular wall. A possible linkage with enhanced allograft arteriosclerosis. *American Journal of Pathology* **144**, 41–50.

Koskinen, P., Lemstrom, K., Mattila, S., Hayry, P. & Nieminen, M.S. (1996) CMV infection associated accelerated heart allograft arteriosclerosis may impair the late function of the graft. *Clinical Transplantation* **10**, 487–493.

Kuroki, T., Nishiguchi, S., Tanaka, M., Enomoto, M. &

Kobayashi, K. (1996) Does GBV-C cause fulminant hepatitis in Japan? *Lancet* **347**, 908.

Lang, P.H. & Niaudet, P. (1991) Update and outcome of renal transplantation patients with human immunodeficiency virus. *Transplantation Proceedings* **23**, 1352–1353.

Lauchart, W., Muller, R. & Pichlmayr, R. (1987) Immunoprophylaxis of hepatitis B virus reinfection in recipients of human liver allografts. *Transplantation Proceedings* **19**, 2387–2389.

Leblond, V., Sutton, L., Dorent, R. *et al.* (1995) Lymphoproliferative disorders after organ transplantation: a report of 24 cases observed in a single center. *Journal of Clinical Oncology* **13**, 961–968.

Leigh, I.M. & Glover, M.T. (1995) Skin cancer and warts in immunosuppresed renal transplant recipients. *Recent Results in Cancer Research* **139**, 69–86.

Linnen, J., Wages, J., Zhang-Keck, Z.Y. *et al.* (1996) Molecular cloning and disease association of hepatitis G virus: a transfusion–transmissible agent. *Science* **217**, 505–508.

Lucas, K.G., Pollok, K.E. & Emanuel, D.J. (1997) Post-transplant EBV induced lymphoproliferative disorders. *Leukaemia and Lymphoma* **25**, 1–8.

McCance, D.J. & Gardner, S.D. (1987) Papovaviruses: papillomaviruses and polyomaviruses. In: *Principles and Practice of Clinical Virology* (eds A.J. Zuckerman, J.E. Banatvala & J.R. Pattison), pp. 479–506. John Wiley and Sons, Chichester.

McCarthy, J.M., Karim, M.A., Krueger, H. & Keown, P.A. (1993) The cost impact of cytomegalovirus disease in renal transplant recipients. *Transplantation* **555**, 1277–1282.

Merigan, T.C. (1981) Immunosuppression and herpesviruses. In: *The Human Herpesviruses. An Interdisciplinary Perspective* (eds A.J. Nahmias, W.R. Dowdle & R.F.Schinazi), p. 309. Elsevier, New York.

Merigan, T.C., Renlund, D.G., Keay, S. *et al.* (1992) A controlled trial of ganciclovir to prevent CMV disease after heart transplantation. *New England Journal of Medicine* **326**, 1182–1186.

Mollison, L.C., Richards, M.J., Johnson, P.D.R. *et al.* (1993) High dose oral aciclovir reduces the incidence of cytomegalovirus infection in liver transplant recipients. *Journal of Infectious Diseases* **168**, 721–724.

Morgan, G. & Superina, R.A. (1994) Lymphoproliferative disease after pediatric liver transplantation. *Journal of Pediatric Surgery* **29**, 1192–1196.

Morris, D.J., Littler, E., Jordan, D. & Arrand, J.R. (1988) Antibody responses to human herpesvirus-6 and other herpesviruses. *Lancet* **2**, 1425–1426.

Muerhoff, A.S., Leary, T.D., Simons, J.N. *et al.* (1995) Genomic organisation of GB viruses A and B: two new members of the flaviviridae associated with GB agent hepatitis. *Journal of Virology* **69**, 5621–5630.

Nadasdy, T., Smith, J., Laszik, Z. *et al.* (1994) Absence of association between CMV infection and obliterative transplant arteriopathy in renal allograft rejection. *Modern Pathology* **7**, 289–294.

Nalesnik, M.A., Jaffe, R.J., Starzl, T.E. *et al.* (1988) The pathology of posttransplant lymphoproliferative disorders occuring in the setting of cyclosporine A—prednisolone immunosuppression. *American Journal of Pathology* **133**, 173–192.

O'Connell, J.B., Renlund, D.G. & Bristow, M.R. (1989) Murine monoclonal CD3 antibody (OKT3) in cardiac transplantation: three year experience. *Transplantation Proceedings* **21** (Suppl. 2), 31–33.

O'Grady, J.G., Alexander, G.J.M., Sutherland, S. *et al.* (1988) Cytomegalovirus infection and donor/recipient HLA antigens: interdependent co-factors in pathogenesis of vanishing bile duct syndrome after liver transplantation. *Lancet* ii, 302–305.

O'Grady, J.G., Smith, H.M. & Davies, S.E. (1992) Hepatitis B reinfection after orthotopic liver transplantation. Serological and clinical implications. *Journal of Hepatology* **14**, 104–111.

Okuno, T., Higashi, K., Shiraki, K. *et al.* (1990) Human herpesvirus 6 infection in renal transplantation. *Transplantation* **49**, 519–522.

Olive, D.M., Simsek, M. & Al-Mufti, S. (1989) Polymerase chain reaction assay for detection of human cytomegalovirus. *Journal of Clinical Microbiology* **27**, 1238–1242.

O'Reilly, R.J., Lee, F.K., Grossbard, E. *et al.* (1981) Papovavirus excretion following marrow transplantation: incidence and association with hepatic dysfunction. *Transplantation Proceedings* **13**, 262–266.

Otero, J., Rodriguez, M., Escudero, D. *et al.* (1990) Kidney transplants with positive anti-hepatitis C virus donors. *Transplantation* **50**, 1086–1087.

O'Toole, C.M., Gray, J.J., Maher, P. & Wreghitt, T.G. (1986) Persistent excretion of cytomegalovirus in heart transplant patients correlates with the inversion of the ratio of T helper/T suppressor-cytotoxic cells. *Journal of Infectious Diseases* **153**, 1160–1162.

Pereira, B.J.G., Milford, E.L., Kirkman, R.L. & Levey, A.S. (1991) Transmission of hepatitis C virus by organ transplantation. *New England Journal of Medicine* **325**, 454–460.

Pereira, B.J.G., Milford, E.L., Kirkman, R.L. *et al.* (1992) Prevalence of hepatitis C virus RNA in organ donors positive for hepatitis C antibody and in the recipients of their organs. *New England Journal of Medicine* **327**, 910–915.

Pirsch, J.D. & Belzer, F.O. (1992) Transmission of HCV by organ transplantation. *New England Journal of Medicine* **326**, 412.

Poli, F., Scalamonga, M., Pizzi, C., Mozzi, F. & Sirchia, G.

(1989) HIV infection in cadaveric renal allograft recipients in the North Italy transplant programme. *Transplantation* 47, 724–725.

Poterucha, J.J., Rakela, J., Lumeng, L. *et al.* (1992) Diagnosis of chronic hepatitis C after liver transplantation by the selection of viral sequences with polymerase chain reaction. *Hepatology* 15, 42–45.

Pouteil-Noble, C., Tandy, J.C., Chossegros, R. *et al.* (1992) Should hepatitis C virus antibody-positive donors be excluded from kidney donation? *Transplant International* 5, S44–S46.

Pouteil-Noble, C., Ecochard, R., Landrivon, G. *et al.* (1993) CMV infection: an etiological factor for rejection? A prospective study in 242 renal transplant patients. *Transplantation* 55, 851–857.

Public Health Laboratory Service Survey (1974) Decrease in the incidence of hepatitis in dialysis units associated with prevention programme. *British Medical Journal* iv, 751–754.

Ragni, M.V., Bontempo, F.A. & Lewis, J.N. (1990) Organ transplantation in HIV-positive patients with haemophilia. *New England Journal of Medicine* 322, 1886–1887.

Rand, K.H., Pollard, R.B. & Merigan, T.C. (1978) Increased pulmonary superinfections in cardiac transplant patients undergoing primary cytomegalovirus infection. *New England Journal of Medicine* 298, 951–953.

Realdi, G., Alberti, A., Rugge, M. *et al.* (1982) Long-term follow-up of acute and chronic non-A, non-B post transfusion hepatitis: evidence of progression to liver cirrhosis. *Gut* 23, 270–275.

Reichard, O., Norkraus, G., Fryden, A. *et al.* (1998) Randomised, placebo-controlled trial of interferon α-2b with and without ribavirin for chronic hepatitis C. *Lancet* 351, 83–87.

Roll, M., Norder, H., Magnius, L.O., Grillner, L. & Lindgren, V. (1995) Nosocomial spread of HBV in a haemodialysis unit confirmed by HBV DNA sequencing. *Journal of Hospital Infection* 30, 57–63.

Rubin, R.H., Jenkins, R.L., Byers, B.W. *et al.* (1987) The acquired immunodeficiency syndrome and transplantation. *Transplantation* 44, 1–4.

Sable, C.A. & Hayden, F.G. (1995) Orthomyxoviral and paramyxoviral infections in transplant patients. *Infectious Disease Clinics of North America* 9, 987–1003.

Salahuddin, S.Z., Ablashi, D.V., Markham, P.D. *et al.* (1986) Isolation of a new virus, HBLV, in patients with lymphoproliferative disorders. *Science* 234, 596–600.

Salt, A., Sutehall, G., Sargaisson, M. *et al.* (1990) Viral and *Toxoplasma gondii* infections in children after liver transplantation. *Journal of Clinical Pathology* 43, 63–67.

Samuel, D., Bismuth, A., Mathieu, D. *et al.* (1991) Passive immunoprophylaxis after liver transplantation in HBsAg positive patients. *Lancet* 337, 813–815.

Samuel, D., Muller, R., Alexander, G. *et al.* (1993) Liver transplantation in HBsAg positive patients: an European experience 1977–90. *New England Journal of Medicine* 329, 1842–1847.

Sandler, E.S., Aquino, V.M., Goss-Shohet, E., Hinrichs, S. & Krisher, K. (1997) BK papovavirus pneumonia following hematopoietic stem cell transplantation. *Bone Marrow Transplantation* 20, 163–165.

Schmidt, N.J., Lennette, E.H., Woodie, J.D. & Ho, H.H. (1965) Immunofluorescent staining in the laboratory diagnosis of varicella-zoster virus infections. *Journal of Laboratory and Clinical Medicine* 66, 403–412.

Shields, A.F., Hackman, R.C., Fife, K.H., Corey, L. & Meyers, J.D. (1985) Adenovirus infection in patients undergoing bone marrow transplantation. *New England Journal of Medicine* 312, 529–533.

Smyth, R.L., Higenbottam, T.W., Scott, J.P. *et al.* (1990) Herpes simplex virus infection in heart–lung transplant recipients. *Transplantation* 49, 735–739.

Smyth, R.L., Scott, L.K., Borysiewicz, L.D. *et al.* (1991a) Cytomegalovirus infection in heart–lung transplant recipients: risk factors, clinical associations, and response to treatment. *Journal of Infectious Diseases* 164, 1045–1050.

Smyth, R.L., Sinclair, J.P., Scott, J.J. *et al.* (1991b) Infection and reactivation with cytomegalovirus strains in lung transplant recipients. *Transplantation* 52, 480–481.

Snydman, D.R., Werner, B.G., Heinze-Lacey, B. *et al.* (1987) Use of cytomegalovirus immune globulin to prevent cytomegalovirus disease in renal transplant recipients. *New England Journal of Medicine* 317, 1049–1054.

Snydman, D.R., Werner, B.G., Tilney, N.L. *et al.* (1988) A further analysis of primary cytomegalovirus disease prevention in renal transplant recipients with a cytomegalovirus immune globulin: interim comparison of a randomized and open-label trial. *Transplantation Proceedings* 20 (Suppl. 8), 24–30.

Stagno, S., Pass, R.F., Reynolds, D.W. *et al.* (1980) Comparative study of diagnostic procedures for congenital cytomegalovirus infection. *Paediatrics* 65, 251–257.

Starzl, T.E., Nalesnik, M.A., Porter, K.A. *et al.* (1984) Reversibility of lymphomas and lymphoproliferative lesions developing under cyclosporine-steriod therapy. *Lancet* i, 583–587.

Stovin, P.G., Wreghitt, T.G., English, T.A.H. & Wallwork, J. (1989) Lack of association between cytomegalovirus infection of the heart and rejection-like inflammation. *Journal of Clinical Pathology* 42, 81–83.

Stratta, R.J., Shaefer, M.S., Cushing, K.A. *et al.* (1991) Successful prophylaxis of cytomegalovirus disease after primary CMV exposure in liver transplant recipients. *Transplantation* 51, 90–97.

Strazzabosco, M., Cornae, B., Iemmolo, R.M. *et al.* (1997) Epstein–Barr virus-associated post-transplant lymphoproliferative disease of donor origin in liver transplant recipients. *Journal of Hepatology* **26**, 926–934.

Summers, J. & Measons, W.A. (1982) Replication of the genome of a hepatitis B-like virus by reverse transcriptase. *Cell* **29**, 403–415.

Sutherland, S., Bracken, P., Wreghitt, T.G. *et al.* (1992) Donated organ as a source of cytomegalorvirus in orthotipic liver transplantation. *Journal of Medical Virology* **37**, 170–173.

Swinnen, L.J., Costanzo-Nordin, M.R., Fisher, S.G. *et al.* (1990) Increased incidence of lymphoproliferative disorder after immunosuppression with the monoclonal antibody OKT3 in cardiac transplant recipients. *New England Journal of Medicine* **323**, 1723–1728.

Tedder, R.S., Mortimer, P.P. & Lord, R.B. (1981) Detection of antibody to varicella-zoster virus by competitive and IgM antibody capture immunoassay. *Journal of Medical Virology* **8**, 89–101.

Tedder, R.S., Briggs, M., Cameron, C.H. *et al.* (1987) A novel lymphotropic herpesvirus. *Lancet* **ii**, 390–392.

The, T.H., van der Bij, W., van den Berg, A.P. *et al.* (1990) Cytomegalovirus antigenemia. *Reviews of Infectious Diseases* **12** (Suppl. 7), S737–S744.

Toyoda, M., Galfayan, K., Galera, O.A. *et al.* (1997) CMV infection induces anti-endothelial cell antibodies in cardiac and renal allograft recipients. *Transplant Immunology* **5**, 104–111.

Turner, D.P.J., Zuckerman, M., Alexander, G.J.M., Waite, J. & Wreghitt, T.G. (1997) Risk of inappropriate exclusion of organ donors by introduction of anti-HBc testing. *Transplantation* **63**, 775–777.

Tzakis, A.G., Cooper, M.H., Dummer, J.S. *et al.* (1990) Transplantation in HIV positive patients. *Transplantation* **40**, 354–358.

Van den Berg, A.P., Klompaker, I.J., Haagsma, E.B. *et al.* (1991) Antigenemia in the diagnosis and monitoring of active cytomegalovirus infection after liver transplantation. *Journal of Infectious Diseases* **164**, 165–170.

Van der Bij, W., Schirm, J., Torensma, R. *et al.* (1988) Comparison between viremia and antigenemia for detection of cytomegalovirus in blood. *Journal of Clinical Microbiology* **26**, 2531–2535.

Ward, K.N., Gray, J.J. & Efstathiou, S. (1989) Brief report: primary human herpesvirus 6 infection in a patient following liver transplantation from a seropositive donor. *Journal of Medical Virology* **28**, 69–72.

Ward, K.N., Sheldon, M.J. & Gray, J.J. (1991) Primary and recurrent cytomegalovirus infections have different effects on human herpesvirus-6 antibodies in immunosuppressed organ graft recipients: absence of virus cross-reactivity and evidence for virus interaction. *Journal of Medical Virology* **34**, 258–267.

Ward, K.N., Gray, J.J., Joslin, M. & Sheldon, M.J. (1993) Avidity of IgG antibodies to human herpesvirus-6

distinguishes primary from recurrent infection in organ transplant recipients and excludes cross-reactivity with other herpesviruses. *Journal of Medical Virology* **39**, 44–49.

Warrell, M.J., Chinn, I., Morrish, P.J. & Tobin, J.O'H. (1980) The effects of viral infections on renal transplants and their recipients. *Quarterly Journal of Medicine* **49**, 219–231.

Webster, R.G. (1968) The immune response to influenza virus III: changes in the avidity and specificity of early IgM and IgG antibodies. *Immunology* **14**, 39–52.

Wendt, C.H., Fox, J.M. & Hertz, M.I. (1995) Paramyxovirus infection in lung transplant recipients. *Journal of Heart and Lung Transplantation* **14**, 479–485.

Winston, D.J., Wirin, D., Shaked, A. & Busuttil, R.W. (1995) Randomised comparison of ganciclovir and high-dose aciclovir for long term cytomegalovirus prophylaxis in liver transplant recipients. *Lancet* **346**, 69–74.

World Health Organization (1985) Acquired immune deficiency syndrome (AIDS): provisional US Public Health Service interagency recommendations for screening donated blood and plasma for antibody to the virus causing AIDS. *Weekly Epidemiological Record* **4**, 21.

Wreghitt, T.G. (1991) Viral and *Toxoplasma gondii* infections in heart, heart–lung, liver and kidney transplant recipients. In: *Transplantation and Clinical Immunology XXII* (eds J.L. Touraine, J. Traeger, H. Betuel *et al.*), pp. 25–32. Excerpta Medica, Amsterdam.

Wreghitt, T.C. & Smith, D.J. (1989) A rapid latex agglutination test for detecting CMV antibody in transplant recipients. In: *Proceedings of the Fifth International Symposium on Rapid Methods and Automation in Microbiology and Immunology* (eds A. Balows, R.C. Tilton & A. Turano), pp. 636–640.

Wreghitt, T.G., Tedder, R.S., Nagington, J. & Ferns, R.B. (1984) Antibody assays for varicella-zoster virus: camparison of competitive enzyme-linked immunosorbent assay (ELISA), competitive radioimmunoassay (RIA), complement fixation and indirect immunofluorescence assays. *Journal of Medical Virology* **13**, 361–370.

Wreghitt, T.G., Gray, J.J. & Chandler, C. (1986a) Prognostic value of cytomegalovirus IgM antibody in transplant recipients. *Lancet* **i**, 1157–1158.

Wreghitt, T.G., Hicks, J., Gray, J.J. & O'Connor, C. (1986b) Development of a competitive enzyme-linked immunosorbent assay for detecting cytomegalovirus antibody. *Journal of Medical Virology* **18**, 119–129.

Wreghitt, T.G., Hakim, M., Cory-Pearce, R., English, T.A.H. & Wallwork, J. (1986c) The impact of donor-transmitted CMV and *Toxoplasma gondii* disease. in cardiac transplantation. *Transplantation Proceedings* **18**, 1375–1376.

Wreghitt, T.G., Gray, J.J., Ward, K.N. *et al.* (1989) Disseminated adenovirus infection after liver transplantation and its possible treatment with ganciclovir. *Journal of Infection* **18**, 88–89.

Wreghitt, T.G., Whipp, J. & Bagnall, J. (1992) Transmission of chickenpox to two intensive care unit nurses from a liver transplant patient with zoster. *Journal of Infection* **20**, 125.

Wreghitt, T.G., Gray, J.J., Allain, J.P. *et al.* (1994) Transmission of hepatitis C virus by organ transplantation in the United Kingdom. *Journal of Hepatology* **20**, 768–772.

Wreghitt, T.G., Whipp, J., Redpath, C. & Hollingworth, W. (1996) An analysis of infection control of varicella-zoster virus infections in Addenbrooke's Hospital, Cambridge over a 5 year period 1987–1992. *Epidemiology and Infection* **117**, 165–171.

Yilmaz, S., Koskinen, P.K., Kallio, E. *et al.* (1996) CMV infection enhanced chronic kidney allograft rejection is linked with intercellular adhesion molecule-1 expression. *Kidney International* **50**, 526–637.

Zahradnik, J.M., Spencer, M.J. & Porter, D.D. (1980) Adenovirus infection in the immunocompromised host. *American Journal of Medicine* **68**, 725–732.

Zipeto, D., Revello, M.G., Silini, E. *et al.* (1992) Development and clinical significance of a diagnostic assay based on the polymerase chain reaction for detection of human cytomegalovirus DNA in blood samples from immunocompromised patients. *Journal of Clinical Microbiology* **30**, 527–530.

# Chapter 17/Bacterial, fungal and parasitic infection after abdominal organ transplantation

MARK FARRINGTON

## Introduction

### General points

Human abdominal organ transplantation was first performed in the 1950s and 1960s; in this early period serious bacterial and fungal infections were common, being the major cause of death of patients. Most of these infections were the result of the intensive and crude immunosuppressive regimens then available.

Today, the 1-year survival of patients receiving kidney transplants from living related donors exceeds 95% with graft survival about 80%; the corresponding figures for cadaveric transplants are about 85% and 55%. Severe infection is less common and less often a direct cause of death (Nicholson & Johnson 1994; Winston *et al.* 1995) and, at least until the past few years (Chang *et al.* 1998), the microbial spectrum has switched towards viral causes. Bacterial infections remain important but early sepsis is now more commonly attributable to technical problems with the transplant operation. Liver transplantation is innately associated with a higher prevalence of fungal and viral infection compared with renal transplantation, mainly as a result of more intense immunosuppression and because of the ubiquitous colonization of both the donor and recipient gastrointestinal tracts with yeasts (Hibbard & Rubin 1994). Combined kidney and pancreas transplantation brings additional technical difficulties with their associated infectious risks. Small-intestinal transplantation, a procedure also frequently combined with other organs, is in its infancy and clearly brings a range of novel problems that are currently being defined. However, survival is improving, in association with developments in intensive care, immunosuppression, organ preservation and many other factors (Park *et al.* 1989). Solution of the remaining problems requires a combined approach involving technical refinements and a careful balance between operative and postoperative antibiotic prophylaxis.

This chapter reviews the range, prevalence, associations and prevention of bacterial, fungal and parasitic infection in recipients of liver, kidney, pancreas and small-bowel transplants. New developments and reports are highlighted, and potential opportunities for clinical progress emphasized. There are difficulties of comparison across time and between centres because techniques and patient acceptance criteria have developed greatly over the past 30 years, and small variations in practice change the spectrum of subsequent infections. In general, immunosuppressive regimens in the UK employ lower doses of fewer agents than regimens popular on the other side of the Atlantic, and this undoubtedly has an effect on the reported patterns of postoperative infection. Risk groups therefore need to be defined with particular care, and factors relevant with one style of immunosuppressive regimen may not be useful elsewhere. Despite refinements in selection and technique, infection remains a major cause of morbidity and mortality in transplant recipients, and each new technical development brings its own novel infectious complications to be overcome. Infection is still found to be the most common cause of death in most studies of transplant outcomes (Washer *et al.* 1983; Park *et al.* 1989).

Many factors common to transplantation of all the abdominal viscera explain much of the patients' general susceptibility to infection and influence the organisms involved. All patients undergoing solid organ transplantation are broadly debilitated, commonly malnourished and frequently suffer from metabolic disturbances that compromise non-specific cellular and humoral immunity. Some of the specific mechanisms behind these effects are being elucidated. Thus, uraemic renal transplant candidates have been shown to have impaired neutrophil chemotaxis and decreased marrow reserves of granulocytes (Salant *et al.* 1976). Hypogammaglobulinaemia was found in 39 of 110 (35.5%) renal transplant recipients, which conferred a significantly greater risk of infectious complications (Pollock *et al.* 1989). Patients undergoing hepatic transplantation for alcoholic liver disease have elevated chemotactic factor inactivator, which inhibits complement factor C5a, also leading to impaired neutrophil chemotaxis (Robbins *et al.* 1987). *Aspergillus* infection is promoted by dysfunction of alveolar macrophages (responsible mainly for inhibition of spore germination) and neutrophils (which mainly act to destroy hyphae), and both cell-mediated and phagocytic deficits promote infection with *Candida* spp. (Khardori 1989; Meunier 1989).

Elderly transplant recipients are especially likely to have cholelithiasis, diverticular disease and chronic obstructive airways disease. Young children receiving organ transplants are at risk of severe infection with capsulate organisms (such as *Streptococcus pneumoniae* and *Haemophilus influenzae*) and they may have only a partially protective response to immunization or be too young to have received a full range of vaccines. Children with biliary atresia and portoenterostomy suffer recurrent cholangitic episodes while awaiting liver transplant, and the recipient's peritoneum is likely to be contaminated with infected bile during the removal of their own liver. Collapse of the right lower lung lobe may predispose liver transplant recipients to bacterial pneumonia (Krowka & Cortese 1985).

## Immunosuppression and infection

Infecting microorganisms may be derived from the patients' own normal flora, supplemented by pre- and postoperatively acquired organisms, and subjected to antibiotic selective pressures from transfused blood and blood products, from the donor organ and from environmental sources. Orr and Gould (1992) have usefully summarized contemporary knowledge about graft-transmitted infection, and extrinsic sources of pulmonary infection in immunocompromised patients are well reviewed by Rhame *et al.* (1984). A small series of multiorgan transplants from donors dying of systemic sepsis published by Little *et al.* (1997) illustrates that, if guidelines for duration of effective antibiotic therapy and clinical status at the time of harvest are followed (Committee on the Microbiological Safety of Human Tissues and Organs used in Transplantation 1996), grafts from such patients have a good outcome.

Advances in immunosuppression may bring novel problems of infection or may complicate its treatment. Thus cyclosporin has important metabolic interactions with ketoconazole (Ferguson *et al.* 1982), amphotericin B (Gerson 1987), erythromycin (Martell *et al.* 1986) and antituberculous drugs (Langhoff & Madsen 1983). Treatment of *Legionella* infections in particular may be complicated by erythromycin raising cyclosporin concentrations and rifampicin reducing them. Fluconazole is partially metabolized via the liver cytochrome-450 system and cyclosporin concentrations are only a little increased (trough levels approximately doubled) after 2 weeks' combination therapy (Canafax *et al.* 1991). Itraconazole may also increase cyclosporin levels (Kwan *et al.* 1987), but is probably less likely to do so than fluconazole. There may be nephrotoxic interactions between cyclosporin and aminoglycosides, amphotericin B and vancomycin, but this is probably significant only if cyclosporin levels are also high.

Enhanced treatment of rejection with immunomodulators other than steroids does not inevitably lead to an increased risk of infection. Thus, Koneru *et al.* (1989) compared the outcome of 27 paediatric liver transplants who received only steroids with that of 53 who received the murine monoclonal antibody OKT3 and found no significant difference in the rates of total, bacterial, fungal or viral infections.

Two recent reports have emphasized the need for stringent aseptic techniques while handling biological products and cells for transplantation in tissue banks or other laboratories. *Enterobacter cloacae* bacteraemias followed infusion of pancreatic islet cells, but the origin of the contamination was not proven (Taylor *et al.* 1994). Ezzedrine *et al.* (1994) described five organ transplant recipients who developed bacteraemia with *Ochrobactrum anthropi* after immunosuppression with a rabbit antithymocyte globulin preparation that had been contaminated with this rare environmental opportunist pathogen. This experience highlights the importance of rigorous process controls during the production of biological immunomodulators and during the processing of human and animal tissues within tissue banks. For example, the deionized water frequently used during preparation of biological reagents and tissues is inevitably colonized with environmental microbes, principally pseudomonads. Such bacteria may contain little lipopolysaccharide and therefore low-level contamination may be undetectable in *Limulus* or other bioassays. There are currently no guidelines recommending use of only autoclave- or filter-sterilized fluids during processing. We have detected consistent low-level contamination of bone grafts with *Pseudomonas cepacia* from water derived from a contaminated deionizer that was repeatedly negative in a *Limulus* assay (Farrington *et al.* 1998). Often only a small percentage of vials may be positive, hence quality control that relies on culture of a few samples may miss contaminated batches, and generally these products do not contain antibacterial preservatives.

## *Pneumocystis carinii* pneumonia

Between 5 and 10% transplant patients not given prophylaxis will suffer *Pneumocystis carinii* pneumonia (PCP) (Rubin & Tolkoff-Rubin 1993). Considerable progress has been made in the management of PCP, mostly in the prophylaxis, diagnosis and treatment of the infection in patients with AIDS (Bartlett & Smith 1991). It is not yet clear how useful some of these techniques will prove in other groups, including solid organ transplant recipients. Laborious microscopical demonstration of cysts in respiratory secretions is still the mainstay of diagnosis in many laboratories. Organism loads are consistently higher in PCP in patients with AIDS than in transplant recipients, and the diagnosis is more readily confirmed in induced sputum in these patients (Limper *et al.* 1989). Immunological stains are probably more sensitive than histochemical ones, but they are expensive and very time-consuming, and experienced microscopists are needed to differentiate between cysts and other bodies, such as yeasts.

Conventional views hold that PCP is largely or entirely the result of reactivation of latent infection acquired in childhood (Rhame *et al.* 1984). A variety of more or less anecdotal reports of transmission of pneumocystis between transplant recipients have been published (Rifkind *et al.* 1966; Singer *et al.* 1975). For example, five cases of PCP occurred over a 22-month period in renal transplant patients treated for graft rejection in a Swiss outpatient unit that also cared for AIDS patients (Chave *et al.* 1991). Although numbers were very small, the authors showed that cases had had more clinical encounters with AIDS patients who had PCP than had matched controls. These associations must remain for the moment unproven, and most authorities would not recommend protective or source isolation for pneumocystis. The marked rise in incidence compared with previous years in PCP among renal transplant recipients in 1991 and 1992 described by Branten *et al.* (1995) remains unexplained, but could be related to an outbreak. It is noteworthy that co-trimoxazole prophylaxis had not been used in these reports, and that Branten *et al.*'s 'outbreak' responded promptly to the institution of prophylaxis.

Arend *et al.* (1996) performed a case–control study of risk factors for PCP pneumonia after renal transplantation without prophylaxis in 15 cases and 95 control patients. They found the relative risks of PCP to be 1.7, 4.8 and 9.5 after one, two and three or more rejection treatments, to be 3.2 if their pretransplant cytomegalovirus (CMV) serology was negative, and to be 5.7 if these patients' donors' serology was positive. Hence it may be possible to define a group who would benefit from co-trimoxazole prophylaxis without exposing the remainder to unnecessary therapy.

## Tropical infections

Tuberculosis and exotic pathogens from abroad, such as *Strongyloides*, *Plasmodium* and *Histoplasma* spp., may emerge under the effects of immunosuppression. These may have been present preoperatively in either donor or recipient. Considering the broad geographical spread of *Strongyloides*, it is surprising that few systemic infections have been reported recently; this may be related to nematocidal activity of cyclosporin (Schad 1986), and a lower threshold for investigation and possibly pre-emptive therapy may be appropriate in patients receiving other immunosuppressive agents.

Stone and Schaffner (1990) reviewed *Strongyloides* hyperinfection and dissemination in transplant recipients, emphasizing its association with periods of increased immunosuppression, its protean manifestations and the wide range of bacteria that may accompany the larvae migrating from the gut, resulting in bacteraemia. Prognosis is clearly correlated with speed of diagnosis and over half of their cases were diagnosed serendipitously during investigations for more conventional pathogens. Nearly 80% cases presented within the first 3 months after transplantation, and over half their cases had normal eosinophil counts. Treatment of established cases is difficult and carries a poor prognosis (nearly half of Stone and Schaffner's cases of hyperinfection died); therefore strenuous efforts should be made to identify faecal larvae and perform serology in prospective transplant recipients to allow eradication before they are immunosuppressed. *Strongyloides* adults can survive for over 30 years in the normal intestine, hence long-standing immigrants may still be at

risk. An interesting view of tropical infections seen during 17 years of renal transplantation in the Philippines is given by Gueco *et al.* (1989).

## Diagnostic issues

Diagnosis and exclusion of bacterial infection in patients with solid organ transplants can be extremely difficult, especially early in the postoperative period. Pneumonia is the most awkward area because there are many non-infectious causes of syndromes presenting with fever, cough and chest X-ray abnormalities, and colonization of conventionally collected sputum with Gram-negative aerobic bacteria is inevitable if selective decontamination therapy is not used. Consequently, about 45% of pneumonias reported in series of solid organ recipients in the 1980s were presumed to be caused by Gram-negative aerobes (Mermel & Maki 1990). More careful investigation, for example of cases of acute pulmonary disease in liver transplant recipients, revealed that up to 64% were really non-infectious in cause (Jensen *et al.* 1986). Development of standardized bronchoscopic techniques, including bronchoalveolar lavage (BAL) and protected specimen brush, has transformed the ability to diagnose bacterial pneumonia specifically (Mermel & Maki 1990). Less clear are the relative efficacies of these techniques because they have rarely been studied in an exclusively transplant population, but BAL has been shown to be more sensitive in one uncontrolled assessment (Johnson *et al.* 1990).

Rubin and Fischman (1996) have recently reviewed the role of radionuclide imaging in immunocompromised patients, emphasizing that these techniques will not come into their own until their speed can be improved by developments which bypass the need to wait at least 24 h after injecting radiolabel before scans can be performed.

## Kidney and pancreas transplantation

### Infections following transplantation

Rubin *et al.* (1981) developed a timetable of infectious complications following renal transplantation that remains useful, although there have been changes of detail and new developments (Rubin & Tolkoff-Rubin 1989). Broadly, the first 4–6 weeks after transplantation are marked by serious bacterial infections, especially of the urinary tract, surgical wound and intravenous lines. Legionellosis is most common shortly after transplantation, presumably because of the combination of maximal immunosuppression with nosocomial exposure. In the next year come a variety of opportunist, often systemic infections with cytomegalovirus, *Nocardia* spp. (Wilson *et al.* 1989), *Listeria monocytogenes*, *Cryptococcus* spp., *Aspergillus* spp. and *Pneumocystis carinii*. Later still, when immunosuppressive regimens are at their weakest, problems with more conventional bacterial pathogens are seen, including pneumococcal pneumonia, influenza, milder urinary tract infections and a continuing risk of listeriosis. Renal transplant patients are not exempt from localized hospital-associated outbreaks; in the past special problems were reported with pseudomonads and other multiply resistant Gram-negative bacilli, *Aspergillus* spp. and legionellosis (Rubin *et al.* 1981). Nowadays, transplant units are particularly concerned by such nosocomial pathogens as methicillin-resistant *Staphylococcus aureus*, aminoglycoside-vancomycin- and penicillin-resistant enterococci, and multiply resistant *Mycobacterium tuberculosis*.

The cyclical peptide cyclosporin, progressively introduced in renal transplantation to replace high-dose prednisolone and azathioprine over a decade ago, is associated with a generally reduced risk of bacterial infective complications (Dummer *et al.* 1983; Najarian *et al.* 1983). For example, renal transplant patients studied by Dummer *et al.* given azathioprine and prednisone had 2.7 times as many non-viral infections as cyclosporin-treated patients during a follow-up period of up to a year (Dummer *et al.* 1983). Much of the reduction was observed in *S. aureus* infections. Similarly, a Canadian multicentre comparative study found fewer infections overall in the cyclosporin group, and opportunist agents caused none of the six cases of pneumonia in the cyclosporin group (Canadian Multicentre Transplant Study Group 1983). These studies have generally not been fully controlled for use of anti-

lymphocyte antibodies and other immunomodulating agents that are less often required with cyclosporin. Kim and Perfect (1989) reviewed 11 reports of randomized comparisons between cyclosporin and azathioprine regimens, mainly in renal transplantation, published between 1982 and 1987. Nine were assessable, of which six reported reduced bacterial infections and five reduced viral infections but, surprisingly, no trial reported fewer fungal infections with cyclosporin.

Possibly because of the ability to reduce steroid doses, infection has been reported to be further reduced in preliminary studies of the use of the macrolide immunosuppressive agent, tacrolimus (Kusne *et al.* 1991). Compared with cyclosporin, historically controlled data suggested that early infections were approximately halved in incidence (total 61% to 33% and non-viral 41% to 21%) after a mean of 152 days follow-up in 63 patients. Forty-one first transplants had a mean of 0.27 infective episodes per patient compared with 0.68 episodes for the 22 repeat transplants.

Despite these advances, over 75% of kidney graft recipients still present with an infectious disease in the first year after transplantation (Rubin & Tolkoff-Rubin 1989) and 70% of all infections occur within the first 3 months (Hibbard & Rubin 1993).

## Spectrum, sites and predisposing conditions

As an example of contemporary practice, Martinez-Marcos *et al.* (1994) reported an interesting study of infection in 50 consecutive renal transplant recipients followed up for 12 months. Patients were given surgical prophylaxis with ampicillin, gentamicin plus cloxacillin, but no other prophylactic agents were used. Overall, 98% of patients suffered one or more infections (mean of 4.5 per patient) and 47% of these occurred within the first 2 months after transplantation. Regular urine screens for infection were performed, which probably explains the high rate of asymptomatic bacteriuria and candiduria that was detected (106 episodes), three times the rate of symptomatic urinary tract infection (UTI). Overall, UTI was seen in 63% of patients, but there were only six episodes of clinical UTI and these apparently responded satisfactorily to outpatient antibiotic treatment. Four patients suffered surgical wound infection, two bacterial pneumonia and one each abdominal abscess and bacteraemia of unknown source. Of the factors assessed, reoperation for haemorrhage and use of antilymphocyte globulin were associated with a higher rate of infection overall, and severe fungal infection (but not severe CMV or bacterial infection) was associated with allograft loss. Interestingly no cases of PCP were seen, and the authors stress the importance of knowing the local incidence of this infection before prophylaxis is necessarily used. However, this is a small study upon which to base recommendations for PCP prophylaxis, and prevention of even one case would have been worthwhile given the safety of intermittent co-trimoxazole regimens. It is also possible that co-trimoxazole might have reduced the observed rate of UTI.

## URINARY TRACT INFECTION

Considering its importance, surprisingly few recent studies have critically addressed the prevalence and associations of UTI after renal transplantation. In the 1960s and 1970s rates of 35–79% were reported (Rubin *et al*. 1981), and there is only a little evidence that early UTI has declined in incidence more recently. *Streptococcus faecalis* UTI has been implicated as a precipitating factor for rejection (Byrd *et al*. 1978). Early UTI is clearly associated with urinary catheterization at the time of operation and with structural abnormalities of the urinary tract, but there is a continuing risk of infection even in 10-year-old grafts (Rao & Anderson 1988). Vesicoureteric reflux in paediatric renal transplant recipients has been associated with a higher rate of postoperative UTI and graft pyelonephritis (Hanevold *et al*. 1987). Stuby *et al*. (1989) found a high rate (85%) of early UTI in patients not given long-term antibiotic prophylaxis. In those receiving cyclosporin A most UTIs occurred in the first 4 weeks, whereas infections later than 1 year after transplantation were only seen in the group treated with azathioprine. Early UTI (within the first 3 months) is more commonly associated with clinical pyelonephritis, bacteraemia and relapse than is UTI presenting later (Rubin *et al*. 1981).

## BACTERAEMIA

Reported rates of bacteraemia have fallen from 26–60% in the late 1960s (Myerowitz *et al*. 1972; Anderson *et al*. 1973) to about 12% in the 1980s (Peterson & Anderson 1986), and more recent studies suggest even lower rates (Wagener & Yu 1992). Most postoperative bacteraemias continue to originate from the urinary tract and frequently involve aerobic Gram-negative bacilli (Neilsen & Korsager 1977) although staphylococci may be increasing in relative importance (Wagener & Yu 1992). More widespread use of co-trimoxazole prophylaxis against PCP and Gram-negative UTI may explain this change. Wagener and Yu (1992) reported that 41% of bacteraemic episodes originated in the urinary tract, 21% from infected dialysis access sites (mostly staphylococci and associated with return to dialysis), only 4% from pneumonia and in only 22% was the source unknown. Fifty-six per cent of bacteraemias occurred more than 12 months after transplantation and 96% involved only one organism. In renal graft recipients the mortality rate was 11.1%. Considering all types of organ transplant recipient (90 episodes of bacteraemia), *Escherichia coli* and other Enterobacteriaceae and *S. aureus* were the most common isolates from community-acquired bacteraemias, whereas the range of species isolated from hospital-acquired infections was much wider with major proportions contributed by *Staphylococcus epidermidis*, *Pseudomonas aeruginosa* and *Enterobacter* spp.

Although its incidence is falling in most countries, *Listeria monocytogenes* remains an important cause of bacteraemia, which may present without accompanying focal sepsis or in association with meningeal or cerebral signs (Rubin 1994). Gastrointestinal sources provide most of the remaining bacteraemias, which characteristically involve large-bowel bacterial flora and frequently involve a mixture of isolates. In particular, these accompany perforations of the stomach and upper small bowel as a result of steroid usage and idiopathic large-bowel infarction and perforation (Han *et al*. 1978). In a series of 116 autopsies performed on renal transplant recipients over a 20-year period, Martino *et al*. (1987) found that 10% had died with gut perforation. Although gut perforation appeared to be common in diabetic patients in this series, this may merely imply that diabetics are more likely to die of the complications. Such perforations remain largely unexplained and were reported in 1.1–2.3% of renal graft recipients in the azathioprine and prednisolone era. More recent data seem not to be available, suggesting that the problem may be less common with cyclosporin. About a quarter were caused by perforation of diverticulae but the remainder appear not to be related to CMV colitis, and the term non-occlusive ischaemia has been coined to explain the characteristic histological appearances (Puglisi *et al.* 1985; Church *et al.* 1986).

PNEUMONIA

Bacterial pneumonia is less common in patients after renal transplantation (1.5%) than in recipients of other solid organ transplants, in whom rates average 20% (Mermel & Maki 1990). Multivariate analysis of risk factors for pneumonia in intensive care units has been successful in elucidating causes in patients without transplants, and these techniques have begun to be applied to the transplant population. Thus, use of prednisone plus azathioprine plus antilymphocyte antibodies rather than prednisone plus cyclosporin (odds ratio (OR) 17.0), use of OKT3 for steroid-resistant rejection (OR 5.0), rejection episodes themselves (OR 3.7) and use of high-dose corticosteroids alone (OR 3.3) have been shown to be independently associated with bacterial pneumonia in renal graft recipients (Webb *et al.* 1978; Hesse *et al.* 1986a; Oh *et al.* 1988). CMV infection, especially primary infection, has been shown in several studies to increase the risk of bacterial pneumonia substantially (Mermel & Maki 1990). BAL is valuable in those who have sufficient pulmonary reserve to tolerate the procedure, and a report by Cahill *et al.* (1991) indicates that it should be considered in transplant patients with acute respiratory illness but without X-ray changes. Fifty-six of 91 consecutive BALs were positive (mainly for *Aspergillus*, CMV and other viruses), 73% of which were from patients whose chest X-rays lacked infiltrates. Unfortunately, the clinical progress of these patients is not given so the contribution made by BAL to their progress and the clinical significance of the isolates recovered are unknown.

Johnson *et al.* (1990) established a bronchoscopic diagnosis team for transplant recipients with signs suggestive of pneumonitis and report the results in 77 renal and three liver transplants. Their findings confirm the rarity of Gram-negative aerobic rod pneumonia when strict criteria are used for diagnosis; only five cases were seen, all diagnosed more than 1 month after transplant. BAL was more sensitive than bronchoscopic brushing, and a diagnosis was made within 1 day by direct staining of aspirated material in 65% of episodes. CMV was the most common isolate (51 cases), mainly occurring between 1 and 4 months postoperatively, but most CMV diagnoses were delayed by the need to culture the virus.

Legionnaires' disease remains a potential problem for all transplant recipients, and the experience of Prodinger *et al.* (1994) of 14 cases over an 8-year period associated with a persistently contaminated water supply emphasizes the importance of good basic design in a modern hospital's services. Preventative maintenance, superheating, hyperchlorination, silver–copper ionization and other proposed control measures for *Legionella* will only be effective if the water system is constructed to a suitable basic standard. As well as its ability to cause pneumonia, *Legionella pneumophila* serogroup 1 has recently been reported as a cause of hepatic infection in a liver graft recipient (Tokunaga *et al.* 1992). Other, less common legionellas continue to be reported as causes of pneumonia in transplant recipients (Jernigan *et al.* 1994). Species and subspecies other than *L. pneumophila* serogroup 1 may not cross-react with the commonly used immunodiagnostic tests, which emphasizes the importance of culture and of referral of serum to specialist laboratories when the diagnosis is suspected but screening serology and urine antigen detection assays are negative.

WOUND INFECTION

In the 1970s, variable but often high rates of wound

infection were reported after renal transplantation, ranging between 1.8 and 56% with a mean of about 15% (Rubin *et al.* 1981; Tillegard 1984; Edelstein *et al.* 1989). Deep wound infection is anatomically synonymous with perinephric infection in a transplanted kidney and such severe infections were associated with loss of the graft in up to 75% of cases (Rubin *et al.* 1981), with mortality rates of up to 30% ensuing from systemic sepsis or rupture of the infected vascular anastomosis (Kyriakides *et al.* 1975). Modern management, however, appears to give better results (Edelstein *et al.* 1989). Some authors have found early (within the first 3 weeks) wound infection usually to be superficial and caused by staphylococci, but later infection to be deep and associated with haematomas, ureterovesical leakage, coliform UTIs and graft dysfunction (Lobo *et al.* 1982). Lobo *et al.* hypothesized from their retrospectively gathered data that perioperative bacteriuria led to colonization and later breakdown of the ureterovesical anastomosis. Others, however, have found staphylococci to be more frequent causes of deep wound infection, and the failure of perioperative antibiotic prophylaxis aimed at urinary coliforms to reduce the incidence of UTI (see below) argues against the general importance of this mechanism.

Leakage of urine from the wound, reoperation for haemorrhage, and wound haematomas have commonly been recognized as precipitating factors for wound infection by all organisms (Kyriakides *et al.* 1975; Muakkassa *et al.* 1983; Tillegard 1984). Indudhara *et al.* (1994) describe a peritransplant lymphocoele, superinfected with *Staphylococcus aureus*, that presented 4.5 months after transplant as an acute abdomen. Some reports have also suggested that grafts from cadaveric donors, recipients with diabetes and implantation of surgical drains are also associated with more infections. Thus the technical quality of the surgery is probably the major factor influencing wound sepsis; Kyriakides *et al.* (1975) reported a wound infection rate of only 1.6% in patients who did not develop a urinary leak or wound haematoma.

In the series of Edelstein *et al.* (1989), seven (0.3%) of 1945 renal transplant recipients developed perinephric abscess between 1975 and 1986. Their literature review suggested that its prevalence has fallen from a mean of 2.3% in transplants performed before 1976 to 0.75% in those after that date. Abscesses presented between 2 weeks and 52 months after transplantation, and were associated with pre-existing haematomas and lymphocoeles. In common with postoperative wound infection, staphylococci were the most frequent isolates (36%), followed by coliforms (32%), anaerobes (28%) and *Candida* spp. (4%). These were usually not also present in the patient's urine, but in two cases the same organisms (*Bacteroides fragilis* and *S. aureus*) had been isolated from blood cultures several months before presentation of the perinephric abscess. Contrary to the experience of Lobo *et al.* (1982), this suggests that organisms were most commonly implanted at operation or haematogenously acquired from other sites, rather than being derived directly from the urinary tract.

Bacterial skin and soft tissue infections not associated with the transplant wound are less common with cyclosporin immunosuppression. Dummer *et al.* (1983) reported similar total rates of skin infections with azathioprine and cyclosporin (27%), but all patients given the latter agent had only minor herpesvirus infections.

### PANCREAS TRANSPLANTATION

Douzdjian *et al.* (1994) compared the outcome of 88 simultaneous pancreas–kidney transplants with that of 65 renal transplants with diabetic end-stage kidney disease. Although kidney graft and patient survival were similar in both groups at 5 years, the combination graft recipients had a higher incidence of sepsis and surgical complications (usually associated with the pancreas transplant) and also vascular and urological problems. Similar results were reported by Smets *et al.* (1997). Five-year patient, kidney and pancreas survival rates of 90.2, 80.3 and 78.6%, respectively, were seen in the 288 simultaneous grafts reported by Sollinger *et al.* (1993). Three infective deaths and 678 infectious episodes (mainly UTIs) occurred. Thirty-five patients required enteric conversion, usually because of leakage of the duodenal segment with associated sepsis.

Involvement of *Candida* spp., bearing in mind that these patients have chronic renal failure plus diabetes mellitus, is unsurprisingly common, and vaginal colonization in recipients may be an important source for infection of the pancreas grafted to the adjacent bladder (Rubin 1994). Host strains will be added to by yeast colonization of the donor duodenum (Potter van Loon *et al.* 1989). *Candida* spp. involvement was seen in 38% of the intra-abdominal infections in Hesse *et al.*'s heterogeneous series of 98 patients (Hesse *et al.* 1986b), but most of the infections were mixed and the role of yeasts in determining outcome (all but five of the 26 intra-abdominal infections resulted in removal of the pancreatic graft) is impossible to assess. Everett *et al.* (1994) document the serious impact of deep wound infection after pancreas transplantation, which frequently resulted in loss of the graft. Barone *et al.* (1996) urge adoption of single-dose antibacterial surgical prophylaxis for pancreas transplantation, rather than multiple-dose regimens, which may well increase risks of *Candida* infection.

Hence, combination grafts have more infectious and other problems than isolated kidney grafts, but patient survival now appears good enough to make the procedure worthwhile in carefully selected patients, and studies should now focus on reducing the special infectious problems that these patients face postoperatively.

FUNGAL INFECTION

*Aspergillus* spp. infections are now uncommon in renal transplant recipients, but patients given high-dose steroids may be especially susceptible to high concentrations of spores released during hospital building work (Rhame *et al.* 1984; Opal *et al.* 1986), and there is one report suggesting a lower rate of *Aspergillus* colonization and invasive disease in renal graft recipients nursed under high-efficiency particulate air (HEPA) filtered air (Rhame *et al.* 1985). At the time of death, aspergillosis after renal transplantation (and after chemotherapy for solid tumours) is more commonly restricted to the lungs than when it follows liver transplantation or chemotherapy for haematological malignancy (Boon *et al.* 1991).

Tang *et al.* (1994) used restriction fragment length polymorphism and random amplified polymorphic DNA analysis to characterize isolates of *Aspergillus fumigatus* from two patients with renal transplants and 11 environmental sites. They suggested that the distinguishable type causing infection was especially pathogenic. It would be interesting to compare the epidemiology of outbreaks in less susceptible patients with that after liver transplantation and haematological malignancy, where less pathogenic strains may be involved. Post-mortem diagnosis remains depressingly frequent; it was first made in 32 of 40 cases reported from one centre during the 1980s (Boon *et al.* 1991) and a sensitive and reliable diagnostic test is still awaited.

Systemic *Candida* infection was involved in up to half of the deaths of renal graft recipients in the 1960s but reduced immunosuppression and, perhaps, careful use of antifungal prophylaxis and early effective treatment have reduced this proportion to about 5% (Paya 1993). Most clinically significant infections occur in the first 6 months after transplantation and involve the urinary tract, although some early systemic infections derive from intravenous line and surgical wound infections, and oesophagitis and other mucosal involvement often accompanies systemic infections. *Candida albicans* is the most common overall isolate, although *C. glabrata* is a relatively more common isolate from the urine, and *C. tropicalis* and *C. parapsilosis* have a propensity to infect plastic catheters and hence are relatively more common as causes of early post-transplant fungaemia. Diagnosis of systemic candidiasis is somewhat eased by the improved ability of modern blood culture systems to grow yeasts more quickly and reliably (normally within 48–72 h), and therapy is now often simplified by the availability of oral azole antifungal agents. Rapid fungal antigen detection systems are yet to be proven of value in the clinical setting (Paya 1993), although there are interesting new developments with ELISAs for detecting *Candida* and *Aspergillus* antigens, which may be more sensitive than PCR for genetic markers (Fujita *et al.* 1995; Stynen *et al.* 1995; Verweij *et al.* 1995). These techniques require further evaluation before they can make a useful clinical impact.

Therefore the decision to begin antifungal therapy

is rarely simple and should be based upon a careful assessment of mucosal, tissue and blood culture results together with the patient's clinical state. In contrast to the position for neutropenic patients with haematological malignancy (Martino *et al.* 1994), prospective studies of the value of screening solid organ transplant recipients for colonization of multiple sites with *Candida* spp. have not been performed. In neutropenic patients, colonization of oropharynx and stool with *C. albicans* was associated with a risk of significant infection, requiring amphotericin therapy about four times that of other patients. Fluconazole prophylaxis, not consistently shown to be valuable when given to all neutropenic patients, may be better reserved for a multiply colonized subgroup, and may be similarly useful in organ transplant recipients. On post-mortem evidence, antirejection therapy and diabetes mellitus have been proposed as predisposing factors for fungal infection in renal transplant recipients (Scroggs *et al.* 1987), and it may therefore be possible to define a risk group on the basis of risk factors plus surveillance cultures.

Prospective assessment of the significance of single or multiple *Candida*-positive blood cultures has not been performed in patients with organ transplants. Single isolates should not be lightly regarded, however, because some studies in neutropenic patients have shown them to have the same prognosis as episodes with multiple positive blood cultures, and complication rates of over 60% have been reported (mainly endophthalmitis).

Antifungal sensitivity testing is difficult to standardize, and speciation even by the newly available commercial test kits is not entirely reliable, therefore important isolates are best referred to a reference laboratory for testing. A rapid distinction between *C. albicans* and other species can usually be made by performance of the 'germ tube' test. Because *Candida* species other than *C. albicans* are more likely to be resistant to azoles, treatment for serious systemic *Candida* infection is best begun with moderate-dose amphotericin (for example, 0.5 mg/kg/day) until a germ-tube-positive result is obtained. Amphotericin is continued for germ-tube-negative isolates until reference laboratory results are obtained; we have had only

very rare problems of toxicity with this restricted dosage regimen. We reserve the expensive liposomal preparations of amphotericin for cases requiring high-dose therapy with proven deteriorating renal function. Earlier distinction between *C. albicans* and other *Candida* spp. in transplant recipients may be achievable by use of selective, indicator, primary isolation media such as the CHROMagar medium described by Pfaller *et al.* (1995). *Cryptococcus neoformans* may cause clinically significant lung infection, meningitis and rare skin and soft tissue infections at any time after renal transplantation (Rubin *et al.* 1981).

## Prevention and treatment

All candidates for solid organ transplantation should have their immunization histories checked and if necessary updated for diphtheria, tetanus, pertussis and inactivated polio vaccines. They should be immunized against *Streptococcus pneumoniae* and annually against influenza A (Mermel & Maki 1990). Fourteen-valent pneumococcal polysaccharide vaccine significantly reduces pneumococcal pneumonia in splenectomized renal transplant recipients, from 6.1 to 0.9% (First *et al.* 1985). Although splenectomy is now rarely performed in transplant recipients, the later 23-valent vaccine should be more effective at reducing pneumococcal sepsis. Whether the new *Haemophilus influenzae* type b vaccines have a role in transplant recipients remains to be proven. Screening for occult infections in donor and recipient, including tropical parasitic and fungal infection in patients who have travelled or resided in endemic areas, is essential and recent reviews have addressed this issue (Orr & Gould 1992; Rubin 1994).

Although culture of cadaveric organ perfusates is commonly positive during renal transplantation (quoted rates range between 2.1 and 23.4% (Mora *et al.* 1991a)), skin commensals and environmental organisms such as *Staphylococcus epidermidis* or *Bacillus* spp. are usually involved, and postoperative sepsis rarely results. Mora *et al.* (1991a) reported two cases in which wound infections (one *S. aureus* and one *E. coli*) were caused by organisms also isolated earlier from perfusates. Overall, the series included 446 operations, with 48 (10.7%) of the perfusates culture-positive.

Antibiotic prophylaxis is potentially attractive for preventing the most common early bacterial complications after renal transplantation. Surprisingly few studies, however, can be marshalled to support its efficacy against postoperative UTI and the best regimen for prophylaxis of local wound sepsis remains unclear.

## WOUND INFECTION

Tilney *et al.* (1978) observed in a retrospective study that a single dose of preoperative ampicillin, oxacillin and gentamicin significantly reduced the wound infection rate from 18 to 1% in 66 patients. Rubin *et al.* (1981) achieved a rate of 2% without prophylaxis, but a later report from their unit implies that prophylaxis has been used more recently and the wound infection rate has been below 0.2% for the past 10 years (Rubin & Tolkoff-Rubin 1993). Townsend *et al.* (1980) prospectively studied only 37 patients and did not demonstrate any difference between perioperative cefamandole plus tobramycin and no prophylaxis.

Novick (1981) introduced prophylaxis with a single intravenous dose of ampicillin, nafcillin and tobramycin at the induction of anaesthesia halfway through a 3-year study period. In the first 89 control patients there was a 10.1% wound infection rate, mostly associated with wound haematoma or urinary leak. Only 1.1% of the following 90 cases who received antibiotics were infected, despite there being a similar incidence of surgical complications. Unfortunately, no details are given of definitions of wound infection or of culture results. In another historically controlled study of 310 patients, Tillegard (1984) found 5 or 2 days of cloxacillin reduced wound infections significantly from 25.6% to 7.8%, which is still high. This observed reduction resulted entirely from a fall in *S. aureus* infections. Wound haematoma was the only complicating factor associated with a higher risk of local sepsis (29.4% risk), but the distribution of this complication between the control and prophylaxis groups is not described, which weakens the value of this report.

Evans *et al.* (1988) found that two doses of co-amoxclav reduced the wound infection rate from 27% to zero in a randomized trial in a heterogeneous range of operations on 46 patients with renal failure, 34 of which were kidney transplants. All six infections in the control group involved co-amoxclav-sensitive *S. aureus*, in one case mixed with sensitive *E. coli*.

Cohen *et al.* (1988) carried out a randomized trial of three doses of cefuroxime plus piperacillin in 53 renal graft recipients. Wound infection was reduced from the extremely high level of 42.3% in the control group to 14.8% in those receiving prophylaxis, which is a significant difference ($P=0.027$). As well as the high baseline rate of wound infection, the patients enrolled in this study had a graft survival of only 60% overall. Including all other infections, the prophylaxis group had a significantly lower rate of infection in the first 5 days, but the difference disappeared if the analysis was extended to 14 days. Importantly, prophylaxis had no effect on the rate of UTI, which was seen in 69.8% of patients overall.

Capocasale *et al.* (1994) reported use of a single dose of the long-half-life, broad-spectrum cephalosporin ceftriaxone in 170 renal transplant recipients and observed no wound infections and a rate of UTI of only 7.1%; however, few details are given and no comparator was included.

We have recently completed a prospective, blinded assessment of perioperative flucloxacillin (1 g with induction and 6-hourly for 24 h postoperatively) vs. no prophylaxis in patients undergoing renal transplantation at Addenbrooke's Hospital, Cambridge. This trial was begun after retrospective analysis revealed a worryingly high rate of wound infection (especially involving *S. aureus*). In this retrospective study, 10 of 33 (30.3%) consecutive patients suffered wound infections, six with different phage types of *S. aureus* and the remainder with various Gram-negative bacteria. Sixty patients (30 given prophylaxis) were recruited to the prospective trial and 57 (28 prophylaxis) satisfied the analysis criteria. Eight suffered wound infections, giving an overall infection rate of 14%. Two of these were in the prophylaxis group (one with flucloxacillin-sensitive *S. aureus*, one with no bacteria isolated) and six in the control group (three with flucloxacillin-sensitive *S. aureus*, one with flucloxacillin-sensitive *S. aureus* plus mixed non-sporing anaerobes and enterococci, one with methicillin-resistant *S. aureus* (MRSA) and one with scanty growth of *S. epidermidis*). These results do not achieve statistical significance because of the lower overall rate of infection during the period of the prospective study, but a trend in favour of anti-staphylococcal prophylaxis is evident. All the *S. aureus* isolates were of different phage types. Postoperative UTI was equally frequent in both prophylaxis and control groups.

Landreneau and McDonald (1987) have reviewed technical aspects of urinary leakage and haematoma formation after renal transplantation, and their effects upon wound infection rates. Recent attempts to reduce the incidence of leakage from the ureteric anastomosis have included use of ureteric stents (Lin *et al.* 1993; Nicol *et al.* 1993). Preliminary experience with these techniques has been favourable and a number of uncommon problems related to stent use or malfunction have usually proved amenable to minimally invasive techniques.

Surgical drainage, combined with modern antibiotic therapy for 3–4 weeks (intravenous for the first week), has improved the results of treatment for deep surgical wound infections, and none of Edelstein *et al.*'s cases required transplant nephrectomy (Edelstein *et al.* 1989).

## URINARY TRACT INFECTION

Early post-transplantation UTI (generally implying infection within the first 2–4 weeks) has generally not been reduced by perioperative antibiotic prophylaxis, and most authorities suggest that treatment of bacteriuria before transplantation and early removal of urinary catheters (at 1–4 days) are the best strategies (Rubin 1994). Early infections (within the first 3 months) are commonly associated with tissue invasion and usually require initial parenteral therapy, which is continued orally for a total of 14 days; some authorities recommend still longer courses for this group (up to 6 weeks with follow-on prophylaxis for those with impaired graft function (Rubin 1994)). Use of

quinolone antibiotics probably allows these course lengths to be markedly reduced because of their excellent tissue penetration and effectiveness against aerobic Gram-negative rods. In contrast, late infection is much more benign, less commonly bacteraemic and can be managed with conventional courses of antibiotics.

By analogy with studies of bacteriuria after transurethral resection of the prostate, perioperative prophylaxis may well reduce bacteriuria in the first few postoperative days but it will have no impact on later bacteriuria, which is much more closely related to the duration of catheterization (Raz *et al.* 1994). One report suggested that culture of the tip of the removed catheter was predictive of clinical infection within the following 2 weeks (Burleson *et al.* 1977), but this work seems not to have been confirmed or repeated with contemporary transplants and is not generally performed. In children with vesicoureteric reflux, surgical procedures such as extravesicular ureteroneo-cystostomy may reduce the rate of postoperative UTI (Hanevold *et al.* 1987). In contrast, prolonged suppressive antibiotic therapy has been used in some centres for many years to reduce later UTI, with apparent success (Peterson *et al.* 1982). Co-trimoxazole has been popular for this indication because one 960 mg tablet nightly for 4 months after removal of the urinary catheter was shown significantly to reduce infections and their severity (Tolkoff-Rubin *et al.* 1982).

Some authorities have been reluctant to adopt this regimen because of possible side effects, interactions with cyclosporin and encouragement of antibiotic resistance. In a double-blind assessment, however, Maki *et al.* (1992) studied 132 patients for 33 876 patient days and found co-trimoxazole prophylaxis to reduce infections of the urinary tract and wound significantly. Patients in the prophylaxis group were not more likely to be colonized by co-trimoxazole-resistant bacteria, but those infections that did occur were with more resistant organisms. *Candida* infection was paradoxically lower in the prophylaxis group, possibly because they received fewer courses of therapeutic broad-spectrum antibiotics. Patients receiving prophylaxis tolerated it well and were not at increased risk of rejection, haematological or liver functional abnormalities, deranged cyclosporin metabolism or persistently impaired renal function. The authors recommended continuing prophylaxis indefinitely in patients judged to be at high risk, but most authorities give co-trimoxazole for the first 6 or 12 months after transplantation (Rubin & Tolkoff-Rubin 1993).

A recently reported Danish study confirmed co-trimoxazole's efficacy (Albrechtsen *et al*. 1990). In 173 patients given 480 mg co-trimoxazole daily for the first 6 months, total infections (24% vs. 39%), infectious mortality (2.9% vs. 6.5%), pneumonia (5% vs. 17%), septicaemia (3% vs. 11%) and PCP (2.7% vs. none) in the first 12 months were significantly lower than in the 600 not given prophylaxis. No effects were seen on wound infection or CMV infection rates. Co-trimoxazole may also reduce the prevalence of *Nocardia* spp. infection in units where this is common (Leaker *et al*. 1989). Ampicillin and cephalexin appear to be possible alternative long-term prophylactic agents (Maddux *et al*. 1989), but lack efficacy against PCP and *Nocardia* sp.

At Addenbrooke's Hospital, low-dose co-trimoxazole prophylaxis (480 mg thrice weekly) has been used since 1988 for 6 months postoperatively, beginning when patients were discharged from hospital to reduce the risk of encouraging antibiotic resistance in the microbial flora of the ward population. Still lower doses of co-trimoxazole, such as 480 mg for 7 days per month, have been recommended in some centres, but the protective effects on other infections have not been reported. Nebulized pentamidine is a possible alternative prophylactic regimen for patients who do not tolerate co-trimoxazole, but breakthrough PCP infections may still be seen, sometimes presenting atypically (Jules-Elysee *et al*. 1990).

### FUNGAL INFECTION

Prophylaxis with conventional oral non-absorbable antifungal agents such as nystatin and amphotericin B has not been subjected to randomized clinical trial in solid organ transplant recipients, but, although amphotericin may be somewhat more effective than oral nystatin in neutropenic patients, some patients remain faecal culture-positive even after high-dose

administration (Paya 1993). Trials are under way to assess the impact of prophylactic intravenous amphotericin and oral fluconazole after liver transplantation (Tollemar *et al*. 1995), but there would seem to be little indication for its assessment in other groups. Candiduria in renal transplant recipients is generally best treated regardless of whether the patient is symptomatic, and 2 weeks of oral fluconazole is the regimen of choice (Rubin & Tolkoff-Rubin 1993). Non-*albicans* isolates should be checked for fluconazole sensitivity, and symptomatic infections treated *ab initio* with low-dose parenteral amphotericin B.

### MYCOBACTERIAL INFECTION

Tuberculosis in transplant recipients occurs about 10 times more frequently than in the general population, and extrapulmonary disease is up to 40 times more common (McWhinney *et al*. 1981; Sinnott & Emmanuel 1990). Rates are highest in patients from recognized risk groups, such as immigrants from the Middle East and the Indian subcontinent and their children, those exposed to relatives with active tuberculosis and those with a past history of tuberculosis. Some units routinely offer isoniazid prophylaxis to these groups and it may presumably be prudent to do so also for those whose donors were at risk. Use of isoniazid for at least 12–18 months is apparently effective after renal transplantation (Samhan *et al*. 1989; Higgins *et al*. 1991), but this must be balanced against the chances of hepatotoxicity. Presentation of active tuberculosis in the transplant recipient is characteristically much more acute than in normal subjects, and a variety of atypical presentations have been described, including bronchial compression, anaemia, leucopenia, polycythaemia and myelofibrosis (Sinnott & Emmanuel 1990). Chest radiographic appearances are highly variable, and tuberculin skin testing is so unreliable as to be useless. Treatment of active tuberculosis after transplantation should be for 1–2 years and is reasonably successful, but graft loss may result from lowered cyclosporin levels through hepatic enzyme induction, and not all groups have reported good overall survival even of renal graft recipients (Samhan *et al*. 1989).

The epidemiology of tuberculosis transmission

can now be investigated with discriminatory typing methods such as restriction fragment length polymorphism, and renal transplant units prove fruitful settings for trying out such techniques, with real outbreaks if open pulmonary cases are admitted (Jereb *et al.* 1993). Management and prophylaxis are complicated in some countries by the recent resurgence in multiple drug-resistant *Mycobacterium tuberculosis* causing cross-infection in hospitals and other closed communities (Hamburg & Frieden 1994). Renal transplantation seems to be associated with a low incidence of infection with the common non-tuberculous mycobacteria such as *Mycobacterium avium-intracellulare*, *M. kansasii* and *M. chelonei*, but the literature suggests that other solid organ transplant recipients have an even lower incidence (Patel *et al.* 1994a). Presentation is usually months or years after transplant, and the most common infections seen are those of skin and soft tissues. Successful responses have followed a combined approach involving reduced immunosuppression, surgical debridement and antimicrobial agents. Drobniewski and Ferguson (1996) review the presentation, transmission, prophylaxis, diagnosis and management of tuberculosis, including multiply resistant strains, in renal units.

NOCARDIA INFECTION

Nine case reports of *Nocardia asteroides* infection in 1255 renal transplant recipients (0.7%) and a literature review, which also noted occasional cases of *Nocardia brasiliensis*, were given by Arduino *et al.* (1993). Cases presented between 32 and 1806 days (mean 586) postoperatively, and five of the nine followed episodes of graft rejection. Historical controls given azathioprine had a higher rate of infection (2.6%) than the current series of patients, who received cyclosporin. Seven of the cases had local involvement only (six pulmonary and one skin), one had successive infections of lung and skin and one had dissemination to lung and brain. All of the cases were diagnosed only on invasive specimens such as skin biopsies and bronchoalveolar lavage fluids, but initial Gram stains of these specimens were positive in all cases. The authors recommended consideration of co-amoxiclav (Aug-

mentin) therapy for *Nocardia* infection in renal transplant recipients because of problems of nephrotoxicity with moderate- to high-dose co-trimoxazole, and they used at least 6 months' treatment for all cases, extended to 12 months or more if there was cerebral involvement. Immunosuppression and graft function was maintained in all cases and there was only one death, in a patient with pulmonary infection. To prevent recurrence King *et al.* (1993) suggested that treated cases of nocardiosis should be given lifelong prophylaxis. Leaker *et al.* (1989) have also published recent experience of seven cases of *Nocardia* infection in kidney transplant recipients, and Chapman and Wilson (1990) review problems of nocardiosis in transplant recipients in general. Weinberger *et al.* (1995) describe a patient who developed pulmonary infection with *N. transvalensis* after liver transplantation. This is only the fifth case of infection with this species to be reported. The diagnosis in the case was delayed and the authors emphasize the importance of considering the possibility of an infective diagnosis in all transplant recipients even when embolic pulmonary disease is strongly suggested clinically.

## Liver transplantation

### Infections following transplantation

Transplantation of organs in continuity with the gastrointestinal viscera brings special problems of bacterial infection because of their inevitable proximity to the dense colonizing flora of these areas in both donor and recipient. In most patients their natural flora has been supplemented by nosocomially acquired microbes, and has been continually under selective pressure from antibiotics given for treatment or prophylaxis.

Few comprehensive studies of infection after liver transplantation have been published recently, and fewer still were prospective, blinded or comparative in design, or have used clear definitions such as those of Kusne *et al.* (1988). Past, current and possible future impacts of changing immunosuppressive regimens on the management of liver transplants, including infectious complications, have been summarized by Calne (1994). Recent general studies of the effects of tacrolimus suggest it is associated with a lower rate of postoperative infection (Alessiani *et al.* 1991), but only one comprehensive, high-quality study focused on infectious outcomes has yet appeared (Chang *et al.* 1998).

## Spectrum, sites and predisposing factors

Early reports of infection after liver transplantation emphasized the high rate of bacteraemia and fungaemia. For example, organisms were grown from the blood during septic episodes in over 70% of the 93 patients of Schroter *et al.* (1976a), and most of these were associated with biliary duct obstruction or leakage. Many of these isolates were aerobic Gram-negative bacilli and mixed bacteraemias were common. In addition to the problems of surgical technique, it is significant that the surgical antibiotic prophylaxis used at that time consisted of agents such as ampicillin and kanamycin with limited Gram-negative spectra and innate activity, and the available immunosuppressive regimens were crude.

Despite developments in the diagnosis and treatment of infection after liver transplantation, the multiple bacterial, viral, fungal and parasitic infections that may strike such patients, especially in the early postoperative days, clearly justify Dr Charles Trey's description of liver transplantation as 'an art as well as a science' (Case Report 1992). This *New England Journal of Medicine* clinicopathological exercise well captures the urgent diagnostic and therapeutic complexity of management of postoperative fever in a patient who turned out to have an EBV-associated B cell lymphoma. Kusne *et al.* (1988) published one of the first comprehensive reviews of infection after liver transplantation in the cyclosporin era, covering 101 consecutive patients transplanted between July 1984 and September 1985, followed up for a mean of 394 days. In comparison with earlier studies of operations between 1981 and 1983, this group found a similar overall infection rate of 81% (83%), but infective deaths were significantly less common (23% vs. 40%, $P < 0.05$). Early bacterial abdominal infections, and consequent bacteraemias, remain closely associated with biliary surgical compli-

cations (McMaster *et al.* 1979; Kusne *et al.* 1988). Winston *et al.* (1995) have published a time chart of infections after liver transplantation that offers interesting contrasts and similarities with the long-established version given by Rubin for infection after renal transplantation (Rubin *et al.* 1981).

When investigating causes of fever and graft dysfunction, rejection is an easier diagnosis to confirm histologically than cholangitis is to prove bacteriologically, especially when a Roux-en-Y anastomosis has been performed or once the T-tube has been removed. Assessment of culture results from abdominal drainage and aspirate fluid is especially complicated if the patient has a Roux-en-Y anastomosis because of inevitable colonization of bile samples with a rich colonic flora. In patients with conventional anastomoses, isolation of faecal anaerobes from peribiliary specimens is often a sign of anastomotic leakage. Surgical complications resulting in biliary tract leakage and haemorrhage into the peritoneum are the most common precursors to peritonitis and abscess formation. Biliary ischaemia will compromise the integrity of the anastomosis, and *Candida* spp. infection of the gallbladder or anastomosis will also predispose to perforation. Mixed infection with aerobic Gram-negative rods, pseudomonads, enterococci, anaerobes and *Candida* spp. results, and such patients frequently used to suffer acute septic episodes with high mortality.

More recently, the availability of broad-spectrum antimicrobial agents with excellent pharmacokinetic properties (including fluoroquinolones and imipenem, and the azole antifungals) and the refinement of radiologically guided aspiration have improved the short-term outlook. Many of these cases now remain febrile for long periods while anastomoses are repaired and abdominal collections are drained, but in our experience cultures of deep aspirates frequently become sterile or contain only coagulase-negative staphylococci and enterococci after the first few days. Careful antibiotic management is required, including resisting the temptation to change therapeutic regimens rapidly in the face of continued fever. Rapid radiological investigations and surgical intervention are more commonly indicated unless there is clear cultural evidence of bacterial or fungal superinfection or the patient has become acutely unwell with signs of systemic infection.

Liver transplant recipients have become one of the more common patient groups suffering colonization and infection with vancomycin-resistant *Enterococcus faecalis* and *E. faecium* (Papanicolaou *et al.* 1996). Although all studies have not reached the same conclusions, vancomycin-resistant enterococcal infection has been associated with heavy usage of vancomycin and quinolone antibiotics on a unit, on prolonged hospital stay and on reoperation, and affected patients have a high mortality (Linden *et al.* 1996; Papanicolaou *et al.* 1996). Choice of antibiotic therapy for such patients is difficult. Although these organisms appear not to be of high virulence, they cannot be ignored in the empirical therapy of a septic, colonized patient, and the choice of agents is often limited to a few older, potentially toxic, antibiotics such as chloramphenicol or tetracycline. Some strains, including most we have seen affecting liver transplant recipients at Addenbrooke's Hospital, remain sensitive to teicoplanin and there are a number of potentially useful investigational agents awaiting full clinical assessment which are currently available on a named patient basis.

Chang *et al.* (1998) have recently published an excellent 2-year prospective study of fever after liver transplantation which suggests that the traditional distribution of causes has changed. Infectious causes accounted for 78% of fevers, with bacteria comprising 62% and viruses only 6%. CMV was distinctly uncommon, with human herpesvirus-6 the predominant viral pathogen. Rejection was the cause of the fever in only 4% of episodes. It remains to be seen whether this picture is common to all centres in the late 1990s.

## BACTERAEMIA

In Wagener and Yu's interesting comparative series of 125 bacteraemias in kidney, heart and liver graft recipients (Wagener & Yu 1992), bacteraemia occurred much earlier after liver grafts than in renal transplant recipients, with about 80% detected during the first 90 days. Just under half the bacteraemias in both groups of recipients were with aerobic Gram-negative rods, with *Enterobacter* spp. and *Pseudomonas* spp. commonly involved after liver transplantation, whereas renal graft recipients more frequently suffered bacteraemia with the generally more antibiotic-sensitive *E. coli* and *Klebsiella* spp. Eleven per cent of bacteraemias in liver transplant recipients were polymicrobial, compared with 7% in kidney recipients and 6% in heart recipients. Overall, Gram-negative bacteraemia and fungaemia carried a mortality rate of 35%, compared with a rate of 8% after Gram-positive bacteraemia. Bacteraemias occurring shortly after transplantation were more commonly fatal than those occurring later, despite many of these presenting out of hospital and hence being subject to delayed treatment. By far the most common source after liver transplantation was the abdomen (27%), but 10% were derived from pneumonias, 7% from the urinary tract, 6% from wounds and 41% were of unknown source. It is likely that many of those of undetermined source were derived from the biliary tree because of the difficulties of confirming the diagnosis of cholangitis in all cases. Broadly similar results were seen in the series of 80 bacteraemias in liver, renal, heart and heart–lung recipients reported by McClean *et al.* (1994).

## PNEUMONIA

Overall, 16.7% of the 180 liver transplant recipients in the series reviewed by Mermel and Maki (1990) developed pneumonia, 64% of which presented in the first postoperative 3 months. Although up to 45% of cases of pulmonary infection in this group have been ascribed to aerobic Gram-negative rods, studies which have employed careful bacterial assessment of cases with invasive techniques and strict definitions have failed to support this figure; many are probably caused by pulmonary collapse and pleural effusion combined with upper airway colonization (Jensen *et al.* 1986). It is likely that elimination of this group erroneously ascribed to Gram-negative bacterial causes would result in a mean date of presentation of true pneumonia markedly later than was suggested in earlier studies, as shown by Johnson *et al.* (1990) in a group of mainly renal transplant recipients.

WOUND AND INTRA-ABDOMINAL INFECTION

Three comprehensive reviews are worthy of especial note. These comprise two reports of bacterial, fungal and parasitic infection after liver transplantation performed in Pittsburgh and Cleveland, USA (Kusne *et al.* 1988; Paya *et al.* 1989), and another which covers only bacterial infection from Memphis, USA (George *et al.* 1991). All are retrospective, but the authors employ careful definitions and give sufficient microbiological and clinical information to allow a comparative assessment of their findings. Together they paint a clear picture of the infective complications of liver transplantation. Table 17.1 summarizes data from the studies of Kusne *et al.* and Paya *et al.*, the main clinical difference between these studies apparently being the use of selective decontamination of the gastrointestinal tract (SDGT) in the latter centre. It is difficult to see a major impact of SDGT on the overall picture of infection or on outcome, although Paya *et al.* highlight the lower rate of aerobic Gram-negative rod infection in their series. This may be a result of reduced colonization or a genuinely reduced infection rate from SDGT, but there are a number of minor differences between the studies—such as in prophylactic co-trimoxazole usage—that may also have been influential.

Kusne *et al.* (1988) report on 101 patients followed for a mean of 394 days; operative prophylaxis comprised 5 days of cefotaxime plus ampicillin, and nystatin was given orally until discharge from hospital. Twenty-six per cent of patients died and 89% of these were associated with infection. Bacterial and fungal infections were most commonly seen in the first month, viral infections during the second month and protozoal infection increased in incidence between months 1 and 6. After 6 months, 94% infections were again bacterial. Thirty-three bacteraemias were detected in 26 patients, of which 33% derived from the abdomen, 21% from UTI and 21% had no obvious source. Fifty-one per cent of bacteraemias involved aerobic Gram-negative rods, 27% aerobic Gram-positive bacteria and 9% anaerobes. Many abdominal infections, especially the 16 intra-and perihepatic abscesses, were related to technical surgical problems and occurred in the first postoperative month. Three-quarters of the 15 pneumonias occurred while still in hospital postoperatively, and usually involved aerobic Gram-negative rods in ventilated patients. Two of the five community-acquired pneumonias involved *Streptococcus pneumoniae*, two *Staphylococcus aureus* and one apparently *E. coli*. Eight of the nine patients with proven cholangitis had suffered technical problems with the anastomosis, and four of the nine were bacteraemic with faecal flora. Fourteen invasive *Candida* spp. infections were seen in 13 patients, all within the first 2 months; 10 of these involved *C. albicans*. Four patients suffered aspergillosis, all of which were fatal, and the 11 cases of PCP all presented around 3 months postoperatively.

Paya *et al.* (1989) studied 53 patients who received single liver transplants and were followed for a minimum of 6 months. Patients were given 48 h of perioperative cefotaxime plus tobramycin, followed by SDGT, and prophylactic co-trimoxazole was used in the later part of the series in those patients given immunosuppressive therapy with OKT3. Five of the 53 patients died (9%), only 8% infected patients died but four of the five deaths were from infective causes. There was a peak in infections at 4 weeks, which is later than the report of George *et al.* (1991), a difference which the authors ascribe to their use of SDGT. It is not possible to compare these times exactly with those in the report of Kusne *et al.* (1988) because different periods are analysed. Overall, 64% of infections involved Gram-positive organisms with only 15% caused by aerobic Gram-negative bacteria, including only one of the 16 bacteraemias. Three cases of PCP presented between 2 and 3 months postoperatively,

**Table 17.1** Comparison of infection rates after liver transplantation between two studies.

|  | Kusne *et al.* (1988) | Paya *et al.* (1989) |
| --- | --- | --- |
| Infected (severe infection) | 83% (67%) | 75% (53%) |
| Bacterial infection (severe) | 59% (54%) | 66% (53%) |
| Fungal infection (severe) | 18% (16%) | 10% (4%) |
| Protozoal infection (severe) | 12% (12%) | 4% (4%) |
| Viral infection (severe) | 53% (24%) | NG (39%) |

NG, information not given in paper.

and two of these patients died of their infections. All 16 patients receiving more than one liver graft suffered major infections, apparently with an especially high incidence of CMV and fungal involvement. Mortality was higher in the multiple transplant group but this was not directly associated with infection.

George *et al.* (1991) describe the bacterial infections in 103 liver transplants performed in 79 patients. The authors carried out a logistic regression analysis to discover independent risk factors for infection and provide an interesting comparative review of the published literature. Cefoxitin alone was given for operative prophylaxis and SDGT was not used. They point out that a high proportion of their patients were transplanted for acute hepatic failure (15.4%) and hepatocellular disease (55%), but these variables were not independently associated with a higher risk of infection. Overall 68% had bacterial infections, 53% of which presented within the first 2 postoperative weeks. Seven patients died of infection (8.9%) and the mortality rate was 13% of infected patients. Thirty per cent of infections involved the abdominal organs, with most of the rest being bacteraemias and wound infections; wound infection occurred occasionally after the first month, sometimes associated with biliary anastomotic leaks. Aerobic Gram-negative bacilli were the most common isolates from abdominal infections and 37% were polymicrobial. Surgical drainage or debridement was required in 59% of the abdominal infections. Isolates resistant to prophylactic cefoxitin were significantly more common in early infections. Logistic regression analysis revealed that the only factors independently associated with bacterial infection were duration of surgery $\geq 8$ h (which carried an independent risk of 49%) and bilirubin $\geq 12$ mg/dL (18%). Patients with both factors had a risk of 70%, and those with neither 10%. Considering only abdominal and wound infection, the influential variables were prolonged duration of surgery, transfusion requirement $\geq 2$ blood volumes and prior hepatobiliary surgery. These factors are, of course, not readily amenable to reduction preoperatively except by patient exclusion and the authors point out that the appropriate response may be to adopt 'an aggressive diagnostic and therapeutic approach when clinical signs suggest infection' in a

**Table 17.2** Risk factors for all types of infection after liver transplantation. (Modified from Kusne *et al.* 1988 and Saliba *et al.* 1994.)

| Timing | Factors |
| --- | --- |
| Preoperative | T-helper/suppressor $\geq 2.8$ (especially associated with viral and protozoal infections) |
| | Alanine aminotransferase >60 IU/L |
| | Encephalopathy |
| | Prolonged prothrombin time |
| | Male sex |
| | Urgent status |
| | Diabetes mellitus |
| | Renal failure |
| | Prolonged antibiotic therapy |
| Perioperative | Operation duration (especially total >12 h) |
| | Repeat abdominal operation |
| | Repeat transplant if Roux-en-Y anastomosis used |
| Postoperative | More than 5 days of antibiotic therapy |
| Rejection | OKT3 use |

patient with one or more of these pointers. Extensive analyses of factors associated with all types of infection have been performed in two studies, one employing univariate analysis (Kusne *et al.* 1988) and the other multivariate analysis (Saliba *et al.* 1994), and the results are combined in Table 17.2.

### PAEDIATRIC LIVER TRANSPLANTATION

In 36 paediatric liver transplant recipients, George *et al.* (1992) found that non-viral infections had a similar epidemiology and range of causative species to those seen in adults. Most infections presented in the first 2 postoperative weeks and were abdominal, but the authors noted that relatively few involved or progressed to peritoneal or hepatic abscess formation which is seen in about half of adult cases. They speculated that this may be a result of age-related depressed phagocyte activity, to differences in the usage of corticosteroids, to reduced intra-abdominal blood collection or to differences in antibiotic prophylaxis. Hepatic artery occlusion and thrombosis have been recognized for many years to be more common in the paediatric liver recipient (Schroter *et al.* 1976a); these are likely to be secondary to physical causes, probably because of the relatively small size of the anastomosis, and hepatic necrosis, abscesses and bacteraemia may result (Rollins *et al.* 1988).

In Cambridge we have seen two cases of *Clostridium perfringens* gas gangrene of the liver after hepatic artery occlusion. Cienfuegos *et al.* (1984) reported a 20% rate of graft infectious complications in paediatric patients, of which the most serious were hepatic abscesses following hepatic artery or portal vein thrombosis. These complications almost always occur within the first 30 postoperative days and a range of organisms, including multiply resistant aerobic Gram-negative rods, yeasts and filamentous fungi, are usually involved. Percutaneous drainage of abscesses, broad-spectrum antimicrobial therapy and urgent retransplantation are the management of choice. In Cambridge we use the combination of intravenous ciprofloxacin, vancomycin, metronidazole and moderate-dose conventional amphotericin B unless cultures indicate microbial resistance; full-dose amphotericin B is used if there are clinical clues to suggest filamentous fungal involvement. Prophylaxis is continued with all four agents for at least 48 h after retransplant even if progress is excellent, and ciprofloxacin is often continued for 5–7 days after the other agents are stopped to provide a period of early gut decontamination in this high-risk population.

## FUNGAL INFECTION

Of all solid organ transplant recipients, patients with liver transplants have the highest risk of serious fungal infection (Boon *et al.* 1991). This was first documented by Schroter *et al.* (1976b) with azathioprine immunosuppression. These carry a poor prognosis once established, an actuarial survival rate of only 55.3% in the first year compared with 84.2% in those without fungal infection. Building work is continuous in many large hospitals today and there are increasing pressures to keep clinical units working with normal patient activity during all but the most major restructuring work. Outbreaks of *Aspergillus* infection from disturbance of fungally colonized insulation materials are well recognized (Opal *et al.* 1986), and a similar outbreak of seven cases of *Nocardia asteroides* infection among patients on a hepatology ward has recently been described (Sahathevan *et al.* 1991). Control measures included improved dust screening, more frequent cleaning of ward areas and formaldehyde fumigation. While building work continued, patients were only moved off the unit after a cluster of cases had occurred: reports such as this may be useful to infection control teams when persuading hospital managers of the risks of exposing immunocompromised patients to airborne dust. Other environmentally acquired systemic fungal infections cannot be blamed on the construction industry; prolonged dry weather has increased human exposure to *Coccidioides immitis* in southern California, with a consequent rise in clinical cases, and Holt *et al.* (1997) describe eight cases in liver transplant recipients.

Dissemination of filamentous fungal infection greatly reduces the chances of therapeutic success, which are probably better than 50% for localized disease (Denning & Stevens 1990). Cerebral aspergillosis has perhaps the most sinister reputation, with prolonged survival being the exception rather than the rule. In a series of 22 cases in organ transplants (13 with liver grafts) alteration of mentation was seen in 86%, seizures in 41% and focal neurological deficit in 32% (Torre-Cisneros *et al.* 1993). Only 19% had signs of meningeal irritation. Fifty-nine per cent of the cases had diabetes mellitus and organ rejection and intensified immunosuppression preceded cerebral signs in most cases. Ante-mortem diagnosis was made in half the cases and post-mortem findings confirmed that the lungs were the likely site of acquisition in all but two. Unexplained cerebral signs and symptoms in a patient after liver transplantation should be vigorously investigated and empirical therapy for aspergillosis should be started immediately if otherwise unexplained radiological lesions are seen in brain and lungs. Full-dose conventional amphotericin probably remains the initial agent of choice and we have had one long-term survival in a culture-proven case who was given prolonged oral follow-on therapy with high-dose itraconazole; others have advocated use of liposomal amphotericin in this condition (Polo *et al.* 1992). Other filamentous fungi may cause the same clinical picture and the prognosis is not universally hopeless; for example, Vukmir *et al.* (1994) describe successful treatment of a liver graft recipient with pulmonary and cerebral involvement with *Dactylaria gallopava* with 8.5 g colloidal amphotericin B followed by oral itraconazole for 12 months. *Cryptococcus neoformans* is the most common fungal cause of subacute meningitis in transplant recipients, usually presenting with fever and headache, but focal signs may occur, although disturbance of consciousness and meningism are less common than in HIV-1 antibody positive individuals (Hibbard & Rubin 1994).

Benedict *et al.* (1992) described five liver transplant recipients with nodular, violaceous skin lesions caused by primary, localized infection with fungi (one each culture-positive for *Aspergillus flavus*, *Paecilomyces* spp. and *Alternaria* spp., two diagnosed only histologically), and reviewed 27 similar cases reported in solid organ transplant recipients. Most presented 3 or more months after transplantation, in contrast to the generally early presentation of disseminated fungal infection. Surgical excision appeared to give the best cure rate (86%), followed by systemic therapy alone with amphotericin B.

In contrast to the picture with other solid organ transplants, several studies have examined the clinical factors associated with fungal infection in liver transplant recipients (Wajszczuk *et al.* 1985; Colonna *et al.* 1988; Castaldo *et al.* 1991; Mora *et al.* 1991b; Singh *et al.* 1997), which are classified in Table 17.3. Not all authors have clearly distinguished between yeast and *Aspergillus* infections, although the identified risk factors are likely to be predictive mainly of *Candida* infections because of their relatively greater prevalence. Most studies have involved few microbiologically, clinically and histologically proven infections. Few of the factors are amenable to alteration — although they may prove useful for defining a group likely to benefit from prophylaxis — and most are not independent variables.

Three studies have employed multivariate analysis to

**Table 17.3** Risk factors for fungal infection after liver transplantation, from studies employing univariate analyses. (Modified from Wajszczuk *et al.* 1985, Kusne *et al.* 1988, Castaldo *et al.* 1991, Mora *et al.* 1991a and Singh *et al.* 1997.)

| Classification | Risk factor |
| --- | --- |
| Preoperative | Urgent status |
| | Administration of steroids and antibiotics |
| | High serum albumin level |
| | Fulminant hepatic failure |
| | Biliary atresia |
| | Chronic active hepatitis |
| | Malnutrition |
| | Age >20 years |
| | Diabetes mellitus |
| | Elevated serum creatinine |
| Perioperative | Transfusion requirement |
| | Roux-en-Y biliary anastomosis |
| | Vascular or gastrointestinal complications |
| | Prolonged operation |
| | Perioperative cholestasis |
| | Duration of ICU stay |
| Postoperative | Reintubation |
| | Requirement for therapeutic antibiotics |
| | Prolonged time in ITU |
| | Re-exploration of abdomen |
| | Renal support required |
| | Parenteral nutrition required |
| | Recurrent hepatitis C |
| Rejection | Steroid dose |
| | Additional immunotherapy |
| | Triple immunosuppression |

assess factors predisposing to fungal infection. In the study of Castaldo *et al.* (1991) involving 303 patients receiving 355 liver grafts, the factors emerging as independently predictive were retransplantation, reintubation, 'urgent' clinical status, high clinical risk score, intraoperative transfusion, Roux-en-Y anastomosis, postoperative steroid usage and bacterial infections, and vascular complications. *Candida* spp. caused 83.5% of the 91 episodes of fungal infection in 72 patients and 78.9% of these were *C. albicans*. Mortality was 50% in those with fungal disease and 16.5% in those without, and actuarial 1-year survival was 55.3% and 84.2%, respectively.

In a fascinating report, Collins *et al.* (1994) retrospectively studied 187 operations in 158 patients for their first 100 postoperative days and documented 34 infections (28 *Candida* spp., five filamentous fungi, one *Candida* plus *Aspergillus* spp.). Five factors were independently associated with fungal infection: creatinine level (hazard ratio (HR) 1.4); length of transplant procedure (HR 1.2); retransplant (HR 3.2); additional abdominal or intrathoracic operations (HR 2.5); and CMV infection (HR 8.5). Early yeast colonization correlated with early invasive disease (within the first 10 days), but not with late disease, and colonization of multiple sites did not correlate with significant infection. A predictive model combining four factors (creatinine >3 mg/dL; operation duration >11 h; retransplantation; early yeast colonization), identified a high-risk group with two or more of these factors with a 65% chance of invasive fungal infection. About 1% of those with no risk factors and 20% with one risk factor developed infections.

Briegel *et al.* (1995) used consecutive logistic regression analysis to study predictors of fungal infection in 186 orthotopic transplant operations performed on 152 patients between 1985 and 1992. The 10 cases of disseminated candidiasis, 11 of aspergillosis and four with combined infections were independently predicted by a model including only the amount of fresh frozen plasma transfused because of poor initial allograft function, and whether the patient had acute renal failure requiring haemofiltration.

Others have shown that prediction of invasive *Candida* spp. infection in liver transplant recipients is not possible from surveillance cultures alone; Tollemar *et al.* (1990) reported colonization of three or more sites to have a sensitivity of only 78% and a specificity of only 50%. Kusne *et al.* (1994) used endoscopic sampling to confirm that *Candida* spp. are common gastrointestinal commensals in patients awaiting liver transplants; not surprisingly, as a normal gut colonist, *C. albicans* was the most common (64% isolates), but 19% grew *C. tropicalis*, 10% *C. krusei* and 7% *C. glabrata*. Stomach samples were reasonably representative of duodenal carriage, which was present in 86% cases, and 53% samples contained high concentrations of yeasts above 300 colony-forming units per millilitre.

Colonization at other body sites did not correlate with positive cultures from any intestinal point. For this work to lead to useful developments it is now necessary to investigate any association between sites or density of carriage and future yeast infections; the work of Collins *et al.* (1994) suggests, however, that this approach may not be fruitful.

## Prevention and treatment

Various regimens for pre- and postoperative screening of patients receiving liver transplants have been published, and the European approach has been summarized by Orr and Gould (1992). I would emphasize the importance of screening for methicillin-resistant *S. aureus* (MRSA) of all patients admitted for liver transplantation who have been inpatients at hospitals with high or unknown rates of MRSA infection. Units using SDGT by absorbed or non-absorbable regimens should screen patients for the appearance of strains resistant to the decontaminating antibiotics and for achievement of decontamination, and inoculation of agar plates containing incorporated selective antibiotics is the most sensitive and efficient way to achieve this. Paya *et al.* (1989) express the US view on screening by recommending preoperative tests for MRSA, invasive fungi (*Cryptococcus*, *Histoplasma*, *Coccidioides* and *Blastomyces* spp. serology), cultures of blood, urine, throat and rectal swabs and a vaccination update (tetanus, diphtheria, pneumococcus, hepatitis B and influenza). Postoperatively they recommend that throat, rectal, abdominal drain and T-tube swabs should be cultured twice weekly for the first 4 weeks, and then repeated as available at 3 and 6 months. Fungal serology should be repeated weekly for 4 weeks, then at 3 and 6 months.

### SURGICAL PROPHYLAXIS

No recent comparative studies of perioperative antibiotic prophylaxis have been reported in liver transplantation. Most units have now adopted a 48-h duration of prophylaxis, but 5-day regimens were popular in the past. With the move in most types of surgery towards single-dose prophylaxis, strictly a 48-h prophylactic course should be considered perioperative prophylaxis plus empirical therapy. The 48-h period allows time for any operation-related sepsis to manifest itself and assures cover if early reoperation for haemorrhage is required. In Cambridge we continue prophylaxis for a further 24 h if the patient appears septic at 48 h or requires reoperation, and then reassess the choice of agents if no improvement is seen. Arnow *et al.* (1992) studied the perioperative pharmacokinetics of cefotaxime and ampicillin in 18 adult liver recipients and confirmed the existing practice in many centres of using high prophylactic doses to account for blood loss and of giving extra intraoperative doses, especially if the operation is prolonged. A centre's choice of prophylactic regimen should be influenced by the range of antibiotic sensitivities observed in the faecal flora of patients admitted for transplantation; colonization with multiply resistant coliforms and pseudomonads is common because of the extensive antibiotic treatment that these patients have usually received. There is considerable variation in choice of antibiotics, but centres often choose either an extended-spectrum cephalosporin (such as cefotaxime) plus ampicillin and sometimes metronidazole, or a single broad-spectrum agent such as meropenem or imipenem. Penicillin-allergic recipients are usually given a quinolone plus vancomycin and metronidazole, but clindamycin plus aztreonam has been used (Chang *et al.* 1998).

## SELECTIVE GUT DECONTAMINATION

Selective decontamination of the gastrointestinal tract (SDGT) has been applied in liver transplantation in an effort to reduce further the incidence of postoperative infection, especially with Gram-negative bacteria. In theory, Gram-negative bacteria and yeasts are cleared from the gastrointestinal tract, while most of the anaerobic (and often the Gram-positive) flora are retained. Left *in situ* they may inhibit recolonization and translocation of pathogens across the gut wall, an effect known as colonization resistance (Van der Waaij 1982).

Non-absorbed antimicrobial agents have been popular for SDGT, but few satisfactory and convincing studies have been published. A preliminary report of 50 patients randomized to receive amphotericin, polymyxin E and tobramycin enterally and as an oral gel showed that endotoxaemia was reduced in frequency, but Gram-negative bacteria were cleared from the faeces in only 75% cases (Badger *et al.* 1991). Antibiotic resistance appeared not to be induced or selected, but more patients must be recruited to establish measurable advantages and disadvantages of this regimen. Wiesner *et al.* (1988; Wiesner 1991) believed that SDGT with polymyxin E, gentamicin and nystatin begun a week or more preoperatively reduced Gram-negative and yeast colonization and infection within the first 30 days in 145 liver transplant recipients, but Gram-positive infections remained. Successful elimination of coliforms was achieved from the gut of most patients, but the study was uncontrolled so the overall results are difficult to interpret. Full definitions of infection that were used in the study are not given, but it is likely that reduction of upper airway colonization with aerobic Gram-negative bacteria by the SDGT regimen would inevitably have reduced the number of chest problems diagnosed as pneumonia. Occasional isolation of gentamicin-resistant coliforms was reported in the stools of patients after SDGT was discontinued.

A study of 52 assessable elective liver transplant recipients randomized to receive SDGT with oral amphotericin, polymyxin E and tobramycin for 5–15 days, or oral nystatin only, failed to show any significant effect on endotoxaemia (measured by LAL assay) during the operation, or on outcome (Bion *et al.* 1994). Gram-negative bacilli were not significantly less often isolated from the faeces of patients receiving SDGT, so the decontamination abilities of the regimen must be questioned and a financial analysis came out in favour of no prophylaxis. Bacterial resistance was not detected during this 16-month study. Gram-negative colonization of the respiratory tract was reduced but specific criteria for pneumonia diagnosis (such as BAL) were not used, thus the incidence of pneumonia in the two groups is difficult to evaluate. Most of the reported reduction in 'clinical infection' was in 'pneumonias' and is therefore not surprising, given the inclusion of isolation of Gram-negative bacteria from sputum in the definition of pneumonia. Interestingly, portal endotoxaemia was not predictive of systemic endotoxaemia, and endotoxaemia in neither circulation correlated with organ system failure.

In an open study Steffen *et al.* (1994) combined Orabase paste (gentamicin, polymyxin and nystatin) with 48-h systemic prophylaxis with cefotaxime, tobramycin and metronidazole in 206 liver graft recipients. Gram-negative decontamination was usually achieved but faecal cultures for yeasts frequently remained positive. Two-year patient survival was excellent at 92% and Gram-positive aerobic organisms were involved in most of the 27.8% patients who suffered postoperative infections. Increased bacterial resistance ascribable to the SDGT regimen was not seen. A similar regimen was used by Paya *et al.* (1989) in 83 patients, with the substitution of cefotaxime plus tobramycin as parenteral prophylaxis. Overall 53% patients were infected, with 65% involving aerobic Gram-positive isolates. In addition, from Germany, Raakow *et al.* (1990) and Rossaint *et al.* (1991) report a comparable experience with 75 grafts in 70 patients; however, the lack of control groups and problems with definition of infection in these studies make firm conclusions about the efficacy and overall impact of SDGT impossible to draw.

A note of caution was added to the SDGT debate by the report of Patel *et al.* (1994b), who described *Lactobacillus* spp. bacteraemia in eight liver transplant recipients given Orabase while intubated plus gentamicin, polymyxin B and nystatin while in hospital. In a case–control study, lactobacillaemia was more common in those with Roux-en-Y anastomoses and may also have been associated with prior vancomycin therapy. Of the 390 transplants performed during the study period, colonization of the bile was seen in a further 28 patients without positive blood cultures and this was more common in those with problems of biliary drainage and Roux-en-Y procedures. *Lactobacillus* spp. are always resistant to gentamicin and polymyxin B, and often also to vancomycin and teicoplanin, but usually sensitive to penicillin. Problems with other glycopeptide-resistant Gram-positive organisms are increasingly reported, especially in liver transplant recipients (Green *et al.* 1991). Some of these infections are serious and the therapeutic opportunities are currently extremely limited; therefore SDGT regimens must be carefully assessed for their tendencies to encourage overgrowth with these organisms and continuous faecal monitoring must be performed for vancomycin-resistant bacteria.

It must be remembered that some authors have reported low rates of total and Gram-negative infection and low infectious mortality without use of SDGT. For example, Pirsch *et al.* (1989) reported only one death from infection among 52 infectious episodes in 41 patients given antibiotics only perioperatively; the infections included 13 bacteraemias and 10 cases of wound sepsis but only eight pneumonias. Similarly, in the series of 21 bacteraemias reported by McClean *et al.* (1994) who did not use SDGT, 62% involved Gram-positive aerobic bacteria and only 24% Gram-negative bacteria.

Some of the variability in efficacy of SDGT regimens to clear Gram-negative aerobic rods from the faeces may be a result of the duration of administration preoperatively (Arnow *et al.* 1992). Thus, Rosman *et al.* (1990) found that only 64% of their 39 patients achieved clearance of most Gram-negative aerobic faecal organisms with oral non-absorbable agents beginning 6–8 h preoperatively, and infection was significantly more common in those who failed to clear. Definitions of infection supplied are scanty, but only one case of pneumonia was seen so the observed difference is probably clinically and microbiologically significant. Prolonged preoperative usage may allow decontamination before operative ileus supervenes, but is difficult to achieve in patients waiting for a graft which will become available at short notice. Systemic antibiotics, especially fluoroquinolones, have theoretical attractions for SDGT in patients after liver transplantation because they are excreted in high concentration to the bile and via the gut wall and decontamination can thereby be extended to the intra- and extrahepatic biliary tree. Reliable clearance of facultative Gram-negative rods from the faeces can generally be achieved and the agents are more palatable than the non-absorbable alternatives. For example, Cuervas-Mons *et al.* (1989) used oral norfloxacin and nystatin in 23 patients who were given 26 liver transplants. Administration began 4–6 h preoperatively and continued until discharge from hospital; aerobic Gram-negative bacteria were eliminated from the gut flora in all cases. Few clinical or microbiological details are given, but it is noteworthy that three of the nine infections in the first month were caused by Gram-negative rods. Well-controlled comparative trials are needed if the relative merits of decontamination regimens in liver transplantation are ever to be established scientifically.

## FUNGAL INFECTION

At the time of transplantation it appears now to be possible to define a high-risk group for serious fungal infection (Collins *et al.* 1994); one limited study of selective amphotericin prophylaxis guided by such criteria has been published and it will be interesting to see further assessments of this approach. In an uncontrolled study, Mora *et al.* (1992) found that low-dose prophylactic amphotericin B (10 mg intravenously for each of the first 10–15 days) used in selected patients resulted in an incidence of fungal infection of only 7.5% with follow-up for between 5 and 26 months. In a controlled trial Tollemar *et al.* (1995) showed a reduced incidence of fungal infection in patients given 1 mg/kg liposomal amphotericin for 5 days, but the drug costs of this regimen were substantial. It remains to be shown whether postoperative prophylaxis or early empirical antifungal therapy is effective, and whether usage of fluconazole (aimed at the much more commonly occurring *C. albicans*), perhaps itraconazole, the potentially toxic but broader-spectrum amphotericin B, or the expensive lipid-complexed formulations of amphotericin B will be the best strategy. Further trials of these regimens are under way; for example, Lumbreras *et al.* (1996) have shown that oral fluconazole (100 mg/day for the first 28 days post-transplant) was significantly better than oral nystatin at reducing *Candida* colonization and infection, and that it was not associated with toxicity or the emergence of resistant strains.

Overall, fungal infection has been reported to have reduced in incidence as experience with liver transplantation has grown (Kusne *et al.* 1988). This is undoubtedly a multifactorial improvement, related to refined immunosuppression, shortened operations, earlier use of empirical amphotericin therapy, greater use of oral antifungal prophylaxis and doubtless other factors. It is unfortunately not possible to relate the resulting alterations in yeast and filamentous fungal infection to changes in autologous risk factors, such as oral azole prophylaxis against yeasts or *Aspergillus*, or intravenous amphotericin usage, and environmental exposure, such as HEPA filtration to reduce *Aspergillus* spore exposure. Accurate dissection of these factors would enable targeting of these expensive, and potentially toxic, prophylactic measures towards those patients most likely to benefit from each, but adequate data are not yet available clearly to guide one's recommendations for solid organ transplant recipients.

The current position has been well reviewed by a Working Party of the British Society for Antimicrobial Chemotherapy (1993), who only recommend antifungal prophylaxis for hepatic graft recipients; fluconazole should be considered for the first postoperative month. If there is a high institutional incidence of aspergillosis, itraconazole should be substituted for fluconazole. If the patient has graft vs. host disease, oral itraconazole should be used for 3 months as long as serum levels are adequate. If adequate levels are not achievable, thrice daily nasal amphotericin spray should be substituted for itraconazole. Beyer *et al.* (1994) have also recently reviewed experience with the available strategies for preventing aspergillosis in susceptible patients, and Zeluff (1990) has summarized causes, predisposing factors, diagnosis and prevention of most of the primarily pathogenic and opportunist fungal infections in transplant recipients. Despite its high capital cost, provision of HEPA-filtered air to areas where patients with hepatic transplants are nursed is likely to reduce greatly the incidence of aspergillosis (Rhame *et al.* 1984). However, filtered air cannot be supplied to all areas to which patients travel for treatment or special investigations, and outbreaks related to environmental exposure within operating theatres and radiology departments have been reported.

Management of systemic yeast infection after liver transplantation is broadly similar to that after renal grafting (see below). The problems with managing infections with non-*albicans Candida* species and *Aspergillus* spp. are well illustrated by the report of

Viviani *et al.* (1992). These authors describe deep *Candida* spp. infections in five and *Aspergillus* spp. infections in 11 of 89 liver transplant recipients given oral amphotericin or oral or intravenous fluconazole prophylaxis. Prophylaxis was successful against *C. albicans*, but prophylaxis and treatment of infection with the other fungi was difficult, with five of the 12 patients infected with non-*C. albicans* fungi dying. Liposomal amphotericin, and other complexed preparations, may prove to have specific roles in treatment of fungal infection in liver graft recipients, but there are currently few data indicating improved efficacy and its high cost mandates its restriction at present to cases with progressive nephrotoxicity from the conventional preparation or failure to respond (Khoo *et al.* 1994). If usage in tertiary referral hospitals with solid organ and bone marrow transplant units is restricted to indications covered in the manufacturer's data sheet, cost savings of several hundred thousand pounds per annum can be expected when compared to similar units without restrictions. Rhinocerebral zygomycosis is one fungal infection where liposomal amphotericin in high daily dosage appears to have an a priori role in combination with surgical debridement, and Munckhof *et al.* (1993) describe the successful therapy of maxillary infection with *Rhizopus arrhizus* in a liver transplant recipient.

## Small-bowel transplantation

Transplantation of the small intestine is known to promote bacterial overgrowth in a rat model, and addition of cyclosporin immunosuppression increases bacterial translocation to mesenteric lymph nodes and further systemic spread (Browne *et al.* 1991). Graft vs. host disease and rejection provide further opportunities for organisms within the gut to spread within the body (Sigalet *et al.* 1992), and preventative measures aimed at these problems have been applied with some apparent success to human small-bowel transplantation.

A limited small-intestinal transplant programme has been performed at the University of Pittsburgh since 1990, with 34 operations performed by January 1993, some combined with liver transplants (Reyes *et al.*

1993). At this unit, surgical antibiotic prophylaxis with cefotaxime, ampicillin and metronidazole was continued for 5 days and SDGT with polymyxin, gentamicin and amphotericin given for 4 postoperative weeks. Oral co-trimoxazole was given for the first year as prophylaxis against PCP. Repeated episodes of bacteraemia and fungaemia were seen, believed to arise by translocation across the graft mucosa during rejection episodes, and quantitative stool bacteriology was performed as a guide to the timing and spectrum of antibiotic pre-emptive therapy. Concentrations of $>10^9$/mL of stoma fluid are considered significant (Browne *et al.* 1991). Intra-abdominal sepsis, requiring repeated laparotomy, was common and five of the seven deaths were infective in cause.

Five small-bowel transplants have been performed in Cambridge at the time of writing. All had had small-bowel resections in the past and were maintained pre-operatively on total parenteral nutrition via central venous access; most had suffered multiple episodes of line infection, usually involving coagulase-negative staphylococci or enterococci.

Donors were given 300 mg of the intravenous preparation of ciprofloxacin and 200 mg of the intravenous preparation of fluconazole preoperatively via nasogastric tube. Recipients received 200 mg ciprofloxacin, 500 mg vancomycin and 500 mg metronidazole 12-hourly intravenously, beginning with the induction of anaesthesia and continued for 48 h. In addition, 0.5 mg/kg intravenous amphotericin B in 100 mL saline was infused over 2 h each day. Orally, patients received 200 mg fluconazole daily plus 400 000 units of nystatin q.d.s. At 48 h, if the patient was stable, the vancomycin and metronidazole were stopped and the ciprofloxacin was converted to 500 mg 12-hourly by mouth, but this was continued intravenously if gut absorptive function was suspect. Once the gut was considered to be reliably functional the amphotericin was stopped. Oral antibacterial and antifungal prophylaxis continued for about a further month, when it was replaced with co-trimoxazole for *Pneumocystis* prevention, but was reinstated during episodes of bowel dysfunction (for example, CMV, enteritis or rejection) (Grant *et al.* 1991).

All patients suffered at least one postoperative bacteraemia with coagulase-negative staphylococci which we assessed as secondary to intravenous catheter infections. One patient, known preoperatively to have extensive large vein thrombosis, suffered recurrent bacteraemias with coagulase-negative staphylococci, *Stenotrophomonas maltophilia* and *C. albicans* apparently of thrombophlebitic origin, and the graft was removed 59 days after transplant. Another patient presented with fever 6 weeks after transplantation which responded to aspiration of an upper abdominal fluid collection from which coagulase-negative staphylococci and *Enterococcus faecalis* were isolated. In the three patients with surviving grafts significant fungal infection has not been seen: use of systemic antifungal agents has not been required on clinical therapeutic grounds, and they have been used only prophylactically during the initial postoperative period and episodes of graft dysfunction. During episodes of bowel rejection stools are screened on ciprofloxacin–vancomycin CLED agar to assess the completeness of decontamination and to guide alternative antibiotic choice, but quantitative culture has not been performed.

More experience will accrue quickly about the special infective problems of patients after small-intestinal transplantation, but our management of these cases has been successful so far, and predicted problems of graft bacterial permeability and rampant fungal infection have been amenable to prophylactic measures. Patients coming to intestinal transplantation who have been maintained on total parenteral nutrition for long periods, with attendent past histories of catheter infection and phlebitis, are likely to pose especially difficult problems.

## Conclusions

Many developments in the prevention, control, diagnosis and analysis of risk factors for infection in immunocompromised patients in general are applicable to solid organ transplant recipients, and important advances should result from these. In particular, observational studies employing logistic regression analysis are defining risk groups more accurately, and it is to be hoped that these will be used to design trials of targeted interventional therapy and prophylaxis especially aimed at fungal infection. Trials will be more easily comparable if standardized definitions are used for infectious complications and in time analyses. It is probably unfortunately now a forlorn hope that well-controlled trials of surgical prophylaxis or SDGT will ever be performed in liver transplantation.

One recent development which will bring new opportunities for infectious complications in transplant recipients is the introduction of organ procurement from transgenic animals, especially pigs, and the potential for direct zoonotic infection from such sources has been recently reviewed by Fishman (1994). Solutions to novel infectious challenges will continually be required in the field of solid organ transplantation.

## References

Albrechtsen, D., Bentdal, O., Berg, K.J. *et al.* (1990) Infections in cyclosporine-treated kidney graft recipients: beneficial effect of cotrimoxazole prophylaxis. *Transplantation Proceedings* **22**, 245–246.

Alessiani, M., Kusne, S., Martin, M. *et al.* (1991) Infections in adult liver transplant patients under FK 506 immunosuppression. *Transplantation Proceedings* **23**, 1501–1503.

Anderson, R.J., Schafer, L.A., Olin, D.B. & Eickoff, T.C. (1973) Septicemia in renal transplant recipients. *Archives of Surgery* **106**, 692–694.

Arduino, R.C., Johnson, P.C. & Miranda, A.G. (1993) Nocardiosis in renal transplant recipients undergoing immunosuppression with cyclosporine. *Clinical Infectious Diseases* **16**, 505–512.

Arend, S.M., Westendorp, R.G.J., Kroon, F.P. *et al.* (1996) Rejection treatment and cytomegalovirus infection as risk factors for *Pneumocystis carinii* pneumonia in renal transplant recipients. *Clinical Infectious Diseases* **22**, 920–925.

Arnow, P.M., Furmaga, K., Flaherty, J.P. & George, D. (1992) Microbiological efficacy and pharmacokinetics of prophylactic antibiotics in liver transplant patients. *Antimicrobial Agents and Chemotherapy* **36**, 2125–2130.

Badger, I.L., Crosby, H.A., Kong, K.L. *et al.* (1991) Is selective decontamination of the digestive tract beneficial in liver transplant patients? Interim results of a prospective randomized trial. *Transplantation Proceedings* **23**, 1460–1461.

Barone, G.W., Hudec, W.A., Sailors, D.M. & Ketel, B.L. (1996) Prophylactic wound antibiotics for combined kidney and pancreas transplants. *Clinical Transplantation* **10**, 386–388.

Bartlett, M.S. & Smith, J.W. (1991) *Pneumocystis carinii*, an opportunist in immunocompromised patients. *Clinical Microbiological Reviews* **4**, 137–149.

Benedict, L.M., Kusne, S., Torre-Cisneros, J. & Hunt, S.J. (1992) Primary cutaneous fungal infection after solid-organ transplantation: report of five cases and review. *Clinical Infectious Diseases* **15**, 17–21.

Beyer, J., Schwartz, S., Heinemann, V. & Siegert, W. (1994) Strategies in prevention of invasive pulmonary aspergillosis in immunosuppressed or neutropenic patients. *Antimicrobial Agents and Chemotherapy* **38**, 911–917.

Bion, J.F., Badger, I., Crosby, H.A. *et al.* (1994) Selective decontamination of the digestive tract reduces Gram-negative pulmonary colonization but not systemic endotoxaemia in patients undergoing elective liver transplantation. *Critical Care Medicine* **22**, 40–49.

Boon, A.P., O'Brien, D. & Adams, D.H. (1991) 10 year review of invasive aspergillosis detected at necropsy. *Journal of Clinical Pathology* **44**, 452–454.

Branten, A.J.W., Beckers, P.J.A., Tiggeler, R.G.W.L. & Hoitsma, A.J. (1995) *Pneumocystis carinii* pneumonia in renal transplant recipients. *Nephrology, Dialysis and Transplantation* **10**, 1194–1197.

Briegel, J., Forst, H., Spill, B. *et al.* (1995) Risk factors for systemic fungal infections in liver transplant recipients. *European Journal of Clinical Microbiology and Infectious Diseases* **14**, 375–382.

Browne, B.J., Johnson, C.P., Edmiston, C.E. *et al.* (1991) Small bowel transplantation promotes bacterial overgrowth and translocation. *Journal of Surgical Research* **51**, 512–517.

Burleson, R.L., Brennan, A.M. & Scruggs, B.F. (1977) Foley catheter tip cultures: a valuable diagnostic aid in the immunosuppressed patient. *American Journal of Surgery* **133**, 723–725.

Byrd, L.H., Tapin, L., Cheigh, J.S. *et al.* (1978) Association between *Streptococcus faecalis* urinary tract infections and graft rejection in kidney transplantation. *Lancet* **ii**, 1167–1169.

Cahill, B., Snyder, L., Woodward, M. & Hertz, M. (1991) Non-bacterial infections in solid organ transplant patients with roentgenographically inapparent lung injury: the diagnostic yield of bronchoalveolar lavage. *American Review of Respiratory Disease* **143** (Suppl.), A113.

Calne, R.Y. (1994) Immunosupression in liver transplantation. *New England Journal of Medicine* **331**, 1154–1155.

Canadian Multicentre Transplant Study Group (1983) A randomized clinical trial of cyclosporin in cadaveric renal transplantation. *New England Journal of Medicine* **309**, 809–815.

Canafax, D.M., Graves, N.M., Hilligoss, D.M. *et al.* (1991)

Increased cyclosporine levels as a result of simultaneous fluconazole and cyclosporine therapy in renal transplant recipients: a double-blind, randomized pharmacokinetic and safety study. *Transplantation Proceedings* **23**, 1041–1042.

Capocasale, E., Mazzoni, M.P., Tondo, S. & D'Errico, G. (1994) Antimicrobial prophylaxis with ceftriaxone in renal transplantation. *Chemotherapy* **40**, 435–440.

Case Report. (1992) Case 8-1992. *New England Journal of Medicine* **326**, 547–559.

Castaldo, P., Stratta, R.J., Wood, R.P. *et al.* (1991) Fungal disease in liver transplant recipients: a multivariate analysis of risk factors. *Transplantation Proceedings* **23**, 1517–1519.

Chang, F.Y., Singh, N., Gayowski, T., Wagner, M.M. & Marino, I.R. (1998) Fever in liver transplant recipients: changing spectrum of etiologic agents. *Clinical Infectious Diseases* **26**, 59–65.

Chapman, S.W. & Wilson, J.P. (1990) Nocardiosis in transplant recipients. *Seminars in Respiratory Infection* **5**, 74–79.

Chave, J.-P., David, S., Wauters, J.-P., van Melle, G. & Francioli, P. (1991) Transmission of *Pneumocystis carinii* from AIDS patients to other immunosuppressed patients: a cluster of *Pneumocystis carinii* pneumonia in renal transplant recipients. *AIDS* **5**, 927–932.

Church, J.M., Braun, W.E., Novick, A.C., Fazio, V.W. & Steinmuller, D.R. (1986) Perforation of the colon in renal homograft recipients. *Annals of Surgery* **203**, 69–76.

Cienfuegos, J.A., Mora, N.B., Coper, J.B. *et al.* (1984) Surgical complications in the postoperative period in liver transplantation in children. *Transplantation Proceedings* **16**, 1230–1235.

Cohen, J., Rees, A.J. & Williams, G. (1988) A prospective randomized controlled trial of perioperative antibiotic prophylaxis in renal transplantation. *Journal of Hospital Infection* **11**, 357–363.

Collins, L.A., Samore, M.H., Roberts, M.S. *et al.* (1994) Risk factors for invasive fungal infections complicating orthotopic liver transplantation. *Journal of Infectious Diseases* **170**, 644–652.

Colonna, J.O., Winston, D.J., Brill, J.E. *et al.* (1988) Infectious complications in liver transplantation. *Archives of Surgery* **123**, 360–364.

Committee on the Microbiological Safety of Human Tissues and Organs used in Transplantation. (1996) *Guidance on the Microbiological Safety of Human Tissues and Organs used in Transplantation.* HSG(96)26. NHS Executive, London.

Cuervas-Mons, V., Barrios, C., Garrido, A. *et al.* (1989) Bacterial infections in liver transplant patients under selective decontamination with norfloxacin. *Transplantation Proceedings* **21**, 3558.

Denning, D.W. & Stevens, D.A. (1990) Antifungal and

surgical treatment of invasive aspergillosis: a review of 2121 published cases. *Reviews of Infectious Diseases* 12, 1147–1201.

Douzdjian, V., Abecassis, M.M., Corry, R.J. & Hunsicker, L.G. (1994) Simultaneous pancreas–kidney versus kidney-alone transplants in diabetics: increased risk of early cardiac death and acute rejection following pancreas transplants. *Clinical Transplantation* 8, 246–251.

Drobniewski, F.A. & Ferguson, J. (1996) Tuberculosis in renal transplant units. *Nephrology, Dialysis and Transplantation* 11, 768–770.

Dummer, J.S., Hardy, A., Poorsattar, A. & Ho, M. (1983) Early infections in kidney, heart and liver transplant recipients on cyclosporine. *Transplantation* 36, 259–267.

Edelstein, H.E., McCabe, R.E. & Lieberman, E. (1989) Perinephric abscess in renal transplant recipients: report of seven cases and review. *Reviews of Infectious Diseases* 4, 569–577.

Evans, C.M., Purohit, S., Colbert, J.W. *et al.* (1988) Amoxycillin-clavulanic acid (Augmentin) antibiotic prophylaxis against wound infections in renal failure patients. *Journal of Antimicrobial Chemotherapy* 22, 363–369.

Everett, J.E., Wahoff, D.C., Statz, C. *et al.* (1994) Characterization and impact of wound infection after pancreas transplantation. *Archives of Surgery* 129, 1310–1317.

Ezzedrine, H., Mourad, M., Van Ossel, C. *et al.* (1994) An outbreak of *Ochrobactrum anthropi* bacteraemia in five organ transplant patients. *Journal of Hospital Infection* 27, 35–42.

Farrington, M., Matthews, I., Foreman, J. & Caffrey, E. (1998) Microbiological monitoring of bone grafts: 2 years' experience at a tissue bank. *Journal of Hospital Infection* 38, 261–271.

Ferguson, R.M., Sutherland, D.E., Simmons, R.L. & Najarian, J.S. (1982) Ketoconazole cyclosporin metabolism and renal transplantation. *Lancet* ii, 882–883.

First, M.R., Linnemann, C.C., Munda, R. *et al.* (1985) Beneficial effect of pneumococcal polysaccharide vaccine in splenectomized renal transplant recipients. *Transplantation Proceedings* 17, 147–150.

Fishman, J.A. (1994) Minature swine as organ donors for man: strategies for prevention of xenotransplant-associated infections. *Xenotransplantation* 1, 47–57.

Fujita, S., Lasker, B.A., Lott, T.J., Reiss, E. & Morrison, C.J. (1995) Microtitration plate enzyme immunoassay to detect PCR-amplified DNA from *Candida* species in blood. *Journal of Clinical Microbiology* 33, 962–967.

George, D.L., Arnow, P.M., Fox, A.S. *et al.* (1991) Bacterial infection as a complication of liver transplantation: epidemiology and risk factors. *Reviews of Infectious Diseases* 13, 387–396.

George, D.L., Arnow, P.M., Fox, A. *et al.* (1992) Patterns of infection after pediatric liver transplantation. *American Journal of the Diseases of Children* 146, 924–929.

Gerson, B. (1987) Cyclosporine controversies. *Clinical and Laboratory Medicine* 7, 669–686.

Grant, D., Hurlbut, D., Zhong, R. *et al.* (1991) Intestinal permeability and bacterial translocation following small bowel transplantation in the rat. *Transplantation* 52, 221–224.

Green, M., Barbadora, K. & Michaels, M. (1991) Recovery of vancomycin-resistant Gram-positive cocci from pediatric liver transplant recipients. *Journal of Clinical Microbiology* 29, 2503–2506.

Gueco, I., Saniel, M., Mendoza, M., Alano, F. & Ona, E. (1989) Tropical infections after renal transplantation. *Transplantation Proceedings* 21, 2105–2107.

Hamburg, M.A. & Frieden, T.R. (1994) Tuberculosis transmission in the 1990s. *New England Journal of Medicine* 330, 1750–1751.

Han, T., van Hook, E.J., Simmons, R.L. & Najarian, J.S. (1978) Prognostic factors of peritoneal infections in transplant patients. *Surgery* 84, 403–416.

Hanevold, C.D., Kaiser, B.A., Palmer, J.A. *et al.* (1987) Vesicoureteric reflux and urinary tract infections in renal transplant recipients. *American Journal of the Diseases of Children* 141, 982–984.

Hesse, U.J., Fryd, D.S., Chatterjee, S.N. *et al.* (1986a) Pulmonary infections: the Minnesota randomized prospective trial of cyclosporine vs. azathioprine-antilymphocyte globulin for immunosuppression in renal allograft recipients. *Archives of Surgery* 121, 1056–1060.

Hesse, U.J., Sutherland, D.E.R., Najarian, J.S. & Simmons, R.L. (1986b) Intra-abdominal infections in pancreas transplant recipients. *Annals of Surgery* 203, 153–162.

Hibbard, P.L. & Rubin, R.H. (1993) Renal transplantation and related infections. *Seminars in Respiratory Infection* 8, 216–224.

Hibbard, P.L. & Rubin, R.H. (1994) Clinical aspects of fungal infection in organ transplant recipients. *Clinical Infectious Diseases* 19 (Suppl. 1), S33–S40.

Higgins, R.M., Cahn, A.P., Porter, D. *et al.* (1991) Mycobacterial infections after renal transplantation. *Quarterly Journal of Medicine* 78, 145–153.

Holt, C.D., Winston, D., Kubak, B. *et al.* (1997) Coccidioidomycosis in liver transplant patients. *Clinical Infectious Diseases* 24, 216–221.

Indudhara, R., Menon, M. & Khauli, R.B. (1994) Posttransplant lymphocele presenting as an 'acute abdomen'. *American Journal of Nephrology* 14, 154–156.

Jensen, W.A., Rose, R.M., Hammer, S.M. *et al.* (1986) Pulmonary complications of orthotopic liver transplantation. *Transplantation* 42, 484–490.

Jereb, J.A., Burwen, D.R., Dooley, S.W. *et al.* (1993) Nosocomial outbreak of tuberculosis in a renal transplant unit: application of a new technique for restriction fragment polymorphism analysis of *Mycobacterium tuberculosis* isolates. *Journal of Infectious Diseases* 168, 1219–1224.

Jernigan, D.B., Sanders, L.I., Waites, K.B. *et al.* (1994) Pulmonary infection due to *Legionella cincinnatiensis* in renal transplant recipients: two cases and implications for laboratory diagnosis. *Clinical Infectious Diseases* 18, 385–389.

Johnson, P.C., Hogg, K.M. & Sarosi, G.A. (1990) The rapid diagnosis of pulmonary infections in solid organ transplant recipients. *Seminars in Respiratory Infection* 5, 2–9.

Jules-Elysee, K.M., Stover, D.E., Zamar, M.B., Bernard, E.M. & White, D.A. (1990) Aerosolized pentamidine: effect on diagnosis and presentation of *Pneumocystis carinii* pneumonia. *Annals of Internal Medicine* 112, 750–757.

Khardori, N. (1989) Host–parasite interaction in fungal infections. *European Journal of Clinical Microbiology and Infectious Diseases* 8, 331–351.

Khoo, S.H., Bond, J. & Denning, D.W. (1994) Administering amphotericin B—a practical approach. *Journal of Antimicrobial Chemotherapy* 33, 203–213.

Kim, J.H. & Perfect, J.R. (1989) Infection and cyclosporine. *Reviews of Infectious Diseases* 11, 677–690.

King, C.T., Chapman, S.W. & Butkus, D.E. (1993) Recurrent nocardiosis in a renal transplant recipient. *Southern Medical Journal* 86, 225–228.

Koneru, B., Scantlebury, V.P., Makowka, L. *et al.* (1989) Infections in pediatric liver recipients treated for acute rejection. *Transplantation Proceedings* 21, 2251–2252.

Krowka, M.J. & Cortese, D.A. (1985) Pulmonary aspects of chronic liver disease and liver transplantation. *Mayo Clinic Proceedings* 60, 407–418.

Kusne, S., Dummer, J.S., Singh, N. *et al.* (1988) Infections after liver transplantation. An analysis of 101 consecutive cases. *Medicine (Baltimore)* 67, 132–143.

Kusne, S., Martin, M., Schapiro, R. *et al.* (1991) Early infections in kidney transplant recipients under FK506. *Transplantation Proceedings* 23, 956–957.

Kusne, S., Tobin, D., Pasculle, A.W. *et al.* (1994) Candida carriage in the alimentary tract of liver transplant candidates. *Transplantation* 57, 398–402.

Kwan, J.T.C., Foxall, P.J.D., Davidson, D.G.C., Bending, M.R. & Eisinger, A.J. (1987) Interaction of cyclosporin and itraconazole. *Lancet* ii, 282.

Kyriakides, G.R., Simmons, R.L. & Najarian, J.S. (1975) Wound infections in renal transplant wounds: pathogenic and prognostic factors. *Annals of Surgery* 182, 770–777.

Landreneau, M.D. & McDonald, J.C. (1987) Genitourinary complications in renal transplantation. *Transplantation Reviews* 1, 59–84.

Langhoff, E. & Madsen, S. (1983) Rapid metabolism of cyclosporin and prednisolone in kidney transplant patient receiving tuberculostatic treatment. *Lancet* ii, 1031.

Leaker, B., Hellyar, A., Neild, G.H. *et al.* (1989) Nocardia infection in a renal transplant unit. *Transplantation Proceedings* 21, 2103–2104.

Limper, A.H., Offord, K.P., Smith, T.F. & Martin, W.J. (1989) Differences in lung parasite number and inflammation in patients with and without AIDS. *American Review of Respiratory Diseases* 140, 1204–1209.

Lin, L.C., Bewick, M. & Koffman, C.G. (1993) Primary use of a double J silicone ureteric stent in renal transplantation. *British Journal of Urology* 72, 697–701.

Linden, P.K., Pasculle, A.W., Manez, R. *et al.* (1996) Differences in outcomes for patients with bacteraemia due to vancomycin-resistant *Enterococcus faecium* or vancomycin susceptible *E. faecium*. *Clinical Infectious Diseases* 22, 663–670.

Little, D.M., Farrell, J.G., Cunningham, P.M. & Hickey, D.P. (1997) Donor sepsis is not a contraindication to cadaveric organ donation. *Quarterly Journal of Medicine* 90, 641–642.

Lobo, P.I., Rudolf, L.E. & Krieger, J.N. (1982) Wound infections in renal transplant recipients—a complication of urinary tract infections during allograft malfunction. *Surgery* 92, 491–496.

Lumbreras, C., Cuervas-Mons, V., Jara, P. *et al.* (1996) Randomized trial of fluconazole versus nystatin for the prophylaxis of *Candida* infection following liver transplantation. *Journal of Infectious Diseases* 174, 583–588.

McClean, K., Kneteman, N. & Taylor, G. (1994) Comparative risk of bloodstream infection in organ transplant recipients. *Infection Control and Hospital Epidemiology* 15, 582–584.

McMaster, P., Herbertson, B.M., Cusick, C. *et al.* (1979) The development of biliary 'sludge' following liver transplantation. *Transplantation Proceedings* 11, 262–266.

McWhinney, N., Khan, O. & Williams, G. (1981) Tuberculosis in patients undergoing maintenance haemodialysis and renal transplantation. *British Journal of Surgery* 68, 408–411.

Maddux, M.S., Veremis, S.A., Bauma, W.D., Pollak, R. & Mozes, M.F. (1989) Effective prophylaxis of early post-transplant urinary tract infections (UTI) in the cyclosporine (CSA) era. *Transplantation Proceedings* 21, 2108–2109.

Maki, D.G., Fox, B.C., Kunz, J., Sollinger, H.W. & Belzer, F. (1992) A prospective, randomized, double-blind study of trimethoprim-sulphamethoxazole for prophylaxis of infection in renal transplantation. *Journal of Laboratory and Clinical Medicine* 119, 11–24.

Martell, R., Heinrichs, D., Stiller, C.R. *et al.* (1986) The effects of erythromycin in patients treated with cyclosporine. *Annals of Internal Medicine* 104, 660–661.

Martinez-Marcos, F., Cisneros, J., Gentil, M. *et al.* (1994) Prospective study of renal transplant infections in 50 consecutive patients. *European Journal of Clinical Microbiology and Infectious Diseases* 13, 1023–1028.

Martino, M.W., Wolfe, J.A., Bollinger, R.R. & Sanfillipo, F. (1987) Cause of death in renal transplant recipients: a review of autopsy findings from 1966 through 1985. *Archives of Pathology and Laboratory Medicine* 111, 983–987.

Martino, P., Girmenia, C., Micozzi, A. *et al.* (1994) Prospective study of *Candida* colonization, use of empiric amphotericin B and development of invasive mycosis in neutropenic patients. *European Journal of Clinical Microbiology and Infectious Diseases* 13, 797–804.

Mermel, L.A. & Maki, D.G. (1990) Bacterial pneumonia in solid organ transplantation. *Seminars in Respiratory Infection* 5, 10–29.

Meunier F. (1989) Candidiasis. *European Journal of Clinical Microbiology and Infectious Diseases* 8, 438–447.

Mora, M., Wilms, H. & Kirste, G. (1991a) Significance of bacterial contamination of cadaver donor renal allografts before transplantation. *Transplantation Proceedings* 23, 2648.

Mora, N.P., Coper, J.B., Solomon, R.M. *et al.* (1991b) Analysis of severe infections (INF) after 180 consecutive liver transplants: the impact of amphotericin B prophylaxis for reducing the incidence and severity of fungal infections. *Transplantation Proceedings* 23, 1528–1530.

Mora, N.P., Klintmalm, G., Soloman, H. *et al.* (1992) Selective amphotericin B prophylaxis in the reduction of fungal infections after liver transplant. *Transplantation Proceedings* 119, 984–991.

Muakkassa, W.F., Goldman, M.H., Mendez-Picon, G. & Lee, H.M. (1983) Wound infections in renal transplant patients. *Journal of Urology* 130, 17–19.

Munckhof, W., Jones, R., Tosolini, F.A. *et al.* (1993) Cure of rhizopus sinusitis in a liver transplant recipient with liposomal amphotericin B. *Clinical Infectious Diseases* 16, 183.

Myerowitz, R.L., Medieros, A.A. & O'Brien, T.F. (1972) Bacterial infection in renal homotransplant recipients: a study of fifty-three bacteraemic episodes. *American Journal of Medicine* 53, 306–314.

Najarian, J.S., Ferguson, R.M., Sutherland, D.E., Ryanasiewicz, J.J. & Simmons, R.L. (1983) A prospective trial of the efficacy of cyclosporine in renal transplantation at the University of Minnesota. *Transplantation Proceedings* 15, 438–441.

Neilsen, H.E. & Korsager, B. (1977) Bacteraemia after renal transplantation. *Scandinavian Journal of Infectious Diseases* 9, 111–117.

Nicholson, V. & Johnson, P.C. (1994) Infectious complications in solid organ transplant recipients. *Surgical Clinics of North America* 74, 1223–1279.

Nicol, D.L., P'Ng, K., Hardie, D.R., Wall, D.R. & Hardie, J.R. (1993) Routine use of indwelling ureteral stents in renal transplantation. *Journal of Urology* 150, 1375–1379.

Novick, A.C. (1981) The value of intraoperative antibiotics in preventing renal transplant wound infections. *Journal of Urology* 125, 151–152.

Oh, C.S., Stratta, R.J., Fox, B.C. *et al.* (1988) Increased infections associated with the use of OKT3 for treatment of steroid-resistant rejection in renal transplantation. *Transplantation* 45, 68–73.

Opal, S.M., Asp, A.A., Cannady, P.B. *et al.* (1986) Efficacy of infection control measures during a nosocomial outbreak of disseminated aspergillosis associated with hospital construction. *Journal of Infectious Diseases* 153, 634–637.

Orr, K.E. & Gould, F.K. (1992) Infection problems in patients receiving solid organ transplants. *Reviews in Medical Microbiology* 3, 96–103.

Papanicolaou, G.A., Meyers, B.R., Mayers, J. *et al.* (1996) Nosocomial infections with vancomycin-resistant *Enterococcus faecium* in liver transplant recipients: risk factors for acquisition and mortality. *Clinical Infectious Diseases* 23, 760–766.

Park, G.R., Lindop, M.J., Klinck, J.R. *et al.* (1989) Mortality during intensive care after orthotopic liver transplantation. *Anaesthesia* 44, 959–963.

Patel, R., Roberts, G.D., Keating, M.R. & Paya, C.V. (1994a) Infections due to nontuberculous mycobacteria in kidney, heart, and liver transplant recipients. *Clinical Infectious Diseases* 19, 263–273.

Patel, R., Cockerill, F.R., Porayko, M.K. *et al.* (1994b) Lactobacillemia in liver transplant patients. *Clinical Infectious Diseases* 18, 207–212.

Paya, C.V. (1993) Fungal infections in solid organ transplantation. *Clinical Infectious Diseases* 16, 677–688.

Paya, C., Hermans, P.E., Washington, J. *et al.* (1989) Incidence, distribution and outcome of episodes offection in 100 orthotopic liver transplantations. *Mayo Clinic Proceedings* 64, 555–564.

Peterson, P.K. & Anderson, R.C. (1986) Infection in renal transplant recipients: current approaches to diagnosis, therapy and prevention. *American Journal of Medicine* 81, 2–10.

Peterson, P.K., Ferguson, R., Fryd, D.S. *et al.* (1982) Infectious diseases in hospitalized renal transplant recipients: a prospective study of a complex and evolving problem. *Medicine (Baltimore)* 61, 360–372.

Pfaller, M.A., Houston, A. & Coffmann, S. (1995) Application of CHROMagar candida for rapid screening of clinical specimens for *Candida albicans, Candida tropicalis, Candida krusei* and *Candida glabrata. Journal of Clinical Microbiology* 34, 58–61.

Pirsch, J.D., Armbrust, M.J., Stratta, R.J. *et al.* (1989) Perioperative infection in liver transplant recipients under a quadruple immunosuppressive protocol. *Transplantation Proceedings* 21, 3559.

Pollock, C.A., Mahony, J.F., Ibels, L.S. *et al.* (1989) Immunoglobulin abnormalities in renal transplant recipients. *Transplantation* **47**, 952–956.

Polo, J.M., Fabrega, E., Casafont, F. *et al.* (1992) Treatment of cerebral aspergillosis after liver transplantation. *Neurology* **42**, 1817–1819.

Potter van Loon, B.J., Lichtendahl, A.T., Mulder, S.S. *et al.* (1989) Microbial contamination of donor duodenum in whole-pancreas transplantation. *Diabetes* **38** (Suppl. 1), 242–243.

Prodinger, W.M., Bonatti, H., Allerberger, F. *et al.* (1994) Legionella pneumonia in transplant recipients: a cluster of cases of eight years duration. *Journal of Hospital Infection* **26**, 191–202.

Puglisi, B.S., Kauffman, H.M., Stewart, E.T. *et al.* (1985) Colonic perforation in renal transplant patients. *American Journal of Radiology* **145**, 555–558.

Raakow, R., Steffen, R., Lefebre, B. *et al.* (1990) Selective bowel decontamination effectively prevents Gram-negative bacterial infections after liver transplantation. *Transplantation Proceedings* **22**, 1556–1557.

Rao, K.V. & Anderson, R.C. (1988) Long-term results and complications in renal transplant recipients. *Transplantation* **45**, 45–52.

Raz, R., Almog, D., Elhanan, G. & Shental, J. (1994) The use of ceftriaxone in the prevention of urinary tract infection in patients undergoing transurethral resection of the prostate (TUR-P). *Infection* **22**, 43–48.

Reyes, J., Tzakis, A.G., Todo, S., Abu-Elmagd, K. & Starzl, T.E. (1993) Post-operative care of bowel transplant recipients. *Care of the Critically Ill* **9**, 193–198.

Rhame, F.S., Streifel, A.J., Kersey, J.H. & McGlave, P.B. (1984) Extrinsic risk factors for pneumonia in the patient at high risk of infection. *American Journal of Medicine* **77**, 42–52.

Rhame, F.S., Striefel, A., Stevens, P. *et al.* (1985) Endemic aspergillus spore levels are a major risk factor for aspergillosis in bone marrow transplant patients. In: *The 25th Intersciences Conference of Antimicrobial Agents and Chemotherapy, Minneapolis*, abstract 147. American Society for Microbiology.

Rifkind, D., Faris, T.D. & Hill, R.B. (1966) *Pneumocystis carinii* pneumonia. *Annals of Internal Medicine* **65**, 943–956.

Robbins, R.A., Zetterman, R.K., Kendall, T.J. *et al.* (1987) Elevation of chemotactic factor inactivator in alcoholic liver disease. *Hepatology* **7**, 872–877.

Rollins, N.K., Andrews, W.S., Currarino, G. *et al.* (1988) Infected bile lakes following pediatric liver transplantation: nonsurgical management. *Radiology* **166**, 169–171.

Rosman, C., Klompmaker, I.J., Bonsei, G.J. *et al.* (1990) The efficacy of selective bowel decontamination as infection prevention after liver transplantation. *Transplantation Proceedings* **22**, 1554–1555.

Rossaint, R., Raakow, R., Lewandowski, K. *et al.* (1991) Strategy for prevention of infection after orthotopic liver transplantation. *Transplantation Proceedings* **23**, 1965–1966.

Rubin, R.H. (1994) Infection in the organ transplant recipient. In: *Clinical Approach to Infection in the Compromised Host* (eds R.H. Rubin & L.S. Young), 3rd edn. Plenum Press, New York.

Rubin, R.H. & Fischman, A.J. (1996) Radionuclide imaging of infection in the immunocompromised host. *Clinical Infectious Diseases* **22**, 414–422.

Rubin, R.H. & Tolkoff-Rubin, N.E. (1989) Infection: the new problems. *Transplantation Proceedings* **21**, 1440–1445.

Rubin, R.H. & Tolkoff-Rubin, N.E. (1993) Antimicrobial strategies in the care of organ transplant recipients. *Antimicrobial Agents and Chemotherapy* **37**, 619–624.

Rubin, R.H., Wolfson, J.S., Cosini, A.B. & Tolkoff-Rubin, N.E. (1981) Infections in the renal transplant recipient. *American Journal of Medicine* **70**, 405–411.

Sahathevan, M., Harvey, F.A., Forbes, G. *et al.* (1991) Epidemiology, bacteriology and control of an outbreak of *Nocardia asteroides* infection on a liver unit. *Journal of Hospital Infection* **18** (Suppl. A), 473–480.

Salant, D.J., Glover, A.M., Anderson, R. *et al.* (1976) Depressed neutrophil chemotaxis in patients with chronic renal failure and after renal transplantation. *Journal of Laboratory and Clinical Investigation* **88**, 536–545.

Saliba, F., Ephraim, R., Mathieu, D. *et al.* (1994) Risk factors for bacterial infection after liver transplantation. *Transplantation Proceedings* **26**, 266.

Samhan, M., Panjwani, D.D., Dadah, S.K. *et al.* (1989) Is tuberculosis a contraindication for renal transplantation? *Transplantation Proceedings* **21**, 2036–2038.

Schad, G.A. (1986) Cyclosporine may eliminate the threat of overwhelming strongyloidiasis in immunosuppressed patients. *Journal of Infectious Diseases* **153**, 178.

Schroter, G.P.J., Hoelscher, M., Putnam, C.W. *et al.* (1976a) Infections complicating orthotopic liver transplantation. *Archives of Surgery* **111**, 1337–1347.

Schroter, G.P.J., Hoelscher, M., Putnam, C.W., Porter, K.A. & Starzl, T.E. (1976b) Fungus infections after liver transplantation. *Annals of Surgery* **186**, 115–122.

Scroggs, M.W., Wolfe, J.A., Bollinger, R.R. & Sanfilippo, F. (1987) Causes of death in renal transplant recipients. *Archives of Pathology and Laboratory Medicine* **111**, 983–987.

Sigalet, D., Kneteman, N.M. & Thomson, A.B.R. (1992) Small bowel transplantation: past, present and future. *Digestive Disease* **10**, 258–273.

Singer, C., Armstrong, D., Rosen, P.P. *et al.* (1975) *Pneumocystis carinii* pneumonia: a cluster of eleven cases. *Annals of Internal Medicine* **82**, 772–777.

Singh, N., Gayowski, T., Wagener, M., Doyle, H. & Marino, I.R. (1997) Invasive fungal infections in liver transplant recipients receiving tacrolimus as the primary immunosuppressive agent. *Clinical Infectious Diseases* 24, 179–184.

Sinnott, J.T. & Emmanuel, P.J. (1990) Mycobacterial infections in the transplant patient. *Seminars in Respiratory Infection* 5, 65–73.

Smets, Y.F.C., van der Pijl, J.W., van Dissel, J.T. *et al.* (1997) Infectious disease complications of simultaneous pancreas kidney transplantation. *Nephrology, Dialysis and Transplantation* 12, 764–771.

Sollinger, H.W., Ploeg, R.J., Eckhoff, D.E. *et al.* (1993) Two hundred consecutive simultaneous pancreas–kidney transplants with bladder drainage. *Surgery* 114, 736–743.

Steffen, R., Reinhartz, O., Blumhardt, G. *et al.* (1994) Bacterial and fungal colonization and infections using oral selective bowel decontamination in orthotopic liver transplantations. *Transplant International* 7, 101–108.

Stone, W.J. & Schaffner, W. (1990) *Strongyloides* infections in transplant recipients. *Seminars in Respiratory Infection* 5, 58–64.

Stuby, U., Kaiser, W., Grafinger, P., Biesenbach, G. & Zazgornik, J. (1989) Urinary tract infection after renal transplantation under conventional therapy and cyclosporine. *Transplantation Proceedings* 21, 2110–2111.

Stynen, D., Goris, A., Sarfati, J. & Latge, J.P. (1995) A new sensitive sandwich enzyme-linked immunosorbent assay to detect galactofuran in patients with invasive aspergillosis. *Journal of Clinical Microbiology* 33, 497–500.

Tang, C.M., Cohen, J., Rees, A.J. & Holden, D.W. (1994) Molecular epidemiological study of invasive pulmonary aspergillosis in a renal transplantation unit. *European Journal of Clinical Microbiology and Infectious Diseases* 13, 318–321.

Taylor, G.D., Kirkland, T., Lakey, J., Rajotte, R. & Warnock, G. (1994) Bacteraemia due to transplantation of contaminated cryopreserved pancreatic islets. *Cell Transplantation* 4, 103–106.

Tillegard, A. (1984) Renal transplant wound infection: the value of prophylactic antibiotic treatment. *Scandinavian Journal of Nephrology* 18, 215–221.

Tilney, N.L., Strom, T.B., Vineyard, G.C. & Merill, J.P. (1978) Factors contributing to the declining mortality rate in renal transplantation. *New England Journal of Medicine* 299, 1321–1325.

Tokunaga, Y., Concepcion, W., Berquist, W.E. *et al.* (1992) Graft involvement by *Legionella* in a liver transplant recipient. *Archives of Surgery* 127, 475–477.

Tolkoff-Rubin, N.E., Cosimi, A.B., Russell, P.S. & Rubin, R.H. (1982) A controlled study of trimethoprim-sulphamethoxazole prophylaxis of urinary tract infection in renal transplant recipients. *Reviews of Infectious Diseases* 4, 614–618.

Tollemar, J., Ericzon, B.-G., Holmberg, K. & Andersson, J. (1990) The incidence and diagnosis of invasive fungal infections in liver transplant recipients. *Transplantation Proceedings* 22, 242–244.

Tollemar, J., Hockerstedt, K., Ericzon, B.G., Jalanko, H. & Ringden, O. (1995) Liposomal amphotericin B prevents invasive fungal infections in liver transplant recipients. *Transplantation* 59, 45–50.

Torre-Cisneros, J., Lopez, O.L., Kusne, S. *et al.* (1993) CNS aspergillosis in organ transplantation: a clinicopathological study. *Transplantation Proceedings* 25, 1062–1063.

Townsend, T.R., Rudolf, L.E., Westervelt, F.B., Mandell, G.L. & Wenzel, R.P. (1980) Prophylactic antibiotic therapy with cefamandole and tobramycin for patients undergoing renal transplantation. *Infection Control* i, 93–96.

Van der Waaij, D.J. (1982) Colonization resistance of the digestive tract. *Journal of Antimicrobial Chemotherapy* 10, 263–270.

Verweij, P.E., Stynen, D., Rijs, A.J. *et al.* (1995) Sandwich enzyme-linked immunosorbent assay compared with Pastorex agglutination test for diagnosing invasive aspergillosis in immunocompromised patients. *Journal of Clinical Microbiology* 33, 1912–1914.

Viviani, M.A., Tortorano, A.M., Malaspina, C. *et al.* (1992) Surveillance and treatment of liver transplant recipients for candidiasis and aspergillosis. *European Journal of Epidemiology* 8, 433–436.

Vukmir, R.B., Kusne, S., Linden, P. *et al.* (1994) Successful therapy for cerebral phaeohyphomycosis due to *Dactylaria gallopava* in a liver transplant recipient. *Clinical Infectious Diseases* 19, 714–719.

Wagener, M.M. & Yu, V.L. (1992) Bacteraemia in transplant recipients: a prospective study of demographics, etiological agents, risk factors and outcomes. *American Journal of Infection Control* 20, 239–247.

Wajszczuk, C.P., Dummer, J.S., Ho, M. *et al.* (1985) Fungal infections in liver transplant recipients. *Transplantation* 64, 555–564.

Washer, G.F., Schroter, G.P., Starzl, T.E. & Weil, R. (1983) Causes of death after kidney transplantation. *Journal of the American Medical Association* 250, 49–54.

Webb, W.R., Gamsu, G., Rohlfing, B.M. *et al.* (1978) Pulmonary complications of renal transplantation: a survey of patients treated by low-dose immunosuppression. *Radiology* 126, 1–8.

Weinberger, M., Eid, A., Schreiber, L. *et al.* (1995) Disseminated *Nocardia transvalensis* infection resembling pulmonary infarction in a liver transplant recipient. *European Journal of Clinical Microbiology and Infectious Diseases* 14, 337–341.

Wiesner, R.H. (1991) Selective bowel decontamination for infection prophylaxis in liver transplantation patients. *Transplantation Proceedings* 23, 1927–1928.

Wiesner, R.H., Hermans, P.E., Rakela, J. *et al.* (1988) Selective bowel decontamination to decrease Gram-negative aerobic bacterial and *Candida* colonization and prevent infection after orthotopic liver transplantation. *Transplantation* **45**, 570–574.

Wilson, J.P., Turner, H.R., Kirchner, K.A. *et al.* (1989) Nocardial infections in renal transplant recipients. *Medicine (Baltimore)* **68**, 38–57.

Winston, D.J., Emmanouilides, C. & Busuttil, R.W. (1995) Infections in liver transplant recipients. *Clinical Infectious Diseases* **21**, 1077–1091.

Working Party of the British Society for Antimicrobial Chemotherapy (1993) Chemoprophylaxis for candidosis and aspergillosis in neutropenia and transplantation: a review and recommendations. *Journal of Antimicrobial Chemotherapy* **32**, 5–21.

Zeluff, B.J. (1990) Fungal pneumonia in transplant recipients. *Seminars in Respiratory Infection* **5**, 80–89.

# Chapter 18/Bacterial, fungal and protozoal infection after transplantation of the heart or lungs

JULIET E. FOWERAKER & SAMUEL W.B. NEWSOM

## Introduction

The initial literature on infections after heart transplant from Stanford (Jamieson *et al.* 1982) now seems horrendous—600 infectious episodes in 227 patients, including 280 infections of the chest, 60 of the urinary tract and 63 bacteraemias. The scene has improved dramatically since then. The 14th International Transplant Registry report in 1997 had details on file for 40 738 heart, 2186 heart–lung and 3939 double and single lung transplants (Hosenpud *et al.* 1997). This report gives data on reason for transplantation, age and procedure. It shows an increase in survival in all transplant groups in recent years. Dummer *et al.* (1995) summarized the experience from Pittsburgh and included an excellent chart of mortality caused by infection after heart transplantation, noting that from 1987 to 1990 this largely occurred within 6 months of the operation, reaching around 4%. By contrast, in the first half of the 1980s, mortality as a result of infection in the first 6 months was nearly 10% rising to 25% by 8 years post-transplant. A major reason for this change was the introduction of cyclosporin for immunosuppression. This markedly reduced infection rates (Kim & Perfect 1989), albeit at the expense of some renal toxicity (McGiffen *et al.* 1985). Sarris *et al.* (1994a) reported on the Stanford experience of cardiac transplantation in the cyclosporin era, and noted a

77% 5-year survival in those given cyclosporin plus OKT3 since 1987. Actuarial freedom from infection-related death after 5 years was 85%, a marked improvement on the 1982 figures.

Better use of prophylaxis has helped to prevent infection transmitted from the donor as well as continuous or reactivated infection in the recipient. Reduction in viral infection, especially cytomegalovirus (see Chapter 16), also means that there are fewer bacterial and fungal infections. Improvements in infection control procedures have reduced the impact of nosocomial infection. Whereas 20 years ago the bacteriologist was repeatedly facing new challenges, heart transplant patients now, although more numerous, provide only the occasional microbiological problem. Furthermore, the transplant programmes preceded the AIDS epidemic so what were quite unusual problems raised by T cell depression, such as toxoplasmosis, pneumocystis or even systemic salmonellosis, are now better understood.

As the technology for heart transplantation improved so the numbers of centres providing a service increased and transplantation has become limited by the availability of donors. The development of bridge-to-transplantation techniques (Johnson *et al.* 1992) using artificial pumps of various types has brought the added hazard of vascular-access device infections (Maki 1994). Further developments include the accumulation of a significant number of retransplant patients and extension of heart transplantation to children (Dunn *et al.* 1987) and the elderly (Olivari *et al.* 1988).

Transplant technology has advanced to include heart–lung and single or double lung transplants. Lobar transplants from dead or living donors can now be used for children and small adults. (For indications and procedures for lung transplantation, see Chapter 11.) Lung transplantation brings with it an increased risk of bacterial infection in that it is a less 'clean' operation—involving an organ exposed to a normal flora and open to airborne contaminants, including fungi. Patients with infective lung diseases such as cystic fibrosis have received many years' antibiotic therapy, so allowing the selection of highly antibiotic-resistant organisms. The methicillin-resistant *Staphylococcus aureus* (MRSA), and *Burkholderia* (previously *Pseudomonas*) *cepacia* are particularly important in this group of patients (Spencer 1995).

The procedure of lung transplantation abolishes the cough reflex distal to the anastomosis, interrupts lymphatic drainage, may compromise blood supply to the anastomosis and reduces mucociliary clearance. Chronic rejection leads to the bronchiolitis obliterans syndrome, which includes bronchiectasis. The lung transplant recipient has therefore more risk of infection in the transplant than does the heart transplant patient. These factors have to be added to the general risk of opportunist infection after immunosuppression.

A recent survey of 44 heart–lung, single and double lung transplant patients who died within the first 30 days found the most common cause of death to be infection (Goddard *et al.* 1998). In the registry data, infection remains the main cause of death in the lung transplant group until after 1 year, when the cause is obliterative bronchiolitis (Hosenpud *et al.* 1997). In this group, however, infection is the terminal event in most patients.

## Preoperative factors

### Recipient

The healthy person has excellent physical and biologi-cal defences to infection: not so the potential heart or lung recipient. Previous hospitalization exposes all patients to an increased risk of infection and possible generation of a more resistant bacterial flora following antibiotic therapy. The two UK National Prevalence surveys have revealed an average 9–10% incidence of nosocomial infection in all inpatients, a risk increasing with time spent in hospital (Meers *et al.* 1981; Emmerson *et al.* 1995). Cardiac failure may be complicated by pulmonary infarction, oedema or infection, and methods for a bridge-to-transplantation for end-stage heart disease, such as the left ventricular assist device, put the patients at further risk of infection. Patients requiring lung transplant for bronchiectasis, cystic fibrosis and to a lesser extent chronic obstructive pulmonary disease will have had repeated chest infections and may carry multiple antibiotic-resistant bacteria selected by long and repeated treatment courses. Those with pulmonary hypertension may have had prolonged therapy involving long-term intravascular access lines, with the risk of bacterial and fungal line infection and septicaemia. In addition, lung damage and antibiotic usage can predispose recipients to yeast and filamentus fungal colonization and infection.

Do other factors in the recipient affect risk of infection? Fabbri *et al.* (1992a) surveyed the effect of gender of both donor and recipient in the Papworth heart transplant programme and concluded that there was no gender-related difference in infection rates. One hundred and fifteen late survivors of heart transplantation during the first year of life were described by Bailey *et al.* (1993); only one in the whole series died of severe infection. Sarris *et al.* (1994b) reviewed the Stanford paediatric heart transplant experience and showed a satisfactory medium-term survival; although after 1 year only 37% were free from any infection, and eight (out of 72) had died from infection, 88% remained free from infection-related death at 5 years. Smyth *et al.* (1989) described early experiences at Papworth with heart–lung transplants for children with terminal respiratory disease; although three of the five had episodes of postoperative infection—including one of staphylococcal pneumonia—all five were alive and well after 17 months. Several groups have presented data on heart transplants in the elderly. Fabbri *et al.* (1992b), for example, presented data on the 46 patients over 55 years old in a Papworth series of 206 transplants. This study showed that the older patients were no more likely to have infectious episodes. Smart *et al.* (1996), however, reviewed the incidence of infection after heart transplant in 30 institutions in the USA and found an increased risk of fatal infection in the young and elderly (over 55 years), use of organs from older donors, longer donor ischaemic time and a recipient on ventilation support at the time of transplant. This group did not look at diabetes, which may be expected to put a patient at increased risk of infection. An encouraging report, however, came from Rhenman *et al.* (1988), who found no difference in medium-term survival of heart transplant recipients between 57 non-diabetic patients and nine with pre-existing diabetes (the latter were, however, carefully selected and had tailored immunosuppression). Lanza *et al.* (1984) found that major infections in patients transplanted for ischaemic heart disease were twice as common in those with cardiomyopathy, while three of eight patients operated on in the presence of pulmonary infarcts developed extensive empyema (Young *et al.* 1986). Patients receiving heart–lung transplants for cystic fibrosis had no more postoperative infections overall than those transplanted for other conditions (Dennis *et al.* 1993). A more recent analysis of the Papworth data, however, has shown a significant increase in bacterial infections in the first 30 days post-transplant for recipients with cystic fibrosis. Selection of recipients and prophylaxis is particularly important in the cystic fibrosis group (Starnes *et al.* 1992).

The recipient of retransplantation has the additional burden of long-term immunosuppression as well as the effects of end-stage organ failure. A survey of 449 retransplants from the Registry of the International Society for Heart and Lung Transplantation (Karwande *et al.* 1992a) showed an overall mortality significantly higher than that for the first transplant, but a similar incidence of infection.

What of pre-existing infection or colonization in the recipient? Anguita *et al.* (1993) described seven cardiac patients who were transplanted with acute bacterial infections with no problems postoperatively. By contrast Murray-Leisure *et al.* (1986) reported an unusual case whose intraoperative cultures following bridging with a balloon pump revealed disseminated infection with *Trichosporon beigelii*, from which the patient later died despite therapy with amphotericin B.

Some centres have refused to accept patients with infection or colonization by MRSA. Outbreaks of nosocomial infection by recently emerged types of MRSA such as EMRSA-16 may be extremely hard to control (Cox *et al.* 1995). This poses a problem both for the individual patient, who has to be isolated from other patients on the cardiothoracic unit, and for the cohort of transplant patients, who will be returning to the unit for check-ups or further therapy for many years. It is therefore crucial to screen potential recipients at assessment and regular intervals while on the waiting list so that MRSA can be covered in the prophylaxis at surgery and the patient barrier-nursed to reduce the risk to others. MRSA is now widespread in many units and there is no significant evidence that carriers do worse as long as correct prophylaxis is prescribed and good postoperative care, including physiotherapy, is given. Many units would now accept MRSA carriers for transplantation.

*Aspergillus* often colonizes the airways of patients requiring double lung or heart–lung transplantation. This is thought to present little risk. Patients with *Aspergillus* extending to the pleural wall, however, would be excluded from transplantation because of the probability of invasive fungal disease after transplantation (De Leval *et al.* 1991; Dennis *et al.* 1993).

*Burkholderia cepacia* is often resistant to many antibiotics. It is commonly found only in patients with cystic fibrosis. Several papers have advanced clinical data to support person-to-person transmission (e.g. Govan *et al.* 1993), to the extent that the Cystic Fibrosis Trust of the UK has issued guidelines for the segregation of colonized patients both in and out of hospital. A recent study from Boston (Steinbach *et al.* 1994) using ribotyping and chromosomal fingerprinting on strains from five double-lung recipients and 17 other patients with cystic fibrosis showed that each harboured a separate clone of bacteria that persisted and reappeared after transplant. Two of the transplant patients had a severe disseminated disease. Cystic fibrosis patients colonized with *B. cepacia* who undergo heart–lung transplant may have a worse outlook than those not colonized. (Ramirez *et al.* 1992; Ryan & Stableforth 1996). Rather than exclude all patients colonized with *B. cepacia*, research is urgently needed to find the host and/or bacterial factors that would enable us to separate the patients who will do badly from the significant number who have an uncomplicated postoperative course in spite of continuing colonization with *B. cepacia*. If patients with *B. cepacia* are operated on they should be kept separate, during both the short- and long-term follow-up, from other patients with cystic fibrosis.

There are also concerns about multidrug-resistant strains of *Pseudomonas aeruginosa* found in the sputum prior to transplantation. Does infection or colonization persist once the old lungs have been removed? Eleven patients with cystic fibrosis had their sensitive strains typed by macrorestriction fragment pattern similarity (Walter *et al.* 1997). Each patient had the same clone of *P. aeruginosa* in the lung 1 week before and 1 week and 6 months after transplantation. The clones from the 11 patients were all different so this was not a problem of cross-infection but reinfection of the new lungs from a reservoir. Patients (usually with cystic fibrosis) who carry pan-resistant *P. aeruginosa*, *Stenotrophomonas maltophila* or *Alcaligenes* spp. as well as *B. cepacia* are usually excluded from transplantation (Egan *et al.* 1995). The difficulty is in defining pan-resistant as antibiotic combinations may need to be tested for synergy and there is no universally accepted method for synergy testing in the laboratory that consistently predicts clinical effect.

The fact that pseudomonads and fungi can still cause infection after the lungs have been removed indicates that other sites of carriage, such as the upper respiratory tract (including paranasal sinus) and the gut, are important. Some groups routinely give sinus washouts to potential recipients (Lewiston *et al.* 1991). Others would drain sinuses if there was clinical or radiological evidence of infection, but accept that it is not known if this is effective (Ramirez *et al.* 1992). Others rely on targeted prophylaxis, both systemic and by inhalation, and early treatment of infection after transplantation (Yacoub *et al.* 1990).

Certain infections remain latent in the recipient but may reactivate after transplantation and cause disease either in the new organ or at other sites; the risk is greatly enhanced by immunosuppression. If there is a past history of tuberculosis the choice is between long-term prophylaxis (isoniazid carries the risks of hepatitis, development of resistance and interaction with cyclosporin) and close observation, rapid diagnosis (use of nucleic acid multiplication and detection systems such as those using polymerase chain reaction and automated liquid culture) with early treatment. A risk of strongyloidiasis would be considered in a patient with a history of exposure—which may have occurred decades ago—or of eosinophilia; stools should be examined and serology may be helpful. Although rarely encountered in the UK, prior infection with some systemic mycoses can present a major risk of reactivation. *Coccidioides immitis*, for example, is endemic in south-west USA so that in Arizona 50% of the population will have had prior infection. Serology and a careful clinical history are required from any patient who has been exposed. Management of such patients is controversial but long-term antifungal treatment appeared to give the best outcome in a study of heart transplant patients (Hall *et al.* 1993b). Chagas' disease cardiomyopathy is the cause of the end-stage heart failure in 20% of patients referred for heart transplantation in São Paulo, Brazil (Almeida *et al.* 1996). There is a significant risk of reactivation. Leishmaniasis may recur post-transplantation—prior exposure, clinical history and positive serology are helpful clues. Virus (especially cytomegalovirus) and *Toxoplasma* reactivation in the donor are dealt with in Chapter 16.

The general approach in recipient management is to consider patients' exposure history and test for diseases that may reactivate with immunosuppression; screen patients for resistant bacteria and fungi that may cause infection postoperatively; give prophylaxis to cover the organisms present; and prevent reactivation of latent infection where the benefit outweighs the risk.

## Donor

Heart and lung transplantation is part of the larger

field of tissue or organ donation, for which the avail-ability of suitable donors is strictly limited. This is even more restricted by the many reports of transmission of viral, bacterial, fungal and protozoal agents following transplantation of organs and tissues. The Department of Health Committee on Microbiological Safety of Blood and Tissues for Transplantation in the UK has produced guidelines (NHS Executive 1996) to try to ensure the microbiological safety of all human tissues and organs used in transplantation, including items such as bone and heart valves as well as organs. Potential donors with human immunodeficiency virus (HIV), hepatitis B and C viruses (HBV, HCV), rabies, Creutzfeldt–Jakob disease, malaria (present or past) or tuberculosis are to be excluded. Testing is required for cytomegalovirus, syphilis and *Toxoplasma* (for heart donation). The document notes that the organ should not have been damaged by infection or transmit difficult-to-treat infection such as that caused by multiresistant bacteria. A list of infections which require specialist microbiological advice is given (see Table 18.1). Further guidance has been prepared by the British Transplantation Society (1998).

As a heart transplant is a 'clean' operation, donor-transmitted bacterial or fungal infection is usually caused by septicaemia or fungaemia in the donor and could be secondary to chest infection, intravascular access lines or diseases with a bacteraemic component such as meningitis. One interesting possibility is translocation of bacteria and endotoxin in the organ donor from the gut into the blood when the organs are harvested. Van Goor *et al.* (1994) looked at 24 donors and found that all had factors that might encourage translocation; endotoxin was found in 19% of periph-eral blood samples. There is, however, no evidence of transmission of infection with faecal-type flora. Pos-sible contamination of a heart with respiratory tract bacteria when the lung block was separated has been described (see p. 510). Protozoa may reside in the heart tissue—the Papworth experience of toxoplasmosis is fully described by Wreghitt *et al.* (1992). A retrospec-tive analysis initiated after two of the first 35 patients developed toxoplasmosis showed that they were the only patients in which a heart from a donor with *Toxo-plasma* antibodies was placed into a recipient without

**Table 18.1** Infections identified in hospital in potential organ and tissue donors which require specialist microbiological advice to determine suitability for transplantation.

| Infections |
| --- |
| Adenovirus, systemic infection |
| Aspergillosis |
| Blastomycosis |
| Brucellosis |
| Candidosis |
| Coccidioidomycosis |
| *Coxiella burnetii* (Q fever) |
| Cryptococcosis |
| Cytomegalovirus |
| Encephalomyelitis, any aetiology |
| Enterovirus, systemic infection |
| Herpes simplex, encephalomyelitis or systemic infection |
| Histoplasmosis |
| HTLV 1, symptomatic or previously diagnosed as positive |
| Listeriosis |
| Lyme borreliosis |
| Measles, systemic infection |
| Melioidosis |
| Meningitis |
| Methicillin-resistant *Staphylococcus aureus* (MRSA) |
| *Mycobacterium leprae* |
| Nocardiosis |
| Paratyphoid |
| Parvovirus B19, systemic infection |
| Septicaemia |
| *Toxoplasma* |
| Typhoid |
| Varicella zoster |

*Toxoplasma* antibodies. Since then pyrimethamine and co-trimoxazole prophylaxis has been used for similar mismatches. *Trypanosoma cruzi*—the cause of Chagas' disease—also resides in heart muscle, but so far there is no record of its transmission from the donor. *Plasmod-ium falciparum* has been transmitted by heart trans-plant. The donor was originally from Cameroon, but had resided in France for 15 months and remained free of fever. She had not been screened for malaria in spite of her country of origin (Babinet *et al.* 1991).

Donor selection for transplantation of lungs is com-plicated by the additional possibilities of chest infec-tion or tracheal contamination with mouth or gut bacteria. Zenati *et al.* (1989, 1990) noted that 78% of cultures of donor trachea at operation grew mouth- or pharyngeal-type flora and so recommended the use of wide-spectrum antibiotic cover. A later study comparing the donor tracheal organisms with those found in 37 recipients noted that, although 16 of the latter developed chest infection within 2 weeks of operation, only in three cases was infection caused by donor organisms. These, however, were from three of the four donors colonized with *Candida* and all the recipients died of invasive candidiasis. A detailed comparison of all the infected and non-infected groups showed that the single statistically significant difference was isolation of mouth flora from donor tracheal cultures. Low *et al.* (1993) extended these findings; their analysis of bronchial washings revealed growth in 97% of donors, commonly with staphylococci or Gram-negative bacteria. They recommended tailoring any prolonged perioperative antibiotics to the culture results. Ciulli *et al.* (1993) documented the Papworth experience. In only two of 125 occasions were the bacteria isolated from the donor trachea subsequently thought to be a cause of infection in the recipient. One case of pneumonia and empyema was caused by *S. aureus* and in the other *Haemophilus influenzae* from the donor was found in a paratracheal abscess that accompanied a tracheal dehiscence 17 days after operation. Both patients died. Although bacteria were isolated from 54% of the donor trachea cultures these bacteria did not cause infection in the recipients. In a histological study of donor lungs not used for transplant for reasons other than infection, a high rate of bronchitis was noted (Stewart *et al.* 1993). The use of perioperative prophylaxis with extension to 7–10 days of treatment if bacteria were grown from donor cultures would therefore appear to be advisable.

The transplantation team assessing a potential donor should look for clinical indicators of infection and any positive microbiology results. If there are severe signs of infection at bronchoscopy the lungs would not be taken; mild signs, however, would be assessed in the context of the whole state of the donor. For Papworth transplants, specimens for culture taken at bronchoscopy and blood cultures are brought back to our microbiology laboratory. Donor trachea is also cultured at transplant. Prophylaxis for the recipient should take into account any positive microbiology results available before transplant.

## Perioperative factors

The perioperative risk factors for infection from transplantation are similar to those of open-heart surgery generally, although without the additional infection risk provided by the leg wounds and vein harvest required for coronary artery surgery. Any postoperative infection is likely to be more difficult to treat, especially during the early enhanced immunosuppression. Simple ways of reducing risk, for example reducing wound infection by best-practice skin preparation and avoiding shaving, are crucial. The skill of the surgeon in limiting the length of operation, bleeding and the need for reoperation all helps to avoid infection. Lung transplants have the additional problem of an airway anastamosis and the maintenance of a good blood supply to this area. Failure of the blood supply may result in at least a dead surface for microbial colonization and at worst a tracheal or bronchial dehiscence. Various techniques, for example pericardial flap-plasty (Haverich *et al.* 1989), have been used to try and overcome this problem.

Antibiotic prophylaxis has always been used for open-heart surgery. The original prophylaxis of benzylpenicillin, flucloxacillin and gentamicin used at Papworth (Newsom 1978) for cardiac transplantation worked well, but needed modification on the arrival of cyclosporin, as there are concerns of nephrotoxicity with use of prophylactic gentamicin. A short period of using flucloxacillin/fucidin was abruptly terminated following an early Gram-negative pneumonia, and cefotaxime was added. Use of cefotaxime and flucloxacillin for cardiac transplantation was documented by Khagani *et al.* (1988). The general use of cefotaxime for surgical prophylaxis has been reviewed (Sader & Jones 1992). The reduction of prophylaxis to single-dose or short courses, so avoiding the risk of inducing or selecting bacterial resistance, was noted. Patients for lung transplantation with pre-existing infection with *Pseudomonas* spp. or other cefotaxime-resistant bacteria may require alternative prophylaxis. Patients with end-stage cystic fibrosis usually have highly resistant strains of infecting bacteria, so that prophylaxis should be tailored to the preoperative recipient culture results. Ceftazidime is often used, but ciprofloxacin, a ureidopenicillin such as azlocillin, a carbapenem such as imipenem, or a combination may be required. In this latter group, prophylaxis may merge into the treatment of early chest infection. It is also common practice to give 7–10 days of appropriate antibiotics if donor cultures are positive. Inhaled antimicrobials, colistin, tobramycin, amphotericin may have a role in early prophylaxis (DeLeval *et al.* 1991; Ramirez *et al.* 1992; Dennis *et al.* 1993).

The presence of highly immunosuppressed patients in the intensive care facility after major surgery initially prompted a strict reverse barrier-nursing regime. Following the Stanford protocol, patients at Papworth were originally kept isolated for 1 month—even their letters and newspapers were gas-sterilized before being admitted to the isolation cubicle. Great care was also taken with food; several beverages were cultured to check for microbial contamination and ice from machines was banned in the light of previous experience (Newsom 1968). Gamberg *et al.* (1987) reported a retrospective review of modified isolation at Stanford and concluded that the intensity of isolation appeared to have no impact on the incidence, morbidity or mortality resulting from infection. Likewise a survey by the American Association of Critical Care Nurses answered by 68 (of 120) cardiac transplant centres noted that older and larger centres used fewer precautions and survival rates appeared unrelated to the precautions used (Lange *et al.* 1992). Most infections in the early transplant period are from the patient's (or donor's) organism. If good infection control procedures are adhered to in the ITU, single-room isolation should not be required. While on the ITU, however, the patient is at risk of bacteraemia from line infection, which could seed the atrial suture line or a dysfunctional tricuspid valve in the heart transplant patient. Intubation increases the risk of pulmonary infection in heart and lung transplant recipients. The patient is, in addition, more likely to be exposed to resistant bacteria in an ITU setting. Length of time ventilated after surgery was one factor associated with infection in the first 30 days in patients after heart–lung transplantation (Ciulli *et al.* 1993). Early extubation and line removal are encouraged.

In view of the ever-present dangers of *Legionella* spp. in institutional water supplies, patients are discouraged from having showers in many transplant units. This is still a controversial issue. The most important ways to reduce the risk of *Legionella* infection are to ensure compliance with the engineering and monitoring recommendations to control Legionnaires' disease in hospital premises. Hospital-acquired *Aspergillus* infection may be associated with building work. Everything possible should be done to reduce dust levels in any patient areas in hospital. In particular, the ventilation systems in theatres and in the ITU should be up to the recommended standards and regularly monitored and maintained. (For more on *Legionella* and *Aspergillus* spp., see pp. 511, 513 and 515.)

## Postoperative problems

The developmental nature of cardiothoracic transplant programmes and the use of immunosuppression has meant that data concerning infection have been carefully collected and tabulated. While chest infections have predominated, as they do in all transplant programmes, the presence of a major thoracic wound has also meant a significant incidence of wound infection and even mediastinitis, and the use of allograft lungs has meant an even greater possibility of chest infection, especially in cystic fibrosis patients. Gentry and Zeluff (1988) noted that the incidence and type of early nosocomial infection were no different in heart transplant patients than in those undergoing cardiothoracic surgery generally, but after the first month these were replaced by opportunistic infections. Dummer *et al.* (1995b) summarized infections occurring in the first year from 150 patients in the Pittsburgh series (119 heart transplants, 31 heart–lung transplants). The heart patients had an average of 1.36 infections accounting for a 15% infection-associated mortality. Of these 13% had bacteraemia, 8% invasive fungal infection and 27% had infections affecting the lungs. For heart–lung transplants the figures were 3.19 infections per patient accounting for 45% infection-associated mortality. Of these 19% had bacteraemia, 23% invasive fungal infection and 57% had chest infections. The experience of 42 patients undergoing heart–lung transplantation from 1985 to 1992 at Papworth (Dennis *et al.* 1993) was that infection occurred most frequently during the first 3 months: 2.26±0.26 events per 100 patient days declining to 0.40±0.08 by the end of the first year. There is a late increase in chest infections in lung transplant patients with the development of obliterative bronchiolitis (Heng *et al.* 1998) and bronchiectasis, an expression of chronic rejection. In this chapter we shall consider infection by system, dealing in particular with the most frequently occurring and those with a significant impact on morbidity and mortality.

## Mediastinitis

Mediastinitis is a rare but serious postoperative complication. It is defined as a retrosternal infectious process with or without sternal instability. It may result from extension of a superficial wound infection or arise deep in the chest from intraoperative contamination or an infected organ or anastomosis. Risk factors include previous sternotomy, especially reoperations to control haemorrhage and prolonged postoperative ventilation (Albat *et al.* 1993). In this series, the mediastinitis rate appeared to decrease following reduction in corticosteroid dose. The most common organism was *S. aureus*, followed by *Staphylococcus epidermidis*. Methicillin-resistant *S. aureus* can cause serious infection and this emphasizes the importance of vancomycin prophylaxis at surgery if donor or recipient carries MRSA. Infections with Gram-negative bacteria—Enterobacteriaceae (e.g. *Escherichia coli*, *Klebsiella* spp.)—and *Pseudomonas* spp. are rare compared with non-transplant cardiac surgery. These organisms are most probably introduced with the leg veins used for coronary artery bypass grafts (Wells *et al.* 1983).

A paper from Texas (Baldwin *et al.* 1992) noted that seven of nine cases were caused by staphylococci and

two by *Enterobacter cloacae*. Toporoff *et al.* (1994) described a case of *Enterobacter* mediastinitis complicated by endocarditis, which required debridement, irrigation and prolonged antibiotic treatment for cure. The infecting organism was also found in the trachea and donor lungs harvested at the same time but used for a different recipient. It was assumed that the heart had been contaminated when the heart–lung block was separated prior to transplant. Karwande *et al.* (1992b) presented 12 cases from their series of 420 cardiac transplants. Again 11 were caused by staphylococci (species and antibiotic sensitivity pattern not given), with one case of infection by *Legionella* sp. They noted that prolonged antibiotic therapy did not work and that debridement plus irrigation used in eight of the 12 patients had a poor response. They strongly favoured debridement and the muscle flap technique, which succeeded in all four of the patients in whom they were used.

The diagnosis will be obvious in many instances in that mediastinitis usually follows sternal wound infection but sometimes may present as a cryptic infection that requires scanning for detection. Quirce *et al.* (1991) described a case caused by *Haemophilus aphrophilus* presenting as fever and leucocytosis that required a gallium scan for elucidation. Aspiration of sternal pus or tissue from debridement is essential for accurate diagnosis and therapy. Blood cultures may also yield the causative agent.

Patients with lung transplants are at greater risk of mediastinitis and may be susceptible to infection with organisms from the respiratory tract, presumably introduced after a minor tracheal or bronchial anastamotic leak (Dauber *et al.* 1990). In this series from 1982 to 1989, eight of 60 patients surviving for more than 2 weeks developed mediastinitis. Causes of early infection were *S. aureus*, *Candida albicans* and *Mycoplasma hominis*. A late cause (at 7 weeks) occurred after a major airway dehiscence and infection with *P. aeruginosa*. *M. hominis* with or without *Ureaplasma urealyticum* is a rare but important cause of a culture-negative infection. The laboratory diagnosis of *Mycoplasma* infections requires a high degree of suspicion because these organisms do not grow on normal culture media. As they lack a cell wall they will not respond to the β-lactam antibiotics commonly used as empirical therapy. The two patients described by Steffenson *et al.* (1987) both died of other causes but, although their cultures had become free of mycoplasmas, the wounds had not healed. Other cases reported did respond to a mixture of debridement with muscle flap coverage and therapy with a tetracycline plus erythromycin (Boyle *et al.* 1993) or doxycycline and clindamycin (Sielaff *et al.* 1996).

A patient from France (Thaler *et al.* 1992) developed mediastinitis caused by *Nocardia asteroides* after heart transplantation and was successfully treated by debridement, sugar in the wound and prolonged antibiotics. *Aspergillus fumigatus* was reported from Belgium as a cause of mediastinitis. The fungus spread into the aorta causing a pseudoaneurysm with subsequent rupture (Byl *et al.* 1993). These authors suggested that seeding of the wound occurred from the air during surgery.

## Chest infections

### PREDISPOSTION

While both heart and lung transplant patients are prone to bacterial chest infections and share the predisposition created by immunosuppression, surgery and ITU care, other risk factors are quite separate. The heart transplant recipient is subjected to a technically less complicated operation and so is less likely to require, for example, prolonged postoperative intubation. The heart transplant patient, however, has the original lungs *in situ* and the previous state of heart failure may have resulted in emboli or pulmonary oedema and lungs therefore at risk of infection. The patient with ischaemic heart disease after smoking may also have a degree of chronic obstructive pulmonary disease with exacerbation caused by *H. influenzae* or *Streptococcus pneumoniae*. The first Papworth long-term survivor had repeated bouts of infection caused by *H. influenzae*, while Amber *et al.* (1990) documented pneumococcal infection in five of 129 cardiac transplant recipients, noting that previous vaccination did not always prevent development of infection. Corensek *et al.* (1988) performed a multivariate analy-

sis of risk factors found in 34 months for the 12 of 50 patients in their series who developed pneumonia and concluded that reintubation and immunosuppression with higher-dose steroids were significant; development of pneumonia was itself a risk factor for mortality.

The development of cytomegalovirus pneumonitis or the enhanced immunosuppression for treating rejection predisposes the heart–lung transplant patient to chest infection. The recipient of a lung allograft has healthy new lungs but many other problems. The role of organisms carried with the donor tissue has been discussed (see pp. 506–508). Peritransplant injury can damage the airway mucosa, reducing mucociliary clearance, and cause oedema because of damage to the alveoli; both of these predispose the lungs to infection. A poor blood supply to the bronchial or tracheal anastomosis can result in ischaemia and infection. These in turn may lead to a collapsing or stenotic airway, which encourages distal infection and may require insertion of a stent (Higgins *et al.* 1994). Dehiscence may occur with complications such as mediastinitis and/or bronchopleural fistula. In addition, there is an abolition of the cough reflex, supplemented by a significant decrease in mucociliary clearance as measured using inhalation of a $^{99m}$Tc-labelled albumin aerosol containing 7.5 μm particles (Herve *et al.* 1993).

An interesting experimental study of other risk factors was performed by Aeba *et al.* (1993), who infected rats by instillation of $10^5$ colony-forming units of *Legionella pneumophila* and then subjected them to various procedures, comparing the lung *Legionella* concentrations 6 days later. Thoracotomy, transplantation procedures and allogeneic (as opposed to isogenic) lung transplants had no effect, but hilar stripping and immunosuppression did. They concluded that immunosuppression, denervation and interruption of lymphatic vessels and bronchial arteries resulted in the early development and increased severity of pneumonia after lung transplantation.

Noyes *et al.* (1991) examined the ability of blood monocytes and alveolar macrophages from lung recipients to moderate lymphocyte responses to mitogens or antigens. They found that the alveolar macrophages worked well but blood monocytes failed to present antigens for processing. Hruban *et al.* (1988) showed that during episodes of rejection the bronchus-associated lymphoid tissue is depleted. Lung allografts from two patients with rejection had a marked depletion of submucosal IgA- and IgG-bearing cells, as shown by immunoperoxidase techniques.

For those with single lung transplants there may be the additional risk of disease in the contralateral lung (Horvath *et al.* 1993); the lung may be a source of infection although it is now practice to use double lung or heart–lung blocks for infective lung disease. An emphysematous lung may also put pressure on the transplant, leading to collapse and a susceptibility to infection. Extension of lung transplants to patients with cystic fibrosis has added further risk factors. By the time the end-stage of this disease is reached the patients will have had many years of antibiotic therapy and prophylaxis so that, in addition to the heavy load of bacteria in their respiratory tract, there will be selection of antibiotic-resistant flora elsewhere, for example in the gut, and so resistant strains of *Pseudomonas aeruginosa*, *B. cepacia* and *Stenotrophomonas* (previously *Xanthomonas*) *maltophila* are to be expected. The overall rate of infection appears no different in patients with or without cystic fibrosis (Dennis *et al.* 1993). There is, however, a significant impact of *B. cepacia* on morbidity and mortality, raising the question of whether patients colonized with *B. cepacia* and other resistant bacteria should be transplanted (see also below). The pattern of pulmonary infection in cystic fibrosis and non-cystic fibrosis lung transplant recipients is well reviewed by Starnes *et al.* (1992), Ramirez *et al.* (1992), Massard *et al.* (1993), Flume *et al.* (1994) and Kurland (1996).

Finally, chronic rejection, manifested by bronchiolitis obliterans syndrome, causes bronchiectasis with repeated chest infection. A similar pattern occurs as seen in cystic fibrosis, with colonization and episodes of infection, primarily with *P. aeruginosa* but also atypical mycobacteria and *Aspergillus* spp. (Heng *et al.* 1998).

### DIAGNOSIS

A reduction in lung function with fever may signal infection or rejection. Maurer *et al.* (1992) followed the infectious episodes in 40 single or double lung transplant recipients over 6 years. They concluded that chest infection is common and problematical and recommend the Papworth approach of patients doing daily spirometry with hand-held spirometers (Otulana *et al.* 1988) for early detection of both impending infection and rejection. Diagnosis is crucial for accurate treatment. Culture should always be carried out as well as histological examination of tissue and lavage. Fibreoptic bronchoscopy with bronchoalveolar lavage (BAL) and transbronchial biopsy is the gold standard for obtaining material in these patients. Higgenbottam *et al.* (1988) reported on its use for differentiating infection and rejection in the first 21 heart–lung transplant recipients at Papworth. Fifteen patients had a total of 43 biopsies. Opportunistic lung infection was diagnosed in eight patients with a sensitivity of 38% and specificity of 100%. Schulman *et al.* (1988) reported a similar study on heart transplant recipients, in whom, as lung rejection was not a problem, BAL gave better results than transtracheal biopsy—namely in 63% of cases as opposed to 46%. Bronchial brushing gave the lowest return (43%).

### EARLY INFECTION

Ciulli *et al.* (1993) documented the incidence of infection within 30 days in a series of 125 patients (42 with cystic fibrosis) undergoing heart–lung transplantation. Nineteen (15.2%) developed early infections, including eight with pneumonia, three with empyema, two with tracheal dehiscence, three with bronchitis, one aortic rupture, one septicaemia (*P. aeruginosa*) and one peritonitis. Six of the eight episodes of pneumonia were caused by *P. aeruginosa* or *B. cepacia*. Deusch *et al.* (1993) described early infections in 29 lung transplant recipients (two with cystic fibrosis), of whom 11 (38%) developed pulmonary infection within 2 weeks of operation. The most common organisms found were *Klebsiella pneumoniae*, *E. coli* and *P. aeruginosa*. Only two were infected with *S. aureus*, although 12 donor cultures had been positive with that organism. Those with early infection had a lower survival rate in the first 3 months. No particular predisposition was found in the infected group. Orr *et al.* (1991) described five patients with nosocomial infection or colonization with *S. maltophila*. A rapid fingerprinting of the strains showed that they were related but not identical; however, during the investigation the unauthorized reuse of cleaned disposable nebulizers was noted. One nebulizer grew the strain of *S. maltophila*. This again serves to emphasize the importance of basic infection control for all inpatients but in particular this vulnerable group.

LATE INFECTION

Causes of late-onset chest infections that may affect all types of transplant patient are *Legionella pneumophila,* mycobacteria (tuberculous and nontuberculous), *Nocardia asteroides* and fungi, including *Pneumocystis carinii, Aspergillus fumigatus,* and rarer species such as *Cryptococcus neoformans* and *C. immitis.*

*Legionella spp.*

Horbach and Fehrenbach (1990) reported on 20 cases of Legionnaires' disease found in a 2-year study of heart transplant recipients and suggest that in a hospital outbreak twice-weekly urinary antigen detection tests should be carried out for early diagnosis. Some patients continued to excrete *Legionella* antigen in the urine for up to 179 days, in contrast to 1–3 weeks in non-immunosuppressed patients. In contrast, Dauber *et al.* (1990) recorded no cases of *Legionella* in his series of transplant patients. It should be possible to avoid cases of nosocomial Legionnaires' disease by the provision of safe water supplies, taking up the many recommendations for ensuring a safe water supply in hospital. There has been a concern that shower nozzles can act as multiplication sites for *Legionella pneumophila*. Showers also generate aerosols that can penetrate the lower respiratory tract. Although the particular role of showers compared with other water sources in causing *Legionella* infection is still a matter of debate, many units would not allow new organ recipients to use a shower in hospital.

*Nocardia spp.*

As with other transplant patients, the recipients of heart and lung transplants may suffer from lung infection with *N. asteroides* but this has become rare since the introduction of co-trimoxazole for *P. carinii* pneumonia prophylaxis. A report from Philadelphia documents a case of pneumonia caused by the newly characterized *Nocardia nova*, which responded to therapy with clarithromycin when sulfisoxazole had failed (Monteforte & Wood 1993).

*Mycobacterium tuberculosis*

Transplant recipients are at risk of tuberculosis from reactivation of disease in the recipient or in the donor tissue or from acquiring the organism for the first time after transplantation. Hospital outbreaks have occurred and, as transplant recipients are at particular risk, it is important that any patient with possible tuberculosis is appropriately isolated until a diagnosis is made and the degree of infectivity assessed.

Tuberculosis after heart or lung transplant has been only rarely reported. Muñoz *et al.* (1995) described three cases (two pulmonary) from 144 recipients of heart transplant occurring 55–102 days after the procedure. The route of infection was not proven in these cases. Dromer *et al.* (1993) described four cases out of 61 patients undergoing single, double or heart–lung transplantation in France. One patient had evidence of reactivation from mediastinal nodes, another had acquired tuberculosis from a room-mate but in the other two the source was uncertain. Tuberculosis had presented between three and 13 months postoperatively and could easily have been missed as the clinical and radiological findings were not typical. The authors experienced the difficulties of maintaining cyclosporin levels when using rifampicin and opted for an alternative regimen (isoniazid, ethambutol, pyrazinamide and streptomycin for 12–18 months).

One asymptomatic donor appeared to infect two single lung recipients in a case study by Ridgeway *et al.* (1996). Both recipients were shown to be infected at 6 weeks by the same strain of *Mycobacterium tuberculosis* (typed by restriction fragment length polymorphism analysis). The authors recommended that candidates for transplantation with evidence of prior exposure (positive tuberculosis skin test) should receive a year's prophylactic isoniazid and that identification of tuberculosis from donor BAL using the polymerase chain reaction should be considered. The use of isoniazid is controversial as there are doubts as to its efficacy and whether its use as monotherapy encourages resistance to develop. Tuberculin skin testing would not be helpful in the UK as many UK residents have received vaccination with BCG in childhood. Polymerase chain reaction (PCR) is not as sensitive a test as first thought for *M. tuberculosis*. Reference laboratories at present find that only 70% of smear-negative sputa that are eventually culture-positive give a positive PCR reaction. A high index of suspicion, early diagnosis and prompt treatment are probably still better than trying to prevent post-transplant tuberculosis. PCR does, however, have a useful role at a very early stage to help discriminate between *M. tuberculosis* and atypical mycobacteria in specimens in which acid-fast bacilli are seen. To get a result within days rather than waiting weeks for culture is helpful because the management of the patient and risks of cross-infection differ radically.

### Non-tuberculosis Mycobacterium spp.

Non-tuberculous or atypical mycobacteria (NTM) are spread in the environment and can cause infection in the immunosuppressed. They are not passed from patient to patient. They may be found as colonizers or cause disease in the lungs of patients with cystic fibrosis. In one study, three of 27 recipients of lung transplants who had cystic fibrosis were colonized with atypical mycobacteria preoperatively but none were culture-positive or needed treatment after transplantation (Flume *et al.* 1994). Patel *et al.* (1994) described one case and summarized the literature on NTM in 22 heart transplant recipients. The time of onset of NTM infection was later than for tuberculosis (on average 74 months, range 3–269 months). The most common organism was *M. kansasii* (nine cases), followed by *M. avium-intracellulare scrofulaceum* complex (seven cases). Half of the patients had pulmonary involvement; half had skin lesions (see p. 519).

In the study by Novick *et al.* (1990), 14 of 508 heart transplant recipients developed infection with NTM. The prevalence of infection decreased after the introduction of cyclosporin. The 14 patients had had a higher rejection rate and therefore more corticosteroids. Eight had disseminated disease, four had localized pulmonary disease and one subcutaneous infection at the previous site of a left ventricular assist device. The most common organisms were again *M. kansasii* and *M. avium-intracellulare*.

In 1989 Trulock *et al.* described the first case of NTM infection in a heart–lung transplant recipient. The patient was suffering from the bronchiolitis obliterans syndrome. Caseating granulomas were seen in the transbronchial biopsy during life and in the lungs at post-mortem, indicating that the NTM (*M. chelonei*) had caused disease rather than being found in the damaged airways as a saprophyte.

Early infection of the pleural space with *M. fortuitum* was described by Baldi *et al.* (1997), with a wide range of potential sources postulated, from use of contaminated ice around the donor organ to an introduction of the organism at insertion of a chest drain. At Papworth Hospital between 1985 and 1996, six of the 316 patients who underwent heart–lung, double lung or single lung transplantation developed infection with NTM, four with *M. kansasii* and two with *M. fortuitum*. The optimal treatment for NTM is still poorly understood although clinical experience from NTM in AIDS has given some guidance.

### Pneumocystis carinii

Pneumonia caused by *P. carinii* (PCP) has been a frequent occurrence in transplant programmes. While an induced sputum examination is often sufficient for diagnosis of PCP in AIDS, fewer organisms are present in transplant patients and bronchial biopsy or examination of BAL is needed. The subject is well reviewed by Hadley and Ng (1995) and by Walzer (1994). Recent developments in molecular biology have shown that *P. carinii* is a fungus, not a protozoan. It is, however, resistant to amphotericin and nystatin, probably because the cell walls lack ergosterol. Much of the epidemiology remains unclear. If sufficiently immunosuppressed, most people will develop infection. Serological studies have shown that 94% of children had antibodies by the age of 2.5 years so the organism must be ubiquitous (Peglow *et al.* 1990). What may appear to be an outbreak of infection in transplant units (e.g. Gryzan *et al.* 1988) is probably reactivation of carriage after immunosuppression rather than nosocomial spread. Gryzan *et al.* monitored 16 lung transplant recipients for pneumocysts by serial examination of BAL samples. The prevalence of pneumocystis infection was 88%, although only six episodes of pneumonia occurred; the other 10 patients had little or no sign of disease.

In Dauber *et al.*'s review (1990) they contrast the experience prior to 1986, when *P. carinii* was found in 15 of 21 recipients, some of whom had recurrent infection and two died, with the later period after institution of prophylaxis, when only three of 25 became infected, none of whom had taken the prophylactic drugs. In Kramer *et al.*'s review (1992) of PCP in heart–lung and lung transplantation, most cases occurred 3–6 months postoperatively and the introduction of prophylaxis reduced the rate of infection from 27% to zero. Late cases of PCP (after 1 year) were associated with the use of high-dose corticosteroids for rejection. The authors felt that 1 year of trimethoprim–sulphamethoxazole prophylaxis was sufficient, but that it should be restarted whenever the immunosuppression was increased.

### Aspergillus spp.

*Aspergillus fumigatus* is a filamentous fungus widespread in the environment which can be grown from the sputum in a significant number of normal people. A review of the detection of antigen or antibodies in diagnosis of invasive aspergillosis (Kurup & Kumar 1991) describes several elegant techniques but concludes that, as the common antigens required for diagnosis remain to be identified, there remains a need for early diagnostic methods. Currently available methods appear promising but may not be sensitive enough. An early indicator may be the isolation of aspergillus spp. from sputum. The usual practice of investigation by bronchoscopy and biopsy or needle aspiration of a suspi-

cious nodule means that most cases of invasive aspergillosis are confirmed by histology. Some patients may arrive for transplant with aspergilli already resident in their lungs; this is particularly true of those with cystic fibrosis. In one study, however, none of the 17 patients with *Aspergillus* spp. in sputum preoperatively had antifungal prophylaxis and none needed treatment after transplantation. Nosocomial aspergillosis has been encountered in the transplant unit (Flume *et al.* 1994). Potential sources include hospital renovations, road construction and fireproofing materials as well as air conditioning; these have been well reviewed by Rhame (1991).

Harmati *et al.* (1993) reported on nine patients with pulmonary nodules caused by *Aspergillus* in 257 cardiac transplant recipients. Invasive aspergillosis was responsible for two fatalities in the 95 heart transplant recipients described by Rabito and Pankey (1992). Recipients of lung or heart–lung transplants develop invasive disease in the lung parenchyma at a higher rate than inpatients receiving heart transplants. In one series the incidence of invasive aspergillosis, mostly pulmonary, was 4.5% for heart transplant recipients but 18% for lung transplants (Guillemain *et al.* 1995). Seven of 42 patients undergoing heart–lung transplantation for cystic fibrosis developed 12 episodes of invasive aspergillosis. *Aspergillus* spp. had not been identified in pretransplant sputum or tracheal cultures. All, however, had had cytomegalovirus pneumonitis and multiple rejection episodes before onset of invasive fungal infection (Dennis *et al.* 1993). In another series of single and bilateral lung transplants, 16% developed invasive aspergillosis with a significant association with cytomegalovirus pneumonitis (Yeldandi *et al.* 1995). Complicated infection and mortality were more common in the single than the double lung recipients in the group described by Westney *et al.* (1996), the native lung being thought to be the source of infection. There may, however, be particular problems at the anastomosis after single lung transplant.

Ulcerative tracheobronchitis is a form of invasive aspergillosis described in lung transplant recipients (Kramer *et al.* 1991). The combination of an ischaemic airway anastomosis, often with necrotic tissue extending distally, and immunosuppression leads to this early complication. The condition can be seen at bronchoscopy and confirmed by culture and biopsy. It is treated as any invasive aspergillosis.

To date amphotericin B remains the best treatment, although some success has been recorded with itraconazole (Denning & Stevens 1990). Amphotericin B is, however, nephrotoxic and likely to interact with cyclosporin. Thus liposomal amphotericin appears attractive in the light of claims for efficacy with reduced renal toxicity (Katz *et al.* 1990; Mannes *et al.* 1995). This is an expensive drug but has had an impressive impact on mortality and morbidity at Papworth.

Is there a role for antifungal prophylaxis? Beyer *et al.* (1994) have shown that amphotericin aerosols delay the onset of invasive aspergillosis in an animal model and that the drug is not absorbed. As the bronchial anastomosis after single lung transplantation in humans is particularly at risk of ischaemia, inhaled amphotericin is given at transplantation and continued until the anastomosis heals to prevent *Aspergillus* ulcerative bronchitis. The use of prophylaxis for all lung transplantation, however, has been questioned (Paradowski 1997). This author reviewed 126 patients who underwent transplantation. Of the 65 with cystic fibrosis, 52% were colonized with *Aspergillus* spp. before surgery and 40% after the operation. None of the colonized patients received prophylaxis and none developed infection. Of the three patients who did develop invasive pulmonary disease none had had preoperative colonization and infection presented 5 months or more after surgery.

Itraconazole may have a role in long-term treatment or prophylaxis of *Aspergillus* infection. Early experience (Faggian *et al.* 1989) showed it could be effective and lacked the nephrotoxicity of conventional amphotericin. It is important that therapeutic levels are achieved and the cyclosporin dose is adjusted down, as itraconazole has a cyclosporin-sparing effect.

### Candida spp.

*Candida* may rarely cause tracheal or bronchial dehiscence but is very unusual as a cause of pneumonia except as part of disseminated disease. It is, however, often cultured from sputum or BAL, where it is a contaminant from the mouth or upper airways. Oral candidiasis may occur, especially if the patient is on broad-spectrum antibiotics. This may be prevented or well controlled by topical antifungals.

### Other fungi: cryptococcosis, coccidioidomycosis, mycoses, etc.

Cryptococcal infection is another cause of nodular lung shadows in transplant recipients. Simultaneous infections with both *Cryptococcus* and *Legionella* were described as an expression of defective cell-mediated immunity in three patients (including one cardiac transplant recipient) from Pittsburgh (Korvick & Yu 1988).

Unlike other fungal infections, coccidioidomycosis is geographically restricted to, for example, the arid south-west states of the USA; Hall *et al.* (1993a) noted that 4.5% of their heart transplant patients from Arizona were affected. However, the infections responded to amphotericin plus later ketoconazole maintenance therapy. Two patients relapsed after the latter was stopped but the actuarial survival at 1 and 5 years after transplant did not differ from the other patients in the series. Coccidioidomycosis may relapse or be acquired (see p. 506).

Other fungi such as *Mucor, Absidia, Rhizopus* spp. (the mucorales) are rare after solid organ transplantation. They are more frequently seen after bone marrow transplantation and other conditions with more profound immunosuppression with neutropenia. Infection with *Mucor* spp. has been described in a heart transplant recipient (Muhm *et al.* 1996). Mucorales as a group can be recognized on biopsy by the irregular hyphae and lack of septae. They do not show the acute-angle branching seen in *Aspergillus* and *Fusarium* spp. and *Pseudoallescheria boydii*. As with all fungi, it is important to distinguish contamination or colonization of the airways from invasive disease. This is particularly important for the mucorales and *Pseudoallescheria boydii*, which are more resistant to amphotericin and can be very difficult to treat, needing higher doses of amphotericin and, if possible, excision of infected necrotic tissue.

## Cardiovascular infections

The patient after heart or heart–lung transplantation is at particular risk of endocarditis because of the atrial and large-vessel suture lines. There may be some degree of tricuspid and mitral regurgitation. Repeated biopsy of the right ventricle may add risk by injury to the tricuspid valve and ventricular endocardium. Any poorly controlled sepsis with *S. aureus* may lead to bacteraemia and seeding of normal valves; hence the importance of early removal of intravascular lines and prompt treatment of infection. In spite of this, there are few cases of endocarditis in the transplant literature.

Khoo *et al.* (1989) reported the first case of *S. aureus* mitral valve endocarditis in a heart recipient, which followed drainage of an abscess in the sternotomy scar some 33 months post-transplantation. Hasan *et al.* (1993) described the first case of endocarditis in a heart–lung recipient, also caused by *S. aureus*. The patient had an apparently free vegetation in the left ventricle, which was removed at operation, and has survived. Mediastinal infection preceded *Enterobacter* endocarditis in the patient described by Toporoff *et al.* (1994) already discussed (see p. 510). Vegetations were seen attached to either side of the atrial septum suture line. A mitral valve endocarditis caused by *Staphylococcus epidermidis* was described by Counihan *et al.* (1991); it occurred 7 months after the operation. Endocarditis in the early postoperative period could be catheter-related and Venditti *et al.* (1993) describe such a case caused by a vancomycin-resistant strain of *Enterococcus faecalis*.

The approach to prophylaxis for endocarditis differs between transplant centres. The suture lines should heal well but valve dysfuntion may continue. Most would consider a patient with cardiac transplantation at risk and would advise prophylaxis according to American Heart Association (Dajani *et al.* 1990) or British Society for Antimicrobial Chemotherapy (Simmons *et al.* 1992) guidelines.

Bacterial myocarditis is an even rarer complication of transplantation. Stamm *et al.* (1990) documented two patients with a *Listeria monocytogenes* myocarditis, in one case coexisting with cerebral infection (q.v.).

Both patients were treated successfully by antibiotics but needed retransplantation. The explanted hearts showed myocarditis with abscess formation and necrosis consistent with bacterial infection. Both patients had positive blood cultures, and one had positive heart muscle cultures. (For further information on the role of *Listeria* in transplant patients, see p. 518.)

*Trypanosoma cruzi* myocarditis (Chagas' disease) is a major cause of heart failure in South America. The disease may reactivate after heart transplantation (Libow *et al.* 1991). The drugs used to treat Chagas' disease have major side effects. In one group's experience, reactivation occurred in only three of 15 infected patients followed up for an average of 16 months. They advised treating recurrence rather than giving all patients post-transplant prophylaxis (Almeida *et al.* 1996).

Knosalla *et al.* (1996) reported three cases of mycotic aortic aneurysm after heart transplant and reviewed a further seven. Two were caused by *C. albicans*, five by *S. aureus*, two by *P. aeruginosa* and one by both bacterial species. Three involved previous cannulation sites and two the aortic suture line. Most were associated with mediastinitis but it is uncertain if infection was by direct extension or following a bacteraemia. *Aspergillus* mediastinitis spreading to the aorta was described by Byl *et al.* (1993). Four out of 66 heart–lung transplant patients in Pittsburgh developed fatal disruption of the aorta at the anastamotic site. *Candida* was either cultured from the suture line or present on the aortic wall at autopsy in three of them (Dowling *et al.* 1990). *Candida* may enter the bloodstream through vascular access sites, but in two of these three cases a heavy growth of *Candida* was cultured from the donor trachea—hence the donor was presumed to be the source of infection. Following this experience, the group added amphotericin B to perioperative prophylaxis and also wrapped both tracheal and aortic anastamoses in omentum.

## Infections of the central nervous system and eye

Hall *et al.* (1989) documented 13 intracranial infections in 417 heart and heart–lung transplant recipients. Infection of the central nervous system in solid organ transplant recipients was reviewed by Conti and Rubin (1988), who noted that three organisms—*Listeria monocytogenes*, *C. neoformans* and *A. fumigatus*—accounted for most of the non-viral infections. The principal factor affecting survival was speed of diagnosis. However, the onset of the disease is often insidious and an aggressive approach, with high-resolution scanning, early lumbar puncture and blood cultures, is recommended for patients with headache and fever or altered states of consciousness.

Infection with *L. monocytogenes* may cause meningitis, diffuse encephalitis or even well-localized abscesses. Early diagnosis may be made by culturing blood as well as cerebrospinal fluid. Heart transplant recipients with listerial infection were recorded by Hall *et al.* (1989), Stamm *et al.* (1990), whose patient also had myocarditis, and Larner *et al.* (1989), who recorded an unusual case with recurrent infection. In the latter case both episodes followed increased doses of corticosteroids for treatment of rejection. These authors note that the source of infection was not identified and at the outset of the transplant programmes the origin of the *Listeria* was indeed a mystery. Some well-publicized outbreaks of listeriosis, such as that attributed to Mexican-style cheese which affected newborn babies of Hispanic mothers in California (Linman *et al.* 1988), other soft cheeses and pâté, have shown it to be food-borne. Transplant patients require appropriate dietary advice similar to that published for pregnant mothers.

The transplant patient may develop the more common forms of bacterial meningitis but appears no more at risk than the general population. Empirical treatment must include penicillin, as cefotaxime—often used as monotherapy in the adult—does not have activity against *L. monocytogenes*.

The central nervous system is affected in about one-third of patients infected by *N. asteroides*. There is usually a cerebral abscess but meningitis may occur, although often in connection with microabscesses. While cerebral involvement is usually in addition to lung disease, it may occur as the only manifestation of disease, often missed until autopsy (Prayson & Estes 1995). There are also reports of nocardial endophthalmitis; Gregor *et al.* (1989) report a case of subvit-real infection diagnosed by transvitreal fine-needle biopsy; Knouse and Lorber (1990) reviewed the literature (10 cases) and also stressed the value of fine-needle biopsy for early diagnosis of this potentially fatal infection.

Fungal infections can be hard to both diagnose and treat and may also involve the central nervous system and eye. *C. neoformans* has long been known to be a cause of meningoencephalitis in the immunosuppressed. The large yeast cells in the cerebrospinal fluid could be mistaken for lymphocytes, but nowadays antisera are used to detect the cryptococcal antigen and so simplify the diagnosis. Korvick and Yu (1988) recorded one cardiac transplant patient in their three cases of combined *Legionella* and cryptococcal infection. Cryptococcal infection may spread from the central nervous system directly to the eye, sometimes with catastrophic results (Rex *et al.* 1993); alternatively an endophthalmitis may be a result of direct spread from the lungs or be the only manifestation of cryptococcal infection.

Cerebral aspergillosis may cause a diffuse spreading lesion or a cerebral abscess. It is usually secondary to bloodstream spread from pulmonary infection (Torre-Cisneros *et al.* 1993). Diagnosis is difficult. Hall *et al.* (1989) were able to localize abscesses by computed tomography but in many cases the infection is only found in autopsy studies, such as that by Prayson and Estes (1995). However, Boriani *et al.* (1989) reported a case of invasive aspergillosis with cerebral and renal abscesses where the patient recovered after a lobotomy, nephrectomy and itraconazole therapy. Invasive aspergillosis may also spread to the eye. Graham *et al.* (1995) reported early endogenous ophthalmitis following lung transplantation and stress the value of fundus photography in patients with visual disturbances as an aid to diagnosis and stimulus to early therapy for the systemic disease. Treatment usually requires removal of infected vitreous and high-dose amphotericin B.

Candidaemia more commonly leads to peripheral seeding in the immunosuppressed transplant patient than the immunocompetent. Endophthalmitis should always be looked for and may require prolonged treatment.

Various other fungi may affect the central nervous system. *C. immitis* is a major cause of meningitis as well as lung infections (Hall *et al.* 1993b); transplant patients may reactivate or acquire infection.

A case of multiple cerebral abscesses caused by *Scedosporium apiospermum* (*Pseudoallescheria boydii*) has been reported (Lopez *et al.* 1998). Although very rare, it is an important organism to identify correctly as it is relatively resistant to amphotericin B. It can look the same as a sensitive *Aspergillus* on tissue section, with septae and acute-angle branching. This underlines the importance of culture as well as histology in the diagnosis of fungal infection.

Any bacteria in the blood may settle in the eye. Pseudomonal endophthalmitis has been described after lung transplantation for cystic fibrosis (Sheares *et al.* 1997). This is of particular interest as the organism was a mucoid strain of *P. aeruginosa* that only rarely causes bacteraemia in the immunocompetent, even in the presence of severe lung infection with the organism. There was no intravascular source (lines, endocarditis, etc.) and the bacteraemia was thought to have originated from the lung.

## Miscellaneous infections (bone, joint, skin and soft tissue)

Isolated instances of bone and joint infection with fungi and *Nocardia* spp. have been reported. *Aspergillus flavus* osteitis of the tibia followed local trauma and required both local debridement and antifungal drugs (De Vuyst *et al.* 1992). Invasive aspergillosis causing spondylodiscitis has been reported in nine immunosuppressed patients by a group in France (Cortet *et al.* 1994). Three were in cardiac transplant recipients and the authors suggest that spondylodiscitis will become more common, should be diagnosed rapidly by percutaneous needle biopsy and will respond to therapy with itraconazole. Reports citing *Nocardia* spp. include patients with arthritis and soft-tissue and skin infections (Simmons *et al.* 1992; Ostrum 1993; Rees *et al.* 1994). These are all recent reports and stress the value of imipenem in treatment. Atypical mycobacteria such as *M. haemophilum* may rarely cause osteomyelitis (Plemmons *et al.* 1997).

*Phaeoannellomyces werneckii* (previously *Exophiala werneckii*) is a brown yeast-like fungus, that is an example of phaeohyphomycosis and as yet an unusual infection involving the skin and subcutaneous tissues (Sudduth *et al.* 1992; Gold *et al.* 1994). Local excision plus antifungal therapy is required.

One case of dermal leishmaniasis was described in a heart transplant patient by Golino *et al.* (1992). Leishmaniasis may be limited to the skin or mucous membranes or may spread to the reticulo-endothelial system. Any immunosuppression may predispose to the development of visceral leishmaniasis (Fernandez-Guerrero *et al.* 1987).

In a detailed description of the dermatological manifestations of infectious disease in transplantation, Gentry *et al.* (1994) reviewed the full spectrum of bacterial, viral, fungal, protozoal and metazoal parasite infections. *Nocardia* spp. may cause local mycetomas and disseminate but has become very rare since the introduction of prophylaxis for *P. carinii*. The risks and signs of reactivation or reinfection with *Strongyloides stercoralis*, *T. cruzi*, coccidioidomycosis or histoplasmosis with their skin manifestation are also considered by Gentry *et al.* (1994).

Skin disease is the most common presentation of infection with the atypical mycobacteria in heart transplant recipients. Fourteen of 502 cardiac transplant recipients at Stanford had non-tuberculous mycobacterial infection—most of those with skin involvement following disseminated disease. Infections occurred in patients with multiple episodes of rejection (Novick *et al.* 1990).

## Conclusions

The study of infection in heart and lung transplant recipients covers almost the entire spectrum of pathogens and has increased our knowledge of the role of the immune response in the handling of these organisms. Early experience in infectious complications after solid organ transplantation helped understanding of problems in the subsequent HIV epidemic. The close cooperation between the experimental and clinical aspects of transplantation has meant that patients have been very carefully followed up in cohorts over a period of time, thus providing many valuable data. The prevention and control of infection after transplantation have allowed an expansion of the techniques available, but the development of antibiotic resistance in common organisms may be a problem for the future.

The microbiologist has an important role in the management of both heart and heart–lung or lung transplant patients by providing rapid and accurate diagnosis, antimicrobial sensitivity testing and advice on the appropriate use of antimicrobial chemotherapy. The rise in antibiotic resistance seen in recent years is of great concern (American Society for Microbiology 1995; House of Commons Select Committee on Science and Technology 1998). The introduction of rapid tests, in particular antigen and nucleic acid amplification and probe methods for organisms and resistance genes, may hold promise for early and effective treatment in this vulnerable group of patients.

# References

Aeba, R., Stout, R.J., Francalancia, N.A. *et al.* (1993) Aspects of lung transplantation that contribute to increased susceptibility to pneumonia. An experimental study. *Journal of Thoracic and Cardiovascular Surgery* **106**, 449–457.

Albat, B., Trinh-Duc, P., Boulfroy, D. *et al.* (1993) Mediastinitis in heart transplant recipients: successful treatment by closed local irrigation. *Cardiovascular Surgery* **1** (6), 657–659.

Almeida, D.R., Carvalho, A.C., Branco, J.N. *et al.* (1996) Chagas' disease reactivation after heart transplantation: efficacy of Allopurinol treatment. *Journal of Heart and Lung Transplantation* **15**, 988–992.

Amber, I.J., Gilbert, E.M., Schiffman, G. & Jacobson, J.A. (1990) Increased risk of pneumococcal infection in cardiac transplant recipients. *Transplantation* **49**, 122–125.

American Society for Microbiology (1995) Report of the ASM Task Force on Antibiotic Resistance. *Antimicrobial Agents and Chemotherapy* **39** (Suppl.), 1–23.

Anguita, M., Arizon, J.M., Valles, F. *et al.* (1993) Results of heart transplantation in recipients with active infection. *Journal of Heart and Lung Transplantation* **12**, 808–809.

Babinet, J., Gay, F., Bustos, D. *et al.* (1991) Transmission of *Plasmodium falciparum* by heart transplant. *British Medical Journal* **303**, 1515–1516.

Bailey, L.L., Gundry, S.R., Razzouk, A.J. *et al.* (1993) Bless the babies: one hundred fifteen late survivors of heart transplantation during the first year of life. *Journal of Thoracic and Cardiovascular Surgery* **105**, 805–814.

Baldi, S., Rapellino, M., Ruffini, E., Cavallo, A. & Mancuso, M. (1997) Atypical mycobacteriosis in a lung transplant recipient. *European Respiratory Journal* **10** (4), 952–954.

Baldwin, R.T., Radovancevic, B., Sweeney, M.S., Duncan, J.M. & Frazier, O.H. (1992) Bacterial mediastinitis after heart transplantation. *Journal of Heart and Lung Transplantation* **11**, 545–549.

Beyer, J., Schwartz, S., Barzen, G. *et al.* (1994) Use of amphotericin B aerosols for the prevention of pulmonary aspergillosis. *Infection* **22**, 143–148.

Boriani, G., Mirri, A., Iacopittii, P. *et al.* (1989) Aspergillosi cerebrale e renale in un paziente con trapianto cariaco ortotopico: diagnosi, trattemento e follow-up. *Cardiologia* **34**, 807–811.

Boyle, E.M., Burdine, J. & Bolman, R.M. (1993) Successful treatment of mycoplasma mediastinitis after heart-lung transplantation. *Journal of Heart and Lung Transplantation* **12**, 508–512.

British Transplantation Society (1998) *Towards Standards for Organ and Tissue Transplantation in the United Kingdom*. British Transplantation Society, London.

Byl, B., Jacobs, F., Antoine, M. *et al.* (1993) Mediastinitis caused by *Aspergillus fumigatus* with ruptured pseudoaneurysm in a heart transplant recipient. *Heart and Lung* **22**, 145–147.

Ciulli, F., Tamm, C., Dennis, C. *et al.* (1993) Donor-transmitted bacterial infection in heart–lung transplantation. *Transplantation Proceedings* **25**, 1155–1156.

Conti, D.J. & Rubin, R.H. (1988) Infection of the central nervous system in organ transplant recipients. *Neurologic Clinics* **6**, 241–260.

Corensek, M.J., Stewart, R.W., Keys, T.F., Mehta, A.C. & McHenry, M.C. (1988) A multivariate analysis of risk factors for pneumonia following cardiac transplantation. *Transplantation* **46**, 860–865.

Cortet, B., Richard, R., Deprez, X. *et al.* (1994) Aspergillus spondylodiscitis: successful conservative treatment in 9 cases. *Journal of Rheumatology* **21**, 1287–1289.

Counihan, P.J., Yelland, A., de Belder, M.A. & Pepper, J.R. (1991) Infective endocarditis in a heart transplant recipient. *Journal of Heart and Lung Transplantation* **10**, 275–279.

Cox, R.A., Conquest, C., Mallaghan, C. & Marples, R.R. (1995) A major outbreak of methicillin-resistant *Staphylococcus aureus* caused by a new phage-type (EMRSA-16). *Journal of Hospital Infection* **29**, 87–106.

Dajani, A.S., Bisno, A.L., Chung, K.J. *et al.* (1990) Prevention of bacterial endocarditis: recommendations by the American Heart Association. *Journal of the American Medical Association* **264**, 2919–2922.

Dauber, J.H., Paradis, I.L. & Dummer, J.S. (1990) Infectious complications in pulmonary allograft recipients. *Clinics in Chest Medicine* 11, 291–308.

De Leval, M.R., Smyth, R., Whitehead, B. *et al.* (1991) Heart and lung transplantation for terminal cystic fibrosis. *Journal of Thoracic and Cardiovascular Surgery* 101, 633–642.

De Vuyst, D., Surmont, J., Verhaegen, J. & Vanhaecke, J. (1992) Tibial osteomyelitis due to *Aspergillus flavus* in a heart transplant patient. *Infection* 20, 48–49.

Denning, D.W. & Stevens, D.A. (1990) Antifungal and surgical treatment of invasive aspergillosis: a review of 2121 published cases. *Reviews of Infectious Diseases* 12, 1147–1201.

Dennis, C., Caine, N., Sharples, L. *et al.* (1993) Heart–lung transplantation for end-stage respiratory disease in patients with cystic fibrosis at Papworth Hospital. *Journal of Heart and Lung Transplantation* 12, 893–902.

Deusch, E., End, A., Grimm, M. *et al.* (1993) Early bacterial infection in lung transplant recipients. *Chest* 104, 1412–1416.

Dowling, R.D., Baladi, N., Zenati, M. *et al.* (1990) Disruption of the aortic anastamosis after heart-lung transplantation. *Annals of Thoracic Surgery* 49, 118–122.

Dromer, C., Nashef, S.A.M., Velly, J.F., Martigne, C. & Couraud, L. (1993) Tuberculosis in transplanted lungs. *Journal of Heart and Lung Transplantation* 12, 924–927.

Dummer, J.S. & Ho, M. (2000) Infections in solid organ transplant recipients. In: *Principles and Practice of Infectious Diseases*, Vol. 2, 5th edn (eds G.L. Mandell, J.E. Bennet & R. Dolin), pp. 3148–3159. Churchill Livingstone, New York.

Dunn, J.M., Cavarocchi, N.C., Balsara, R.K. *et al.* (1987) Paediatric transplantation at St Christopher's Hospital for Children. *Journal of Heart Transplantation* 6, 334–421.

Egan, T.M., Detterbeck, F.C., Mill, M.R. *et al.* (1995) Improved results of lung transplantation for patients with cystic fibrosis. *Journal of Thoracic and Cardiovascular Surgery* 109, 224–235.

Emmerson, A.M., Enstone, J.E. & Kelsey, M.C. (1995) The Second National Prevalence Survey of Infection in Hospitals. *Journal of Hospital Infection* 30, 7–30.

Fabbri, A., Bryan, A.J., Sharples, L.D. *et al.* (1992a) The influence of recipient and donor gender on outcome after heart transplantation. *Journal of Heart and Lung Transplantation* 11, 701–707.

Fabbri, A., Sharples, L.D., Mullins, P. *et al.* (1992b) Heart transplants in patients over 54 years of age with triple drug immunotherapy immunosuppression. *Journal of Heart and Lung Transplantation* 11, 929–932.

Faggian, G., Livi, U., Bortolotti, U. *et al.* (1989) Itraconazole therapy for acute invasive pulmonary aspergillosis in heart transplantation. *Transplantation Proceedings* 21, 2506–2507.

Fernandez-Guerrero, M.L., Aguado, J.M., Buzon, L. *et al.*

(1987) Visceral leishmaniasis in immunocompromised hosts. *American Journal of Medicine* 83 (6), 1098–1102.

Flume, P.A., Egan, T.M., Paradowski, L.J. *et al.* (1994) Infectious complications of lung transplantation: impact of cystic fibrosis. *American Journal of Respiratory Critical Care Medicine* 149, 1601–1607.

Gamberg, P., Miller, J.L. & Lough, M.E. (1987) Impact of protection isolation on the incidence of infection after heart transplantation. *Journal of Heart Transplantation* 6 (3), 147–149.

Gentry, L.O. & Zeluff, B.J. (1988) Nosocomial and other difficult infections in the immunocompromised cardiac transplant patient. *Journal of Hospital Infection* 11 (Suppl. A), 21–28.

Gentry, L.O., Zeluff, B. & Keilhofner, M.A. (1994) Dermatologic manifestations offectious diseases in cardiac transplant patients. *Infectious Disease Clinics of North America* 8, 637–654.

Goddard, M.J., Stewart, S., Foweraker, J., McNeil, K. & Wallwork, J. (1998) A post-mortem audit of 30 day mortality following heart–lung and lung transplantation. *Journal of Heart and Lung Transplantation* 17, 47.

Gold, W.L., Vellend, H., Salit, I.E. *et al.* (1994) Successful treatment of systemic and local infections due to *Exophiala* species [see comments]. *Clinical Infectious Diseases* 19 (2), 339–341.

Golino, A., Duncan, R.M., Zeluff, B. *et al.* (1992) Leishmaniasis in a heart transplant patient. *Journal of Heart and Lung Transplantation* 11, 820–823.

Govan, J.R.W., Brown, P.H., Maddison, J. *et al.* (1993) Evidence for transmission of *Pseudomonas cepacia* by social contact in cystic fibrosis. *Lancet* 342, 15–19.

Graham, D.A., Kinyoun, J.L. & George, D.P. (1995) Endogenous aspergillus endophthalmitis after lung transplantation. *American Journal of Ophthalmology* 119, 107–109.

Gregor, R.J., Chong, C.A., Augsburger, J.J. *et al.* (1989) Endogenous *Nocardia asteroides* subretinal abscess diagnosed by transvitreal fine-needle aspiration biopsy. *Retina* 9, 118–121.

Gryzan, S., Paradis, I.L., Zeevi, A. *et al.* (1988) Unexpectedly high incidence of *Pneumocystis carinii* infection after lung–heart transplantation. *American Review of Respiratory Disease* 137, 1268–1274.

Guillemain, R., Lavarde, V., Amrein, C. *et al.* (1995) Invasive aspergillosis after transplantation. *Transplantation Proceedings* 27 (1), 1307–1309.

Hadley, W.K. & Ng, V.L. (1999) Pneumocystis. In: *Manual of Clinical Microbiology*, 7th edn (eds P.R. Murray, E.J. Baron, M.A. Pfaller, F. Tenover & R.H. Yolken), pp. 1200–1211. American Society for Microbiology, Washington.

Hall, K.A., Sethi, G.K., Rosado, L.J. *et al.* (1993a) Coccidiomycosis and heart transplantation. *Journal of Heart and Lung Transplantation* 12, 525–526.

Hall, K.A., Copeland, J.G., Zukoski, C.F., Sethi, G.K. & Galgiani, J.N. (1993b) Markers of coccidioidomycosis before cardiac or renal transplantation and the risk of recurrent infection. *Transplantation* **55**, 1422–1424.

Hall, W.A., Martinez, A.J., Dummer, J.S. *et al.* (1989) Central nervous infections in heart and heart–lung transplant recipients. *Archives of Neurology* **46**, 173–177.

Harmati, L.B., Schulman, L.L. & Austin, J. (1993) Lung nodules and masses after cardiac transplantation. *Radiology* **188**, 491–497.

Hasan, A., Hamilton, J.R., Au, J. *et al.* (1993) Surgical management of infective endocarditis after heart–lung transplantation. *Journal of Heart and Lung Transplantation* **12**, 320–321.

Haverich, A., Frimpong-Boateng, K., Wahlers, T. & Schafers, H.J. (1989) Pericardial flap-plasty for protection of the tracheal anastamosis in heart–lung transplantation. *Journal of Cardiac Surgery* **4**, 136–139.

Heng, D., Sharples, L.D., McNeil, K. *et al.* (1998) Bronchiolitis obliterans syndrome: incidence, natural history, prognosis and risk factors. *Journal of Heart and Lung Transplantation* **17**, 1255–1263.

Herve, P., Silbert, D., Cerrina, J., Simmoneau, G. & Dartevelle, P. (1993) Impairment of bronchial mucociliary clearance in long-term survivors of heart/lung and double lung transplantation. *Chest* **104**, 681–685.

Higgenbottam, T., Stewart, S., Penketh, A. & Wallwork, J.W. (1988) Transbronchial lung biopsy for the diagnosis of rejection in heart-lung transplant patients. *Transplantation* **46**, 532–539.

Higgins, R., McNeil, K., Dennis, C. *et al.* (1994) Airway stenosis after lung transplantation: management with expanding metal stents. *Journal of Heart and Lung Transplantation* **13**, 774–778.

Horbach, I. & Fehrenbach, F.J. (1990) Legionellosis in heart transplant recipients. *Infection* **18**, 361–363.

Horvath, J., Dummer, J.S., Loyd, J. *et al.* (1993) Infection in the transplanted and native lung after single lung transplantation. *Chest* **103**, 59–63.

Hosenpud, J.D., Bennett, L.E., Keck, B.M., Fiol, B. & Novick, R.J. (1997) The Registry of the International Society for Heart and Lung Transplantation: Fourteenth Official Report. *Journal of Heart and Lung Transplantation* **16**, 691–712.

House of Commons Select Committee on Science and Technology (1998) *Resistance to Antibiotics and Other Antimicrobial Agents.* HMSO, London.

Hruban, R.H., Beschorner, W.E., Baumgartner, W.A. *et al.* (1988) Depletion of bronchus-associated lymphoid tissue associated with lung allograft rejection. *American Journal of Pathology* **132**, 6–11.

Jamieson, S.W., Oyer, P.E., Reitz, B.A. *et al.* (1982) Cardiac transplantation at Stanford. *Heart Transplantation* **1**, 86–91.

Johnson, K.E., Prieto, M., Joyce, L.D., Pritzker, M. & Emery, R.W. (1992) Summary of the clinical use of the Symbion total artificial heart. *Journal of Heart and Lung Transplantation* **11**, 103–161.

Karwande, S.V., Ensley, R.D., Renlund, D.G. *et al.* (1992a) Cardiac retransplantation: a viable option? *Annals of Thoracic Surgery* **54**, 840–844.

Karwande, S.V., Renlund, D.G., Olson, S.L. *et al.* (1992b) Mediastinitis in heart transplantation. *Annals of Thoracic Surgery* **54**, 1039–1045.

Katz, N.M., Pierce, P.F., Anzeck, R.A. *et al.* (1990) Liposomal amphotericin B for treatment of pulmonary aspergillosis in a heart transplant patient. *Journal of Heart Transplantation* **9**, 14–17.

Khagani, A., Martin, M., Fitzgerald, M. *et al.* (1988) Cefotaxime and flucloxacillin as antibiotic prophylaxis in cardiac transplantation. *Drugs* **35** (Suppl. 2), 124–126.

Khoo, D.E., Zebro, T. & English, T.A. (1989) Bacterial endocarditis in a transplanted heart. *Pathology Research and Practice* **185**, 445–447.

Kim, J.H. & Perfect, J.R. (1989) Infection and cyclosporine. *Reviews of Infectious Diseases* **11**, 677–690.

Knosalla, C., Weng, Y., Warnecke, H. *et al.* (1996) Mycotic aortic aneurysms after orthotopic heart transplantation: a three-case report and review of the literature. *Journal of Heart and Lung Transplantation* **15**, 827–839.

Knouse, M.C. & Lorber, B. (1990) Early diagnosis of *Nocardia asteroides* endophthalmitis by retinal biopsy: case report and review. *Reviews of Infectious Diseases* **12**, 393–398.

Korvick, J. & Yu, V.L. (1988) Simultaneous infection with *Cryptococcus neoformans* and *Legionella pneumophila*. In vivo expression of common defects in cell-mediated immunity. *Respiration* **53**, 132–136.

Kramer, M.R., Denning, D.W., Marshall, S.E. *et al.* (1991) Ulcerative tracheobronchitis after lung transplantation: a new form of invasive aspergillosis. *American Review of Respiratory Disease* **144**, 552–556.

Kramer, M.R., Stoehr, C., Lewiston, N.J., Starnes, V.A. & Theodore, J. (1992) Trimethoprim-sulfamethoxazole prophylaxis for *Pneumycistis carinii* infections in heart–lung and lung transplantation—How effective and for how long? *Transplantation* **53**, 586–589.

Kurland, G. (1996) Pediatric lung transplantation: indications and contraindications. *Seminars in Thoracic and Cardiovascular Surgery* **8** (3), 277–285.

Kurup, V.P. & Kumar, A. (1991) Immunodiagnosis of aspergillosis. *Clinical Microboiological Review* **4**, 439–456.

Lange, S.S., Prevost, S., Lewis, P. & Fadol, A. (1992) Infection control practises in cardiac transplant recipients. *Heart and Lung* **21**, 101–105.

Lanza, R.P., Cooper, D.K., Boyd, S.T. & Barnard, C.N. (1984) Comparison of patients with ischemic, myopathic, and rheumatic heart disease as cardiac transplant recipients. *American Heart Journal* 107, 8–12.

Larner, A.J., Conway, M.A., Mitchell, R.G. & Forfar, J.C. (1989) Recurrent *Listeria monocytogenes* meningitis in a heart transplant recipient. *Journal of Infection* 19, 263–266.

Lewiston, N., King, V., Umetsu, D. *et al.* (1991) Cystic fibrosis patients who have undergone heart–lung transplantation benefit from maxillary sinus antrostomy and repeated sinus lavage. *Transplantation Proceedings* 23 (1/2), 1207–1208.

Libow, L.F., Beltrani, V.P., Silvers, D.N. & Grossman, M.E. (1991) Post transplantation reactivation of Chagas' disease diagnosed by skin biopsy. *Cutis* 48, 37–40.

Linman, M.J., Mascola, L., Lou, X.D. *et al.* (1988) Epidemic listeriosis associated with Mexican-style cheese. *New England Journal of Medicine* 319, 823–828.

Lopez, F.A., Crowley, R.S., Wastila, L., Valantine, H.A. & Remington, J.S. (1998) *Scedosporium apiospermum (Pseudallescheria boydii)* infection in a heart transplant recipient: a case of mistaken identity. *Journal of Heart and Lung Transplantation* 17, 321–324.

Low, D.E., Kaiser, L.R., Haydock, D.A., Trulock, E. & Cooper, J.D. (1993) The donor lung: infectious and pathologic factors affecting the outcome in lung transplantation. *Journal of Thoracic and Cardiovascular Surgery* 106, 614–621.

McGiffen, D.C., Kirklin, J.K. & Naftel, D.C. (1985) Acute renal failure after transplantation and cyclosporine. *Journal of Heart Transplantation* 4, 396–399.

Maki, D.G. (1994) Infections caused by intravascular devices used for infusion therapy: pathogenesis, prevention and management. In: *Infections Associated with Indwelling Medical Devices* (eds A.L. Bisno & F.A. Waldvogel), pp. 155–213. American Society for Microbiology, Washington.

Mannes, G.P.M., van der Bij, W., de Boer, W.J. & Groningen Lung Transplantation Group (1995) Liposomal amphotericin B in three lung transplant recipients. *Journal of Heart and Lung Transplantation* 14, 781–784.

Massard, G., Shennib, H., Metras, D. *et al.* (1993) Double-lung transplantation in mechanically ventilated patients with cystic fibrosis. *American Thoracic Surgery* 55, 1087–1092.

Maurer, J.R., Tullis, E., Grossman, R.F. *et al.* (1992) Infectious complications following isolated lung transplantation. *Chest* 101, 1056–1059.

Meers, P.D., Ayliffe, G.A.J., Emmerson, A.M. *et al.* (1981) Report on National Survey of Infection in Hospitals. *Journal of Hospital Infection* 2 (Suppl.), 1–53.

Monteforte, J.S. & Wood, C.A. (1993) Pneumonia caused by *Nocardia nova* and *Aspergillus fumigatus* after cardiac transplantation. *European Journal of Clinical Microbiology and Infectious Diseases* 12, 112–114.

Muhm, M., Zuckermann, A., Prokesch, R. *et al.* (1996) Early onset of pulmonary mucormycosis with pulmonary vein thrombosis in a heart transplant recipient. *Transplantation* 62, 1185–1187.

Muñoz, P., Palomo, J., Muñoz, R. *et al.* (1995) Tuberculosis in heart transplant recipients. *Clinical Infectious Diseases* 21, 398–402.

Murray-Leisure, K.A., Aber, R.C., Rowley, L.J. *et al.* (1986) Disseminated *Trichosporon beigelii* infection in an artificial heart recipient. *Journal of the American Medical Association* 256, 2995–2998.

Newsom, S.W.B. (1968) Hospital infection from contaminated ice. *Lancet* ii, 620–622.

Newsom, S.W.B. (1978) Antibiotic prophylaxis for open-heart surgery. *Journal of Antimicrobial Chemotherapy* 4, 389–391.

NHS Executive (1996) *Guidance on the Microbiological Safety of Human Tissues and Organs used in Transplantation.* Department of Health, London.

Novick, R.J., Moreno-Cabral, C.E., Stinson, E.B. *et al.* (1990) Nontuberculous mycobacterial infections in heart transplant recipients: a seventeen-year experience. *Journal of Heart Transplantation* 9, 357–363.

Noyes, B.E., Paradis, I.L. & Dauber, J. (1991) Accessory cell function of blood monocytes and alveolar macrophages after human lung transplantation. *American Review of Respiratory Disease* 144, 606–611.

Olivari, M.T., Antolick, A., Kaye, M.P., Jamieson, S.W. & Ring, W.S. (1988) Heart transplantation in elderly patients. *Journal of Heart Transplantation* 7, 258–264.

Orr, K., Gould, F.K., Sisson, P.R. *et al.* (1991) Rapid inter-strain comparison by pyrolysis mass spectrometry in nosocomial infection with *Xanthomonas maltophilia*. *Journal of Hospital Infection* 17, 187–195.

Ostrum, R.F. (1993) Nocardia septic arthritis of the hip associated with avascular necrosis. A case report. *Clinical Orthopaedics* 288, 282–286.

Otulana, B.A., Higgenbottam, T.W., Hutter, J. & Wallwork, J. (1988) Close monitoring of lung function in heart–lung transplant allows detection of pulmonary infection and rejection. *American Review of Respiratory Disease* 137, A245.

Paradowski, L.J. (1997) Saprophytic fungal infections and lung transplantation revisited. *Journal of Heart and Lung Transplantation* 16, 524–531.

Patel, R., Roberts, G.D., Keating, M.R. & Paya, C.V. (1994) Infections due to nontuberculous mycobacteria in kidney, heart and liver transplant recipients. *Clinical Infectious Diseases* 19, 263–273.

Peglow, S.L., Smulian, L.J., Linke, C.L. *et al.* (1990) Serologic response to specific *Pneumocystis carinii* antigens in health and disease. *Journal of Infectious Diseases* 161, 296–306.

Plemmons, R.M., McAllister, C.K., Garces, M.C. & Ward, R.L. (1997) Osteomyelitis due to *Mycobacterium haemophilum* in a cardiac transplant patient: case report and analysis of interactions among clarithromycin, rifampicin and cyclosporine. *Clinical Infectious Disease* 24, 995–997.

Prayson, R.A. & Estes, M.L. (1995) The neuropathology of cardiac allograft transplantation. *Archives of Pathology and Laboratory Medicine* 11, 59–63.

Quirce, R., Serano, J., Arnal, C., Banzo, I. & Carril, J.M. (1991) Detection of mediastinitis after heart transplantation by gallium-67 scintigraphy. *Nuclear Medicine* 32, 860–861.

Rabito, F.J. & Pankey, G.A. (1992) Infections on orthotopic heart transplant patients at the Oschner Medical Institutions *Medical Clinics of North America* 76, 1125–1134.

Ramirez, J.C., Patterson, G.A., Winton, T.L. *et al.* (1992) Bilateral lung transplantation for cystic fibrosis. *Journal of Thoracic and Cardiovascular Surgery* 103, 287–294.

Rees, W., Schuler, S., Hummel, M. & Hetzer, R. (1994) Primar kutane *Nocardia farcinia* infektion nach Hertztransplantation. *Deutsche Medizinische Wochenschrift* 119, 1276–1280.

Rex, J.R., Larsen, J.A., Dismukes, W.E. *et al.* (1993) Catastrophic visual loss due to *Cryptococcus neoformans* meningitis. *Medicine* 72, 207–224.

Rhame, F. (1991) Prevention of nosocomial aspergillosis. *Journal of Hospital Infection* 18 (Suppl. A), 446–472.

Rhenman, M.J., Rhenman, B., Icenogle, T., Christensen, R. & Copeland, J.A. (1988) Diabetes and heart transplantation. *Journal of Heart Transplantation* 7, 356–358.

Ridgeway, A.L., Warner, G.S., Phillips, P. *et al.* (1996) Transmission of *Mycobacterium tuberculosis* to recipients of single lung transplants from the same donor. *American Journal of Respiratory Critical Care Medicine* 153, 1166–1168.

Ryan, P.J. & Stableforth, D.E. (1996) Referral for lung transplantation: experience of a Birmingham adult cystic fibrosis centre between 1987 and 1994. *Thorax* 51, 302–305.

Sader, H.S. & Jones, R.N. (1992) Cefotaxime is extensively used for surgical prophylaxis. *American Journal of Surgery* 164 (Suppl. 4A), 28–38.

Sarris, G.E., Moore, K.A., Schroder, J.S. *et al.* (1994a) Cardiac transplantation: the Stanford experience in the cyclosporin era. *Journal of Thoracic and Cardiovascular Surgery* 108, 240–251.

Sarris, G.E., Smith, J.A., Bernstein D. *et al.* (1994b) Paediatric cardiac transplantation: the Stanford experience. *Circulation* 90, 1152–1155.

Schulman, L.L., Smith, C.R., Drusin, R., Rose, E.A. & Enson, Y. (1988) Utility of airway endoscopy in the diagnosis of respiratory complications of cardiac transplantation. *Chest* 93, 960–971.

Sheares, B.J., Prince, A.S., Quittell, L.M., Neu, N.M. & Bye, M.R. (1997) *Pseudomonas aeruginosa* endophthalmitis after lung transplantation for cystic fibrosis. *Paediatric Infectious Disease Journal* 16, 820–821.

Sielaff, T.D., Everett, J.E. & Shumway, S.J. (1996) *Mycoplasma hominis* infections occurring in cardiovascular surgical patients. *Annals of Thoracic Surgery* 61 (1), 99–103.

Simmons, B.P., Gelfand, M.S. & Roberts, G. (1992) *Nocardia otidiscaviarum (caviae)* infection in a heart transplant patient presented as having a thigh abscess (Madura Thigh). *Journal of Heart and Lung Transplantation* 11, 824–826.

Smart, F.W., Naftel, D.C., Costanzo, M.R. *et al.* (1996) Risk factors for early, cumulative and fatal infections after heart transplantation: a multiinstitutional study. *Journal of Heart and Lung Transplantation* 15, 329–341.

Smyth, R.L., Higgenbottam, T.W., Scott, J.P. *et al.* (1989) Early experience of heart-lung transplantation. *Archives of Diseases in Childhood* 64, 1225–1229.

Spencer, R.C. (1995) The emergence of epidemic, multiple-antibiotic-resistant *Stenotrophomonas (Xanthomonas) maltophilia* and *Burkholderia (Pseudomonas) cepacia*. *Journal of Hospital Infection* 30 (Suppl.), 453–464.

Stamm, A.M., Smith, S.H., Kirklin, J.K. & McGiffen, D.C. (1990) Listerial myocarditis in cardiac transplantation. *Review of Infectious Diseases* 12, 820–831.

Starnes, V.A., Lewison, N., Theodore, J. *et al.* (1992) Cystic fibrosis: target population for lung transplantation in North America in the 1990s. *Journal of Thoracic and Cardiovascular Surgery* 103, 1008–1114.

Steffenson, D.O., Dummer, J.S., Granick, M.S. *et al.* (1987) Sternotomy infections with *Mycoplasma hominis*. *Annals of Internal Medicine* 106, 204–208.

Steinbach, S., Sun, L., Jiang, R.J. *et al.* (1994) Transmissibility of *Pseudomonas cepacia* infection in clinic patients and lung transplant recipients with cystic fibrosis. *New England Journal of Medicine* 331, 981–987.

Stewart, S., Ciulli, F., Wells, F. & Wallwork, J. (1993) Pathology of unused donor lungs. *Transplantation Proceedings* 25, 1167–1168.

Sudduth, E.J., Crumbley, A.J. & Farrar, W.E. (1992) Phaeohyphomycosis due to *Exophilia species*: clinical spectrum of disease in humans. *Clinical Infectious Diseases* 15, 639–644.

Thaler, F., Gotainer, B., Teodori, G., Dubois, C. & Loirat, P. (1992) Mediastinitis due to *Nocardia asteroides* after cardiac transplantation. *Intensive Care Medicine* 18, 127–128.

Toporoff, B., Rosado, L.J., Appleton, C.P., Sethi, G.K. & Copeland, J.G. (1994) Successful treatment of early infective endocarditis and mediastinitis in a heart transplant recipient. *Journal of Heart and Lung Transplantation* 13, 546–548.

Torre-Cisneros, J., Lopez, O.L., Kusne, S. *et al.* (1993) CNS aspergillosis in organ transplantation: a clinicopathological study. *Journal of Neurology, Neurosurgery and Psychiatry* **56**, 188–193.

Trulock, E.P., Bolman, R.M. & Genton, R. (1989) Pulmonary disease caused by *Mycobacterium chelonae* in a heart–lung transplant recipient with obliterative bronchiolitis. *American Review of Respiratory Disease* **140**, 802–805.

Van Goor, H., Rosman, C., Grond, J. (1994) Translocation of bacteria and endotoxin in organ donors. *Archives of Surgery* **129** (10), 1063–1066.

Venditti, M., Biavasco, F., Macchiarelli, A. *et al.* (1993) Catheter-related endocarditis due to glycopeptide-resistant *Enterococcus faecalis* in a transplanted heart. *Clinical Infectious Diseases* **17**, 524–525.

Walter, S., Gudowius, P., Boßhammer, J. *et al.* (1997) Epidemiology of chronic *Pseudomonas aeruginosa* infections in the airways of lung transplant recipients with cystic fibrosis. *Thorax* **52**, 318–321.

Walzer, P.D. (1994) *Pneumocystis Pneumonia*. Marcel Dekker, New York.

Wells, F.C., Newsom, S.W.B. & Rowland, C. (1983) Wound infection in cardiothoracic surgery. *Lancet* **i**, 1209–1210.

Westney, G.E., Kesten, S., de Hoyos, A. *et al.* (1996)

*Aspergillus* infection in single and double lung transplant recipients. *Transplantation* **61**, 915–919.

Wreghitt, T.G., Gray, J.J., Pavel, P. *et al.* (1992) Efficacy of pyrimethamine for the prevention of donor-acquired *Toxoplasma gondii* infection in heart and heart–lung recipients. *Transplant International* **5**, 197–200.

Yacoub, M.H., Banner, N.R., Khaghani, A. *et al.* (1990) Heart–lung transplantation for cystic fibrosis and subsequent domino heart transplantation. *Journal of Heart Transplantation* **9**, 459–467.

Yeldandi, V., Laghi, F., McCabe, M.A. *et al.* (1995) Aspergillus and lung transplantation. *Journal of Heart and Lung Transplantation* **14**, 883–890.

Young, J.N., Yazbeck, J., Esposito, G. *et al.* (1986) The influence of acute pre-operative pulmonary infarction on the results of heart transplantation. *Journal of Heart Transplantation* **5**, 20–21.

Zenati, M., Dowling, R.D., Armitage, J.M. *et al.* (1989) Organ procurement for pulmonary transplantation. *Annals of Thoracic Surgery* **48**, 882–886.

Zenati, M., Dowling, R.D., Dummer, J.S. *et al.* (1990) Influence of the donor lung on development of early infections in lung transplant recipients. *Journal of Heart Transplantation* **9**, 502–508.

# Chapter 19/Infection in bone marrow transplant patients

J. PETER DONNELLY

## Introduction

Bone marrow transplantation (BMT) has become a life-saver for many thousands of patients throughout the world suffering from haematological and other malignancies as well as diseases, such as thalassaemia, severe aplastic anaemia, inborn errors of metabolism and other genetically determined diseases. The procedure is also being considered for treating other conditions, including rheumatic diseases and AIDS. Before receiving a transplant, the recipient's immunity has to be demolished because the progenitor or haematopoietic stem cells that give rise to all the blood cells have to be replaced by healthy ones, either from the recipient, autologous, or from a donor, allogeneic (Fig. 19.1). Allogeneic haematopoietic stem cell transplants, and syngeneic transplants in the case of genetically identical siblings, are used for all types of recipient, whereas autologous haematopoietic stem cell transplants are given mainly as part of the intensive treatment for lymphoma, multiple myeloma and solid tumours (Gratwohl & Hermans 1994). Although most often derived from bone marrow aspirates, haematopoietic stem cells isolated from the peripheral blood are increasingly being used for autologous haematopoietic stem cell transplants and are also beginning to be used for allogeneic transplants (Bensinger et al. 1995).

The normal human individual is equipped with an impressive array of defences which protect him or her from microbial foes and friends alike and allow him or her to distinguish between them. Millions of microorganisms inhabit the nooks and crannies of the body, covering all of the skin and every square centimetre of the oral cavity and alimentary tract. Bacteria are by far the most numerous microorganisms and that so few of the several hundred species are pathogenic is a testimony to the body's defences. In addition, we encounter many more species and strains in our everyday lives, of

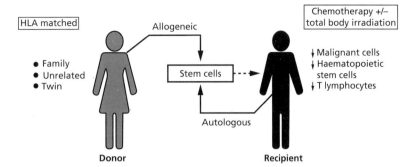

**Fig. 19.1** Stem cell transplantation.

which most remain harmless although some infect us and cause disease. Yet, apart from the more well-known professional pathogens, such as *Mycobacterium tuberculosis* and *Streptococcus pneumoniae*, our bodies invariably manage to regain their immunological equilibrium, mostly without any need for any antimicrobial treatment. How this is achieved is the result of a complex and dynamic interplay between a balanced microbial flora and effective local and systemic defence mechanisms. Each of these elements is damaged to a variable extent by the haematopoietic stem cell transplant procedure.

## Transplant procedure

### Conditioning therapy

The preparation for a haematopoietic stem cell transplant requires that the bone marrow be ablated, which is usually achieved by treatment with cytostatic agents, such as cyclophosphamide, together with irradiation. Once haematopoiesis ceases, the patient becomes entirely dependent upon the blood cells in the circulation. Short-lived cells, such as platelets and neutrophils, rapidly become depleted, leaving the patient profoundly thrombocytopenic and neutropenic. In order to prepare for an allogeneic haematopoietic stem cell transplant, the numbers of circulating T cell lymphocytes have also to be reduced to minimize the risk of graft rejection and so recipients are exposed to high doses of irradiation, usually of the entire body. The residual B cell lymphocytes, monocytes and

macrophages, survive this assault but the patient is bereft of a major line of defence, namely phagocytosis. Moreover, the rapidly dividing cells of the integument, i.e. the skin and the mucosa of the oropharynx and alimentary tract, lose their capacity to repair minor traumas, such as cuts and abrasions, brought about by normal activities.

## Perturbations to the immunity as a result of the transplantation procedure

Each component of the host defences is, to a varying extent, dependent upon another in attaining maximum efficacy. For instance, without IgA and other secretory substances, the skin and mucosa would prove less effective as barriers. Moreover, the surfaces of the human body exhibit a clear propensity to interact with the resident commensal resident flora, which is composed of normally avirulent microorganisms that protect the human host from invasion of more professional pathogens by competing for binding sites on the cell surfaces and for the available nutrients. The success of the defences depends upon the integration of each individual component, including the physical barriers, into an amalgamated coordinated defence system. However, such a complex system is vulnerable to profound perturbations brought about by the haematopoietic stem cell transplant process.

The inner and outer surfaces of our bodies are inhabited by a myriad of microorganisms representing some 700 different species. It is estimated that the microbial flora contains in excess of $10^{14}$ microorganisms, equivalent to several grams, most of which are concentrated in the oral cavity and large bowel, where every variety of microorganism can be found, including spirochaetes, spore-formers, bacilli and cocci. By contrast, the skin is colonized by only a few Gram-positive genera which are able to withstand desiccation.

Resident bacteria probably grow as a biofilm rather than the more familiar planktonic growth that occurs under laboratory conditions. Biofilm consists of microcolonies enmeshed in a complex matrix, mostly composed of carbohydrates and known as glycocalyx (Costerton *et al.* 1987), and provides a distinct and separate niche for each species while affording protection against the elements as well as against antimicrobial agents (Costerton & Marrie 1983). Many of the resident bacteria also produce bacteriocins to keep closely related microorganisms at bay and allow the individual species to establish and maintain their own territory.

### Erosion of the skin integument

The skin of an adult has an estimated surface area of 1.5–2.3 m$^2$ and is a hostile environment for most microorganisms. Rapid cell turnover limits the opportunities for transient organisms to adhere as the indigenous flora are adept at attaching avidly and quickly. The surface temperature is about 5°C lower than that of the internal organs and there is little water available for microorganisms as a result of the lipophilic substances found in sebum, e.g. triglycerides. The resident microbial flora also releases a variety of long- and short-chain fatty acids in the sebaceous secretions, resulting in a hydrophobic acid milieu. Thus, only those microorganisms that can withstand these hostile conditions and compete successfully for binding sites and nutrients are able to establish a permanent and intimate attachment to the epidermis (Roth & James 1988). The flora is therefore much simpler than that of the mucosal surfaces and embraces the coagulase-negative staphylococci, particularly *Staphylococcus epidermidis*, *Corynebacterium jeikeum* and other coryneforms and *Propionibacterium* spp.

The skin's ability to act as a defence barrier is impaired by cuts and abrasions as well as needle punctures. Minor breaches in the integument can lead to

local infection and associated exudates may provide a reservoir that assists further spread to other body surfaces, including the oral cavity, via the fingers. Imbalance between the cutaneous defences and resident flora around the hair follicles can lead to inflammation, folliculitis. The fibronectin released after trauma may also facilitate colonization with *Staphylococcus aureus* and other changes facilitate colonization with Gram-negative bacilli, such as *Acinetobacter baumanii* and enterobacteria.

Transplant recipients usually require a central intravascular catheter for venous access, which can offer a ready portal of entry for potential pathogens. Moreover, many bacteria, particularly the coagulase-negative staphylococci, e.g. *S. epidermidis* and some yeasts, e.g. *Candida parapsilosis*, adhere readily to the plastic and can migrate along the external surface of the device, leading to local infection, which can provide a nidus for dissemination. Apart from readily adapting their biofilm existence to plastic surfaces, such as those provided by intravascular catheters, staphylococci always have a mutant clone at hand for each and every antimicrobial agent, whether antibiotic or not, that enables the species to exploit any sudden selective advantage afforded by antimicrobial treatment.

The skin barrier can also be undermined in more subtle ways. Topical antimicrobial agents and those secreted in sweat will disturb the microbial ecology, rendering the surface vulnerable to colonization by exogenous potential pathogens. The agents will also inhibit or kill susceptible members of the resident flora, giving selective advantage to more resistant species and strains. For example, resistance to ciprofloxacin emerges among *S. epidermidis* within a few days of starting treatment with ciprofloxacin as a result of the drug being secreted with sweat (Høiby *et al.* 1995, 1997). Chemotherapy and irradiation also exert a profound effect by halting normal cell replacement, resulting in hair loss, dryness and reduced sweat production. Steroids are used to treat graft vs. host disease (GVHD) and alter sebum secretions.

### Effect of chemotherapy and irradiation on the oral cavity

Cytostatic chemotherapy and irradiation interrupt cell

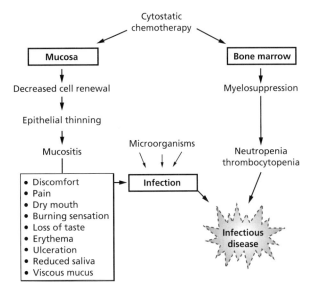

**Fig. 19.2** Impact of chemotherapy on the body's defences. It is universally understood that neutropenia is a risk factor for infectious complications but it is gradually becoming clearer that cytostatic chemotherapy simultaneously induces mucosal barrier injury not just to the oral cavity (known as mucositis or stomatitis) but also to the gut. (Modified from Sonis 1989.)

division, leading to breakdown in integrity because of mechanical damage. The production of saliva may be impaired, leading to a dry mouth, and, if mucin is produced, it may be extremely viscous and difficult to either swallow or expectorate. Periodontal disease may be exacerbated and minor oral cuts and abrasions may become inflamed and ulcerated. The non-keratinized surfaces of the mouth, including the underside of the tongue, the roof of the mouth and the cheeks, may become red, inflamed and swollen, limiting the intake of both food and drink (Kolbinson *et al.* 1988; Weisdorf *et al.* 1989; Donnelly *et al.* 1992; Rocke *et al.* 1993; Duenas-Gonzalez *et al.* 1996). This phenomenon is now generally referred to as mucositis although some prefer the older term, stomatitis.

Most important of all is the fact that myelotoxicity and integumental toxicities occur simultaneously so the patient is deprived of two major lines of defence (Fig. 19.2). Moreover, mucosal changes normally progress to a peak severity, which coincides with the nadir of bone marrow aplasia, and recovery only begins as haematopoiesis returns (Fig. 19.3) (Kolbinson *et al.* 1988; Weisdorf *et al.* 1989; Donnelly *et al.* 1992; Rocke *et al.* 1993; Duenas-Gonzalez *et al.* 1996). Ulcers that persist beyond this time often signify oral GVHD (Woo *et al.* 1993). The risk of other toxici-

ties, such as hepatic veno-occlusive disease, is more frequent in patients suffering mucositis than in those who remain free of this complication (Wingard 1990).

Herpes simplex infection usually develops within 7–11 days of the transplant (Wade *et al.* 1984; Shepp *et al.* 1985; Engelhard *et al.* 1988) as a result of reactivation induced by conditioning treatment for transplantation. Herpes simplex I infection may also be a risk factor for candidosis as has been shown to be the case following cytostatic chemotherapy (Beattie *et al.* 1989). Patients who are irradiated before transplant are more likely to develop marked mucositis and fever than are those who are not irradiated (Callum *et al.* 1991). Before prophylaxis with aciclovir became the norm, activated herpes simplex I infection was frequently involved in mucositis (Redding 1990) but now this complication rarely occurs. However, infections caused by aciclovir-resistant thymidine-kinase-deficient virus can occur, causing severe infection, including fatal pneumonia (Ljungman *et al.* 1990).

When mucositis is present, the mouth loses its normal ability to dilute foreign bacteria. The microecology will also be profoundly altered during the mucosal changes associated with mucositis. In addition, exposing oral commensal flora to the antimicrobial agents used for prophylaxis and local antisepsis

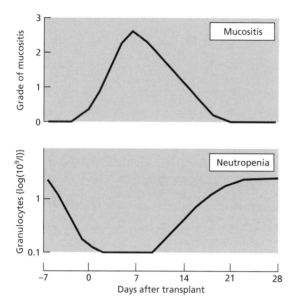

**Fig. 19.3** Schematic representation of the course of oral mucositis in relation to neutropenia. The course of neutropenia and mucositis run parallel. The first phase reflects the initial damage done by cytostatic chemotherapy. Tissue damage to the mucosa generally peaks during the nadir of neutropenia. Haematopoiesis may precede or coincide with healing of the mucosa but usually mucositis only resolves completely some time after adequate bone marrow function has been established. (Compiled from Kolbinson *et al.* 1988, Weisdorf *et al.* 1989, Donnelly *et al.* 1992, Rocke *et al.* 1993 and Duenas-Gonzalez *et al.* 1996.)

will inevitably select the more resistant species. Very susceptible bacteria, such as the oral *Neisseria* spp., are suppressed by a wide range of antimicrobial agents, whereas others that are marginally susceptible, if at all, to agents frequently used, such as co-trimoxazole, penicillin and fluoroquinolones, will thrive. This partly explains why the viridans streptococci have become one of the most frequent causes of bacteraemia in neutropenic patients who have undergone cytostatic chemotherapy for leukaemia or who have received a bone marrow transplant, although the type of cytostatic chemotherapy may be a more important factor, especially when it induces severe mucosal damage (Donnelly *et al.* 1995). One particular viridans streptococcus species, *Streptococcus mitis*, many of which are

actually *Streptococcus oralis* (Ferretti *et al.* 1987; Weisdorf *et al.* 1989; Meurman *et al.* 1991), is causing concern as its appearance in the bloodstream can be associated with sepsis syndrome and adult respiratory distress syndrome (ARDS). Bacteraemia caused by other unusual oral commensals, such as *Stomatococcus mucilaginosus*, *Capnocytophaga* spp. and *Leptotrichia buccalis*, are likely to be selected for by quinolones as they are also only marginally susceptible, and there have been reports of gingivitis being the source of bacteraemia caused by *S. epidermidis* (Schuster 1992; Bronchud 1993).

The chlorhexidine mouthwashes used to minimize infective complications arising from the oral toxicity induced by cytostatics also influence the microflora (Ferretti *et al.* 1987; Weisdorf *et al.* 1989; Meurman *et al.* 1991). The oral flora may also change as a direct result of chemotherapy (Bergmann 1991) and it is likely that more intensive conditioning regimens will aggravate oromucositis, leading to a commensurate increase in the number of unusual bacteria.

Use of the growth factors G-CSF and GM-CSF (Schuster 1992; Bronchud 1993) does not appear to have any influence on oromucositis (De Witte *et al.* 1993). Therefore haematopoietic stem cell transplant recipients will continue to experience varying degrees of mucosal damage, depending upon the nature of their conditioning therapy (Sable & Donowitz 1994), because some, e.g. melphalan, produce extensive damage, often with the production of thick mucus (McGuire *et al.* 1993). Oromucositis can also be particularly severe when anthracyclines are combined with total body irradiation and cyclophosphamide to condition patients for an allogeneic transplant (Raemaekers *et al.* 1989), resulting in a commensurate increase in bacteraemia caused by viridans streptococci. Fortunately, the morbidity associated with Gram-positive infections is usually mild and the attributable mortality is negligible (Rubin *et al.* 1988; EORTC International Antimicrobial Therapy Cooperative Group 1990; EORTC International Antimicrobial Therapy Cooperative Group & National Cancer Institute of Canada 1991; Awada *et al.* 1992; Devaux *et al.* 1992; Menichetti 1992). Moreover, bacteraemia with resident oral commensal flora might actually represent 'spillover' from a local infection rather than metastatic infection of the major organs (Donnelly *et al.* 1993).

## Effect of chemotherapy and irradiation on the intestinal tract

The ecology of the bowel flora will be altered markedly by diarrhoea induced by radiation and cytostatic chemotherapy, by GVHD (Guiot *et al.* 1987) and by total body irradiation (Callum *et al.* 1991) and can be exacerbated by viral infection (Yolken *et al.* 1982). Intensive chemotherapy can induce toxicity to the caecum, causing typhlitis or neutropenic enterocolitis, which is associated with the Gram-negative bacilli, particularly *Pseudomonas aeruginosa* and more recently *Clostridium septicum* (Johnson *et al.* 1994). Gut permeability also increases following conditioning therapy for BMT (Fegan *et al.* 1990; Johansson & Ekman 1997) as well as viral infection of the gut (Fegan *et al.* 1990). This may explain why the aminoglycosides, gentamicin and tobramycin, can be absorbed in patients with acute GVHD reactions and severe mucositis to yield serum concentrations within the therapeutic range when under normal circumstances absorption is negligible (Rohrbaugh *et al.* 1984). Gut motility will be reduced during parenteral nutrition because of the low amounts of fibre and reduced microbial biomass which result in dilute faeces.

## Impact of antimicrobial agents on colonization resistance of the alimentary tract

The anaerobic recesses of the bowel and the gingival crevices provide the ideal niche for those commensal bacteria, particularly the anaerobic Gram-positive non-sporing lactic acid-producing bacilli, such as *Bifidobacterium* spp., that contribute to the so-called colonization resistance (Donnelly 1993), i.e. the facility to withstand the establishment of exogenous or allochthonous organisms which is known as colonization resistance (Van der Waaij 1989; Vollaard & Clasener 1994). These bacteria are also the most vulnerable to the action of cell-wall-active antimicrobial agents, such as the penicillins, as well as other agents,

such as clindamycin, exposure to which radically perturbs the microbial ecology of the mucosal surfaces. However, the integrity of the mucosa, the production of saliva and mucus, peristalsis, gastric pH, bile acids, digestive enzymes and the levels of secretory IgA also have an important role in maintaining colonization resistance (Van der Waaij 1989). This balanced milieu is considered responsible for keeping the numbers of endogenous Gram-negative bacilli, e.g. *Escherichia coli*, in check while restricting the ability of other exogenous species that are regularly ingested in food and drink, e.g. *Klebsiella pneumoniae* and *P. aeruginosa*, from establishing a foothold.

The few commensal species that do infect immunosuppressed individuals, e.g. the oral viridans streptococci, are actually poorly adapted to the environment within the body proper. When infection does develop, it is usually the combined result of treatment with antimicrobial agents generating selective pressure favouring species such as *S. oralis* and the loss of integrity manifested by mucositis induced by chemotherapy, resulting in bacteraemia.

In addition to carrying bacteria many of us harbour yeasts, usually *Candida albicans*, on the mucosal surfaces of the oral cavity and bowel. Some also carry less common so-called non-*albicans Candida* species such as *Candida* (*Torulopsis*) *glabrata* and *Candida krusei*. *Candida parapsilosis* is a lipophilic relative of *C. albicans* and is found on the skin of some individuals around the apocrine secretions of the axilla. *Pityrosporum ovale* (*Malassezia furfur*) also inhabits the skin of some individuals. None of these yeasts are professional pathogens but all can and do cause opportunistic infections.

Exposure to a variety of antimicrobial agents, including penicillins, cephalosporins, rifamycin, clindamycin, erythromycin, bacitracin and vancomycin, will impair, if not destroy, colonization resistance, resulting in overgrowth of yeasts and enterococci (Van der Waaij 1984; Donnelly 1993). Consequently, cell surfaces may become vacant, allowing exogenous bacteria such as *P. aeruginosa* to establish themselves permanently, rendering the individual vulnerable to invasion and systemic dissemination when the mucosal barrier is damaged, e.g. by chemotherapy. Other β-lactam antibiotics, for example the carbapenems and the quinolones, e.g. ciprofloxacin, appear to have a much less deleterious effect on colonization resistance, although this may only be true when the gut functions normally. Antibiotics such as ceftazidime and piperacillin that individually appear to spare colonization resistance might have a marked impact when given in combination (Meijer-Severs & Joshi 1989). Prophylaxis with the fluoroquinolones, such as ofloxacin and ciprofloxacin, is safe and effective in preventing infection caused by Gram-negative bacilli of the Enterobacteriaceae, as well as *P. aeruginosa*, but resistance has been reported to have emerged among the indigenous *E. coli* of neutropenic patients (Cometta *et al.* 1994; Kern *et al.* 1994; Zinner *et al.* 1994).

Given its dependence on normal gut function, it is doubtful whether colonization resistance will remain intact following conditioning treatment for haematopoietic stem cell transplantation. Thus, the recipient will run the risk of acquiring nosocomial bacilli, e.g. *K. pneumoniae* and *P. aeruginosa*, from the environment unless isolated to some extent from the hospital environment and given only a low microbial-content diet.

## Impact on non-specific systemic host defences

### INHIBITORY SUBSTANCES IN NATURAL SECRETIONS

Lysozyme is a potent enzyme found in saliva, plasma, tears and inside phagocytic cells and cleaves *N*-acetyl muramic acid, which is a vital component of the bacterial cell wall. Production of the enzyme is impaired during bone marrow aplasia because of neutropenia and when the amount of saliva is reduced after irradiation. Its absence in body fluids could conceivably play a part in the occurrence of the Gram-positive cocci that predominate during this time, as Gram-positive bacteria are usually the most vulnerable to enzyme action, not being protected by an outer membrane of lipid as are the Gram-negative bacilli.

Tuftsin is a small peptide that binds to the Fc portion of IgG and becomes involved in activating phagocytes after being released from the immunoglobulin by leucokinase, which is bound to the membranes of neutrophils and macrophages, and tuftsin endocarboxypeptidase, which is produced in the spleen. Recipients of allogeneic haematopoietic stem cell transplants will therefore be deficient in tuftsin as they are functionally asplenic.

Allogeneic haematopoietic stem cell transplantation also leads to a less efficient complement system as there is less of the complement factor properdin, rendering patients more at risk for bacterial infections. Moreover, a lack of C3b, which normally induces phagocytosis, and C3a, which interacts with mast cells to induce inflammation, will further exacerbate immunosuppression and result in the well-known muted response to infection.

### COMMUNICATION MOLECULES (CYTOKINES)

#### IL-6

IL-6 is an inducer of the acute-phase response (hence a proinflammatory cytokine) and appears to be involved in the pathogenesis of several disease states, including GVHD, following allogeneic bone marrow transplantation. Serum levels of IL-6 are elevated after haematopoietic stem cell transplantation at a time when most patients suffer from mucositis and are febrile. Levels of IL-6 closely mirror changes in serum C-reactive protein (CRP) but are not predictive for non-infectious major transplant-related complications (Chasty *et al.* 1993). The concentrations of the cytokine peaks about 10 days after transplantation when platelet engraftment takes place (Steffen *et al.* 1997). At the same time concentrations of cyclosporin and one of its metabolites increase, suggesting that the variable pharmacokinetics of cyclosporin frequently observed after transplant might be the result of an inflammatory reaction brought about by endogenous IL-6 inhibiting cytochrome P450 3A-dependent enzyme activities (Chen *et al.* 1994). Besides being involved in the induction of acute-phase proteins, IL-6 stimulates haematopoietic stem cell growth and thrombopoiesis.

A functional haematopoietic system is clearly not necessary for regular production of the cytokine because patients continue to mount an inflammatory response during the aplastic phase following transplantation. Indeed, the levels of IL-6 are no different from those of other febrile patients and it is thought that cells other than those of the monocyte lineage contribute to its production.

### Other cytokines

While there is a clear association between elevated IL-6 levels and an elevated body temperature and CRP levels, there is no connection with tumour necrosis factor (TNF) production, which is usually only detectable in a few patients and not associated with infection (Pechumer *et al.* 1995). By contrast, an increase in soluble TNF receptor levels appears to be associated with transplant-related complications (Chasty *et al.* 1993).

Elevated TNF levels are not specific for infection *per se* but, as with IL-6, are associated with inflammatory disorders in general. Moreover, plasma concentrations of IL-1α, IL-1β and TNFα are more elevated during GVHD than at other times post-transplant although there is no correlation between the plasma concentrations and clinical manifestations of acute GVHD. However, when peripheral blood cells rather than plasma are used for monitoring cytoplasmic IL-1α and IL-1β, there is a better correlation with acute GVHD (Rowbottom *et al.* 1993). When human recombinant IL-1 is used clinically to shorten the duration of neutropenia the side effects of treatment include fever, chills and hypotension, suggesting that cytokine is involved naturally in these processes (Nemunaitis *et al.* 1994).

### ACUTE-PHASE REACTANTS

### C-reactive protein

Serum CRP, so called because it was found to bind to the phosphocholine moiety of the C-protein of *S. pneumoniae*, is one of the acute-phase reactants induced by IL-1, TNF and IL-6 in response to inflammation. CRP coats bacteria, resulting in opsonization and the fixing of complement. Levels above 100 mg/L have been associated with bacterial infection, but not with GVHD or viral or fungal infection (Walker *et al.* 1984a). However, others disagree, as there is no difference in CRP concentrations in the presence of GVHD with or without infection (Rowe *et al.* 1984). CRP levels may also be elevated in response to mucositis, which is often associated with bacteraemia, particularly with Gram-positive bacteria, such as viridans streptococci (Donnelly *et al.* 1993). Severe GVHD involving the entire surface area of the skin and the gastrointestinal tract may also be associated with similarly high levels of CRP, as found with bacterial infection and systemic candidosis (Pinter & Krivan 1996). In fact, CRP is produced in response to a wide variety of non-infectious inflammatory conditions as diverse as burns (Nijsten *et al.* 1987), pancreatitis (Viedma *et al.* 1992; Heath *et al.* 1993), ulcerative colitis (Raab *et al.* 1994), stress (Dugue *et al.* 1993), head injury (McClain *et al.* 1991) and myocardial infarction (Haq *et al.* 1993). However, when timed properly and interpreted together with clinical and microbiological findings, CRP measurements can be a valuable aid in the management of fever after BMT, especially as a negative predictor (De Bel *et al.* 1991).

Apart from opsonizing bacteria and fixing complement, CRP stimulates the production of IL-1 and TNF by mononuclear phagocytes *in vitro* and may do so at inflammatory sites where alterations of capillary permeability combined with an increased serum level lead to enhanced local concentrations of this acute-phase protein (Ballou & Lozanski 1992; Galvederochemonteix *et al.* 1993).

### Other acute-phase reactants

Mannose-binding protein serum amyloid A protein and α1-acid glycoprotein are also produced in large amounts in response to inflammation whereas other substances are only produced in moderate amounts, including α1 proteinase inhibitors, α1-antichymotrypsin, which inhibit bacterial protease, complement factors C2, C9 and factor B, which augment complement function, caeruloplasmin, which is a reactive oxygen intermediate scavenger, fibronectin, which permits cell-to-cell binding, as well as fibrinogen, α2-macroglobulin, angiotensin and haptoglobulin. Levels of β2-microglobulin fall initially after conditioning therapy and gradually recover after the haematopoietic stem cell transplant takes. Concentrations of $\beta_2$-microglobulin are elevated by acute and chronic GVHD and by reactivation of herpes simplex virus, varicella-zoster virus and cytomegalovirus (CMV) infections but not by bacterial infections. A fall in levels of $\beta_2$-microglobulin can be used to monitor the success of treating chronic GVHD (Norfolk *et al.* 1987).

## Phagocytic cells

### MONONUCLEAR PHAGOCYTES

The monocytes that are still in the circulation have a short half-life of 3 days whereas those which have already migrated into the tissues may remain viable for several weeks. Thus, once the haematopoietic stem cell pool is ablated, no new monocytes will be generated. However, those in tissue continue to function, albeit less efficiently because they require the cooperation of activated T lymphocytes for the optimal killing of intracellular microorganisms.

### POLYMORPHONUCLEAR LEUCOCYTE OR NEUTROPHIL

Virtually all cytotoxic drugs used in the treatment of malignant diseases have a more or less dose-dependent deleterious effect on the proliferation of normal haematopoietic progenitor cells, particularly those of the myeloid series. Consequently, the conditioning regimens used to prepare for a transplant all result in depletion of the marrow pool reserve and neutropenia of several days or even weeks ensues. Cytotoxic chemotherapy and irradiation also interfere with those cells already in the circulation by diminishing their capacity for chemotaxis, phagocytosis and intracellular killing.

Even after the graft takes and the bone marrow begins to recover, the neutrophilic granulocytes may find themselves in a hostile environment created by glucocorticosteroids used to manage GVHD. These drugs will mobilize the marginal as well as marrow pool reserve but they will impede migration to any site of inflammation by reducing the neutrophil's response to chemotaxis and its capacity to adhere to, ingest and kill microorganisms in a dose-dependent fashion. Several other drugs, including antimicrobial agents, are also known to interfere adversely with the generation of granulocytes. For instance, co-trimoxazole can delay neutrophil recovery (Imrie *et al.* 1995; Lew *et al.* 1995). Others, e.g. ceftazidime and meropenem, can impair neutrophil function at least *in vitro* by reducing the production of the reactive oxygen intermediates hypochlorite, superoxides, singlet oxygen, hydroxyl radicals and hydrogen peroxide (Matera *et al.* 1995; Mathyhartert *et al.* 1995), while the fluoroquinolones may actually enhance function (Kubo *et al.* 1994). The lack of neutrophils will also mean lower levels of lactoferrin and bacterial permeability-increasing factor, therefore leaving more iron available to any potential pathogens and decreasing the capacity for mopping up circulating endotoxin.

Neutropenia is thought to be the single most important factor in the increased risk of infection because there is an inverse correlation between the number of circulating neutrophils and the frequency of infection. Moreover, virtually all patients with profound neutropenia (neutrophil count of $<0.1\times10^9$/L for more than 3 weeks) will develop an infectious complication (Bodey *et al.* 1966). The risk for further infections also increases proportionally with the duration of neutropenia, as does the attributable mortality. It is therefore not surprising that the haematopoietic growth factors recombinant human granulocyte colony-stimulating factor (rhG-CSF) and recombinant human granulocyte–macrophage colony-stimulating factor (rhGM-CSF) have been investigated for their potential to shorten neutropenia. Treatment with these CSFs does accelerate recovery of peripheral neutrophil counts after haematopoietic stem cell transplantation, thereby reducing the duration of neutropenia by a few days without either increasing the rate of relapse or the incidence and severity of GVHD, as was initially feared (Frampton & Faulds 1996; Locatelli *et al.* 1996), and this treatment can be used to overcome graft failure (Grant & Heel 1992). Furthermore, because of the shorter neutropenia, less intravenous treatment with antimicrobial agents and other therapies, such as packed red blood cell transfusions, are required so patients can be discharged that much earlier (Martin Algarra *et al.* 1995). The infection-related mortality also appears somewhat lower (De Witte *et al.* 1991). G-CSF appears well tolerated but can cause fatigue and has been reported to cause ARDS when there are pre-existing pulmonary infiltrates (Demuynck *et al.* 1995), whereas GM-CSF induces mild to moderate flu-like symptoms and fever and can cause fluid retention. Moreover, the savings in costs are only marginal (Souetre *et al.* 1996) so these agents tend to be used for specific indications, such as for reversing the prolonged neutropenia associated with the use of methotrexate to prevent GVHD (Martin Algarra *et al.* 1995), and may prove worthwhile adjuncts to therapy for fungal and other infections (Bodey *et al.* 1994; Maher *et al.* 1994; Peters *et al.* 1996).

The availability of G-CSF has led to a resurgence in interest in giving leucocyte transfusions to infected patients because this drug increases the granulocyte count in donors, thereby permitting large numbers of mature myeloid cells to be collected by leucophaeresis (Grigg *et al.* 1996). The drug is well tolerated by most donors although fatigue appears a common complaint after a second collection. However, these infusions only help septic patients who have neither multiorgan dysfunction nor extensive pulmonary infection.

THROMBOCYTOPATHY

Thrombocytopenia and decreased function of existing thrombocytes invariably result from irradiation and cytostatic chemotherapy, leading to an increased susceptibility to infection and a lesser capacity to repair damaged tissues. Thrombocytopenia is also an independent risk factor for bacteraemia (Viscoli *et al.* 1994) and diffuse alveolar haemorrhage frequently has a role in fatal infections (Agusti *et al.* 1995).

## Suppression of the humoral response

The humoral system recognizes a plethora of bacterial or viral microorganisms as well as the soluble proteins they release. IgM is secreted early and plasma cells become committed during differentiation to producing the other classes of immunoglobulin, namely IgG, IgA, IgE and IgD (Van der Meer 1994). The specific functions of IgG and IgM include neutralization of the antigen, activation of complement and opsonization. Radiotherapy combined with chemotherapy results in lower antibody levels and increased susceptibility to infections with the encapsulated bacteria, particularly *S. pneumoniae* and *Haemophilus influenzae*, probably because, in the absence of opsonizing antibodies, complement and tuftsin, the capsule enables the bacteria to elude phagocytosis. In both allogeneic and autologous haematopoietic stem cell transplant recipients the greatest risk for infections by these bacteria occurs during the first 1–2 years after transplant (Parkkali *et al.* 1996) and their susceptibility to pneumococcal disease may also be related to lowered concentrations of antibody to pneumococci after engraftment (Giebink *et al.* 1986). Serum and salivary levels of each IgA, IgG and IgM diminish after transplant. IgM recovers around 6 months post-transplant whereas both IgA and IgG only do so after 1 year (Norhagen *et al.* 1994). By contrast, serum IgE concentrations are elevated during episodes of infection and GVHD (Walker *et al.* 1984b).

Secretory IgA, which is found on mucosal surfaces, is not an opsonin but it inhibits the motility of bacteria, neutralizes their toxins and prevents their adherence to epithelial cells. Serum and salivary IgA levels are low during the first 6 months after allogeneic haematopoietic stem cell transplant and take as long as 2 years before returning to normal (Abedi *et al.* 1990). Children have lower IgA levels at 3 and 6 months post-transplant than do adults; this is not dependent upon the age of the donor. Prophylaxis with either methotrexate or cyclosporin alone for GVHD results in markedly lower IgA levels than are found in patients given both drugs or in those transplanted with T cell-depleted marrow, but mean IgA levels are within the normal range 3 months after BMT. Patients with grade II or III acute GVHD maintain lower levels between 3 and 24 months after transplantation and IgA levels in those with chronic GVHD remain low for 1 or 2 years after haematopoietic stem cell transplant. Severe acute GVHD seems to be the main reason for IgA deficiency although other factors, such as CMV infection and donor status, might also play a part (Abedi *et al.* 1990). Circulating IgA probably has only a minor role in host defence and such concentrations of secretory IgA as are available may be further reduced by IgA1 proteases which are elaborated by the oral commensals *S. mitis* biovar 1, *Streptococcus sanguis* and *Haemophilus parahaemolyticus* as well as *Haemophilus influenzae* and *S. pneumoniae* (Kilian *et al.* 1995).

## Suppression of cell-mediated responses

The cellular immune system is charged with eliminating cells that present a 'foreign' immunological profile, such as those infected with intracellular microbial pathogens, including viruses. Both specific cells, such as T helper and cytotoxic T cells, and non-specific cells, including macrophages, neutrophils and natural killer (NK) cells, are required for the system to fulfil its function. Thus cell-mediated immunity is severely impaired following haematopoietic stem cell transplant, especially when the recipient has been irradiated.

Normal macrophages have a limited capacity for killing ingested microorganisms and various organisms, e.g. *Toxoplasma gondii*, *Pneumocystis carinii*, *Cryptococcus* spp., *Listeria* spp., *Salmonella* spp. and *Legionella* spp., are able to survive and replicate inside the cell, unless the macrophage becomes activated. The activation of macrophages is a complex process which is primarily under the control of cytokines. IFN-γ, produced by NK cells and Th cells, is the most important player in the field but the presence of TNFα is also required. The activated macrophage is characterized by morphological changes, expression of certain antigens, increased oxygen consumption and a marked up-regulation of both oxygen-dependent and nitric oxide-based microbicidal mechanisms, enabling the cell to kill intracellular pathogens.

The lack of cytotoxic effector cells means that lysis of virus-infected or foreign lymphocytes and macrophages is impaired and the reduced number of helper T cells leads to dysfunctional delayed-type hypersensitivity reactions. Moreover, any antigen that is presented on the surface of macrophages and dendritic cells will not be recognized. The lack of helper T cells will also mean the induction of TNFα and IL-12

will not proceed because of the lack of helper T cells, and so the NK cells will not be activated to produce interferon (IFN-γ). Consequently, there will be no activation of macrophage nitrate synthase and no reactive oxygen metabolites produced, which are essential for killing microorganisms.

A lack of the helper T cells that produce IL-2, IL-3, GM-CSF and IFN-γ will lead to fewer cytokine-producing T cells and IL-12 and TNFα will be less efficient in stimulating NK cells to produce IFN-γ. In the absence of this interferon, the extravasation of monocytes and other non-specific inflammatory cells will be impaired because the necessary changes in nearby endothelial cells cannot take place as normal and there will be fewer cellular adhesion molecules and no IL-8 secreted. Without these reactions there will be no influx of neutrophils and monocytes into the site of infection. However, macrophages that do manage to become activated will begin to produce IL-10 but will be unable to initiate negative feedback in the absence of NK cells and the lack of specific T cells will mean little cellular response to infection.

## Disarray of the immune response

Thus, by the time the haematopoietic stem cell transplant takes place, the immune system is in complete disarray. The risk for infection and the types of microorganisms are more or less commensurate with the summation of the individual immune defects (Fig. 19.4). The professional pathogens have a freer rein to advance their own survival, with the encapsulated bacteria gaining a distinct advantage in the absence of opsonizing immunoglobulins and the intracellular pathogens enjoying a much less hostile environment because of the lack of functioning T lymphocytes. The opportunistic pathogens that inhabit the mucosal surfaces find themselves able to invade relatively easily because the altered permeability and damaged integument enhance their translocation and the absence of neutrophils allows their dissemination. Finally, those microorganisms that are able to set up home on the surfaces of an intravascular device can now take full advantage of the ready access afforded by the device.

The remnants of the immune system may also prove

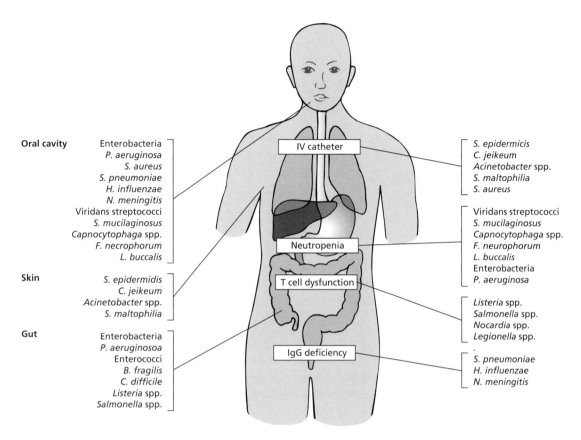

**Oral cavity**
Enterobacteria
*P. aeruginosa*
*S. aureus*
*S. pneumoniae*
*H. influenzae*
*N. meningitis*
Viridans streptococci
*S. mucilaginosus*
*Capnocytophaga* spp.
*F. necrophorum*
*L. buccalis*

**Skin**
*S. epidermidis*
*C. jeikeum*
*Acinetobacter* spp.
*S. maltophilia*

**Gut**
Enterobacteria
*P. aeruginosoa*
Enterococci
*B. fragilis*
*C. difficile*
*Listeria* spp.
*Salmonella* spp.

IV catheter

*S. epidermicis*
*C. jeikeum*
*Acinetobacter* spp.
*S. maltophilia*
*S. aureus*

Viridans streptococci
*S. mucilaginosus*
*Capnocytophaga* spp.
*F. neurophorum*
*L. buccalis*
Enterobacteria
*P. aeruginosa*

Neutropenia

T cell dysfunction

*Listeria* spp.
*Salmonella* spp.
*Nocardia* spp.
*Legionella* spp.

IgG deficiency

*S. pneumoniae*
*H. influenzae*
*N. meningitis*

**Fig. 19.4** Immune defects and infecting organisms. The nature of infecting organisms is determined partly by their habitat, e.g. skin or mucous membranes, and partly by the host defences mobilized against them. Knowledge of the resident microflora of a particular habitat and the nature of the immune defect can provide a clue to the likely cause of infection but is insufficient to allow an accurate prediction. Enterobacteria includes *Escherichia coli* and other members of the Enterobacteriaceae.

damaging. For instance, the local production of pro-inflammatory cytokines might give rise to the development of pulmonary oedema (Quabeck 1994) and an initial exaggerated pulmonary inflammatory response that, if it persists unabated over time, can result in ARDS (Meduri *et al.* 1995). Just as important, the development of fever and the triggering of an acute-phase response are no longer reliable heralds of an infectious process but instead may reflect inflammation induced by other processes, such as mucositis or GVHD, rather than active infection. Moreover, the use of high doses of glucocorticosteroids to treat GVHD will often cause a drop in temperature.

Remnants of the immune system can also lead to other complications associated with the transplant, such as renal failure associated with haemolytic uraemic syndrome, in which complement and IgM accumulate in the kidneys.

## Infectious complications

Infectious complications can be divided into four relatively distinct phases in relation to the transplant:
1 pretransplant;
2 the engraftment or neutropenic phase;
3 early postengraftment, covering the first 100 days

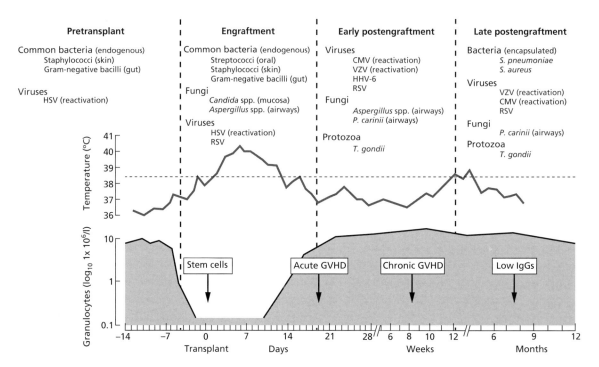

**Fig. 19.5** Infectious phases following transplant. The *pretransplant phase* corresponds with conditioning treatment and usually includes the insertion of a ventral intravenous catheter of 1 or 2 lumens. The neutropenia and mucosal barrier injury that occur place the patient in double jeopardy since the damage to the integument allows access to bacteria and yeasts that reside on the mucosal and cutaneous surfaces, and the lack of phagocytic cells permits their further invasion and spread. In addition, radiotherapy reactivates herpes simplex which can exacerbate mucositis, extend to the oesophagus as well as predispose to oral and oesophageal candidosis. During the entire *engraftment phase*, the patient remains profoundly neutropenic, thrombocytopenic and has oral and intestinal mucositis. Hence, local infections can lead to systemic disease, and certain organisms such as *Escherichia coli* can translocate from the mucosal surfaces to the bloodstream leading to sepsis. The initial period of risk of

bacterial and fungal infection resolves with recovery of the granulocytes after which the autologous stem cell transplant recipient is usually no longer at risk of infection. By contrast, the allogeneic stem cell transplant recipient remains vulnerable to developing infectious complications *postengraftment* depending upon the pace of reconstitution of the various components of the immune system and the development and treatment of graft-versus-host disease (GVHD). Bacteria seldom cause infectious disease during GVHD, being largely replaced by fungi, particularly *Aspergillus fumigatus*, and viruses as pathogens. Once GVHD has resolved, or is at least under control, the patient remains hypogammaglobulinaemic for months if not years and is unable to opsonize bacteria effectively so is vulnerable to infections of the respiratory tract due to encapsulated organisms such as *Streptococcus pneumoniae*.

after transplant and coinciding with the onset of acute and chronic GVHD; and

4 late postengraftment, the period thereafter (Fig. 19.5), which corresponds with the reconstitution of the immune system and is characterized by hypogammaglobulinaemia.

## Infections before transplant

There are few infectious complications before transplant, possibly because most patients have already been heavily treated with broad-spectrum antimicrobial therapy during previous courses of chemotherapy and are relatively free of potential pathogens. Moreover the full toxicity of the conditioning treatment is usually not yet manifest.

REMOVAL OF THE GRAFT

The graft and its procurement are a potential source of infection for the recipient but this rarely occurs in the case of bacteria because bone marrow is normally sterile. Potential contamination of bone marrow allografts can occur during their manipulation *in vitro*, when T cells are depleted either physically or by immunological means to minimize the risk of GVHD, but the incidence is low (Prince *et al.* 1995), being 1–2% for harmless commensal flora and less than 0.2% for potentially pathogenic Gram-negative bacilli. However, one of the earliest outbreaks of bacteraemia caused by viridans streptococci was attributed to contamination of the graft (Henslee *et al.* 1984; Mascret *et al.* 1984) even though the likelihood of this happening was remote, given that these bacteria originate from the oral cavity and are usually only transferred by droplets produced by coughing or sneezing.

## Sequence of events during neutropenia

Profound neutropenia and mucosal damage usually develop about a week after the start of cytoreductive chemotherapy and oral mucositis can be particularly severe when anthracyclines are combined with total body irradiation and cyclophosphamide (Raemaekers *et al.* 1989). There are usually other toxicities, particularly those affecting the alimentary tract. Nausea and vomiting are commonplace symptoms of extramedullary side effects of conditioning regimens during the first week of treatment. Serotonin (5-hydroxytryptamine) receptor antagonists are at least as effective in preventing and treatment of emesis than traditional remedies, such as chlorpromazine, and, because they result in less sedation and are better tolerated, their use has improved the outlook for most patients markedly (Tiley *et al.* 1992; Bosi *et al.* 1993; Roberts & Priestman 1993; Schwella *et al.* 1994; Spitzer *et al.* 1994; Agura *et al.* 1995; Barbounis *et al.* 1995). Nausea and diarrhoea can also be signs of gut toxicity, which is associated with permeability changes which begin within 12 days of initiating cytotoxic conditioning therapy, but they only become clinically apparent 4–7 days post-transplant, i.e. 10–14 days after starting chemotherapy (Johansson & Ekman 1997). The nausea and diarrhoea reach their peak about 1 week after transplant, which is when most damage to the oral mucosa occurs, as evidenced by severe oral mucositis (Sable & Donowitz 1994). This also coincides with maximum gut permeability, which might explain the severe diarrhoea experienced by recipients of autologous bone marrow transplants conditioned by total body irradiation (Callum *et al.* 1991).

Bacterial complications differ widely between the different types of transplant recipient. Almost all bone marrow transplant recipients develop fever within a few days after receiving the graft (Menichetti *et al.* 1989; De Pauw *et al.* 1990; Callum *et al.* 1991; Wimperis *et al.* 1991; Schmeiser *et al.* 1993). However, infectious complications invariably coincide with the worsening of oral mucositis and the increase in gut permeability, with fever developing around 3–4 days after transplant (Fig. 19.6). Bacteraemia caused by organisms other than coagulase-negative staphylococci also tend to occur at the same time. By contrast, intraluminal colonization by coagulase-negative staphylococci of intravascular catheters tends to become established a few days later and may appear as a superinfection if the staphylococci are not cultured earlier. The risk of cutaneous infections related to the central venous device tends to increase with the length of time that the catheter has been in place and signs and symptoms usually manifest themselves during the first few days of fever, i.e. after 72 h or during the first week after transplant. Infectious complications related to the lung tend to occur a few days later, often being recognized only after 5–6 days of fever. The period of risk of bacterial and fungal infection diminishes with recovery of the granulocytes when the clinical manifestations of tissue infections may be temporarily exacerbated before finally resolving. However, GVHD, particularly its chronic form, can lead to a recurrence of neutropenia with the attendant increase in the risks of infection.

The duration of neutropenia corresponds closely

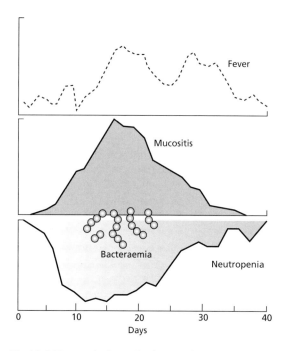

**Fig. 19.6** Temporal relationship between bacteraemia, fever, neutropenia and mucositis. This schematic representation is based on the author's original data. During a study of oral mucositis in 52 consecutive allogeneic BMT recipients, mucositis was scored daily and the neutrophil count was determined from the start of conditioning therapy. Blood was also obtained for culture each morning to detect bacteraemia. Oral viridans streptococci were detected in the blood of 32 patients within 8 days of the transplant when mucositis was already present but was not yet severe. There were no cases of bacteraemia before mucositis was present and none after mucositis began to subside.

with the incidence of infectious complications. An infectious complication rate of the order of 30–35% is not unusual although fever remains unexplained in two out of every three episodes. With the regular occurrence of mucositis and the use of fluoroquinolones and intravascular catheters, bacteraemia mostly involves the viridans streptococci, mostly *S. oralis* and *S. mitis*, and *S. epidermidis*. Localized infections are less frequent, complicating less than 5% of transplants, and are either related to the catheter in the form of an exit site or tunnel infection or to the lung.

### INFECTIONS CAUSED BY RESIDENT ORAL MICROFLORA

Although there are over 40 different bacterial species that reside on the epithelia of the upper respiratory tract and oral cavity, very few are capable of successful translocation into the bloodstream and fewer still of establishing disseminated infection (Table 19.1). During the course of a normal day the acts of chewing and teeth brushing lead to transient bacteraemia caused, mainly, by viridans streptococci but most of the species capable of causing any kind of infection do so only to a limited extent, leading to local necrosis and inflammation.

Mucositis is associated with bacteraemia caused by oral viridans streptococci, particularly *S. oralis* and *S. mitis* (Classen *et al.* 1990; De Pauw *et al.* 1990; Bochud *et al.* 1994a), and usually develops within 5–7 days of transplant (Valteau *et al.* 1991; Donnelly *et al.* 1993; Engelhard *et al.* 1995). The incidence is 5–10% but can be as high as 60% following conditioning with a regimen causing particularly severe mucositis (Donnelly *et al.* 1993). Prophylactic quinolones may actually increase the risk of bacteraemia caused by the oral viridans streptococci, which raises concern in haematopoietic stem cell transplant recipients because of the

**Table 19.1** Bacteraemia related to oral mucositis.

| Enterobacteria |
| --- |
|    *Escherichia coli* |
|    *Klebsiella pneumoniae* |
|    *Enterobacter cloacae* |
| Non-fermenting Gram-negative bacilli |
|    *Pseudomonas aeruginosa* |
| Viridans streptococci |
|    *Streptococcus oralis* |
|    *Streptococcus mitis* |
| Coagulase-negative staphylococci |
|    *Staphylococcus epidermidis* |
| Other Gram-positive cocci |
|    *Stomatococcus mucilaginosus* |
| Anaerobic bacteria |
|    *Leptotrichia buccalis* |
|    *Fusobacterium* spp. |
|    *Prevotella* spp. |
|    *Capnocytophaga* spp. |

putative risk of developing ARDS and sepsis syndrome, which appears to affect approximately 1 in 10 patients following both autologous (Steiner *et al.* 1993) and allogeneic haematopoietic stem cell transplantation (Martino *et al.* 1995). Other risk factors for streptococcal bacteraemia include age under 18 years and acute lymphocytic leukaemia (Villablanca *et al.* 1990). It is also likely that, as conditioning regimens become more intensive, oromucositis will increase, leading to a commensurate increase in the number of unusual bacteria causing bacteraemia, especially Gram-positive oral commensals, such as *S. mucilaginosus* (Weers-Pothoff *et al.* 1989; McWhinney *et al.* 1992), and anaerobes, such as *Capnocytophaga* spp. (Bilgrami *et al.* 1992). Moreover, while bone marrow recovery can be accelerated by the use of the growth factors G-CSF and GM-CSF (Schuster 1992; Bronchud 1993), these agents do not appear to have any influence on oromucositis (De Witte *et al.* 1993). However, despite the frequent morbidity associated with Gram-positive infections the attributable mortality is negligible.

Approximately half of patients are carriers of *C. albicans* before transplant, which rises to almost every patient by the end of neutropenia (Chandrasekar *et al.* 1994). Colonization of both the oral cavity and gut or persistent colonization at one or other of these sites is a risk factor for candidosis (Verfaillie *et al.* 1991). Oral mucositis also appears to be a major risk factor. Prolonged treatment with azole antifungal agents, such as fluconazole, reduces carriage of *C. albicans* but selects naturally resistant species, such as *C. krusei* and *C. glabrata* (Goodman *et al.* 1992; Chandrasekar *et al.* 1994; Wingard 1994).

### INFECTIONS CAUSED BY RESIDENT GUT MICROFLORA

The alimentary tract is the major reservoir of Gram-negative bacilli which are endogenous, e.g. *E. coli* (Schimpff 1993). Other Gram-negative bacilli, such as *P. aeruginosa*, *Enterobacter cloacae* and *Stenotrophomonas* (*Xanthomonas*) *maltophilia*, are exogenous organisms found in the environment, particularly soil and unwashed vegetables, but once acquired may establish themselves as part of the resident flora, which will increase the risk that the carrier will become infected by them. Carriage will normally be detected by surveillance cultures of the oral cavity and intestinal tract, but it is by no means certain that this will inevitably lead to infection.

*Escherichia coli*, *Enterobacter cloacae* and *P. aeruginosa* are know to cause infections during the neutropenia that follows BMT (Winston 1993). Consequently, many centres give fluoroquinolone as prophylaxis, which effectively suppresses these bacteria and has virtually eradicated infection caused by Gram-negative bacilli (Menichetti *et al.* 1989; De Pauw *et al.* 1990; Schmeiser *et al.* 1993). However, selective oral antimicrobial prophylaxis has little or no positive impact in reducing infections caused by Gram-positive bacteria in recipients of haematopoietic stem cell transplants (Menichetti *et al.* 1989; De Pauw *et al.* 1990); indeed, these agents may actually increase them.

### CUTANEOUS INFECTIONS

Cutaneous infections in the immunocompromised patient can also develop from needle punctures but the insertion of catheters provides the single most effective means of breaching the skin barrier and creating ready access for microorganisms to both the stratum corneum and the bloodstream. Intravenous catheters are often essential for the successful management of immunocompromised patients because they provide ready and safe access to the bloodstream with minimal trauma and discomfort. With good technique the complications resulting from inserting indwelling catheters, such as the Hickman device, are minimal.

The use of intravenous catheters allows skin commensals a portal of entry into the bloodstream, while other devices, such as urinary catheters and ventilators, introduce further opportunities for nosocomial infection. Colonization of intravenous catheters with skin staphylococci, particularly *S. epidermidis*, is probably virtually universal (Raad & Bodey 1992) and affects mainly the catheter lumen. These organisms have a predilection for hydrophobic surfaces and a proclivity to form biofilms. The incidence of such bacteraemia, which some consider as a catheter-related infection, appears to depend upon whether or not access to the device is achieved by an implanted port, as well as how frequently (Groeger *et al.* 1993; Alnor *et al.* 1994), reflecting the fact that the hub is the most likely source of contamination (Salzman *et al.* 1993). This is thought to be the common route of infection by other, normally minor, residents of the skin flora, e.g. *Corynebacterium urealyticum*, which are given a selective advantage by antimicrobial agents (Wood & Pepe 1994) because they are frequently multiply resistant and only appear to cause catheter-related infections. Exotic saprophytic bacteria, such as Gram-negative non-fermentative bacilli *Comomonas acidovorans* (Castagnola *et al.* 1994), *Ochrobactrum anthropi* and *Agrobacterium* spp. (Alnor *et al.* 1994), as well as the more common and familiar species of Gram-negative bacilli, including *P. aeruginosa*, that are found in aqueous environments, also gain access this way. In fact, the ability to attach to the plastic used to make catheters and to grow in biofilms producing copious amounts of slime seems to be a prerequisite for colonization of the device and, under such circumstances, antibiotic treatment rarely achieves a complete cure, necessitating removing the catheter (Table 19.2).

**Table 19.2** Microbaemia related to intravascular catheters.

---

Coagulase-negative staphylococci
  *Staphylococcus epidermidis*
  *Staphylococcus haemolyticus*
Other Gram-positive bacteria
  *Corynebacterium jeikeum*
  *Stomatococcus mucilaginosus*
Gram-negative bacilli
  *Pseudomonas aeruginosa*
  *Stenotrophomonas maltophilia*
  *Acinerobacter* spp.
  *Enterobacter* spp.
Miscellaneous bacteria
  *Mycobacerium* spp.
Yeasts
  *Candida parapsilosis*
  *Candida albicans*

---

Microbaemia is a term coined to avoid the impression of there being a bloodstream infection simply because a given microorganism has been detected in blood which has, in fact, simply served as a means of transporting the microorganism from one place to another.

By contrast, colonization of the external surface of a catheter may lead to infection of the catheter–tissue interface at the exit site, which occasionally extends along the track, causing cellulitis when a tunnelled device, such as the Hickman catheter, is involved, or phlebitis. These infections occur much less frequently than does intraluminal colonization and tend to involve other resident Gram-positive bacteria, including *C. jeikeum* and *S. mucilaginosus* and occasionally some exogenous Gram-negative bacilli, e.g. *Enterobacter cloacae*, *Acinetobacter* spp. and *Stenotrophomonas maltophilia*, which have established colonization beforehand. The catheter is also a portal of entry for fungi, including *C. parapsilosis* and other candida (Lecciones *et al.* 1992), and can be for moulds, such as *Aspergillus* spp. and *Rhizopus* spp. Once established, such truly cutaneous infections are very difficult to treat without removing the device.

Infections associated with intravenous catheters more often than not represent colonization of the lumen, which gives rise to bacteraemia and therefore presents a therapeutic dilemma. On the one hand, treatment with drugs administered intraluminally seldom succeeds in sterilizing the device, while on the other hand intraluminal colonization rarely poses a threat to the patient and metastatic infection with *S. aureus*, *Candida* spp. and Gram-negative bacilli has been rarely encountered. Persistent colonization with coagulase-negative staphylococci or *C. jeikeum* often leads to repeated episodes of bacteraemia, which may only be noticed when the patient experiences shaking chills, tachycardia, hypotension and peripheral cyanosis after the line is manipulated, the classic manifestations of intraluminal colonization. However, persistent bacteraemia caused by *S. epidermidis* is more usually little more than a manifestation of intraluminal colonization which can appear to be eradicated during treatment with glycopeptides only to rebound once therapy is discontinued or even a few hours after the drug has been infused through the line in a vain attempt to flush the organism out (Fig. 19.7). Needless to say catheter-related infections remain a fertile ground for hot controversy and for further investigations for prevention and management.

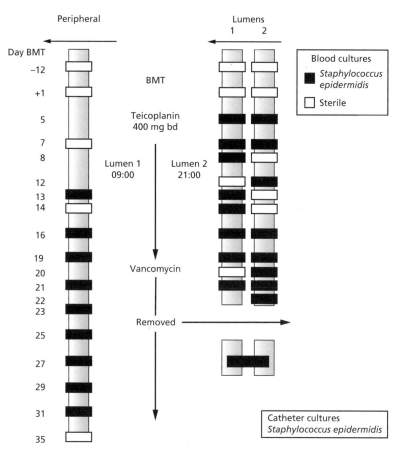

**Fig. 19.7** Catheter colonization and bacteraemia. The case of catheter-related bacteraemia depicted in this figure is not unusual and illustrates the difficulty in trying to sterilize a catheter *in situ*. The patient had received a double-lumen subclavian catheter 13 days before transplant and blood was obtained from each lumen twice weekly to detect colonization. *Staphylococcus epidermidis* was duly detected from both lumens 5 days after insertion and again 2 days later. It was therefore decided to administer the glycopeptide teicoplanin to each lumen every 24 h to try to eliminate the bacteria. This manoeuvre failed as the same bacteria were recovered repeatedly from venous blood as well as blood drawn through the catheter and another glycopeptide drug, vancomycin, was tried for 4 days. This too failed to eliminate the colonization so the catheter was removed altogether. The bacteria were recovered from cultures of the device and the patient remained bacteraemic for a further 2 weeks indicating that the vein in which the catheter had been lodged was also infected.

## Influence of other forms of supportive care

### IMMUNOSUPPRESSION TO PREVENT HOST REJECTION OF THE GRAFT AND VICE VERSA

Prophylaxis against GVHD has become an integral part of the standard protocols for allogeneic haematopoietic stem cell transplantation. Almost without exception, the regimen consists of cyclosporin with or without methotrexate (Ruutu *et al.* 1997b). However, among participants of the European Group for Blood and Marrow Transplantation wide variations existed between the parenteral dose, which ranged from 1 to 20 mg/kg/day with a mean of

3 mg/kg/day, and oral doses, from 2 to 12.5 mg/kg/day with a mean of 10 mg/kg/day. Treatment starts just before transplant and, while two-thirds of centres continue for approximately 12 weeks and then stop, the remainder may continue cyclosporin for 5–6 months. Treatment with cyclosporin alone results in a lower transplant-related mortality than is seen with the combination with methotrexate but is associated with increased risk for acute and chronic GVHD in recipients of grafts not depleted of T lymphocytes, as well as relapse of acute lymphocytic leukaemia (Bortin *et al.* 1993). Exposure to the drugs primarily causes impairment of cell-mediated immunity, leading to a reduction in the number and functions of various T cell subsets, including CD4 and CD8 cells, a decrease in IL-2 and the blastogenic response to CD4 cells and a lowered response to recall antigens. Depletion of IgG and IgM also occurs, the response of IgA to antigenic stimuli is attenuated and the pneumococcal polysaccharide is less immunogenic (Sable & Donowitz 1994). Neutrophils are less mobile and the alveolar macrophages become indifferent to chemotactic stimuli, ingest fewer bacteria and fungi and kill them less efficiently.

BLOOD AND BLOOD PRODUCTS

Blood and blood products intended for CMV-negative recipients are usually irradiated before infusion to minimize the risk of primary CMV infection.

## Infections after engraftment

### Graft vs. host disease

Graft vs. host disease remains the major complication of allogeneic BMT. T cells in the donor bone marrow recognize and react against host alloantigens and thereby initiate the disease, but it is not known exactly how the host tissues become damaged. There is a growing body of evidence to suggest that inflammatory cytokines act as mediators of acute GVHD and that most of the clinical manifestations can be accounted for by the unregulated production of cytokines by T cells and other inflammatory cells. Instead of an orderly cascade, perturbation of the cytokine network

induces a 'cytokine storm' which culminates in the rapid onset of severe, acute GVHD (Ferrara *et al.* 1993). By contrast, chronic GVHD may be an autoimmune disease and therefore quite different from acute GVHD (Parkman 1993).

ACUTE GRAFT VS. HOST DISEASE

Acute GVHD follows a sequence involving first the skin, resulting in a maculopapular rash, often on the palms and soles of the feet, then the gastrointestinal tract, causing diarrhoea, and finally the biliary tree, manifested by hyperbilirubinaemia and elevated alkaline phophatase and transaminases (Barrett 1989). The disease can also extend to the mucous membranes and the airways. In the small and the large intestine GVHD produces extensive destruction of mucosal tissue. Endocrine cells seem to be less vulnerable to the effects of GVHD than epithelial cells and are spared (Bryan *et al.* 1991).

The disease appears to be the result of donor T4 helper and T8 suppressor lymphocytes recognizing major histocompatibility antigens (the CD4 and CD8 accessory surface molecules of MHC class I and II, respectively). This results in the production of IL-2, which 'fuels the fire' of GVHD by clonally expanding the graft vs. host reactive cell population and both activating and inducing proliferation of NK cells, which are thought to have a prominent role in killing target cells, together with cytotoxic T lymphocytes and macrophages. TNF is also thought to be actively involved in the damage.

The severity of the disease is graded from I to IV according to the degree of damage to the skin, gastrointestinal tract and liver. Because the disease is all but inevitable except for syngeneic transplants, prophylaxis is universal and consists of daily cyclosporin with or without intermittent methotrexate. Depletion of T cells is also practised by some centres, using physical means of counterflow elutriation or immunological means, using antibodies such as CAMPATH-1.

Risk factors for acute GVHD include disparity between the histocompatibility and sex of the donor and recipient, their ages, lack of T cell depletion of the graft and of GVHD prophylaxis, the intensity of the conditioning treatment, reactivation of herpesvirus infections, particularly CMV and possibly human herpesvirus 6 (Appleton *et al.* 1995).

Treatment with methylprednisolone or an equivalent glucocorticosteroid is mostly given for grade II–IV GVHD but not grade I. There is wide variation in dosage, ranging from 0.5 mg/kg/day to 20 mg/kg/day and even higher (Ruutu *et al.* 1997b), even though there is no evidence that higher doses are more effective and doses in excess of 15 mg/kg/day carry a significant risk for aspergillosis. The steroids are thought to exert a non-specific anti-inflammatory effect and, when this fails, alternative treatments can include azathioprine and thalidomide as well as antithymocyte globulin and monoclonal antibodies to IL-2. Both acute GVHD and its treatment delay immunological recovery and prolong immunodeficiency, rendering the recipient vulnerable to all types of infections, whether reactivation, e.g. varicella-zoster virus (VZV), extracellular pathogens, e.g. Gram-negative bacilli, or intracellular pathogens, such as *P. carinii* and *T. gondii*.

### CHRONIC GRAFT VS. HOST DISEASE

Chronic GVHD is characterized by progression to scleroderma-like skin involvement, with hyperkeratosis, reticular hyperpigmentation, atrophy with ulceration and fibrosis with limitation of joint movement. Sicca syndrome, idiopathic interstitial pneumonitis and infectious complications are frequent, with DNA virus infections being prominent. A spectrum of immune abnormalities is observed, including hypergammaglobulinaemia, immunoglobulin M (IgM) paraprotein, elevated circulating immune complexes, plasma cell hyperplasia, lymphocytotoxic antibodies and autoantibodies to autologous or donor lymphocytes. Chronic GVHD appears to be a syndrome of disordered immune regulation with features of immunodeficiency and autoimmunity (Graze & Gale 1979).

Corticosteroids are still the mainstay for treating chronic GVHD but other remedies include ultraviolet irradiation with or without psoralen, penicillamine or azathioprine, thalidomide and, perhaps, the antimycobacterial drug clofazimine (Vogelsang *et al.* 1985; Lee *et al.* 1997)

## Infections during the early postengraftment phase

### BACTERIAL INFECTIONS

While receiving immunosuppression for the treatment or prevention of GVHD, allogeneic haematopoietic stem cell transplant recipients will be susceptible to intracellular pathogens, including mycobacteria. However, in one large series there were only nine (0.6%) of 1486 allograft haematopoietic stem cell transplant recipients and two (0.3%) of 755 autograft recipients affected. *Mycobacterium tuberculosis* and *Mycobacterium avium intracellulare* accounted for two cases each and the remainder involved the rapidly growing atypical mycobacteria *Mycobacterium fortuitum* and *Mycobacterium chelonae*, all but one of which was responsible for catheter-related tunnel infections (Roy & Weisdorf 1997).

Any patients treated in hospitals with inadequately maintained hot water supply and air conditioning units are at risk of becoming infected with *Legionella* spp. (Gentry & Zeluff 1988) although infection is very infrequent (Harrington *et al.* 1996).

Haematopoietic stem cell transplant recipients with deficient cell-mediated immunity can also be at risk for infection caused by other intracellular pathogens, including *Salmonella typhimurium*, *Nocardia* spp. and *Listeria monocytogenes* (Long *et al.* 1993). Infection with *S. typhimurium* can result from food poisoning and, because many eggs are infected, consumption of foodstuffs made from raw eggs should be avoided. Nocardiosis occurs in isolated cases (Freites *et al.* 1995) but outbreaks have occurred among renal transplant recipients and therefore exposure of all similarly immunosuppressed individuals should be avoided by placing infected individuals in isolation to prevent airborne transmission (Hellyar 1988). Patients with a predilection for soft cheeses made from unpasteurized milk are also at greater risk of becoming infected with *Listeria* spp., especially during the summer, and are advised to avoid these foodstuffs.

GVHD and its treatment has an even more profound effect because it often coincides with CMV infection, compromising the patient even further (Meyers *et al.*

1986). Such patients are again at risk of infection with the same range of pathogens encountered during neutropenia entering through the same portals of entry, namely the oral mucosa, gut and catheter, if one is present (Meyers 1986). The onset of infection may also be so abrupt that sepsis is already well established before fever develops, thereby increasing the likelihood of fulminant sepsis.

## VIRAL INFECTIONS

By the time we reach adulthood most of us have already been infected with most herpesviruses, including herpes simplex virus, CMV, Epstein–Barr virus, VZV and herpesvirus 6. Infected recipients of haematopoietic stem cell transplants are prone to reactivation of these viruses as a result of cytostatic chemotherapy, irradiation, GVHD and hypogammaglobulinaemia. Moreover, active infection with CMV and human herpesvirus 6 is itself immunosuppressive and can exacerbate GVHD. CMV infection probably induces myelosuppression by suppressing the production of IL-6, GM-CSF and G-CSF by the cells of the marrow microenvironment (Lagneaux *et al.* 1994).

## CYTOMEGALOVIRUS INFECTION

Cytomegalovirus disease manifested as interstitial pneumonitis remains a major complication of allogeneic haematopoietic stem cell transplantation. The development of the disease depends upon reactivation of infection in seropositive recipients and primary infection of seronegative recipients. However, other factors also play a part. For instance, donor CMV seropositivity appears protective against disease supporting the hypothesis that immunity against CMV can be adopted from donor T cell-depleted marrow (Webster *et al.* 1993). The development of GVHD is an independent risk factor and measures that reduce this disease, such as cyclosporin prophylaxis and T cell depletion, also result in a lower incidence of CMV interstitial pneumonitis (Griffiths 1993). Infection with CMV is also associated with an increase in the number of CD8+ T cell counts and a decrease in the relative proportion of CD4+ T cells and CD20+ B cells, as are

found during acute GVHD. The use of aciclovir to prevent herpes simplex infection also significantly reduces the risk both of CMV infection and disease in seropositive allogeneic bone marrow transplant (Meyers *et al.* 1988; Balfour 1990). Hyperimmunoglobulin does not prevent CMV infection or disease in CMV seronegative allogeneic haematopoietic stem cell transplant recipients who receive a transplant from a seropositive donor or who receive blood products unscreened for CMV during the treatment (Ruutu *et al.* 1997a). However, this approach does improve the outcome for seropositive recipients (Snydman 1990; Bass *et al.* 1993) although it has been largely superseded by the use of acyclovir as prophylaxis for herpes simplex infection. The use of blood products from CMV seronegative donors reduces the risk of primary CMV infection (Goodrich *et al.* 1994) but does not appear necessary for recipients of T-cell-depleted grafts (De Witte *et al.* 1990).

CMV interstitial pneumonitis is frequently fatal and failure of treatment to inhibit CMV infection markedly increased the risk of mortality (Neiman *et al.* 1977). There has, however, been marked progress in the diagnosis and treatment of CMV infection after allogeneic BMT. Seventy centres from 20 countries responded to a survey conducted by the European Group for Blood and Marrow Transplantation. Most centres rely on high-dose acyclovir for prophylaxis although some employ ganciclovir, even though this may prolong neutropenia. None the less, two-thirds still give hyperimmunoglobulin. Almost all centres routinely attempt diagnosis of CMV using blood, most with an isolation technique. However, just over half of them also look for antigens in leucocytes or employ polymerase chain reaction. Two-thirds of centres start treatment preemptively with ganciclovir when cytomegalovirus or its pp65 antigen is detected in the blood (Ljungman *et al.* 1993); a 3-week course of ganciclovir appears to offer the best balance between efficacy and toxicity (Singhal *et al.* 1995). However, the presence of CMV viraemia cannot be relied upon to predict CMV pneumonitis, which may be the result of local rather than disseminated CMV infection (Webster *et al.* 1993). Most centres obtain bronchoalveolar lavage but most do not wait for a result, preferring to treat suspected CMV interstitial pneumonitis and gastrointestinal disease with ganciclovir and intravenous immunoglobulin (Ljungman *et al*. 1993). Thus, a strategy of prophylactic acyclovir combined with pre-emptive treatment with ganciclovir when surveillance detects the pp65 antigen of CMV is likely to provide the best approach for reducing the risk of developing CMV disease in allogeneic CMV seropositive HLA-matched haematopoietic stem cell transplant recipients (Prentice & Kho 1997).

FUNGAL INFECTIONS

*Pulmonary aspergillosis*

The incidence of invasive pulmonary aspergillosis among recipients of haematopoietic stem cell transplants varies from 3 to 16%, depending upon whether or not complications have developed (Allan *et al*. 1988; McWhinney *et al*. 1993; Saugier Veber *et al*. 1993; Morrison *et al*. 1994; O'Donnell *et al*. 1994; Jantunen *et al*. 1997). Autologous haematopoietic stem cell transplants tend to develop the infection during neutropenia whereas recipients of allogeneic haematopoietic stem cell transplants are just as likely to develop the disease after engraftment when they are no longer in any form of protective isolation (Wingard *et al*. 1987; McWhinney *et al*. 1993; Morrison *et al*. 1994). Pulmonary disease is the most common manifestation and is sometimes accompanied by cerebral abscess, and *Aspergillus fumigatus* predominates (Morrison *et al*. 1994). Radiographic abnormalities can involve one or both lungs and infiltrates are usually alveolar but can be interstitial or mixed. Cavitary lesions are usually seen less frequently and later, after engraftment. The occurrence of alveolar or nodular pulmonary infiltrates during neutropenia or treatment for GVHD strongly suggests invasive mycosis (Allan *et al*. 1988). Mortality tends to be high, typically 60–80%, and the diagnosis is usually only confirmed post-mortem (Allan *et al*. 1988; Morrison *et al*. 1994).

Risk factors include those relating to the haematopoietic stem cell transplant recipient, such as underlying disease, particularly myelodysplastic syndrome (MDS), chronic myelogenous leukaemia and aplastic anaemia, and older age; those relating to the donor, namely matched-unrelated donor, or the procedure, e.g. allogeneic transplant, conditioning treatment; and those relating to the graft, namely delayed engraftment or prolonged granulocytopenia, or graft rejection. Factors relating to GVHD include the use of high-dose corticosteroids for prophylaxis as well as the presence of grade II–IV GVHD or extensive chronic GVHD and its treatment (Morrison *et al*. 1994; Jantunen *et al*. 1997). However, many of these factors assume less importance after multivariate analysis. For example, when only allogeneic recipients are considered, seropositive CMV status, delayed engraftment and age of 18 years or older are independent risk factors for fungal infection (Morrison *et al*. 1994).

Early diagnosis remains an intractable problem and the infection is still frequently confirmed at post-mortem. Specific antibodies are of no help but *Aspergillus* galactomannan antigen can be detected in serum at an early stage and may allow treatment to be started promptly before the disease has reached an advanced stage. The inability to obtain tissue poses the main difficulty in making a diagnosis and this is not overcome by bronchoalveolar lavage because this technique only seems useful for identifying those with diffuse pulmonary disease caused by *Aspergillus* infection (McWhinney *et al*. 1993).

More effective antifungal prophylaxis and therapy, earlier diagnosis and transplant regimens that result in a shorter period of neutropenia may substantially reduce the incidence and clinical impact of these infections (Morrison *et al*. 1994).

Patients who undergo surgical resection as part of the treatment for invasive aspergillosis are at no greater risk of recurrent aspergillosis than other haematopoietic stem cell transplant recipients are of primary infection (McWhinney *et al*. 1993; Hoover *et al*. 1997).

*Other mould infections*

Other moulds, such as *Fusarium* spp., *Alternaria* spp., *Rhizopus* spp., are much less common than is *Aspergillus fumigatus* in causing pulmonary infection but CMV is often also involved (Allan *et al*. 1988; Morrison *et al*. 1994).

*Pneumocystis carinii*

Long considered to be a protozoon, *P. carinii* is now accepted as a fungus, despite being susceptible to co-trimoxazole and pentamidine and not to the polyenes or azole antifungal agents. The incidence of infection with this organism is now less than 1%, most probably as a result of the widespread use of co-trimoxazole as prophylaxis. Indeed, patients who develop the disease are just those who, for one reason or another, are not taking the drug (Hoyle & Goldman 1994).

Pneumonia typically occurs within the first 6 months post-transplant and most patients have a history of graft rejection or relapsed malignancy. Symptoms include cough, dyspnoea and fever and diffuse alveolointerstitial infiltrates are seen on chest X-ray. On computed tomography (CT) scan there are areas of homogeneous attenuation having a 'ground-glass' appearance. Patients are hypoxic and half require mechanical ventilation. An increased percentage of lymphocytes, often accompanied by blasts, is seen in bronchoalveolar lavage samples (Leskinen *et al.* 1990) and diagnosis is established by detecting cysts in methenamine silver-stained preparations, although both direct fluorescence monoclonal antibody and calcofluor white provide acceptable alternatives for staining (Aslanzadeh & Stelmach 1996). Coinfection with CMV is common and *Aspergillus fumigatus* can also be involved. Mortality remains about one in three with the only variable with prognostic significance being the need for mechanical ventilation.

*Candidosis*

Resident flora, such as *Candida* spp., can establish a superficial infection, often as a result of reactivation of herpes simplex (Beattie *et al.* 1989; Bergmann 1992), marked by the presence of pseudomembranes over the ulcerated tissue, but can also initiate local invasion and progressive spread to the oesophagus and gastrointestinal tract, resulting in disseminated candidosis. While *C. albicans* predominates, other species may become more prominent as exposure to fluconazole begins to exert selective pressure, because some *Candida* species, such as *C. krusei* and *C. glabrata*, are naturally resistant to the azole. There has been a steady decline in the incidence of disseminated candidosis among haematopoietic stem cell transplant recipients, which may be the result of aciclovir prophylaxis or the increasing use of fluconazole for both prevention and early treatment.

## Infections during the late postengraftment phase

The process of reconstructing the immune system usually takes weeks and, in the case of allogeneic transplants, can take months or even years before becoming complete. During the often arduous journey the recipient has to be led through several periods of risk for infection and protected against the worst of the opportunistic pathogens. Therefore, one of the best ways of starting this journey is to ensure that the recipient is as healthy as possible, virtually free of the malignant disease and has no grumbling foci of infection that might erupt, multiply, spread throughout the body and overwhelm the remnants of the immunity. Clearly, any measures that can be taken to bolster residual defences should be adopted but one first has to look at the normal defences to understand the process from an infective perspective.

Following an allogeneic haematopoietic stem cell transplant, recovery of immune function takes up to a year, during which time patients are at high risk from CMV and VZV infections and also from *P. carinii* pneumonia. The response to vaccines is also likely to be poor. Patients with chronic GVHD have an increased susceptibility to bacterial, fungal and viral infections. Most patients who are free of chronic GVHD recover immune function fully and develop antibodies to specific recall antigens.

DYSFUNCTIONAL CELL-MEDIATED IMMUNITY

The absolute numbers of T lymphocytes are reduced in recipients of CAMPATH-1 T-cell-depleted allografts at 3 and 6 months and their proliferative capacity *in vitro* is markedly reduced. The number of CD4+ cells remains low for at least a year, whereas CD8+ cells regenerate more rapidly, reaching normal levels after 6 months. NK cell activity is raised during the first month after transplant and B cells recover rapidly and maintain normal numbers thereafter (Parreira *et al.* 1987).

Similar results are found for children after undergoing T-lymphocyte-depleted haematopoietic stem cell transplants from either closely matched unrelated donors or partially matched familial donors, except that reconstitution takes somewhat longer (Kook *et al.* 1996). Total lymphocyte counts as well as CD3+ and CD4+ T cell counts remain depressed until 2–3 years post-transplant, whereas CD8+ T cell counts normalize by 18 months, resulting in an inverted CD4:CD8 ratio until 12 months post-transplant. The absolute number of NK cells remains unchanged early post-transplant although their relative proportion is higher. CD20+ B cells are depressed until 12–18 months post-transplant. Younger patients tend to have higher total lymphocyte counts post-transplant. Higher marrow cell doses were not associated with hastened immunophenotypic recovery. GVHD and its treatment significantly delay the immune reconstitution of CD3+, CD4+ and CD20+ cells.

Allogeneic haematopoietic stem cell transplantation brings about a long-lasting dysfunction of T and B cells, and the opportunistic infection caused by these defects may become manifest long after transplantation and recovery from neutropenia. The most prominent example is VZV infection, which occurs in up to 50% of haematopoietic stem cell transplant recipients in some series (Han *et al.* 1994), mostly between 5 and 12 months after haematopoietic stem cell transplantation when immune reconstitution is still under way (Dix & Wingard 1996). Herpes zoster (shingles) is more common than primary infection (varicella) and is complicated in approximately one-third of cases. Varicella-zoster virus infections occur more frequently among seropositive patients, the onset is earlier and often more complicated and they suffer disseminated infection more frequently (Han *et al.* 1994). Recipients older than 10 years who receive radiation as part of their conditioning therapy have an incidence of 44% by 3 years, whereas children aged 10 years or less who have had no radiotherapy and are VZV-seronegative have a zero incidence (Han *et al.* 1994). Autologous haematopoietic stem cell transplant recipients are as likely to develop VZV infection as their allogeneic counterparts but infection develops 2 months earlier and is rarely associated with complications (Wacker *et al.* 1989). Prophylaxis with acyclovir is advocated by many centres for the first 9 months after transplant but is probably not required as most patients respond to therapy with this drug and suffer minimal morbidity. It is doubtful whether or not VZV should be treated at all but patients with zoster clearly benefit from treatment, the rash and pain associated with shingles are attenuated, the risk of post-herpetic neuralgia is reduced and ocular involvement is prevented altogether (Wagstaff *et al.* 1994).

The lymphocyte transformation response to VZV antigen has been shown to be depressed following haematopoietic stem cell transplantation and parellels periods of increased susceptibility to VZV infection (Meyers *et al.* 1980). However, the test has never been applied in practice.

Chronic GVHD and the immunosuppressive agents used for its treatment further render these patients at risk for infection with VZV, *Aspergillus* spp. and *P. carinii*.

### HYPOGAMMAGOBULINAEMIA

Most recipients of haematopoietic stem cell transplants lose the protective immunity to tetanus and poliovirus as a result of hypogammaglobulinaemia, particularly of IgG2. Immunization with tetanus and diphtheria toxoids, inactivated poliovirus vaccine and influenza vaccine is therefore recommended for both allogeneic and autologous haematopoietic stem cell transplant recipients (Fielding 1994). However, when questioned, only two-thirds of member centres of the European Group for Blood and Marrow Transplantation routinely immunized recipients of allogeneic haematopoietic stem cell transplants, mostly only with tetanus toxoid and inactivated poliovirus vaccine, and only just over one-third offered immunization to recipients of autologous haematopoietic stem cell transplants (Ljungman *et al.* 1995).

Patients are also at risk for infections caused by polysaccharide-encapsulated organisms, particularly *S. pneumoniae* and *H. influenzae* type b, and respond poorly to polysaccharide vaccines. Male haematopoietic stem cell transplant recipients are more likely to develop infection caused by *S. pneumoniae* than are females, as are those of either gender with abnormally low or high serum IgG and IgM levels. Serum opsonic activity for *S. pneumoniae* is decreased and patients with impaired opsonic activity also tend to have low serum antibody levels for the capsular polysaccharide, and some also have low serum complement activity (Winston *et al*. 1979). Prophylactic penicillin (Schwella *et al*. 1993) or pneumococcal vaccination should be considered to protect against infection caused by *S. pneumoniae*.

Immunizing patients with *H. influenzae* type b conjugate, tetanus toxoid and polysaccharide pneumococcal vaccines before harvesting the haematopoietic stem cells enhances the early recovery of specific antibody to *H. influenzae* type b and increases antibody concentrations to tetanus toxoid by the end of 3 months post-transplant but not to *S. pneumoniae*. This approach may be worthwhile considering for those at risk for *H. influenzae* type b, such as children (Molrine *et al*. 1996). Other vaccines, particular the live attenuated ones, should be considered on an individual basis and those to *H. influenzae* type b and *S. pneumoniae* should not be given later than 6–8 months post-transplant (Parkkali *et al*. 1996). Ideally, antibody titres should be measured to allow selective reimmunization but universal vaccination may be a more viable alternative (Fielding 1994).

Autologous haematopoietic stem cell transplantation is also characterized by defects in B and T cell function and loss of specific antibody although immune reconstitution usually gets under way rapidly, eventually becoming complete. Patients immunized against *H. influenzae* type b, tetanus toxoid and polysaccharide pneumococcal vaccines before an autologous transplant do have higher antibody titres to *H. influenzae* type b and tetanus toxoid but not pneumococci during the first 2 years post-transplant than is seen with similar patients immunized for the first time at a later stage (Molrine *et al*. 1996). None the less, routine reimmunization is usually thought unnecessary because immune deficiency is by and large short-lived.

Hypogammaglobulinaemia may be partly compensated for by giving either hyperimmune or conventional immunoglobulin as prophylaxis because this results in a significant reduction in fatal CMV infection, interstitial pneumonitis whether caused by CMV or not, as well as in the total mortality. However, prophylaxis does not reduce the incidence of acute GVHD or that of symptomatic CMV infection in seropositive recipients (Bass *et al*. 1993).

INFECTIVE PULMONARY COMPLICATIONS

## Virus infections

During the winter months community respiratory virus infection is as common among haematopoietic stem cell transplant recipients as it is among normal hosts. Respiratory syncytial virus (RSV) is responsible for half and influenza virus, picornaviruses, parainfluenza virus and adenovirus account for the remainder of infections. Clinical symptoms included low-grade fever, non-productive cough, rhinorrhea or nasal congestion, and radiographic evidence of interstitial infiltrates and sinusitis (Englund *et al*. 1988). More than half of infections can be complicated by pneumonia with an associated mortality of 50%. Patients who acquired the RSV infection before engraftment tend to develop pneumonia more frequently than do engrafted patients (Harrington *et al*. 1992) and, although the pneumonia remains almost exclusively a viral infection, the mortality is 100% unless treated promptly with antiviral agents, such as ribavarin. Both haematopoietic stem cell transplant recipients and their family members as well as employees may be infected at the same time. By contrast, pneumonia caused by other viruses either tends to be self-limiting viral pneumonia or becomes complicated by secondary bacterial or fungal infection (Whimbey *et al*. 1996). Early recognition of influenza A virus infection and prompt treatment with amantadine may prevent pneumonia and therefore other complications (Whimbey *et al*. 1994). Patients with other respiratory virus infections may benefit from treatment with ribavarin although no clinical trials have been conducted (Wendt & Hertz 1995).

## Bacterial infections

Late bacterial pneumonia caused by *S. pneumoniae* and *P. aeruginosa* may occur more than 6 months after transplant because of prolonged immunodeficiency brought about by chronic GVHD and functional asplenia (Hoyle & Goldman 1994). As pneumonia can, to some extent, be anticipated after transplant, prophylaxis should be considered an essential part of the supportive care of the haematopoietic stem cell transplant recipient at greatest risk. While prophylaxis with penicillin is recommended to prevent infection with *S. pneumoniae*, little is known about what drug, if any, would provide protection against infection caused by *P. aeruginosa*, although a fluoroquinolone such as ciprofloxacin may prove effective, provided compliance is good. Adoptive transfer of antibody responses to *P. aeruginosa* is also feasible as this can be achieved by immunizing haematopoietic stem cell transplant recipients and their donors with a polyvalent O-polysaccharide–toxin A conjugate vaccine. Antibody titres, primarily of the IgG1 and IgG2 subclasses, to all polysaccharide components increase to levels shown to be protective in animal models of Gram-negative sepsis (Gottlieb *et al.* 1990).

Quite why haematopoietic stem cell transplant recipients should be at greater risk of infection caused by Gram-negative bacilli postengraftment is not known, though it is probably because prophylaxis is mostly stopped altogether after engraftment. However, it has been observed that the rate at which Gram-negative bacilli were isolated from oral gargle specimens of renal transplant recipients is significantly higher in CMV-positive recipients than that found in samples of CMV-negative recipients (Mackowiak *et al.* 1991). If Gram-negative bacilli are actively carried by a recipient with chronic GVHD, infection might occur in a similar setting to that found following cytotoxic chemotherapy, namely impaired mucosal integument and myelosuppression, causing functional if not actual neutropenia. The risk for infection may also be augmented by the presence of hypoglobulinaemia, which results in impaired opsonization.

*Legionella* spp. seldom develop after haematopoietic stem cell transplantation and in a large series the incidence was less than 1% over a period of 6 years (Harrington *et al.* 1996). *Legionella pneumophila*, *L. feeleii*, *L. micdadei* and *L. bozemanii* were almost equally represented among the 10 cases, making diagnosis by direct fluorescent antibody assays unreliable (Harrington *et al.* 1996). Five of the seven patients infected with non-*pneumophila* species recovered from their pneumonia, whereas all three patients infected with *L. pneumophila* died. All six allogeneic haematopoietic stem cell transplant recipients had GVHD and three of the four autologous haematopoietic stem cell transplant recipients developed infection during neutropenia.

### PARANASAL SINUSITIS

When considering respiratory complications associated with haematopoietic stem cell transplantation, most attention has been devoted to the oral cavity and the lower respiratory tract. Sinusitis has attracted much less interest even though it is common after allogeneic haematopoietic stem cell transplantation. The nasal respiratory epithelium is frequently abnormal after transplant, with either squamous metaplasia or heterogeneous axonemal defects of peripheral and central microtubules, although these appear to have no relationship to the presence of acute or chronic sinusitis, previous irradiation, GVHD or immunosuppressive therapy (Cordonnier *et al.* 1996). Nevertheless, it seems likely that defects in the nasal defences will predispose to paranasal sinusitis. Paranasal sinusitis is characterized by fluid, opacification or marked mucosal thickening. Most episodes will occur during the early postengraftment phase although some occur during neutropenia. Hypoglobulinaemia may be present and most cases will have some degree of acute GVHD and many will have the chronic form of the disease so most patients will be receiving corticosteroids (Savage *et al.* 1997). Specific pathogens are seldom isolated although parainfluenza virus, *P. aeruginosa* and moulds, such as *Aspergillus* spp., including *A. fumigatus* and *A. flavus*, and other moulds, such as *Fusarium* spp. and *Mucor* spp., are associated with invasive fungal sinusitis, which can prove fatal unless aggressively treated with surgical debridement and antifungal therapy (Drakos *et al.* 1993; Morrison & McGlave 1993). Other fungi, such as *Alternaria* spp., can also cause sinusitis but without dissemination (Morrison & Weisdorf 1993). The infection is most likely to begin before engraftment and signs and symptoms of sinusitis may be absent or muted initially. However, the discovery of nasal lesions should be viewed with suspicion and receive prompt histological and mycological investigation. As with other fungal sinusitis, treatment requires both systemic antifungal therapy and surgical debridement. When treatment is effective, paranasal sinusitis is seldom fatal but can become chronic in many cases (Savage *et al.* 1997).

### BRAIN ABSCESS

Brain abscess is an infrequent but usually fatal complication of allogeneic haematopoietic stem cell transplantation, almost invariably caused by a fungus; *Aspergillus* spp. predominate, followed by *Candida* spp. Other fungi, including *Rhizopus* spp., *Absidia* spp., *Scopulariopsis* spp. and *Pseudallescheria* spp., and bacteria, such as *Stenotrophomonas maltophilia*, *P. aeruginosa*, *Enterobacter cloacae* and *Clostridium* spp. and *T. gondii*, only occur sporadically. Cerebral abscesses caused by *Aspergillus* spp. are usually accompanied by pulmonary disease and those caused by *Candida* spp. often occur together with fungaemia or neutropenia. Almost two-thirds of abscesses develop during GVHD 9–11 weeks after transplant; however, no other specific risk factors were identified (Hagensee *et al.* 1994).

Toxoplasmosis of the brain is rare, affecting an estimated 0.4% of allogeneic haematopoietic stem cell transplants, and is invariably fatal (Slavin *et al.* 1994). Given that an estimated 15% of allogeneic transplant recipients are seropositive for *T. gondii*, the risk of developing infection has been estimated to be around 2%. Infection is detected 7–14 weeks after transplant and most patients have grades II–IV acute GVHD. As with other brain abscesses, diagnosis is confirmed mostly at post-mortem. Tachyzoites can be seen in brain, heart and lung tissue, whereas cysts are only found in the heart and lungs.

## Transplant-related mortality

A decade ago almost half of haematopoietic stem cell transplant recipients died from causes directly related to the procedure. Today transplant-related mortality has been reduced to 25% amongst allogeneic haematopoietic stem cell transplant recipients treated for acute leukaemia and allografted in first complete remission and appears attributable to the use of cyclosporin for preventing GVHD. Improvements have also been brought about by the use of less total body irradiation for conditioning and by ensuring that the interval between achieving remission and receiving a transplant is shorter. Other factors resulting in lower transplant-related mortality probably include better patient care, particularly the use of more potent antibacterial agents for both prophylaxis and treatment (Frassoni *et al.* 1996).

Older patients are at greater risk than are younger recipients although the causes of death are similar and mainly related to toxicity associated with the conditioning regimen rather than relapse of leukaemia (Miller *et al.* 1996). Male recipients of grafts from a female donor are also at greater risk, as are allogeneic haematopoietic stem cell transplant recipients with chronic myeloid leukaemia (Gratwohl & Hermans 1996) and autologous haematopoietic stem cell transplant recipients.

The three most common primary causes of transplant-related mortality are interstitial pneumonitis, GVHD and veno-occlusive disease, with infection coming fourth (Frassoni *et al.* 1996), accounting for about one in 10 deaths amongst adult recipients, irrespective of age (Ringden *et al.* 1993). However, adducing the cause of death is often far from straightforward as infection may contribute to interstitial pneumonitis and GVHD and vice versa.

### AUTOPSY EVIDENCE

One of the best ways of corroborating clinical estimates of infection is to review autopsy data. In a series involving 56 patients who had undergone BMT at the Detroit Medical Center during 1988–92, at least one infection was identified in 25 of 40 (63%) allogeneic and four of 16 (25%) autologous BMT recipients. Bacteria were identified as the sole cause of infection in only four cases, whereas CMV infection was found in 14 cases, i.e. 25% of autopsies, half of which also involved fungi. In all, yeasts were found in 13 patients and *Aspergillus* in six patients. Infections caused by bacteria were more likely to be recognized antemortem than were those caused by fungi and viruses. Abnormalities of the lungs and the gastrointestinal tract predominated and were confirmed, respectively, by the presence of diffuse alveolar damage, interstitial pneumonia and bronchopneumonia, and by ulcerations and haemorrhages of the oesophagus, stomach, small and large intestines (Chandrasekar *et al.* 1995).

INTERSTITIAL PNEUMONITIS

The lung appears to be particularly vulnerable to damage by cytostatic chemotherapy and irradiation and is exquisitely susceptible to infection. Total body irradiation is itself a risk factor because autologous haematopoietic stem cell transplant recipients who receive it are more likely to develop pulmonary complications, including interstitial pneumonitis, than are those who only receive cytostatic chemotherapy (Carlson *et al.* 1994).

Interstitial pneumonitis occurs in up to 50% of patients after haematopoietic stem cell transplant and is the main cause of mortality. Previous treatment and infections, transplant conditioning, the particular regimen for GVHD prophylaxis as well as prolonged severe immunosuppression are all risk factors and the period of greatest risk is within 3 months of transplant. The most common infectious aetiologies are aspergillosis and CMV infection, although idiopathic, non-infectious interstitial pneumonia may be the result of toxicity to the conditioning regimen (Cunningham 1992).

Immunopathological reactions mediated by the pulmonary macrophages that survive chemotherapy can lead to various other syndromes, including respiratory distress. Lung haemorrhage as a result of profound thrombocytopenia will further imperil the lung, increasing the risk of infection. However, the risk of invasion and dissemination is high when the integrity of the mucosa is impaired, the ecology of resident flora is disturbed and an exogenous microorganism, such as a Gram-negative bacillus or another potential pathogen, gains a foothold and establishes colonization. Aspiration and inhalation of spores and hyphal elements of *Aspergillus* spp. and other moulds permit colonization of the sinuses and bronchial tree, which may extend into the alveolar spaces, resulting in invasive disease which is often fatal.

Chronic GVHD involving the sinuses and respiratory tract can be associated with idiopathic interstitial pneumonitis as well as infections, including aspergillosis and also sinusitis involving *Zygomyces* moulds. Whether or not infection is involved, allogeneic T cell-depleted bone marrow haematopoietic stem cell transplant recipients who develop interstitial pneumonitis appear to have an excess of CD8 suppressor/cytotoxic type T lymphocytes that express activation markers indicating an aggressive local immune response (Milburn *et al.* 1990). Oedema, pulmonary haemorrhage, bacterial infection and ARDS are more likely causes of interstitial pneumonitis during neutropenia than are infection with CMV or *P. carinii* (Winer Muram *et al.* 1996). CMV interstitial pneumonitis used to prove invariably fatal but treatment with the combination of ganciclovir and immunoglobulin has significantly reduced mortality. By contrast, there has been little success in treating interstitial pneumonitis involving *Aspergillus* infection.

## Preventing infection

### General principles

There are almost as many protocols for prevention of infection as there are centres and there is no obvious consensus. Although the total isolation advocated 20 years ago has been abandoned in favour of single rooms and high-efficiency particulate air (HEPA) filtered air, many autologous haematopoietic stem cell transplant recipients are treated in an open ward. Isolation measures range from full surgical hygiene to simply removing outer clothing and hand washing. Sterile foods are barely palatable and have given way to low-microbial-content diets typically supplied by the

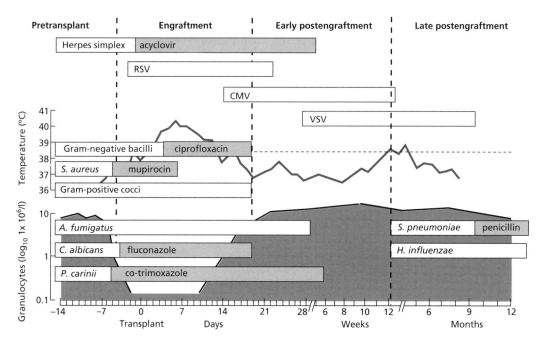

**Fig. 19.8** Prophylactic scheme for allogeneic BMT recipients. The scheme presented here is one of many variations on a common theme. Prophylaxis provides effective protection against a limited number of infectious complications, e.g. herpes simplex by acyclovir, enteric Gram-negative bacilli by ciprofloxacin, *Pneumocystis carinii* by co-trimoxazole, *Candida albicans* by fluconazole. There is no effective prophylaxis against mould infections such as those caused by *Aspergillus fumigatus*, CMV infections and respiratory viral infections.

hospital kitchen, which are perfectly safe provided fresh vegetables such as lettuce are avoided. Patients usually follow a special programme for oral care but otherwise normal standards of personal hygiene are expected. Some centres advocate disinfectant soaps and antibiotic toothpastes while others have no such requirements. Contact with the outside world also varies widely, with some centres relying on two-way telephones while others allow personal contact with close relatives. Whatever the local practices and rituals most centres agree that the goal of such measures is to prevent the recipient from acquiring a nosocomial potential pathogen. Protocols to protect the patient from extrinsic potential pathogens range from simple isolation in a single room to laminar air flow units (LAFs) with HEPA filtration to afford protection against aspergillosis (Fenelon 1995).

However, physical means of preventing infection are considered inadequate and so antimicrobial agents are commonly used to secure prevention against either infections that are rapidly fulminant, such as those caused by the Gram-negative bacilli *P. aeruginosa* and *E. coli*, or those that increase morbidity, e.g. herpes simplex infections (Fig. 19.8). Whichever regimen is used, even one containing only a fluoroquinolone, antimicrobial prophylaxis is a trade-off between suppressing more dangerous potential pathogens and inevitably selecting ones that are less virulent but more resistant to the agents used.

## Antibacterial prophylaxis against bacterial infections

The original intention of total decontamination of the oral and alimentary tracts has long since given way to the use of fluoroquinolones for preventing infection caused by Gram-negative bacilli, whether indigenous, e.g. *E. coli*, or exogenous and acquired, e.g. *P. aerugi-*

*nosa*. This approach has been largely superseded by prophylactic regimens containing a single fluoro-quinolone, as the patient finds it easier to comply with taking one or two relatively tasteless tablets a day instead of the noxious cocktails required for total decontamination. However, the dramatic fall in rates of Gram-negative sepsis has been accompanied by a commensurate rise in the incidence of bacteraemia caused by Gram-positive cocci, particularly the viridans streptococci and coagulase-negative staphylococci. Consequently there are still those who advocate patients swallowing solutions of aminoglycosides and vancomycin 'to extend the antimicrobial cover to Gram-positive cocci' even though there is absolutely no evidence that this is effective and considerable evidence that this practice runs the risk of selecting resistant bacteria, such as vancomycin-resistant *Enterococcus faecium* (Centers for Disease Control 1996).

Mupirocin is effective in suppressing carriage of *S. aureus* (Lamb 1991). However, prolonged use can lead to selection of clones amongst the coagulase-negative staphylococci that already have plasmids carrying the resistance determinant (Connolly *et al.* 1993). As might be expected, resistance can be transferred to *S. aureus in vitro* and therefore this is possible *in vivo*.

## Prophylaxis against candidosis

Prophylaxis with fluconazole has been shown to be effective against candidosis (Goodman *et al.* 1992; Slavin *et al.* 1995) although it is still not clear whether every patient should be given the drug or whether its use should be restricted to those who are at risk, namely carriers of *Candida* spp. Moreover, exposure to the drug is likely to lead to the selection of any natively resistant *Candida* spp. such as *C. krusei* and *C. glabrata* already harboured by the patient (Wingard *et al.* 1993; Chandrasekar *et al.* 1994; Hoppe *et al.* 1994; Behre *et al.* 1995; Epstein *et al.* 1996). Therefore, as with antibacterial prophylaxis, the use of fluconazole reduces one reservoir of infection while encouraging the emergence of another.

## Prophylaxis against aspergillosis

Even when the endogenous potential pathogens have

been successfully suppressed, the whole procedure of haematopoietic stem cell transplantation increases the risk of aspergillosis developing, particularly in a setting of thrombocytopenia, pulmonary toxicity, GVHD and its treatment with corticosteroids. *Aspergillus fumigatus* is a saprophyte and its spores are found in all manner of dust, whether derived from dried plant material, such as pepper, tea, straw, hay, cardboard and paper, or from building activities. Infection is acquired almost exclusively by inhaling spores. Thus the risk of infection can be reduced markedly by minimizing exposure. This can be achieved by accommodating haematopoietic stem cell transplant recipients in single rooms equipped with whole-wall HEPA filtration units delivering a horizontal laminar flow (Sherertz *et al.* 1987), which can reduce the number of aerial spores to less than 0.01 colony-forming units/m$^3$. Further measures include the avoidance of items contaminated with *Aspergillus* spores. Inhaling amphotericin B is thought by many to help lower the chance of inhaling viable spores still further but the evidence is not compelling. Low-dose amphotericin (5–10 mg/day) begun the day after transplant and continuing for 2–3 months reduces the incidence of fungal infections without renal toxicity, although cyclosporin levels are lower, leading to an increase in the rate of GVHD (O'Donnell *et al.* 1994).

Although devastating, aspergillosis affects only 5–10% of patients and these are just those whose outlook is often dismal because of graft rejection (McWhinney *et al.* 1993) or severe GVHD (Meyers 1990). The potential factors that influence the incidence of aspergillosis comprise both host factors and aerial spore counts, which are affected by, among other things, building activity. Inhalation of the spores is virtually the only route of infection and the use of LAFs appears to be the best means of affording protection against aspergillosis (Fenelon 1995). LAFs are considered expensive to run but they can and do lower the risk of aspergillosis markedly and might prove to be cost-effective. By contrast, inhaling amphotericin B (Jeffery *et al.* 1991; Behre *et al.* 1995) or administering low doses of the drug parenterally (Rousey *et al.* 1991; Perfect *et al.* 1992) have never been widely adopted because of doubts about their true effectiveness.

## Other prophylactic measures

In a survey of 18 UK centres, 17 routinely gave co-trimoxazole at various doses for periods varying between 3 and 12 months, or sometimes longer if chronic GVHD was present, and six centres gave nebulized pentamidine to patients intolerant of co-trimoxazole to prevent *P. carinii* infection. Six centres gave penicillin for 1–3 years to allograft patients to prevent infection by *S. pneumoniae*. Thirteen centres gave only CMV-negative blood products to CMV-seronegative patients, one centre gave CMV immuno-globulin and five centres continued acyclovir for 6 months. Despite these measures, 113 (6.2%) of 1825 autologous and allogeneic haematopoietic stem cell transplant recipients required readmission to hospital for severe infections, mostly pulmonary and involving CMV in one in five cases, with *P. carinii*, *S. pneumoniae*, *Aspergillus* spp. and *P. aeruginosa*. Some patients with severe infections were not taking 'appropriate' prophylaxis, which may be especially important when immunosuppression persists (Hoyle & Goldman 1994).

## Treatment of infection

### General principles

The general principle guiding treatment during the last decade is that during neutropenia therapy should be started promptly as soon as fever occurs, i.e. empirically, with a regimen that possesses broad-spectrum bactericidal activity against pathogens that can cause potentially fatal infections. Hitherto only a combined regimen of a β-lactam antibiotic and an aminoglyco-side was thought adequate but recently monotherapy with ceftazidime and the so-called fourth-generation cephalosporins, such as cefepime and cefpirome, has come into its own. It has also become more widely accepted that the empirical period covers the first 3–4 days of fever and that after this time subsequent infections can occur, requiring the original regimen to be adapted accordingly. Thus the approach is becoming one of empirical therapy until such time as the cause of fever is known, then attempting to tailor the regimen according to individual circumstances. Thus the initial regimen may remain unchanged or might be replaced by a more appropriate one but usually complementary treatment is begun to deal with specific problems that arise during the course of neutropenia. At other times postengraftment, a diagnosis should be attempted before deciding upon whether or not treatment is required and with what regimen.

### Empirical or pathogen-directed therapy?

How infection is treated is as important as which agents are used. In certain circumstances, notably BMT recipients with fever during neutropenia, therapy is begun empirically because it is considered hazardous to wait the 24–48 h for microbiological results, as infection with Gram-negative bacilli can rapidly escalate to septic shock and death. However, prophylaxis with flu-oroquinolones will virtually eliminate this risk because these agents effectively suppress colonization. More-over, the development of resistance among Gram-negative bacilli has yet to be reported as a significant reason for failure of prophylaxis. It therefore seems illogical, at least at first glance, to assume that the occurrence of fever during quinolone prophylaxis heralds Gram-negative sepsis. On the other hand, com-pliance to oral regimens is influenced by the extent of nausea, oromucositis and gut toxicity and it seems prudent to provide broad-spectrum systemic therapy against the most lethal putative pathogens by switching to intravenous agents, such as the traditional amino-glycoside–β-lactam regimens. However, aminogly-cosides are considered unsafe for BMT recipients receiving cyclosporin because of the potential for nephrotoxicity, and so initial monotherapy with a cephalosporin, such as ceftazidime (Verhagen *et al.* 1986) or cefepime (Okamoto *et al.* 1994), is preferred. Monotherapy appears successful provided that treat-ment is complemented as and when required, for instance, with a glycopeptide for infections caused by Gram-positive bacteria, amphotericin B for mould mycosis, fluconazole for candidosis and so on.

Alternatively, the same fluoroquinolone used for prophylaxis could be continued orally or given par-enterally to sustain cover against Gram-negative bacilli provided there was no evidence of colonization with resistant strains. A ureidopenicillin and a glycopeptide might be given to complement the fluoroquinolone to afford better activity against the Gram-positive cocci (Warren *et al.* 1990). In fact, the same argument can be applied to any of the empirical regimens as none is the optimal choice for treating persistent bacteraemia or infection with Gram-positive cocci, including coagulase-negative staphylococci, which are the most common indication to add a glycopeptide. Similarly, supplementing the empirical regimen with antimicrobial agents, such as penicillin, to treat oral viridans streptococcal bacteraemia has been advocated (Bochud *et al.* 1994b) but quickly leads to the selection of resistant oral streptococci (Guiot *et al.* 1994). The addition of clindamycin to ceftazidime also failed to influence the clinical course of fever even though all the streptococci had been eradicated from the blood (Donnelly 1993). Giving penicillin prophylactically to those receiving selective oral prophylaxis might be a more reasonable approach because it prevents bacteraemia (Gerson *et al.* 1984; Guiot *et al.* 1992) but the clinical course appears unaltered and resistance is likely to emerge (Bochud *et al.* 1994a).

The primary assumption underlying empirical therapy is that fever is caused by infection. The problem is that not all infections are caused by bacteria. It should also be borne in mind that an empirical approach to therapy is not without risk. If only the onset of fever is used to initiate therapy, infected patients being treated with steroids will not be treated until clinical infection becomes manifest. Thus, by the time treatment is begun the infection might very well be advanced. On the other hand, if everyone who is either febrile or being treated with steroids is given empirical therapy most may be put at risk of unnecessary drug toxicity. Another drawback of the empirical approach is that the temptation to escalate therapy by adding more drugs automatically becomes almost irresistible when cultures fail to yield a pathogen and fever persists. Empirical treatment can also instil a false sense of security, precisely because the regimens chosen offer such broad-spectrum activity, encouraging the belief that further attempts at diagnosis can be abandoned. Therefore, once started, empirical treatment should only be complemented when there is an objectively verifiable reason for doing so, such as drug toxicity, evidence of deterioration, persistence or progression of a primary microbiologically defined infection or the occurrence of a new microbiologically or clinically defined infection.

## Conclusions

The human defence system is able to cope with a tremendous number of insults before it finally begins to show the first signs of collapse. Any qualitative or quantitative defect in one of the components of the human defence system will predispose to infection, but haematopoietic stem cell transplantation leads to impairment of all elements of the immune defences, to some extent making infection inevitable. The greatest risk of infection occurs before and immediately after transplant because the aggressive treatment necessary to prepare the recipient for the graft vitiates the integrity of the integument and induces bone marrow aplasia. Moreover, therapeutic interventions to manage infection, GVHD and other complications will inevitably conspire to inflict further damage on the fragile remains of the immune system and impede its reconstruction, thereby prolonging the risks of infection. Haematopoietic stem cell transplantation tilts the balance firmly in favour of both the professional and opportunistic pathogen and returns the host for a time to a state of immunological naïvety. None the less, much progress has been made and more recipients are surviving free of disease and in good health. The next hurdle will be to understand how to refine the whole process such that the immune system is barely disturbed at all, infections do not occur and the new graft can slip quietly into place without being noticed.

## References

Abedi, M.R., Hammarstrom, L., Ringden, O. & Smith, C.I. (1990) Development of IgA deficiency after bone marrow transplantation. The influence of acute and chronic graft-versus-host disease. *Transplantation* 50, 415–421. (Published erratum appears in *Transplantation* 51, 285.)

Agura, E.D., Brown, M.C., Schaffer, R., Donaldson, G. & Shen, D.D. (1995) Antiemetic efficacy and pharmacokinetics of intravenous ondansetron infusion during chemotherapy conditioning for bone marrow transplant. *Bone Marrow Transplantation* 16, 213–222.

Agusti, C., Ramirez, J., Picado, C. *et al.* (1995) Diffuse alveolar hemorrhage in allogeneic bone marrow transplantation. A postmortem study. *American Journal of Respiratory Critical Care Medicine* 151, 1006–1010.

Allan, B.T., Patton, D., Ramsey, N.K. & Day, D.L. (1988) Pulmonary fungal infections after bone marrow transplantation. *Pediatric Radiology* 18, 118–122.

Alnor, D., Frimodt-Moller, N., Espersen, F. & Frederiksen, W. (1994) Infections with the unusual human pathogens *Agrobacterium* species and *Ochrobactrum anthropi*. *Clinical Infectious Diseases* 18, 914–920.

Appleton, A.L., Sviland, L., Peiris, J.S. *et al.* (1995) Human herpes virus-6 infection in marrow graft recipients: role in pathogenesis of graft-versus-host disease. Newcastle upon Tyne Bone Marrow Transport Group. *Bone Marrow Transplantation* 16, 777–782.

Aslanzadeh, J. & Stelmach, P.S. (1996) Detection of *Pneumocystis carinii* with direct fluorescence antibody and calcofluor white stain. *Infection* 24, 248–250.

Awada, A., Van Der Auwera, P., Meunier, F., Daneau, D. & Klastersky, J. (1992) Streptococcal and enterococcal bacteremia in patients with cancer. *Clinical Infectious Diseases* 15, 33–48.

Balfour, H.H. Jr (1990) Management of cytomegalovirus disease with antiviral drugs. *Reviews of Infectious Diseases* 12, 0862–0886.

Ballou, S.P. & Lozanski, G. (1992) Induction of inflammatory cytokine release from cultured human monocytes by C-reactive protein. *Cytokine* 4, 361–368.

Barbounis, V., Koumakis, G., Vassilomanolakis, M. *et al.* (1995) A phase II study of ondansetron as antiemetic prophylaxis in patients receiving high-dose polychemotherapy and stem cell transplantation. *Support Care Cancer* 3, 301–306.

Barrett, A.J. (1989) Graft versus host disease—clinical features and biology. *Bone Marrow Transplantation* 4, 18–21.

Bass, E.B., Powe, N.R., Goodman, S.N. *et al.* (1993) Efficacy of immune globulin in preventing complications of bone marrow transplantation: a meta-analysis. *Bone Marrow Transplantation* 12, 273–282.

Beattie, G., Whelan, J., Cassidy, J. *et al.* (1989) Herpes simplex virus, *Candida albicans* and mouth ulcers in neutropenic patients with non-haematological malignancy. *Cancer Chemotherapy and Pharmacology* 25, 75–76.

Behre, G.F., Schwartz, S., Lenz, K. *et al.* (1995) Aerosol amphotericin B inhalations for prevention of invasive pulmonary aspergillosis in neutropenic cancer patients. *Annals of Hematology* 71, 287–291.

Bensinger, W.I., Weaver, C.H., Appelbaum, F.R. *et al.* (1995) Transplantation of allogeneic peripheral blood stem cells

mobilized by recombinant human granulocyte colony-stimulating factor (see comments). *Blood* 85, 1655–1658.

Bergmann, O.J. (1991) Alterations in oral microflora and pathogenesis of acute oral infections during remission-induction therapy in patients with acute myeloid leukaemia. *Scandinavian Journal of Infectious Diseases* 23, 355–366.

Bergmann, O.J. (1992) Oral infections in haematological patients—pathogenesis and clinical significance. *Danish Medical Bulletin* 39, 15–29.

Bilgrami, S., Bergstrom, S.K., Peterson, D.E. *et al.* (1992) Capnocytophaga bacteremia in a patient with Hodgkin's disease following bone marrow transplantation: case report and review (see comments). *Clinical Infectious Diseases* 14, 1045–1049.

Bochud, P.Y., Calandra, T. & Francioli, P. (1994a) Bacteremia due to viridans streptococci in neutropenic patients: a review. *American Journal of Medicine* 97, 256–264.

Bochud, P.Y., Eggiman, P., Calandra, T. *et al.* (1994b) Bacteremia due to viridans streptococcus in neutropenic patients with cancer—clinical spectrum and risk factors. *Clinical Infectious Diseases* 18, 25–31.

Bodey, G.P., Buckley, M., Sathe, Y.S. & Freirich, E.J. (1966) Quantitative relationships between circulating leucocytes and infection in patients with acute leukaemia. *Annals of Internal Medicine* 64, 328–340.

Bodey, G.P., Anaissie, E., Gutterman, J. & Vadhanraj, S. (1994) Role of granulocyte–macrophage colony-stimulating factor as adjuvant treatment in neutropenic patients with bacterial and fungal infection. *European Journal of Clinical Microbiology and Infectious Diseases* 13, S18–S22.

Bortin, M.M., Horowitz, M.M., Rowlings, P.A. *et al.* (1993) 1993 Progress Report from the International Bone Marrow Transplant Registry Advisory Committee of the International Bone Marrow Transplant Registry. *Bone Marrow Transplantation* 12, 97–104.

Bosi, A., Guidi, S., Messori, A. *et al.* (1993) Ondansetron versus chlorpromazine for preventing emesis in bone marrow transplant recipients: a double-blind randomized study. *Journal of Chemotherapy* 5, 191–196.

Bronchud, M. (1993) Can hematopoietic growth factors be used to improve the success of cytotoxic chemotherapy? *Anti-Cancer Drugs* 4, 127–139.

Bryan, R.L., Antonakopoulos, G.N., Newman, J. & Milligan, D.W. (1991) Intestinal graft versus host disease. *Journal of Clinical Pathology* 44, 866–867.

Callum, J.L., Brandwein, J.M., Sutcliffe, S.B., Scott, J.G. & Keating, A. (1991) Influence of total body irradiation on infections after autologous bone marrow transplantation. *Bone Marrow Transplantation* 8, 245–251.

Carlson, K., Backlund, L., Smedmyr, B., Oberg, G. & Simonsson, B. (1994) Pulmonary function and complications subsequent to autologous bone marrow transplantation. *Bone Marrow Transplantation* **14**, 805–811.

Castagnola, E., Tasso, L., Conte, M. *et al.* (1994) Central venous catheter-related infection due to *Comamonas acidovorans* in a child with non-Hodgkin's lymphoma. *Clinical Infectious Diseases* **19**, 559–560.

Centers for Disease Control (1996) Recommendations for preventing the spread of vancomycin resistance: Recommendations of the Hospital Infection Control Practices Advisory Committee (HICPAC). *Morbidity and Mortality Weekly Report* **44**, 1–12.

Chandrasekar, P.H., Gatny, C.M. and the Bone Marrow Transplantation Team. (1994) The effect of fluconazole prophylaxis on fungal colonisation in neutropenic cancer patients. *Journal of Antimicrobial Chemotherapy* **33**, 309–318.

Chandrasekar, P.H., Weinmann, A. & Shearer, C. (1995) Autopsy-identified infections among bone marrow transplant recipients: a clinico-pathologic study of 56 patients. *Bone Marrow Transplantation* **16**, 675–681.

Chasty, R.C., Lamb, W.R., Gallati, H. *et al.* (1993) Serum cytokine levels in patients undergoing bone marrow transplantation. *Bone Marrow Transplantation* **12**, 331–336.

Chen, Y.L., Levraux, V., Leneveu, A. *et al.* (1994) Acute-phase response, interleukin-6, and alteration of cyclosporine pharmacokinetics. *Clinical Pharmacology and Therapeutics* **55**, 649–660.

Classen, D.C., Burke, J.P., Ford, C.D. *et al.* (1990) *Streptococcus mitis* sepsis in bone marrow transplant patients receiving oral antimicrobial prophylaxis. *American Journal of Medicine* **89**, 441–446.

Cometta, A., Calandra, T., Bille, J. & Glauser, M.P. (1994) *Escherichia coli* resistant to fluoroquinolones in patients with cancer and neutropenia. *New England Journal of Medicine* **330**, 1240–1241.

Connolly, S., Noble, W.C. & Phillips, I. (1993) Mupirocin resistance in coagulase-negative staphylococci. *Journal of Medical Microbiology* **39**, 450–453.

Cordonnier, C., Gilain, L., Ricolfi, F. *et al.* (1996) Acquired ciliary abnormalities of nasal mucosa in marrow recipients. *Bone Marrow Transplantation* **17**, 611–616.

Costerton, J.W. & Marrie, T.J. (1983) The role of the bacterial glycocalyx in resistance to antimicrobial agents. In: *Medical Microbiology*, Vol. 3. (ed. C.A.S. Easmon), pp. 64–85. Academic Press, London.

Costerton, J.W., Cheng, K.J., Geesey, G.G. *et al.* (1987) Bacterial biofilms in nature and disease. *Annual Reviews of Microbiology* **41**, 435–464.

Cunningham, I. (1992) Pulmonary infections after bone marrow transplant. *Seminars in Respiratory Infection* **7**, 132–138.

De Bel, C., Gerritsen, E., De Maaker, G., Moolenaar, A. & Vossen, J. (1991) C-reactive protein in the management of

children with fever after allogeneic bone marrow transplantation. *Infection* **19**, 92–96.

De Pauw, B.E., Donnelly, J.P., De Witte, T., Novakova, I.R. & Schattenberg, A. (1990) Options and limitations of long-term oral ciprofloxacin as antibacterial prophylaxis in allogeneic bone marrow transplant recipients. *Bone Marrow Transplantation* **5**, 179–182.

De Witte, T., Schattenberg, A., Van Dijk, B.A. *et al.* (1990) Prevention of primary cytomegalovirus infection after allogeneic bone marrow transplantation by using leukocyte-poor random blood products from cytomegalovirus-unscreened blood-bank donors. *Transplantation* **50**, 964–968.

De Witte, T., Gratwohl, A., Van der Lely, N. *et al.* (1991) Recombinant human granulocyte-macrophage colony stimulating factor (rhGM-CSF) reduces infection-related mortality after allogeneic T-cell depleted BMT. *Bone Marrow Transplantation* **2**, 0268–3369.

De Witte, T., Van Der Lely, N., Muus, P., Donnelly, J.P. & Schattenberg, T. (1993) Recombinant human granulocyte macrophage colony stimulating factor (rhGM-CSF) accelerates bone marrow recovery after allogeneic T-cell depleted bone marrow transplantation. *L'Ospedale Maggiore* **87**, 42–46.

Demuynck, H., Zachee, P., Verhoef, G.E.G. *et al.* (1995) Risks of rhG-CSF treatment in drug-induced agranulocytosis. *Annals of Hematology* **70**, 143–147.

Devaux, Y., Archimbaud, E., Guyotat, D. *et al.* (1992) Streptococcal bacteremia in neutropenic adult patients. *Nouvelle Revue Française D Hématologie* **34**, 191–195.

Dix, S.P. & Wingard, J.R. (1996) Management of viral infections in bone marrow transplant recipients. *Clinical Immunotherapeutics* **6**, 352–382.

Donnelly, J.P. (1993) Selective decontamination of the digestive tract and its role in antimicrobial prophylaxis. *Journal of Antimicrobial Chemotherapy* **31**, 813–829.

Donnelly, J.P., Muus, P., Schattenberg, A. *et al.* (1992) A scheme for daily monitoring of oral mucositis in allogeneic BMT recipients. *Bone Marrow Transplantation* **9**, 409–413.

Donnelly, J.P., Muus, P., Horrevorts, A.M., Sauerwein, R.W. & De Pauw, B.E. (1993) Failure of clindamycin to influence the course of severe oromucositis associated with streptococcal bacteraemia in allogeneic bone marrow transplant recipients. *Scandinavian Journal of Infectious Diseases* **25**, 43–50.

Donnelly, J.P., Dompeling, E.C., Meis, J.F. & de Pauw, B.E. (1995) Bacteremia due to oral viridans streptococci in neutropenic patients with cancer: cytostatics are a more important risk factor than antibacterial prophylaxis. *Clinical Infectious Diseases* **20**, 469–470.

Drakos, P.E., Nagler, A., Or, R. *et al.* (1993) Invasive fungal sinusitis in patients undergoing bone marrow transplantation. *Bone Marrow Transplantation* **12**, 203–208.

Duenas-Gonzalez, A., Sobrevillacalvo, P., Friasmendivil, M. *et al.* (1996) Misoprostol prophylaxis for high-dose chemotherapy-induced mucositis: a randomized double-blind study. *Bone Marrow Transplantation* **17**, 809–812.

Dugue, B., Leppanen, E.A., Teppo, A.M., Fyhrquist, F. & Grasbeck, R. (1993) Effects of psychological stress on plasma interleukin-1-beta and interleukin-6-beta, C-reactive protein, tumour necrosis factor-alpha, anti-diuretic hormone and serum cortisol. *Scandinavian Journal of Clinical and Laboratory Investigation* **53**, 555–561.

Engelhard, D., Morag, A., Or, R. *et al.* (1988) Prevention of herpes simplex virus (HSV) infection in recipients of HLA-matched T-lymphocyte-depleted bone marrow allografts. *Israeli Journal of Medicine Science* **24**, 145–150.

Engelhard, D., Elishoov, H., Or, R. *et al.* (1995) Cytosine arabinoside as a major risk factor for *Streptococcus viridans* septicemia following bone marrow transplantation: a 5-year prospective study. *Bone Marrow Transplantation* **16**, 565–570.

Englund, J.A., Sullivan, C.J., Jordan, M.C. *et al.* (1988) Respiratory syncytial virus infection in immunocompromised adults. *Annals of Internal Medicine* **109**, 203–208.

EORTC International Antimicrobial Therapy Cooperative Group (1990) Gram-positive bacteraemia in granulocytopenic cancer patients. *European Journal of Cancer* **26**, 569–574.

EORTC International Antimicrobial Therapy Cooperative Group and National Cancer Institute of Canada (1991) Vancomycin added to empirical combination antibiotic therapy for fever in granulocytopenic cancer patients. *Journal of Infectious Diseases* **163**, 951–958.

Epstein, J.B., Ransier, A., Lunn, R. *et al.* (1996) Prophylaxis of candidiasis in patients with leukemia and bone marrow transplants. *Oral Surgery, Oral Medicine, Oral Pathology, Oral Radiology and Endodentronics* **81**, 291–296.

Fegan, C., Poynton, J.A. & Whittaker, J.A. (1990) The gut mucosal barrier in bone marrow transplantation. *Bone Marrow Transplantation* **5**, 373–377.

Fenelon, L.E. (1995) Protective isolation: who needs it? *Journal of Hospital Infection* **30**, 218–222.

Ferrara, J.L., Abhyankar, S. & Gilliland, D.G. (1993) Cytokine storm of graft-versus-host disease: a critical effector role for interleukin-1. *Transplantation Proceedings* **25**, 1216–1217.

Ferretti, G.A., Ash, R.C., Brown, A.T. *et al.* (1987) Chlorhexidine for prophylaxis against oral infections and associated complications in patients receiving bone marrow transplants. *Journal of the American Dental Association* **114**, 461–467.

Fielding, A.K. (1994) Prophylaxis against late infection

following splenectomy and bone marrow transplant. *Blood Review* **8**, 179–191.

Frampton, J.E. & Faulds, D. (1996) Filgrastim: a reappraisal of pharmacoeconomic considerations in the prophylaxis and treatment of chemotherapy induced neutropenia. *Pharmacoeconomics* **9**, 76–96.

Frassoni, F., Labopin, M., Gluckman, E. *et al.* (1996) Results of allogeneic bone marrow transplantation for acute leukemia have improved in Europe with time—a report of the acute leukemia working party of the European Group for Blood and Marrow Transplantation (EBMT). *Bone Marrow Transplantation* **17**, 13–18.

Freites, V., Sumoza, A., Bisotti, R. *et al.* (1995) Subcutaneous *Nocardia asteroides* abscess in a bone marrow transplant recipient. *Bone Marrow Transplantation* **15**, 135–136.

Galvederochemonteix, B., Wiktorowicz, K., Kushner, I. & Dayer, J.M. (1993) C-reactive protein increases production of IL-1-alpha, IL-1-beta, and TNF-alpha, and expression of messenger RNA by human alveolar macrophages. *Journal of Leukocyte Biology* **53**, 439–445.

Gentry, L.O. & Zeluff, B.J. (1988) Nosocomial and other difficult infections in the immunocompromised cardiac transplant patient. *Journal of Hospital Infection* **11**, 21–28.

Gerson, S., Talbot, G., Huwitz, S. *et al.* (1984) Prolonged granulocytopenia: the major risk factor for invasive pulmonary aspergillosis in patients with acute leukemia. *Annals of Internal Medicine* **100**, 345–351.

Giebink, G.S., Warkentin, P.I., Ramsay, N.K. & Kersey, J.H. (1986) Titers of antibody to pneumococci in allogeneic bone marrow transplant recipients before and after vaccination with pneumococcal vaccine. *Journal of Infectious Diseases* **154**, 590–596.

Goodman, J.L., Winston, D.J., Greenfield, R.A. *et al.* (1992) A controlled trial of fluconazole to prevent fungal infections in patients undergoing bone marrow transplantation. *New England Journal of Medicine* **326**, 845–851.

Goodrich, J.M., Boeckh, M. & Bowden, R. (1994) Strategies for the prevention of cytomegalovirus disease after marrow transplantation. *Clinical Infectious Diseases* **19**, 287–298.

Gottlieb, D.J., Cryz, S.J. Jr, Furer, E. *et al.* (1990) Immunity against *Pseudomonas aeruginosa* adoptively transferred to bone marrow transplant recipients. *Blood* **76**, 2470–2475.

Grant, S.M. & Heel, R.C. (1992) Recombinant granulocyte–macrophage colony-stimulating factor (RGM-CSF)—a review of its pharmacological properties and prospective role in the management of myelosuppression. *Drugs* **43**, 516–560.

Gratwohl, A. & Hermans, J. (1994) Bone marrow transplantation activity in Europe 1992: report from the European Group for Bone Marrow Transplantation (EBMT). *Bone Marrow Transplantation* **13**, 5–10.

Gratwohl, A. & Hermans, J. (1996) Allogeneic bone marrow transplantation for chronic myeloid leukemia. Working Party Chronic Leukemia of the European Group for Blood and Marrow Transplantation (EBMT). *Bone Marrow Transplantation* 17 (Suppl. 3), S7–9.

Graze, P.R. & Gale, R.P. (1979) Chronic graft versus host disease: a syndrome of disordered immunity. *American Journal of Medicine* 66, 611–620.

Griffiths, P.D. (1993) Current management of cytomegalovirus disease. *Journal of Medical Virology* 1, 106–111.

Grigg, A., Vecchi, L., Bardy, P. & Szer, J. (1996) G CSF stimulated donor granulocyte collections for prophylaxis and therapy of neutropenic sepsis. *Australian and New Zealand Journal of Medicine* 26, 813–818.

Groeger, J.S., Lucas, A.B., Thaler, H.T. *et al.* (1993) Infectious morbidity associated with long-term use of venous access devices in patients with cancer. *Annals of Internal Medicine* 119, 1168–1174.

Guiot, H.F.L., Biemond, J., Klasen, E. *et al.* (1987) Protein loss during acute graft-versus-host disease: diagnostics and clinical significance. *European Journal of Haematology* 38, 187–196.

Guiot, H.F.L., Van der Meer, J.W.M., Van den Broek, P.J., Willemze, R. & Van Furth, R. (1992) Prevention of viridans-group streptococcal septicemia in oncohematologic patients—a controlled comparative study on the effect of penicillin-G and co-trimoxazole. *Annals of Hematology* 64, 260–265.

Guiot, H.F.L., Corel, L.J.A. & Vossen, J.M.J.J. (1994) Prevalence of penicillin-resistant viridans streptococci in healthy children and in patients with malignant haematological disorders. *European Journal of Clinical Microbiology and Infectious Diseases* 13, 645–650.

Hagensee, M.E., Bauwens, J.E., Kjos, B. & Bowden, R.A. (1994) Brain abscess following marrow transplantation: experience at the Fred Hutchinson Cancer Research Center, 1984–1992. *Clinical Infectious Diseases* 19, 402–408.

Han, C.S., Miller, W., Haake, R. & Weisdorf, D. (1994) Varicella zoster infection after bone marrow transplantation: incidence, risk factors and complications. *Bone Marrow Transplantation* 13, 277–283.

Haq, M., Haq, S., Tutt, P. & Crook, M. (1993) Serum total sialic acid and lipid-associated sialic acid in normal individuals and patients with myocardial infarction, and their relationship to acute phase proteins. *Annals of Clinical Biochemistry* 30, 383–386.

Harrington, R.D., Hooton, T.M., Hackman, R.C. *et al.* (1992) An outbreak of respiratory syncytial virus in a bone marrow transplant center. *Journal of Infectious Diseases* 165, 987–993.

Harrington, R.D., Woolfrey, A.E., Bowden, R., McDowell, M.G. & Hackman, R.C. (1996) Legionellosis in a bone marrow transplant center. *Bone Marrow Transplantation* 18, 361–368.

Heath, D.I., Cruickshank, A., Gudgeon, M. *et al.* (1993) Role of interleukin-6 in mediating the acute phase protein response and potential as an early means of severity assessment in acute pancreatitis. *Gut* 34, 41–45.

Hellyar, A.G. (1988) Experience with *Nocardia asteroides* in renal transplant recipients. *Journal of Hospital Infection* 12, 13–18.

Henslee, J., Bostrom, B., Weisdorf, D. *et al.* (1984) Streptococcal sepsis in bone marrow transplant patients. *Lancet* i, 393.

Høiby, N. & Johansen, H.K. and the Copenhagen Study Group on Antibiotics in Sweat (1995) Ciprofloxacin in sweat and antibiotic resistance. *Lancet* 346, 1235.

Høiby, N., Jarløv, J.O., Kemp, M. *et al.* (1997) Excretion of ciprofloxacin in sweat and multiresistant *Staphylococcus epidermidis*. *Lancet* 349, 167–169.

Hoover, M., Morgan, E.R. & Kletzel, M. (1997) Prior fungal infection is not a contraindication to bone marrow transplant in patients with acute leukemia. *Medical and Pediatric Oncology* 28, 268–273.

Hoppe, J.E., Klingebiel, T. & Niethammer, D. (1994) Selection of *Candida glabrata* in pediatric bone marrow transplant recipients receiving fluconazole. *Pediatric Hematological Oncology* 11, 207–210.

Hoyle, C. & Goldman, J.M. (1994) Life-threatening infections occurring more than 3 months after BMT. 18 UK Bone Marrow Transplant Teams. *Bone Marrow Transplantation* 14, 247–252.

Imrie, K.R., Prince, H.M., Couture, F., Brandwein, J.M. & Keating, A. (1995) Effect of antimicrobial prophylaxis on hematopoietic recovery following autologous bone marrow transplantation: ciprofloxacin versus co-trimoxazole. *Bone Marrow Transplantation* 15, 267–270.

Jantunen, E., Ruutu, P., Niskanen, L. *et al.* (1997) Incidence and risk factors for invasive fungal infections in allogeneic BMT recipients. *Bone Marrow Transplantation* 19, 801–808.

Jeffery, G.M., Beard, M.E., Ikram, R.B. *et al.* (1991) Intranasal amphotericin B reduces the frequency of invasive aspergillosis in neutropenic patients. *American Journal of Medicine* 90, 685–692.

Johansson, J.E. & Ekman, T. (1997) Gastro-intestinal toxicity related to bone marrow transplantation: disruption of the intestinal barrier precedes clinical findings. *Bone Marrow Transplantation* 19, 921–925.

Johnson, S., Driks, M.R., Tweten, R.K. *et al.* (1994) Clinical courses of seven survivors of *Clostridium septicum* infection and their immunologic responses to a-toxin. *Clinical Infectious Diseases* 19, 761–764.

Kern, W.V., Andriof, E., Oethinger, M. *et al.* (1994) Emergence of fluoroquinolone-resistant *Escherichia coli* at a cancer center. *Antimicrobial Agents and Chemotherapy* **38**, 681–687.

Kilian, M., Husby, S., Host, A. & Halken, S. (1995) Increased proportions of bacteria capable of cleaving IgA1 in the pharynx offants with atopic disease. *Pediatric Research* **38**, 182–186.

Kolbinson, D.A., Schubert, M.M., Fluornoy, N. & Truelove, E.L. (1988) Early oral changes following bone marrow transplantation. *Oral Surgery, Oral Medicine, Oral Pathology* **66**, 130–138.

Kook, H., Goldman, F., Padley, D. *et al.* (1996) Reconstruction of the immune system after unrelated or partially matched T-cell-depleted bone marrow transplantation in children: immunophenotypic analysis and factors affecting the speed of recovery. *Blood* **88**, 1089–1097.

Kubo, S., Matsumoto, T., Takahashi, K. *et al.* (1994) Enhanced chemiluminescence response of polymorphonuclear leukocytes by new quinolone antimicrobials. *Chemotherapy* **40**, 333–336.

Lagneaux, L., Delforge, A., Snoeck, R., Stryckmans, P. & Bron, D. (1994) Decreased production of cytokines after cytomegalovirus infection of marrow-derived stromal cells. *Experimental Hematology* **22**, 26–30.

Lamb, Y.J. (1991) Overview of the role of mupirocin. *Journal of Hospital Infection* **19**, 27–30.

LaRocco, M.T. & Burgert, S.J. (1997) Infection in the bone marrow transplant recipient and the role of the microbiology laboratory in clinical transplantation. *Clinical Microbiology Reviews* **10**, 277–297.

Lecciones, J.A., Lee, J.W., Navarro, E.E. *et al.* (1992) Vascular catheter-associated fungemia in patients with cancer: analysis of 155 episodes. *Clinical Infectious Diseases* **14**, 875–883.

Lee, S.J., Wegner, S.A., McGarigle, C.J., Bierer, B.E. & Antin, J.H. (1997) Treatment of chronic graft-versus-host disease with clofazimine. *Blood* **89**, 2298–2302.

Leskinen, R., Taskinen, E., Volin, L. *et al.* (1990) Use of bronchoalveolar lavage cytology and determination of protein contents in pulmonary complications of bone marrow transplant recipients. *Bone Marrow Transplantation* **5**, 241–245.

Lew, M.A., Kehoe, K., Ritz, J. *et al.* (1995) Ciprofloxacin versus trimethoprim/sulfamethoxazole for prophylaxis of bacterial infections in bone marrow transplant recipients: a randomized, controlled trial. *Journal of Clinical Oncology* **13**, 239–250.

Ljungman, P., Ellis, M.N., Hackman, R.C., Shepp, D.H. & Meyers, J.D. (1990) Acyclovir-resistant herpes simplex virus causing pneumonia after marrow transplantation. *Journal of Infectious Diseases* **162**, 244–248.

Ljungman, P., De Bock, R., Cordonnier, C. *et al.* (1993) Practices for cytomegalovirus diagnosis, prophylaxis and treatment in allogeneic bone marrow transplant recipients: a report from the Working Party for Infectious Diseases of the EBMT. *Bone Marrow Transplantation* **12**, 399–403.

Ljungman, P., Cordonnier, C., de Bock, R. *et al.* (1995) Immunisations after bone marrow transplantation: results of a European survey and recommendations from the infectious diseases working party of the European Group for Blood and Marrow Transplantation. *Bone Marrow Transplantation* **15**, 455–460.

Locatelli, F., Pession, A., Zecca, M. *et al.* (1996) Use of recombinant human granulocyte colony-stimulating factor in children given allogeneic bone marrow transplantation for acute or chronic leukemia. *Bone Marrow Transplantation* **17**, 31–37.

Long, S.G., Leyland, M.J. & Milligan, D.W. (1993) Listeria meningitis after bone marrow transplantation. *Bone Marrow Transplantation* **12**, 537–539.

McClain, C., Cohen, D., Phillips, R., Ott, L. & Young, B. (1991) Increased plasma and ventricular fluid interleukin-6 levels in patients with head injury. *Journal of Laboratory and Clinical Medicine* **118**, 225–231.

McGuire, D.B., Altomonte, V., Peterson, D.E. *et al.* (1993) Patterns of mucositis and pain in patients receiving preparative chemotherapy and bone marrow transplantation. *Oncology Nursing Forum* **20**, 1493–1502.

Mackowiak, P.A., Goggans, M., Torres, W. *et al.* (1991) Relationship between cytomegalovirus and colonization of the oropharynx by Gram-negative bacilli following renal transplantation. *Epidemiology and Infection* **107**, 411–420.

McWhinney, P.H.M., Kibbler, C.C., Gillespie, S.H. *et al.* (1992) *Stomatococcus mucilaginosus*: an emerging pathogen in neutropenic patients. *Clinical Infectious Diseases* **14**, 641–646.

McWhinney, P.H.M., Kibbler, C.C., Hamon, M.D. *et al.* (1993) Progress in the diagnosis and management of aspergillosis in bone marrow transplantation — 13 years experience. *Clinical Infectious Diseases* **17**, 397–404.

Maher, D.W., Lieschke, G.J., Green, M. *et al.* (1994) Filgrastim in patients with chemotherapy-induced febrile neutropenia — a double-blind, placebo-controlled trial. *Annals of Internal Medicine* **121**, 492–501.

Martin Algarra, S., Bishop, M.R., Tarantolo, S. *et al.* (1995) Hematopoietic growth factors after HLA-identical allogeneic bone marrow transplantation in patients treated with methotrexate-containing graft-vs.-host disease prophylaxis. *Experimental Hematology* **23**, 1503–1508.

Martino, R., Manteiga, R., Sanchez, I. *et al.* (1995) Viridans streptococcal shock syndrome during bone marrow transplantation. *Acta Haematologica* **94**, 69–73.

Mascret, B., Maraninchi, D., Gastaut, J.A. *et al.* (1984) Risk factors for streptococcal septicaemia after marrow transplantation. *Lancet* **i**, 1185–1186.

Matera, G., Berlinghieri, M.C. & Foca, A. (1995)

Meropenem: effects on human leukocyte functions and interleukin release. *International Journal of Antimicrobial Agents* 5, 129–133.

Mathyhartert, M., Debydupont, G., Deby, C. *et al.* (1995) Cytotoxicity towards human endothelial cells, induced by neutrophil myeloperoxidase: protection by ceftazidime. *Mediators and Inflammation* 4, 437–443.

Meduri, G.U., Kohler, G., Hendley, S. *et al.* (1995) Inflammatory cytokines in the BAL of patients with ARDS: persistent elevation over time predicts a poor outcome. *Chest* 108, 1303–1314.

Meijer-Severs, G.J. & Joshi, J.H. (1989) The effect of new broad-spectrum antibiotics on faecal flora of cancer patients. *Journal of Antimicrobial Chemotherapy* 24, 605–613.

Menichetti, F. (1992) Gram-positive infections in neutropenic patients—glycopeptide antibiotic choice. *Journal of Antimicrobial Chemotherapy* 29, 461–462.

Menichetti, F., Felicini, R., Bucaneve, G. *et al.* (1989) Norfloxacin prophylaxis for neutropenic patients undergoing bone marrow transplantation. *Bone Marrow Transplantation* 4, 489–492.

Meurman, J.H., Laine, P., Murtomaa, H. *et al.* (1991) Effect of antiseptic mouthwashes on some clinical and microbiological findings in the mouths of lymphoma patients receiving cytostatic drugs. *Journal of Clinical Periodontology* 18, 587–591.

Meyers, J.D. (1986) Infection in bone marrow transplant recipients. *American Journal of Medicine* 81, 27–38.

Meyers, J.D. (1990) Fungal infections in bone marrow transplant patients. *Seminars in Oncology* 17, 10–13.

Meyers, J.D., Flournoy, N. & Thomas, E.D. (1980) Cell-mediated immunity to varicella-zoster virus after allogeneic marrow transplant. *Journal of Infectious Diseases* 141, 479–487.

Meyers, J.D., Flournoy, N. & Thomas, E.D. (1986) Risk factors for cytomegalovirus infection after human marrow transplantation. *Journal of Infectious Diseases* 153, 478–488.

Meyers, J.D., Reed, E.C., Shepp, D.H. *et al.* (1988) Acyclovir for prevention of cytomegalovirus infection and disease after allogeneic marrow transplantation. *New England Journal of Medicine* 318, 70–75.

Milburn, H.J., Du Bois, R.M., Prentice, H.G. & Poulter, L.W. (1990) Pneumonitis in bone marrow transplant recipients: results from a local immune response. *Clinical and Experimental Immunology* 81, 232–237.

Miller, C.B., Piantadosi, S., Vogelsang, G.B. *et al.* (1996) Impact of age on outcome of patients with cancer undergoing autologous bone marrow transplant. *Journal of Clinical Oncology* 14, 1327–1332.

Molrine, D.C., Guinan, E.C., Antin, J.H. *et al.* (1996) *Haemophilus influenzae* type B (HIB)-conjugate immunization before bone marrow harvest in autologous bone marrow transplantation. *Bone Marrow Transplantation* 17, 1149–1155.

Morrison, V.A. & McGlave, P.B. (1993) Mucormycosis in the BMT population. *Bone Marrow Transplantation* 11, 383–388.

Morrison, V.A. & Weisdorf, D.J. (1993) Alternaria: a sinonasal pathogen of immunocompromised hosts. *Clinical Infectious Diseases* 16, 265–270.

Morrison, V.A., Haake, R.J. & Weisdorf, D.J. (1994) Non-*Candida* fungal infections after bone marrow transplantation: risk factors and outcome. *American Journal of Medicine* 96, 497–503.

Neiman, P.E., Reeves, W., Ray, G. *et al.* (1977) A prospective analysis interstitial pneumonia and opportunistic viral infection among recipients of allogeneic bone marrow grafts. *Journal of Infectious Diseases* 136, 754–767.

Nemunaitis, J., Ross, M., Meisenberg, B. *et al.* (1994) Phase I study of recombinant human interleukin-1 beta (rhIL-1 beta) in patients with bone marrow failure. *Bone Marrow Transplantation* 14, 583–588.

Nijsten, M.W.N., De Groot, E.R., Ten Duis, H.J. *et al.* (1987) Serum levels of interleukin-6 and acute phase responses. *Lancet* ii, 921.

Norfolk, D.R., Forbes, M.A., Cooper, E.H. & Child, J.A. (1987) Changes in plasma beta 2 microglobulin concentrations after allogeneic bone marrow transplantation. *Journal of Clinical Pathology* 40, 657–662.

Norhagen, G., Engstrom, P.E., Bjorkstrand, B.L.H., Smith, C.I.E. & Ringden, O. (1994) Salivary and serum immunoglobulins in recipients of transplanted allogeneic and autologous bone marrow. *Bone Marrow Transplantation* 14, 229–234.

O'Donnell, M.R., Schmidt, G.M., Tegtmeier, B.R. *et al.* (1994) Prediction of systemic fungal infection in allogeneic marrow recipients—impact of amphotericin prophylaxis in high-risk patients. *Journal of Clinical Oncology* 12, 827–834.

Okamoto, M.P., Nakahiro, R.K., Chin, A., Bedikian, A. & Gill, M.A. (1994) Cefepime—a new fourth-generation cephalosporin. *American Journal of Hospital Pharmacology* 51, 463–477.

Parkkali, T., Kayhty, H., Ruutu, T. *et al.* (1996) A comparison of early and late vaccination with *Haemophilus influenzae* type B conjugate and pneumococcal polysaccharide vaccines after allogeneic BMT. *Bone Marrow Transplantation* 18, 961–967.

Parkman, R. (1993) Is chronic graft versus host disease an autoimmune disease? *Current Opinion in Immunology* 5, 800–803.

Parreira, A., Smith, J., Hows, J.M. *et al.* (1987) Immunological reconstitution after bone marrow transplant with Campath-1 treated bone marrow. *Clinical and Experimental Immunology* 67, 142–150.

Pechumer, H., Wilhelm, M. & Zieglerheitbrock, H.W.L. (1995) Interleukin-6 (IL-6) levels in febrile children during maximal aplasia alter bone marrow transplantation (BMT) are similar to those in children with normal hematopoiesis. *Annals of Hematology* **70**, 309–312.

Perfect, J.R., Klotman, M.E., Gilbert C.C. *et al.* (1992) Prophylactic intravenous amphotericin-B in neutropenic autologous bone marrow transplant recipients. *Journal of Infectious Diseases* **165**, 891–897.

Peters, B.G., Adkins, D.R., Harrison, B.R. *et al.* (1996) Antifungal effects of yeast-derived rhu-GM-CSF in patients receiving high-dose chemotherapy given with or without autologous stem cell transplantation: a retrospective analysis. *Bone Marrow Transplantation* **18**, 93–102.

Pinter, E. & Krivan, G. (1996) Diagnostic value of C-reactive protein levels in children with bone marrow transplantation. *Orvosi Hetilap* **137**, 1259–1262.

Prentice, H.G. & Kho, P. (1997) Clinical strategies for the management of cytomegalovirus infection and disease in allogeneic bone marrow transplant. *Bone Marrow Transplantation* **19**, 135–142.

Prince, H.M., Page, S.R., Keating, A. *et al.* (1995) Microbial contamination of harvested bone marrow and peripheral blood. *Bone Marrow Transplantation* **15**, 87–91.

Quabeck, K. (1994) The lung as a critical organ in marrow transplantation. *Bone Marrow Transplantation* **14**, 0268–3369.

Raab, Y., Hallgren, R. & Gerdin, B. (1994) Enhanced intestinal synthesis of interleukin-6 is related to the disease severity and activity in ulcerative colitis. *Digestion* **55**, 44–49.

Raad, I.I. & Bodey, G.P. (1992) Infectious complications of indwelling vascular catheters. *Clinical Infectious Diseases* **15**, 197–210.

Raemaekers, J., De Witte, T., Schattenberg, A. & Van Der Lely, N. (1989) Prevention of leukaemic relapse after transplantation with lymphocyte-depleted marrow by intensification of the conditioning regimen with a 6-day continuous infusion of anthracyclines. *Bone Marrow Transplantation* **4**, 167–171.

Redding, S.W. (1990) Role of herpes simplex virus reactivation in chemotherapy-induced oral mucositis. *National Cancer Institutes Monograph* **9**, 103–105.

Ringden, O., Horowitz, M.M., Gale, R.P. *et al.* (1993) Outcome after allogeneic bone marrow transplant for leukemia in older adults [see comments]. *Journal of the American Medical Association* **270**, 57–60.

Roberts, J.T. & Priestman, T.J. (1993) A review of ondansetron in the management of radiotherapy-induced emesis. *Oncology* **50**, 173–179.

Rocke, L.K., Loprinzi, C.L., Lee, J.K. *et al.* (1993) A randomized clinical trial of two different durations of oral cryotherapy for prevention of 5-fluorouracil related stomatitis. *Cancer* **72**, 2234–2238.

Rohrbaugh, T.M., Anolik, R., August, C.S., Serota, F.T. & Koch, P.A. (1984) Absorption of oral aminoglycosides following bone marrow transplantation. *Cancer* **53**, 1502–1506.

Roth, R.R. & James, W.D. (1988) Microbial ecology of the skin. *Annual Review of Microbiology* **42**, 441–464.

Rousey, S.R., Russler, S., Gottlieb, M. & Ash, R.C. (1991) Low-dose amphotericin B prophylaxis against invasive *Aspergillus* infections in allogeneic marrow transplantation. *American Journal of Medicine* **91**, 484–492.

Rowbottom, A.W., Riches, P.G., Downie, C. & Hobbs, J.R. (1993) Monitoring cytokine production in peripheral blood during acute graft-versus-host disease following allogeneic bone marrow transplantation. *Bone Marrow Transplantation* **12**, 635–641.

Rowe, I.F., Worsley, A.M., Donnelly, J.P. *et al.* (1984) Measurement of serum C-reactive protein concentration following bone marrow transplantation. *Journal of Clinical Pathology* **37**, 263–266.

Roy, V. & Weisdorf, D. (1997) Mycobacterial infections following bone marrow transplantation: a 20 year retrospective review. *Bone Marrow Transplantation* **19**, 467–470.

Rubin, M., Hathorn, J.W., Marshall, D. *et al.* (1988) Gram-positive infections and the use of vancomycin in 550 episodes of fever and neutropenia. *Annals of Internal Medicine* **108**, 30–35.

Ruutu, T., Ljungman, P., Brinch, L. *et al.* (1997a) No prevention of cytomegalovirus infection by anti cytomegalovirus hyperimmune globulin in seronegative bone marrow transplant recipients. *Bone Marrow Transplantation* **19**, 233–236.

Ruutu, T., Niederwieser, D., Gratwohl, A. & Apperley, J.F. (1997b) A survey of the prophylaxis and treatment of acute GVHD in Europe: a report of the European Group for Blood and Marrow Transplantation (EBMT). *Bone Marrow Transplantation* **19**, 759–764.

Sable, C.A. & Donowitz, G.R. (1994) Infections in bone marrow transplant recipients. *Clinical Infectious Diseases* **18**, 273–281.

Salzman, M.B., Isenberg, H.D., Shapiro, J.F., Lipsitz, P.J. & Rubin, L.G. (1993) A prospective study of the catheter hub as the portal of entry for microorganisms causing catheter-related sepsis in neonates. *Journal of Infectious Diseases* **167**, 487–490.

Saugier Veber, P., Devergie, A., Sulahian, A. *et al.* (1993) Epidemiology and diagnosis of invasive pulmonary aspergillosis in bone marrow transplant patients: results of a 5-year retrospective study. *Bone Marrow Transplantation* **12**, 121–124.

Savage, D.G., Taylor, P., Blackwell, J. *et al.* (1997) Paranasal sinusitis following allogeneic bone marrow transplant. *Bone Marrow Transplantation* **19**, 55–59.

Schimpff, S.C. (1993) Gram-negative bacteremia. *Support Care Cancer* 1, 5–18.

Schmeiser, T., Kern, W.V., Hay, B., Hertenstein, B. & Arnold, R. (1993) Single-drug oral antibacterial prophylaxis with ofloxacin in BMT recipients. *Bone Marrow Transplantation* 12, 57–63.

Schuster, M.W. (1992) Granulocyte–macrophage colony-stimulating factor (GM-CSF) — what role in bone marrow transplantation? *Infection* 20, S95–S99.

Schwella, N., Schwerdtfeger, R., Schmidt Wolf, I., Schmid, H. & Siegert, W. (1993) Pneumococcal arthritis after allogeneic bone marrow transplantation [see comments]. *Bone Marrow Transplantation* 12, 165–166.

Schwella, N., Konig, V., Schwerdtfeger, R. *et al.* (1994) Ondansetron for efficient emesis control during total body irradiation. *Bone Marrow Transplantation* 13, 169–171.

Shepp, D.H., Dandliker, P.S., Flournoy, N. & Meyers, J.D. (1985) Once-daily intravenous acyclovir for prophylaxis of herpes simplex virus reactivation after marrow transplantation. *Journal of Antimicrobial Chemotherapy* 16, 389–395.

Sherertz, R.J., Belani, A., Kramer, B.S. *et al.* (1987) Impact of air filtration on nosocomial *Aspergillus* infections. Unique risk of bone marrow transplant recipients. *American Journal of Medicine* 83, 709–718.

Singhal, S., Mehta, J., Powles, R. *et al.* (1995) Three weeks of ganciclovir for cytomegaloviraemia after allogeneic bone marrow transplantation. *Bone Marrow Transplantation* 15, 777–781.

Slavin, M.A., Meyers, J.D., Remington, J.S. & Hackman, R.C. (1994) *Toxoplasma gondii* infection in marrow transplant recipients: a 20 year experience. *Bone Marrow Transplantation* 13, 549–557.

Slavin, M.A., Osborne, B., Adams, R. *et al.* (1995) Efficacy and safety of fluconazole prophylaxis for fungal infections after marrow transplantation — a prospective, randomized, double-blind study. *Journal of Infectious Diseases* 171, 1545–1552.

Snydman, D.R. (1990) Cytomegalovirus immunoglobulins in the prevention and treatment of cytomegalovirus disease. *Review of Infectious Diseases* 12 (Suppl. 7), S839–848.

Souetre, E., Qing, W. & Penelaud, P.F. (1996) Economic analysis of the use of recombinant human granulocyte colony stimulating factor in autologous bone marrow transplantation. *European Journal of Cancer* 7, 1162–1165.

Spitzer, T.R., Bryson, J.C., Cirenza, E. *et al.* (1994) Randomized double-blind, placebo-controlled evaluation of oral ondansetron in the prevention of nausea and vomiting associated with fractionated total-body irradiation. *Journal of Clinical Oncology* 12, 2432–2438.

Steffen, M., Dürken, M., Pichlmeier, U. *et al.* (1997) Serum interleukin 6 levels during bone marrow transplantation:

impact on transplant-related toxicity and engraftment. *Bone Marrow Transplantation* 40, 301–307.

Steiner, M., Villablanca, J., Kersey, J. *et al.* (1993) Viridans streptococcal shock in bone marrow transplantation patients. *American Journal of Hematology* 42, 354–358.

Tiley, C., Powles, R., Catalano, J. *et al.* (1992) Results of a double blind placebo controlled study of ondansetron as an antiemetic during total body irradiation in patients undergoing bone marrow transplantation. *Leukemia and Lymphoma* 7, 317–321.

Valteau, D., Hartmann, O., Brugieres, L. *et al.* (1991) Streptococcal septicaemia following autologous bone marrow transplantation in children treated with high-dose chemotherapy. *Bone Marrow Transplantation* 7, 415–419.

Van der Meer, J. (1994) Defects in host defense mechanisms. In: *Current Approaches to Infection in the Compromised Host.* (eds R. Rubin & L. Young), pp. 33–66. Plenum Medical, New York.

Van der Waaij, D. (1984) Effect of antibiotics on colonization resistance. In: *Medical Microbiology*, Vol 4. (ed. C.S. Easmon), pp. 227–237. Academic Press, London.

Van der Waaij, D. (1989) The ecology of the human intestine and its consequences for overgrowth by pathogens such as *Clostridium difficile*. *Annual Review of Microbiology* 43, 69–87.

Verfaillie, C., Weisdorf, D., Haake, R. *et al.* (1991) *Candida* infections in bone marrow transplant recipients. *Bone Marrow Transplantation* 8, 177–184.

Verhagen, C., De Pauw, B.E., De Witte, T. *et al.* (1986) Ceftazidime does not enhance cyclosporin A nephrotoxicity in febrile bone marrow transplantation patients. *Blut* 53, 333–339.

Viedma, J.A., Perezmateo, M., Dominguez, J.E. & Carballo, F. (1992) Role of interleukin-6 in acute pancreatitis — comparison with C-reactive protein and phospholipase-A. *Gut* 33, 1264–1267.

Villablanca, J.G., Steiner, M., Kersey, J. *et al.* (1990) The clinical spectrum of infections with viridans streptococci in bone marrow transplant patients. *Bone Marrow Transplantation* 6, 387–393.

Viscoli, C., Bruzzi, P., Castagnola, E. *et al.* (1994) Factors associated with bacteraemia in febrile, granulocytopenic cancer patients. *European Journal of Cancer* 30A, 430–437.

Vogelsang, G.B., Hess, A.D., Berkman, A.W. *et al.* (1985) An *in vitro* predictive test for graft versus host disease in patients with genotypic HLA-identical bone marrow transplants. *New England Journal of Medicine* 313, 645–650.

Vollaard, E.J. & Clasener, H.A.L. (1994) Colonization resistance. *Antimicrobial Agents and Chemotherapy* 38, 409–414.

Wacker, P., Hartmann, O., Benhamou, E., Salloum, E. & Lemerle, J. (1989) Varicella-zoster virus infections after autologous bone marrow transplantation in children. *Bone Marrow Transplantation* 4, 191–194.

Wade, J.C., Newton, B., Flournoy, N. & Meyers, J.D. (1984) Oral acyclovir for prevention of herpes simplex virus reactivation after marrow transplantation. *Annals of Internal Medicine* 100, 823–828.

Wagstaff, A.J., Faulds, D. & Goa, K.L. (1994) Aciclovir: a reappraisal of its antiviral activity, pharmacokinetic properties and therapeutic efficacy. *Drugs* 47, 153–205.

Walker, S.A., Rogers, T.R., Riches, P.G., White, S. & Hobbs, J.R. (1984a) Value of serum C-reactive protein measurement in the management of bone marrow transplant recipients. Part I: early transplant period. *Journal of Clinical Pathology* 37, 1018–1021.

Walker, S.A., Rogers, T.R., Perry, D., Hobbs, J.R. & Riches, P.G. (1984b) Increased serum IgE concentrations during infection and graft versus host disease after bone marrow transplantation. *Journal of Clinical Pathology* 37, 460–462.

Warren, R.E., Wimperis, J.Z., Baglin, T.P., Constantine, C.E. & Marcus, R. (1990) Prevention of infection by ciprofloxacin in neutropenia. *Journal of Antimicrobial Chemotherapy* 26, 109–123.

Webster, A., Blizzard, B., Pillay, D. *et al.* (1993) Value of routine surveillance cultures for detection of CMV pneumonitis following bone marrow transplantation. *Bone Marrow Transplantation* 12, 477–481.

Weers-Pothoff, G., Nováková, I.R.O., Donnelly, J.P. & Muytjens, H.L. (1989) Bacteraemia caused by *Stomatococcus mucilaginosus* in a granulocytopenic patient with acute lymphocytic leukaemia. *Netherlands Journal of Medicine* 35, 143–146.

Weisdorf, D.J., Bostrom, B., Raether, D. *et al.* (1989) Oropharyngeal mucositis complicating bone marrow transplantation: prognostic factors and the effect of chlorhexidine mouth rinse. *Bone Marrow Transplantation* 4, 89–95.

Wendt, C.H. & Hertz, M.I. (1995) Respiratory syncytial virus and parainfluenza virus infections in the immunocompromised host. *Seminars in Respiratory Infection* 10, 224–231.

Whimbey, E., Elting, L.S., Couch, R.B. *et al.* (1994) Influenza A virus infections among hospitalized adult bone marrow transplant recipients. *Bone Marrow Transplantation* 13, 437–440.

Whimbey, E., Champlin, R.E., Couch, R.B. *et al.* (1996) Community respiratory virus infections among hospitalized adult bone marrow transplant recipients. *Clinical Infectious Diseases* 22, 778–782.

Wimperis, J.Z., Baglin, T.P., Marcus, R.E. & Warren, R.E. (1991) An assessment of the efficacy of antimicrobial prophylaxis in bone marrow autografts. *Bone Marrow Transplantation* 8, 363–367.

Winer Muram, H.T., Gurney, J.W., Bozeman, P.M. & Krance, R.A. (1996) Pulmonary complications after bone marrow transplantation. *Radiology Clinics of North America* 34, 97–117.

Wingard, J.R. (1990) Oral complications of cancer therapies. Infectious and noninfectious systemic consequences. *National Cancer Institutes Monographs* 9, 21–26.

Wingard, J.R. (1994) Infections due to resistant candida species in patients with cancer who are receiving chemotherapy. *Clinical Infectious Diseases* 19, S49–S53.

Wingard, J.R., Beals, S.U., Santos, G.W., Merz, W.G. & Saral, R. (1987) *Aspergillus* infections in bone marrow transplant recipients. *Bone Marrow Transplantation* 2, 175–181.

Wingard, J.R., Merz, W.G., Rinaldi, M.G. *et al.* (1993) Association of *Torulopsis glabrata* infections with fluconazole prophylaxis in neutropenic bone marrow transplant patients. *Antimicrobial Agents and Chemotherapy* 37, 1847–1849.

Winston, D.J. (1993) Prophylaxis and treatment of infection in the bone marrow transplant recipient. *Current Clinical Topics in Infectious Diseases* 13, 293–321.

Winston, D.J., Gale, R.P., Meyer, D.V. & Young, L.S. (1979) Infectious complications of human bone marrow transplantation. *Medicine (Baltimore)* 58, 1–31.

Woo, S.B., Sonis, S.T., Monopoli, M.M. & Sonis, A.L. (1993) A longitudinal study of oral ulcerative mucositis in bone marrow transplant recipients. *Cancer* 72, 1612–1617.

Wood, C.A. & Pepe, R. (1994) Bacteremia in a patient with non-urinary tract infection due to *Corynebacterium urealyticum*. *Clinical Infectious Diseases* 19, 367–368.

Yolken, R.H., Bishop, C.A., Townsend, T.R. *et al.* (1982) Infectious gastroenteritis in bone-marrow-transplant recipients. *New England Journal of Medicine* 306, 1010–1012.

Zinner, S.H., Calandra, T., Meunier, F. *et al.* (1994) Reduction of fever and streptococcal bacteremia in granulocytopenic patients with cancer—a trial of oral penicillin V or placebo combined with pefloxacin. *Journal of the American Medical Association* 272, 1183–1189.

# Index

Page references in *italics* refer to figures or their captions; those in **bold** refer to tables.